Manual of Standardized Methods for Veterinary Microbiology

Manual of Standardized Methods for Veterinary Microbiology

Prepared by
The Subcommittee on Standardized Methods for Veterinary Microbiology,
Committee on Animal Health, Board on Agriculture and Renewable Resources,
National Academy of Sciences–National Research Council, Washington

EDITED BY **GEORGE E. COTTRAL**

Research Veterinarian (Retired), Plum Island Animal Disease Center,
Agricultural Research Service, United States Department of Agriculture;
Senior Research Fellow, Australian National Animal
Health Laboratory, Commonwealth Scientific and
Industrial Research Organization

COMSTOCK PUBLISHING ASSOCIATES a division of

CORNELL UNIVERSITY PRESS / Ithaca and London

Copyright © 1978 by Cornell University

All rights reserved. Except for brief quotations in a review, this book, or parts thereof, must not be reproduced in any form without permission in writing from the publisher. For information address Cornell University Press, 124 Roberts Place, Ithaca, New York 14850. This work may be reproduced in whole or in part, however, for the official use of the U.S. Government.

First published 1978 by Cornell University Press.
Published in the United Kingdom by Cornell University Press Ltd.,
2–4 Brook Street, London W1Y 1AA.

International Standard Book Number 0-8014-1119-X
Library of Congress Catalog Card Number 77-90900
Printed in the United States of America by Vail-Ballou Press, Inc.
Librarians: Library of Congress cataloging information appears on the last page of the book.

Preface

In 1963 the Biologics Committee of the Council on Biological and Therapeutic Agents of the American Veterinary Medical Association recognized the need for a source of laboratory procedures and practices that were generally accepted by the scientific community for the manipulation of pathogenic microorganisms of animals. The council endorsed the recommendation of the Biologics Committee. In a series of ad hoc committee meetings cosponsored by the American Veterinary Medical Association and the National Academy of Sciences–National Research Council (NAS–NRC) the original concept was broadened to encompass pertinent information on pathogenic agents and agent-host interactions. To these ad hoc meetings, representatives were invited from those organizations that would have the greatest interest and need for a handbook on standardized methods in veterinary microbiology. These organizations included the American College of Veterinary Microbiologists; American Veterinary Medical Association; Animal and Plant Health Inspection Service, Agricultural Research Service, United States Department of Agriculture; Committee on Biologics, United States Animal Health Association; Conference of Veterinary Laboratory Diagnosticians; National Academy of Sciences–National Research Council; National Institutes of Health; Veterinary Biologics Licensees Committee, Animal Health Institute; and Western Hemisphere Committee on Animal Virus Characterization, which was affiliated with the Research Reference Reagents Committee of the National Institute of Allergy and Infectious Diseases, National Institutes of Health, with the United States Animal Health Association, with the Eastern Hemisphere Committee on Animal Virus Characterization, and with the World Health Organization.

As a result of the endorsement of these organizations and of financial support from the Agricultural Research Service, United States Department of Agriculture, the Division of Biology and Agriculture of NAS–NRC in 1967 created a subcommittee of its Committee on Animal Health to review, evaluate, and select acceptable standardized procedures in veterinary microbiology. Subsequently, the United States Agency for International Development also contributed to the subcommittee's support. Members of the subcommittee were C.J. York, chairman, F.R. Abinanti, R.A. Bankowski, V.J. Cabasso, G.E. Cottral, H.W. Dunne, J.H. Gillespie, D.P. Gustafson, K.L. Heddleston, D.L. Huxsoll, J.P. Newman, G.V. Peacock, A.C. Pier, and W.L. Sippel.

Responsibility for completing the manuscript was accepted by the Committee on Animal Health of the newly organized Board on Agriculture and Renewable Resources in 1974. The members of the committee were R.P. Hanson, chairman, C.W. Beard, H. DeGraff, W.L. Fishel, N.M. Konnerup, W.M. Moulton, J.A. Pino, and G.C. Poppensiek.

In the performance of its charge, the subcommittee used the talents of many United States and foreign scientists in the preparation, review, and editing of a publication that it feels reflects the present thinking of veterinary experts. The publication represents an earnest effort to set forth practical, effective, and substantive procedures to be used in the identification and study of pathogenic microorganisms of animals. The book should be read, however, with an awareness of human fallibility and of the fact that new information becomes available at unpredictable moments.

The subcommittee continued to function until 1972, when funds were exhausted and the subcommittee was discharged. The completed first draft was held until 1974, when a service contract was issued by the Plum Island Animal Disease Center, ARS, USDA, to George E. Cottral to revise, update, and edit the manuscript.

THE SUBCOMMITTEE

Washington, D.C.

Acknowledgments

Members of the Subcommittee on Standardized Methods for Veterinary Microbiology were responsible for preparing various sections of the manual, selecting authors, consultants, and reviewers, and approving the submitted manuscripts. The chairman, C.J. York, had the additional responsibility of collecting and assembling the manuscripts and giving guidance to the subcommittee. Without the help of the many authors, consultants, and reviewers, the manual could not have been written; most of them are specialists on the pathogens and diseases they covered.

The subcommittee gratefully acknowledges the financial support of the United States Department of Agriculture, Agricultural Research Service, Office of the Administrator, T.W. Edminster, and the support of the Commonwealth Scientific and Industrial Research Organization (CSIRO), Division of Animal Health, Australian National Animal Health Laboratory, W.A. Snowdon, Officer-in-Charge, in granting the editor time and facilities to complete the manual. It acknowledges the assistance of three individuals whose initial and continued efforts have made the publication of this manual possible: Jerry J. Callis, Director, Plum Island Animal Disease Center, ARS, USDA; William R. Hinshaw, Consultant, National Academy of Sciences; and James H. Gillespie, Professor and Chairman, Department of Veterinary Microbiology, New York State College of Veterinary Medicine, Cornell University. It also acknowledges the help of Dorsey W. Bruner, Professor Emeritus, New York State College of Veterinary Medicine, Cornell University, who read the entire manuscript. Finally, it acknowledges the typing and proofreading assistance of Leone Dalton and Stella Chan of Melbourne, Victoria, and Roberta Jaklevic of Cutchogue, New York, and the help of the CSIRO library staff, especially Janet Hills and Elizabeth Davy.

GEORGE E. COTTRAL, EDITOR
(FOR THE SUBCOMMITTEE)

Melbourne, Victoria, Australia

Contents

Preface ... 5
Acknowledgments ... 7
Authors ... 13
Consultants and Reviewers ... 17

PART ONE: GENERAL LABORATORY METHODS

1. Introduction ... 21
2. Laboratory Safety ... 23
3. Collection and Processing of Specimens ... 35
4. Biologic Test Systems ... 47
5. Serology ... 60
6. Preservation and Inactivation of Microorganisms ... 94
7. Biochemical, Biophysical, and Histochemical Tests ... 102

PART TWO: VIROLOGY

8. Adenoviruses (Adenoviridae) ... 112
   bovine, 112; canine (infectious canine hepatitis), 114; porcine, 115; simian, 116
9. Coronaviruses (Coronaviridae) ... 119
   avian infectious bronchitis virus, 119; transmissible gastroenteritis virus of swine, 123
10. Herpesviruses (Herpetoviridae) ... 126
    infectious bovine rhinotracheitis virus, 127; equine rhinopneumonitis virus, 129; pseudorabies virus, 131; canine herpesvirus, 134; feline rhinotracheitis virus, 136; malignant catarrhal fever virus, 138; bovine herpes mammillitis virus, 142; Marek's disease virus, 143; avian infectious laryngotracheitis virus, 146; duck plague virus, 148; swine cytomegalovirus, 150; guinea pig cytomegalovirus, 152; pigeon herpesvirus, 153; cottontail rabbit herpesvirus, 155; channel catfish herpesvirus, 156; simian herpesviruses, 158
11. Leukoviruses (Retroviridae, subfamily Oncovirinae) ... 167
    avian leukosis-sarcoma viruses, 167; murine leukemia viruses, 177

12. Orbiviruses (Reoviridae)   187
    bluetongue virus, 187; African horsesickness virus, 192; Ibaraki disease virus, 196; epizootic hemorrhagic disease virus of deer, 197
13. Orthomyxoviruses (Orthomyxoviridae)   199
    influenza viruses of humans, swine, horses, and birds (fowl plague)
14. Papovaviruses (Papovaviridae)   204
    papilloma, polyoma, and vacuolating viruses (deer fibroma, K virus of mice, simian vacuolating virus)
15. Paramyxoviruses (Paramyxoviridae)   212
    parainfluenza-3 virus, 213; Newcastle disease virus, 216; canine distemper virus, 219; rinderpest virus, 225; peste des petits ruminants virus, 229
16. Parvoviruses (Parvoviridae)   231
    rodent parvoviruses, 232; feline panleukopenia virus, 236; porcine parvovirus, 240; bovine parvovirus, 243; adeno-associated viruses, 244
17. Picornaviruses (Picornaviridae)   248
    foot-and-mouth disease virus, 248; swine vesicular disease virus, 253; equine rhinovirus, 254; porcine enteroviruses, 255; bovine enteroviruses, 258; simian enteroviruses, 260; vesicular exanthema of swine virus, 263; feline picorna respiratory viruses, 266; encephalomyocarditis virus, 268
18. Poxviruses (Poxviridae)   273
    orthopoxviruses (variola-vaccinia), 273; parapoxviruses (Orf), 278; capripoxviruses (sheeppox), 282; avipoxviruses (fowlpox), 284; leporipoxviruses (myxoma), 285; molluscum contagiosum, 289; swinepox, 290
19. Reoviruses (Reoviridae)   292
    orphan viruses of three serotypes
20. Rhabdoviruses (Rhabdoviridae)   299
    vesicular stomatitis virus, 299; rabies virus, 301; bovine ephemeral fever virus, 307
21. Togaviruses (Togaviridae)   309
    equine encephalomyelitis viruses, 309; Wesselsbron disease virus, 310; hog cholera virus, 311; bovine viral diarrhea–mucosal disease virus, 318; equine arteritis virus, 321
22. Bunyamwera Group Viruses (Bunyaviridae)   325
    Rift Valley fever virus, 325; Akabane virus, 326
23. Unclassified Viruses   330
    African swine fever virus, 330; equine infectious anemia virus, 333; Borna disease virus, 338
24. Viruses of Chronic Degenerative Diseases   340
    visna and maedi viruses (Retroviridae, subfamily Lentivirinae), 340; transmissible mink encephalopathy virus, 344; scrapie virus, 345; sheep pulmonary adenomatosis "virus," 348

PART THREE: BACTERIOLOGY

25. Enteric Organisms   349
    Escherichia, 351; Shigella, 357; Salmonella and Arizona (fowl typhoid, pullorum disease), 358; Klebsiella, 366; Alcaligenes, 368

Contents

26.	Mima	371
27.	Pseudomonas (glanders, melioidosis)	373
28.	Staphylococcus (suppurative lesions)	380
29.	Streptococcus (respiratory infections, mastitis)	389
30.	Brucella (brucellosis)	395
31.	Bordetella (respiratory infections, pertussis)	404
32.	Haemophilus (swine influenza and polyserositis, avian coryza)	408
33.	Pasteurella, Yersinia, and Francisella (fowl cholera, hemorrhagic septicemia, tularemia) Pasteurella, 413; Yersinia, 419; Francisella, 422	413
34.	Listeria (meningoencephalitis, abortion, neonatal death)	425
35.	Erysipelothrix (erysipeloid, septicemia, arthritis)	429
36.	Bacillus (anthrax)	437
37.	Moraxella (conjunctivitis, corneal ulcers)	445
38.	Haemobartonella (parasitism of erythrocytes)	449
39.	Actinobacillus (joint ill, actinobacillosis)	452
40.	Campylobacter and Vibrio (venereal genital vibriosis, abortion, blackscours, seafood poisoning)	461
41.	Mycoplasma (bovine and caprine pleuropneumonia, contagious agalactia, arthritis, synovitis, sinusitis)	472
42.	Chlamydia (psittacosis, ornithosis, pneumonitis, polyarthritis, abortion, encephalomyelitis, conjunctivitis, enteritis, lymphogranuloma venereum, trachoma)	485
43.	Leptospira (leptospirosis, renal infection)	494
44.	Borrelia (spirochetosis)	502
45.	Clostridia (hemoglobinuria, enterotoxemia, malignant edema, botulism, tetanus, blackleg, wound infections)	509
46.	Nonsporeforming Anaerobes (foot infections of sheep, cattle footrot, liver abscesses, navel ill, liver granulomas of turkeys)	526
47.	Mycobacterium (tuberculosis)	537
48.	Corynebacterium (purulent processes, lymphangitis, cystitis, pneumonia, arthritis, abortion, mastitis)	544
49.	Actinomyces (actinomycosis, lumpy jaw)	553
50.	Dermatophilus (cutaneous streptothricosis)	559
51.	Nocardia (respiratory infections, mastitis)	562
52.	Rickettsia (Q fever, heartwater, tick-borne fever, canine ehrlichiosis, contagious ophthalmia, salmon poisoning, Jembrana disease)	566

PART FOUR: MYCOLOGY

53.	Aspergillus (avian aspergillosis, bovine mycotic abortion)	583
54.	Blastomyces (blastomycosis)	588
55.	Candida (candidiasis, moniliasis, thrush)	593
56.	Coccidioides (coccidioidomycosis of arid areas)	598
57.	Cryptococcus (cryptococcosis, torulosis)	605
58.	Dermatophytes (ringworm, favus of chickens)	610
59.	Geotrichum (geotrichosis)	631
60.	Histoplasma (histoplasmosis, epizootic lymphangitis)	633

61. Phycomycetes (phycomycosis)	639
62. Prototheca (protothecosis, mastitis)	649
63. Sporotrichum (sporotrichosis)	651
64. Trichosporon (trichosporosis, mastitis)	654
65. Fungi Associated with Tumors or Wartlike Lesions (mycetoma, chromomycosis)	655
66. Mycotoxins (aflatoxicosis, facial eczema, slobber factor, ergotism, paspalum staggers, estrogenism, mold nephrosis)	659

APPENDIXES

A. Media, Reagents, and Special Techniques	671
B. Stains	695

ABBREVIATIONS 702

Index of Scientific Names	711
General Index	717

Authors

F.R. Abinanti, College of Veterinary Medicine, Washington State University, Pullman
M. Appel, James A. Baker Institute for Animal Health, Department of Microbiology, New York State College of Veterinary Medicine, Cornell University, Ithaca, N.Y.
P.K.C. Austwick, School of Veterinary Medicine, University of Cambridge, England
P.A. Bachmann, Institut für Mikrobiologie und Infektions-krankheiten der Tiere, Ludwig Maximilians University, Munich, West Germany
R.A. Bankowski, School of Veterinary Medicine, University of California, Davis
M.S. Bergdoll, Food Research Institute, Madison, Wis.
L.N. Binn, Division of Veterinary Medicine, Walter Reed Army Institute of Research, Washington
J.L. Bittle, Pitman-Moore, Inc., Washington Crossing, N.J.
B.O. Blackburn, National Animal Disease Center, APHIS, USDA, Ames, Iowa
H.G. Blobel, University of Giessen, Giessen, West Germany
E.H. Bohl, Department of Veterinary Science, Ohio Agricultural Research and Development Center, Wooster
S.S. Breese, Plum Island Animal Disease Center, ARS, USDA, Greenport, N.Y.
J.H. Bryner, National Animal Disease Center, ARS, USDA, Ames, Iowa
R.J. Byrne, National Institute of Allergy and Infectious Diseases, NIH, Bethesda, Md.
V.J. Cabasso, Microbiological Research, Cutter Laboratories, Berkeley, Calif.
J.J. Callis, Plum Island Animal Disease Center, ARS, USDA, Greenport, N.Y.
E.A. Carbrey, National Animal Disease Center, APHIS, USDA, Ames, Iowa
L.E. Carmichael, James A. Baker Institute for Animal Health, Department of Microbiology, New York State College of Veterinary Medicine, Cornell University, Ithaca, N.Y.
H.L. Chute, Department of Animal Science, University of Maine, Orono
K.D. Claus, National Animal Disease Center, APHIS, USDA, Ames, Iowa
L. Coggins, Department of Pathology, New York State College of Veterinary Medicine, Cornell University, Ithaca, N.Y.
J.R. Collier, Department of Microbiology, Colorado State University, Fort Collins
G.E. Cottral, Australian National Animal Health Laboratory, Division of Animal Health, CSIRO, Melbourne, Vic., Australia. Retired from Plum Island Animal Disease Center, Greenport, N.Y.
C.H. Cunningham, Department of Microbiology, College of Veterinary Medicine, Michigan State University, East Lansing
A.H. Dardiri, Plum Island Animal Disease Center, ARS, USDA, Greenport, N.Y.
A.J. Della Porta, Animal Health Research Laboratory, Division of Animal Health, CSIRO, Parkville, Vic., Australia
D.P. Dennet, Animal Health Research Laboratory, Division of Animal Health, CSIRO, Parkville, Vic., Australia

H.W. Dunne, Department of Veterinary Science, Pennsylvania State University, University Park (deceased)
B.C. Easterday, Department of Veterinary Sciences, University of Wisconsin, Madison
B.E. Eddy, Division of Biologics Control, NIH, Bethesda, Md. (retired)
E.M. Ellis, National Animal Disease Center, APHIS, USDA, Ames, Iowa
K.A. Eugster, Texas Veterinary Medical Diagnostic Laboratory, College Station
D.H. Evans, Defence Research Board, Department of National Defence, Ottawa, Ont., Canada
J. Fabricant, Department of Avian and Aquatic Medicine, New York State College of Veterinary Medicine, Cornell University, Ithaca, N.Y.
M. Forbes, Lederle Laboratories, Pearl River, N.Y.
M.L. Frey, Veterinary Medical Research Institute, Iowa State University, Ames
C. Gale, Greenfield Laboratories, Eli Lilly and Company, Greenfield, Ind.
L.K. Georg, Mycology Section, Center for Disease Control, Atlanta, Ga. (retired)
G.L. Gilardi, Hospital for Joint Disease Microbiology, New York
J.H. Gillespie, Department of Veterinary Microbiology, New York State College of Veterinary Medicine, Cornell University, Ithaca, N.Y.
P.J. Glantz, Department of Veterinary Microbiology, University of Saskatchewan, Saskatoon, Sask., Canada
M.A. Gordon, Division of Laboratories and Research, New York State Health Department, Albany, N.Y.
J.H. Graves, Plum Island Animal Disease Center, ARS, USDA, Greenport, N.Y.
D.P. Gustafson, Department of Veterinary Microbiology, Pathology, and Public Health, School of Veterinary Science and Medicine, Purdue University, West Lafayette, Ind.
A.J. Hackett, Naval Biomedical Research Laboratory, Naval Supply Center, Oakland, Calif.
L.E. Hanson, College of Veterinary Medicine, University of Illinois, Urbana
D.L. Harris, Veterinary Medical Research Institute, Iowa State University, Ames
R.L. Heberling, Southwest Foundation for Research and Education, San Antonio, Tex.
R.J. Heckly, Naval Biomedical Research Laboratory, Naval Supply Center, Oakland, Calif.
K.L. Heddleston, National Animal Disease Center, ARS, USDA, Ames, Iowa
J.B. Henson, Department of Veterinary Pathology, Washington State University, Pullman
W.P. Heuschele, Department of Veterinary Preventive Medicine, Ohio State University, Columbus
R.J. Hidalgo, Department of Veterinary Microbiology, Texas A & M University, College Station
M.S. Hofstad, Veterinary Medical Research Institute, Iowa State University, Ames
L.V. Holdeman, Anaerobe Laboratory, Virginia Polytechnic Institute and State University, Blacksburg
R. Hugh, Department of Microbiology, George Washington University Medical School, Washington
D.E. Hughes, National Animal Disease Center, ARS, USDA, Ames, Iowa
R.N. Hull, Biological Research Division, Lilly Research Laboratory, Eli Lilly and Company, Indianapolis, Ind.
R.F. Kahrs, Department of Preventive Medicine, College of Veterinary Medicine, University of Florida, Gainesville
W. Kaplan, Mycology Section, Center for Disease Control, Atlanta, Ga.
V.R. Kaschula, Veterinary Laboratory and Research Institute, FAO, UN, Abu Ghraib, Baghdad, Iraq
A.B. Larsen, National Animal Disease Center, ARS, USDA, Ames, Iowa
A.J. Luedke, Agricultural Research Service, USDA, Denver, Colo.
M.E. Macheak, National Animal Disease Center, APHIS, USDA, Ames, Iowa
S.H. Madin, School of Public Health, University of California, Berkeley
S. McConnell, Department of Veterinary Microbiology, College of Veterinary Medicine, Texas A & M University, College Station
D.G. McKercher, Department of Veterinary Microbiology, School of Veterinary Medicine, University of California, Davis
W.L. Mengeling, National Animal Disease Center, ARS, USDA, Ames, Iowa
R.W. Menges, Environmental Health Surveillance Center, University of Missouri, Columbia (deceased)
M.E. Meyer, Department of Microbiology, School of Veterinary Medicine, University of California, Davis

Authors

E.A. Mirand, Roswell Park Memorial Institute, Buffalo, N.Y.
W.E.C. Moore, Anaerobe Laboratory, Virginia Polytechnic Institute and State University, Blacksburg
A.C. Moran, Department of Microbiology, Oregon State University, Corvallis
E.C. Osborn, Departments of Medicine and Metabolic Medicine, Welsh National School of Medicine, Cardiff Royal Infirmary, Cardiff, Wales, U.K.
J.W. Osebold, Department of Veterinary Microbiology, School of Veterinary Medicine, University of California, Davis
Y. Ozawa, Food and Agriculture Organization, UN, Rome
L.A. Page, National Animal Disease Center, ARS, USDA, Ames, Iowa
A.C. Pier, National Animal Disease Center, ARS, USDA, Ames, Iowa
W. Plowright, Department of Pathology, Royal Veterinary College, London
G.H. Purchase, National Programs Staff, ARS, USDA, Beltsville, Md.
R.E. Reed, Department of Veterinary Science, University of Arizona, Tucson
J.L. Richard, National Animal Disease Center, ARS, USDA, Ames, Iowa
M. Ristic, Department of Pathology and Hygiene, College of Veterinary Medicine, University of Illinois, Urbana
L.L. Roach, Lee Laboratories, Grayson, Ga.
L. Rosen, Pacific Research Section, National Institute of Allergy and Infectious Diseases, NIH, Honolulu, Hawaii
R.F. Ross, Veterinary Medical Research Institute, Iowa State University, Ames
K.R. Schell, Federal Vaccination Laboratory, Basel
F.W. Scott, Department of Veterinary Microbiology, New York State College of Veterinary Medicine, Cornell University, Ithaca, N.Y.
G.R. Sharpless, Lederle Laboratories, Pearl River, N.Y.
R.D. Shuman, National Animal Disease Center, ARS, USDA, Ames, Iowa (retired)
K. Sikes, Public Health Division, Georgia Department of Human Resources, Atlanta
W.L. Sippel, Texas Veterinary Medical Diagnostic Laboratory, College Station
E. Small, College of Veterinary Medicine, University of Illinois, Urbana
J.M.B. Smith, Department of Microbiology, University of Otago, Dunedin, New Zealand
O.H.V. Stalheim, National Animal Disease Center, ARS, USDA, Ames, Iowa
R.A. Steeves, Department of Developmental Biology and Cancer, Albert Einstein College of Medicine, New York
H.G. Stoenner, Rocky Mountain Laboratory, NIH, Hamilton, Mont.
W.P. Switzer, College of Veterinary Medicine, Iowa State University, Ames
R. Trautman, Plum Island Animal Disease Center, ARS, USDA, Greenport, N.Y.
J.G. Tully, Bacterial Diseases Laboratory, National Institute of Allergy and Infectious Diseases, NIH, Bethesda, Md.
G.E. Wessman, National Animal Disease Center, ARS, USDA, Ames, Iowa
R.P. Williams, Department of Microbiology, Baylor University Medical School, Houston, Tex.
A.J. Winters, Department of Large Animal Medicine and Surgery, New York State College of Veterinary Medicine, Cornell University, Ithaca, N.Y.
R.L. Witter, Regional Poultry Research Laboratory, ARS, USDA, East Lansing, Mich.
R.L. Wood, National Animal Disease Center, ARS, USDA, Ames, Iowa
C.J. York, School of Medicine, University of California, San Diego, La Jolla, Calif.
Y.C. Zee, Department of Microbiology, School of Veterinary Medicine, University of California, Davis

Consultants and Reviewers

A.D. Alexander, Department of Veterinary Microbiology, Chicago College of Osteopathic Medicine, Chicago

G.G. Alton, Animal Health Research Laboratory, Division of Animal Health, CSIRO, Parkville, Vic., Australia

C.A. Brandly, College of Veterinary Medicine, University of Illinois, Urbana (retired)

R.W. Brown, National Animal Disease Center, ARS, USDA, Ames, Iowa

B.R. Burmester, Regional Poultry Research Laboratory, ARS, USDA, East Lansing, Mich. (retired)

B.L. Clark, Animal Health Research Laboratory, Division of Animal Health, CSIRO, Parkville, Vic., Australia

B.L. Deyoe, National Animal Disease Center, ARS, USDA, Ames, Iowa

S.K. Dinka, Plum Island Animal Disease Center, ARS, USDA, Greenport, N.Y.

F. Fenner, Centre for Research and Environmental Studies, Australian National University, Canberra, A.C.T., Australia

E.L. French, Animal Health Research Laboratory, Division of Animal Health, CSIRO, Parkville, Vic., Australia (retired)

L.C. Grumbles, Department of Microbiology, College of Veterinary Medicine, Texas A & M University, College Station

W.R. Hinshaw, Consultant, National Academy of Sciences–National Research Council, Washington

K.L. Hughes, School of Veterinary Science, University of Melbourne, Parkville, Vic., Australia

D.L. Huxsoll, Division of Veterinary Medicine, Walter Reed Army Institute of Research, Washington

A.G. Karlson, Mayo Clinic, Rochester, Minn.

L. Kemeny, National Animal Disease Center, ARS, USDA, Ames, Iowa

A.W.D. Lepper, Animal Health Research Laboratory, Division of Animal Health, CSIRO, Parkville, Vic., Australia

I.R. Littlejohns, Veterinary Research Station, Glenfield, N.S.W., Australia

L.C. Lloyd, Animal Health Research Laboratory, Division of Animal Health, CSIRO, Parkville, Vic., Australia

P.D. McKercher, Plum Island Animal Disease Center, ARS, USDA, Greenport, N.Y.

M.N. Mickelson, National Animal Disease Center, ARS, USDA, Ames, Iowa

J.P. Newman, Department of Microbiology, Michigan State University, East Lansing

R.A. Packer, Department of Veterinary Microbiology, Iowa State University, Ames

G.V. Peacock, Animal and Plant Health Inspection Service, USDA, Hyattsville, Md.

J.E. Peterson, Animal Health Research Laboratory, Division of Animal Health, CSIRO, Parkville, Vic., Australia

J.C. Ramage, Department of Medicine and Surgery, College of Veterinary Medicine, Texas A & M University, College Station
T.O. Roby, Agricultural Research Service, USDA, Beltsville, Md.
M. Rogul, Division of Veterinary Medicine, Walter Reed Army Institute of Research, Washington
R.E. Shope, Yale Arbovirus Research Unit, School of Medicine, Yale University, New Haven, Conn.
W.A. Snowdon, Australian National Animal Health Laboratory, CSIRO, Melbourne, Vic., Australia
J.R. Songer, Safety Staff, National Animal Disease Center, ARS, USDA, Ames, Iowa
J. Storz, Department of Microbiology, Colorado State University, Fort Collins
R. Uskavitch, Plum Island Animal Disease Center Library, ARS, USDA, Greenport, N.Y.
A.G. Wedum, Division of Microbiological Safety, Fort Detrick, Frederick, Md. (deceased)
J.E. Williams, Poultry Disease Research Center, ARS, USDA, Athens, Ga.
R. Yedloutschnig, Plum Island Animal Disease Center, ARS, USDA, Greenport, N.Y.

Manual of Standardized Methods for Veterinary Microbiology

PART ONE: GENERAL LABORATORY METHODS

1. Introduction

The success of laboratory procedures in providing data for an accurate diagnosis of a disease depends upon many factors. The three most important factors are (1) selection and preservation of an adequate number of specimens that are aseptically taken from the most advantageous anatomic sites at the proper stage of the disease for the isolation or demonstration of pathogens, (2) collection of serum samples at a time when a diagnostic titer of antibodies could be expected, and (3) the knowledge and skill of the laboratory workers, who must select the appropriate laboratory methods from their knowledge of the similar diseases under suspicion, and who must skillfully conduct these procedures using adequate controls and safeguards.

The laboratory workers must have complete confidence in their equipment, media, cell cultures, embryonating eggs, test animals, solutions, reagents, antigens, antisera, and stains. In order to maintain this confidence, they must exercise strict quality and sterility controls. In addition, the laboratory must frequently train its personnel, have all materials and equipment readily available, and test this equipment often. The old adage "Nothing succeeds like success" very aptly applies to laboratory procedures. However, the price of success is constant preparedness and attention to details. At this stage in the development of the laboratory art we no longer can rely on chance to help us detect the pathogens.

There are many laboratory pitfalls ready to trap the unwary. Worthless and misleading results may be obtained when the equipment and materials are not properly sterilized. Traces of detergents and other toxic or inhibitory chemicals on glassware or rubber stoppers may get into media and prevent growth or destroy microorganisms or cell cultures. Cell cultures may have latent infections that may be reactivated to produce confounding cytopathic effect (CPE) or plaques. Pure cultures may become contaminated and, in subsequent passages, may be replaced by an overgrowth of the invader. Antisera prepared from inadequately pretested host animals may contain antibodies for disease agents other than the known one inoculated, and thus may give reactions that result in a wrong diagnosis. In stained preparations, artifacts may masquerade as bacteria, fungi, or inclusion bodies.

Serious laboratory disasters are caused by accidents or by disregard for microbiological laboratory safety, and may result in infection of laboratory workers, escape of disease agents, and infection of nearby animals, as well as spread of infection by means of contaminated biologics. Another potential disaster may result from failure to recognize or suspect an exotic disease soon enough to prevent its spread. Clinicians, field diagnosticians, and laboratory workers can be assisted in their preliminary assessment of the disease through the provision of an accurate history and through the pooling of knowledge regarding the diseases current in the animal population of the area.

In order to prevent this manual from becoming too voluminous, many topics have had to be condensed or omitted. Thus, Part One: General Laboratory Methods applies to the three types of pathogens treated in this manual, that is, the viral, bacterial, and mycotic disease agents. In the text for each pathogen, the specific test procedures commonly used are listed and, if the procedure differs from the accepted standardized method, that difference is noted. Another form of condensation is the liberal use of abbreviations, which are explained at the end of the text. The appendixes mainly apply to bacterial and mycotic pathogens. The scientific names mentioned in the text are listed in a special index. The virology family names are taken from the International Committee on Taxonomy of Viruses: F. Fenner, The classification and nomenclature of viruses, *Intervirology* 6:1–12, 1975/76.

2. Laboratory Safety

Precautions for working with disease agents should be used by every microbiological laboratory to prevent one or more of the following: (1) accidental infection or cross-contamination within the laboratory, which would nullify or confuse experimental results; (2) contamination or spread of infection to adjacent farms, communities, or larger areas; (3) infection of laboratory personnel; and (4) spread of infection through released biologics.

All microbiological laboratories have probably experienced cross-contamination either in the form of mixed cultures of bacteria or as unwanted or mixed infections of experimental animals and tissue cultures. Readjustments from such accidents are costly and time consuming. Numerous examples of the escape of disease agents from veterinary laboratories have been reported or privately admitted.[15] This type of disaster threatens both animal and human health and can cause great economic loss.

The worldwide literature contains references to approximately 6000 cases of accidental infection of laboratory workers, and undoubtably thousands more were not reported.[21,23,24] In studies of laboratory-acquired infections, the percentages by types of agents were as follows: bacteria 49.1, viruses 31.6, rickettsias 11.3, fungi 5.7, and parasites 2.3.[21] The percentages for the outcomes of the infections were: complete recovery 70, permanent disability 26, and death 4. In a supplementary study with 16.2% deaths, the fatality percentages for the types of agents were: viruses 7.3, bacteria 4.0, rickettsias 2.6, fungi 2.3, and parasites 0.[23] Among all these infections, the specific accident or infecting event was identified for only about 20% of the cases. Part of the other 80% of the cases where the cause was not found may have been due to the unsuspected release of infectious aerosols.[23]

Many of the laboratory-acquired infections are due to zoonoses—disease agents of animals transmissible to humans (Table 2.1).[10] These infections may result from handling the disease agents in the laboratory or from contact with infected animals, their tissues, or excretions. Latent infections with B-virus in Asiatic macaques and with Marburg virus in African green monkeys render these animals and tissues cultures prepared from them potentially hazardous.[8]

Inadequately safety-tested biologic materials and vaccines shipped or released from

Table 2.1. The main animal diseases transmissible to humans (zoonoses), excluding protozoan diseases*

Diseases	Hosts	Human hazard classification[22]
Viral zoonoses		
Rabies	Mammals	3
Rift Valley fever	Sheep, cattle	3†
Equine encephalomyelitis	Horses, birds	
Venezuelan		4†
Eastern and western		3
Vesicular stomatitis	Horses, cattle, swine	3
Cowpox	Cattle	2
Milker's nodules	Cattle	2
Horsepox	Horses	2
Camelpox	Camels	2†
Contagious ecthyma (Orf)	Sheep	2
Papular stomatitis	Cattle	2
Foot-and-mouth disease	Cloven-hoofed animals	2†
Newcastle disease	Poultry	2
Louping ill	Sheep	3†
Wesselsbron disease	Sheep	3†
Sendai influenza	Mice, swine	3
Swine influenza	Swine	2
Swine vesicular disease	Swine	2
Nairobi sheep disease	Sheep	2†
Yellow fever	Monkeys, rodents	4
Measles	Monkeys	2
Mumps	Monkeys	2
Chicken pox	Chimpanzees	3
B-virus infection	Monkeys, rodents	4
Marburg virus disease	Monkeys	4
Kyasanur Forest disease	Monkeys	4
Ilheus	Monkeys	2
Salivary gland virus infection	Monkeys	3
Russian spring-summer encephalitis	Rodents	4
Central European encephalitis	Rodents, goats	4
St. Louis encephalitis	Birds	3
Japanese B encephalitis	Birds, horses	4
Murray Valley encephalitis	Birds	4
West Nile fever	Birds	4
Mokola virus disease	Shrews	4
Omsk hemorrhagic fever‡	Muskrats (*Ondatra zibetica*)	4
Encephalomyocarditis	Rodents, pigs, primates	3
Bacterial zoonoses		
Tuberculosis	Cattle	3
Anthrax	Cattle, sheep	4
Brucellosis	Cattle, swine, goats	3
Erysipeloid	Swine (erysipelas)	2
Salmonelloses	Various animals, birds	2
Glanders	Horses, mules, asses	3
Melioidosis	Rats, dogs, cats, horses	3§
Tularemia	Rabbits, sheep, squirrels	3
Plague (bubonic, sylvatic)	Rodents (vector, fleas)	3
Leptospirosis	Rodents, various other animals	2
Relapsing fevers	Rodents (vector, lice)	2
Ratbite fever	Rodents, dogs, cats	2
Dermatophilosis	Cattle, sheep, horses	2
Rickettsial zoonoses		
Murine typhus	Rodents (vector, fleas)	3
Rocky Mountain spotted fever	Rodents (vector, ticks)	3
Tsutsugamushi	Rodents (vector, mites)	3
Rickettsial pox	Mice (vector, mites)	3

Diseases	Hosts	Human hazard classification[22]
Boutonneuse fever	Dogs (vector, ticks)	3
Q fever	Rodents, ruminants (vector, ticks)	3
Chlamydial zoonoses		
Psittacosis-ornithosis	Birds	3
Cat scratch disease[ll]	Cats	3
Louisiana pneumonitis	Birds	3
Enzootic abortion of ewes	Sheep	3
Fungal zoonoses#		
Dermatophytoses	Various animals, birds	2

*For protozoan zoonoses see E.J.L. Soulsby (ed.), *Parasitic Zoonoses: Clinical and Experimental Studies.* Proc. 6th Internat. Conf. World Ass. Advancement Vet. Parasit., Vienna, Sept. 1973. Academic Press, New York, 1974.

†These disease agents are also placed in class 5 for exotic pathogens that are restricted from the United States by USDA regulations for protection of livestock. Class 2 represents low risk, class 3 medium risk, and class 4 high risk of human infection and degree of microbiological safety precautions that must be taken with specific pathogens.

‡Signs and lesions have not been reported in suspected host reservoirs for the other hemorrhagic fevers, e.g. Dengue, Bolivian, Argentinian, Korean, and Crimean, nor for California encephalitis.

§USDA import permit required (class 5 exotic pathogen).

ll The etiology is uncertain; it may be a viral disease.[10]

#While only dermatophytoses can be classed with the zoonoses, many of the other mycotic disease agents are hazardous to humans when inhaled as aerosols.

microbiological laboratories have been the source of infection in some instances. Foot-and-mouth disease infections have been traced to smallpox vaccine and pituitary extract. A released fowlpox vaccine was contaminated with Newcastle disease virus. During World War II many servicemen contracted hepatitis from infectious serum used in conjunction with formulation of yellow fever vaccine, and more recently there was the tragic episode with polio vaccine.

Classification of Safety Measures

The host and its geographic range, the degree of pathogenicity and contagiousness, and the volume of the microorganisms handled in a laboratory generally determine the extent to which safety measures should be used.[25] A laboratory that deals only with organisms nonpathogenic to living things would still need basic safety precautions to insure purity of its cultures. Another laboratory that handles large volumes of a contagious foreign pathogen of special hazard to humans and animals would need many special safety precautions. Between these two extremes there are various degrees of safety measures that may be applied (Table 2.2).

The United States Public Health Service has developed a classification of disease agents based on the human risk involved, and from this a laboratory may be classified according to its ability to deal safely with the organisms.[22,23]

Class 1. Agents of no or minimum hazard under ordinary conditions of handling. This class has unrestricted distribution to any bona fide laboratory, teaching, or research institution.

Class 2. Agents of ordinary hazard. This class includes agents that may produce

Table 2.2. Types of microorganisms listed according to the degree of safety precautions required

Type and hazard of organisms	Host range	Examples
Widespread nonpathogen, no hazard	Normal flora	L. acidophilus
Widespread pathogen, low hazard	Humans, animals	E. coli
Indigenous animal pathogen, low hazard	Dogs, wild animals	Canine distemper virus
Zoonosis, low human hazard	Humans, birds	Newcastle disease virus
Exotic animal pathogen, special hazard	Ruminants	Rinderpest virus
Exotic zoonosis, special hazard	Humans, animals	Rift Valley fever virus

human or animal disease from accidental inoculation or injections or other means of cutaneous penetration, but which can be contained by ordinary laboratory techniques. Distribution is restricted to qualified individuals in universities, research and industrial institutions, and diagnostic and other suitable laboratories.

Class 3. Agents involving special hazard or agents derived from outside the United States that require a federal permit for importation, excluding those specified for a higher classification. This class includes pathogens that require special conditions for containment.

Class 4. Agents that require the most stringent conditions for their containment because they are extremely hazardous to laboratory personnel or may cause serious epidemic and/or epizootic disease. This class includes class 3 agents from outside the United States when they are employed in entomological experiments or when other entomological experiments are conducted in the same laboratory area.

Class 5. Foreign animal pathogens that are excluded from the United States by law or whose entry is restricted by USDA (U.S. Department of Agriculture) administrative policy. The etiologic agents of the following diseases are included in this class: African horsesickness, African swine fever, Besnoitia infection, Borna disease, bovine infectious petechial fever, camelpox, contagious agalactia of sheep, contagious bovine pleuropneumonia, East Coast fever, ephemeral fever, foot-and-mouth disease, fowl plague, goatpox, heartwater, hog cholera, louping ill, lumpy skin disease, Nagana, Nairobi sheep disease, Newcastle disease (Asiatic strains), peste des petits ruminants, pseudofarcy, Rift Valley fever, rinderpest, sheeppox, swine vesicular disease, Teschen disease, Theileriosis, vesicular exanthema, and Wesselsbron disease. If any of these diseases are suspected in an outbreak, they should be promptly reported to state and federal authorities.

Safety precautions should pervade all facets of a microbiological laboratory's operations, including administration, location, structural and mechanical design, utilities, air supply and exhaust, introduction of supplies, movement of personnel and animals, laboratory techniques and operation of equipment, disinfection and sterilization, removal of wastes, acquisition and disposal of animals, and testing and packaging of biologics.[3,6,17,18,19,20]

Safety measures should be practical and logical to encourage compliance and offer a minimum of impedance to the work effort. However, they should be applied in multiples where possible to avoid dependence on a single measure. For example, personnel may be required to avoid animals susceptible to a disease being studied in the laboratory when they are away from work, in case their personal decontamination procedures are ever inadequate.[3]

Laboratory Design and Construction

The laboratory should be located with due regard for the adjacent community and the proximity of hosts susceptible to the disease agents studied. Prevailing winds, surface water drainage, and sewage outfall may effect site selection. Reliability of utilities is important; a modern microbiological laboratory can not safely function without full electrical power or an adequate water supply.

The built-in safety features, convenience of floor plan, and efficiency of mechanical equipment for handling wastes and air all contribute to a successful safety operation.[4,13,15,17] Safety problems are greatly magnified by design deficiencies, which are costly to correct at a later date.

General Design

Laboratories of class 1 or 2 may be buildings of conventional or ordinary construction. However, laboratories of class 3, 4, or 5 should be specially constructed for the intended purposes.[17] A safety-designed laboratory building should be constructed so that it is virtually fireproof and so that each floor and room is virtually waterproof, airtight, and insect- and verminproof. Thus only the controlled entrances and intakes and exits and exhausts would need continual surveillance for trouble on the outside or between floors. All windows should be sealed shut and all expansion joints and pipe sleeves should be filled with a pliable material that continually makes a seal. Ideally, the building should be "a box within a box," so that the highly contaminated rooms are the inner box. (This is the design concept for the new Australian National Animal Health Laboratory, Division of Animal Health, CSIRO.)

The interior walls, floors, and ceilings should be made of materials that are smooth and easily cleaned.[16] They also should withstand disinfection, including use of either alkaline or acid solutions.

Electrical conduits, piping, and duct work should be confined to machinery areas and enclosed spaces to eliminate extra cleaning. However, if hollow spaces between walls exist, they should be sealed between rooms and floors and should not be penetrated by unsealed electrical conduits and boxes, piping, or duct work. If conventional construction were allowed, air movement between walls or through electrical conduits could carry pathogens from one infected area to another or to clean areas; this is particularly important in animal rooms and all contaminated areas.[7]

Other built-in safety features include double-door autoclaves, pass-through disinfectant traps, conveniently located steam and water supply stations for wash down and cleaning, air locks, showers, and storage facilities for sterilized clothing and special equipment.

Traffic

A class 3, 4, or 5 laboratory should have a carefully designed floor plan with definite flow patterns for movement into buildings and between areas for personnel, animals, feed, supplies, and equipment. The admittance of personnel into laboratories and the introduction or removal of materials should be accomplished only by trained personnel familiar with all safety precautions for the entire operation.

Entrance and exit facilities for personnel should consist of inner and outer change rooms with a shower area or stalls interposed between them. When leaving the laboratory (class 3, 4, or 5), all personnel should be required to remove laboratory clothing, scrub hands, clean fingernails, and take a complete shower before entering outer change room. Laboratory clothing and towels should be sterilized and sent to the laboratory laundry before redistribution.

Air locks that may be disinfected after use are suitable for movement of animals, feed, equipment, and supplies into the laboratory areas. Built-in autoclaves with doors at each end may be used for introduction of materials (cold) or for removal of materials from the laboratory after sterilization.[2,16]

All animal carcasses and burnable trash should be incinerated. Nonburnable materials should be autoclaved prior to removal from laboratory. Gas sterilization may be used for books, instruments, and other materials that could be harmed by heat or chemical disinfectants. Chemical disinfection of materials being removed from the laboratory may be done in air locks.

Sewage and Air Control

Sewage, liquid wastes, and blood from necropsy rooms, especially of class 3, 4, and 5 laboratories, should be heated or treated with chemicals and then diluted to inactivate the disease agents prior to discharge into a sewage disposal plant or leaching field.[7]

Air pressure in the laboratory should be controlled so that air flows from the outside through buffer zones and then into contaminated areas.[4] The animal rooms, necropsy room, and safety hood or cabinet work areas should have a lower air pressure than adjacent corridors or laboratory rooms, all of which should be considered as potentially contaminated.

The incoming air should be filtered to remove dust, and heat tempered or air conditioned as necessary. The exhaust air of class 4 and 5 laboratories ideally should be zoned according to degree of potential contamination. All exhaust air from contaminated or potentially contaminated areas should be passed through HEPA (high efficiency particulate air) filters.[13] A plan must be carefully devised for sterilization, removal, disposal, and replacement of air filters. Before installation, each HEPA filter should be given a challenge test with di-octyl-phthallate (DOP) of known particle size to prove the filter's integrity. The integrity of the seal around the filters is also important in making replacements. The air system should be carefully monitored so that clogged filters do not upset the air balance. Exhaust air stacks or ports should be located as far as possible from air intakes. (See Appendix A, "Filter Test Techniques," for other tests.)

Animal and Necropsy Rooms: Personnel Entry and Exit

There are at least nine methods for controlling disease agents in relation to personnel entry and exit to and from animal quarters. The choice of the method will be determined by the class of agent that is being studied and the nature of the work.

1. *Covering garments.* Clothing and footwear that may be laundered or decontaminated are worn over street clothes and footware.
2. *Laboratory clothing.* Street clothing and footwear are not permitted in animal rooms; only laboratory apparel is permitted.
3. *Clothing and footwear change without shower.* A complete change in garments from that worn in the laboratory area is made.
4. *Clothing and footwear change with shower.* A complete change in garments from that worn in the laboratory area is made and a shower is taken before exit from animal room. Entrance showers could also be required.
5. *Nude with boots and gloves.* Several laboratories have operated animal rooms that require the personnel to wear only boots and gloves and shower before exit.
6. *Rubber or plastic garments.* Laboratory clothing is removed and personnel don sterilized protective clothing, which is disinfected before exit.
7. *Rooms with special animal cages.* Contamination within an animal room may be partially controlled by use of special isolation cages, such as Horsfall-Bauer units[9] or laminar airflow cage racks.[5]
8. *Complete external and respiratory protection.* Personnel wear sterilized protective clothing that has its own or an outside air supply through a hose. The suit is disinfected prior to exit.
9. *Remote manipulation and telemetry.* A system of animal cages is operated within enclosed safety cabinets by means of gloved ports or remote mechanical manipulation. Telemetry may be used to monitor the vital signs of the animals.

Animal Restraint

Many minor and some serious laboratory injuries and infections of personnel result from inadequate or improper restraint of animals. One of these is accidental inoculation of fingers or hands because the animal made a sudden move at the moment an operator was poised with a needle and syringe. In one survey about 26% of accidental human infections involved needle puncture, while in another survey it was only 4%.[18,24] With proper restraint or use of anesthetics this type of accident can be avoided. Humane treatment of the animals also should be a major consideration.

Exposure of Animals

All infectious materials and equipment necessary for animal inoculation or exposure should be taken into animal rooms in closed metal carrying cases. Thus if the material is dropped enroute, the general area is not contaminated. The animal room should be considered potentially contaminated from a microbiological safety standpoint at the moment when vials or containers of infectious material are opened or pierced with a hypodermic needle. From this moment, all decontamination procedures for leaving the room would be in effect. The used equipment may be replaced in the carrying case for removal from the room and sterilization before unloading. Surplus biologic materials may be retrieved from the carrying case prior to sterilization by use of a safety cabinet.

Necropsy Rooms

Necropsy examinations may be performed in designated rooms or in safety cabinets when small animals are involved. Provisions must be made for transporting small animals to the necropsy room and from there to an autoclave and to the incinerator in containers that can be exteriorly disinfected. For large animals, the necropsy rooms should be adjacent to animal room corridors and also should have a convenient means of access to the incinerator area for disposal of carcasses. Animal rooms and corridors along the route that the infected animals are moved should have tight-fitting doors to preserve the isolated integrity of any room not involved. The necropsy room should have only the bare necessities, since everything in the room and adjacent corridors involved in the procedure should be washed and decontaminated before re-use or opening to other laboratory areas. In some instances necropsy examinations may be performed in the animal room. This results in the need for closed containers for the removal of carcasses. When dead animals are to be stored, a closed container should be used to prevent contamination of refrigerator or freezer. These general provisions should apply to all classes of agents; necropsy rooms should not become the unsanitary eyesore of any laboratory.

Decontamination

The decontamination of animal rooms and corridors may consist of any or all of the following, depending upon the disease agent: (1) washing with running water to remove excreta, feed debris, and dust; (2) scrubbing the entire room and contents with a detergent solution; (3) rinsing to remove detergent; (4) spraying the room with a disinfectant approved for the disease agent and flooding the floor with disinfectant if necessary; (5) disinfecting and removing surplus items from the room; and (6) rinsing to remove disinfectant.

In the case of dangerous human pathogens, gas sterilants may be used at the beginning of the procedure.[14,16] The room may be again disinfected and rinsed immediately before re-use. Formaldehyde vapor is an economical and practical disinfectant for various kinds of rooms or enclosed cabinets.[20]

Laboratory Safety Techniques

Laboratory safety techniques may be applied in various degrees, from the bench-top aseptic methods used by general bacteriologists to the completely enclosed system used for extremely hazardous human pathogens. Common sense rules should be followed in handling infectious materials in the laboratory. Before beginning any of the many procedures common to microbiological laboratories, the investigators and their technicians should review their operations from a safety standpoint to determine what safeguards are needed. Their safety objectives should be to provide containment and decontamination procedures that avoid danger from aerosols, drop-spilling of infectious materials, contamination of objects by contact with used equipment, and aspiration or movement of infectious materials through equipment beyond control points. If safety techniques are not used, the laboratory room, personnel, and equipment all may become grossly contaminated, and the disease agent may be spread throughout the laboratory building.

Laboratory Safety

How Accidental Infection Occurs

Common manipulations with the inoculating needle, pipette, syringe, centrifuge, lyophilizer, and blender create bacteria- or virus-laden aerosolized particles suitable for inhalation.[1,4] Table 2.3 shows the number of such particles that may be recovered at a distance of 2 ft (60.96 cm) from the work area. Because most bacteria in the air occur in clumps, these amounts can contain a human infectious dose, particularly if the operation is repetitious.[25] Common laboratory accidents likewise liberate organisms into the air. Accidents with petri plates, lyophilized ampules, or a centrifuge may create microbial aerosols that can cause infection in persons stationed in other parts of the building one or more floors away.[1,24]

Table 2.3. Bacteria recovered by air sampling within 2 ft (60.96 cm) of the site of common procedures[18,25]

Procedure	Colonies obtained per operation
Removing tight cover of standard Waring blender immediately after mixing culture	Too numerous to count
Opening lyophile culture tube	86
Decanting centrifuged fluid into flask	17
Inserting hot loop in culture flask	9
Removing dry cotton plug from shaken flask	5
Pipetting 1 ml of inoculum to poured agar petri plate	3
Pipetting 1 ml of culture into 50 ml of broth	1

General Techniques for All Microorganisms

1. Establish a minimum standard that will be at least equivalent to the techniques taught in general microbiology courses, which are aimed at obtaining and maintaining standard or pure cultures.

2. Maintain a work area that is not cluttered and provides protection against any dropping or spilling of microorganisms.

3. Decontaminate the work area and disinfect or sterilize all equipment used with or potentially contaminated with microorganisms. It is good practice to resterilize items that were in the work area but were not actually used before replacing them in the sterile supply area.

4. Label clearly all preparations of microorganisms and store materials to be frozen in containers capable of withstanding the thermal shock of freezing and thawing. Freezers are difficult to decontaminate. Periodically clean deep-freeze and dry-ice chests in which cultures or serum samples are stored to remove any broken ampules or tubes. Use rubber gloves during this cleaning.

5. Whenever possible, hold or carry infectious materials so that the bottom of the tube, vial, or flask rests against the palm of hand.

6. Carry all infectious materials to and from distant instruments or animal rooms in closed metal containers, not in open trays.

7. Wear rubber gloves and protective clothing when handling infectious material and decontaminate exposed parts after completion of the operation.

8. Avoid the mouth pipetting technique with infectious agents or toxic fluids. Use only pipettes plugged with cotton. Do not blow infectious fluids out of pipettes.

9. Before centrifuging, inspect tubes for cracks. Inspect the inside of the trunnion cup for rough walls caused by erosion or adhering matter. Carefully remove all bits of glass from the rubber cushion. A germicidal solution added between the tube and the trunnion cup not only disinfects the surfaces of both of these, but also provides an excellent cushion against shocks that otherwise might break the tube. For better protection use sealable centrifuge cups.[25]

10. Use only syringes that lock onto the needle.

11. If protective garments are worn over laboratory clothing, give preference to use of operating-room gowns fastened at the back.[24]

12. Decontaminate laboratory room floors and bench tops frequently.

Special Techniques for More Hazardous Pathogens

1. The microbiological safety cabinet is the most useful primary barrier. The cabinet will contain accidentally produced aerosols or spills and thus prevent contamination of the laboratory room.[1,4,25] The laminar flow biohazard cabinet provides HEPA filtered air within the cabinet and an air curtain downward across the opening of the cabinet.[11,12,25] It protects the worker and also the experimental materials from contamination. Each cabinet must be tested at its exact point of use to establish an optimum balance between the inward and downward airflow at the front opening and the filtered airflow within the cabinet over the work area. All exhaust air from the cabinet should be passed through a HEPA filter. All seams and utility entry points must be checked for leaks.[25]

2. Use a lyophile apparatus that has provision for internal decontamination and controlled exhaust through air filters.

3. Provide isolation rooms with exit decontamination facilities for personnel and materials when using large-volume repetitive techniques with organisms that have a low human hazard but high animal hazard (e.g., inoculation of large numbers of tissue cultures or embryonating eggs). Such a room also may be used to house the ultracentrifugation apparatus, which is bulky and often produces aerosols.

4. When an agent is used in entomological experiments, the room must be insect-proof. Provide screened vestibules and have pyrethrum insecticide or other suitable insect-killing devices available for entry and exit of personnel and animals.

5. Provide air locks with remote control spraying devices for disinfectants.

Personnel Health Program

Personnel assigned to work in areas where they may be exposed to disease agents of human hazard should be vaccinated if immune prophylaxis is available.[7,13] Pregnant women and children under age 15 should never be permitted to enter such areas.[8] Future reference serum should be taken from all personnel before they are permitted to start work in areas where zoonoses or other human pathogens are being studied. Vaccination for tetanus should be encouraged and provided for all persons handling animals, especially large animals.[3]

Establishing a Microbiological Safety Program

The microbiological safety of a laboratory is the responsibility of the laboratory director. However, he or she cannot carry out this responsibility without a planned safety program, the cooperation of every employee, and the help of a safety officer and/or a safety committee of key supervisors. Larger laboratories also should have a safety force and security guards. Furthermore, the director must have the backing of the higher echelons of management to implement and enforce such a program.[3]

The microbiological safety program should be set forth in the form of written regulations and instructions. All employees should read this material and receive training so that they will know what is expected of them. The unit supervisors must be responsible for updating the training, monitoring employee work habits, and enforcing the safety regulations.[7] The microbiological safety program will not succeed, however, without penalties for willful violations or complete disregard of the established safety procedures.[3] The penalties for infractions of safety rules could range from a reprimand to reassignment, partial withholding of pay, or dismissal.[3]

The laboratory should also have plans to cover emergencies such as fires, explosions, infection of animals outside of laboratory, and evacuation of sick, injured, or dead employees. All of these events pose major microbiological safety problems.

Equipment or systems relied upon for microbiological safety should be regularly tested for operational efficiency, using simulant agents if necessary. This would include safety cabinets, air handling and filtration units, sewage decontamination equipment, disinfectants, and sterilizers.

A trained employee should accompany laboratory visitors at all times to assure compliance with all safety regulations.

References

1. Barbeito, M.S., and L.A. Taylor. Containment of microbial aerosols in a microbiological safety cabinet. *Appl. Microbiol.* 16:1225–1229, 1968.
2. Brewer, J.H. *Lectures on Sterilization.* Duke University Press, Durham, N.C., 1973.
3. Callis, J.J., and G.E. Cottral. Methods for containment of animal pathogens at the Plum Island Animal Disease Laboratory. In *Methods in Virology,* K. Maramorosch and H. Koprowski (eds.), vol. 4, pp. 465–480. Academic Press, New York, 1968.
4. Chatigny, M.A., and D.I. Clinger. Contamination control in aerobiology. In *An Introduction to Experimental Aerobiology,* R.L. Dimmick and A.B. Akers (eds.), pp. 194–263. Wiley, New York, 1969.
5. Cook, R.O. New ventilated isolation cage. *Appl. Microbiol.* 16:762–771, 1968.
6. Darlow, H.M. Safety in the microbiological laboratory. In *Methods in Microbiology,* J.R. Norris and D.W. Ribbons (eds.), pp. 169–204. Academic Press, New York, 1969.
7. Hellman, A. (ed.). *Biohazard Control and Containment in Oncogenic Virus Research.* HEW Publication no. (NIH) 73-459, 1973.
8. Hellman, A., M.N. Oxman, and P. Pollack (eds.). *Biohazards in Biological Research.* Cold Spring Harbor Laboratory, Cold Spring Harbor, N.Y., 1973.
9. Horsfall, F.L., and H.H. Bauer. Individual isolation of infected animals in a single room. *J. Bact.* 40:569–580, 1940.
10. Hubbert, W.T., W.F. McCulloch, and P.R. Schnurrenberger. *Diseases Transmitted from Animals to Man.* 6th ed. Thomas, Sprinfgield, Ill., 1975.
11. Korcyznski, M.S., W.S. Holden, and R.F. Schmitt. Microbial evaluation of a sterility test laminar airflow cabinet. *J. Am. Air Contamination Control* 3:13–18, 1971.
12. Kukla, H.E. Evaluation of a vertical airflow microbiological cabinet. *J. Am. Air Contaimination Control* 3:5–10, 1971.

13. Lennette, E.H., E.H. Spaulding, and J.P. Truant (eds.). *Manual of Clinical Microbiology*. 2d. ed. American Society of Microbiology, Washington, 1974.
14. Perkins, J.J. *Principles and Methods of Sterilization in Health Sciences*. 2d. ed. Thomas, Springfield, Ill., 1970.
15. Phillips, G.B. *Microbiological Safety in U.S. and Foreign Laboratories*. Technical Study no. 35. Industrial Health and Safety Division, U.S. Army Biological Laboratories, Frederick, Md., 1961.
16. Phillips, G.B., and W.S. Miller. *Industrial Sterilization*. Duke University Press, Durham, N.C., 1973.
17. Phillips, G.B., and R.S. Runkle. Design of facilities for microbiological safety. In *Handbook of Laboratory Safety*, N.V. Steere (ed.), pp. 393–399. Chemical Rubber Co., Cleveland, 1967.
18. Reitman, M., and A.G. Wedum. Microbiological safety. *Public Health Rep.* 71:659–665, 1956.
19. Runkle, R.S., and G.B. Phillips. *Microbial Contamination Control Facilities*. Van Nostrand Reinhold, New York, 1969.
20. Songer, J.R., D.T. Braymen, R.G. Mathis, and J.W. Monroe. The practical use of formaldehyde vapor for disinfection. *Health Lab. Sci.* 9:46–55, 1972.
21. Sulkins, S.E. Laboratory-acquired infections. *Bact. Rev.* 25:203–209, 1961.
22. U.S. Public Health Service, Ad Hoc Committee. *Classification of Etiological Agents on the Basis of Hazard*. 4th ed. HEW, Atlanta, 1974.
23. U.S. Public Health Service, Environmental Services Branch. *National Institutes of Health Biohazards Safety Guide*. HEW, Washington, 1974.
24. Wedum, A.G., and R.H. Kruse. *Assessment of Risk of Human Infection in the Microbiological Laboratory*. Misc. Pub. 19. Department of Army, Fort Detrick, Md., 1966.
25. Wedum, A.G., W.E. Barkley, and A. Hellman. Handling of infectious agents. *J. Am. Vet. Med. Assoc.* 161:1557–1567, 1972.

3. Collection and Processing of Specimens

It is important that a sample be collected and handled in a manner that will permit a high rate of recovery of any microorganisms present. The species of animal involved and the history of the individual animal will provide a basis for selection of specimens and procedures for detection of etiologic agents. In order to avoid failure to isolate a significant microorganism, laboratory diagnosticians should routinely culture a wide range of tissues by screening methods that will detect all pathogenic bacteria, viruses, and fungi.

Collection of Specimens

The selection of a valid sample is a problem for the field veterinarian. Since this manual is written as a guide for laboratory workers, the field aspects of this subject will be given only cursory consideration.

Very often the value of laboratory test results are directly dependent on the selection, preparation, handling, and shipment of specimens. It is important to have for examination an animal, or specimens from an animal, that is typically affected with the condition in question. If the selection is left to the owner rather than the veterinarian, often a chronically ill animal will be selected instead of a more representative sample.

In the case of a herd problem, the best specimen to receive at the laboratory is a live animal typically affected with the disease in question (not a cull). The laboratory personnel can then obtain blood and other specimens desired prior to euthanasia. A complete necropsy can be performed, lesions observed, and specimens for various laboratory examinations collected. It is very desirable to have the caretaker of the animals accompany them to the laboratory. This individual's account of the circumstances surrounding the illness, in addition to the history supplied by the veterinarian, will usually be helpful in deciding what diseases should be considered and what tests performed. The second best choice of specimens is an animal that died shortly before being brought to the laboratory.

A necropsy by the field veterinarian, while often most instructive to him, is the third choice of samples submitted for examination, since it is necessary to depend upon his knowledge of selection and handling of specimens for the laboratory tests desired.

Because he may never have been actively engaged in laboratory work, his choices of material may be inappropriate for the disease in question. However, because the majority of specimens received in a laboratory will probably come from a field necropsy, it is important for laboratory workers to continually aid practicing veterinarians in the selection and shipment of the appropriate specimens.

Each instance of an improperly selected, prepared, or shipped specimen should be called to the attention of the sender. Some laboratories send a printed form to each individual who has submitted improperly selected, prepared, or shipped specimens. These forms enumerate the deficiencies and explain why some other method is preferred. Few people intentionally send poor specimens and most will react favorably to such suggestions.

All specimens should be accompanied by an adequate history of the disease (and necropsy findings if available), as observed by the veterinarian. It is recommended that laboratories have forms prepared for this purpose. These can be distributed to field veterinarians, and can help improve the accuracy and availability of a history.

If a clinical diagnosis has been made and confirmation is desired, the researcher should consult the discussion of the suspected disease found elsewhere in this text in order to find the preferred specimens for examination. If a specific diagnosis has not been made, specimens from diseased animals should be collected for bacteriological, virological, and mycological examination. The specimens desired are the same in both live and dead animals but the availability is more limited in the case of live animals.

For recovery of bacterial or viral agents, specimens should be collected from animals at the height of the febrile state or as early in the acute phase of the disease as possible. If there is strong evidence of a certain disease or group of diseases, such as might be exhibited by an animal with a central nervous system (CNS) disturbance, the specimens submitted can be rather selective. However, as few clinical signs are truly pathognomonic, it is always safer to select a full complement of tissues for microbiological isolation attempts.

In summation, the person who obtains the specimens should: (1) use animals that have not been subjected to therapy, if possible; (2) collect specimens aseptically from anatomic sites most likely to contain the suspected pathogen; (3) select animals in the early or acute stages of the disease, rather than those chronically affected (except for serum samples); (4) submit a meaningful history of the disease outbreak; and (5) offer a tentative clinical diagnosis based on the animals observed and a knowledge of diseases in the area.

Specimens for Bacterial Isolation
Specimens from Live Animals

Specimens of defibrinated blood for culture should be obtained from animals in the febrile stage of a disease. Immediate plating on blood agar or other suitable media is preferred but seldom possible in the field.

If a nasal exudate is present, a swab can be used to collect a specimen from deep in the nasal passage. Pharyngeal swabs or saliva are desirable for some diseases. A cup probang may be used to collect oesophageal-pharyngeal (OP) fluid specimens.[7]

Under proper circumstances, spinal fluid can be obtained from living animals for culture. The specimen should be collected with aseptic technique through the foramen magnum or lumbosacral space. This technique is a surgical procedure, not without danger to the animal, and is not used frequently for these reasons.

Urine can be obtained by bladder tap, catheterization, or at urination, in that order of preference. Uterine, cervical, or vaginal swabs are procured in the same manner as nasal material. Collection of semen material may be necessary at times.

When swabs are collected, there is a danger of their drying out. Therefore, they should be placed immediately in a fluid transport media, such as Leibovitz media, sucrose solution, or broth, to prevent loss of infectious agents in shipment. The peptides, amino acids, or sugars in these solutions aid in the preservation of viruses and bacteria. All specimens should be refrigerated as soon as possible. If not, contaminants frequently encountered under field conditions may overgrow the etiologic agent and make its isolation difficult or impossible.

For bacterial recovery, inoculation of freshly prepared solid media in the field has the advantage of providing information on the number and types of bacteria present. This solid media technique is especially useful for the evaluation of cervical or uterine cultures. Such preparations can be incubated by the practitioner, and those with no growth or with colonies readily recognized need not be sent to the laboratory.

Feces specimens to be examined for bacteria or viruses can be obtained from large animals by insertion of the hand and arm into the rectum, protected by a disposable plastic sleeve. The sleeve can then be turned inside out over the specimen, tied shut at the wrist, and the glove portion used as a container. The sleeve part is cut off and discarded. An identifying number can be written on a paper enclosed with the specimen or written on masking tape applied to the glove. Another method is the insertion of a large tongue depressor into the rectum. The depressor is pressed down slightly, thus allowing the inflation of the rectum with air and stimulating defecation. Again, use sterile plastic bags. Collection of feces even from small animals is desirable directly from the rectum. If this is not possible, fresh droppings should be collected and handled in a similar manner.

Necropsy Specimens

Ample-sized portions of the following (up to 300 g) should be placed individually in polyethylene bags or other suitable leakproof containers: spleen, liver, kidney, lung, tonsil, portions of any abnormal-appearing muscle, a mesenteric, a pharyngeal, and a medistinal lymph node, a longitudinal half of the brain, a tied-off section of intestine containing the ileocecal valve and adjacent lymph node, and a gut section showing lesions if possible. If reproductive problems, abortions, or weak births have occurred, the uterus or its secretion, the placenta, or, in an aborted fetus, the tied-off fetal stomach and contents, should be submitted. If enterotoxemia is suspected, intestinal contents from the affected portion should be removed from the gut, placed in a plastic or glass container and shipped to the laboratory, frozen or well refrigerated, as quickly as possible. Tissue enzymes in the gut wall inactivate the toxin if not removed promptly, making identification of the toxin impossible. If the carcass is too decomposed for reliable results by culture of the tissues listed above, a long bone or rib can be collected for culture of the marrow. Specimens from other tissues or organs that appear abnormal should be included in addition to the above, such as joint, abdominal, pericardial, and spinal fluids, and urine or purulent material.

Specimens for Virus Isolation

In many instances, the same specimens can be used for bacterial and viral isolation attempts. Therefore, the following comments are basically supplemental to the procedures described earlier. Table 3.1 lists a series of preferred specimens that should be considered, depending on the disease suggested.

Specimens from Live Animals

When a suitable animal is not available for necropsy, all available specimens should be collected. Jugular blood should be obtained, including samples allowed to clot and those mixed with an anticoagulant. Up to 50 ml of each are desired. Whole blood for serum should be collected from both acute-stage and convalescent animals when available. The blood containing anticoagulant should not be frozen. Deep nasal swabs, pharyngeal swabs, and saliva can be obtained with a sterile cotton swab or the cup probang, in a manner similar to that described for bacteria.[7] Conjunctival swabs can be obtained by inserting a cotton swab into the lower conjunctival sac and rotating it while moving it laterally through the sac. The swabs should be placed in sterile screw-capped tubes of transport media, as already described. Urine samples collected by sterile bladder tap, catheterization, or other method, and shipped in a sterile jar with leakproof lid, should be obtained. A feces sample can be obtained as described under collection of specimens from live animals for bacterial culture. Vesicle fluid should be collected with a syringe and a 22-gauge needle. Where vesicles have ruptured, the epithelium around the vesicle should be peeled off with forceps and shipped as described for conjunctival swabs. Portions of any other exanthematous or poxlike lesions (scabs) should be collected when available and shipped in the same manner. Spinal fluid may be of value in the diagnosis of certain CNS viral diseases and can be collected as outlined under collection of bacterial specimens from live animals.

It is usually desirable to add antibiotic to the fluids used for transporting swabs for virus isolation, e.g. 500 units of penicillin, 500 μg of streptomycin, or 500 units of mycostatin or fungizone per ml. All specimens for virus isolation should be shipped under refrigeration by liquid nitrogen, dry ice, or (least preferable) wet ice.

Necropsy Specimens

If an animal is available for necropsy, a wider selection of specimens can be obtained, but it should include all of the above. Animals in the febrile or acute stage of the disease are preferred. Tissues collected should include a longitudinal half of the brain (shared with the bacteriologist); conjunctiva; tonsillar tissue; lung; pharyngeal, mediastinal, and mesenteric lymph nodes; heart; muscle; spleen; liver; kidney; adrenal gland; tied-off portions of small intestine and lower bowel, including contents; testicles; uterus; and placenta when available. Urine and any other available secretions or excretions should also

Table 3.1. Suggested specimens for isolation of viruses (see key below)

	Equine	Bovine	Ovine	Porcine	Canine	Feline	Avian
Adenoviruses		5, 12		2, 5, 21	25		1, 5, 11, 18
Bunyamwera viruses							
Rift Valley fever		1	1				
Coronaviruses							
Transmissible gastroenteritis				5, 8			
Herpesviruses							
Pseudorabies	12, 13, 15,* 16, 22	3, 4, 12, 13,† 15, 16, 22		2, 3, 15, 16, 21	15, 25‡	12, 16,§ 22	1, 5,‖ 10, 13, 22
Malignant catarrhal fever	2, 10, 16	2, 10, 16			2, 10, 16	2, 10, 16	
Bovine herpes mammillitis		1, 16, 18					
		23					
Orthomyxoviruses (influenza)	12, 13, 22	13, 22		12, 13, 22			5, 12, 13
Paramyxoviruses (PI-3, ND)	13, 22			13			4, 12, 18, 22
Rinderpest, distemper		4, 5, 7, 13, 14	4, 5, 13, 14	4, 5, 13, 14	25		
Papovaviruses (papilloma)		10			10		
Parvoviruses		5, 7, 16		15		1, 5, 7, 16	
Picornaviruses (enteroviruses)		5, 6, 7		2, 5, 6, 7, 15	5, 7	4, 5, 7, 19	2, 5, 7
Rhinovirus	13, 22	13					
Vesicular exanthema	10, 21, 24	10, 21, 24	10, 21, 24	10, 21, 24			
Foot-and-mouth disease		10, 21, 24	10, 21, 24	10, 21, 24			
Poxviruses	10	10	10	10			10
Reoviruses		5, 7, 13			5, 13		5, 13
Orbiviruses							
African horsesickness	1, 10, 13						
Bluetongue		1, 10, 16	25				
Rhabdoviruses							
Rabies	2, 17	2, 17	2, 17	2, 17	2, 17	7, 21	
Vesicular stomatitis	1, 16, 24	1, 16, 24		1, 16, 24			
Togaviruses (VEE, EEE, WEE, louping ill)	1, 2, 3, 13, 26	1, 2	1, 2, 3	1			
Equine arteritis	1, 13, 15, 16, 18						
Hog cholera, bovine viral diarrhea–mucosal disease		5, 7, 13, 14, 16		25			
Unclassified viruses							
African swine fever				25			
Equine infectious anemia	1, 18						

*Equine rhinopneumonitis. †Infectious bovine rhinotracheitis. ‡Hemorrhagic disease of pups.
§Feline rhinotracheitis. ‖Marek's disease, infectious laryngotracheitis, duck plague.

1. Blood whole
2. Brain
3. Cerebrospinal fluid
4. Conjunctival secretions
5. Feces
6. Heart
7. Intestinal mucosa
8. Jejunum-ileum
9. Kidney
10. Lesion material
11. Liver
12. Lung
13. Nasal and pharyngeal secretions
14. Peyer's patches
15. Placenta-fetus
16. Regional lymph nodes
17. Salivary gland
18. Spleen
19. Stomach
20. Tongue
21. Tonsil (OP fluid)
22. Tracheal mucosa
23. Udder-teat, milk
24. Vesicular fluid
25. Virtually all organs and secretions
26. Pancreas

be collected. All specimens should be collected in individual containers and frozen on dry ice or by liquid nitrogen. If dry ice or liquid nitrogen are not available, wet ice can be used. A poor substitute for using ice is placing tissue specimens in 50% neutral buffered glycerol.

Fixed Specimens for Histologic Examination

In many instances, fixed specimens for histologic examinations, such as determining types of cell changes, presence of inclusion bodies, or infiltration of lymphocytes, can be of considerable aid in arriving at a diagnosis. Therefore, 10% Formalin–preserved specimens about 1–2 mm square should be collected in parallel with the fresh material.

Specimens from Mycotic Infections

Diagnoses of ringworm and other dermatophytes are made most easily when skin scrapings direct from the animal are placed in fresh selective media, such as Sabouraud's (see Appendix A) or a transport media, and mailed in this media to the laboratory. Often, recoveries are increased severalfold when this technique is used in comparison with mailing dry skin scrapings to the laboratory in an envelope or other container. Some laboratories, however, prefer to receive both dry and wet specimens in order that digestion of dry scrapings with 10% potassium hydroxide can be used for a rapid diagnostic attempt.

When a systemic mycosis is suspected, pieces of affected tissue can be sent to the laboratory, refrigerated, in a plastic bag. Sputum, feces, urine, milk, or purulent material from the involved area may be used if necropsy specimens are not available. Biopsies and any additional specimens from the involved area should also be submitted for histopathologic examination in 10% Formalin whenever possible.

Specimens of moldy feed can be submitted in sealed containers for examination for aflatoxin or other fungal toxins, and for feeding trials in laboratory animals, dermal toxicity tests, or other techniques.[4]

Packaging of Material for Shipment

Preparation of Specimens

Great care should be devoted to preparation of specimens for shipment to the laboratory in order to insure that the specimens do not deteriorate excessively or damage the mail by leakage. Specimens for viral recovery should be sent frozen with dry ice or liquid nitrogen whenever possible. If blood samples are included, the serum should be separated aseptically before freezing in sealed screw-capped vials. The exception is blood with anticoagulant, which should not be frozen but shipped on ice. If dry ice is not available, wet ice can be used but is not as efficient in preserving viruses.

For specimens for bacterial culture, wet ice is preferred, as frozen specimens must be allowed to thaw before they can be processed, thus causing delay. In the thawing process, tissues tend to become soft and mushy and therefore should not be considered for histopathologic examination. Do not freeze specimens in Formalin.

Refrigerant (wet or dry ice) should constitute 50% of the weight of the contents of the

Collection and Processing of Specimens

package. Wet ice should be placed in leakproof plastic bags. Conversely, dry ice should not be packed in containers from which the carbon dioxide cannot escape after sublimation.

Styrofoam boxes, adequately protected from damage by outer coverings of wood or sturdy cardboard, are preferred for shipping refrigerated specimens.

Legal Responsibility

If, during shipment, spillage occurs that damages mail, equipment, or personnel, the shipper may face prosecution, even though the material involved was not infectious or otherwise hazardous. Damon states: "The Criminal Statute—18 USC 1716—is of interest to all shippers of diagnostic materials, whether potentially pathogenic or not. In fact, it is most important in the latter case since in-transit damage from laboratory specimens has involved blood for serologic tests or urine for chemical examination yet free from pathogenic organisms. Thus, if spillage occurs so as to injure or damage mail, equipment or personnel, the shipper may face prosecution even though there be no question of hazard from an infectious agent. The value of meticulous packaging with sufficient absorbing material around the specimen to absorb any leaking fluid extends well beyond the major concern of preventing accidental infection."[3] For this reason, a capable individual should supervise the packaging.

If agents infectious to man are shipped, the container should be wrapped in absorbent material soaked in 4% Formalin and then sealed in a plastic bag or other leakproof container. Glass containers, tubes, etc., should have *tight-sealing* screw-cap lids and should be placed in a box inside an outer sturdy container. If several tubes are included they should be wrapped individually in paper. These should be placed in a refrigerator box, such as a styrofoam box (thick-walled semen shipping containers are excellent), with adequate packing provided to prevent excessive jostling of the contents and to allow for the melting or sublimation of the refrigerant. The outside of the container should be labeled "Perishable," "Refrigerated Biologic Materials," "Biologic Specimen," etc. If sent by mail, it should go by special delivery. If sent by bus, parcel delivery service, or express, the recipient's telephone number should be placed on the outside with the request to "Call on Arrival." When necessary, the consignee should be notified by telephone or wire how and when the specimen will arrive.

Routine Procedures for Processing General Unknowns

If tissues are received with a request to culture for a specific bacterial, viral, or fungal agent, the choice of media and techniques is narrowed down considerably. (See indexes for references to specific microorganisms.) However, most tissues will be sent to the laboratory for assistance in determining the etiologic agent, leaving the choice of procedures to the diagnosticians. These individuals are expected to use procedures that will result in the isolation and identification of all organisms in the tissues submitted. In order for a laboratory to be effective, it must have routine procedures that will meet this goal as nearly as possible in a minimum time.

Bacteria

Impression Smears

Impression smears stained with Gram's stain are often very helpful in suggesting a group of organisms likely to be involved. Smears from any abnormal-appearing tissues such as swollen liver or reddened intestine or muscle may be used. Information gained by this simple procedure may allow shortcuts to recovery of the specific agent but should not eliminate the general use of the standard procedures for recovery of bacterial, fungal, or viral agents.

Preparing Tissues for Culture

The surface of the tissue should be seared with a soldering iron or heated spatula and the specimen removed for culture with a Pasteur pipette. (Sterile disposable pipettes are available commercially.) No tissues or other specimens should be discarded until findings are reported to the consignor of the material. Appropriate storage, by freezing or otherwise, is necessary. Tissues or other specimens should be cultured on a preliminary basis as outlined in Table 3.2. Information regarding the individual bacteria under examination, including enterotoxemia, may be found in the section "Bacteriology."

Table 3.2. General scheme for isolation and identification of pathogens

Mycoplasma	Aerobic bacteria	Anaerobic bacteria	Fungi	Viruses
PPLO broth	Trypticase Blood agar	Blood agar Thioglycollate Brain-heart infusion	Microscopic exam KOH preparation Lactophenol blue PVA	Lab animals Avian embryos Cell cultures Serology
Transfer 2× in PPLO broth and agar	Blood agar Restrictive media	Anaerobic jar Liver infusion shake	Blood agar slant 37°C Sabouraud dextrose slant 25°C Sabouraud C & C slant 25°C	Microscopic examination for inclusions and FA
Typical colonies	Incubate 37°C in 10% CO$_2$ atmosphere Isolated colonies Differential media Biochemical reactions	Isolate colonies Thioglycollate or cooked meat medium Biochemical reactions in thioglycollate basal medium Gas chromatography		

Fungi

The initial step in the examination of clinical material for fungi should be direct microscopic examination.[2] When dermatophytes are suspected, the material is prepared for examination by placing a portion in a drop of 10% potassium hydroxide on a slide and covering with a coverslip. A Giemsa or Wright's stain is usually satisfactory for direct examination when other fungi are suspected.

Culture of material suspected of containing a fungus should entail inoculation of slants of Sabouraud dextrose agar, Sabouraud agar (containing cycloheximide 0.5 mg/ml and chloramphenicol 0.05 mg/ml), and blood agar. The first two media are incubated at 25°C, whereas the blood agar is incubated at 37°C. Cultures should be incubated for at least 4 weeks before discarding.

For identification of fungal isolates, observations of the front and reverse colony characteristics should be made. A portion of colony is placed on a slide in one drop of lactophenol cotton blue. A coverslip is added and the organisms are observed microscopically for characteristic morphologic details.[1] After making preliminary observations, the reader can find details regarding specific fungi in the section "Mycology."

Viruses

There are two basic approaches to the detection of viruses. One is the cytologic method, that is, the observation of typical cellular changes in the affected tissues, and the other is the isolation of the virus.

Cytologic Methods

These include ordinary light microscopy, ultraviolet light microscopy, and electron microscopy. Histopathologic methods using ordinary light microscopy have a narrow application in virology since there are very few pathognomonic lesions that allow an etiologic diagnosis. Histopathologic methods are helpful, though, in giving the microbiologist a lead that may allow him to concentrate on a certain area such as bacteriology, mycology, or virology. Among the instances where histopathologic methods help identify the causative agent are the presence of Negri bodies in the brain, the presence of intranuclear inclusions in the fetal liver tissues of foals aborted due to equine rhinopneumonitis, poxvirus inclusions, intranuclear inclusions in the liver of dogs with viral hepatitis, and cytoplasmic inclusions in canine distemper. The examination of histologic preparations can also be carried out by the fluorescent antibody (FA) technique, because inclusions are not always present or are present in different stages and may therefore not be detectable with routine histologic methods. The FA test is immunologically specific, sensitive, and less time-consuming than the preparation of conventional paraffin-embedded sections. The test can be applied to either impression smears or frozen sections. As a rule, the tissues that are preferred for virus isolation (see Table 3.1) are also most suitable for the FA test. Labeled antisera, many against viruses of domesticated animals, are not presently available commercially. Some labeled antisera are available through federal agencies (NADC and CDC) to qualified laboratories. In some instances, the indirect FA test can be used successfully, which eliminates the rather laborious procedure of conjugating specific viral antisera. (See Chapter 5 for detailed procedures for the FA test.)

Isolation of Viruses

The three basic methods used to isolate viruses are inoculation of cell cultures, inoculation of laboratory animals, and inoculation of embryonating chicken eggs. The possibility of virus recovery will increase as the number of animals, routes of inoculation, and types of cell cultures increase. Blind passages are recommended for all initially negative cultures. Negative isolation results, however, do not necessarily exclude a particular virus. Depending on the stage of the disease, the virus may no longer be present in the animal tissues, even though it was etiologically involved in the infection. Some viruses, such as those responsible for malignant catarrhal fever, equine viral arteritis, or virus diarrhea are difficult to isolate and their successful recovery can depend to a great deal on the technical facilities available and the experience of the investigator.

Conversely, the mere recovery of a virus does not necessarily establish that it is responsible for the disease. The isolation of a virus must be evaluated in terms of the clinical picture of the animal and the history of the virus. Serologic surveys indicate that many common animal viruses have a tendency to produce inapparent infections. Similarly, the isolation of an enterovirus or adenovirus from the feces of an animal may not implicate these agents in the disease in question. An animal also can harbor two or more pathogenic organisms at the same time.

If a virus is isolated, the researcher should make sure that it was actually recovered from the specimens examined and is not a virus of the test host system. Laboratory animals and tissue culture systems, especially primary cell cultures, may contain latent viruses that may become activated by inoculation of the material under examination.

Preparation of specimens. The tissues and body fluids useful for isolating a particular virus are listed in Table 3.1. Homogenates of tissue specimens are prepared in sterile buffered saline or transport media containing serum or other proteins. Antibiotic mixtures are added to the homogenates or body fluids to reduce unwanted bacterial contamination. Penicillin (200 units), streptomycin (200 μg), neomycin (50 μg/ml), polymyxin B sulfate (50 μg/ml) and fungizone (2.5 μg/ml) are commonly used. Most viruses pass a 0.45 μm filter while most bacteria are retained. A 0.22 μm filter also can be used. However, some larger viruses such as poxvirus may be partially retained on this filter. Centrifugation under refrigeration should be chosen as the next step to reduce contamination. Coarse material and the larger bacteria can be eliminated with low speeds from 1000 to 5000 $\times g$ for 10–15 minutes. It is possible to filter the material before or after centrifugation through cellulose-type filters at 0.45 μm porosity size. A 0.22 μm filter may be used if one is sure large viruses such as pox are not involved. However, virus concentrations are often lowered dramatically on filtration. The amount of proteinaceous material, the pH, and the volume to be filtered all make a difference. Successful filtration is best achieved if 50–100 ml or even more is filtered. High-speed centrifugation is sometimes used to concentrate the virus in a pellet. Some viruses that are not affected by ether or fat solvents may be mixed with a fluorocarbon, homogenized in a blender, and then centrifuged. This treatment sediments bacteria, mucus, and cellular debris, leaving the virus in the upper aqueous phase of the centrifuge tube. The technique was developed for isolation of foot-and-mouth disease (FMD) virus in OP fluids.[6]

Sedimentation coefficients of viruses lie in the range of 140–750 S. Papilloma virus, which is one of the smaller viruses (40–55 nm in diameter), is completely sedimented after 70 minutes at 40,000 $\times g$. Differential centrifugation has the disadvantage that the pellet is always contaminated with other particles and that there is usually a loss of infectivity. These disadvantages can be largely avoided through density gradient centrifugation using cesium, rubidium chloride, or sucrose. Chromatography such as diethylaminoethyl (DEAE) cellulose ion exchange has recently also been used successfully in the purification of viruses (see Chapter 7).

Selection of laboratory host system. Although embryonating eggs and laboratory animals are used for virus isolation, tissue culture cells are being used increasingly in virology laboratories. The use of tissue cultures has allowed the discovery of many viruses. However, some are not yet readily isolated or propagated in tissue culture cells. Therefore, use of embryonating eggs and laboratory animals cannot be abandoned in diagnostic laboratories whose specific aim is the speedy recovery of viruses. For example, certain arboviruses causing encephalitis, influenza viruses, poxviruses, and bluetongue virus are more frequently recovered in chicken embryos than in tissue culture.

Detection of viral multiplication. Some viruses produce a typical CPE that may provide a clue to which group the virus belongs. For example, herpesviruses, such as infectious bovine rhinotracheitis (IBR), produce giant cells and syncytia. Picornaviruses usually produce a very rapid cell death with cells rounding up and detaching from the glass. Parvoviruses are mitolytic viruses and require actively growing cells for their replication. Some viruses, such as certain bovine viral diarrhea–mucosal disease (BVD-MD) strains, are noncytopathic. Their presence may be checked by either the FA test or the back-challenge test with a cytopathic BVD-MD strain.

In isolating a virus from clinical specimens, nonspecific or toxic cell degeneration can occur. One or two subpassages of the material usually dilutes out the toxic effect of an inoculum. After preliminary observations, the researcher can carry out various biochemical-biophysical tests to narrow the identification of the isolate down to a specific virus group following the scheme provided in Table 3.3. Final identification of individual viral isolates is done by serologic means.

Table 3.3. Scheme for partial identification of viral isolates[5]

DNA limiting pore size (nm)						RNA limiting pore size (nm)					
>100		50–100		<50		>100		50–100		<50	
Res.	Sens.	Res.	Sens.	Res.	Sens.	Res.	Sens.	Res.	Sens.	Res. pH 3 sens.	Sens. pH 3 res.
Pox	Herpes	Adeno		Papova			Myxo	Reo		Rhino (also FMD)	Entero Arbo

Res., resistant to ether; sens., sensitive to ether; pH 3 res., resistant to pH 3; pH 3 sens., sensitive to pH 3.

References

1. Ajello, L., L.K. George, W. Kaplan, and L. Kaufman. *Laboratory Manual of Medical Mycology.* U.S. Government Printing Office, Washington, 1963.
2. Carter, G.R. *Diagnostic Procedures in Veterinary Bacteriology and Mycology.* 2d ed. Thomas, Springfield, Ill., 1973.

3. Damon, S.R. *Collection, Handling, and Shipment of Diagnostic Specimens*. Public Health Service (HEW) Pub. no. 976, p. 5, 1963.
4. Forgacs, J., and W.T. Carll. Mycotoxicoses. In *Advances in Veterinary Science,* C.A. Brandly and E.L. Jungherr (eds.), vol. 7, pp. 272–383. Academic Press, New York, 1962.
5. Hsiung, G.D. *Diagnostic Virology,* p. 26. Yale University Press, New Haven, Conn., 1964.
6. Sutmoller, P., and G.E. Cottral. Improved techniques for the detection of foot-and-mouth disease virus in carrier cattle. *Arch. ges. Virusforsch.* 21:170–177, 1967.
7. Sutmoller, P., G.E. Cottral, and J.W. McVicar. A review of the carrier state in foot-and-mouth disease. *Proc. 71st Ann. Mtg. U.S. Livestock Sanitary Ass.* 386–395, 1967.

4. Biologic Test Systems

There are two basic biologic test systems: cultivation of pathogens in embryonating avian eggs and cultivation in tissue cultures. These techniques are of primary importance in virology but only of minor importance in bacteriology, except for certain organisms. The use of live animals as biologic test systems is mentioned in the text for each pathogen and will not be covered here.

Embryonating Avian Eggs

The embryonating avian egg is a valuable and widely used medium for the cultivation of many viruses and certain other microbiological agents. The embryo offers an economical and convenient method for primary isolation and identification of viruses, maintenance of stock cultures, and production of vaccines.[7] Growth of a virus in embryo culture may be determined by several methods: (1) sampling of the virus in embryonic fluids and membranes or embryo proper for quantitative infectivity assay, (2) pathologic investigations, (3) serologic tests, (4) hemagglutination, and (5) determination of immunogenic properties.[7,6]

Embryonating chicken eggs are commonly used because of their relative freedom from extraneous contamination. However, consideration must be given to the possible presence of viruses, e.g. avian adenovirus 1 (CELO), avian encephalomyelitis, avian leukosis, and Newcastle disease, in eggs laid during the active stages of the disease, as well as bacterial agents such as mycoplasmas and salmonellae.[2] Antibodies may also be found in eggs laid by specifically immune hens. Only eggs from vigorous, healthy, disease-free breeder stock should be used. Embryonating eggs from other species, e.g. quail, duck, turkey, may also be used.

Some of the factors influencing the growth of viruses in embryonating chicken eggs are: (1) age of embryo, (2) route of inoculation, (3) dilution and volume of inoculum, (4) temperature of incubation, and (5) time of incubation following inoculation.[3] The eggs are incubated at 35.5–37.1°C throughout the entire period. Lower temperatures may be required in certain instances.[3]

Routes of Inoculation

The procedures outlined below are a compilation of methods found to work in the laboratory.[1,3,6,7] Certain modifications would be required for mass production of viral vaccines in order to minimize expenses.

Allantoic Cavity (A1C)

Method A

1. Candle the egg and mark the edge of the air sac membrane.
2. With a sharp, pointed instrument, drill or punch a small hole through the shell 6–7 mm above the edge of the air sac membrane, but do not pierce the shell membrane. Use 9–11-day-old embryonated eggs.
3. Apply a suitable disinfectant to the hole and allow to dry.
4. Using a syringe fitted with a 22–24-gauge, 1-inch (2.54 cm) needle, insert the needle perpendicularly through the hole to a depth of at least 1.5 cm and deposit the inoculum. Withdraw the needle.
5. After the eggs have been inoculated, seal the hole in the egg with melted paraffin or another suitable liquid adhesive.

Method B

1. Candle the egg and select an area of the chorioallantoic membrane (CAM) that is distant from the embryo and amnionic cavity (AmC), free of large blood vessels, and about 3 mm below the base of the air cell. Make a pencil mark at the point for inoculation.
2. Drill or punch a small hole through the shell at the mark but do not pierce the shell membrane.
3. Apply a suitable disinfectant to the holes and allow to dry.
4. Using a 1 ml tuberculin syringe fitted with a 27-gauge, 0.5-inch (1.27 cm) needle, insert the needle through the hole in the side of the egg to a depth of about 6–7 mm and deposit the inoculum. Withdraw the needle.
5. Seal the hole in the egg with melted paraffin or another suitable liquid adhesive.

Amnionic Cavity (AmC)

1. Candle the egg and make a pencil mark on the shell at the base of the air sac, locating the embryo. Use 9–12-day-old embryonated eggs.
2. Draw a circle parallel to and about 5 mm above the base of the air cell.
3. Using a small carborundum disc, cut through the shell at the circle but do not pierce the shell membrane.
4. Apply a suitable disinfectant to the cut and allow it to dry.
5. Using forceps, remove the cap of shell over the air cell.
6. Apply a few drops of sterile, light mineral oil or saline solution to the shell membrane over the embryo to make the membrane transparent. Use only the minimum amount of oil necessary for transparency. An amount to cover more than one-fourth of the shell membrane will interfere with respiration and may result in death of the embryo.
7. Using a 1 ml tuberculin syringe fitted with a 27-gauge, 1-inch (2.54 cm) needle, insert the needle into the AmC and deposit the inoculum. Withdraw the needle.

8. Close the opening in the shell over the air cell by sealing a disc of sterile, heavy paper (preferably white bond) to the shell with melted paraffin or other suitable liquid adhesive. Wide strips of Scotch tape may also be used. The egg may be inverted on the paper to facilitate sealing.

Chorioallantoic Membrane (CAM)[5]

Method A. The simplest method of inoculating infectious material onto the CAM involves the diffusion of a solution from the normal air sac membrane of an embryonating egg to the CAM directly below the air sac. Basically, the air sac membrane is brittle, and once a hole is made it will not close. The CAM consists of living cells and any small hole made in it will immediately close once the penetrating object is removed.

1. Candle an embryonating egg, 9–11 days of age, and with a pencil mark the location of the air sac.
2. Position the egg so that the air sac is upright. If the air sac is completely off center, discard the egg.
3. Following disinfection of the surface of the egg shell with an alcohol-iodine solution or other suitable germicide, penetrate the shell at the center of the air sac with a sharp, pointed instrument or a drill.
4. Deposit through this hole, approximately 6–7 mm beneath the shell, the desired inoculum in either 0.01 ml or 0.02 ml amounts, using a 1-inch (2.54 cm) needle.
5. While the needle is still penetrating the shell wall and after the deposit has been made on the shell membrane, push the needle completely through the air sac membrane and the CAM. Withdraw the needle.
6. Creating a hole between the air sac membrane and the CAM will allow for diffusion of the solution through the hole of the air sac membrane and onto the surface of the CAM.
7. The egg shell hole may be closed with Scotch tape or a paraffin-Vaseline mixture.

Method B. With this method an artificial air cell is produced to make sure that all of the inoculum is deposited on the CAM.

1. Candle the egg and mark the position of the embryo. Use eggs 9–11 days of age.
2. With the long axis of the egg in the horizontal plane and the embryo uppermost, mark one of the following equidistant between the ends of the egg: (a) an area about 1 cm square, or (b) a triangle about 1 cm on each side.
3. Using a small carborundum disc, cut *through the shell* at the marks but *do not pierce the shell membrane*. Also make a short cut (1-2 mm) through the shell over the air cell.
4. Apply a suitable disinfectant to the grooves cut by the disc and allow to dry.
5. With a teasing needle or forceps remove the square or triangle of shell to expose the shell membrane. When removing the triangle of shell, the researcher should elevate it at one of the points rather than at one of the sides to prevent pressing of a point through the shell membrane and possible rupture of the CAM.
6. Using a teasing needle, pierce the exposed shell membrane over the air cell and on the side of the egg but do not pierce the CAM.
7. Create a slight vacuum with a small rubber bulb at the cut over the air cell. Air

will pass through the larger opening in the shell membrane on the side of the egg, permitting the CAM to drop from the shell membrane. The embryo, membrane, and fluids will fill the normal air cell space, thus creating an artificial air cell on the side of the egg. In some instances, the CAM will drop of its own accord and the vacuum need not be employed if the shell membrane over the air cell is pierced first.

8. Using a 1 ml tuberculin syringe fitted with a 27-gauge, 0.5-inch (1.27 cm) needle, insert the needle, bevel down, through the shell membrane over the artificial air cell and deposit the inoculum on the CAM. Withdraw the needle.

9. Close the square or triangular opening in the shell by applying suitable lengths of adhesive tape or Scotch tape. Seal the cut over the normal air cell space with melted paraffin or another suitable liquid adhesive.

Yolk Sac (YS)
Method A
1. Candle the egg and note the center of the air sac. Use 6–8-day-old embryonated eggs.
2. Drill or punch a small hole through the shell at the center of the air sac. If the air sac is off center, position the egg so that the long axis of the egg lines up with the center of the air sac.
3. After disinfecting the hole, use a syringe with a 22–24-gauge, 0.5-inch (1.27 cm) needle. Insert the needle approximately 3.2 cm into the center of the egg, parallel to its long axis. The exact depth of penetration depends on the size of the egg. Deposit anywhere from 0.1 to 0.5 ml of inoculum.
4. Seal the hole with paraffin or other adhesive material.

Method B
1. Candle the egg with the long axis in the horizontal plane and locate the yolk sac. Make a pencil mark on the shell over the yolk sac about halfway from the small end of the egg to the apex of the curvature of the shell.
2. Drill a small hole through the shell at the mark but do not pierce the shell membrane.
3. Apply a suitable disinfectant to the hole and allow to dry.
4. With the long axis of the egg in the horizontal plane, and using a syringe fitted with a 22–24-gauge, 0.5-inch (1.27 cm) needle, insert the needle full-length through the hole and deposit the inoculum. Seal the hole in the egg with melted paraffin or another suitable liquid adhesive.

Intravenous (IV)
This route does not have wide practical application but is employed in specific cases to increase chances of successful isolation or detection of agents and in hematologic studies.[4] Embryos at 10–12 days incubation are most suitable.

1. Candle the egg as previously described and mark an area 1–1.5 cm square around a fairly large straight vein embedded in the CAM.
2. Drill through the marked shell and remove the shell, as described for the CAM, method B.

3. Illuminate the egg from above in a dark room by using an aperture at the base of an opaque perpendicular cylinder containing a 60-watt electric bulb. The injection is made by inserting a 27-gauge, 0.75-inch (1.91 cm) needle attached to a 1 ml tuberculin syringe at an acute angle while the egg is held in the other hand beneath the light source. Resting the elbows on the bench helps to steady the hands. This technique outlines the veins clearly and also permits observation of blood displacement in the vein when the inoculum is introduced. The amount of inoculum may vary from 0.02–0.05 ml.

4. The opening in the shell is closed as previously described in step 8 for inoculation of the AmC.

Intracerebral (IC)

Intracerebral inoculation of embryos can be performed in 8–14-day-old embryos. The amount of inoculum will vary from 0.01–0.02 ml. This route may be employed in the studies of pathologic alterations of the brain following infection. The viruses of herpes simplex and rabies may be cultivated by this route.

Incubation of Embryonating Eggs

Embryos are incubated for 1–6 days during which time they are candled daily. Deaths before 24 hours may be due to bacterial or traumatic causes. Some arboviruses kill embryos within 24 hours, while Newcastle disease virus kills embryos in 2–6 days. Some do not kill but produce lesions on the CAM or multiply in the allantoic fluids. Serial blind passages may be necessary at times for detecting the virus.

Embryos should be removed from the incubator as soon after death as possible to prevent tissue changes or thermal inactivation of the virus. Embryos are often chilled for several hours or overnight before collection of embryonic fluids.

Collection of Specimens from Embryonating Chicken Eggs

Embryonic fluids and yolk are collected with a 5 or 10 ml syringe fitted with a 20-gauge, 1-inch (2.54 cm) needle. The membranes and embryo are collected with forceps.

Allantoic Fluid

1. Apply a suitable disinfectant to the shell over the air cell. Crack the shell over the air cell with forceps and remove the shell to within 5 or 10 mm of the base of the air cell.

2. Insert the needle into the AlC and aspirate the fluid. The amount collected per egg will vary with the age of the embryo, but from a 12-day embryo one may expect an average of 5 ml per egg.

Amnionic Fluid

1. Remove the covering from the air cell end of the egg.

2. Collect the allantoic fluid as described above. Apply a few drops of saline solution to the shell membrane to render it partially transparent. The shell membrane and the CAM may be removed from the base of the air cell to permit a better view of the am-

nion. Using another syringe and needle, insert the needle into the AmC and aspirate the fluid.

Chorioallantoic Membrane

This method is applicable whether the membrane has been inoculated via the air sac or through an artificial window cut into the side of the shell.

1. Apply a suitable disinfectant over the surface of the shell.
2. With the edge of a spatula or a small kitchen knife, cut off the bottom end of the egg below the midpoint, using a sharp blow.
3. Discard the fluids, YS, and embryo. The CAM will adhere to the shell.
4. With forceps, pull the CAM from the shell into a petri dish or other suitable receptacle.
5. The CAM can then be examined by spreading it over the surface of the glass or suspending it in a small amount of physiological saline.

Yolk Sac

1. For harvesting the YS from the embryo, disinfect the surface of the egg shell with a suitable germicide.
2. With the edge of a spatula or knife, and using a sharp blow, cut off the bottom end of the egg shell below the midpoint.
3. Deposit the YS, embryo, and fluids from the egg into a petri dish.
4. With a set of forceps, the YS can then be readily separated from the embryo, drained of excessive yolk material, and transferred to a clean petri dish or other receptacle for examination.

References

1. Blaskovic, D., and B. Styk. Laboratory methods of virus transmission in multicellular organisms. In *Methods in Virology,* K. Maramorosch and H. Koprowski (eds.), vol. 1. Academic Press, New York, 1967.
2. Cottral, G.E. Endogenous viruses in the egg: The chicken embryo in biological research. *Ann. N.Y. Acad. Sci.* 55:221–234, 1952.
3. Cunningham, C.H. *A Laboratory Guide in Virology.* 6th ed. Burgess, Minneapolis, 1966.
4. Goldsmit, L., and E. Barzilai. An improved method for the isolation and identification of blue tongue virus by intravenous inoculation of embryonating chicken eggs. *J. Comp. Path.* 78:477, 1968.
5. Gorham, J.R. A simple technique for the inoculation of the chorio-allantoic membrane of chicken embryos. *Am. J. Vet. Res.* 18:691–692, 1957.
6. Lennette, E.H., and N.J. Schmidt (eds.). *Diagnostic Procedures for Viral and Rickettsial Diseases.* 3d ed. American Public Health Association, New York, 1964.
7. Subcommittee on Avian Diseases, Committee on Animal Health, Agricultural Board, National Research Council. *Methods for Examining Poultry Biologics and for Identifying and Quantifying Avian Pathogens.* National Academy of Sciences, Washington, 1971.

Tissue Cultures

Although tissue cultures have been used since 1908, they did not become widely used until the developments of the past few decades. Foremost among these were: (1) the discovery that tissue fragments could be dispersed into individual cell components through the use of proteolytic enzymes and chelating agents, permitting the cultivation of cells in a fluid on a solid surface; (2) the development of suitable media for in vitro cell growth;

(3) the growth of cells in suspension culture; (4) the discovery that viruses could be propagated in cultured cells in such a way that they produced demonstrable cytologic changes, thus providing methods for viral study. The availability of suitable antibiotics for inhibiting bacterial contamination greatly facilitated the work of the cell culturist. Since innumerable works give tissue culture methods and applications in detail,[1,2,3,4,6] this chapter will describe only the more widely used and acceptable procedures that yield results in the laboratory without the necessity of elaborate procedures or a variety of culture media. Where exceptions to this general scheme exist, they will be noted in specific chapters on viral or other microbial agents.

Types of Tissue Culture

The basic types of tissue culture in current use are: Maitland, primary monolayer, secondary or tertiary, continuous cell lines, and organ culture. Formulas for media or other solutions referred to in this text may be found in catalogues from several commercial companies supplying tissue culture products (such as Kansas City Biological Co., Lenexa, Kan., or Grand Island Biological Co., Grand Island, N.Y.).

Maitland Tissue Culture

This type of culture, now infrequently employed, is used only when monolayer cultures would not be satisfactory. The method consists basically of the suspension of small fragments of an appropriate tissue in a fluid medium. The tissue is generally minced aseptically by use of scalpels or sharp scissors into 1–2 mm pieces. A petri dish with a small piece of sterile hardwood for a cutting board is useful for this. The pieces are washed gently with buffered physiological saline or balanced salt solution (BSS) to remove damaged cells and debris. The pieces are then suspended in a tissue culture medium such as Eagle's minimum essential medium (MEM) or Earle's lactalbumin hydrolysate, each with a serum supplement (generally 10–20% serum) and appropriate antibiotics. Approximately three to four tissue pieces are suspended per ml of final medium. This suspension is then placed in any one of a number of containers: a small flask; a tube laid horizontally; a small, flat container with a narrow neck, known as a Maitland flask; or a flat-sided plastic flask especially prepared for tissue culture (BioQuest, Lockeysville, Md.). Incubation temperatures range from 33–37°C depending on the purpose of the culture. The best all-purpose temperature is 35°C. Cultures may remain stationary or be shaken gently on a continuous rotating or horizontal shaker. Either procedure is satisfactory although the latter increases the yield of virus being propagated. In the latter method, the cells generally do not proliferate from the edges of the tissue and the tissues survive to allow for virus growth. After 2–4 days, the spent medium is decanted and replaced with a fresh one either supplemented with serum or unsupplemented.

Primary Monolayer Cultures

In this widely used cell culture system, the chosen tissue is removed from the animal and dispensed into individual cells or very small tissue fragments that serve as an inoculum for monolayer cell growth. Various organs such as kidney, thymus, thyroid, lymph nodes, lung, spleen, and others have been used, both from fetal and adult sources. The organs supplying the tissues should be processed as soon as possible after their availability. However, if stored in either tissue culture nutrient fluid or phosphate-buffered saline (PBS), they may be kept for 12–48 hours at 4°C. If a longer period of storage is anticipated, the tissues should be cut into relatively small pieces before suspension in one of the above-mentioned fluids. To initiate monolayer cultures, cut the selected tissues into small pieces 2–4 mm square. One simple way of mincing is to use curved iris scissors in a petri dish, or to cut the tissue in scissorlike fashion with two scalpels. For larger amounts of tissue, two long straight scissors can be used with the tissue in a 50 ml round-bottom centrifuge tube. Wash the minced tissues three times with cold calcium-magnesium–free (CMF) PBS to remove tissue debris, blood, etc.; discard the washings. Then transfer the pieces to a "trypsinization flask" containing a Teflon-covered magnetic stirring bar. Add approximately 100–200 ml of sterile stock trypsin solution (0.25% trypsin at anywhere between 22 and 37°C) to the flask. The amount of trypsin solution added is dependent on the amount of tissue, but 1 part of tissue pieces to 3–5 parts of the trypsin solution can be used. Place the suspension over a magnetic stirrer and allow to stir gently 10–15 minutes. Allow the fragments to settle and remove and discard the supernatant fluid. To the same flask add a similar volume of trypsin solution and stir for another 15 minutes. Allow the tissue particles to settle to the bottom and decant the supernatant fluid containing the cells into a large centrifuge tube, or other suitable container, to be held at 4°C or in an ice bath. Add additional trypsin solution to the tissue particles and repeat the process 2–6 times. For example, chick embryo tissue may be completely separated into a cell suspension in 2–3 steps, while a bovine kidney or similar tissues may take 5–6 steps. The white strands of tissue appearing as the trypsinizing progresses is connective tissue and should be discarded. Following trypsinization, pour this cell suspension through a sterile funnel containing stainless-steel wire cloth of about 70 mesh (Standard Wire Gauge #37 with wire diameter of 0.173 mm and opening size of 0.1905 mm, about 28% open space), or through a sterile funnel containing three or four layers of cheese cloth, to remove coarse debris. Sediment the cells in a centrifuge tube (500–600 rpm for 10 minutes) and decant the trypsin solution. Then wash the cells in approximately 50–100 ml of CMF-PBS and centrifuge them at the same rate of speed. The washing process may be repeated 2–3 times although generally twice is sufficient. At the time of the final washing, the cells should be packed by centrifugation at 800 rpm for 10 minutes in a calibrated centrifuge tube, using a centrifuge with a 6–7-inch (15.24–17.78 cm) radius arm. Adjust accordingly for other sizes. Note the volume of the packed cells and resuspend them in the selected tissue culture medium at approximately 0.5% suspension. A more accurate standardization may also be attempted by staining a small aliquot of cells with 0.5% crystal violet solution, or 1% methylene blue, and counting in a hemacytometer. The cell concentration should then be adjusted to approximately $10^{5.7}$ cells per ml with appropriate medium and dispensed into the culture flask or tube. Growth medium of the following composition may be used (per 100 ml): (1) lactalbumin hydrolysate 0.5 g, (2) calf serum 5–10 ml, (3) sodium bicarbonate solution (1.4%) 2.5 ml, and (4) Hanks' BSS, to make a total of 100 ml. Earle's BSS with reduced $NaHCO_3$ is often used rather than Hanks'. Penicillin and streptomycin are added to the medium at final concentrations of 100 units and 100 μg/ml, respectively. If heavily contaminated tissue is being processed, the concentrations of antibiotic may be increased up to 500 units without damaging cells. Increasingly, laboratories are also using Eagle's MEM with serum supplement and antibiotics. Medium 199 may also be used in the same manner. In order to have a uniform cell suspension, the mixture should be agitated by repeated pipetting or stirring (without foaming) before dispensing into containers. Cells can be disbursed into any number of containers:

1. Tissue culture test tubes, approximately 16 mm × 100–150 mm in size, either screw-capped or rubber-stoppered (virgin white rubber or silicone-rubber formulation), can be used. Generally 1 ml of cell suspension is dispensed into each tube and the tubes are kept stationary until a cell sheet is at least partially established (4–7 days). Replacement of the initial medium with a fresh one after 48 hours often results in growth stimulation. Cells that appear degenerated will frequently grow and therefore should not be discarded prematurely. Generally, confluent monolayers are obtained after 5–7 days of incubation at 35–37°C. At that time, a maintenance medium may be substituted for the initial growth medium; it may consist of media with a reduced level of serum (2%) or Eagle's MEM without serum.

2. Flat-sided prescription bottles or flat plastic tissue-culture flasks of varying sizes are used when large quantities of cells are needed. Similar media, times of medium renewal, and incubation temperatures, as described in (1) above, are used. The cell suspension should cover the bottom of the bottle or flasks and be about 10 mm deep. For example, a 75 sq cm plastic flask should contain 20 ml of cell suspension. Flasks or bottles must be tightly stoppered or fitted with screw caps unless the cultures are maintained in an environment of 5% CO_2 and air.

3. Petri dishes, glass or plastic ones especially prepared for tissue culture, are also widely used, especially for virus plaque work. Methods and medium are the same as above. Generally, 5 ml of cell suspension is dispersed in a 21 sq cm plastic petri dish. However, in order to maintain proper pH, the plates must be incubated in a humid atmosphere of 5% CO_2.

Alternate method of preparing primary monolayer cell cultures. A simpler method of trypsinizing tissues that is in widespread use consists of the same initial preparations; however, after one initial washing with trypsin solution for 10–15 minutes, a larger volume of trypsin is added (usually double the initial amount) and the trypsinizing flask suspended over a magnetic stirrer in a cold room or refrigerator, where it is allowed to stir overnight (or at least 6–7 hours for softer tissues) at 4°C. This procedure alleviates the necessity of repeated trypsin changes. However, washing, filtration, and other steps are identical. Care must be exercised to either suspend the flask above the magnetic stirrer or place a piece of asbestos between the flask and stirrer to prevent heating the solution and tissues. In addition, somewhat larger pieces of tissue, 4–8 mm square, can be used.

Secondary or Tertiary Cell Cultures

In order to have cell preparations that are free of debris or that have more uniform cell types, the primary cultures can be trypsinized and transplanted, as described in the next section for continuous cell lines.

Continuous Cell Lines

A variety of mammalian cells, both from malignant and nonmalignant or normal animal sources, can be subcultured continuously over a period of months or years, although some, known as diploid cell strains, usually are limited to only 40–60 subcultures. The advantage of these continuous cell lines is the fact that they are relatively easy to propagate and can be stored in a frozen state for use when desired without having to resort to the preparation of primary cells. The continuous cell lines multiply quite rapidly, making it possible to have large populations of cells for preparing antigens or large numbers of cultures for use in diagnostic or research efforts. A repository of these cells is now available, the American Type Culture Collection (ATCC), and most cells can be obtained there. Procedures for routine handling of these cells are not unlike those described for the primary cultures. The cells are removed from the surface of the container (whether it be a tube, flask, or plate) through the use of a trypsin-Versene mixture, trypsin alone, or by scraping off the cells with a physical agent such as a rubber policeman. After removal from the container, the cells may be washed one or two times by centrifugation in the culture medium or buffered physiological saline, counted in a hemacytometer or automatic cell counter or similar apparatus, suspended in the appropriate growth medium at an average of 500,000 cells per ml, and dispensed in tubes, bottles, or flasks as described for primary cells. The exact number of cells depends on the culture used and the purpose. Rapidly growing cells can be used with as little as 50,000 cells per ml and slow ones up to 5,000,000 per ml. The medium used is generally the same as for primary cultures. A great majority of investigators now employ Eagle's MEM with a 5–10% serum supplement; however, some cells such as the strain-L mouse cell can be adapted to grow in chemically defined media without serum supplements.

Virus plaque procedures. This is a method of cell preparation whereby an agar overlay is placed on the cell sheet after the virus is added to the cells, confining each area of virus propagation to a small area. The destruction of cells at the spot produces small holes or plaques in the cell sheet. Basically, the preparation of cells is the same as for tubes or bottles. However, the secret to good plaquing of viruses is to seed either 3 oz (89 ml) prescription bottles or small plastic tissue-culture petri dishes with a heavy cell suspension (for a continuous cell line, use no less than 500,000–1,000,000 cells per ml of media). This will allow for rapid development of a confluent sheet of cells without holes in the cell layer.

After about two days of incubation in a 5% CO_2 incubator, remove the media from the cell sheet. Add the virus suspension in appropriate dilutions to the cell sheet and allow adsorption of the virus for 1 hour at incubator temperature. Then overlay onto the cell sheet a half and half mixture of a double concentration of MEM and a 3% suspension of purified agar cooled to about 45°C. Add enough to the cell sheet to form a thickness of 2–3 mm, generally about 4–5 ml of the agar mixture per petri dish. Allow the agar to harden and then incubate the bottles or dishes in the 5% CO_2 incubator. After virus multiplication (see individual virus chapters for specifics on the agent under question), fix the cell sheet by adding a 2% HCl–70% alcohol mixture for 5 minutes.

Remove the agar overlay, wash the cell sheet with distilled water, stain for 2 minutes with hematoxylin, wash again, and air dry. The plaques will appear as clear zones against a blue background.

Cells in suspension. A number of continuous cell lines can be propagated in liquid medium without being attached to a glass or plastic sheet.[1,5] Due to the size of animal cells, some method of agitation is required to keep them in suspension. Various methods have been employed, but the most common has been the use of a rotary stirrer or a shaker. A specialized flask with a stirring device consisting of a Teflon-coated magnet is available (Bellco Glass Co., Wheaton Glass Co.). By use of a magnetic stirrer, variations in the speed of rotation of the shaft are possible. The continual adjustment of pH, the introduction of fresh media, and other adjustments can be made through side arms on these flasks. The suspension culture methods are particularly well suited for large scale production of cells, virus propagation studies of cell nutrition, and metabolism studies. The growth of cells in suspension varies considerably depending on the cell types used. Some cells grow in evenly dispersed cultures while others grow in small clumps or clusters. Diploid cell lines, as opposed to continuous lines of indefinite life span, have not as yet been grown regularly in suspension culture. The media used for suspended cells are generally the same as for monolayer cultures. Eagle's MEM and Medium 199 with a protein supplement (e.g. serum, peptone, tryptose phosphate) are commonly used. The addition of methylcellulose at a final concentration of 0.12% generally improves cell growth. It is employed principally in media that are not supplemented with serum. Some new synthetic mediums are being studied that eliminate all serum supplements and the problems inherent with their use.[1]

Organ Culture Methods

The intent in tissue culture is basically to try to bridge the gap between in vitro and in vivo cell growth. Continuous cell cultures, although useful for many purposes, do not resemble the in vivo situation in terms of organization or the number of cell types present. One effort to bridge this gap is the method of organ culture. It involves the in vitro cultivation of pieces of organs, or even entire embryonic organs. In this manner, the researcher attempts to study normal tissue relationships as they exist in the body but divorced from the complexities of organ interactions. The techniques used are designed to try to inhibit outgrowth of cells from the explant, in contrast to standard cell culture procedures. Explants for organ cultures should be obtained aseptically and as rapidly as possible from the animal source. In general, the younger the animal the more successfully the tissue can be maintained. The pieces of tissues should be on the order of 1–2 sq mm in size. It is vital that the tissue pieces be cut and not fragmented, hence the need for using sharp scalpels or scissors. Cutting the tissues with the aid of a dissecting microscope helps considerably. The architecture of the tissue used should be kept in mind in cutting the pieces. The cuts should be made so that each explant has a normal complement of the cell types of which that particular organ is composed. Initially, organs or organ pieces were cultured on the surface of plasma coagulated by embryo extract. More recently, however, tissues are cultivated on a fluid medium on the surface of a stainless steel grid, an inert sponge, or on a small raft of lens paper. The grids or rafts should be approximately 25–30 sq mm in size. The metal grid method is the one most commonly used; it allows the tissues to be positioned at the gas-medium interface. In order to use the stainless steel mesh, a special organ culture dish with a center well is employed. After cutting, the tissues are washed carefully in BSS, pipetted onto the stainless steel grid, and placed carefully over the center well. Approximately 1 ml of medium is added to the center well, making sure that the raft and tissue *are in contact with the medium but not submerged,* since it is important that oxygen be allowed to diffuse into the tissues. Several media have been employed in organ culture and the medium of choice depends largely upon the tissue being cultivated. Mammary tissue, for instance, may require certain hormonal additives to the medium for growth. Since high oxygen tensions can be toxic for embryonic tissues and organs, tissues obtained from embryonic sources are usually incubated in normal atmospheric air and 5% CO_2 but adult organ tissues are incubated in an atmosphere of 95% O_2 and 5% CO_2. Cultures are generally fed every 2–4 days by aspirating medium from below the raft and replacing with fresh medium. Trowell medium T8, Biggers medium BGJ, or Eagle's MEM with serum may be used for organ cultures.

Method of Choice in Tissue Culture

Because of the large number of methods that have been described in the literature, as well as the assortment of media, it is difficult to maintain all the different cell types and ingredients in laboratories, especially small ones. Accordingly, the following is proposed as a single method that has the broadest application in a virological laboratory.

1. For the animal species that are most often studied, maintain at least one cell line from each host species in 5–20% glycerol at $-70°C$, or preferably in 5–10% dimethy sulfoxide in liquid nitrogen. Even secondary or tertiary subcultured primary cells can be successfully stored in liquid nitrogen and used in routine procedures.

2. Use the trypsin-Versene process or a rubber policemen for transferring cells from one subculture to another or in preparation for freezing.

3. One of the most widely used media is Eagle's MEM fortified with 10% fetal calf serum. If the viruses under investigation are from bovine sources or from animals that may be infected with bovine viruses, the maintenance medium for the cells, after initial outgrowth, should be Eagle's MEM with 2–5% agamma serum or Eagle's MEM without a serum supplement to eliminate the presence of bovine viral antibodies.

4. The medium can be fortified with 100 units of sodium penicillin G per ml and 100 μg of streptomycin sulfate per ml to inhibit bacterial growth. However, it is sometimes desirable to maintain stock cultures (those to be held frozen) antibiotic-free since antibiotics may simply be holding down a contaminant that can reappear and cause loss of the cells being maintained. Also antibiotics may affect cellular functions if heavily contaminated material is to be inoculated. Other antibiotics such as oxytetracycline, neomycin sulfate, and bacitracin may be used. The addition of fungizone (amphotericin B), 2.5–5 μg/ml, or mycostatin (nystatin), 20–50 μg/ml, is often used to inhibit contamination with mold. Kanamycin at 200–400 μg/ml can be used to inhibit mycoplasma.

5. The use of phenol red as an indicator for pH changes in the tissue culture media is a common procedure. However, phenol red has mild toxicity for some tissues, espe-

cially primary cells. Outgrowth of such cells often will be achieved in a more satisfactory manner if phenol red is not added until after the first medium change. In addition, phenol red has a tendency to enhance the inactivation of certain viruses such as measles and canine distemper when the cultures are exposed to light. Accordingly, tissue cultures containing phenol red should be kept away from the light as much as possible, exposing them only during the necessary periods for media change or for examination under the microscope.

6. In determining the inoculum size for subculture, follow the directions for the cell type being studied. Information from the ATCC is available for each cell type.

7. The preferred incubation temperature is 35°C for most virus cell studies.

8. When centrifuging cells, a centrifugation speed of 800 rpm with a centrifuge arm of 6–7 inches (15.24–17.78 cm) can be used for washing cells and for final packing of cells for resuspension and counting.

References

1. Higuchi, K. Cultivation of animal cells in chemically defined media: A review. In *Advances in Applied Microbiology,* D. Perlman (ed.), vol. 16, pp. 111–136. Academic Press, New York, 1973.
2. Kruse, P.F., Jr., and M.K. Paterson. *Tissue Culture Methods and Application.* Academic Press, New York, 1973.
3. Merchant, J., R.K. Kahn, and W.H. Murphy, Jr., *Handbook of Cell and Organ Culture.* Burgess, Minneapolis, 1969.
4. Paul, J. *Cell and Tissue Culture.* E. & S. Livingston, Edinburgh, 1970.
5. Telling, R.C., and P.J. Radlett. Large scale cultivation of mammalian cells. In *Advances in Applied Microbiology,* D. Perlman (ed.) vol. 13, pp. 91–119. Academic Press, New York, 1970.
6. Willmer, E.N. *Cells and Tissues in Culture.* Academic Press, New York, 1965.

5. Serology

The immunologic response of an animal to natural invasion by a pathogen, or to deliberate exposure to antigenic preparations of a microorganism, can be measured by a number of serologic procedures, or by direct challenge of the animal with a virulent culture of the specific microorganism.

General Considerations

By far the greatest number of tests in a microbiological laboratory are carried out by serologic techniques. These are based on the ability of an antibody to react with its corresponding antigen,[2] and the use of an indicator system to visualize the antibody-antigen reaction.

A microorganism isolated from a sick animal may be identified by matching it against a battery of known antibody preparations. Conversely, the presence of an antibody in a convalescing or vaccinated animal may be determined by reacting its serum with a number of predetermined antigens. The reaction can also be used to quantitate or titrate the amount of antigen contained in a culture or preparation of the organism, or the level of antibody in a specimen of serum.

The two indispensable elements of a serologic technique are the serum and the antigen. The obtaining, handling, and shipment of samples or sera for laboratory testing are described elsewhere.

The several serologic procedures available to the microbiologist are generally designated according to the type of indicator system employed. The most widely used tests are the complement fixation (CF), hemagglutination inhibition (HI), and virus neutralization (VN) tests. Also used in certain cases are the hemadsorption (HAd), hemadsorption inhibition (HAdI), hemagglutination (HA), precipitation, flocculation, agar (gel) diffusion (AD), and fluorescent antibody (FA) techniques.[17]

Antibody titers obtained by most serologic procedures are generally expressed as the reciprocal of the highest dilution of serum causing the effect expected from that procedure. This is particularly true for the tests based on the interaction of antibody with a nonviable antigen, such as the CF, HI, agglutination, precipitation, and flocculation tests. For tests such as the VN, which is based on the ability of an antibody to inhibit multiplication of the homologous infectious agent in tissue culture, chicken embryos, or animals, the level of antibody can be expressed in either of two ways: as the neutralization index (NI), or as the highest dilution which protects 50% of the test host from the expected effect. The latter is referred to as the 50% serum-neutralizing (or virus-neutralizing) endpoint (SN_{50} or VN_{50}).

Complement Fixation Test

The CF procedure is perhaps the most frequently used technique in the diagnostic laboratory. Routine testing is done with many viral and rickettsial antigens. The test is relatively easy to perform and the results are usually very helpful to the clinician.

Complement, a heat-labile substance in normal serum, has the ability to combine with antigen-antibody complexes under controlled conditions. Two distinct antigen-antibody systems are involved in complement fixation. If antigen is reacted with homologous antibody in the presence of complement, a complex consisting of antigen-antibody and complement will be formed.

Complement that has fixed in the primary antigen-antibody system will not be available to produce lysis in a second system composed of sheep erythrocytes and rabbit antisheep hemolysin. No hemolysis is a positive result. Complete hemolysis is negative, indicating that complement did not combine with antigen-antibody in the first reaction, but remained free to help in the lysis of the hemolysin-sensitized sheep cells in the second system.

Antibodies capable of combining with homologous antigen to fix complement are usually detectable in the serum of infected subjects within 3 weeks after infection, although the time may vary depending on the virus, the severity of infection, and other factors. Whenever possible, sera from both acute and convalescent phases of infection should be examined in parallel. A fourfold rise in titer between the two sera is generally significant.

Test Components

There are six variables involved in the CF procedure: antigen, antibody, diluent, complement, antisheep heolysin, and sheep erythrocytes.

Antigen

Many viral antigens can be readily secured from commercial sources, or they can be prepared by standard procedures described in microbiology texts. Any viral antigen should be titrated by the user with the appropriate reagent. The potency of an antigen should be established in order to calculate the volume or units necessary for a given test. This may be accomplished by a checkerboard titration (see "Test Procedure" below). The label on a commercial antigen will generally show the optimal titer or dilution. This figure can be misleading, however, because the techniques or the reagents used by the producing and using laboratories to establish this titer may vary.

Viral antigens are produced from various animal tissues. Positive reactions obtained with a given antigen must be checked against the corresponding normal (uninfected) tissue antigen, processed in a manner similar to the viral antigen, to discover any reactions caused by normal tissue that might obscure results.

Viral antigens, like most proteins in solution, are subject to denaturation and loss of potency. They can also develop anticomplementary characteristics (the ability to fix complement nonspecifically) on aging. Such antigens are generally unsuitable for CF tests.

Antibody

Serum to be tested should be separated from clotted blood, preferably no later than 24 hours after drawing, to avoid hemolysis. Serum should be collected aseptically and stored frozen until it is tested. Occasionally lipid separation in a serum will cause anticomplementary reactions. If this happens, 1 volume of serum may be added to 1.5 volumes of chloroform. The mixture is emulsified by shaking vigorously and is chilled overnight. The serum is recovered by centrifugation. Some workers prefer to draw blood from fasting subjects to minimize the lipid content of serum. The use of sera contaminated with bacteria should be avoided, because complement may be fixed by the bacterial contaminants. The use of a bactericide is recommended for serum that is to be used for extended periods of time.

Diluent

Many diluents have been used, and the selection of a diluent for the complement fixation procedure depends on the test. The worker must bear in mind that several characteristics of a diluent may affect the results. Among these are pH and ionic concentrations of magnesium and calcium salts. A diluent that has been used successfully in routine testing is Kolmer saline,[16] which contains 0.85% sodium chloride and 0.1% magnesium sulfate (anhydrous). This solution may be prepared daily or in a relatively large volume, filtered, sterilized, and stored at 4°C.

If a given test system requires a diluent with more buffering capacity or additional calcium, a Veronal-buffered saline is recommended. One Veronal diluent has been used successfully.[35] A stock solution may be prepared as follows: 4.6 g of 5,5-diethylbarbituric acid is dissolved in hot distilled water and added to a second solution composed of the following reagents—sodium chloride 83.8 g, sodium bicarbonate 2.52 g, sodium 5,5-diethylbarbiturate 3 g, magnesium chloride ($MgCl_2 \cdot 6H_2O$) 1 g, and calcium chloride ($CaCl_2 \cdot 2H_2O$) 0.2 g.

The volume is adjusted to 2 liters and the pH to 7.3. This stock solution may be stored in the cold for extended periods of time. For testing, 1 part of Veronal diluent is added to 4 parts distilled water. This diluent may be further modified by the addition of protein. Bovine albumin 0.1 or 0.2% gelatin have been used. The diluent must be isotonic and the same preparation used for all dilution purposes throughout the test.

Complement

Guinea pig complement is available from several commercial sources or may be prepared as follows: bleed healthy adult guinea pigs by heart puncture, using aseptic techniques. Allow the blood to clot in prechilled petri dishes. Refrigerate the clots (4°C) for a few hours to allow retraction, and collect the serum. To avoid loss of complement titer, the procedure should be completed in 1 day, and the samples stored at $-20°C$ or lower. A common source of error in CF procedures is the presence of natural antibodies in the complement. Each lot of complement should be prescreened with each antigen it is to be used with.

Complement activity must be titrated on each day of testing to establish the units necessary for a given procedure. Unless the antigen being tested is known to be anticomplementary, the complement titration should include antigen. The use of either hyperactive or hypoactive complement should be avoided.

Antisheep Hemolysin

Rabbit antisheep hemolysin is available commercially or can be produced. Several methods have been described; here is one method found by the CDC to furnish consistently satisfactory hemolysins. Inoculate young rabbits weighing approximately 2 kg intracutaneously with whole sheep's blood (defibrinated) according to the following schedule of days and amounts: day 1, 0.5 ml; 3, 1 ml; 5, 1.5 ml; 7, 2 ml; 9, 2.5 ml; and inoculate intravenously (IV) with 20% suspension of washed cells on day 12, 1 ml, and day 15, 1 ml. Wash the sheep cells and dilute with Kolmer saline. Bleed the rabbits 3 days after the last inoculation. Animals showing a hemolysin titer of 1:5000 or greater should be exsanguinated and their serums pooled. Hemolysin may be diluted with equal parts glycerol and stored at 2-8°C. Glycerinated hemolysin is remarkably stable and can be held for several years without appreciable loss in titer.

Many laboratories prefer to make a 1:100 working dilution of hemolysin as follows: Kolmer saline (0.85% NaCl and 0.1% $MgSO_4$) 94 ml, phenol solution (5% phenol in Kolmer saline) 4 ml, 50% glycerinated hemolysin 2 ml. The phenol solution should be mixed well with the saline before hemolysin is added. This preparation is relatively stable when stored at 2-8°C. Titration should be performed each day before testing to establish the units of hemolysin needed for the test system.

Sheep Erythrocytes

Sheep blood suitable for use in complement fixation may be purchased from commercial sources or may be drawn by the user and defibrinated. It may also be mixed with an anticoagulant at the time of collection. One method that has been used successfully by the CDC follows.[5] Graduate a 2-liter heavy-walled Erlenmeyer flask to contain 880 ml. Close the flask with a two-holed rubber stopper. Adapt one outlet with a delivery tube and needle for drawing blood, and the other outlet with a suction mouthpiece. Add 480 ml of 3.8% sodium citrate solution to the flask and sterilize the closed assembly. Using aseptic procedures, collect blood from the jugular vein of a sheep directly into the citrate solution. It is advisable to use only the blood from one sheep, and not to form a pool. Blood should be filtered through sterile gauze, dispensed in workable amounts, and stored at 2-10°C, it must remain free from bacterial contamination. Occasionally, sheep cells are too fragile or too resistant for use in CF tests. As a general rule, cells are satisfactory if they show no hemolysis after three successive washings in diluent and overnight storage in the refrigerator.

Test Procedure

Although numerous techniques and modifications for the CF test have been published, only one will be described in detail, the Kolmer One-Fifth Volume Technique.[16] Remember that the *same diluent* must be used throughout the test procedure.

Serum

Separate the serum from the blood clot and centrifuge to remove the red cells. Heat fresh serum specimens at 56°C for 30 minutes. If the specimen has been heated previously, reheat at 56°C for 10 minutes before testing.

Sheep Cell Suspension

1. Filter blood through multiple layers of gauze into a round-bottomed 50-ml centrifuge tube.
2. Add 2–3 volumes of diluent to the blood.
3. Centrifuge tubes at a speed sufficient to form a firm cell pack within 5 minutes (International Equipment Co., Boston, centrifuge no. 1, centrifuge radius 8 inches [20.32 cm], 2000 rpm).
4. Remove supernatant fluid by suction, taking off the white buffy coat (white cells) on top of the cell pack.
5. Fill tube with diluent, suspend by gently inverting the tube several times, and repeat steps 3, 4, and 5 three times. Supernatant should be clear and free from hemolysis at this point.
6. Transfer red cells to a graduated conical 15-ml centrifuge tube by carefully resuspending cell pack in a small volume of diluent. Centrifuge the tube for 10 minutes at the speed indicated in step 3.
7. Read the volume of packed cells and remove the supernatant.
8. Prepare a 2% cell suspension by adding 49 volumes of diluent to the cell pack.
9. Recheck the 2% cell suspension by centrifuging 15 ml in a 15-ml graduated conical centrifuge tube. Adjust suspension if necessary to give a cell pack of 0.3 ml ± 0.01 ml per 15 ml of red cell suspension. Photometric measurement may be used to prepare the 2% suspension if greater accuracy is desired.
10. Store cell suspension in a stoppered flask in the refrigerator. Carefully resuspend cells immediately before (and during) dispensing.

Hemolysin and Complement Titrations

1. These titrations may be performed simultaneously in the same rack.
2. Place ten 13 × 100 mm master dilution tubes (labeled 1–10) in one row. Prepare a 1:1000 dilution of hemolysin in tube 1 by adding 0.5 ml of a 1:100 stock hemolysin dilution to 4.5 ml of diluent. Mix well and discard pipette.
3. Add 0.5 ml of 1:1000 hemolysin dilution to master dilution tubes 2–5.
4. Add the following volumes of diluent (ml) to master dilution tubes 2–10: 2, 0.5; 3, 1.0; 4, 1.5; 5, 2.0; 6, 0.5; 7, 0.5; 8, 0.5; 9, 0.5; 10, 0.5.
5. Place ten 12 × 75 mm hemolysin titration tubes (labeled 1–10) directly in front of the 13 × 100 mm master dilution tubes. Prepare hemolysin dilutions in the master dilu-

Serology

Table 5.1. Hemolysin dilutions

Master dilution tube			Hemolysin titration tube	Resultant hemolysin dilution
1	Mix, add	0.1 ml to	1	1:1000
2	Mix, add	0.1 ml to	2	1:2000
3	Mix, transfer 0.5 ml to dil. tube 6, add 0.1 ml to		3	1:3000
4	Mix, transfer 0.5 ml to dil. tube 7, add 0.1 ml to		4	1:4000
5	Mix, transfer 0.5 ml to dil. tube 8, add 0.1 ml to		5	1:5000
6	Mix, transfer 0.5 ml to dil. tube 9, add 0.1 ml to		6	1:6000
7	Mix, transfer 0.5 ml to dil. tube 10, add 0.1 ml to		7	1:8000
8	Mix,	0.5 ml to dil. tube 10, add 0.1 ml to	8	1:10,000
9	Mix,	add 0.1 ml to	9	1:12,000
10	Mix,	add 0.1 ml to	10	1:16,000

tion tubes as indicated in Table 5.1 and add 0.1 ml of each dilution to the corresponding hemolysin titration (12×75 mm) tubes.

6. Remove hemolysin master dilution tubes from the rack.

7. Prepare a 1:30 dilution of complement by adding 0.1 ml of complement to 2.9 ml of diluent. Mix well and add 0.1 ml of 1:30 complement dilution to each of the hemolysin titration tubes. Note that complement should be thawed (if frozen) or reconstituted (if dried) with cold diluent immediately before use. Complement should be stored in the refrigerator at all times when not in use.

8. Prepare a 1:10 complement dilution. Then prepare master dilutions of complement by adding the amounts of 1:10 complement and diluent shown in Table 5.2.

Table 5.2. Master dilutions of complement

Tube	Add 1:10 complement (ml)	Add diluent (ml)	Dilution
1	0.2	0.3	1:25
2	0.2	0.4	1:30
3	0.2	0.5	1:35
4	0.2	0.6	1:40
5	0.2	0.7	1:45
6	0.2	0.8	1:50

9. Place six 12×75 mm complement titration tubes, numbered 1–6, behind the hemolysin titration tubes and add 0.1 ml of each complement dilution shown above to the corresponding 12×75 mm tubes.

10. Add 0.3 ml of diluent to each tube of the hemolysin titration.

11. Add 0.3 ml of diluent to each tube of the complement titration.

12. Add 0.1 ml of 2% sheep cell suspension to each tube of the hemolysin titration. The tubes at this point should contain the reagents shown in Table 5.3. Incubate the rack containing the hemolysin and complement titrations for 1 hour at 37°C.

13. Remove the rack from the water bath and read the hemolysin titration. One unit of hemolysin is defined as 0.1 ml of the highest dilution that gives complete hemolysis. Calculate the amount of hemolysin necessary and prepare a dilution containing 2 units of hemolysin per 0.1 ml. If tube 7 (1:8000 hemolysin dilution) is the last tube of the hemolysin titration that shows complete hemolysis, then 0.1 ml of a 1:8000 dilution

Table 5.3. Titration of hemolysin and complement

	Tube									
	1	2	3	4	5	6	7	8	9	10
Back row complement titration										
Complement (0.1 ml)	1:25	1:30	1:35	1:40	1:45	1:50				
Diluent (ml)	0.3	0.3	0.3	0.3	0.3	0.3				
Front row hemolysin titration										
Hemolysin (0.1 ml)	1:1000	1:2000	1:3000	1:4000	1:5000	1:6000	1:8000	1:10,000	1:12,000	1:16,000
Complement (1:30, ml)	0.1	0.1	0.1	0.1	0.1	0.1	0.1	0.1	0.1	0.1
Diluent (ml)	0.3	0.3	0.3	0.3	0.3	0.3	0.3	0.3	0.3	0.3
2% sheep cells (ml)	0.1	0.1	0.1	0.1	0.1	0.1	0.1	0.1	0.1	0.1

equals 1 unit of hemolysin. Two units of hemolysin will therefore be contained in 0.1 ml of a 1:4000 dilution.

14. Add 0.1 ml of hemolysin solution (containing 2 units) to each tube of the complement titration.
15. Add 0.1 ml of 2% sheep cell suspension to the complement titration tubes.
16. Incubate the complement titration in a water bath for 30 minutes at 37°C.
17. Remove the rack from the water bath and read the complement titration. One unit of complement is 0.1 ml of the highest dilution that gives complete hemolysis at the end of the incubation period. If tube 4 (1:40 complement dilution) is the last tube of the complement titration that shows complete hemolysis, then one unit of complement is contained in 0.1 ml of a 1:40 dilution. Two exact units of complement (contained in 0.2 ml) are used in the test. Two exact units will be contained in 0.2 ml of a 1:40 complement dilution.

Complement Fixation Test

Reagents should be added in the sequence shown in Table 5.4 (from left to right). Tubes should be mixed thoroughly by gently shaking the rack after each reagent is added.

1. Prepare serial twofold dilutions of the serum (sera) to be tested in diluent.
2. Pipette 0.1 ml of the appropriate serum dilutions into 12 × 75 mm tubes.
3. Pipette 0.1 ml of the 1:4 serum dilution into tube 7, the serum control tube.
4. Prepare serial dilutions of a positive control serum. Select a serum of known titer to the antigen being used and prepare appropriate dilutions that will show the serum endpoint. Pipette 0.1 ml of each dilution into 12 × 75 mm tubes. Prepare a serum control tube.
5. Prepare a negative control serum. Select a known negative serum and add 0.1 ml of the appropriate dilution to two tubes for the test and control respectively.
6. Prepare antigen dilution to contain 2 units of antigen per 0.1 ml. Antigens must be titrated to establish optimal titer. Table 5.5 shows a typical checkerboard titration used to establish antigen unitage. One unit of antigen is defined as the smallest amount of antigen (contained in 0.1 ml) that gives maximum fixation with the control serum. In the

Serology

Table 5.4. Tube contents for CF test

Controls	Tube	Serum	Antigen (2 units, ml)	Diluent (ml)	Complement (2 units, ml)
	1	0.1 ml of 1:4 dil.	0.1	0	0.2
	2	0.1 ml of 1:8 dil.	0.1	0	0.2
	3	0.1 ml of 1:16 dil.	0.1	0	0.2
	4	0.1 ml of 1:32 dil.	0.1	0	0.2
	5	0.1 ml of 1:64 dil.	0.1	0	0.2
	6	0.1 ml of 1:128 dil.	0.1	0	0.2
Serum	7	0.1 ml of 1:4 dil.	0	0.1	0.2
Antigen	8	0	0.1	0.1	0.2
Hemolytic	9	0	0	0.2	0.2
Cell	10	0	0	0.4	0
Pos. ser.	11	0.1 ml of appropriate dil. of known pos.	0.1	0	0.2
Neg. ser.	12	0.1 ml known neg.	0.1	0	0.2

example above 1 unit of antigen is contained in 0.1 ml of a 1:32 dilution. Two units would therefore be contained in 0.1 ml of a 1:16 dilution.

7. Add 0.1 ml (2 units) of antigen to the specified tubes.
8. Prepare an antigen control tube and add 0.1 ml of antigen (2 units).
9. Prepare a hemolytic system control tube and add 0.2 ml of diluent.
10. Prepare a cell control tube and add 0.4 ml diluent.
11. Add the specified amounts of diluent to the appropriate tubes.
12. Allow the tubes to incubate for at least 10 minutes at room temperature.
13. Add 0.2 ml of complement (2 units) to every tube except the cell control.
14. Prepare a series of tubes containing 2 units of complement, 1 unit of complement, 0.5 units of complement, and 0.25 units of complement respectively, each contained in a 0.2 ml volume. Add 0.1 ml (2 units) of each antigen to be tested to one or more sets of complement control tubes. Add 0.1 ml of normal antigen control to a second series of tubes. Add 0.1 ml of diluent to a third series. Add 0.1 ml of diluted serum (1:4 dilution) to a fourth set of tubes. Adjust the volume in the complement control tubes to 0.4 ml with diluent. The complement controls measure the amount of fixation

Table 5.5. An example of a checkerboard titration

Antigen dilution	Positive serum dilution						Negative serum	Antigen control
	1:4	1:8	1:16	1:32	1:64	1:128	1:4	1:16
1:4	4*	4	4	3	1	0	0	0
1:8	4	4	4	4	2	0	0	0
1:16	4	4	4	4	3	0	0	0
1:32	4	4	3	4	3	0	0	0
1:64	4	3	2	1	0	0	0	0
1:128	0	0	0	0	0	0	0	0
Norm. antigen control	0	0	0	0	0	0	0	0
Ser. control	0	0	0	0	0	0	0	0

*Degree of CF as defined in Table 5.6.

that has taken place during overnight fixation and will also show the effect of each variable on the hemolytic system.

15. After all reagents have been added, incubate the test overnight (approximately 18 hours) at 2–8°C.

16. Remove the test from the refrigerator and allow it to stand at room temperature for 15 minutes.

17. Prepare a hemolysin dilution and add 0.1 ml of appropriate dilution (2 units) to all tubes.

18. Resuspend 2% sheep cell suspension and add 0.1 ml of 2% cell suspension to each tube. Note that sheep cell suspension may be sensitized with an equal volume of hemolysin dilution containing 2 units of hemolysin per 0.1 ml. If this is done, allow mixture to stand at room temperature for 15 minutes and add 0.2 ml of the sensitized cells to each tube.

19. Incubate the test in a 37°C water bath. The time of incubation depends on the controls. Test should remain in the water bath for at least 10 minutes after the antigen control and hemolytic control have cleared (100% hemolysis). Complement controls should show complete hemolysis with 2 units and 1 unit of complement, partial to complete hemolysis with 0.5 units, and no hemolysis with 0.25 units. Some workers prefer to leave the test at 37°C until the positive control serum reaches a predetermined pattern of hemolysis. The time of incubation should not exceed 1 hour.

20. Remove the test and read the percentage of hemolysis. Report as in Table 5.6.

Table 5.6. Reporting the test

Degree of CF (+)	% hemolysis	Interpretation
4	0	Positive
3	25	Positive
2	50	Positive
1	75	Positive
±	90	Weakly positive
0	100	Negative

21. Tests on anticomplementary serum specimens (those giving fixation in the absence of antigens) should be repeated, using freshly drawn serum if possible.

Interpretation of Results

Accuracy in measurement is an absolute necessity in the CF technique. The test consists of five variables, and is open to overall error greater than the error caused by each of the variables. The minimal rise of antibody titer considered diagnostically significant is fourfold, a change which is detectable and valid only if every step of the procedure has been carried out precisely.

Nonspecific Reactions

Nonspecific reactions may occur at any time. Each serum should have a control not only for anticomplementary activity but also for nonspecific reactivity. The nonspecific control consists of testing the lowest dilution of serum against an antigen prepared from

Serology

normal tissue or against an antigenically unrelated viral antigen processed in the same way as the test antigen. Since a high proportion of nonspecific reactions may occur with very low serum dilutions, an initial dilution of 1:8 is satisfactory in the test procedure.

Anticomplementary Reactions

Anticomplementary reactions can be troublesome. The sera from some animals can be anticomplementary, or the anticomplementary action can arise from chemical or bacterial contamination of the specimen. Anticomplementary activity can be eliminated by several methods. One is the addition of 1 volume of guinea pig complement to 4 volumes of serum. The mixture, held overnight at 4°C, is warmed in a water bath at 37°C for 30 minutes. Diluent is added to give a 1:4 dilution, and the specimen is inactivated at 60°C for 30 minutes.

Microtechnique Complement Fixation Test

The complement fixation test can also be carried out by microtitration. This has the advantage of saving time and materials, and the results agree well with those obtained with macrotests. A recommended procedure for the microtechnique CF test involves the LBCF (Laboratory Branch Complement Fixation) test. In 1962, the Laboratory Branch of the CDC published this highly standardized macrotechnique test.[32] In 1965, the Public Health Service (HEW) issued its Monograph no. 74, which supplements an exposition of the LBCF test with a description of its adaptation to microtechnique.[33]

Hemagglutination and Hemagglutination Inhibition Procedures

Certain viruses contain hemagglutinins that clump erythrocytes from various species of animals. This is the basis for the HA test. The HI test depends on the ability of an immune serum to specifically inhibit its homologous hemagglutinin from agglutinating these erythrocytes.

Following reports that influenza virus possessed hemagglutinative activity,[13] researchers found that a number of other viruses possessed HA activity, including poxviruses, adenoviruses, myxoviruses, reoviruses, infectious bronchitis virus, African swine fever virus, picornaviruses (enteroviruses), arboviruses, certain papovaviruses, and parvoviruses (Table 5.7).

Hemagglutinin has been shown to be an integral part of the virus particle in certain viruses. The hemagglutinin of the poxviruses, arboviruses, and the chlamydia agents is a soluble phospholipid-protein complex separable from intact virus particles by ultracentrifugation. Myxoviruses attach to specific receptor sites on the surfaces of red blood cells and cause HA by forming bridges between adjacent cells. This reaction is mediated by an enzyme, a sialidase or neuraminidase termed receptor-destroying enzyme (RDE), whose action results in elution of the virus as a consequence of erythrocyte receptor-site destruction. The enzyme is produced commercially and is obtained from culture filtrates of *Vibrio cholerae* (*comma*) or *Clostridium perfringens*. In contrast, other viruses having an insoluble HA do not produce this enzyme. However, treatment of adenoviruses, arboviruses, and reoviruses with potassium periodate prevents agglutination, and picornavirus HA is abolished by treatment of erythrocytes with reagents known to react with

Table 5.7. Animal virus hemagglutination

Virus groups	Erythrocyte type preferred	Conditions
Myxoviruses*	Human-O, guinea pig, fowl	4°C, wide pH range, elution at 37°C
Arboviruses*	Chick or goose	37°C, pH 6–7, lipid inhibitors in serum
Poxviruses*	Fowl, other species	37°C, no elution, wide pH range
Reoviruses	Human-O, bovine (reovirus type 3)	Wide temperature and pH range
Polyoma rat virus	Guinea pig, other species	4°C, pH 5.4–8.4, elution at 37°C, inhibitors in serum and tissue extracts
Enteroviruses	Human-O	Great type and strain variation, 4°C, elution at 37°C
Adenoviruses	Variety of species: rat and rhesus monkey for human types; guinea pig, human-O, or fowl for others	4–37°C, wide pH range

*These viruses (but not all arboviruses) also produce hemadsorption of infected tissue culture cells.

sulfhydryl groups, indicating that -SH groups are vital to the attachment of enterviruses to erythrocytes.[27] Viruses inactivated by Formalin or heat cause HA, but they do not elute from erythrocytes.

Factors that influence viral HA have been reported in detail,[29] and, for the virus, they include: strain, titer/HA activity, passage level, and host cell of propagation. The erythrocyte factors are: species, age, sex, and individual differences of donors; and duration of cell storage. The test reaction environmental factors are: temperature, pH, certain cations, and inhibitors of HA.

Applications of the HA reaction in experimental and diagnostic virology include confirmation of isolates and a first step in virus identification; virus classification and grouping on the basis of the nature of the HA reaction, such as the RDE activity of myxoviruses; detection and titration of viral antibody by specific inhibition (the HI test); and virus purification and concentration. In addition, the antigenic mass of viral suspensions or vaccine is commonly assayed by HA tests.

Hemagglutination Inhibition Test

Several variations of this test have been described in the literature. To illustrate one of the most widely accepted methods, the use of the test with parainfluenza-3 (PI-3, shipping fever of cattle) will be described in detail. The mechanics of the HI test consist of interacting an immune serum with its corresponding hemagglutinin in the presence of an appropriate erythrocyte system. The results will vary depending on pH, the species of erythrocyte used, and the temperature and time of incubation.[29] Another factor to be considered is the presence in many sera of nonspecific inhibitors of viral hemagglutinins, which must be removed to permit determination of the level of specific antibody or the correct identity of a virus isolate. A number of methods have been suggested for the removal of nonspecific inhibitors from serum. These methods entail treatment of the

Serology

serum with *Vibrio comma,* RDE, trypsin, kaolin, sodium periodate, acetone, or carbon dioxide, and are described in subsequent chapters under the individual diseases.

Materials

1. Tubes (Wasserman 13×100 mm) and pipettes that are scrupulously clean. The pipettes should be 1 ml and 2 ml, graduated in hundredths, and 5 ml and 10 ml, divided into tenths.
2. A 0.5% suspension of washed bovine red blood cells (RBC) in PBS solution (disodium phosphate 1.069 g, monosodium phosphate 0.315 g, sodium chloride 8.5 g, distilled water 1 liter, pH 7.2).
3. Virus antigen.
4. Serum from a normal animal known to contain HI antibodies specific for the virus used.
5. Suspected serum or paired serum samples taken before and 10 days to 3 weeks or more after infection.
6. Suitable racks with 0.25-inch (64 mm) coarse mesh wire bottoms, through which the bottoms of the tubes are clearly visible.
7. A two-tube fluorescent lamp (Dazor Floating Fixture no. 23, 24, or 16) to provide illumination from above.
8. A mirror 15×30 cm for viewing the bottoms of the tubes in the racks.

Virus Antigen

Propagate parainfluenza-3 virus in monolayer cultures of primary embryonic bovine kidney cells. Harvest the medium after the CPE of the virus is well marked and store the medium frozen. The antigen may be obtained from the National Animal Disease Center (NADC), Ames, Iowa.

Preparation of Red Blood Cell Suspension

1. Bleed appropriate animals by means of a syringe containing a volume of 5% sodium citrate equivalent to one-fifth of its mixture with blood (e.g., a 20 ml syringe would have 4 ml of citrate and 16 ml of blood). Blood also may be collected aseptically from the heart (chickens) or by venipuncture (bovine, etc.) into heparin at a concentration slightly in excess of 0.3 mg/ml of blood. Guinea pig, human 0, or sheep cells may be used in testing mammalian serums.
2. Wash the cells three times with PBS. The ratio of cells to saline should be at least two or three to one in each washing, and the cells should be centrifuged at 1500 rpm (head radius 20 cm) for 10-15 minutes.
3. Pour off the PBS after the last washing. Store the packed cells in 3 volumes of PBS in the refrigerator. These cells will keep in suitable condition for 4-5 days at 4-9°C. It is customary to prepare the RBC suspension on the first day of each week and discard the remaining cells at the end of the week. Cells that are too old may self-hemagglutinate.
4. Suspend 1 ml or more (depending upon the number of tests to be conducted) of the packed cells in 2 ml of PBS in a graduated, conical centrifuge tube and centrifuge at 100 rpm for 10 minutes. The supernatant saline solution should then be removed and the

cells resuspended in PBS to make a 0.5% (by volume) cell suspension. This suspension should be used only on the same day it is made.

Serum

In HI tests employing RBC from the same species as the serum being tested, adsorption to remove nonspecific agglutination generally is not required. Examples are diagnostic influenza and parainfluenza, in which human serums are tested with human O cells, or HI tests conducted with chicken antiserums prepared with influenza or parainfluenza viruses using chicken RBC. However, if an antiserum to a virus is prepared in rabbits and used in the HI test in which chicken erythrocytes are used, nonspecific agglutination of the RBC may occur, and therefore the serum should be adsorbed with chicken erythrocytes. In addition, all serums that show nonspecific agglutination in the serum control tubes also should be treated. The following procedure of adsorption should be followed: (1) Prepare a 1:10 dilution of the test serum in PBS (0.1 ml serum plus 0.9 ml PBS). (2) Add 0.1 ml of washed 50% suspension of erythrocytes per ml of the starting serum dilution. (3) Mix and hold at 4°C for 1 hour. Resuspend the cells or the agglutinated RBC pellet several times during the incubation period. (4) Recover the serum after 5 minutes centrifugation at 1800 rpm. Infrequently, a second RBC adsorption may be necessary.

Nonspecific reactions may be observed particularly in testing bovine serum for PI-3 antibodies. The method of treatment with kaolin and heat inactivation of bovine serum for the PI-3 HI test is as follows: (1) Mix 0.3 ml of each serum to be tested with 1.2 ml of PBS in a test tube (1:5 dilution). (2) Add 0.1 g of acid-washed kaolin (commercially available, e.g. Fisher Scientific Co., Springfield, N.J.), and agitate (kaolin is easily picked up on a small narrow spatula with a blade 5×12 mm). Allow adsorption to take place for 10 minutes at room temperature (22–24°C). (3) Centrifuge at 1500 rpm for 10 minutes (20 cm head radius). (4) Remove the serum from above the packed kaolin with a pipette and place in a water bath at 56°C for 30 minutes. The inactivated serum, which has been diluted 1:5, is now ready for the HI test.

Hemagglutination Test

The preliminary step in the HI test is to determine the HA titer of the virus. This is necessary because the HA activity of the various strains of virus may differ. The activity also varies with the concentration of RBC suspension and may vary with the strain of virus. The HA titer of the virus should be determined each day and the solution should be used immediately after dilution.

1. Place a row of 10 clean tubes in a rack and pipette 0.8 ml of PBS in the first tube and 0.5 ml in the rest of the tubes.

2. Pipette 0.2 ml of stock virus suspension into the first tube and mix thoroughly.

3. Make a series of doubling dilutions of virus, ranging from 1:5 to 1:1280 by transferring 0.5 ml from tube 1 to tube 2, then 0.5 ml from tube 2 to tube 3, and so on. Use a clean and dry pipette for each transfer and thoroughly mix the contents of the tube before the 0.5 ml is withdrawn. Discard the 0.5 ml of the ninth tube.

4. Add 0.25 ml of 0.5% RBC suspension to each of the 10 tubes and shake the rack

Serology

vigorously. On occasion RBC of certain individual animals will self-hemagglutinate (in tube 10), indicating that the RBC are unsuited for the test.

5. Hold tubes at 4°C overnight. Alternately, the test can be held at room temperature (22–24°C) or at 37°C for 30–90 minutes, depending on the rapidity of settling of the erythrocytes.

In negative tubes, the erythrocytes will be arranged in a sharply demarcated disc or button. In positive tubes the erythrocytes will form a uniform blanket covering the bottom of the tube (++++ reaction); an incomplete HA may appear as a small central disc surrounded by a granular area of agglutinated cells (++ reaction), etc. At times, HA will not be found in the first one or two tubes, but a normal pattern will be seen in the second or third tube and continue to its endpoint in the higher serial dilutions. This is due to elution of virus from the RBC. This may be seen with some strains of Newcastle disease virus, particularly in higher concentrations.

The highest dilution of virus that gives a +++ or ++++ reaction is considered as the HA titer of the virus, or as 1 hemagglutination unit in 0.5 ml of virus suspension.

Hemagglutination Inhibition Test

1. Determine the volume of viral suspension needed to perform the desired number of HI tests.
2. Make a dilution of virus that will contain 8 HA units in 0.5 ml (equivalent to 4 HA units in 0.25 ml). Prepare the dilution in PBS from the original or undiluted virus suspension. *Example:* If the 1:640 dilution of virus contained 1 HA unit in 0.5 ml, then a 1:80 dilution (640 ÷ 80) would contain 8 HA units in 0.5 ml. Because 0.25 ml of virus is used in the HI test, each tube in the serial diluted sample of serum contains 4 HA units of virus. (A back titration of the antigen can be conducted to assure that the diluted antigen dose contains 4 HA units per 0.25 ml.)
3. Place 10 clean test tubes in a rack for each serum.
4. Leaving tube 1 empty, place 0.25 ml of PBS into tubes 2–10.
5. Add 0.25 ml of suspected inactivated serum previously diluted 1:5 into tube 1, tube 2, and tube 10. The latter will serve as a serum control.
6. Make a series of doubling dilutions of serum by mixing the contents of tube 2 with a pipette and transferring 0.25 ml to tube 3. Continue the dilution process and discard the 0.25 ml from tube 9.
7. Make a similar series of serum dilutions using known normal serum and a positive serum, which will serve as negative and positive serum controls respectively.
8. Add to each row of 9 tubes, 0.25 ml of the dilution of virus containing 8 units of virus in 0.5 ml as determined in the titration above.
9. Add 0.25 ml of PBS to tube 10 of each row of diluted serum.
10. Shake the racks well and allow the reaction to proceed for 1 hour at room temperature.
11. Add 0.25 ml of RBC suspension to each tube and agitate.
12. Let the racks stand at 4°C overnight and examine for HA the following day. Room temperature (22–24°C) or 37°C for 30–90 minutes, as mentioned for the HA test, can also be used.

If a serum does not contain HI antibodies, a +++ or ++++ reaction occurs in all tubes. This is a negative HI test.

When a serum contains antihemagglutinins, no agglutination of RBC will occur in one or more of the tubes. The highest dilution of serum that completely inhibits hemagglutination is designated as the HI titer of the serum (see below).

Confirmation of Disease

Titers in the range of 1:10 to 1:40 indicate previous exposure to PI-3 virus but may not be related to recent infection. Since HI titers have been observed to increase about 2 weeks after infection, the best results can be obtained by using the technique on both acute and convalescent serum samples. A fourfold or greater increase in the HI titer may be considered confirmation of a recent infection with PI-3 virus. Cattle having a clinical response to infection develop HI titers of 1:320 or greater.

Hemagglutination Inhibition Microtest

This is carried out with microtiter kits that are available from several commercial sources. Instead of tubes, the system requires Plexiglas or plastic plates that have rows of V-shaped cups. The test proper is identical to that described for the macrotiter system, except that serum and virus volumes are reduced to 0.025 ml each, the volume of the 0.5% erythrocyte suspension is reduced to 0.05 ml, and shaking is done with a mechanical shaker after the cups have been sealed with tape supplied with the kit (BioQuest, Lockeysville, Md.).

Interpretation of Results

The following applies to either of the two systems described above. The HI titer of a test serum is the highest dilution of that serum that inhibits completely the formation of a salmon-colored film at the bottom of the tube. For the results of a test set to be valid, serum and erythrocyte control tubes must exhibit the smooth, red, round, flowing erythrocyte buttons; all tubes used for the titration of known negative serum must show the typical salmon-colored film of HA; and the titer of the known immune serum must fall within twofold of its label value. For the serologic diagnosis, a conversion from negative to positive, or an increase in titer of at least fourfold, must be obtained when antibody levels in paired sera are compared. For strain identification, similar results must be obtained with the test and a reference strain against a known immune serum; conversely, an antiserum prepared with the test strain must yield comparable titers against it and against a reference strain of virus. Preferably, a crisscross titration should be carried out.

Hemadsorption Test

Cells infected in tissue culture with certain viruses, whether cytopathology is evident or not, have the capacity to adsorb erythrocytes from various animal species.[34] Viruses that agglutinate erythrocytes in vitro generally possess this attribute of hemadsorption; however, there are notable exceptions, such as certain echoviruses and the Coe virus, that agglutinate erythrocytes in vitro but fail to cause infected cells to hemadsorb.

The phenomenon of HAd has been used to advantage for the titration in tissue culture of viruses that produce little or no distinct cytopathology. Moreover, even with some cytopathogenic viruses, HAd may demonstrate a higher infective titer than that derived from cytopathology. One such virus is bovine PI-3; the titration is as follows. Dilute the virus preparation in 10-fold steps, and inoculate each dilution into 2–4 tubes of bovine kidney or embryonic bovine muscle cultures, each tube receiving 0.1 ml of the appropriate dilution. Following their incubation for 5–7 days at 35–37°C, observe the tubes for CPE and then empty their medium. Wash the monolayers three times with chilled PBS, then add to each tube 1 ml of a 0.1% guinea-pig erythrocyte suspension prepared by the procedure described previously for the HI test. Hold the tubes at 4°C for 30 minutes, with the erythrocyte suspension covering the monolayer, then examine for the typical adherence of the erythrocytes to and around virus-infected cells. Infective titers by either CPE or HAd can then be calculated by the Reed-Muench or Kärber methods. In a typical titration of a bovine PI-3 virus preparation, the infective titer endpoint may appear to be $10^{-3.5}$ per 0.1 ml by CPE, but it may amount to $10^{-5.5}$ per 0.1 ml by HAd.

Hemadsorption Inhibition Test

Prior treatment of infected PI-3 virus cultures with the corresponding antiserum will inhibit HAd upon the subsequent introduction of guinea pig erythrocytes. A quantitative antibody determination by HAdI is carried out as follows: 5–7 days after virus inoculation, empty an appropriate number of infected tissue culture tubes of their medium, and wash them three times with chilled PBS. Dilute a test serum in twofold steps with PBS, over a range determined from previous experience. The serum should not be heat-inactivated before dilution. Then introduce each serum dilution into two washed tissue culture tubes, 0.1 ml per tube. Hold the tubes at room temperature (22–24°C) for 30 minutes in a position allowing the serum dilution to bathe the entire monolayer. At the end of the half-hour remove the serum dilutions from the tubes, and to each tube add 1 ml of a 0.1% guinea-pig erythrocyte suspension. Following incubation at 4°C for 30 minutes, examine the tubes microscopically for HAd. Appropriate controls, comprising known antibody-free and immune sera, should be included in each test set. The HAdI titer is the highest dilution of serum that completely inhibits adherence of the erythrocytes to the cells of the monolayer.

Virus Neutralization Test

The VN test is based on the fact that a virus is rendered noninfective by combination with its specific antibody. The test is used in the serologic diagnosis of viral infections, the identification of viral isolates, the study of antigenic relationships between viral strains, the evaluation of the immunogenicity of vaccines, the production of immune sera, and the determination of the presence of antibodies in the sera of laboratory animals intended for experimental studies.

Procedures for neutralization tests vary depending on the virus. The basic method consists of mixing the virus with serum, incubating the mixture, and inoculating the mixture into a susceptible host or tissue culture system to determine the extent to which the serum has neutralized the infectivity of the virus.

Stock Virus

Virus preparations of relatively high infectivity are required. A virus isolated from an infected animal must be grown and passed several times in embryonated eggs, tissue cultures, or laboratory animals. Stock virus may be prepared from the CAM, embryonic fluids, or infected tissues of animals (e.g. brains or lungs). The tissues are harvested when the virus has reached its highest titer and are ground in sterile broth, and suspensions are clarified by centrifugation at low speed. Stock virus from tissue cultures is prepared from the culture fluids or by scraping the infected monolayers from the walls of the vessel, disrupting the cells by repeated cycles of freezing and thawing, and clarifying the suspension by centrifugation at low speed. The supernatant fluid is the stock virus. It is dispensed in ampules, shell frozen, and stored at $-70°C$. Since dead virus may combine with the antibody and thus interfere with the neutralization test, the storage period depends on the stability of the virus.

Sera

Sera to be assayed for antibody content are obtained from the infected animals. For diagnostic purposes it is desirable to obtain serum samples during both the acute and convalescent phases of the disease. For typing of virus, immune sera against known viruses are used. Such sera also may be used as positive serum controls in testing unknown sera. Since the neutralizing capacity of mammalian sera may drop at refrigerator temperatures (0–4°C), serum should be removed promptly from the clot and stored in the frozen state. In addition, sera may contain heat-labile nonspecific viral inhibitors that interfere with the neutralization test; therefore, common practice is to heat sera at 56°C for 30 minutes before use.

Antisera prepared by immunizing animals with virus grown in tissue culture may contain antibodies against tissue culture cells, which may interfere with neutralization tests carried out in tissue cultures. They may show CPE or inhibit viral growth. The antibodies may be removed by adsorption with homologous blood cells or the proper tissue cells. Usually their titer is relatively low, and the antisera may be used without the adsorption step at dilutions where anticellular antibodies no longer interfere.

Virus-Serum Mixtures

One of two procedures is commonly followed to determine the neutralizing capacity of a serum. The first procedure, which involves the mixing of constant amounts of serum with varying dilutions of virus, is used primarily for virus identification, and to a lesser extent for detection of cross-reactions with heterologous virus types and strains, and for comparison of antibody levels of sera obtained during acute and convalescent phases of infection. In the second procedure, the amount of virus is constant and is mixed with serial dilutions of serum. This technique is frequently employed to determine the antigenicity of vaccines or the potency of antisera. In either case, the virus-serum mixtures are inoculated into susceptible animals or cultures, following incubation for times and at temperatures that depend on the virus, although opinions differ on whether incubation is required in all cases.[18]

A special immuno-inactivation test has been developed by which low levels of neutralizing antibody can be detected.[9] In this test, constant amounts of virus in varying serum dilutions are incubated for 6 hours at 37°C followed by overnight incubation at 4°C. During this period, viral infectivity disappears slowly from the mixture of virus and immune serum. The process is distinct from the more rapid initial combination of antibody and virus, and may represent a second step in the virus-antibody interaction.

Host Systems

After incubation, virus-serum mixtures are inoculated into a susceptible host system to detect the presence of nonneutralized infective virus in the mixtures. The host systems employed may be embryonated eggs, animals, or tissue cultures.

The neutralizing capacity of the serum is determined in eggs from its ability to prevent viral effects such as death of the embryo, pocklike lesions on the CAM, and the formation of hemagglutinins in the allantoic fluid or the membrane.

Mice are the laboratory animals most commonly used. The neutralizing capacity of a serum is usually measured by its ability to reduce the infective titer of the virus as indicated by mortality or paralysis.

In tissue cultures, neutralizing antibodies are evaluated from the degree of CPE, metabolic inhibition, or plaque formation. In tests based on CPE, constant virus-varying serum dilutions are inoculated into the monolayers of sensitive cells. The cytopathic changes after incubation indicate to what extent the virus was neutralized. The metabolic inhibition test is carried out in cell suspensions, and is based on changes in the pH of the medium, which are reflected by the color of an indicator. Infection with a cytopathogenic virus inhibits cellular metabolism and the medium remains neutral or slightly alkaline; when the virus is neutralized, normal cellular metabolism produces acid. In the plaque test, monolayers of susceptible cells are inoculated with virus-serum mixtures and then overlaid with agar. A significant reduction in the number of plaques compared to the control indicates neutralization of the virus.

A variation of the plaque test consists of inoculating monolayers with virus only and, after overlaying the cells with agar, placing paper discs impregnated with serum on the agar surface. The virus neutralizing capacity of the serum is determined from the size of the zone of inhibition of viral growth (plaque formation) around the discs.

Certain viruses do not produce plaques or cytopathic changes. Their presence can be detected by indirect means, such as hemadsorption, interference, and FA staining. Antibody may be assayed by the same methods.

Micromethods

The microtitration method has been adapted to most serologic procedures, including the neutralization test.[30] The tests are carried out in wells in disposable plastic plates with micropipettes and wire loops calibrated to deliver volumes as small as 0.025 ml (Cooke Engineering Co., Alexandria, Va.). Virus-serum mixtures are prepared using the loops to dilute the serum in tissue culture medium and the micropipettes to add the virus suspension. After appropriate incubation, tissue culture cells are added to each well and the plates are sealed with tape. Final volumes are usually from 0.05 to 0.1 ml. After further incubation the cultures are examined for evidence of infection, which indicates the presence of nonneutralized virus in the virus-serum mixtures. The microtests afford savings in time and materials, and results agree well with those obtained with macrotests.

Infectivity Titer

The antibody content of a serum is determined by the viral infectivity it neutralizes. The infectivity of a virus suspension is expressed in terms of the dilution of the suspension that causes death in 50% of inoculated animals (lethal dose 50%, LD_{50}), signs of infection in 50% of inoculated tissue cultures (tissue culture infecting dose 50%, $TCID_{50}$), or signs of infection in embryonating eggs (embryo infecting dose 50%, EID_{50}). The 50% endpoints are determined by inoculating dilutions of stock virus in animals, tissue cultures, or embryonating eggs and observing mortality or other signs of infection over an appropriate test period, and then calculating with one of several methods.

Fifty Percent Endpoints

There are several rapid methods for estimation of LD_{50}. That of Reed and Muench (R & M method)[28] is the most popular, although it does not give accurate estimates unless the infecting doses bracket the 50% response point symmetrically, a condition that cannot be guaranteed. The Spearman-Kärber method (S-K method)[14,31] is simpler and has been reported to give more accurate estimates of LD_{50} than the R & M procedure, and it also permits calculation of a standard error. Graphic methods such as those proposed by Litchfield and Wilcoxon[20] and Miller and Tainter[22] also permit the determination of a standard error. However, these methods require skill on the part of the investigator in plotting dose-response curves; they give accurate estimates of endpoints in the hands of those experienced in bioassay.

Access to a computer is common today, and advantage should be taken of this to calculate endpoints by the probit or similar method. This will provide standard deviations and slopes and, in some situations, lead to the use of more efficient designs, which eliminate the doses giving 0% and 100% responses (required by the R & M and S-K methods).

Antibody Titer

The antibody titer of a serum may be expressed in two ways, depending on the technique used to determine it. When varying dilutions of serum are tested for their ability to neutralize a constant amount of virus, the antibody titer is expressed as the *50% endpoint* of the serum. The 50% endpoint is that dilution of serum which, when mixed with the test dose of virus and inoculated into susceptible animals, embryonating eggs, or tissue cultures, results in the survival of 50% of the animals or embryos, or in the absence of signs of infection in 50% of the tissue cultures or eggs.

When a constant amount of serum is tested for its ability to neutralize varying dilutions of virus, the antibody titer is expressed as a *neutralization index*. The index is the ratio between the 50% endpoints of the virus stock in the presence of the test serum and in the presence of the negative control serum.

Serology

Constant Virus–Varying Serum Dilutions

This example will compare the neutralizing capacity of a test antiserum against infectious canine hepatitis (ICH) virus with that of a standard antiserum. Dilutions of the test serum and of the standard serum should each be mixed with equal volumes of ICH virus suspension, incubated, and then inoculated into dog kidney tissue cultures. Then simultaneously titrate the virus stock in order to establish the number of $TCID_{50}$ of virus in the virus-serum mixtures. The mixtures should contain between 100 and 1000 $TCID_{50}$ of virus per 0.1 ml. After incubation, examine the cultures for viral CPE. The 50% endpoint dilutions of the test serum and the standard serum can be calculated from the titration results, as follows.

Diluent. Prepare all dilutions in Earle's BSS supplemented with 0.5% lactalbumin hydrolysate, 50 units of penicillin, 50 μg of streptomycin, and 50 units of neomycin per ml.

Stock virus. Seed the ICH virus in monolayers of dog kidney cells. When the CPE is evident, usually about 40 hours after inoculation, harvest the culture fluids, dispense in ampules, and store at $-70°C$.

Sera. The test serum should be a pool of sera obtained from a number of dogs immunized with ICH vaccine. The standard serum is issued by the NADC. Substances that may interfere with the test can be inactivated by heating the sera at 56°C for 30 minutes.

Serum dilutions. Dilute both standard and test sera as shown in Table 5.8. In tubes 1 and 2 place 4.5 ml of diluent and in tubes 3, 4, 5, and 6 place 1.5 ml of diluent. Using a 1 ml pipette, add exactly 0.5 ml of serum to tube 1. With a fresh pipette, mix the suspension in tube 1 by drawing and expelling in and out of the pipette several times. Then transfer 0.5 ml of the mixture to tube 2. With a 2 ml pipette, mix the suspension in tube 2, and transfer 1.5 ml to tube 3. Continue the procedure with all the tubes, using a fresh pipette each time.

Table 5.8. Dilutions of standard and test sera

Tube	Dilution	Mixture in test tube
1	1:10	0.5 ml of serum + 4.5 ml diluent
2	1:100	0.5 ml of 1:10 + 4.5 ml diluent
3	1:200	1.5 ml of 1:100 + 1.5 ml diluent
4	1:400	1.5 ml of 1:200 + 1.5 ml diluent
5	1:800	1.5 ml of 1:400 + 1.5 ml diluent
6	1:1600	1.5 ml of 1:800 + 1.5 ml diluent

Virus dilutions. A dilution of stock virus is required so that after it is mixed with the serum about 100–1000 $TCID_{50}$ of virus will be contained in 0.1 ml of the mixtures. On the basis of previous titrations, a 1:500 dilution of stock virus will probably be needed. Make the dilutions as shown in Table 5.9. Place the diluent in test tubes. With a syringe and a needle, transfer 0.5 ml of the thawed and well-mixed virus stock suspension to tube 1. With a 1 ml pipette, mix the suspension in tube 1 by drawing and expelling the suspension in and out of the pipette several times, and then transfer 0.5 ml to tube 2. With a fresh pipette, mix the suspension in tube 2 and transfer 1 ml to tube 3.

Virus-serum mixtures. Set up two rows of five tubes each. In each of the tubes place

Table 5.9. Dilutions of stock virus

Tube	Dilution	Mixture in test tube	
1	1:5	0.5 ml stock virus suspension	+2.0 ml diluent
2	1:50	0.5 ml 1:5 dilution	+4.5 ml diluent
3	1:500	1.0 ml 1:50 dilution	+9.0 ml diluent

0.5 ml of the appropriate dilution (from 1:200 through 1:1600) of standard or test serum, using a fresh pipette for each dilution. Shake the tubes and incubate them in a water bath at 37°C for 1 hour.

To dilute the virus for titration, add 0.5 ml of diluent to 0.5 ml of the 1:500 dilutions of stock virus. Then incubate the 10^{-3} dilution of stock virus thus prepared in a water bath at 37°C for 1 hour. After incubation, further dilute the virus stock as shown in Table 5.10.

Table 5.10. Further dilutions of stock virus

Tube	Dilution of stock virus	Mixture in test tube
1	10^{-4}	0.5 ml of 10^{-3} dilution + 4.5 ml diluent
2	10^{-5}	0.5 ml of 10^{-4} dilution + 4.5 ml diluent
3	10^{-6}	0.5 ml of 10^{-5} dilution + 4.5 ml diluent
4	10^{-7}	0.5 ml of 10^{-6} dilution + 4.5 ml diluent

Inoculation in tissue cultures. Inoculate monolayers of dog kidney cells with 0.1 ml of each of the virus-serum mixtures and 0.1 ml of each of the virus dilutions from 10^{-4} through 10^{-7}. Use six tubes (or prescription bottles) of tissue culture per dilution. Hold six noninoculated cultures as controls. Incubate the cultures at 37°C for 7 days and then examine for evidence of CPE. Results of a sample virus titration are shown in Table 5.11.

Calculation of virus titer by the Reed and Muench method. The data in Table 5.11 are arranged for the application of the R & M method, which uses the total number of tissue cultures rather than only those bracketing the 50% endpoint. The accumulated values are obtained by adding the number of infected cultures starting at the highest virus dilution on the assumption that they would be infected at the lower virus dilutions. Similarly, the noninfected cultures are added starting at the lower dilutions on the assumption that they would be noninfected at the higher dilutions. The 50% endpoint is between 10^{-5} and

Table 5.11. Titration of virus

	Observed results				Accumulated results			
	Cultures with CPE		Cultures with		Cultures with		Cultures with CPE	
Dilutions of stock virus	Ratio	%	CPE	No CPE	CPE	No CPE	Ratio	%
10^{-4}	6/6	100	6	0	13	0	13/13	100
10^{-5}	5/6	83	5	1	7	1	7/8	88
10^{-6}	2/6	33	2	4	2	5	2/7	29
10^{-7}	0/6	0	0	6	0	11	0/11	0

Serology

10^{-6} (between 29 and 88% in Table 5.11). The formula to determine the proportionate distance of the 50% endpoint is:

$$\text{Proportionate distance} = \frac{\%\text{ infected at next dilution giving more than 50\% response} - 50\%}{\left(\begin{array}{c}\%\text{ infected at next dilution giving more}\\ \text{than 50\% response}\end{array}\right) - \left(\begin{array}{c}\%\text{ infected at next dilution giving less}\\ \text{than 50\% response}\end{array}\right)}$$

$$\text{Proportionate distance} = \frac{88\% - 50\%}{88\% - 29\%} = \frac{38\%}{59\%} = 0.64$$

Log of the 50% endpoint = Log of next dilution giving more than 50% response
 − (Proportionate distance × Log of the dilution factor)

Log $TCID_{50}$ = log 10^{-5} − (0.64)(log 10^1) = −5.00 − (0.64) (1) = −5.64

Thus $TCID_{50} = 10^{-5.64}$; the virus stock contains $10^{5.64}$ $TCID_{50}$ per 0.1 ml. In the neutralization mixtures, 0.5 ml of a 1:500 dilution of stock virus was mixed with 0.5 ml of serum resulting in a 10^{-3} dilution of the stock virus. The mixtures thus contained $10^{5.64} \times 10^{-3} = 10^{2.64}$ $TCID_{50}$ or 430 $TCID_{50}$ per 0.1 ml.

Calculation of the virus titer by the Spearman-Kärber method. This method does not use accumulated data. It should, however, be used only with data including 100% response or with data for which it would be reasonable to expect 100% response at the next higher dose level. The formula is:

$$\begin{array}{l}\text{Log of the}\\ \text{50\% end point}\end{array} = \begin{array}{l}\text{Log of dilution}\\ \text{giving 100\%}\\ \text{response}\end{array} - \left(\frac{\text{Sum of \% mortality at each dilution}}{100} - 0.50\right)\left(\begin{array}{c}\text{Log of the}\\ \text{dilution factor}\end{array}\right)$$

Log $TCID_{50}$ = log 10^{-4} − $\left(\frac{100 + 83 + 33}{100} - 0.50\right)$ (log 10^1) = −4.00 − (1.66) (1) = −5.66

$TCID_{50} = 10^{-5.66}$; the virus stock contains $10^{5.66}$ $TCID_{50}$ per 0.1 ml. Calculated by this method, the virus-serum mixtures thus contained $10^{5.66} \times 10^{-3} = 10^{2.66}$ $TCID_{50}$ or 450 $TCID_{50}$ per 0.1 ml. Results obtained with sample virus-serum mixtures are shown in Table 5.12.

Calculation of the antibody titer by the Reed and Muench method. Now we wish to determine the serum dilution *protecting* 50% of the cultures. For the test serum:

$$\text{Proportionate distance} = \frac{88\% - 50\%}{88\% - 29\%} = 0.64$$

$$\begin{array}{l}\text{Log of the 50\%}\\ \text{endpoint}\end{array} = \begin{array}{l}\text{Log of dilution}\\ \text{giving more than}\\ \text{50\% response}\end{array} + \left(\begin{array}{c}\text{Proportionate}\\ \text{distance}\end{array} \times \begin{array}{c}\text{Log of the}\\ \text{dilution factor}\end{array}\right)$$

(Note the + sign in the formula when dealing with *protection*.)

Log of the 50% endpoint = log $10^{-2.90}$ + (0.64) (log 2) = −2.90 + (0.64) (0.30) = −2.71

The 50% neutralizing dilution is $10^{-2.71}$ or 1:500. (*Note:* The antilog of −2.71 is 0.002, and the reciprocal of 0.002 is 500; therefore the dilution protecting 50% of the cultures is 1:500.) For the standard serum:

Proportionate distance $= \dfrac{70\% - 50\%}{70\% - 12\%} = \dfrac{20}{58} = 0.34$

Log of the 50% endpoint $= -2.90 + (0.34)(0.30) = -2.80$

The 50% neutralizing dilution is $10^{-2.80}$ or $1:630$.

The ratio of the 50% neutralizing dilution of the test serum to the 50% neutralizing dilution of the standard serum is $500/630 = 0.79$. (Specifications for an antiserum may require that this ratio equal 0.67 or more after challenge with 100–1000 $TCID_{50}$ of virus, determined by a simultaneous titration.)

Calculation of the antibody titer by the Spearman-Kärber method. For the test serum:

Log of the 50% endpoint $= \log 10^{-3.50} + \left(\dfrac{100 + 100 + 83 + 33}{100} - 0.50 \right) (\log 2)$
$= -3.50 + (3.16 - 0.50)(0.30) = -2.70$

The 50% neutralizing dilution is $10^{-2.70}$ or $1:500$. For the standard serum:

Log of the 50% endpoint $= \log 10^{-3.50} + \left(\dfrac{100 + 100 + 67 + 17}{100} - 0.50 \right) (\log 2)$
$= -3.50 + (2.84 - 0.50)(0.30) = -2.80$

The 50% neutralizing dilution is $10^{-2.80}$ or $1:630$.

The ratio of the 50% neutralizing dilution of the test serum to the 50% neutralizing dilution of the standard serum is $500/630 = 0.79$. The conclusion is that the test serum passes specifications.

Table 5.12. Neutralization test: Constant virus–varying serum dilutions

Final dilution of serum in virus-serum mixtures	Observed results				Accumulated results			
	Cultures with CPE Ratio	Cultures With CPE	Cultures No CPE		Cultures With CPE	Cultures No CPE	Cultures with CPE Ratio	%
Test serum								
1:200 ($10^{-2.3}$)	0/6	0	6		0	11	0/11	0
1:400 ($10^{-2.6}$)	2/6	2	4		2	5	2/7	29
1:800 ($10^{-2.9}$)	5/6	5	1		7	1	7/8	88
1:1600 ($10^{-3.2}$)	6/6	6	0		13	0	13/13	100
1:3200 ($10^{-3.5}$)	6/6	6	0		19	0	19/19	100
Standard serum								
1:200 ($10^{-2.3}$)	0/6	0	6		0	13	0/13	0
1:400 ($10^{-2.6}$)	1/6	1	5		1	7	1/8	12
1:800 ($10^{-2.9}$)	4/6	4	2		5	2	5/7	70
1:1600 ($10^{-3.2}$)	6/6	6	0		11	0	11/11	100
1:3200 ($10^{-3.5}$)	6/6	6	0		17	0	17/17	100

Constant Serum–Varying Virus Dilutions

This example will determine the presence or absence of antibodies to canine distemper virus (CDV) in a dog's serum. First mix dilutions of CDV suspension with the dog's serum, or control serum, and allow to neutralize. Then inoculate the mixtures onto the CAM of embryonating eggs. After incubation, examine the membranes for lesions typical of CDV infection. Then determine the neutralization index of the serum.

Serology

Sera. Allow the blood from the dog to be tested to stand at room temperature for a few hours to permit the serum to separate from the clot. Then centrifuge the serum at 2500 rpm for 20 minutes. Serum from a dog or horse free of antibodies to CDV should serve as control. Also, a known positive control serum should be included in the test. Substances that may interfere with neutralization can be inactivated by heating the sera in a water bath at 56°C for 30 minutes.

Virus. Thaw a recently prepared stock of CDV grown in chicken embryo tissue cultures. Dilute the virus stock suspension in sterile brain-heart infusion broth containing 50 units of penicillin and 50 μg of streptomycin per ml, as shown in Table 5.13.

Table 5.13. Dilution of virus stock suspension in BHI broth

Tube	Dilution of stock virus	Mixture in test tube	
1	2×10^{-1}	1 ml stock virus	+ 4 ml broth
2	2×10^{-2}	1 ml 2×10^{-1}	+ 9 ml broth
3	2×10^{-3}	1 ml 2×10^{-2}	+ 9 ml broth
4	2×10^{-4}	1 ml 2×10^{-3}	+ 9 ml broth
5	2×10^{-5}	1 ml 2×10^{-4}	+ 9 ml broth

Virus-serum mixtures. Set up three rows of 4 tubes each. Into each tube of the first row place 0.6 ml of the test serum; into each of the second row place 0.6 ml of control serum. To each tube then add 0.6 ml of the appropriate dilution (10^{-2} to 10^{-5}) of the stock virus suspension. Mix the virus-serum suspensions and incubate in the refrigerator (3–5°C) for 4 hours. A simultaneous titration of the virus stock diluted in broth is also usually carried out to ascertain that the control serum is free of antibodies.

Inoculation of eggs. Candle 6–8-day-old embryonating eggs and drill a hole in the top of the egg above the air sac. Swab the drilled holes with 70% alcohol prior to inoculating. With a 2 ml syringe and a 23-gauge, five-ninths inch (1.41 cm) needle, deposit 0.2 ml of each of the mixtures onto the CAM. Use five eggs for each virus-serum mixture. Seal the holes with collodion and incubate the eggs for 7 days at 35°C. Discard eggs with dead embryos. Harvest the CAM of the surviving eggs as follows: With a pair of scissors cut the egg shell around the egg just below the air sac. Remove the CAM with a pair of forceps and spread it on a glass plate. Count the lesions. Each CAM is graded as positive if it has three or more lesions; a CAM with two or less lesions is negative. Results are shown in Table 5.14.

Table 5.14. Neutralization test: Constant serum–varying virus dilutions

Dilutions of stock virus in	Eggs with positive CAM/Eggs inoculated with the following dilutions of stock virus				EID_{50}
	10^{-2}	10^{-3}	10^{-4}	10^{-5}	
Test serum	5/5	1/5	0/5	0/5	$10^{-2.70}$ (1:500)
Control serum	4/4	5/5	5/5	0/5	$10^{-4.50}$ (1:31,600)

Calculation of the neutralization index. This test consists of parallel titrations of the virus in the presence of test serum and in the presence of control serum. The EID_{50} of the virus are determined readily by the Spearman-Kärber method as follows:

$$\text{Test serum} = -2.00 - \left(\frac{100+20}{100} - 0.50\right)(\log 10^1) = -2.70$$

$$\text{Control serum} = -2.00 - \left(\frac{100+100+100}{100} - 0.50\right)(\log 10^1) = -4.50$$

The NI is the ratio between the 50% endpoint dilution of the virus in test serum (1:500) and the 50% endpoint dilution of the virus in control serum (1:31,600): log 4.50 − log 2.70 = log 1.80, or 63 EID_{50} of virus neutralized. A reduction in the viral titer in the presence of test serum of 1.5 log units or more (i.e. an index of 32 or more) is usually considered significant. The conclusion is that the dog's serum contains antibodies against canine distemper virus.

Variations

The constant serum–varying virus dilutions neutralization test for certain other viruses may require some variations from the example given. For example, in tests with FMD virus, the test and control serums should be diluted initially 1:10 or 1:20 (1:20 or 1:40 final dilution when an equal part of viral suspension is added).[6] If this is not done, a clear-cut endpoint may not be found. Likewise, a known positive control serum of high antibody titer to the homologous virus type may require as much as an initial dilution of 1:160 (1:320 final). After the log titers are obtained and the log of the negative control serum is subtracted from the log of the test serum and from the log of the positive control serum, a correction factor for dilution of the serum may be added. For a test serum diluted 1:40 final the factor is log 1.6, and for a serum diluted 1:320 final it is 2.5. With this variation of the test, NI of log 2.9 or more would be considered significant in tests with FMD virus. In this test, the virus suspension is initially diluted 1:5 before the 10-fold dilutions are made. The serum and virus mixtures are incubated in a water bath at 37°C for 1 hour, and the test system is litters of suckling mice 6–8 days old.[6]

Fluorescent Antibody Technique

The FA technique, like other serologic reactions, is based on the specific union of antigen and antibody. Its uniqueness and its advantages are a consequence of the way in which the union is made evident. The FA technique is a sensitive and rapid serologic procedure for identifying a variety of antigens. In veterinary microbiology, as in other disciplines, FA has been used extensively in research to help solve fundamental problems. Many investigations have also established its value in the diagnosis of both infectious and noninfectious diseases. Because our concern here is with diagnosis, most of the chapter is devoted to methods by which FA can be prepared and used to identify either pathogenic microorganisms or abnormal proteins associated with disease processes. Specific diagnostic applications will be discussed elsewhere in this manual.

Briefly, the procedure is as follows: The antibody-containing globulin fraction of an antiserum is labeled (conjugated) with a fluorescent dye, i.e. a fluorochrome. When the labeled (fluorescent) antibody is reacted with homologous antigen, a complex of antigen, antibody, and fluorochrome is formed. After washing away unreacted globulins, the complex is identified by examining the preparation under dark-field microscopy with

Serology

UV light. Fluorochrome molecules excited by UV light emit a longer wavelength of light (color) that is characteristic for the particular fluorochrome.[4,24]

Preparation of Fluorescent Antibody

The preparation of fluorescent antibody involves serum fractionation, labeling, purification, sorption, and standardization. Although various methods may be used to accomplish some of the steps, only one is presented here in detail; reference is made to several alternate methods and modifications. Even when not specifically stated, environmental conditions that minimize denaturation of proteins should be maintained.

Serum Fractionation with Ammonium Sulfate

The observation that nonspecific staining usually occurs significantly less with labeled globulins than with homologous labeled whole serum has resulted in the inclusion of serum fractionation as the initial step in the preparation of most fluorescent antibody. Comparisons of several methods of fractionation have indicated the ammonium sulfate technique as the best method.[19]

Procedure

1. To 2 volumes of chilled serum slowly add 1 volume of a saturated solution of ammonium sulfate (see "Preparation of Reagents" below) at room temperature. (Note that this procedure results mainly in the precipitation of gamma globulins. When antibodies are also part of the beta globulins, it may be desirable to mix equal volumes of a saturated solution of ammonium sulfate and serum to precipitate total globulins.) During the addition of ammonium sulfate the serum should be kept chilled and continuously stirred.

2. Centrifuge the precipitated globulins for 30 minutes at $2000 \times g$. Decant the supernatant fluid and redissolve the globulins in a sufficient volume of distilled water to restore the volume of the globulin solution to the original serum volume.

3. Using the globulin solution in place of the serum, repeat the above procedures twice more, but with one exception. After the last centrifugation, redissolve the globulins in as small a volume of distilled water as possible so that the subsequent adjustment of protein concentration suggested for labeling with fluorochrome can be made by dilution.

4. Dialyze the globulin solution against several changes of a 0.85% NaCl solution at 4°C until it is free of residual ammonium sulfate.

Ammonium sulfate readily diffuses into the dialysate and can be identified by mixing a small volume of dialysate with an equal volume of a saturated solution of barium chloride, whereupon the formation of a precipitate indicates the presence of sulfate.[15]

Labeling Serum Proteins with Fluorescein Isothiocyanate

Because of its bright, yellow-green fluorescence and simplicity of conjugation, fluorescein isothiocyanate is used most frequently for labeling serum proteins. Other fluorochromes are available, however, and may be used to advantage in special cases.[24]

Procedure

1. Determine the protein concentration of the globulin solution by a standard procedure such as the Biuret method.

2. Adjust the protein concentration to 10 mg/ml by dilution with a 0.85% NaCl solution, or by concentration.

3. For each mg of protein of the globulin solution dissolve 0.05 mg of fluorescein isothiocyanate powder in cold (4°C) carbonate-bicarbonate buffer (pH 9) (see "Preparation of Reagents" below). The volume of buffer should be one-tenth that of the globulin solution.

4. Slowly add the fluorescein-containing buffer to the globulin solution at 4°C with constant stirring and allow the conjugation reaction to proceed overnight (16 hours) in the cold.

Purification of Labeled Proteins by Gel Filtration

Following the overnight conjugation reaction there will be many molecules of fluorescein isothiocyanate that have not attached to protein. Because unreacted fluorescein molecules contribute to nonspecific background fluorescence, it is necessary that they be separated from labeled proteins. An efficient and rapid method of separation is by column chromatography with Sephadex gel.[12] Sephadex gels are composed of cross-linked dextran molecules. The frequency of cross-linking determines pore size and thus the size of the molecules that can penetrate the gel. A gel with a pore size that allows unreacted fluorescein isothiocyanate molecules to enter but excludes the larger protein molecules should be selected, e.g. Sephadex gel types G-25 and G-50.

Procedure. The following procedure illustrates the separation of a 25 ml mixture of labeled protein and unreacted fluorescein with Sephadex gel type G-25 coarse. For separation of other volumes, the volume of the gel bed would have to be altered correspondingly.

1. Hydrate 15 g of Sephadex G-25 coarse in 250 ml of PBS, pH 7.2, for the length of time necessary for complete swelling of the gel (specified by manufacturer). This amount will provide an approximately 2×17–20 cm column of settled gel.

2. Pour the slurry of Sephadex into a chromatographic column (2 cm by at least 50 cm). Allow the excess PBS to flow through the column until all the Sephadex has been added and has settled above the column support. Place a filter paper disc, just less than 2 cm in diameter, on the surface of the gel to help prevent disturbance of the surface during the subsequent addition of PBS and the mixture to be separated. Flush the column several times with PBS. Do not allow the fluid level to go below the surface of the gel during any of the above or subsequent procedures. Chill the column.

3. Adjust the fluid level to the level of the surface of the gel and then add the mixture. When the last of the mixture is just at the surface of the gel, start the elution process by adding the PBS. Continue adding PBS until the labeled protein has been eluted from the column and collected. Soon after the elution process is started the separation of the unreacted fluorescein and the labeled protein will become obvious. The yellow band that moves rapidly through the column is labeled protein. The yellow band that remains at the top of the column contains unreacted fluorescein molecules that have penetrated the gel and move slowly through the column because of their more tortuous route.

Sorption with Rabbit Liver Powder

Even after removal of unreacted fluorescein most preparations of FA still contain elements that cause an unacceptable amount of nonspecific background fluorescence. Apparently this is caused by the marked affinity that some labeled serum proteins with a high net negative charge have for positively charged tissues. The resulting attachment is referred to as nonspecific staining in contrast to specific staining, which results from the union of labeled antibody with homologous antigen. Some of the procedures that have been found suitable for selectively removing elements responsible for nonspecific staining are sorption with tissue powders, sorption with tissue homogenates, and ion exchange chromatography.[21] Sorption with rabbit liver powder as described below has been found satisfactory for reducing nonspecific staining of various tissues and for use with globulins from different species. If, however, nonspecific staining is not reduced sufficiently by this procedure, one or more variables may be altered; for example, more than one sorption may be necessary, or another method may be more appropriate, e.g. tissue homogenate or ion exchange.

Procedure. (1) For each mg of labeled protein weigh out 20–30 mg of rabbit liver powder (see "Preparation of Reagents" below). Hydrate the liver powder with 2.5 ml of PBS for each g of powder. (2) Add the labeled protein to the slurry of liver powder. Stir or shake (in either case avoid foaming) the mixture overnight (16 hours) at 4°C. (3) Sediment the bulk of the liver powder by centrifugation at $2000 \times g$ for 30 minutes. Sediment the remaining liver powder by centrifugation at $78,000 \times g$ for 1 hour. Carefully aspirate the supernatant fluid from the sediment so as not to reintroduce any fluorescein-coated particles of liver powder.

Standardization and Storage

As a final step, each preparation of fluorescent antibody should be evaluated to determine the maximum dilution that gives bright specific staining. The time of staining and volume should be the same as used in routine application because, within certain limits, these variables affect both the intensity of specific staining (particularly in the more dilute solutions) and the amount of background fluorescence. When FA is prepared from high-titered antiserum, some dilution can usually be made without significantly altering the intensity of specific staining. Besides the economy, this means that any nonspecificity remaining is rapidly diminished by the dilution.

The FA can be stored for a long period (usually years) without significant loss of potency if kept frozen. If it is necessary to store FA for only a few weeks, it usually may be kept satisfactorily at $-5°C$, especially if thimerosal (1:10,000) is added to inhibit microbial growth.

Preparation of Reagents

1. For saturated solution of ammonium sulfate, dissolve 750 g of ammonium sulfate in 1000 ml of distilled water.
2. For carbonate-bicarbonate buffer, pH 9, 0.5 M, dissolve 1.093 g of $NaHCO_3$ in 80

ml of distilled water and add distilled water to bring the solution to 100 ml. Determine the pH of the solution; it should be between 8.9 and 9.1.

3. For rabbit liver powder, remove omentum and gallbladders from fresh rabbit livers and homogenize the livers in a blender. Wash 1 volume of homogenized liver in 4 volumes of acetone by stirring briefly and allowing the liver to settle. Decant the supernatant fluid and repeat the washing twice more. Then collect the acetone-treated liver on a filter paper in a Buchner funnel and dry the liver with suction until most of the acetone has evaporated. Break up the cake of liver that has formed on the filter paper and dry overnight at 37°C with adequate ventilation. Finally, homogenize the dried liver to a powder in a blender.

Application to Diagnosis
Processing Specimens for Examination

In most instances, specimens are fixed before they are reacted with FA. Depending on the antigen involved, acetone, methanol, ethanol, Formalin, and heat have been used with variable degrees of success. Some fixatives destroy or diminish the reactivity of some antigens. Consequently, the kind of fixative as well as the time and temperature of fixation most suitable for a particular antigen must be selected from previous experience or by trial.

The following is an outline of steps involved in processing a specimen for examination by fluorescent microscopy. In general, the sequence applies equally for specimens containing bacterial, viral, or other antigens. A cell culture monolayer is used here as a sample specimen in order to emphasize several points on the handling of coverslips. For brevity, the direct staining procedure is presented.

Remove one corner of the coverslip for identification of the "cell side" during processing. Corners can be removed before coverslips are unpackaged by grinding with an emery disc backed by a stainless steel disc attached to a small hand drill. The slips are always oriented in Leighton tubes in the same way, so that with the removed corner to the upper left or lower right, the cell surface is uppermost.

For working with only a few specimens, a satisfactory combination of staining rack and humid chamber is provided by a covered petri dish with a damp filter paper over the bottom of the dish. Two swab sticks will support coverslips or microscope slides above the damp filter paper.

A staining rack with a greater capacity can be made inexpensively from a $1 \times 6 \times 45$ cm board and two pieces of plastic tubing 3 mm in diameter and about 48 cm long. When the rack is used for coverslips, apply a *very thin* coating of silicone grease to the tubing so that the light coverslips will adhere to the tubing and not move about while FA is spread over their surface. A $5 \times 30 \times 50$ cm stainless steel pan will provide a humid chamber to accommodate four staining racks. Keep a shallow layer of water in the bottom of the pan, and hold the racks above the water with rubber mesh. A glass cover resting on weather stripping around the lip of the pan will maintain the humid atmosphere.

Types of Staining Procedures

Besides direct staining of antigen there are several variations by which fluorescent antibody may be used as a diagnostic test. The choice depends mainly on whether antigen or antibody is to be identified and on the required sensitivity of the test. Similar controls apply to all procedures. Omission of a reactant or substitution of a homologous with a heterologous reactant will preclude a positive test result.

Direct staining. This method involves the fewest reactants and is completed in a single step: antigen + labeled antibody = labeled complex. It thus provides the least chance for nonspecific reactions. For these reasons, it is the procedure most frequently used for identification of antigen. Antibody also may be identified by direct staining by labeling serum of unknown antibody content and then reacting it with known antigen; however, other staining procedures are better suited for this purpose. The procedure for identification of antigen is as follows: (1) Apply a thin layer of labeled antibody over the prepared specimen. (2) Incubate for 30 minutes at 37°C in a humid chamber. (3) Rinse the specimen for 5 minutes in PBS and then briefly in distilled water, and then allow it to air dry. (4) Mount the specimen in PBS-glycerol and examine by fluorescent microscopy. Specific fluorescence indicates the presence of the antigen in question.

Inhibition of staining. This method allows for the rapid identification of antibody.[9] It is based on blocking the reactive sites of antigen to labeled antibody by prior or concomitant exposure of antigen to unlabeled antibody. Perhaps the most effective procedure to demonstrate inhibition is to mix labeled and unlabeled antibody and then apply the mixture to antigen: antigen + unlabeled antibody + labeled antibody = partially labeled complex.[23] The number of labeled antibody molecules that attach to antigen (and thus the intensity of fluorescence) depends on the relative concentrations of labeled and unlabeled antibody. Because the identification of antibody by this procedure is made by a percentage reduction of intensity of fluorescence, it is important that normal serum as well as known unlabeled antibody are mixed with labeled antibody to provide negative and positive controls for comparison with the serum in question. The procedure for identification of antibody is as follows: (1) Mix labeled antibody with normal serum, antiserum, and the serum in question. Apply a thin layer of each of these mixtures over prepared specimens that contain the homologous antigen. (2) Incubate for 30 minutes at 37°C in a humid chamber. (3) Rinse the specimen for 5 minutes in PBS and then briefly in distilled water, and then allow it to air dry. (4) Mount the specimen in PBS-glycerol and examine by fluorescent microscopy. The inhibition of fluorescence by the serum in question (i.e., more than with normal serum) indicates the presence of antibody.

Indirect staining. This is a two-step procedure. In the first step (primary reaction) unlabeled antibody is reacted with its homologous antigen: antigen + unlabeled antibody = unlabeled complex. In the second step (secondary reaction) the unlabeled antibody of the first step serves as antigen and is reacted with its labeled homologous antibody (labeled antiglobulin): unlabeled complex + labeled antiglobulin = labeled complex. Indirect staining allows for the identification of either antibody or antigen by using either known antigen or known antibody, respectively, in the primary reaction. Because of the layering of unlabeled antibody around antigen in the primary reaction, indirect staining provides an increased number of reactive sites for the subsequent attachment of labeled antibody. Consequently, it is more effective than direct staining for identifying small amounts of antigen. In the secondary reaction, a labeled antispecies globulin can be used for all primary reactions involving antibody from that species. In effect, the latter also applies to complement staining,[11] which is similar to indirect staining in that it is a two-step procedure allowing for the identification of either antigen or antibody. Complement staining differs from indirect staining in that complement is included as one of the reactants in the primary reaction, and labeled anticomplement is used in the secondary reaction to identify the antigen-antibody complex.

The test procedure for identification of either antigen or antibody is as follows: (1) Except for steps 1a and 1b, the general procedure is the same. (a) For identification of antigen, apply a thin layer of unlabeled antibody over the prepared specimen of unknown antigen content. (b) For identification of antibody, apply a thin layer of serum of unknown antibody content over a prepared specimen known to contain the antigen. (2) Incubate for 30 minutes at 37°C in a humid chamber. (3) Rinse the specimen for 5 minutes in PBS and then drain or carefully blot excess moisture from the surface of the specimen. (4) Apply a thin layer of labeled antiglobulin (prepared for globulin of the species from which the antibody [1a] or serum [1b] was obtained) over the specimen. (5) Incubate for 30 minutes at 37°C in a humid chamber. (6) Rinse the specimen for 5 minutes in PBS and then briefly in distilled water and then allow it to air dry. (7) Mount the specimen in PBS-glycerol and examine by fluorescent microscopy. Specific fluorescence indicates the presence of the antigen (1a) or antibody (1b) in question.

Agar (Gel) Diffusion Test

The various AD techniques are especially useful for qualitative analysis of antigen-antibody systems. The techniques are dependent on the use of a medium that prevents convection currents but allows diffusion of antigens and antibodies in aqueous solution. They are, of course, based on the phenomenon of precipitation, which limits their application to antibody populations that participate in aggregative reactions. Also, reactants must be present in sufficient amount to form visible lines of precipitation.

Several substances can be used as the medium in this test, including agar, pectin, cellulose acetate, and acrylamide gels. Washed and purified agar is the most commonly used medium (e.g. Ionagar, from Consolidated Lab., Chicago; Noble Agar, from Difco Lab., Detroit; and Agarose, from Mann Research Lab., New York).

As the agar forms a gel, it produces a meshlike structure with an average pore size that regulates the rate of molecular diffusion. Pore size is inversely proportionate to gel concentration. The agar concentration commonly varies from 0.3% in Oudin tubes for single diffusion studies to 0.7–1.5% in Ouchterlony plates for double diffusion. The liquid phase usually contains an electrolyte such as physiological saline or a suitable buffer. When chicken antibodies are used in the analysis, 10% NaCl solution is recommended. A neutral or somewhat alkaline pH is desirable although results may be obtained between pH 6 and 9. A preservative such as 1:10,000 Merthiolate is commonly incorporated in the gel. To avoid artifacts, tests should be incubated in a humid atmosphere not subject to abrupt changes in temperature.

The techniques of immunodiffusion comprise methods of simple diffusion and double diffusion. The Oudin tube method exemplifies simple diffusion in one dimension. Simple diffusion has not been used extensively in microbiological research, however, and will not be dealt with here.[7,8,26]

Double Diffusion Technique

The techniques of double diffusion have wide application in veterinary microbiology. The multiple-cup plate technique of Ouchterlony illustrates the phenomenon of double diffusion and will be described below.[8,25] Immunoelectrophoresis is another technique of great value that makes use of double diffusion. Antigens are first separated by electrophoresis, then double diffusion in gels produces the delineation of antigen-antibody systems as arcs of precipitation.

The Ouchterlony procedure is commonly performed in dishes that are approximately 55 mm in diameter or as a micromethod using conventional microscope slides. In either case, the glass surface is first coated with a thin layer of agar (0.1%), which is allowed to dry. Then approximately 6–8 ml of 1% melted agar is added to the Ouchterlony plate or 2 ml of agar is added to the surface of the microscope slide. If plastic dishes are used, the first step of coating the surface with agar is not necessary.[7] In either case, cutting dies are used to prepare wells in the agar after it has gelled. The dies are available from several commercial suppliers (Gelman Instrument Co., Ann Arbor, Mich.; Consolidated Lab., Chicago) and are arranged in patterns depending upon the purpose. After the wells have been punched with the cutting dies the core of agar is removed by gentle suction, using a cannula attached by tubing to a water faucet vacuum source.

When antigen and antibody reagents are added to the wells, the processes of diffusion begin immediately. Both antigen and antibody migrate toward a common reaction area before they begin to precipitate. Usually the balance between the two reactants is not exact but moderate differences are compensated for as they meet. A steep gradient of each reactant tends to form on either side of the precipitation zone. The initially stronger reactant forces its way across the developing precipitate and thus dilutes itself and encounters rapidly increasing quantities of the opposite reactant. As a result, the zone of precipitation shifts slightly toward the weaker reactant and then becomes stabilized. Hence, double diffusion systems tend to adjust themselves to balanced conditions. Diffusion may be considered the tendency for a substance to spread uniformly through the space available to it. The net movement of a species of molecules will be from an area of high concentration to one of lower concentration. The rate at which a substance diffuses increases with its initial concentration, with an increase in temperature, and with a decrease in the molecular weight. The reverse conditions would, of course, decrease the rate of diffusion. These factors come into play and are in great part responsible for the position and shape of arcs as they occur in the reaction area.

A commonly performed test is the comparison of two or more antigens with respect to a reference antiserum. Interpretation of the results requires that investigators exercise caution and use their knowledge of the precipitation phenomenon.

References

1. Aalund, O., J.W. Osebold, and F.A. Murphy. Isolation and characterization of ovine gamma globulins. *Arch. Biochem. Biophys.* 109:142–149, 1965.
2. Bordet, J. Les leucocytes et les propriétés actives du serum chez les vaccines. *Ann. Inst. Pasteur* 9:462–506, 1895.
3. Brown, F., and J. Crick. Application of agar-gel diffusion analysis to a study of the antigenic structure of inactivated vaccines prepared from the virus of foot-and-mouth disease. *J. Immunol.* 82:444–447, 1959.
4. Cherry, W.B., M. Goldman, T.R. Carski, and M.D. Moody. *Fluorescent Antibody Techniques in the Diagnosis of Communicable Diseases.* Public Health Service Pub. no. 729. U.S. Gov. Printing Office, Washington, 1961.
5. Communicable Disease Center. *Serologic Tests for Syphilis.* Public Health Service (HEW), 1959.
6. Cottral, G.E. Foot-and-mouth disease virus neutralization test cross reactions. *Bull. Off. Internat. Epiz.* 77(7–8):1239–1261, 1972.
7. Cowan, K.M. Immunochemical studies of FMD. IV. Preparation and evaluation of antisera specific for virus, virus protein sub-unit, and the virus-infection-associated-antigen. *J. Immunol.* 101:1183–1191, 1968.
8. Crowle, A.J. *Immunodiffusion.* Academic Press, New York, 1961.
9. Gard, S. Immunological strain specificity within type 1 poliovirus. *Bull. WHO* 22:235–242, 1960.
10. Goldman, M. Staining *Toxoplasma gondii* with fluorescein-labeled antibody. II. A new serologic test for antibodies to *Toxoplasma* based upon inhibition of specific staining. *J. Exp. Med.* 105:557–573, 1957.
11. Goldwasser, R.A., and C.C. Shepard. Staining of complement and modification of fluorescent antibody procedures. *J. Immunol.* 80:122–131, 1958.
12. Gordon, M.A., M.R. Edwards, and V.N. Tompkins. Refinement of fluorescent antibody by gel filtration. *Proc. Soc. Exp. Biol. Med.* 109:96–99, 1962.
13. Hirst, G.K. The agglutination of red cells by allantoic fluid of chick embryos infected with influenza virus. *Science* 94:22–23, 1941.
14. Kärber, G. Beitrage zur kollectiven behandlung pharmakologischer reihenversuche. *Arch. Exp. Path. Pharm.* 162:480–483, 1931.
15. Kaufman, L., and W.B. Cherry. Technical factors affecting the preparation of fluorescent antibody reagents. *J. Immunol.* 87:72–79, 1961.
16. Kolmer, J.A., E.H. Spaulding, and H.W. Robinson. *Approved Laboratory Technique.* 5th ed. Appleton-Century-Crofts, New York, 1951.
17. Kwapinski, J.B. *Methods of Serological Research.* Wiley, New York, 1965.
18. Lennette, E.H., and N.J. Schmidt. *Diagnostic Procedures for Viral and Rickettsial Diseases.* 3d ed. American Public Health Association, New York, 1964.
19. Lewis, V.J., W.L. Jones, J.B. Brooks, and W.B. Cherry. Technical considerations in the preparation of fluorescent-antibody conjugates. *Appl. Microbiol.* 12:343–348, 1964.
20. Litchfield, J.T., Jr., and F. Wilcoxon. A simplified method of evaluating dose-effect experiments. *J. Pharm. Exp. Ther.* 96:99–113, 1949.
21. McDevitt, H.O., J.H. Peters, L.W. Pollard, J.G. Harter, and A.H. Coons. Purification and analysis of fluorescein-labeled antisera by column chromatograph. *J. Immunol.* 90:634–642, 1963.
22. Miller, L.C., and M.L. Tainter. Estimation of the ED_{50} and its error by means of logarithmic-probit graph paper. *Proc. Soc. Exp. Biol. Med.* 57:261–264, 1944.
23. Moody, M.D., M. Goldman, and B.M. Thomason. Staining bacterial smears with fluorescent antibodies. I. General methods for *Malleomyces pseudomallei. J. Bact.* 72:357–361, 1956.
24. Nairn, R.C. *Fluorescent Protein Tracing.* E. & S. Livingstone, Edinburgh, London, 1962.
25. Ouchterlony, O. Gel-diffusion techniques. In *Immunological Methods,* J.F. Ackroyd (ed.), pp. 55–78. Davis, Philadelphia, 1964.
26. Oudin, J. Specific precipitation in gels and its application to immunochemical analysis. *Meth. Med. Res.* 5:335–378, 1952.
27. Philipson, L., and P.W. Choppin. On the role of virus sulfhydrl groups in the attachment of enteroviruses to erythrocytes. *J. Exp. Med.* 112:455–478, 1960.
28. Reed, L.J., and H. Muench. A simple method of estimating fifty per cent endpoints. *Am. J. Hyg.* 27:493–497, 1938.
29. Rosen, L. Hemagglutination. In *Techniques in Experimental Virology,* R.I.C. Harris (ed.), pp. 257–276. Academic Press, London, 1964.
30. Sever, J.L. Application of a microtechnique to viral serological investigations. *J. Immunol.* 88:320–329, 1962.

31. Spearman, C. The method of right and wrong cases (constant stimuli) without Gauss' Formulae. *Brit. J. Psychol.* 2:227–242, 1908.
32. U.S. Dept. of Health, Education, and Welfare, Public Health Service. *Diagnostic Complement Fixation Method (LBCF)*. CDC Laboratory Branch Training Manual, 1962.
33. U.S. Dept. of Health, Education, and Welfare, Public Health Service. *Standardized Diagnostic Complement Fixation Method and Adaptation to Micro-Test*. Monograph no. 74. U.S. Government Printing Office, Washington, 1965.
34. Vogel, J., and A. Shelokov. Adsorption-hemagglutination test for influenza virus in monkey kidney tissue culture. *Science* 126:358–359, 1957.
35. Wallace, A.L., A.G. Olser, and M.M. Moyer. Quantitative studies of complement fixation. V. Estimation of complement fixing potency of immune sera and its relation to antibody-nitrogen content. *J. Immunol.* 65:661–673, 1950.

6. Preservation and Inactivation of Microorganisms

Preservation of Microorganisms

Because of the diverse characteristics of microorganisms, no blanket rules apply to their preservation. In general, two methods are employed: (1) lowering the storage temperature by either refrigeration or freezing, or (2) dehydration by lyophilization or other means. Regardless of the method selected, inclusion of various substances in the suspending medium enhances retention of viability. Useful substances include proteinaceous materials such as serum, skim milk, and gelatin; protein digests of casein, gelatin, and meat; colloids such as dextran or polyvinylpyrrolidone; sugars such as sucrose and lactose; and polyhydric alcohols such as glycerol, sorbitol, and mannitol. The suspending medium is usually buffered with phosphate but citrate buffers may be useful in some instances. The chloride ion is harmful to many viruses but may be used with most bacteria and fungi.

Preservation of Bacteria and Fungi

The method employed will be determined by the characteristics of the organism and the length of time storage is desired. The least complicated procedure should be tried first. For prolonged storage, lyophilization is usually most effective but some organisms will not withstand freezing.

CAUTION: *Organisms are readily aerosolized during lyophilization;* hence closed ventilating hoods should be used on lyophilization apparatus and other safety precautions should be observed. *Histoplasma capsulatum* and *Coccidioides immitis* are particularly hazardous to personnel and should be lyophilized only if extreme precautions are exercised.

Preservation by Refrigeration

1. *Storage in distilled water*. Suspensions of mature colonies of pathogenic fungi stored in sterile distilled water at room temperature or in the refrigerator will remain viable for months.

2. *Storage under oil*. When growth is established on an agar slant by streaking or stab inoculation, sterile neutral white-paraffin oil is added to completely cover the agar.

Storage may be at room temperature or in a refrigerator. This procedure is useful for 1 year or less. It is advisable to use the same medium for recovery as that used to grow the organism prior to storage.

Preservation by Freezing

1. *Freezing on agar slant.* Cultures of fungi on agar slants may be held for long periods at $-20°C$. If the cap is slightly loose the culture will dry slowly. Actinomycetes have remained viable under these conditions for more than 10 years. Some of the Phycomycetes (*Mucor, Rhizopus, Absidia*) do not survive well under these conditions, and *Histoplasma capsulatum* in the yeast phase will not survive freezing.

2. *Freezing in suspension.* Bacteria and fungi may be preserved for long periods when frozen in suspension. (a) *Suspending medium.* There is no medium that is best for all organisms. Many will survive well in a tryptose-phosphate broth. Survival is prolonged for others in 5% sucrose or lactose with or without 5% gelatin. Skim milk is excellent for some fungi and bacteria. Serum 5–40% is helpful for many bacteria. In any case the pH should approximate 7 and phosphate or citrate may be used as buffer. (b) *Freezing.* Many organisms will withstand rapid freezing in dry ice and alcohol. Others are more fastidious and require slow freezing (1–5°C per minute). Some type of protective substance such as serum, sorbitol, protein digests, or combinations of these substances may prove useful. (c) *Holding temperature.* Temperature should be -10 to $-20°C$ in freezers, -70 to $-80°C$ in mechanical or dry ice freezers, and -170 to $-196°C$ in liquid nitrogen or liquid nitrogen vapor containers. Usually the coldest temperature provides the best preservation, but some organisms, actinomycetes for example, have remained viable at $-20°C$ for more than 10 years. (d) *Containers.* Rubber-stoppered or screw-capped vials or bottles are satisfactory for mechanical refrigeration. Glass-sealed ampules should be used for liquid nitrogen or dry ice. A mechanical seal is unreliable for liquid nitrogen; it will allow the refrigerant to enter and will result in a violent explosion when warmed. Even glass-sealed ampules must be shielded when warmed in order to guard against explosions caused by an imperfect seal. (e) *Recovery.* Rapid thawing in a water bath at 37–40°C is advisable. Many organisms lose viability during thawing and it is best to thaw them as rapidly as possible.

Preservation by Lyophilization

1. A mature culture (approaching the stationary phase of growth) is more likely to withstand freezing and drying. However, some organisms, such as those of pertussis, may be lyophilized successfully as an actively growing 18-hour culture.

2. The suspending media and methods of freezing are those described under the heading "Preservation by Freezing."

3. Lyophilization is accomplished under high vacuum. The final pressure should be 10 μm Hg or less although early in the cycle pressure it may climb to 50 μm Hg. The condenser should be kept as cold as possible ($-80°C$ or less); equipment providing the shortest mean free path will perform most efficiently. Drying time depends upon the size and shape of container, thickness of ice layer, nature of suspending medium, and amount of heat applied to the drying sample.

4. In breaking vacuum, dry nitrogen is most satisfactory. However, ampules or vials sealed under vacuum provide a means for determining if the seal is perfect. The amount of residual moisture that provides best stability is unknown for most organisms and is related to the suspending medium. Sorbitol or glycerol will retain moisture and the dried product will be stable with 1% or less. Some products will be less stable with 0.1% moisture than with 0.3%.

5. Storage of dried material at room temperature has been satisfactory for some products but as a rule survival is best prolonged by lower temperatures.

Preservation of Fastidious Organisms

Organisms such as *Leptospira* do not readily withstand freezing. However, viability has been maintained by slow freezing of blood from infected animals. In addition, cotton gauze soaked with infected blood or infected culture medium has been dried successfully at room temperature without freezing. The precautions employed in freezing mammalian cells should also be applied to fastidious organisms.

Preservation of Viruses

The principles observed for bacteria and fungi in general apply also for viruses. Most viruses withstand freezing, and while many retain full infectivity for long periods when held at -10 to $-20°C$, others are more stable at lower temperatures such as $-80°C$ (dry ice) or -170 to $-196°C$ (liquid nitrogen vapor or liquid).

Preservation by Refrigeration

While refrigeration (4–10°C) is ordinarily employed only for short periods, certain viruses may survive for long periods. Myxomatosis virus–infected tissues and arboviruses such as bluetongue virus are examples. The addition of various chemicals will enhance virus survival.

1. Glycerol 40–50% is a viral preservative and also an inhibitor of bacterial growth. It is commonly used to preserve specimens collected in the field under circumstances where refrigeration is not possible.

2. Mannitol or sorbitol 10%, with 1% sodium glutamate, works well with some myxoviruses. Viruses are usually most stable near pH 7 and thus a buffered medium is recommended.

3. Crystal violet 0.25–0.5% has been used for some viruses even though it is also used to inactivate hog cholera virus.

Preservation by Freezing

1. *Containers*. (a) Rubber-stoppered or screw-capped vials may be used. (b) Heat-sealed glass ampules are recommended for all occasions, are essential for liquid nitrogen, and are the safest for dry ice.

CAUTION: When thawing, protect against explosion of ampules that have been stored in liquid nitrogen.

2. *Suspending media components*. (a) *Proteins*. Serum 5–20% or gelatin 1–5% may be used (skim milk is useful for some *Rickettsia*). (b) *Colloids*. Dextran 5% or polyvi-

nylpyrrolidone 5–15% are recommended. (c) *Protein digests*. Peptone to 5%, NZ (enzymatic) amine to 5%, or lactalbumin hydrolysate to 5% are all good. (d) *Polyhydric alcohols* (moisture stabilizers). Glycerol 1–20%, sorbitol to 10%, and mannitol 5–10% may be used. (e) *Buffers*. Phosphate or citrate 0.02–0.1 m are recommended. (f) *Sugars*. Sucrose 5–10% or lactose 5–10% may be used, but avoid other reducing sugars such as glucose. (g) *Carbonyl group neutralizers*. Protein digests or sodium glutamate 0.5–1% are sometimes used. The medium will usually consist of a buffer along with one or two of the above components such as a protein digest and/or a polyhydric alcohol.

3. *Freezing*. Rapid freezing is usually most effective. A dry ice–alcohol or acetone bath is most convenient. Liquid nitrogen or liquid air are useful if means are provided for dissipating the layer of gas that is volatilized around the container and acts as an insulator. For some fastidious viruses, for example those strongly cell associated, a controlled rate of freezing will retain more viable virus. For these viruses, rapid thawing is also advisable. For other viruses the thawing rate is not so critical.

Preservation by Lyophilization

Because storage temperature is not so critical, freeze-drying of viruses is a means of storing them economically for long periods. The process is the same as described for bacteria and fungi. The media used are similar to those used for freezing. However, no more than 1–2% glycerol should be used, and sorbitol up to 5% is preferred. Some viruses such as polio are not readily lyophilized. They can be dried successfully from the wet, unfrozen state or they may be lyophilized if most of the inorganic salts are removed from the medium.

Inactivation of Microorganisms

Inactivation is defined as rendering an organism incapable of reproduction. The method employed will depend upon the site of the organism and the purpose of the inactivation.

Physical Procedures
Heat

1. *Incineration*. Animal carcasses and excreta, and disposable and broken glass and plastic laboratory ware, as well as air entering and leaving infectious areas, may be sterilized by incineration. However, to avoid the escape of contaminated aerosols, all gases leaving the incinerators must be heated to at least 730°C. Therefore, the laboratory should provide adequate air supply and provide a secondary combustion chamber heated to greater than 730°C.

2. *Dry heat oven*. This procedure may be used for noncombustible materials that can withstand 170°C for extended periods. The method of packaging, loading of the oven, and heat conductivity of the material all influence the effectiveness of the treatment. A recording thermometer or other monitoring device should be placed in the center of the load. Two to four hours at 160–170°C from the time this temperature is reached should suffice. Disadvantages are poor control of hot-air flow and dependence upon thermoconductivity of material being sterilized.

3. *Boiling in water.* Small instruments and equipment can usually be sterilized by boiling for 15–20 minutes. However, certain soil bacilli have not been inactivated by more than 20 hours of boiling. Since temperature is dependent upon atmospheric pressure, the temperature should approach 100°C.

4. *Pasteurization.* Virulent mycobacteria and *Brucella abortus* are inactivated by heating to 60°C for 30 minutes or to 70°C for 2–3 minutes. The procedure has been effective in destroying these infectious agents in milk without seriously affecting flavor or nutritive quality.

5. *Arnold sterilization.* Materials such as mucin and some bacterial media will not withstand the high temperature of an autoclave. These materials have been sterilized by heating in the Arnold sterilizer (live steam) for 30 minutes on 3 successive days.

6. *Autoclaving.* Because saturated steam under pressure conducts heat readily, this is the most dependable means of sterilization. As with the dry heat chamber, the load must be arranged to allow for penetration of steam to all parts. The most effective steam penetration will result if the air is evacuated before steam is admitted. Steam under 15 lb/sq in (103.35 kPa) pressure will result in a temperature of about 121°C. Thirty to forty-five minutes at this pressure and temperature is sufficient for most materials. One drawback to this method is that materials toxic to cells may be volatilized and deposited on glassware and equipment. These toxic materials may come from "dirty steam," paper wrapping, untreated cotton, or even the plastic marking that is now sometimes used on glassware in place of etching.

7. *Selective inactivation.* Some heat-sensitive microorganisms may be inactivated with minimum denaturation of their antigenic proteins. Certain ions such as Ca^{++} and Mg^{++} may affect inactivation rates. However, with viruses, the heat stability of the nucleic acids (the reproductive component) tends to be greater than that of the antigen-containing protein coat. Heat is therefore mostly employed in combination with other inactivants in order to speed reactions rather than as an inactivant itself when minimum denaturation of antigens is required.

Radiation

1. *Ultraviolet radiation.* Ultraviolet (UV) radiation (nonionizing) has been shown to be an inactivant for various viruses and bacteria, and it has a minimum denaturing action on their antigenic proteins. Because ultraviolet is so readily absorbed, however, its degree of penetration into a suspension of microorganisms cannot be controlled with precision. Direct exposure of a thin film of the suspension to UV is most effective. UV has been used in various situations as a space decontaminant. It is effective only if the source is emitting the expected amount of radiation and if it is a short distance (60–90 cm) from the surface to be sterilized. Air circulation must be minimal and UV output must be checked frequently. For air sterilization by UV, the air must be free of particulate matter and circulate close to the UV source.

2. *Photodynamic inactivation (photosensitization).* Microorganisms stained with dyes such as methylene blue, toluidine blue, acridine orange, eosin, neutral red, or acriflavine will be inactivated in the presence of oxygen when exposed to visible light. How-

ever, the process is difficult to control and has not been useful in preparing inactivated vaccines.

3. *Ionizing radiation.* Gamma rays are high energy emissions from certain radioactive isotopes such as cobalt-60. They have excellent penetrability and permit sterilization in glass or metal containers even in the frozen state. Serum for tissue culture has been sterilized in this manner and many microorganisms have been effectively inactivated without loss of antigencity. X rays have good penetration but are not readily absorbed and thus have limited value. Beta rays inactivate microorganisms but they show variable ionization efficiencies at different depths of the matter irradiated and thus are impossible to precisely control.

Other Physical Methods

1. *Ultrasonic waves.* Many bacteria and fungi are readily disrupted by ultrasonic waves. Viruses as a group are resistant to sonification but some with rodlike structures and some bacteriophages can be disrupted. The procedure has been most useful in research or in procedures for preparations of cell components.

2. *Pressure.* Sudden release of high atmospheric pressure or changes in osmotic pressure have not effectively inactivated viruses, but some bacteria have been disrupted by this means.

Chemical Procedures
Liquid Decontaminants and Inactivants

In order to enhance their penetration, some germicidal solutions contain surface-active agents. Temperature, pH, and amount of organic matter affect germicidal action.

1. *Oxidizing agents.* Chlorine, iodine, and hypochlorite are effective inactivants of microorganisms. Iodine in 70% alcohol in a proportion of 2:100 has proved to be very effective. Hydrogen peroxide and potassium permanganate are less effective in the presence of protein. While the halogens are very effective, they are corrosive to metals.

2. *Acids, alkalies, aldehydes.* (a) *Peracetic acid.* This has been used effectively in maintenance of gnotobiotic animals. A 2% solution with a surfactant effectively sterilizes plastics but is corrosive to metals. It evaporates more readily at 25°C or higher. The vapors are highly irritating. (b) *Other acids and alkalies.* Hydrochloric, nitric, sulfuric, citric, and boric acids have been used for particular conditions. Alkalies for the most part are not very effective decontaminants, although sodium hydroxide (2% solution), quick lime, and soda ash may be useful under certain conditions, particularly for foot-and-mouth disease virus. (c) *Formaldehyde.* Formaldehyde solution U.S.P. (also known as Formalin) is of great practical importance in the preparation of toxoids, bacterins, and inactivated virus vaccines. With some of the clostridia, apparent inactivation is reversible when there is suffient protein to gradually react with all of the formaldehyde. Reversal does not occur when there is free formaldehyde present. The same phenomenon may occur with some toxoids. While formaldehyde combines with amino groups, denaturation of antigenic proteins does not occur when the concentration of formaldehyde is low. An apparent exception is rabies virus, in which formaldehyde destroys antigenicity. As a

space decontaminant, formaldehyde is effective and has had wide use. However, a white film of polymerized formaldehyde is difficult to remove and is particularly noticeable on stainless steel. Formaldehyde gas can be generated by mixing 1.2 ml of formaldehyde solution U.S.P with 0.6 g of potassium permanganate per cubic foot (0.028 cu m) of space to be disinfected, or by heating in an electric frying pan 0.3 g of paraformaldehyde per cubic foot. (An electric pan can be turned on remotely and is therefore safer.)

3. *Alkylating agents.* (a) *Nitrogen and sulfur mustards.* These will inactivate viruses and bacteria. However, they are strong vesicants and their effectiveness is reduced by organic materials, with which they combine readily. They are not recommended. (b) *Ethylene oxide.* In liquid form ethylene oxide is an excellent sterilizing substance, and as a 1% solution in water it inactivates various viruses and bacteria with good retention of antigenicity. it combines readily with chloride ions to form ethylene chlorhydrin and thus makes the suspension alkaline, although adjustment of the pH is necessary if the medium contains sodium chloride. It hydrolyzes fairly rapidly, and because of its low boiling point (10.7°C), excess can be removed readily under reduced pressure. Ethylene oxide as a gas has been used extensively for sterilization of equipment and materials that are heat sensitive. Because it is explosive in the presence of oxygen, it is mixed with carbon dioxide as a 10% ethylene oxide–90% CO_2 mixture, or with Freon. Material being sterilized must be arranged to allow contact with the gas, and air must be evacuated as well. Sterilization is accomplished most readily in the presence of some moisture (30–40% humidity) and preferably at a temperature of 25°C or higher (56°C is commonly used). Exposure for 3–6 hours allows sufficient time for the gas to penetrate most materials if the chamber has been properly loaded. (c) *Beta-propiolactone.* Bacterial and viral suspensions are quickly inactivated by 0.2–0.5% beta-propiolactone (BPL) with retention of antigenicity. The optimum concentration varies with the amount of protein in the suspension. BPL hydrolyzes quickly (half-life 30 minutes at 37°C or 24 hours at 4°C) and the hydrolytic product (beta-hydroxy-propionic acid) is a natural by-product of fat metabolism. BPL has been used for sterilization of areas that cannot be steam-sterilized and where toxic residues cannot be tolerated, such as vacuum chambers used for lyophilization. As a concentrate it is irritating to skin and may be carcinogenic.

4. *Quaternary ammonia compounds.* Various ammonia compounds have been used as germicides but they are not highly effective against either viruses or bacteria, although they have low toxicity. They are most effective in combination with other agents; being surface active they assist in promoting contact between other active materials and microorganisms.

5. *Organic solvents.* (a) *Ethyl-ether.* Ether will inactivate viruses or bacteria that contain lipids as an integral part of the cell wall or virus coat. It is used as a research tool principally. (b) *Alcohol (ethanol, methanol, propinol).* These alcohols are mild germicides at room or body temperature. They are useful as solvents for iodine. (c) *Acetone.* Acetone has been used as an inactivating agent in preparing some bacterial vaccines such as typhoid. (d) *Chloroform.* The action of chloroform is similar to that of ethyl-ether but chloroform is more effective than ether on some viruses.

6. *Phenol.* Dating back to Lister (1867), phenol and numerous phenolic compounds have been used for decontamination and disinfection. Phenol is used in numerous paren-

teral biologic products to maintain sterility. For many years it was the only inactivating agent used in preparing rabies vaccine (Semple vaccine). At a concentration of 0.5%, it slowly inactivates (as long as 1 week at room temperature) rabies virus in suspensions of rabies-infected brain. Antigenicity of the virus is retained in the presence of 0.2–0.3% phenol for periods of a year or more at 4°C. Phenol has also been used to extract nucleic acid from plant and mammalian viruses.

7. *Mercury salts*. Mercury bichloride is an effective germicide. A 1.7% solution will inactivate anthrax spores in a few minutes. Phenyl mercuric borate, acetate, and nitrate along with thimerosal are used as germicides for surfaces, and at concentrations of 1:10,000 are used in vaccines as bactericides or inhibitors. They are not effective at this concentration in serum or other high-protein products. Thimerosal has been used to inactivate *Leptospira* for vaccines.

8. *Other chemicals*. Many other chemicals have been used, including arsenicals, resorcinols, chaulmoogra oil, some alkaloids, salts of fatty acids, saponin, bile acids, and sodium lauryl sulfate.

Biologic Procedures

Specific antibody is an effective inactivant of viruses, bacteria, and toxins. Antivenoms, antitoxins, and various antisera are also used extensively. Combinations of antiserum and bacteria or toxins have been used effectively for immunization. Simultaneous administration of antiserum and virus as was used for many years with hog cholera is an example. In vitro inactivation with antibody may be reversible if excess antibody has not been used. Dilution, incubation at low pH or with 0.1 M buffer, or addition of fluorocarbons followed by homogenization and centrifugation promotes dissociation of the antigen-antibody complex.

Bacteriophages destroy bacteria for which they are specific.

Nonspecific Inhibitors

A number of soluble host materials normally present in the body are capable of inhibiting microorganism activity. Mucoproteins, glycoproteins, or mucopolysaccharides may inhibit activity of viruses, possibly by covering the combining sites on the viral protein coat. A lipoprotein from susceptible cells reduces the infectivity of polio virus. Lecithinlike lipids in serum reduce or inhibit the infectivity of some myxoviruses and the psittacosis agent. Interferons—proteins produced by cells in response to various types of stimulation—act on susceptible cells in some undetermined manner to render them nonsusceptible to infection by a number of viruses. All these nonspecific inhibitors are found in normal animals, but with present knowledge their use is limited to experimental procedures.

7. Biochemical, Biophysical, and Histochemical Tests

During the last two decades many biochemical, biophysical, and histochemical characteristics of animal viruses have been discovered. This chapter will describe several methods that are used to broadly delineate different types of viral agents. The laboratory tests outlined below can be routinely employed to evaluate the following criteria: type of viral nucleic acid, possession of essential lipids, susceptibility to physical and chemical agents (heat and pH), particle size, and morphology.

Nucleic Acid Determination
Indirect Methods
Metabolic Inhibitors[9,13]

Metabolic inhibitors such as the halogenated nucleosides (5-bromo- and 5-fluoro-2'-deoxyuridine) are often used to differentiate between the types of nucleic acid (DNA or RNA) in animal viruses. Although 5-bromo-2'-deoxyuridine (BUDR) and 5-fluoro-2'-deoxyuridine (FUDR) inhibit the replication of DNA viruses, they have no effect on the multiplication of most RNA viruses. They do exert an inhibitory effect on the replication of RNA leukoviruses because early DNA synthesis is required for the replication of these viruses. Their effect is reversible by thymidine.

Several things have to be kept in mind when using metabolic inhibitors: first, the toxic level of BUDR or FUDR on a specific cell system must be predetermined to eliminate nonspecific inhibitory effects; second, dosage levels of inhibitors and thymidine may vary depending on the type of cell system and virus being tested; and third, adequate controls of known RNA and DNA viruses must be included with the test virus.

Materials. The test requires tubes of appropriate cell cultures for viral titration, growth medium deficient in thymidine, BUDR or FUDR, thymidine, a DNA virus (herpes simplex or adeno) and a RNA virus (polio or Coxsackie B-5), and the unknown virus.

Procedure. (1) Treat cell cultures with growth medium that is deficient in thymidine and contains 50 μg/ml of BUDR. (2) Decant the media from cultures after incubation at 37°C for 24 hours. Inoculate four cultures with each corresponding virus. Incubate the cultures at 37°C for 1 hour and remove the unadsorbed virus by washing each tube with

5 ml of phosphate buffer. Add 5 ml of growth medium with 20 μg/ml of thymidine per tube to half of the cultures and 5 ml of growth medium containing 50 μg/ml BUDR per tube to the other half of the cultures. Include another two tubes of infected but untreated cultures as controls. (3) Incubate cultures at 37°C and examine daily for CPE. When CPE becomes apparent in tubes with the growth medium containing thymidine (the time of which will depend on the type of virus), harvest both sets of cultures as well as the control cultures and titrate for viral infectivity.

Acridine Orange Staining [7,8]

Acridine orange staining of virus-infected cells gives rise to characteristic colors when the stain is observed under a microscope with UV light. Intracellular aggregates of RNA viruses stain flame-red while those of DNA viruses stain yellow-green.

Materials. This test requires normal and virus-infected cell cultures on a coverslip, acetic acid–ethanol (1:3) fixative, phosphate buffer pH 7, and 0.05% acridine orange solution with the pH adjusted to 1.5–3.5 by addition of 1 N HCl.

Procedure. (1) Fix normal and virus-infected cell cultures on coverslips with an acetic acid–ethanol (1:3) fixative at room temperature for 30 minutes. (2) Pour off the fixative and allow the coverslips to air dry before staining. Coverslips can be stained immediately or kept at 4°C for several days before staining. (3) Stain the coverslips with 0.05% acridine orange solution at room temperature for 30 minutes. Wash the coverslips twice with phosphate buffer before mounting them on slides with a drop of the phosphate buffer. The edges of the coverslips can be sealed with wax. (4) Examine the coverslips under the UV microscope.

Direct Method: Radioisotopic Labeling

Direct determination of the type of nucleic acid possessed by a virus requires that the virus suspension be sufficiently purified so that cellular nucleic acids do not interfere with interpretation of the experimental results.

The fact that RNA differs constitutionally from DNA, in that RNA incorporates uridine while DNA incorporates thymidine, affords a simple method to directly distinguish an RNA-containing virus from one containing DNA. Basically, the virus-synthesizing cell is incubated with radiosotopically labeled uridine or thymidine, and the virus synthesized during that period is analyzed for the presence of the isotopic marker.

Materials. The materials required are: cell cultures infected with the unknown virus, as well as others infected with a known virus suspected to be similar to the unknown agent; tritiated uridine (^{3}H-5-uridine, 20 Ci/μmol) and tritiated thymidine (^{3}H-thymidine, 20 Ci/μmol) in sterile water; perchloric acid (0.5%) in distilled water; ethanol (95%); chromatographic paper, size 3 MM Chr, 0.33 mm thick, 3 cm wide (Whatman, Clifton, N.J.); and PPO-POPOP scintillator in toluene (Beckman Instruments, Palo Alto, Calif.).

Procedure. (1) Incubate replicate cultures of cells infected with the known and unknown viruses as well as uninfected control cultures for 8 hours in the presence of ^{3}H-5-uridine or ^{3}H-thymidine, which should be added directly to the tissue culture medium to give a final concentration of 10 μCi/ml. (It is critical that viral nucleic acid synthesis be proceeding during this interval.) (2) Recover and purify the virus from the infected cells and/or from tissue culture fluids by suitable procedures. Treat uninfected control cell cultures in an identical manner. (3) Absorb a given volume (up to four drops) of virus and control cell suspensions into 9 cm strips of the Whatman chromatographic paper that have been marked with pencil designating the sample applied. (4) Place the papers in individual beakers and add 150 ml of cold (4°C) 0.5% perchloric acid. The papers need not be completely dry. Refrigerate the beakers for 30 minutes. (5) Discard the perchloric acid into the liquid radioactive waste container and add 30 ml of cold (4°C) 95% ethanol to the beaker. The ethanol is then discarded as was the perchloric acid. (6) To each beaker add 150 ml of cold (4°C) 95% ethanol and return the beaker to the refrigerator for at least 2 hours during which time the 150 ml of alcohol should be discarded and replaced with another volume of 150 ml of cold alcohol. (7) Discard the final alcohol wash and permit the chromatographic papers to dry. (8) Place the dried chromatographic paper strips into liquid scintillation vials to which is added sufficient scintillator fluid (PPO-POPOP in toluene) to cover the papers. If the papers show a color, it is caused by the perchloric acid that was not entirely removed during the ethanol washes. (9) Then close the vials and measure the radioactivity in a liquid scintillation counter.

Essential Lipid Determinations

Lipid solvents remove essential lipids from the nucleocapsid or outer envelope of viruses possessing such materials, thereby destroying the infectivity of these agents. Most animal viruses that have envelopes surrounding their nucleocapsids are sensitive to lipid solvents such as ether or chloroform.

Chloroform Sensitivity[4]

Materials. Reagent-grade chloroform, the virus to be tested, and appropriate cell cultures for the titration of the test virus are needed.

Procedure. (1) Mix chloroform with viral suspension to a concentration of 4.8% at 4°C for 10 minutes. (2) Centrifuge the mixture at $500 \times g$ for 5 minutes. (3) Remove the upper aqueous layer and titrate for viral infectivity. (4) Viral suspensions without chloroform treatment should be titrated as controls. Dilution factors for chloroform should be included in the calculation of viral titers. (5) A decrease in viral titer of 1.0 log or more in the treated sample suggests susceptibility to chloroform.

Ether Sensitivity[1]

Materials. Diethyl ether, reagent grade, the virus to be tested, and appropriate cell cultures for viral titration are required.

Procedure. (1) Mix 4 parts of viral suspension to 1 part of ether and incubate the mixture at 4°C for 24 hours. (2) Centrifuge the mixture at $1000 \times g$ for 20 minutes. (3) Remove the aqueous layer and titrate for viral infectivity. (4) Viral suspensions without ether treatment should be titrated as controls. A decrease in viral titer of 1.0 log or more in the treated sample suggests susceptibility to diethyl ether.

Deoxycholate Sensitivity[14]

Materials. This test requires sodium deoxycholate solution (0.2% with 0.75% bovine albumin), the virus to be tested, appropriate cell cultures for viral titration, and phosphate buffer at pH 7.

Procedure. (1) Prepare 0.2% sodium deoxycholate solution with 0.75% bovine albumin added. The solution can be stored at 4°C but should be warmed to 37°C before use. (2) Centrifuge viral suspension at $5000 \times g$ for 1 hour. (3) Mix 1 part of clarified viral suspension with 1 part of 0.2% sodium deoxycholate solution. For control, mix 1 part of clarified viral suspension with 1 part of growth medium. (4) Incubate the mixtures at 37°C for 1 hour. (5) Dialyze the mixture against phosphate buffer, pH 7, at 4°C for 24 hours to remove deoxycholate salts that are toxic to cells. (6) Titrate the dialysate for viral infectivity.

Physical and Chemical Determinations

Heat Inactivation[5,10]

Some animal viruses are susceptible to heat, 50°C for 30 minutes. However, heat susceptibility may be influenced by the concentration of certain substances in the medium, such as L-cysteine and L-cystine. Therefore, standardization of the conditions for heat inactivation studies is extremely important.

Materials. Use the viral suspension to be tested and appropriate cell cultures for viral titration.

Procedure. (1) Place 2 ml of viral suspension in a tube and incubate in a water bath at 50°C for 30 minutes. (2) Incubate an equal amount of viral suspension at 4°C for 30 minutes as the control. (3) Titrate both samples for viral infectivity and compare the differences.

pH Lability

Exposure of viruses to pH 3 for 30 minutes reduces the infectivity of some viruses (human rhinoviruses) while it exerts no effect on others (human enteroviruses). Viruses can be characterized as acid labile (loss of 1.0 log or more) or acid stable (no loss in titer or loss of less than 1.0 log).

Materials. Use growth medium adjusted to pH 3 and 7.2 with Tris buffer, the viral suspension to be tested, and appropriate cell cultures for viral titration.

Procedure. (1) Mix 1 part of viral suspension with 9 parts of growth medium either at pH 3 or 7.2. (2) Allow the mixture to stand at 25°C for 2 hours. (3) Titrate both samples for viral infectivity.

Cationic Stabilization[17,18]

High concentrations of divalent cations such as magnesium chloride stabilize certain viruses (human enteroviruses, reoviruses) when they are subjected to 50°C for 1 hour, while they increase thermo-inactivation of other viruses (adenoviruses, herpes simplex, vaccinia).

Materials. Use 1 M $MgCl_2$, the viral suspension to be tested, and appropriate cell cultures for viral titration.

Procedure. (1) Dilute viral suspension 10-fold in 1 M $MgCl_2$ and another suspension in distilled water (control). (2) Incubate the tubes in a water bath at 37°C for 1 hour. (3) Titrate both samples for viral infectivity.

Determination of Size and Morphology

Several methods are available for the determination of viral particle size; they include electron microscopy, filtration, and ultracentrifugation. A variety of biophysical factors that enter into these methods permit only an estimate of actual virion size. In electron microscopy, fixation, staining, and dehydration may lead to alteration in virus size. During filtration, adsorption of virus to the filter membrane can lead to appreciable errors in viral particle size estimates. Size estimation by ultracentrifugation requires information or assumptions regarding virus buoyant density, extent of hydration, and permeability of the virus to the solutes through which it sediments, as well as other factors that determine the sedimentation properties of the virus. (For dealing with photographs of viruses, see "Magnification Formulas" in Appendix A.)

Electron Microscopy[3,6,12]

Negative Staining

During recent years negative staining has been the most common technique for the determination of size and shape of viral particles. The method involves the embedding of viral particles in a layer of electron-dense material, such as phosphotungstate, phosphomolybdate, tungstoborate, or uranyl formate, so that the specimen is viewed as a light object against the dark background. Surface structures of viral particles can be demonstrated by this technique because the negative stains can penetrate gaps in the viral structure.

Materials. (1) *Virus.* It is best to use a partially purified and concentrated viral suspension for negative staining; however, crude viral preparations or even clinical specimens may be used if the preparation has a high concentration of viral particles. (2) *Negative stain.* There are several negative stains available but only phosphotungstic acid (PTA) will be described here. Make up a 1.5% phosphotungstic acid solution by dissolving potassium phosphotungstate in distilled water, and then adjust the pH of the solution to 7.2 by using 1 N KOH. The PTA should be made fresh and filtered. (3) *Grids.* Use copper grids (200–400 mesh) coated with either Formvar or parlodion and carbonized.

Procedure. (1) Place the Formvar-coated carbonized grids on a piece of clean wax paper. Using a bacteriological platinum loop, place one drop of viral suspension on each grid and allow to stand at room temperature for 2–3 minutes. (2) Remove the excess viral suspension from the grids by touching the edge with a piece of filter paper. (3) Place one drop of 1.5% PTA onto each grid and allow to stand at room temperature for 1–2 minutes. Remove the excess stain with a piece of filter paper. (4) Let the grids dry in a covered petri dish on a piece of clean filter paper before examining them in the electron microscope.

Thin Sectioning

The advantage offered by thin sectioning of fixed and embedded virus-infected cells is the opportunity to observe various stages of viral morphogenesis and morphologic changes of the host cell in response to the viral infection. The disadvantage is the difficulty of demonstrating fine surface detail of viral particles in thin sections. In determining the size and shape of viral particles, it is important to integrate the information gained by the examination of thin sections with that of other techniques, such as negative staining. Thin sectioning also may be applied to bacteria and fungi.

Materials

1. *Fixative.* Use phosphate buffer and osmium (1%) stock solutions: (a) 0.066 M dibasic sodium phosphate ($Na_2HPO_4 \cdot 2H_2O$), 11.876 g per liter; (b) 0.066 M monobasic potassium phosphate (KH_2PO_4), 9.078 g per liter; and (c) osmium tetroxide (OsO_4), 1 g ampules. *Fixative constituents:* $Na_2HPO_4 \cdot 2H_2O$, 78 ml; KH_2PO_4, 22 ml; and OsO_4, 1 g; pH should be 7.4.

2. *Embedding media.* Epon resins have become very popular because they are a softer plastic and are easier to cut than araldite. Epon plastics are more electron transparent, offering a higher contrast to specimens embedded in them. *Components:* The individual component (the accelerator) may be kept in stoppered bottles at room temperature, but the two solutions, A and B, should be kept in the refrigerator until needed (up to 6 months). Allow the solutions to come to room temperature before using in order to avoid water condensation. Solution A is made of 62 ml of epon resin 812 and 100 ml of hardener DDSA (dodecyl succinic anhydride). Solution B is made of 100 ml epon resin 812 and 89 ml of hardener NMA (nadic methyl anhydride). Immediately before use, add the accelerator, DMP-30 (2,4,6-dimethylaminomethyl phenol), to the resin mixture (1.5% up to 3% of the accelerator as it ages) and stir thoroughly. Note that two different hardeners are used and that no plasticizer is required because of the softer plastic. Blocks of various hardness can be obtained by using different mixtures of solutions A and B. Pure solution A will produce a soft block, while pure solution B will produce a hard block. The recommended mixture is as follows: solution A, 7 ml; solution B, 3 ml; DMP-30, 0.15 ml.

3. *Stains.* Use lead hydroxide chelated with citrate preparation. In a 50 ml volumetric flask add: lead nitrate ($Pb[NO_3]_2$), 1.33 g; sodium citrate, 1.76 g; distilled water, 30 ml. Shake vigorously for about 1 minute and then frequently for the next 30 minutes. Add 8 ml of 1 N sodium hydroxide at which time the solution will become clear. Use only freshly made, carbonate-free NaOH solution. Add distilled water up to the 50 ml mark and mix by inverting.

Uranyl Acetate Stain

An excess of uranyl acetate is placed in a small (5–20 ml) dark bottle containing 50% ethanol. The uranyl acetate will dissolve slowly and form a saturated solution in about 24 hours. As the solution is used, it can be replenished by adding more 50% ethanol to the bottle. However, the solution should be allowed an additional 24 hours to again reach saturation before use. The stain should be stored at room temperature away from light.

Procedure. In order for the researcher to obtain thin sections to be examined by the electron microscope, the pathogen-infected cell cultures or tissue fragments have to be fixed, dehydrated, infiltrated, embedded, sectioned, mounted on copper grids, stained, and dried.

1. *Fixation.* Place the tissue in the phosphate buffer and osmium fixative solution, starting at 4°C and allowing the solution to come to room temperature. This will take about 3 hours.

2. *Dehydration.* Dehydration may be performed with 10% steps of ethanol, with 15 minutes of soaking at each step interrupted by aspiration during the 30%, 40%, and 50% steps. After two 15-minute changes in dry absolute alcohol, the tissue is then transferred into propylene oxide for 30 minutes each in solutions of the following proportions—1:3, 1:1, and 3:1 propylene oxide to ethanol. Finally, the tissue is held for two 30-minute changes in 100% propylene oxide. *Rapid schedule:* Some investigators recommend starting dehydration at the 30% ethanol level, going through 50, 70, 90, and 100% ethanol, and then directly to 100% propylene oxide. Each step should last about 5 minutes. This procedure avoids prolonged exposure of tissues to solvents, which may cause swelling of the tissues. However, some tissues will collapse with too rapid a dehydration schedule.

3. *Infiltration and embedding.* After dehydration the tissue is placed in a 1:1 mixture of plastic resin and propylene oxide for from 1 hour to overnight at room temperature with occasional swirling to prevent the tissue from sticking to the bottom. After draining on filter paper, the specimen is transferred into fresh plastic mixture for about 30 minutes at room temperature. This is repeated at least once and can be done under a weak vacuum to remove trapped gas bubbles. Embedding is accomplished by draining the specimen on filter paper and placing it in fresh plastic mixture (in capsules or small beakers) in a 60°C oven for overnight polymerization.

4. *Sectioning.* Mount the small blocks of embedded tissues on holders and cut the thin sections using the ultramicrotome. Then mount the sections on copper grids.

5. *Staining.* The grids bearing the tissues can be stained by floating them section side down on single drops of the stain solution for 5–30 minutes on a covered wax surface. After staining, the grids should be rinsed in alternate streams of 0.02 N NaOH and distilled water for the lead hydroxide stain, or rinsed in two changes of distilled water for the uranyl acetate stain. Using lead citrate stain after uranyl acetate stain gives an added effect, as though the uranyl acetate were acting as a mordant for the lead stain. This double staining procedure is recommended for a beginning student. Allow the stained grids to dry in a covered petri dish before examining with the electron microscope.

Filtration[2,16]

With the wide distribution and availability of the electron microscope, filtration as a means of viral particle size determination has become less important. Nevertheless, under appropriate conditions, virus-sizing by filtration does permit a bracketing of a virion diameter and has the important advantage over electron microscopy that it allows an estimate not just of particle size but of infectious particle size. The latter distinction could be of considerable significance when testing crude preparations that may contain more than one type of virus.

Estimation of viral particle size essentially involves sequential dispensing of a virus-containing solution through filters of successively smaller pore size and assaying aliquots of the filtrates at each subsequent step. Two problems encountered when estimating virus size by this means are: (1) the virus adsorbing to the filter membrane, and (2) virus transit through the filter being restricted to particles less than 1.25–1.55 times smaller than the average pore diameter of the filter, although virus adsorption onto filter membranes can be effectively eliminated by pretreatment with protein-containing solutions.

Two types of filters have been used for virus size determination. One is the collodion or Gradacol membrane filter (available from St. Mary's Hospital, London). The other is the mixed cellulose ester or Millipore M-F filter (available from Millipore Corp., Bedford, Mass.). The filtration procedure to be described will deal with Millipore filters only, since they are readily available and represent the normal complement of materials in most virology laboratories.

Materials. The following materials are required: (1) Millipore 25 mm filter holder (Swiney or Swinnex); (2) Millipore 25 mm filters—mean pore sizes of 650, 450, 300, 220, 100, 50, and 25 nm; (3) Millipore 90 mm filter holder; (4) Millipore 90 mm filters—300, 220, 100, and 50 nm mean pore diameter, and a (fiberglass) prefilter (AP); (5) 10% fetal calf serum (FCS) in distilled water; and (6) 10 × Earle's saline or equivalent.

Procedure

1. *Membrane filter assembly and sterilization.* The procedure for assembly is that given in Millipore instructions; the following comments are for the 25 mm filter assembly. (a) Place the membrane on the holder support pad with the glossy side of the filter up. (b) Place the O-ring on top of the filter and screw the cap on loosely. (c) Wrap in suitable paper and autoclave at 121°C for 15 minutes.

2. *Preparation of FCS pretreatment solution.* (a) Filter the 10% FCS through the prefilter. (b) Pass the 10% FCS filtrate through 90 mm filters of 300, 220, 100, and 50 nm pore size in series. (c) Adjust 50 nm filtrate to isotonicity with 10× Earle's saline.

3. *Pretreatment of 25 mm filters.* (a) Tighten the sterilized filter holder assembly. (b) Draw 5 ml of the pretreatment solution into a sterile Luer-Lok syringe and attach syringe to filter holder. Do not at any time attempt to draw back on ther syringe as this will rupture the filter membrane. The pretreatment should permit nearly total recovery of viruses whose diameter is approximately half that of mean pore diameter.

4. *Filtration of virus suspension.* (a) Clarify the virus suspension to be tested by centrifugation at $5000 \times g$ for 10 minutes. (b) Transfer the supernatant to a sterile tube and draw 5–10 ml into a Luer-Lok syringe. (c) Filter the virus suspension sequentially through each of the pretreated filters beginning with that of the largest pore size. Retain a small aliquot of the starting sample and of each successive filtrate for bioassay.

5. *Decontamination.* (a) Sterilize by placing the intact filter holder into boiling distilled water for 10 minutes or by autoclaving the intact assembly at 121°C for 15 min-

utes. (b) Disassemble the filter holder and discard the old filter and rinse the filter holder parts with distilled water before reassembly and resterilization.

Ultracentrifugation[11,15]

Ultracentrifugation is an important biophysical technique that is exceedingly useful in virology for both the description of agents, including their subunits and antibodies, and for their partial purification and concentration. The basic molecular variables involved are size, shape, and mass, but the practical variables are sedimentation coefficient (universally called s-rate), with units of Svedbergs (S), and buoyant density, with units of g/ml usually specifying the medium used, e.g. CsCl or sucrose. The larger the s-rate the larger or more nearly spherical the particle of a given density. Typical values are under 20 S for antibodies, under 100 S for nucleic acids, and over 100 S for whole viruses. The buoyant density reflects the relative composition in terms of water of hydration, lipid, protein, nucleic acid, and salt, listed here in order of increasing constituent density. Typical values are less than 1.2 g/ml for large viruses with membranes, 1.3–1.5 for nucleoprotein cores, and over 1.7 for nucleic acids.

The so-called preparative ultracentrifuge can be used to determine the s-rate and the buoyant density of any agent in an impure state provided there is a specific bioassay available. The technique is to assay each of several fractions taken from the centrifuge tube after a spin of known rpm, time, temperature, and solvent in order to determine how much the agent has moved. After the s-rate and buoyant density are known for *both* the agent and the major contaminants, appropriate preparative ultracentrifugation procedures can be designed to partially purify and/or concentrate the agent.

The so-called analytic ultracentrifuge uses a nonspecific optical assay to reveal locations of material in a special centrifuge cell. It is rarely used now in virology, but has been important in the development of centrifugation concepts and in characterizing pure materials. Most text books in virology, immunology, and biophysics have chapters on centrifugation techniques. Especially valuable is the bibliography of methods published by Beckman Instruments.[15] A recent conference honored the fiftieth anniversary of the first publication of The Svedberg's investigation on the ultracentrifuge, and the proceedings should be consulted for the latest references and concepts.[11]

References

1. Andrewes, C.H., and D.M. Hockman. The susceptibility of viruses to ethyl ether. *J. Gen. Microbiol.* 3:290–297, 1945.
2. Black, F.L. Relationship between virus particle size and filterability through Gradacol membranes. *Virology* 5:391–392, 1958.
3. Dawes, C.J. *Biological Techniques in Electron Microscopy*. Barnes and Noble, New York, 1971.
4. Feldman, H.A., and S.S. Wang. Sensitivity of various viruses to chloroform. *Proc. Soc. Exp. Biol. Med.* 106:736–740, 1961.
5. Hampanian, V.V., M.R. Hilleman, and A. Ketler. Contributions to characterization and classification of animal viruses. *Proc. Soc. Exp. Biol. Med.* 112:1040–1050, 1963.
6. Hayat, M.A. *Principles and Techniques of Electron Microscopy*, vol. 1. Van Nostrand Reinhold, New York, 1970.
7. Mayor, H.D. Cytochemical and fluorescent antibody studies on the growth of polio virus in tissue culture. *Texas Rep. Biol. Med.* 19:106–122, 1961.
8. Mayor, H.D., and A.R. Diman. Studies on the acridine orange staining of two purified RNA viruses: Polio virus and tobacco mosaic virus. *Virology* 14:74–82, 1961.

9. Plowright, W., F. Brown, and J. Parker. Evidence for the type of nucleic acid in African swine fever virus. *Arch. ges. Virusforsch.* 19:289–304, 1966.
10. Pohjanpelto, P. Stabilization of polio virus by cystine. *Virology* 6:472–487, 1958.
11. *Proceedings, Conference on Fifty Years of the Utracentrifuge,* Feb. 1975, Bethesda, Md. Cosponsored by the Division of Computer Research and Technology and the John E. Fogarty International Center for Advanced Study in the Health Sciences, Public Health Service, National Institutes of Health. (To be published.)
12. Sjostrand, R.S. *Electron Microscopy of Cells and Tissues,* vol. 1. Academic Press, New York, 1967.
13. Tamm, I., and H.J. Eggos. Specific inhibition of replication of animal viruses. *Science* 142:24–33, 1963.
14. Theilen, M. Action of sodium desoxycholate on arthropod-borne viruses. *Proc. Soc. Exp. Biol. Med.* 96:380–382, 1957.
15. *Ultracentrifuge Applications, 1970–1971: A Continuing Bibliography,* comp. Phyllis M. Browning, pp. 1–208. Spinco Division, Beckman Instruments, Palo Alto, Calif.
16. Ver, B.A., J.L. Melnick, and C. Wallis. Efficient sizing of viruses with membrane filters. *J. Virol.* 2:21–25, 1968.
17. Willis, G.C., and J.L. Melnick. Cationic stabilization: A new property of enteroviruses. *Virology* 16:504–505, 1962.
18. Zee, Y.C., and A.J. Hackett. The influence of cations on the thermal inactivation of vesicular exanthema of swine virus. *Arch. ges. Virusforsch.* 20:473–476, 1967.

PART TWO: VIROLOGY

8. Adenoviruses

Adenoviruses form a large and widespread group of viruses that infect humans and many other species of mammals and birds.[13] More than 50 distinct antigenic types have been isolated from humans, chimpanzees, monkeys, cattle, dogs, swine, mice, opossum, and birds. With few exceptions, adenoviruses do not produce overt disease in conventional laboratory animals, so their recognition was delayed until tissue cultures came into general use. The mammalian adenoviruses have been placed in the genus *Mastadenovirus* and the avian in *Aviadenovirus*.

The following criteria establish membership in the adenovirus group: (1) possession of deoxyribonucleic acid (DNA); (2) virion size of 60–85 nm, the virion consisting of a DNA core enclosed in a protein coat comprised of 252 capsomeres arranged in icosahedral symmetry; (3) replication in the host cell nucleus with formation of intranuclear inclusions and production of characteristic cytopathology, indicated by rounding of affected cells and aggregation in grapelike clusters; (4) relative host specificity, both in vivo and in vitro, often with inapparent infection and persistence of virus in host tissues; (5) production of a group-specific soluble CF antigen (not the avian adenoviruses though); (6) agglutination of RBC of homologous or heterologous animal species (many, but not all, adenoviruses); and (7) ether-resistance.

The human adenoviruses are not described here but are well reviewed elsewhere.[1,13] Likewise, the avian adenoviruses (serotype 1: CELO, quail bronchitis virus, GAL [*Gallus* adeno-like] 3 and 4, no. 93, and Ote; and serotype 2: GAL 1, no. 65, and no. SR-48) are reviewed and referenced in the NAS publication *Methods for Examining Poultry Biologics* (Washington, 1971). Here we are concerned only with the bovine, canine, porcine, and simian adenoviruses.

Bovine Adenoviruses

Three bovine adenovirus serotypes have been authenticated. By international agreement, they have been designated with a prototype strain as follows: type 1 (Klein's bovine no. 10), type 2 (Klein's bovine no. 19),[20] and type 3 (Darbyshire's strain WBR-1).[10] Two additional serotypes, types 4 and 5, have been suggested but not confirmed.[10] Although frequency of infection of cattle is high, bovine adenoviruses are not known to infect other animal species. The role they play in natural disease is unclear, but infections of the respiratory and intestinal tracts have consistently been produced in colostrum-deprived calves by experimental exposure. Certain serotypes may prove to possess a greater predilection for intestinal than for respiratory tract tissues.[10] Respiratory tract lesions in calves after experimental infection are confined to the lungs, which may show areas of collapse, consolidation, and emphysema. There also may be proliferative bronchiolitis and necrosis with bronchiolar occlusion. Intranuclear inclusions are often found in cells of the lungs, tonsils, trachea, and lymph nodes.

Specimens

Swabs taken from the conjunctivas, noses, and rectums of experimentally infected calves have yielded virus isolates for as long as 10–11 days after infection. Viremia was not detected.[10] Virus may be recovered quite consistently from the lungs and trachea, but less consistently from other tissues including lymph nodes.[10] Virus was not found in calves killed 3 months after experimental infection.[10]

Laboratory Procedures

Cultures. Bovine adenoviruses apparently can grow only in bovine cells. Calf kidney and testicle cultures are the systems of choice. Cell cultures inoculated with virus materials for primary isolation must be observed for at least 2 weeks because the CPE is slow to develop with bovine adenoviruses. Even after several passages CPE may not be evident for 5 or 6 days, and then it is seldom complete. Infective titers rarely exceed 1000 $TCID_{50}$ per ml.

Animal inoculation. None of the bovine adenoviruses have produced infection in chicken embryos, suckling or adult mice, guinea pigs, hamsters, or rabbits.[20] Type 3, strain WBR-1, induced tumors in newborn hamsters, but no infectious virus could be isolated from the tumors.[10]

Immunology and serology. Types 1 and 2 bovine adenoviruses agglutinate rat erythrocytes, and type 2 also agglutinates mouse erythrocytes. However, agglutination test results were negative with the RBC of chickens, guinea pigs, sheep, human group O, and even cattle. The type 3 virus agglutinates rat red cells very poorly and mouse cells only irregularly.[10]

A new viral isolate can be identified as an adenovirus by CF or AD tests, using the infected TC fluid against a serum possessing adenovirus group antibody, such as rabbit antiserum to strain "adenoid 75" (American Type Culture Collection [ATCC] VR-5). The new isolate can be assigned to bovine types 1 or 2 by VN tests using monospecific immune serums.

Infected cattle develop adenovirus group–specific antibodies that can be detected by CF or AD tests, using any mammalian adenovirus. Such serums can further be identified as to bovine type in VN tests or by agglutination of tanned RBC onto which a bovine adenovirus has been adsorbed, such as type 1, strain bovine no. 10 (ATCC VR-313), or type 2, strain bovine no. 19 (ATCC VR-314).[29]

Canine Adenovirus

Only one canine adenovirus is currently recognized. The same virus causes infectious canine hepatitis (ICH) and fox encephalitis, and a varient (Toronto A-26 strain) causes canine laryngotracheitis (kennel cough).[11] The Toronto A-26 strain differs from the classic ICH strains in virulence, structure of the soluble antigen, erythrocyte agglutination spectrum, and neutralization kinetics. However, the Toronto A-26 strain successfully immunizes dogs against virulent ICH virus strains. It is not known whether natural infection with this virus occurs in other members of the Canidae family (e.g. wolves, coyotes, jackals), but members or other animal families that have been tested are essentially insusceptible to ICH virus.

The disease in foxes primarily involves the CNS, and clinical signs of illness are usually related to brain and spinal cord damage. Mortality rates are usually from 10 to 25%, but go as high as 40% in some outbreaks.[15] Mortality is higher in young foxes than in adults. In dogs, the disease has a variety of forms: fulminating and fatal, severe but not fatal, mild, or inapparent.[23] There are several good reviews on ICH viral infections.[2,3,27] Lymphadenopathy is a constant finding in ICH since there is general infection of the reticuloendothelial system. A transient corneal opacity may occur after clinical recovery, and this may be a manifestation of Arthus-type ocular hypersensitivity.[4] Changes in the levels of serum enzymes, particularly glutamine–oxalacetic transaminase and glutamine–pyruvic transaminase may be of value for early diagnosis of ICH.[14] There also is a prolonged blood clotting time.[14]

Specimens

In dogs, virus is present in the blood and virtually all organs and body fluids at the time of death. Viremia may be detected as early as 24 hours after infection and may persist for 6–8 days. Virus may remain in the liver after clinical recovery,[21] and it has been found in the urine for as long as 6 months after infection.[25] Specimens may be taken from the spleen, liver, lymph nodes, kidney, or blood. Intranuclear inclusions are common in liver parenchymal and Kupffer cells and in kidney glomerular endothelial cells in dogs with ICH. In foxes, the inclusions may be primarily in the vascular endothelium, meningeal, and hepatic cells.[7] High concentrations of viral antigen have been demonstrated in the inclusion masses by FA techniques.[9]

Laboratory Procedures

Cultures. Canine adenovirus grows readily in cultures of dog kidney cells, which should be used for primary isolations. Dog testicle, lung, liver, and spleen cell cultures also may be used for passages of the virus. Good plaque formation can be attained in dog or swine kidney cell cultures if the viral inhibitors in serums used for the agar overlay media are eliminated.[3] Viral inhibitors are present in the serums of many animal species.[5] Another problem is that primary dog cell cultures may harbor latent ICH virus, which can confuse results unless controls are used.

ICH virus in dog kidney cell cultures causes a typical adenovirus CPE and produces intranuclear inclusions. The time of appearance of CPE is related to the viral dose; CPE may occur as early as 30 hours or as long as 7 days after inoculation. Canine herpesvirus produces CPE that is somewhat similar to that of ICH virus, but with some experience a person can see differences between the two.

Animal inoculation. Guinea pigs are susceptible to inoculation with large doses of ICH virus.[28] The other conventional laboratory animals and chicken embryos are not susceptible. Susceptible dogs (and probably foxes) are readily infected by subcutaneous (SC), intraperitoneal (IP), oral, or IV inoculations of ICH virus, but the intraocular (IO) route appears to be the most sensitive.[3]

Immunology and serology. A new ICH virus isolate may be identified by CF, VN, AD, FA, or direct HI tests. In the HI test, rat or human group O erythrocytes are used. For the detection of ICH antibodies in serums, the VN, CF, HI, or FA tests may be used with reference ICH virus strain such as Utrecht (ATCC VR-293). However, the VN test is the most practical and reproducible procedure. A serum VN titer as low as 1:4 is indicative of past host experience with ICH virus infection. The CF test is not very reliable for the detection of serum antibodies. The FA test is adequate for qualitative but not quantitative estimations with serums. The HI test yields reliable results, but has not been used extensively.

Dogs that recover from ICH are immune to reinfection for long periods of time; dogs maintained in isolation have proved immune after 5 years. Passive immunity to ICH is transferred to puppies from the mother mainly by the colostrum, and the half-life of this immunity is 8.6 days.[6] Immune animals withstand challenge with virulent virus. The Lederle 255 strain of ICH virus (ATCC VR-133) may be used as a challenge virus. Monotypic ICH antiserum is available from the Research Reference Branch, NIH.

Porcine Adenoviruses

The first porcine adenovirus (isolate 25R) came from a rectal swab of a piglet (12 days old) with diarrhea.[16] Subsequently, adenoviruses were frequently isolated from kidneys of pigs obtained at slaughterhouses in Germany,[22] and from the brain of a pig (10 weeks old) in the United States.[19] To date, three serologically distinct porcine adenoviruses have been recognized.[8]

Preliminary indications are that porcine adenoviruses are only mildly virulent but may persist in infected tissues. Although adenoviruses were recovered from piglets with diarrhea and encephalitis, it is not known whether these viruses were primarily responsible for the associated disease.[19] Only swine are known to be naturally infected with these viruses.

Specimens

Rectal swabs, feces, brain, and kidney tissues have yielded porcine adenoviruses.

Laboratory Procedures

Cultures. Porcine adenoviruses grow readily in primary swine kidney cell cultures derived from embryos or young pigs (1–3 weeks old). On primary viral isolation, CPE is slow to develop and often requires 2 weeks incubation. After serial passage of the virus, CPE may occur within 18 hours. At least one blind passage should be made before results are considered negative. Characteristic CPE suggests the isolation of an adenovirus. Replication of the virus in bovine embryonic kidney cell cultures has been demonstrated. Intranuclear inclusions are found in infected cells.

Animal inoculation. The usual laboratory animals are not susceptible to porcine adenoviruses.

Immunology and serology. A new isolate may be identified as an adenovirus by CF, AD, and VN tests, using a serum with adenovirus group antibody.[10] The VN test with monospecific antiserums is used to determine the porcine adenovirus type. Strain 25R will agglutinate rat but not rhesus monkey erythrocytes.[16] The Kasza strain performs similarly but in addition it agglutinates fowl erythrocytes, and to a lesser degree guinea pig, hamster, and mouse cells.[19] Reactions were optimal at room temperature. Antibodies to porcine adenoviruses can be detected by CF, AD, and VN tests. An HI test also may be used, employing chicken or rat red cells.[19] About 25% of pigs tested in Great Britain had precipitating antibodies in their serums that reacted with both human type 5 and ICH adenoviruses.[10] There are no reports on immunity to challenge or duration of immunity. The Kasza strain (ATCC VR-359) may be obtained for conducting tests.

Simian Adenoviruses

Simian viruses, among them adenoviruses, were discovered in cultures of rhesus and cynamolgus monkey kidney tissues used for poliovirus replication and testing of inactivated virus vaccines.[18] To date 12 serotypes of simian adenoviruses have been differentiated by cross VN tests.[24] No association between the various adenovirus serotypes and primate disease has been well established, but a few instances of disease that may be attributable to natural adenovirus infection have been reported. An adenovirus was isolated from nasal and conjunctival secretions of patas monkeys living in captivity and suffering from a disease resembling the pharyngoconjunctival fever of humans.[30] Several other isolates were recovered during an outbreak among rhesus monkeys of a disease characterized by conjunctivitis and pneumonia, from a chimpanzee suffering from a mild upper respiratory infection, and from the ocular discharge of a monkey with conjunctivitis.[12,17]

Specimens

The following specimens have yielded simian adenoviruses: nasal and conjunctival secretions, throat swabs, feces, and kidney and tonsilar tissues.

Laboratory Procedures

Cultures. Simian adenoviruses multiply readily in primary cultures of monkey kidney tissue. Most also will grow in established strains of monkey cells, but not as well as in primary cultures. An established line of rabbit kidney cells (RK-13) also may be used. The CPE of simian adenoviruses is similar to that of other adenoviruses. It becomes evident 3–4 days after infection and progresses slowly until the whole cell sheet has degenerated. Hematoxylin and eosin (H & E) staining of infected cultures reveals intranuclear inclusions. They appear as small eosinophilic bodies throughout the nucleus, some surrounded by an unstained halo and others as vacuoles near the nuclear membrane and nucleoli. The chromatin in a few cells may be massed in or near the center of the nucleus and surrounded by an unstained halo.

Animal inoculation. The only animals susceptible to simian adenoviruses appear to be those in which natural infection occurs. The viruses are not pathogenic for guinea pigs, rabbits, suckling or weanling hamsters or mice, or chicken embryos. However, tumors were induced in newborn hamsters by 5 of the 17 virus strains that were inoculated.[17] Following inoculation of normal monkeys with adenoviruses by the IC, intramuscular (IM), or other routes, only those inoculated IC with large amounts of certain viruses became ill.[18] Some monkeys died in 4–6 days and others eventually became prostrate. In each instance, virus of the type inoculated was readily recovered from brain and cord tissues. The histopathology was limited to complete or nearly complete destruction of the choroid plexus and surrounding epithelial cells, with no damage to nerves.

Immunology and serology. Like most adenoviruses, the simian viruses agglutinate a variety of RBC, although the species of erythrocytes agglutinated and the conditions for optimal HA vary with the serotype of virus tested.[26] On the basis of HA properties, four groups of simian adenoviruses have been distinguished.[26]

Simian adenoviruses share a common CF antigen among themselves and with human adenoviruses, and the CF test is useful for confirming the adenovirus nature of a new virus isolate. However, typing of the virus must be accomplished with the VN test, using type specific antiserums. The FA test also can be used to detect infection of cells. Reference strains of the various serotypes of simian adenoviruses may be obtained from ATCC.

References

1. Brandon, F.B., and I.W. McLean. Adenovirus. In *Advances in Virus Research,* K.M. Smith and M.A. Lauffer (eds.), vol. 9, pp. 157–193. Academic Press, New York, 1962.
2. Bruner, D.W., and J.H. Gillespie. Infectious canine hepatitis *and* Epizootic fox encephalitis. In *Hagan's Infectious Diseases of Domestic Animals,* pp. 922–931. 5th ed. Cornell University Press, Ithaca, N.Y., 1966.
3. Cabasso, V.J. Infectious canine hepatitis virus. *Ann. N.Y. Acad. Sci.* 101:498–514, 1962.
4. Carmichael, L.E. The pathogenesis of ocular lesions of infectious canine hepatitis. I. Pathology and virological observations. *Path. Vet.* 1:73–95, 1964.
5. Carmichael, L.E., G.F. Atkinson, and F.D. Barnes. Conditions influencing virus-neutralizing tests for infectious canine hepatitis antibody. *Cornell Vet.* 53:369–388, 1963.
6. Carmichael, L.E., D.S. Robson, and F.D. Barnes. Transfer and decline of maternal infectious canine hepatitis antibody in puppies. *Proc. Soc. Exp. Biol. Med.* 109:677–681, 1962.
7. Chaddock, T.T., and W.E. Carlson. Fox encephalitis (infectious canine hepatitis) in the dog. *N. Am. Vet.* 31:35–41, 1950.
8. Clarke, M.C., H.B.A. Sharpe, and J.B. Darbyshire. Some characteristics of three porcine adenoviruses. *Arch. ges. Virusforsch.* 210:91–97, 1967.
9. Coffin, D.L., A.H. Coons, and V.J. Cabasso. A histologic study of infectious canine hepatitis by means of fluorescent antibodies. *J. Exp. Med.* 98:13–20, 1953.
10. Darbyshire, J.H. Bovine adenoviruses. *J. Am. Vet. Med. Ass.* 152:786–792, 1968.
11. Ditchfield, J., L.W. Macpherson, and A. Zbitnew. Association of a canine adenovirus (Toronto A 26/61) with an outbreak of laryngotracheitis ("kennel cough"): A preliminary report. *Can. Vet. J.* 3:238–247, 1962.
12. Gavrilov, V.I., N.N. Dodonova, L.N. Kuborina, E.S. Voronin, and E.A. Shchekochikina. A study of adenovirus infection in Macaca rhesus monkey. *Voprosy Virusologii,* no. 4, pp. 475–480, 1963.
13. Ginsberg, H.S., and J.H. Dingle. Adenoviruses. In *Viral and Rickettsial Infections of Man,* F.L. Horsfall, Jr., and I. Tamm (eds.), pp. 860–891. 4th ed. Lippincott, Philadelphia, 1965.

14. Goret, P., M. Compagnucci, C. Pilet, and A. Chevet. Enzyme activity as a diagnostic aid in canine virus hepatitis. *Rec. Med. Vet.* 138:1035–1059 (in French), 1962.
15. Green, R.G. Epizootic encaphalitis of foxes. II. General consideration of fur-range epizootics. *Am. J. Hyg.* 13:201–223, 1931.
16. Haig, D.A., M.C. Clarke, and M.S. Pereira. Isolation of an adenovirus from a pig. *J. Comp. Path.* 74:81–84, 1964.
17. Hull, R.N., I.S. Johnson, C.G. Culbertson, C.B. Reimer, and H.F. Wright. Oncogenicity of simian adenoviruses. *Science* 150:1044–046, 1965.
18. Hull, R.N., J.R. Minner, and C.C. Mascoli. New viral agents recovered from tissue cultures of monkey kidney cells. III. Recovery of additional agents both from cultures of monkey tissues and directly form tissues and excreta. *Am. J. Hyg.* 68:31–44, 1958.
19. Kasza, L. Isolation of an adenovirus from the brain of a pig. *Am. J. Vet. Res.* 27:751–758, 1966.
20. Klein, M. The relationship of two bovine adenoviruses to human adenoviruses. *Ann. N.Y. Acad. Sci.* 101:493–497, 1962.
21. Larin, N.M. The mechanism of immunity in canine virus hepatitis. *Brit. Vet. J.* 115:35–45, 1959.
22. Mahnel, H., and B. Bibrach. Isolierung von Adenoviren aus Zellkulturen von nieven normaler Schlachtschwein. *Zentralblatt Bakt.* 199:329–338, 1966.
23. Parry, H.B., and N.M. Larin. The natural history of virus hepatitis of dogs (Rubarth's disease). *Vet. Rec.* 63:833–846, 1951.
24. Pereira, H.G., R.J. Huebner, H.S. Ginsberg, and J. Van der Veen. A short description of the adenovirus group. *Virology* 20:613–620, 1963.
25. Poppensiek, G.C., and J.A. Baker. Presistence of virus in urine as factor in spread of infectious hepatitis in dogs. *Proc. Soc. Exp. Biol. Med.* 77:279–281, 1951.
26. Rapoza, N.P. A Classification of simian adenoviruses based on hemagglutination. *Am. J. Epidemiol.* 86:736–745, 1967.
27. Rubarth, S. An acute virus disease with liver lesions in dogs (*hepatitis contagiosa canis*): A pathologic-anatomical and etiological investigation. *Acta Path. Microbiol. Scand.*, supp. 69, 1947.
28. Salenstedt, C.R. Studies on the virus of *hepatitis contagiosa canis* (HCC). II. Susceptibility of guinea pigs to experimental infection with HCC virus. *Arch. ges. Virusforsch.* 8:600–609, 1959.
29. Tribe, G.W., and K.F. Pullen. A rapid test for the estimation of bovine adenovirus 3 serum antibody. *Vet. Rec.* 82:442–443, 1968.
30. Tyrrell, D.A.J., F.E. Buckland, M.C. Lancaster, and R.C. Valentine. Some properties of a strain of SV17 virus isolated from an epidemic of conjunctivitis and rhinorrhea in monkeys (*Erythrocebus patas*). *Brit. J. Exp. Path.* 41:610–616, 1960.

9. Coronaviruses

Coronaviruses received their name from the fringe of petal-like projections about 20 nm long that can be seen around the surface of the virion, giving the viral particle the appearance of a crown. The viruses of avian infectious bronchitis, transmissible gastroenteritis of swine, hemagglutinating encephalomyelitis of pigs, and mouse hepatitis are included in this group. However, only the first two viruses will be discussed.

Avian Infectious Bronchitis Virus

Avian infectious bronchitis (AIB) is an acute, highly contagious, ubiquitous respiratory disease of the chicken, which is the only known natural host.[1,4] Vectors are not a part of the ecosystem and AIB is of no known public health importance. Initial introduction of the virus (IBV) into a flock is usually by direct airborne transmission, with the trachea and upper respiratory tract of susceptible chickens being the primary target of infection. Transmission may also be by contaminated feed and utensils and by movement of persons from infected to susceptible flocks.

A presumptive clinical diagnosis may be made after the disease has progressed sufficiently so that the history of the disease is of some value. The signs of pneumonic involvement resemble those of other respiratory diseases of chickens and there are no definitive pathognomonic or differential features. The morbidity rate in a flock is high but mortality usually occurs only in chicks less than 6 weeks of age. Serous or catarrhal exudate in the nasal passages, sinuses, lower trachea, and bronchi; congestion and edema of the lungs; and fibrinous inflammation of air-sac membranes are the common lesions at necropsy. The principal histologic lesions of the respiratory tract are cellular infiltration and edema of the mucosa and submucosa, hyperplasia, and vacuolation of the epithelium. The tracheal mucosa undergoes cyclic changes in acute, reparative, and immune phases for 18–21 days following tracheal infection with final restoration of the epithelium. Fluid egg yolk material may be in the abdominal cavity but if it is in layers this is not an abnormality specifically related to AIB. Nephritis, nephrosis, and uremia with distension of the ureters by urate crystals may also be associated with AIB.

Although AIB is recognized clinically as a respiratory disease, pathogenic virus is not solely or specifically restricted to the respiratory tract, but is disseminated from this primary target via a viremia as a generalized systemic infection with localization and replication in organs of other systems. The oviduct, which may be permanently damaged by the virus, and the intestinal tract are secondary targets. Abdominal viscerotropism is reflected in the susceptibility of the kidneys to the nephrosis- and nephritis-inducing Australian T virus, which produces transient respiratory signs followed by a terminal uricemia and acute renal disfunction. Virus of low clinical pathogenicity usually remains localized in the respiratory tract without invasion of the abdominal viscera.

The major economic loss is due to infection of and damage to the oviduct. In laying flocks there is a precipitous depression of egg production and there may be complete cessation within 1 week. Some 6 or 8 weeks or more may elapse before production returns to the preinfection level. In most cases, however, this is never attained. The first few eggs may be small, soft-shelled, malformed, and abnormal in quality. Some flocks are so severely affected that even after clinical recovery the flock is not an economic unit and must be replaced. Signs of infection persist in some flocks for several weeks or months. The debilitating nature of the disease results in poor utilization of feed especially when chickens are infected at an early age.

Virus can reside in the respiratory and intestinal tracts of clinically recovered chickens and be transmitted to cohabitating chickens for as long as 6–8 weeks after primary infection under controlled isolation conditions and for much longer under less effective isolation, with possible continuous reinfection. The chicken is probably an immune carrier rather than a true carrier resulting from primary infection.

The AIB virus is the prototype of the coronaviruses. It is generally spherical but is moderately pleamorphic. Its characteristic corona of pedunculated, petal- or club-shaped surface projections makes the overall diameter of the extracellular virus 80–120 nm. The projections, which may be extensions of the outer layer of the envelope of the virus, are easily detached, leaving breaks in the envelope.

The virus contains discontinuous, single-stranded RNA marked by extreme heterogeneity in the size of the fragments.[9] The largest two classes of fragments are (1) a large class, 75–85% of the total RNA, consisting of heterogeneous fragments of high molecular weight; and (2) a smaller class, 9–20% of the total RNA, with a size approximately that of 4 S ribosomal RNA. The nucleocapsid, 7–8 nm diameter, is loosely wound and probably of helical symmetry. Surrounding the genome are the 7–8 nm outer shell, the 9–17 nm inner shell, and the 4 nm peripheral layer of the envelope, all of which are derived from cytoplasmic material during morphogenesis of the virus. Replication occurs solely within the cytoplasm.

Specimens

Infectious bronchitis virus can be readily isolated from lungs, trachea, and bronchi collected from chickens during the incubation and throughout the respiratory phase of the disease, but only occasionally for as long as 10–14 days after infection.[1,4,8] Carriers may, however, shed virus for as long as 49 days and perhaps longer. Virus can be isolated from viscera, especially the kidney, oviduct, and bursa, but only in low concentration. Blood is not a common source of the virus as the viremic stage of the disease is brief and transient.

Specimens should be collected in the laboratory if possible, processed immediately, and tested for virus. If organs and tissues have to be sent to the laboratory they should be maintained in a frozen state. It is possible to send specimens in a 50% solution of glycerol without refrigeration, but this is not recommended.

Laboratory Procedures

Chicken embryos. Host-origin IBV is fastidious in its requirements for primary isolation in, and adaptation to, the chicken embryo before being transferred to, and secondarily adapted in, avian cell and tracheal organ cultures.[8] Suspension of the specimens suitably treated with appropriate antibiotics are generally inoculated via the allantoic sac of 9–11-day-old chicken embryos. On the initial passage and for the first few subpassages, the predominant features of infection are curling and dwarfing of the embryo, thickening and fibrosis of the amniotic membrane, and presence of urates in the mesonephros after 5 or 6 days incubation. Embryo mortality is variable and generally low for the first few passages, although different isolates of the virus vary in this respect.

Allantoic fluid should be collected from a few living embryos 48–72 hours after inoculation for use as inoculum for subpassage, if necessary. If there was a presumptive clinical diagnosis of AIB and there were no positive responses of the chicken embryo indicative of the virus on the fifth or sixth day of the first passage of host-origin inoculum, the sample of allantoic fluid should be used for the subpassage. If positive responses are not produced following three or four subpassages, the virus is presumed not to have been present in the original inoculum.

Successive passage of the virus in embryos is accompanied by a parallel decrease in virulence, pathogenicity, antigenicity, and immunogenicity for the natural host with a progressive increase in lethality for the embryo. Embryo mortality alone is the criterion of infection by "embryo-adapted" virus, of which the Beaudette virus is the classic example.[3]

Cell and organ culture. A variety of cell cultures of avian origin support replication of IBV, but whole chicken embryo fibroblast, chick kidney, and chicken embryo kidney cell cultures are most commonly employed. The plaque technique may also be used. The main CPE of the virus is the development of syncytia, which increase in size and number with terminal necrosis.

Embryo-adapted IBV has been cultivated in certain mammalian cells, principally Vero (African green monkey) cells, but these are not commonly employed media.

Rounding and sloughing of ciliated epithelial cells and complete cessation of ciliary movement in tracheal organ cultures is the specific cytopathic effect produced by IBV.

Animal inoculation. Suspensions of the specimens used for initial inoculation of chicken embryos, as well as samples of allantoic fluid collected from the embryos, can be used as inoculum for susceptible chicks for infectivity and cross-immunity tests. Tracheal rales and respiratory distress will develop within 24–36 hours in susceptible chicks. Chickens are generally not used for diagnostic purposes because of the usual limitations of isolation facilities.

Some chicken embryo-adapted isolates of IBV have been adapted to intracerebral cultivation in suckling mice and rabbits, but this is not a suitable method for primary isolation of the virus.[1]

Immunology and serology. The AD, FA, and CF tests can be used to identify IBV and its antibody, but they do not have the sensitivity of the VN test for quantitative analysis of the antigenic relationship of different isolates of the virus.[2,3,7]

The VN test performed with chicken embryos generally uses five 9–11-day-old embryos per dilution. The test by the decreasing virus–constant serum method uses 10-fold dilutions of the virus. The test by the constant virus–decreasing serum method generally uses 100 doses of virus and dilutions of serum less than 10 fold. The quantal dose response is used to calculate the NI. Positive response are embryo lethality with highly embryo-adapted virus such as the Beaudette virus, and gross lesions and lethality for less well-adapted viruses. A NI of 100 or more neutralizing doses is considered positive.[1] Plaque reduction of 80% or more by the constant virus–decreasing serum (2-fold dilutions of serum) method in chicken embryo kidney cell culture is considered a positive test. Tracheal organ cultures are receiving attention as the indicator system for VN tests of IBV.[6] Direct hemagglutination is not a property of IBV and the HI test cannot be employed.

It is generally agreed that Massachusetts and Connecticut IBV are the only distinct serotypes in the United States and that others, such as Georgia, Delaware, Iowa 97, Iowa 609, and New Hampshire EF, are tentative candidates with antigenic variants within the serotypes. The Australian T virus is distinct from the above viruses. Standard procedures and reagents are needed to develop a system of nomenclature to adequately describe antigenic and immunogenic types of the virus.[5]

Immunity to IBV must be assessed from the pathogenesis of the disease, the antigenic and immunogenic determinants of the virus, and the type and availability of immunoglobulins to protect against reinfection.[3] Modified or attenuated live IBV vaccines administered either in the drinking water or by aerosol induce better protection against reinfection than do the inactivated IBV vaccines. Maternal antibody is effective as passive immunity for about 2 weeks after the chick is hatched. The efficacy of vaccines has been interpreted from a variety of criteria including (1) clinical response, residence, and dissemination of the virus; (2) in vivo and in vitro response of tracheal epithelium; (3) protection against challenge with virulent homologous and heterologous types of the virus; and (4) induced secretory and humoral antibody.

References
1. Cunningham, C.H. Avian infectious bronchitis. In *Advances in Veterinary Science and Comparative Medicine,* C.A. Brandly and E.L. Jungherr (eds.), vol. 14, pp. 105–148. Academic Press, New York, 1970.
2. Cunningham, C.H. Immunity to avian infectious bronchitis. In *Developments in Biological Standardization.* International Symposium on Immunity to Infections of the Respiratory System in Man and Animals, London, 1974. International Association of Biological Standardization. Vol. 28, pp. 546–562. S. Krager, Basel, 1975.
3. Cunningham, C.H. Avian infectious bronchitis: Characteristics of the virus and antigenic types. *Am. J. Vet. Res.* 36:522–523, 1975.
4. Hofstad, M.S. Avian infectious bronchitis. In *Diseases of Poultry,* M.S. Hofstad, B.W. Calnek, C.F.

Helmboldt, W.M. Reid, and H.W. Yoder, Jr. (eds.), pp. 586–606. 6th ed. Iowa State University Press, Ames, 1972.
5. Hopkins, S.R. Serological comparisons of strains of infectious bronchitis virus using plaque-purified isolates. *Avian Dis.* 18:231–239, 1974.
6. Johnson, R.B., and W.W. Marquardt. The neutralizing characteristics of strains of infectious bronchitis virus as measured by the constant-virus variable-serum method in chicken tracheal cultures. *Avian Dis.* 19:82–90, 1975.
7. Marquardt, W.W. Infectious bronchitis: Detection of viral antigen in eggs and antibodies in chicken serum by complement-fixation. *Avian Dis.* 18:105–110, 1974.
8. Subcommittee on Avian Diseases, Committee on Animal Health, Agricultural Board. *Methods for Examining Poultry Biologics and for Identifying and Quantifying Avian Pathogens.* National Research Council, Washington, 1971.
9. Tannock, G.A. The nucleic acid of infectious bronchitis virus. *Arch. ges. Virusforsch.* 42:1–10, 1973.

Transmissible Gastroenteritis Virus of Swine

Transmissible gastroenteritis (TGE) is a highly contagious, viral, enteric infection of swine resulting in a very high mortality in pigs under 2 weeks of age.[3] In the densely swine-populated areas of the midwestern United States, TGE is one of the major causes of diarrhea and death in young pigs. It is not known to produce disease in animals other than swine, although the virus has been isolated from dogs, foxes, and starlings following experimental inoculation, and TGE antibodies have been detected in dogs.[1]

The disease occurs in the United States mainly in the winter. This may be caused by (1) the ability of the virus to survive better in cold than warm weather, and (2) the spread of the virus by starlings or other birds, which tend to congregate in great numbers around swine in winter in search of food.

After ingestion, the virus propagates rapidly in the small intestine and, at least in young pigs, results in a rapid and extensive loss of epithelial cells. A marked shortening of the villi of the small intestine occurs in young pigs.[4] The altered function of the intestine impairs digestion and absorption, resulting in a severe diarrhea. Vomiting is usually present in the early phase of the disease. Dehydration and an electrolyte imbalance quickly follow, and in pigs under 10 days of age, mortality may approach 100%.

Although swine of all ages are susceptible to infection, the severity of clinical signs usually decreases as the animal matures. Diarrhea may be present for only 1 or 2 days, and subclinical infections occur. Lactating sows, however, may become very sick, with an elevated temperature, agalactia, vomiting, inappetence, and diarrhea. The disease is often undiagnosed or unreported in feeding, finishing, and breeding swine.[1]

Very little virus is excreted in feces by most swine after the feces become firm,[8] and the longest recorded period of excretion was for 8 weeks after inoculation.[6] TGE virus has also been isolated from porcine lungs.[11] The ability of TGE virus to cause lung lesions or to be transmitted via the respiratory tract—especially from carrier animals—has not been clarified.

As a member of the coronavirus group,[10] TGE virus is characterized as follows: it contains RNA, is of medium size (80–120 nm), is moderately pleomorphic, bears pear-shaped surface projections, and is ether and chloroform labile.[1,5,7] In addition, it is trypsin resistant, stable at pH 3, relatively stable in pig bile, and photosensitive.[5]

When TGE occurs in a totally susceptible population, an accurate diagnosis can usually be made from clinical signs and history. TGE is the only swine disease as yet described that has the following characteristics on a herd basis: it produces a liquid diarrhea of short duration occurring in swine of all ages, spreads rapidly within the herd, and results in almost a 100% mortality in newborn pigs but almost no mortality in pigs older than 8 weeks. When TGE occurs in immune or partially immune swine an accurate diagnosis can be difficult, even by laboratory methods.[1] This is especially true in pigs nursing immune sows, in which case the clinical signs and epidemiological characteristics of the disease will be modified.

Specimens

The highest concentration of TGE virus occurs in the small intestine during the first few days following infection.[4] Thus scrapings or contents of the small intestine collected early in the disease are the preferred specimen for detecting the virus. From living animals, fecal samples would be the appropriate specimen. Several days after infection, viral isolations will be more successful from jejunal scrapings or contents than from feces.[8]

Laboratory Procedures

Laboratory procedures for the diagnosis of TGE usually consist of one or a combination of the following: (1) inoculation of the virus followed by the appearance of typical clinical signs in susceptible pigs, (2) isolation of virus by cell culture, (3) presence of villous atrophy, (4) FA tests, and (5) serology.

Cultures. Primary porcine kidney cells, thyroid and salivary gland cells, and a continuous line of porcine testis cells have been used for the initial isolation and for propagation of TGE virus.[1,7,12] The CPE produced by field strains can be transient or negligible in early passages, depending on the susceptibility of the cell culture used and probably on the field strain. The plaque technique has also been useful for isolating and titrating the virus.[1] Identification of an isolated virus is accomplished by VN with specific anti-TGE serum.

Animal inoculation. Probably the most sensitive method for detecting the presence of TGE virus is the oral administration of the specimen to susceptible piglets, preferably only a few days old. If TGE virus is present, vomiting will often be the first clinical sign, followed in a few hours by a severe diarrhea, then dehydration and usually death.

Marked shortening and blunting of the villi of the jejunum and/or ileum occurs in piglets infected with TGE virus.[4] This lesion can be detected with a hand lens or a dissecting microscope at magnifications of 5–10 times. However, villous atrophy should not be considered pathognomonic for TGE.

Immunology and serology. The FA technique can be used to detect TGE viral antigen in infected cell cultures and in tissues (sections or smears of the small intestines) from infected pigs.[9] This diagnostic technique can be especially useful with tissues obtained in the first few days of the disease.

The VN test, using cell cultures as the indicator system, is highly satisfactory for detecting TGE antibodies.[1] The constant virus–varying serum test is the one most commonly used: it can demonstrate an inhibition of CPE or a plaque reduction (PR), using a cytopathic strain of TGE virus. The test is also reliable for the diagnosis of TGE, especially if acute and convalescent serum samples are used. Antigenic comparisons of TGE virus isolates have revealed no major differences among them.

Swine that have recovered from TGE are usually clinically protected when re-exposed. However, immunity to reinfection or to clinical signs may not be complete, especially if the initial infection is in young pigs and if the viral challenge is severe and given months later. Circulating antibodies alone provide little if any immunity. This is true whether antibodies are passively or actively acquired.

Sows that have recovered from the disease provide passive immunity to their suckling pigs through neutralizing antibodies in the sow's colostrum and milk. Ingested antibodies in the lumen of the gut apparently neutralize any ingested virus and thus protect the highly susceptible epithelial cells of the intestinal tract. This immune mechanism has been termed "latogenic immunity."[4] For antibodies to be most effective they should be almost continually present in the alimentary tract and should be of the IgA class.[2] TGE antibodies in mammary secretions can be of the IgA and/or IgG classes. The former provides better passive immunity and apparently occurs only as a consequence of an antigenic stimulation of the gastrointestinal tract.[2] A modified live virus vaccine is commercially available for vaccinating pregnant swine, so as to provide passive immunity to suckling pigs. This vaccine is of limited effectiveness, however, partially because the stimulated antibodies in mammary secretions are primarily of the IgG class.[2]

References
1. Bohl, E.H. Transmissible gastroenteritis. In *Diseases of Swine,* H.W. Dunne (ed.), pp. 158–176. 3d ed. Iowa State University Press, Ames, 1970.
2. Bohl, E.H., and L.J. Saif. Passive immunity in transmissible gastroenteritis of swine: Immunoglobulin characteristics of antibodies in milk after inoculating virus by different routes. *Infec. Immunity* 11:23–32, 1975.
3. Doyle, L.P., and L.M. Hutchings. A transmissible gastroenteritis in pigs. *J. Am. Vet. Med. Ass.* 108:257–259, 1946.
4. Haelterman, E.O., and B.E. Hooper. Transmissible gastroenteritis of swine as a model for the study of enteric disease. *Gastroenterology* 53:109–113, 1967.
5. Harada, K., T. Kaji, T. Kumagai, and J. Sasahara. Studies on transmissible gastroenteritis in pigs. IV. Physicochemical and biological properties of TGE virus. *Nat. Inst. Anim. Health Q.* 8:140–147, 1968.
6. Lee, K.M., M. Moro, and J.A. Baker. Transmissible gastroenteritis in pigs. *Am. J. Vet. Res.* 15:364–370, 1954.
7. McClurkin, A.W., and J.O. Norman. Studies on transmissible gastroenteritis of swine. II. Selected characteristics of a cytopathogenic virus common to five isolates from transmissible gastroenteritis. *Can. J. Comp. Med. Vet. Sci.* 30:190–198, 1966.
8. Morin, M., L.G. Morehouse, R.F. Solorzana, and L.D. Olson. Transmissible gastroenteritis in feeder swine: Role of feeder swine in the epizootiologic features. *Am. J. Vet. Res.* 35:251–255, 1974.
9. Pensaert, M.B., E.O. Haelterman, and T. Burnstein. Transmissible gastroenteritis of swine: Virus-intestinal cell interactions. I. Immunofluorescence, histopathology and virus production in the small intestine through the course of infection. *Arch. ges. Virusforsch.* 31:321–334, 1970.
10. Tajima, M. Morphology of transmissible gastroenteritis virus of pigs: A possible member of coronaviruses. *Arch. ges. Virusforsch.* 29:105–108, 1970.
11. Underdahl, N.R., C.A. Mebus, E.L. Stair, M.B. Rhodes, L.D. McGill, and M.J. Twiehaus. Isolation of transmissible gastroenteritis virus from lungs of market-weight swine. *Am. J. Vet. Res.* 35:1209–1216, 1975.
12. Witte, K.H., and B.C. Easterday. Isolation and propagation of the virus of transmissible gastroenteritis of pigs in various pig cell cultures. *Arch. ges. Virusforsch.* 20:327–350, 1967.

10. Herpesviruses

The rootword designating this group of viruses (Greek, *herpein*) means "to creep" and especially describes the lesions of epithelial tissue of persons affected with herpes simplex virus (HSV). Many other viruses have important physical and chemical similarities to HSV and have been classified in a group named herpesviruses. All viruses of this group contain DNA, are rather large with similar morphology, are assembled in the nucleus of a host cell, and cause the formation of an eosinophilic intranuclear inclusion. These viruses are quite sensitive to lipolytic agents. The virions are coated with an outer membrane, which makes precise definition of their diameter difficult.

Some biologic characteristics are common among herpesviruses. Most of the group tend to produce latent infections that have been considered to be related to intranuclear replication, although the mechanism of latency has not been established. In cell culture and on embryonating chicken membranes, the members of the group for which there is information produced focal cytopathic effects in the form of plaques or pocks. In several instances the member viruses cause focal lesions in epithelial tissues.

All herpesviruses have cuboidal symmetry. The virus particle is an icosahedral capsid having a diameter of about 100 nm and is constructed of 162 subunits or capsomeres. Each capsomere is about 9 nm across and 12.5 nm deep; the central cavity is about 75 nm in diameter and contains the double-stranded DNA molecule. The molecular weight of the nucleic acid for the members of the viral group ranges from 51×10^6 to 84×10^6 daltons.

Few cross-neutralizing serologic relationships have been found among herpesviruses. However, relatively few investigations have been made considering the number of viruses in the group and the rapidity with which new members have been proposed in recent years. The only cross-neutralizations reported between viruses from different host species have been between HSV and B-virus of monkeys and between HSV and canine herpesvirus; the tests indicate that there is a sharing of antigens between these viruses. In somewhat similar fashion, infectious bovine rhinotracheitis (IBR) and equine rhinopneumonitis (ER) viruses have been shown to be related by a common antigen through CF and AD tests, but reciprocal neutralization has not been observed. Pseudorabies virus (PrV), HSV, and B-virus have been found in AD tests to share what may be a group antigen and is suggestive of a structural antigen; yet all are distinct immunologically from a neutralization viewpoint. Negative results were obtained by several workers in various tests between PrV and the following herpesviruses: infectious laryngotracheitis virus, ER virus, virus III of rabbits, herpes zoster, and varicella.

Electron microscopy studies of herpesviruses are useful in helping to identify unknown viruses as members of the group. The enveloped capsid is the mature infective form of the virus and the morphology is similar for the group. Observation of a naked cuboidal capsid containing 162 capsomeres in a field with enveloped particles strengthens the possibility of the presence of a herpesvirus.

Herpesviruses are considered to be poor producers of interferon. Few positive reports have been made; however, it is possible that not much interferon is required to contain these infections or that the cell-associated resistance systems operating in herpesvirus infections are not detectable with current methods.

Infectious Bovine Rhinotracheitis Virus

Infectious bovine rhinotracheitis (IBR) is also called pustular vulvovaginitis. Cattle are the primary hosts. Mule deer often have naturally acquired virus-neutralizing antibodies in their serum, and they are susceptible to the virus under experimental conditions,[4] as are young goats.[12]

Infectious bovine rhinotracheitis is an acute febrile disease accompanied by an intense inflammation of the upper respiratory passages and trachea.[7] In many instances, conjunctivitis is the only sign of illness.[1,9] In young cattle, encephalitis is occasionally a sequela.[8] In diary herds the disease also produces pustules on the mucosal surface of the vulva and vagina.[5,6] Abortions may occur and significant lesions can be found in fetuses.[11,14,16]

In severe cases the changes are intensified and the exudate is copious and of catarrhal character, even to becoming a pseudomembrane extending to the larynx or down the trachea to the bronchi. Petechiation and ecchymosis appear in the frontal sinus and trachea. The mucosa of the muzzle becomes hyperemic and there is a tendency for it to crack and peel.[3,11,12,14,16] In the vulva, pustules circumscribed by hyperemic areas appear above the lymphatic follicles. As pustules coalesce a purulent exudate forms.[10,17] Histopathologic changes are consistent with those found in any acute catarrhal inflammation.[5] Typical herpesvirus eosinophilic intranuclear inclusions occur in epithelial cells of the respiratory tract.

Specimens

The specimens to be collected vary with the signs of illness in a given outbreak. Nasal washings or swabs from the nares, conjunctival sacs, or vagina should be used, depending on the situation. If signs of encephalitis have occurred, brain tissue from different locations should be used.[7] In cases of abortion, virus has been isolated from thoracic cavity fluid of the fetus and from cotyledons, although not with high frequency. Virus is most readily found in specimens obtained during the febrile period of the infection. However, virus can be isolated several months after cessation of clinical signs from some animals.

Laboratory Procedures

Cultures. Primary or secondary cell cultures of bovine kidneys, fetal bovine kidneys, or bovine testicular tissue are frequently employed for virus isolation. However, continuous cell cultures such as Madin-Darby bovine kidney (MDBK) or bovine tracheal cells (BTC) are equally useful. The virus can also be propagated in kidney cells of swine, goats, sheep, rabbits, and horses. Cell cultures derived from rabbit testicles, human amnions, and bovine lymph nodes will support viral replication also. Typical cytopathology becomes apparent after 24–30 hours of incubation, with destruction of the cell sheet in about 4 days. The rapidity of cell destruction is dose dependent. Various overlays may be used for the plaque assay technique.

Animal inoculation. Reference hyperimmune serums have been produced in rabbits,[3] guinea pigs,[15] and steers.[13] A variety of regimens have been employed. Usually, about 10^6 $TCID_{50}$ of virus are injected IV or IM 2–6 times at weekly intervals. Serum is collected about a week after the last injection.

Immunology and serology. All isolates of IBR virus that have been tested have been found to be immunologically identical. The VN test is used to identify IBR virus and antibodies. The LA strain is available for reference (ATCC VR-188). Both direct and indirect FA tests have been used to detect the virus in tissues, cell cultures, and impression smears; the direct method is most commonly employed. Viral antigens have been found in many tissues such as spleen and tonsils.[2]

Modified live virus vaccines are commercially available and the limits of their application are provided in the literature accompanying them. The duration of immunity provided by them is not clearly recognized. Cattle, after recovery from the disease, are resistant to challenge with virulent virus by any route. Following vaccination, intranasal (IN) challenge of immunity with virulent virus may elicit a mild response.

References

1. Abinanti, F.R., and G.J. Plummer. The isolation of infectious bovine rhinotracheitis virus from cattle infected with conjunctivitis: Observation on experimental infection. *Am. J. Vet. Res.* 22:13–17, 1961.
2. Bocciarelli, D.S., Z. Orfel, G. Mandino, and A. Persechino. The core of a bovine herpes virus. *Virology* 3:58–61, 1966.
3. Burroughs, A.L. Viral infection in commercial feedlot cattle. *Am. J. Vet. Res.* 28:365–371, 1967.
4. Chow, T.L., and R.W. Davis. The susceptibility of mule deer to infectious bovine rhinotracheitis. *Am. J. Vet. Res.* 25:518–519, 1964.
5. Curtis, R.A., A.A. Van Dreumel, and J. Ditchfield. Infectious bovine rhinotracheitis: Clinical, pathological, and virological aspects. *Can. Vet. J.* 7:161–168, 1966.
6. Gillespie, J.H., K. McEntee, J.W. Kendrick, and W.C. Wagner. Comparison of infectious pustular vulvovaginitis virus with infectious bovine rhinotracheitis virus. *Cornell Vet.* 49:288–297, 1959.
7. Griffin, T.P., W.F. Howells, R.A. Crandell, and F.D. Maurer. Stability of the virus of infectious bovine rhinotracheitis. *Am. J. Vet. Res.* 18:990–992, 1958.
8. Hall, W.T.K., G.C. Simmons, E.L. French, W.A. Snowdon, and M. Asdell. The pathogenesis of encephalitis caused by the infectious bovine rhinotracheitis virus. *Austral. Vet. J.* 42:229–237, 1966.
9. Hughes, J.P., H.J. Olander, and M. Wada. Keratoconjunctivitis associated with infectious bovine rhinotracheitis. *J. Am. Vet. Med. Ass.* 145:32–39, 1964.
10. Kahrs, R.F., and R.S. Smith. Infectious bovine rhinotracheitis, infectious pustular vulvovaginitis and abortion in a New York dairy herd. *J. Am. Vet. Med. Ass.* 146:217–220, 1965.
11. Kendrick, J.W., and O.C. Straub. Infectious bovine rhinotracheitis–infectious pustular vulvovaginitis virus infection in pregnant cows. *Am. J. Vet. Res.* 28:1269–1292, 1967.

12. McKercher, D.G. Infectious bovine rhinotracheitis. In *Advances in Veterinary Science,* C.A. Brandley and E.L. Jungherr (eds.), vol. 5, pp. 299–328. Academic Press, New York, 1959.
13. Mohanty, S.B., and M.G. Lillie. A quantitative study of infectious bovine rhinotracheitis neutralization test. *Am. J. Vet. Res.* 26:892–896, 1965.
14. Molelio, J.A., T.L. Chow, N. Owen, and R. Jensen. Placental pathology. V. Placental lesions of cattle experimentally infected with infectious bovine rhinotracheitis virus. *Am. J. Vet. Res.* 27:907–909, 1966.
15. Sabina, L.R. Studies of infectious bovine rhinotracheitis virus. *Can. J. Microbiol.* 11:887–892, 1965.
16. Sattar, S.A., E.H. Bohl, and M. Senturk. Viral causes of bovine abortion in Ohio. *J. Am. Vet. Med. Ass.* 147:1207–1210, 1965.
17. Studdart, M.J., E.M. Wada, W.M. Kortum, and F.A. Groverman. Bovine infectious pustular vulvovaginitis in the Western United States. *J. Am. Vet. Med. Ass.* 144:615–619, 1964.

Equine Rhinopneumonitis Virus

Equine rhinopneumonitis (ER) is currently the most common term used to describe a disease of equines that has also been called equine abortion disease. A more recent name given in an effort to organize the herpesvirus group nomenclature is equine herpesvirus 1. The disease is usually manifested as an infection of the upper respiratory tract of weanling horses but may affect adult horses in a similar manner. Abortions may occur in infected mares without producing respiratory problems. Equine species are apparently the only natural hosts for the virus.

The febrile response peak is usually 105–106°F (40.5–41°C). Neutropenia develops during the febrile period and lasts from 2 to 7 days.[9] While it is possible to develop long-lasting immunity to the abortive aspects of the infection, the immunity to the respiratory infection lasts only about 3 months. Older horses having experienced a series of exposures to the virus may become resistant to clinical disease. Mares not recently exposed to the virus may abort fetuses 30–90 days after an exposure. Most abortions occur near the eighth month of pregnancy. The mares who abort generally do not show other signs of the disease, and the genital tract is not damaged; the mares breed again in normal fashion.[2] Abortion occurs shortly after in utero fetal death. The mucous membranes of the fetus show punctate hemorrhages and the lungs are edematous. The surface of the liver may show small discrete areas of necrosis.[5] Intranuclear inclusion bodies can be found in the cells surrounding such lesions and in other tissues, including spleen, lymph nodes, and the epithelium of the ethmoid turbinates.

The ER virus (ERV) has some chemical characteristics that set it apart from the other herpesviruses. The guanine-cytosine base content of the viral nucleic acid is 55 moles per 100 moles phosphorus. The DNA density is 1.714 g/ml.[14] The enveloped virion is approximately 121–146 nm in diameter; the nucleoid 25–45 nm. The virus has some antigenic relationship to IBR, but complete reciprocal neutralization of virus with antiserum does not occur with members of the herpesvirus group.[3]

Specimens

Nasal washings obtained during the febrile period of the disease are the most commonly used specimen for virus isolation. Virus may also be isolated from blood, nasal mucosa, turbinates, spleen, and kidneys.[10] In cases of abortion, the lungs of aborted fetuses are the specimen of choice; however, virus may be isolated from other internal organs, notably the liver and spleen.[10]

Laboratory Procedures

Cultures. The virus will replicate in baby hamsters, cell cultures, and embryonating hens' eggs.[8] Two-day-old hamsters inoculated IP with a 20% suspension of equine fetal lung in BSS have been useful for cultivation of the virus.[7,16]

The virus can be cultivated in a wide variety of primary and established cell cultures. Primary cultures of kidney cells of porcine, bovine, equine, hamster, feline, and ovine origin, and established cultures of Earle's L-cells, human amnion cells, and HeLa cells have been used for growth of the virus.[4,13] The CAM, AmC, and YS routes of inoculation in 10-day embryonating chicken eggs have been successfully used to cultivate the virus.[8]

Animal inoculation. Newborn hamsters may be used as laboratory animals.

Immunology and serology. The VN test is conducted by the commonly accepted methods on any of the susceptible cell cultures mentioned.[1] However, plaque assay and PR tests are the most precise means of assaying virus-neutralizing antibodies. HA and HI tests using horse or guinea pig erythrocytes are conducted using the commonly accepted methods.[11,15] The CF test may be conducted using lung tissue from aborted fetuses as the source of antigen.[6] Indirect FA tests are applicable, using infected cell cultures. Hyperimmune serum produced in rabbits is adsorbed to the cell cultures followed by an overlay of fluorescein-labeled, lyophilized antirabbit serum of commercial origin.[12]

Abortion due to ERV rarely occurs in the same mare in two successive seasons, suggesting that an immunity develops after initial exposure. Vaccination with a hamster-adapted live virus vaccine has been found useful. All horses on a given premise should be vaccinated. The first inoculation should be given late in June or early in July and a second dose in October. The vaccine is administered intranasally. Mature horses do not react visibly but young ones often have mild febrile reactions accompanied by nasal discharge.

References

1. de Boer, G.F. Distribution of neutralizing antibodies against equine rhinopneumonitis virus in Dutch horse sera as measured by a plaque assay method with fluid overlay. *Arch. ges. Virusforsch.* 19:23–31, 1966.
2. Bryans, J.T. Viral respiratory disease of horses *J. Am. Vet. Med. Ass. Proc. Ann. Mtg.*, pp. 112–121, 1964.
3. Carmichael, L.E., and F.D. Barnes. The relationship of infectious bovine rhinotracheitis virus to equine rhinopneumonitis virus. *Proc. U.S. Livestock Sanitary Ass.* 65:384–388, 1961.
4. Darlington, R.W., and C. James. Biological and microbiological aspects of the growth of equine abortion virus. *J. Bact.* 92:250–259, 1966.
5. Dimock, W.W., P.R. Edwards, and D.W. Bruner. Infections observed in equine fetuses and foals. *Cornell Vet.* 37:89–99, 1947.
6. Doll, E.R., W.H. McCollum, M.E. Wallace, J.T. Bryans, and M.G. Richards. Complement-fixation reactions in equine virus abortion. *Am. J. Vet. Res.* 14:40–45, 1953.
7. Doll, E.R., M.G. Richards, and M.E. Wallace. Adaptation of equine abortion virus to suckling Syrian hamsters. *Cornell Vet.* 43:551–558, 1953.
8. Doll, E.R., and M.E. Wallace. Cultivation of equine abortion and equine influenza viruses on the chorioallantoic membrane of chicken embryos. *Cornell Vet.* 45:454–461, 1954.
9. Doll, E.R., M.E. Wallace, and M.G. Richards. Thermal, hematological, and serological responses of weanling horses following inoculation with equine abortion viruses: Its similarity to equine influenza. *Cornell Vet.* 44:181–190, 1953.

10. Jones, T.C., C.A. Gleiser, F.D. Maurer, M.W. Hale, and T.O. Roby. Transmission and immunization studies on equine influenza. *Am. J. Vet. Res.* 9:243–253, 1948.
11. McCollum, W.H., E.R. Doll, and J.T. Bryans. Agglutination of horse erythrocytes by tissue extracts from hamsters infected with equine abortion virus. *Am. J. Vet. Res.* 17:267–275, 1956.
12. Metzger, J.F., C.W. Smith, and M.D. Hoggan. A model for the purification of viruses for the production of specific immune serum. *Biochem. Biophys. Acta* 115:230–232, 1966.
13. Randall, C.C., and L. Lawson. Adaptation of equine abortion virus to Earle's L-cells in serum-free medium with plaque formation. *Proc. Soc. Exp. Biol. Med.* 110:487–489, 1962.
14. Russell, W.C., and L.V. Crawford. Properties of the nucleic acids from some herpes group viruses. *Virology* 22:288–291, 1964.
15. Semerdjiev, B. Hemagglutination of the virus of mare abortion. *Zentralblatt Bakt.* 185:316–324, 1962.
16. Sharp, D.G., and E.C. Bracken. Quantitation and morphology of equine abortion virus in hamsters. *Virology* 10:419–431, 1960.

Pseudorabies Virus

Pseudorabies, Aujeszky's disease, infectious bulbar paralysis, and "mad-itch" are synonyms for a disease that has been observed in a wide range of animal life. Most commonly the disease occurs in swine, cattle, sheep, dogs, and cats.

The pseudorabies virus (PrV) has a molecular weight of 70×10^6 daltons, and enveloped infectious particles have an average diameter of 186 nm.[5,7] The nucleic acid has a guanine-cytosine base composition of 73 moles per 100 moles phosphorus.[2,8]

Pseudorabies virus (PrV) causes an acute nonsuppurative meningoencephalitis. In those instances in which virus invasion occurs peripherally through trauma, the virus probably passes through the epineural lymph to the dorsal root ganglion, apparently resulting in intense itching at the site of introduction, and the animal responds accordingly. The crucial infection occurs in the mesencephalon and rhombencephalon. In swine there are three common routes of infection of the CNS. Since the epithelial cells of the nasopharynx are susceptible to infection, infection results in the release of virus, which assures ample virus for invasion of the first cranial nerve via the olfactory epithelium, then to the bipolar nerve cells, then through the cribiform plate of the ethmoid bone to the olfactory lobe of the telencephalon, from which the infection spreads caudally. Simultaneously, the fifth and ninth cranial nerves also become involved, as evidence of infection can be found at the Gasserian ganglion and at the solitary nucleus in the medulla, from which the infection spreads rostrally and caudally.

In cattle, sheep, dogs, and cats, evidence of pruritus is almost always present at some site. If dogs or cats have eaten infected tissue and become infected, evidence of pruritus often is manifested by excessive licking and chewing of the oral margins, sometimes until blood is extravasated. Cattle and sheep usually rub some site until it becomes raw and swollen. This activity occurs just prior to and during the CNS signs.

In swine, PrV is sometimes confused with hog cholera or enterovirus infections. Pseudorabies infections differ in the following ways in swine: (1) leukopenia does not occur; (2) convulsions are brief, and as many as three may occur within 10 minutes; after each, the pig arises and moves about somewhat unsteadily but in control for the most part; (3) in the initial phases, fine tremors of the tail can be observed about the time of the onset of the febrile response, which is followed closely by anorexia and constipation; (4) histopathologic findings may reveal polymorphonuclear leukocytes in the meninges covering the frontal areas of the cerebrum as a result of bacterial invasion following destruction of tissue barriers at the olfactory epithelium and the cribiform plate of the ethmoid bone.

Pseudorabies virus infections have occurred naturally in several kinds of animals and may be induced in many more. Swine probably are the primary host because they seem to be more resistant than the other common natural hosts, namely cattle, sheep, cats, dogs, and sometimes rats. The evidence suggesting natural infections in horses is not great and experimental infections have not been uniformly successful. Human infections have been reported outside the United States but the evidence is not entirely convincing.[4] The relative insusceptibility of swine and possibly rats, as compared with cattle, sheep, dogs, and cats, seems to provide the environment in which latent infections and shedder states occur. Infected cattle, sheep, dogs, and cats do not endanger other animals in their environment.

Specimens

Virus may be isolated from the olfactory epithelium and olfactory bulb 24 hours after infection of swine. Probably the best tissues for virus isolation during the febrile period would be from the midbrain, pons, and medulla in any of the susceptible species. Viremia is transient and blood is not a specimen of choice. Urine and feces are likewise unlikely to yield virus.

Asymptomatic swine having recovered from the disease may shed the virus for varying periods. Virus may be obtained from them by rinsing the nasopharynx. A balanced salt solution of 30 ml can be steadily forced from a syringe through a plastic cannula inserted into nostrils of pigs of nearly any size for recovery in an open receptacle. These nasal washings occasionally have been found to contain virus and have been considered to be evidence of the carrier-shedder swine. Some workers have found swabbing of the oral pharynx useful. Specimens to be stored should be frozen and kept as cold as possible. Those which are to be kept for long periods should be chopped into fine pieces and mixed with glycerol to 20% by volume and frozen for storage.

Laboratory Procedures

Cultures. Pseudorabies virus replicates and produces type A Cowdry intranuclear inclusion bodies in a wide variety of mammalian cell cultures. Cell lines derived from kidneys of swine have been most widely used for the isolation of PrV from tissue specimens. Cell lines derived from monkey kidney, fetal swine lymph node, ovine leukocyte, ovine brain, human peritoneal fluid, and ovine choroid plexus have been used for experimental purposes.[9] Primary cell cultures from rabbit, swine, and bovine kidney have also been found to be useful.

Fresh materials, mechanically chopped fine, may be mixed with BSS and centrifuged. The amount of BSS may be varied to meet the experimental requirements. Tissue suspensions of 10–50% have been used. The supernatant fluids in 0.1 ml amounts should be added to cell cultures in 16×125 mm tubes and allowed to incubate at 37°C for 1 hour prior to adding 1 ml of cell culture medium.[9]

Frozen tissue specimens may be triturated using a cold mortar and pestle in an acetone and dry ice bath. Subsequent handling procedures are the same as with fresh specimens.

Frozen and stored specimens which had been minced and mixed with glycerol (20–50%) may be thawed and centrifuged and the supernatant fluid applied to cell cultures as in the case of fresh specimens.

Specimens containing much virus and suffering little loss in preparation for assay may cause CPE to be visible under low-power microscopy in as little as 18 hours. The usual incubation period for satisfactory expression of CPE is 48 hours and in fluids with low viral content changes may not be convincing until 96 hours. In the latter case, fixation with an acid fixative and H & E staining is recommended to show the characteristic intranuclear inclusions.

Plaque assay systems give values of greater precision than tube dilution titrations. This technique also provides the means for cloning virus populations and the means for differentiating between some strains. Virulent strains invariably cause the formation of very small plaques while modified strains cause larger plaques, sometimes as large as 8–10 mm in diameter.[6]

Many years ago it was found that PrV would replicate in embryonating chicken eggs. Plaques on the CAM appear about 4 days after exposure and precede invasion of the CNS of the embryo.[1]

Animal inoculation. Experimental infections have been established in rabbits, guinea pigs, mice, goats, horses, asses, foxes, hedgehogs, monkeys (*M. mulatta*), marmoset monkeys, porcupines, opossum, pigeons, geese, ducks, buzzards, sparrow hawks, chickens, and jackals.[4] Cats seem to be more susceptible than rabbits.

Rabbits, mice, guinea pigs, and rats are susceptible to the disease and may be used to test for the presence of PrV in an inoculum. Subcutaneous inoculation in the flank should result in a satisfactory test. The period of the syndrome in rabbits is often rather short; most commonly an inoculated rabbit will be found dead, with hair from the site of inoculation in its mouth, having torn it out in response to a CNS signal that the area itched severely. The rabbits usually respond to the inoculation about 36–48 hours later and die within a few hours. However, occasionally the syndrome is delayed and death may occur as late as the seventh day. Guinea pigs, mice, and rats are much less susceptible to subcutaneous inoculation. One hundred to one thousand times as much virus is necessary to cause the disease in guinea pigs, and rats and mice are even more resistant to this route of exposure.[4]

Immunology and serology. Of the naturally infected animals, only swine have been found to recover. Consequently, VN tests are most often conducted with swine sera. The reference virus strain Aujeszky is available (ATCC VR-135). Screening tests for the presence of VN antibodies are conducted on cell cultures exposed to a preincubated mixture of 0.1 ml of a virus dilution containing approximately 50 $TCID_{50}$ per 0.1 ml and 0.1 ml of a 1:2 dilution of serum. The mixture should be incubated at 37°C for 1.5 hours prior to the test on cell cultures. The inoculum is 0.2 ml per tube with a minimum of four tubes per test. Endpoints are obtained by doubling dilutions of serum against the constant virus value. Values in serums from recovered swine usually range from 1:8 to 1:64 when tested against approximately 100 $TCID_{50}$ of virus.

PR tests of serum provide more precise evaluation of virus neutralizing capacity. The values obtained by the tube method are roughly comparable. Monolayer agar overlay, monolayer-methylcellulose overlay,[10] and cells-suspended-in-agar[3] techniques may be used to assay virus or VN titer of serum. The monolayer agar overlay technique is most widely used.

Direct FA testing procedures are commonly used for diagnostic purposes. Cell cultures are prepared in Leighton tubes and exposed to suspected virus-containing tissue extracts. The test is conducted without major differences from the protocols presented elsewhere.

No significant neutralization of PrV has been observed with either B-virus antiserum or type 1 herpesvirus antiserum.[11]

References

1. Bang, F.B. Experimental infection of the chick embryo with the virus of pseudorabies. *J. Exp. Med.* 76:263–270, 1942.
2. Ben-Porat, T., and A.S. Kaplan. The chemical composition of herpes simplex and pseudorabies viruses. *Virology* 16:261–266, 1962.
3. Cooper, P.D. An improved agar cell suspension plaque assay for poliovirus: Some factors effecting efficiency of plating. *Virology* 13:153–157, 1961.
4. Galloway, I.A. Aujeszky's disease. *Vet. Rec.* 50:745–762, 1938.
5. Kaplan, A.S., and T. Ben-Porat. Mode of replication of pseudorabies virus DNA. *Virology* 23:90–95, 1964.
6. Mayer, V., and R. Skoda. The behavior of modified and virulent strains of pseudorabies (Aujeszky disease) virus at different temperatures. *Acta Virol.* 6:95–99, 1962.
7. Melnick, J.L. Editorial note and summary of classification of animal viruses. *Prog. Med. Virol,* 9:483–485, 1967.
8. Plummer, G. Comparative virology of the herpes group. *Prog. Med. Virol.* 9:302–340, 1967.
9. Saunders, J.R., D.P. Gustafson, H.J. Olander, and R.K. Jones. An unusual outbreak of Aujeszky's disease in swine. *67th Ann. Mtg. Proc. U.S. Livestock Sanitary Ass.,* pp. 256–265, 1963.
10. Tytell, A.A., and R.E. Neuman. A medium free of agar, serum and peptone for plaque assay of herpes simplex virus. *Proc. Soc. Exp. Biol. Med.* 113:343–346, 1963.
11. Watson, D.H., P. Wildy, B.A.M. Harvey, and W.I.H. Sheddon. Serological relationships among viruses of the herpes group. *J. Gen. Virol.* 1:134–141, 1967.

Canine Herpesvirus

Canine herpesvirus is a typical type A herpesvirus. Isolations have been made in the United States, Great Britain, France, and Japan. In neonatal dogs the virus causes a fatal disseminated infection.[3,7] Puppies die 6–9 days following exposure. Signs of illness usually appear 1 or 2 days prior to death. Inappetence, abdominal tenderness, rapid shallow respiration, and finally incoordination mark this period.[2] Older dogs may have an inapparent infection or show only a few signs of the disease. Although the virus has been recovered both from dogs with nonfatal and with fatal respiratory disease, the virus' relationship to these clinical signs has not been resolved.[1,4]

The possibility of canine herpesvirus infection should be considered in cases of abortion or neonatal death in puppies. At necropsy, hemorrhages and focal necrosis of visceral organs are common, especially in the kidneys. Lungs are hyperemic and edematous, the heart valves are swollen and petechiated, and all lymphoid organs are enlarged and hyperemic. Microscopically the main changes in the CNS and peripheral nervous system are those of disseminated nonsuppurative meningoencephalitis with focal and diffuse mononuclear cell infiltration.[5] In other organs the fundamental lesion is disseminated necrosis. Hemorrhage resulting in necrosis of adjacent parenchyma is present in the lung, auricles of the heart, liver, kidney, lamina propria of the intestine, and lymphoid organs.[2]

Specimens

Virus may be recovered from the tissues of neonatal pups at necropsy. Kidney, liver, lung, and spleen are tissues of choice. From older dogs, nasal, oropharyngeal, and vaginal secretions can be used. All specimens should be placed in a protective medium prior to storage at $-70°C$ or colder temperature.

Laboratory Procedures

Cultures. Canine herpesvirus has been propagated in vitro only in cultures of canine cells. Isolations of virus are made in primary canine kidney or lung cell cultures. The virus-containing fluids are inoculated into cell cultures and incubated at 35–37°C. Specimens containing large multiplicities of virus may produce CPE within 24 hours; however, minimal multiplicities may delay the appearance of the CPE by as much as 7 days. The cell changes are characteristic of the herpesvirus group. Cultures without CPE should be subcultured once before the specimens are considered free of virus. Canine herpesvirus has been recovered from primary uninoculated canine cell cultures. Five to ten percent of the cultures should be held as uninoculated controls whenever primary or secondary cells are being used. Plaque methods are also readily applicable.

Animal inoculation. The usual laboratory animals are not susceptible. Rabbits are used for production of immune serum.

Immunology and serology. Using a reference strain of virus (strain D-004, ATCC VR-552), neutralizing antibodies can be detected in the serum of dogs. Such antibodies may be detected up to 10–14 days after infection and are usually low in titer, being 1:2 to 1:32. Approximately 100 $TCID_{50}$ per 0.1 ml of virus is mixed with serial two- or fourfold dilutions of heat-inactivated serum and incubated for 1 hour at room temperature. Primary or line dog kidney cell cultures are inoculated with 0.2 ml per tube of the serum-virus mixtures. The cell cultures are incubated at 36°C for 6 days. A reference serum and virus titration should be included in each test. VN tests provide a more precise evaluation of the serum protective capacity than the tube tests. The antibody titers of the serum may be two- to fourfold higher in the plaque test.

The virus can be identified by a combination of attributes: neutralization by specific immune rabbit serum, characteristic type A inclusion bodies in vivo or in vitro, and biochemical characteristics such as the presence of DNA as indicated by the use of halogenated deoxyuridines.[6]

References

1. Binn, L.M., G.A. Eddy, E.C. Lazar, J. Helms, and T. Murnane. Viruses recovered from laboratory dogs with respiratory disease. *Proc. Soc. Exp. Biol. Med.* 126:140–145, 1967.
2. Carmichael, L.E., R.A. Squire, and L. Krook. Clinical and pathologic features of a fatal viral disease of newborn pups. *Am. J. Vet. Res.* 26:803–814, 1965.
3. Carmichael, L.E., J.D. Strandberg, and F.D. Barnes. Identification of a cytopathogenic agent infectious for puppies as a canine herpes virus. *Proc. Soc. Exp. Biol. and Med.* 120:644–650, 1965.
4. Karpas, A., F.G. Garcia, F. Calvo, and R.E. Cross. Experimental production of canine tracheobronchitis

(kennel cough) with canine herpes virus isolated from naturally infected dogs. *Am. J. Vet. Res.* 29:1251–1257, 1968.
5. Percy, D.H., J.F. Munnel, H.J. Olander, and L.E. Carmichael. Pathogenesis of canine herpesvirus encephalitis. *Am. J. Vet. Res.* 31:145–156, 1970.
6. Spertzel, R.O., D.L. Huxsoll, S.J. McConnell, L.N. Binn, and R.H. Yagar. Recovery and characterization of a herpes-like virus from dog kidney cell cultures. *Proc. Soc. Exp. Biol. Med.* 120:651–655, 1965.
7. Stewart, S.E., J. David-Ferreira, E. Lovelace, J. Landon, and N. Stock. Herpes-like virus isolated from neonatal and fetal dogs. *Science* 148:1341–1343, 1965.

Feline Rhinotracheitis Virus

Feline rhinotracheitis (FR) is an acute upper respiratory disease of cats that has a herpesvirus as the etiologic agent. The initial isolation of the causative agent was made in 1957 from an outbreak of the disease occurring in young kittens.[6] A number of herpesviruses have since been isolated from the cat, and all appear to be closely related to the prototype strain, C-27.[2,5,9] The virus is widespread, having been isolated from cats in many regions of the United States and Europe.[2,5,14,18] Feline rhinotracheitis has been found to be unrelated to other herpesviruses, including IBRV, HSV, and bovine herpes mammilitis virus (BHMV). No serologic relationship has been demonstrated between feline rhinotracheitis and other feline viruses, including feline panleukopenia and the feline picornaviruses.[1,2,4,15]

Electron microphotographs of feline rhinotracheitis grown in RK-13 cells show the virus to have a diameter of 100 nm with 162 capsomers, each measuring 10 nm in diameter.[10] Ultrafiltration studies through graded collodion membranes suggest a particle size of about the same size.[13] The virus is sensitive to 5-bromodeoxyuridine and to 5-iodo-2-deoxyuridine,[3,8,9] indicating that it is a DNA-type virus. It is rapidly inactivated at a pH below 4, inactivated slowly at pH 5, pH 8, and pH 9, and most stable at pH 6 and pH 7.[11] Suspensions of the virus containing approximately 10^6 $TCID_{50}$ per 0.1 ml in Hanks' BSS with 0.5% lactalbumin hydrolysate added were completely inactivated at 56°C in 4.5 minutes, at 37°C in 35 hours, at 25°C in 33 days, and at 4°C in 155 days.[16]

The mortality rate in young kittens may be as high as 50%. Older cats appear to be more resistant and therefore have a lower mortality rate. The morbidity rate in susceptible cats is very high, approaching 100%. The onset of signs occurs approximately 48 hours after exposure and includes temperature elevation, sneezing, and excessive salivation. Rhinitis and conjunctivitis develop and usually become severe, resulting in mucopurulent discharges from the eye and nasal cavities. There is inappetence and depression during the early stages. The signs may subside after a week, or the disease may develop into a chronic form. A cough and labored breathing often occur. Also associated with the chronic form is a sinusitis that may produce a unilateral or bilateral tenacious nasal discharge. A chronic conjunctivitis is common with this disease. Infected cats also show a leukocytosis that parallels the temperature response. In uncomplicated infections, the leukocytosis may last 2–10 days, wth leucocyte counts reaching 30,000–50,000 cells per cu mm. In the chronic disease, the leukocytosis may persist for longer periods.

Intranuclear inclusion bodies are consistently found in the epithelial cells of the upper respiratory tract following infection with feline rhinotracheitis. The inclusions occur early in the course of the disease and may be found in epithelial cells of the nasal septum, tonsils, epiglottis, trachea, and nictatating membranes. The inclusions are found by swabbing the nasopharyngeal region or conjunctiva with a cotton swab and smearing the exudate on a slide. After drying, the cells may be fixed and stained with H & E. Hepatic focal necrosis, as seen with other herpesvirus infections, has been demonstrated in young neonatal kittens infected with feline rhinotracheitis.

Specimens

Virus can be isolated from the nasopharyngeal region and from the conjunctival membranes for long periods (more than 30 days) after infection. The virus has also been recovered from the liver, lung, spleen, kidney, salivary gland, and brain 9 days after the onset of clinical signs.[15] The virus is most readily recovered by applying moist, sterile swabs to the mucous membranes of the conjunctiva and nasopharyngeal region. The swabs should be placed directly into primary feline kidney tissue culture tubes containing broad spectrum antibiotics and gently squeezed against the side of the tube opposite the monolayer. After 2 hours at 37°C the media should be replaced with fresh maintenance media.

Laboratory Procedures

Cultures. Feline kidney cells are used for growth of the virus. The only other cells shown to support growth of the virus are rabbit kidney cells.[9] The virus produces a characteristic herpeslike cytopathology in feline kidney tissue cultures. Small foci of degeneration with rounding cells are observed 24 hours after inoculation, and this continues until the entire monolayer is destroyed. Intranuclear inclusion bodies may be demonstrated in stained cultures. The inclusion is acidophilic and is usually oval or spherical and separated from the nuclear membrane by a clear halo.[6] Supernatant tissue culture fluids contain approximately the same quantity of extracellular virus as found in cell-associated virus culture fluids.[10] Like other viruses in the herpes group, it is not highly stable. Unless properly stabilized and held at low temperature, the virus infectivity will deteriorate rapidly. Ten percent fetal bovine serum will improve virus stability, and storage temperatures below $-60°C$ should always be used.

Animal inoculation. The cat is the only species that has been shown to be susceptible to this virus.[17] Susceptibility may be demonstrated by the absence of VN antibodies. Young, unexposed kittens are in general more susceptible than older cats. Cats may be infected from exposure by various routes, including IN, IO, SC, IM, and IV. The symptoms, consisting of upper respiratory signs, begin within 48 hours with a temperature elevation that may persist for 6–10 days. Rabbits and goats may be hyperimmunized by repeated inoculation of high titer antigen by the IV route.

Immunology and serology. Cats that recover from feline rhinotracheitis develop VN antibody titers between 1:2 and 1:16, although titers as high as 1:64 have been reported. There is evidence to suggest that the antibody titers do not persist for long periods and reinfection may occasionally take place,[7] although careful epidemiological data to support this is not available.

The serum neutralization test is performed by mixing twofold dilutions of serum with virus calculated to contain approximately 100 $TCID_{50}$ per 0.2 ml. The mixture is incubated at room temperature (approximately 25°C) for 2 hours, and 0.2 ml of each serum virus mixture is inoculated into four feline kidney tissue culture tubes. The tubes are incubated at 37°C and readings made at 5 and 7 days.

HA and HAd by three isolates of the virus, including the Crandell strain, have been described. The hemagglutination titers of the tissue-cultured viruses ranged from 1:2 to 1:8. If the HA titer of the virus is high enough, a HI test can be used for routine serology.[11] A CF test has been reported, but is not routinely used.[12]

References

1. Bartholomew, P.T., and J.H. Gillespie. Feline viruses. I. Characterization of four isolates and their effect on young kittens. *Cornell Vet.* 58:248–265, 1968.
2. Bittle, J.L., C.J. York, J.W. Newberne, and M. Martin. Serologic relationship of new feline cytopathogenic viruses. *Am. J. Vet. Res.* 21:547–550, 1960.
3. Burki, F., S. Lindt, and V. Freudiger. Enzootischer, virusbedingter Katzenschnupfen in einen tierheim. II. Mittelung: Virologisher and Experimenteller teil. *Zentralblatt Veterinärmedizin* 11:110, 1964.
4. Crandell, R.A., and J.R. Ganaway. A study of the antigenic relationships between feline and human viruses. *Virology* 11:649–651, 1960.
5. Crandell, R.A., J.R. Ganaway, W.H. Niemann, and F.D. Maurer. Comparative study of three isolates with the original feline viral rhinotracheitis virus. *Am. J. Vet. Res.* 21:504–506, 1960.
6. Crandell, R.A., and F.D. Maurer. Isolation of a feline virus associated with intranuclear inclusion bodies. *Proc. Soc. Exp. Biol. Med.* 97:488–490, 1958.
7. Crandell, R.A., J.A. Rehkemper, W.H. Niemann, J.R. Ganaway, and F.D. Maurer. Experimental feline viral rhinotracheitis. *J. Am. Vet. Med. Ass.* 138:191–196, 1961.
8. Crandell, R.A., and G.R. Weddington. Effects of nucleic acid analogues on the multiplication and cytopathogenicity of feline viral rhinotracheitis virus *in vitro. Cornell Vet.* 57:38–42, 1967.
9. Ditchfield, J., and I. Grinyer. Feline rhinotracheitis virus: A feline herpesvirus. *Virology* 26:504–506, 1965.
10. Ebner, F.F., and R.A. Crandell. Growth of feline viral rhinotracheitis virus in cultures of feline renal cells. *Proc. Soc. Biol. Med.* 105:153–56, 1960.
11. Gillespie, J.H., A.B. Judkins, and F.W. Scott. Feline viruses. XII. Hemagglutination and hemadsorption tests for feline herpesvirus. *Cornell Vet.* 61:159–171, 1971.
12. Hersey, D.F., and F.D. Maurer. Immunological relationship of selected feline viruses by complement fixation. *Proc. Soc. Exp. Biol. Med.* 107:645–646, 1961.
13. Johnson, R.H. Feline panleucopaenia virus. III. Some properties compared to a feline herpesvirus. *Res. Vet. Sci.* 7:112–115, 1966.
14. Johnson, R.H., and R.G. Thomas. Feline viral rhinotracheitis in Britain. *Vet. Rec.* 79:188–190, 1966.
15. Karpas, A., and J.K. Routledge. Feline herpesvirus: Isolations and experimental studies. *Zentralblatt Veterinärmedizin,* ser. B, 15:599–606, 1968.
16. Miller, G.W., and R.A. Crandell. Stability of the virus of feline viral rhinotracheitis. *Am. J. Vet. Res.* 23:351–353, 1962.
17. Ott, R.L. Viral diseases. In *Feline Medicine and Surgery,* E.J. Catcott, ed., pp. 71–98. American Veterinary Publications, Wheaton, Ill., 1964.
18. Piercy, S.E., and J. Prydie. Feline influenza. *Vet. Rec.* 75:86–89, 1963.

Malignant Catarrhal Fever Virus

Malignant catarrhal fever (MCF) is often considered a specific disease of cattle, but in actuality it may be a collection of diseases sharing similar clinical and pathologic signs. There is little data to indicate that the disease is produced by the same etiologic agent in different parts of the world. Epidemiologic evidence indicates that the disease in cattle is obtained by contact with sheep carrying an inapparent infection,[1,11,12,13] with the exception of sub-Saharan Africa where the disease is commonly associated with contact between cattle and wildebeest.[3,9,10] However, even in these areas of Africa sheep probably play a role in the epidemiology of the disease.[6] Most of the experimental work with malignant catarrhal fever has been carried out with the wildebeest virus, with limited correlations to virus of sheep origin.

The natural hosts of wildebeest strains of malignant catarrhal fever virus are wildebeest of two species, *Connochaetes taurinus* and *Connochaetes gnu*. Infection occurs via the placenta in latently infected dams or early in the life of the calf, but no clinical signs are produced.[7] Only wildebeest calves in the early stages of infection can transmit infection to cattle. Neutralizing antibody has been found in some other wild ungulates including Thompson's gazelle (*Gazella thompsonii*) and topi (*Damaliscus korrigum*). Experimentally, the eland (*Taurotragus oryx*) is susceptible to malignant catarrhal fever (wildebeest strains) but sheep and African buffaloes are not. The mortality rate in cases of malignant catarrhal fever in cattle is probably over 95%, death occurring on average about the eighth day. Cattle that survive the infection remain carriers of the virus for months or even years.

The sheep strains of virus are assumed on epizootiological grounds to be derived only from sheep but there may be other natural hosts with inapparent infection that harbor the same virus as sheep. The disease outside Africa occurs naturally in cattle and domestic buffaloes and has been reported in deer (*Elaphurus davidianus*)[2] and elk.

In cattle and buffalo, malignant catarrhal fever is a highly lethal infection characterized by fever, generalized lymph node enlargement and congestion, and necrosis and erosion of the oral, nasal, and vaginal mucosae. The conjunctival and scleral vessels become intensely congested very early in the course of the disease and by the second or third days of pyrexia there usually is a peripheral corneal opacity that extends centripetally and often eventually involves the whole cornea. There are slight seromucoid nasal and ocular discharges early in the clinical course, which later become more profuse and mucopurulent and account for the usual names applied to the disease. The muzzle is at first hot, later becoming dry, cracked, and covered with exudate.

Areas of painful exudative dermatitis occur in some animals and others show symptoms of a laminitis and/or inflammation of the horn cores, which may lead to the shedding of the horns. The CNS may also be involved; symptoms concerning it include hyperaesthesia, muscle tremors, incoordination of movement, high stepping, or even torticollis.

Specimens

Direct transmission of the disease from bovine to bovine is difficult. Whole blood collected during the height of the disease and treated with 0.5% versene has given the best results. Even then, large quantities of blood must be used, injected IV into the test animal. Lymphoid tissue from the infected animal may also be used and may be the tissue of preference in tissue culture isolation attempts. Any delay in collecting material from postmortem cases should not be more than 1–2 hours. Lymph node biopsies may also provide suitable material for virus recovery.

Both solid tissues and blood should be kept on ice or in a refrigerator at 4°C from the time of harvest. Wildebeest strains will retain infectivity for up to 10–12 days under these conditions, although it is preferable to have the materials processed as soon as possible. It should be stressed that storage of field specimens at -20 or at $-70°C$ results in a complete loss of infectivity in a relatively short time, presumably due to association with cell death. Osmotic disruption, dessication, or lyophilization have a similar effect.[5] However, strains of wildebeest virus can be stored at $-70°C$, provided the suspensions of either bovine tissue or tissue culture cells are contained in a media consisting of 10% glycerol and 20% serum. After the virus has been adapted to tissue cultures and transferred in cell cultures for a number of passages, free or released virus can be obtained in the tissue culture fluids, which can be preserved either at $-70°$ C or by lyophilization.

Laboratory Procedures

Cultures. The wildebeest strains of the virus have been cultivated most readily by inoculation of calf thyroid tissue culture cells.[8] Where work has been conducted with cattle isolates of the sheep-associated strains of malignant catarrhal fever, this has also been used as the tissue culture cell of choice. However, there are no well-documented reports of initial isolation of sheep-associated strains of MCF virus in cell cultures. The techniques for propagating virus in tissue culture from field specimens or experimentally infected cattle are as follows. For the blood: (1) Centrifuge 10–20 ml of blood (with 0.5% versene) in narrow tubes for 20–30 minutes at 2500–3000 rpm. (2) Discard the supernatant plasma and aspirate the buffy-coat (leukocyte) layer into a Pasteur pipette. Expel the contents of the pipette into about 10–20 ml of 0.85% NaCl or PBS in a clean centrifuge tube and mix well. (3) Deposit the cells by spinning at 2500 rpm for 10 minutes; resuspend and disperse well in sufficient tissue culture maintenance medium. Replace the fluid in a series of tube cultures of primary calf thyroid cells with this infected cell suspension. (4) Roll the tube cultures at about 8rph and wash them well with PBS after 18–24 hours to eliminate erythrocytes and other unattached residues. Replace the medium completely every 3 days for a further 18–20 days and examine all parts of the monolayer as frequently as possible for evidence of a cytopathogenic agent. (5) The CPE of MCF virus in bovine thyroid cells will appear after 3–14 days or more and are characterized by the formation of syncytia in which clumps of nuclei are usually visible in living preparations. The syncytia often enlarge considerably, becoming vacuolated and retracting centrally but expanding slowly into the normal cell sheet at the periphery. With small infective inocula only a few cytopathic foci are present and these do not increase in numbers on prolonged incubation. Sometimes foci may be partially or completely eliminated by the growth of resistant, fibroblastlike cells. Cultures of primary bovine adrenal cells or some lines of serially cultivated calf kidney cells have also been found to be susceptible to the virus. For the lymphoid tissues: (1) Chop the infected tissue into small pieces, about 1–2 mm diameter, with crossed scalpels or scissors. (2) Homogenize to produce a 10% (weight to volume) suspension in tissue culture maintenance medium, using an all-glass tissue grinder (Ten Broeck) and no abrasive. (3) Prepare two- to tenfold dilutions of the suspension in maintenance medium and inoculate into calf thyroid monolayers. Concentrated suspensions (10%) are often cytotoxic. A 10^{-2} suspension, or even higher dilutions of the suspension, may have to be used to reduce the cytotoxicity. (4) Incubate and observe the cultures as outlined above.

The serial transfer of virus isolated in bovine thyroid cells can be carried out by the subinoculation of infected viable tissue culture cells into fresh tissue culture cells. The detachment of infected monolayers can be accomplished by mechanical means, using a rubber policeman, or by the use of versene and/or trypsin in concentration of 0.02 or 0.01%. During the early stages, it is necessary to mix infected cells with the normal bovine thyroid cells at the ratio of one part infected cells to three parts normal cells at the time of seeding the new culture tubes. This is because initially the virus is almost entirely cell associated, with little if any free virus found. Significant amounts of cell-free virus can generally by obtained in somewhere between 7 and 20 passages of infected cells. There is evidence that use of roller tube cultures will enhance the rate of virus propagation and the degree of cytopathogenic effects in contrast to use of stationary cultures.

Observations or tests that indicate propagation of the virus in tissue cultures, excluding serology, are as follows: (1) cytopathology, including discrete syncytium formation, with formation of DNA-positive intranuclear inclusions and sometimes irregular cytoplasmic inclusions of which a proportion at least is also DNA-positive; (2) the absence or virtual absence of cell-free infectivity in early culture passages, although transmission is easy with intact cells; (3) the production of typical MCF in susceptible cattle inoculated parenterally with intact cells, with an incubation period in the range of 10–60 days and death in some animals after 5–10 days (recovery is possible).

Animal inoculation. Rabbits can be infected easily with the wildebeest virus strain by parenteral routes and react after 9–60 days. They invariably die, with characteristic lesions, particularly of lymphoid tissues.[4] The experimental host range of the sheep strains of virus includes also the rabbit and red deer, both of which develop a severe, fatal disease.[2] However, the sheep-associated MCF virus is more difficult to transmit to rabbits than is the wildebeest-associated MCF virus.

Immunology and serology. After the virus in the tissue culture systems starts to be liberated through serial passages, the free virus can be used in conventional VN tests with immune serum obtained from cattle that have recovered from the disease. The serologic method of choice is the constant virus–variable serum test, using approximately 100 $TCID_{50}$ of virus. Antibodies appear only late in the convalescence of the disease and do not reach high titers. Therefore, two- or fourfold dilutions of serum are recommended. The serum-virus mixtures are incubated overnight at 4°C prior to inoculation into the susceptible tissue cultures. The AD test may also be used as a serologic method, provided there are high titers of virus obtained from the tissue culture system.

Cattle that recover from infection with one wildebeest strain of virus are completely resistant to challenge by any other virulent isolate for periods up to at least 7 years.[6] The usual methods of challenge are by the SC inoculation of lymph node suspensions (5 ml of 10^{-1} suspension) or the IV inoculation of 5 ml of blood freshly harvested from infected cattle. It is assumed that these observations are true also for sheep virus infections although experimental data are lacking. A proportion of cattle that receive high-passage, cell-free culture virus develop neutralizing antibody and resist challenge without showing any clinical reaction.

References
1. Blood, D.C., H.C. Roswell, and M. Savan. An outbreak of bovine malignant catarrh in a dairy herd. II. Transmission experiments. *Can. Vet. J.* 2:319–325, 1961.

2. Huck, R.A., A. Shand, P.J. Allsop, and A.B. Paterson. Malignant catarrh of deer. *Vet. Rec.* 73:457–465, 1961.
3. Piercy, S.E. Studies in bovine malignant catarrh: Experimental infection in cattle. *Brit. Vet. J.* 103:35–47, 1952.
4. Piercy, S.E. Studies in bovine malignant catarrh. VI. Adaptation in rabbits. *Brit. Vet. J.* 111:484–491, 1955.
5. Plowright, W. Studies on the virus of malignant catarrhal fever in Africa. *Proc. 17th World Vet. Cong.* (Hannover) 1:519–523, 1963.
6. Plowright, W. Studies on malignant catarrhal fever of cattle. D.V.Sc. thesis, University of Pretoria, South Africa, 1964.
7. Plowright, W. Malignant catarrhal fever in East Africa. II. Observations on wildebeest calves at the laboratory and contact transmission of the infection to cattle. *Res. Vet. Sci.* 6:69–83, 1965.
8. Plowright, W., and R.D. Ferris. The preparation of bovine thyroid monolayers for use in virological investigations. *Res. Vet. Sci.* 2:149–152, 1961.
9. Plowright, W., R.D. Ferris, and G.R. Scott. Blue wildebeest and the aetiological agent of malignant catarrhal fever. *Nature* 188:1167–1169, 1960.
10. Plowright, W., R.F. Macadam, and J.A. Armstrong. Growth and characterization of the virus of bovine malignant catarrhal fever in East Africa. *J. Gen. Microbiol.* 39:253–266, 1965.
11. Rinjard, P. Contribution à l'étude experimentale du coryza gangreneux. *Recueil Med. Vet.* 111:335–356, 1935.
12. Roderick, L.M. Malignant catarrhal fever. *Vet. Med.* 54:509–512, 1959.
13. Storz, H. Comments on malignant catarrhal fever. *J. Am. Vet. Med. Ass.* 152:804–806, 1968.

Bovine Herpes Mammillitis Virus

Bovine herpes mammillitis (BHM) is a viral, ulcerative infection primarily affecting teats and udders of lactating cows. The virus can invade other areas of the skin and infection is related to trauma. Transmission of the disease within a herd may be via milkers' hands or milking machines. The disease occurs more frequently during late fall and winter. Experimentally, calves and baby mice can be infected.

Generally the infection causes extensive swelling of the teat wall. The skin over the affected areas becomes soft and may slough within 48 hours leaving deep, irregularly shaped, painful ulcers, which may exude serous fluid until a scab is formed. Uncomplicated cases show no clinical signs of systemic illness. Mastitis may occur as a complication, often resulting when the lesions are so severe that milking is impossible, or when the swelling affects the teat sphincter muscles.

The virus produces Cowdrey type A eosinophilic intranuclear inclusions in the cells of the epidermis. Electron microscopy of epidermal specimens reveals that the replication and extracellular extrusion of the mature BHM virus is most widespread about 8 days after inoculation. Also, many cytoplasmic inclusions may be found adjacent to infected nuclei of epidermal cell syncytia.[1]

The BHM virus, in electron microscopy, appears as a spherical capsid, which in the complete particle is surrounded by a loose envelope. The virion has the same appearance and diameter as the duck plague virus.

Specimens

The BHM virus has been isolated from lesion biopsies and the fluid exudate of lesions. The virus titer in milk samples is usually very low.[3] It is important to select early lesions for virus isolation.[1]

Laboratory Procedures

Cultures. Fetal calf kidney and baby hamster kidney cell cultures may be used for virus isolation. The virus produces a CPE and multinucleated syncytia are found.[4] Intranuclear inclusions may be found in the infected tissue culture cells. A cell line of feline lung cells also will support viral replication.[5]

Animal inoculation. Calves and baby mice can be used as laboratory animals. Calves inoculated with BHM virus may have an inflamed raised plaque in the skin at the site of inoculation in about 6 days.[2] Superficial ulceration may occur and the lesion may heal within a week. Virus can be recovered from such lesions.

Immunology and serology. BHM viral isolates have been made in Great Britain, the United States, and Italy. All of these isolates as well as the Allerton herpesvirus (AHV) (see lumpy skin disease) appear to be serologically identical. No serologic relationships were found between these viruses and herpes simplex virus.[2] The VN test has been used for both virus and serum identification.[5]

Natural infection of individual animals shows the severity of the disease decreasing as the infection progresses through the herd. Where such active immunity is present, field observations reveal that clinical BHM does not occur over a period of at least 2 years, and actual resistance to reinfection may be of a much longer duration.[6] The most practical vaccine is a nonattenuated live virus given IM; the TV strain of BHM was used for this purpose in Great Britain.[6] The vaccine was safely used in pregnant cows, there was no evidence of transmission to susceptible contact animals, and resistance to challenge was evident in about a week and lasted for at least 8 months.[6] The live virus vaccine was superior to inactivated virus vaccines that were tested.[6]

References

1. Lepper, A.W.D., D.A. Haig, and J. Wilcox. Cellular pathology of calves experimentally infected with bovine herpes mammillitis virus. *J. Comp. Path.* 79:489–494, 1969.
2. Martin, W.B., B. Martin, D. Hay, and I.M. Lander. Bovine ulcerative mammillitis caused by a herpesvirus. *Vet. Rec.* 78:495–497, 1966.
3. Martin, W.B., Z. James, I.M. Lauder, M. Murray, and H.M. Pirie. Pathogenesis of bovine mammillitis virus infection in cattle. *Am. J. Vet. Res.* 30:2151–2166, 1969.
4. Rweyemamu, M.M, and R.H. Johnson. Bovine herpes mammillitis virus: I. *In vitro* behavior of the virus. *Brit. Vet. J.* 123:482–491, 1967.
5. Rweyemamu, M.M., and R.H. Johnson. Bovine herpes mammillitis virus: II. Standardization of an *in vitro*. neutralization test. *Brit. Vet. J.* 124:9–15, 1968.
6. Rweyemamu, M.M, and R.H. Johnson. The development of a vaccine for bovine herpes mammillitis. *Res. Vet. Sci.* 10:419–427, 1969.
7. Rweyemamu, M.M., A.D. Osborne, and R.H. Johnson. Observations on the histopathology of bovine herpes mammillitis. *Res. Vet. Sci.* 10:203–207, 1969.

Marek's Disease Virus

Neural lymphomatosis, range paralysis, fowl paralysis, and skin leukosis are all synonyms for Marek's disease (MD). The chicken is the primary host for the virus, but turkeys, pheasants, and possibly quail can also be infected. Clinical signs and lesions similar to those of MD have been reported in ducks, geese, pigeons, canaries, budgerigars, and swans.[3,8]

Marek's disease is caused by a herpesvirus belonging to the B group of cell-associated herpesviruses. The virions are 85–100 nm in diameter and the capsid is composed of 162 hollow cylindrical capsomeres. Virus particles from the feather follicles have a similar morphology but usually have a loose irregular envelope up to 400 nm in diameter. DNA extracted from the virus has a high guanine-cytosine content similar to that of cytomegaloviruses. All isolates so far examined have cross-reacted in the AD and FA tests;[4,7] however, some isolates passaged in cell culture have been altered antigenically. By cross-absorption and use of FA or AD tests, some pathogenic isolates can be differentiated from some nonpathogenic field isolates. A herpesvirus isolated from turkeys (HVT) is antigenically related to Marek's disease virus but is distinguishable from it in AD and FA tests and is nonpathogenic for chickens and turkeys.[6,11]

Marek's disease is a lymphoproliferative disease that primarily affects the nervous system, but visceral organs and other tissues may also be involved.[1,3,8] The mildest or classic form of Marek's disease is characterized by paresis or paralysis of one or more of the extremities, but any nerve may be affected, so the clinical signs vary. The wings, tail, neck, or eyelids may droop and birds sometimes gasp. All degrees of severity may be encountered.[9] In the most acute forms, the disease may affect birds as early as 6–8 weeks of age, but the disease also occurs in older birds. The only antemortem signs may be depression and anorexia. Morbidity and mortality may exceed 50% of the flock and birds that die have lymphoid tumors, which affect most commonly the gonads, liver, kidney, heart, lungs, and skin.

The visceral tumors of MD and lymphoid leukosis cannot be distinguished by gross examination alone; however, the history, symptoms, gross and microscopic pathology, and cytology are of assistance. (These two diseases are compared in the section in this manual on leukosis.) The peripheral nerves and ganglia may be infiltrated with pleomorphic lymphocytes. Tumors composed of pleomorphic lymphocytes may occur in the visceral organs, skin, and muscle. There occasionally may be a diffuse enlargement of the bursa of Fabricius due to interfollicular accumulation of lymphoid cells; however, an atrophy of this organ or no change is a more common finding.[9] Characteristic inclusion bodies are sometimes observed in the epithelial lining of the feather follicles.

Specimens

Virus can be readily isolated from diseased chickens and from many normal-appearing chickens once infection is established in a flock.[12] Infection persists in a bird for long periods, possibly for the rest of its life. Congenital infection probably does not occur, so embryos and young chicks are free of virus. Tumor cells, kidney cells, and whole blood are the specimens of choice. Since the virus is highly cell-associated in these tissues, whole cells must be used as inoculum and storage of specimens for virus isolation should be under conditions that preserve the viability of the cells, that is, addition of dimethyl sulfoxide, slow freezing, and storage at $-196°C$. Enveloped virus has been demonstrated in the feather follicles.[2] These may be the only places where complete virus is produced, and this production is probably responsible for the infectivity of dander, litter, and poultry house dust. Feces and oral and nasal washings have been shown to be infectious, but are not good sources of virus.

Herpesviruses

Laboratory Procedures

Cultures. The virus may be demonstrated by the inoculation of laboratory animals, cell cultures, or embryonating chicken eggs. Pathogenic strains of virus produce symptoms and lesions in genetically susceptible chicks, such as line 7 or Cornell S, in 18–21 days when chicks are inoculated intra-abdominal (IAb) at 1 day of age.[1] Gross or microscopic lesions in the nerves and/or viscera, the presence of specific antigen in the feather follicles, virus isolation in cell culture, and detection of antibody are all suitable criteria of infection.

Marek's disease virus produces characteristic plaques in duck embryo fibroblast and chick kidney cell cultures.[5,10] Plaques that appear in 6–14 days consist of rounded and fusiform refractile cells and polykaryocytes that have Cowdry type-A, DNA-containing intranuclear inclusion bodies. Direct cultivation of kidney cells from test chickens is the most sensitive method of isolation of the virus; however, inoculation of cell cultures with whole blood, or suspension of tumor, spleen, kidney, or buffy-coat cells of blood, is also suitable. Virus isolation in cell culture is from tenfold to more than a thousandfold less sensitive than chicken inoculation.

The virus produces pocks on the CAM of embryonating eggs inoculated by the YS or CAM routes at 4–6 or 10–11 days respectively.

Identification of the virus may be based on both the in vivo response and cell culture changes. The presence of infection in a bird may be confirmed serologically or by examination of the feather follicles for immunofluorescent antigen or for virus particles. In cell culture, the characteristic cytopathologic response may be prevented by inhibitors of viral DNA synthesis.

Animal inoculation. Other than chickens and turkeys, the usual laboratory animals cannot be used.

Immunology and serology. Antibody can be demonstrated in the sera of exposed or recovered birds by the AD or indirect FA tests. Antigen for the AD test consists of chick kidney or duck embryo fibroblast cultures. It can also be prepared by homogenizing the skin of feather tracts from infected birds. The antigen is placed in a well in an agar layer containing 8% NaCl and the antibody in an adjacent well. Precipitin lines develop after 24–72 hours. More than one line may develop. The major line produced by antigen, which is present in cell culture supernates and skin extracts, has been referred to as the A precipitin line, and the others have been lettered alphabetically. The A line is absent in laboratory-attenuated strains.

Antigen for the indirect FA test is usually prepared by growing infected chick kidney cells on coverslips.[7] After fixation in acetone, the coverslips are reacted with a dilution of chicken serum and the excess is washed off. They are then stained with fluorescein-conjugated antichicken globulin and examined. If the serum is positive, antigen in both the nucleus and cytoplasm of the infected cells will fluoresce.

The AD test is most widely used for the detection of antibody to MD virus and for distinguishing between the virulent and tissue culture–attenuated strains.[4] The indirect FA test has been used to distinguish between MD virus and HVT.[6,11]

Most birds and almost all flocks of chickens have antibody to MD by the time they reach sexual maturity, whether or not the flock has suffered losses from MD. Thus the presence of antibody is only an indication of past infection and is of no value in determining the cause of death.

There is no effective immunity to virus infection; however, the resistance of birds to tumor formation may be affected by the genetic line of chickens, the age at which exposure occurs, the antibody status of the dam, and exposure to avirulent viruses. The resistance of chickens may be evaluated by the IAb inoculation of virulent virus or by contact exposure to infected chickens. Depending on the nature of the challenge virus, the age when inoculated, and the resistance of the chickens, a satisfactory response may be obtained in 6–20 weeks.

Passive immunity will delay the onset and reduce the incidence of disease in birds challenged at 1 day of age by a natural route, but it has little effect when birds are challenged by IAb inoculation. The protective effect is lost by the time birds are 3 weeks of age.

Commercial vaccines to be administered IAb during the first day of life are available. Attenuated or nonpathogenic strains of MD or HVT are effective in markedly reducing the clinical form of Marek's disease.[6]

References

1. Biggs, P.M., and L.N. Payne. Studies on Marek's disease. I. Experimental transmission. *J. Nat. Cancer Inst.* 39:267–280, 1967.
2. Calnek, B.W., and S.B. Hitchner. Localization of viral antigen in chickens infected with Marek's disease herpesvirus. *J. Nat. Cancer Inst.* 43:935–949, 1969.
3. Calnek, B.W., and R.L. Witter. Marek's disease. In *Diseases of Poultry,* M.S. Hofstead, B.W. Calnek, C.F. Helmboldt, W.M. Reid, and H.W. Yoder (eds.), pp. 470–502. 6th ed. Iowa State University Press, Ames, 1972.
4. Chubb, R.C., and A.E. Churchill. Precipitating antibodies associated with Marek's disease. *Vet. Rec.* 83:4–7, 1968.
5. Churchill, A.E., and P.M. Biggs. Agent of Marek's disease in tissue culture. *Nature* 215:528–530, 1967.
6. Okazaki, W., H.G. Purchase, and B.R. Burmester. Protection against Marek's disease by vaccination with a herpesvirus of turkeys (HVT). *Avian Dis.* 14:413–429, 1970.
7. Purchase, H.G. Immunofluorescence in the study of Marek's disease. I. Detection of antigen in cell culture and an antigenic comparison of eight isolates. *J. Virol.* 3:557–565, 1969.
8. Purchase, H.G. Recent advances in the knowledge of Marek's disease. In *Advances in Veterinary Science and Comparative Medicine,* C.A. Brandly and E.L. Jungherr (eds.), vol. 16, pp. 223–258. Academic Press, New York, London, 1972.
9. Purchase, H.G., and P.M. Biggs. Characterization of five isolates of Marek's disease. *Res. Vet. Sci.* 8:440–449, 1967.
10. Solomon, J.J., P.A. Long, and W. Okazaki. Procedures for the *in vitro* assay of viruses and antibody of avian lymphoid leukosis and Marek's disease. ARS Agriculture Handbook no. 404, p. 18. U.S. Government Printing Office, Washington, 1971.
11. Witter, R.L., K. Nazarian, H.G. Purchase, and G.H. Burgoyne. Isolation from turkeys of a cell-associated herpesvirus antigenically related to Marek's disease virus. *Am. J. Vet. Res.* 31:525–538, 1970.
12. Witter, R.L., J.J. Solomon, and G.H. Burgoyne. Cell culture techniques for primary isolation of Marek's disease–associated herpesvirus. *Avian Dis.* 13:101–118, 1969.

Avian Infectious Laryngotracheitis Virus

Infectious laryngotracheitis (ILT) is an acute respiratory disease primarily involving adult chickens.[11] The disease was first described in the United States in 1925.[10] Later it was identified in Canada, Great Britain, Europe, Australia, and Finland. The disease was identified as infectious bronchitis by some workers but the name was later established as ILT.[1]

ILT virus causes an acute epizootic disease in chickens that is characterized by gasping, coughing, and moist rales and serous exudation from the nostrils. The coughing may be so severe that it results in expulsion of bloody mucus. Death results from asphyxiation when the trachea and bronchi become occluded by tissue exudates and clotted blood. The most extensive tissue changes occur in the trachea and bronchi. The first changes are edema and cellular infiltration of the mucosa. Later necrosis of cellular elements of the mucosa and hemorrhage are followed by desquamation of large areas of tracheal mucosa. Intranuclear inclusions appear in the epithelial cells of the trachea during the first few days of clinical illness, but the cells containing the inclusions are often absent at time of death due to desquamation of the mucosa.

ILT is most likely to be confused with Newcastle disease and infectious bronchitis. Distinguishing characteristics of ILT are as follows: (1) only respiratory signs are produced; (2) coughing with expulsion of mucus and blood occurs; (3) depression of egg production is less severe than in Newcastle disease and infectious bronchitis infections; (4) plaques are consistently produced on the CAM of inoculated embryonating eggs; (5) intranuclear inclusions can be consistently demonstrated in the affected cells.

Specimens

The virus can be most consistently isolated from tracheal and lung tissue removed aseptically from affected birds. Tracheal swabs can be used to isolate virus from acutely ill birds or from some chickens during the carrier stage following clinical recovery. Some birds may remain carriers as long as 2 years following the acute illness. The tracheal and lung tissue or swab suspensions can be stored in 50% glycerol-saline solution at −20 or −70°C for extended periods prior to inoculation of embryonating eggs or cell culture.

Laboratory Procedures

Cultures. ILT virus is easily cultivated in 10-day-old embryonating chicken eggs inoculated by either the CAM or the allantoic routes.[3] The virus causes proliferation of groups of cells on the CAM, with the formation of plaques and usually the death of the embryos in 5–12 days. Embryos do not always die, however, especially during the initial passage. Intranuclear inclusions can be observed in histologic sections of the CAM plaques after one or more days of incubation. Inoculation of chicken embryo kidney cell cultures with ILT virus results in the formation of giant cells, intranuclear inclusions, and necrosis.[5] Cell changes may be observed as early as 12–18 hours but are most marked at 24–48 hours. Cell culture cultivation of ILT virus is most readily accomplished with 10% suspensions of infected CAM.

Animal inoculation. ILT infections occur naturally only in chickens. The reservoir of infections appears to result from the presence of recovered or vaccinated chickens. Pheasants are susceptible to inoculations and to contact exposure.[8,9] Turkeys are also susceptible to inoculation of ILT virus, but natural infections have not been demonstrated.[12] Inoculation of the infraorbital sinus of the chicken with ILT virus results in swelling of the sinus and discharge of serous fluids,[6] but this procedure is not definitive since *Mycoplasma gallisepticum* can cause similar signs. Detection of the etiologic agent of ILT can be made by suspending ground trachea or tracheal exudates in 50% glycerol-saline solution and inoculating susceptible chickens intratracheally (IT). Inflammation of the larynx develops in 49 hours, followed by necrosis and occlusion of the opening by the fourth or fifth day. Similarly, the suspension can be brushed on the abraded surface of the bursa of Fabricius of a sexually immature bird. The bursa becomes markedly inflamed about the second day and reaches its height of reaction on the fourth or fifth day. Chickens inoculated on the bursa do not die. Identification of ILT can be made 10–20 days later by demonstrating resistance to a challenge inoculation of virulent virus IT or into the infraorbital sinuses. No respiratory symptoms should develop. The Lederle strain (ATCC VR-23) is available for this purpose.

Immunology and serology. Generally, VN tests have been used to demonstrate the presence of antibodies in chicken sera.[4] The test is conducted in 9–12-day-old embryonating eggs, the serum is mixed with tenfold dilutions of ILT virus, and the virus and serum mixtures are incubated at room temperature for 30 minutes before inoculation of the eggs. About 6 days later, the EID_{50} is determined by examination of the CAM for plaque formation. Neutralization tests can also be conducted in chicken kidney cell cultures.[5,7] The test can be conducted in culture tubes and evaluations made by neutralization of cell changes or in monolayer agar overlay cultures by the PR test.

References

1. Beach, J.R. Infectious bronchitis of fowls. *J. Am. Vet. Med. Ass.* 68:570–580, 1926.
2. Brandly, C.A. Some studies of laryngotracheitis: the continued propagation of the virus upon the CAM of the hen's egg. *J. Infec. Dis.* 57:201–206, 1935.
3. Burnet, F.M. The propagation of the virus of ILT on the CAM of the developing egg. *Brit. J. Exp. Path.* 15:52–55, 1934.
4. Burnet, F.M. Immunological studies with the virus of ILT of fowl using the developing egg technique. *J. Exp. Med.* 63:685–701, 1936.
5. Chang, P.W., V.J. Yates, A.H. Dardiri, and D.E. Fry. Some observations on the propagation of ILT in tissue culture. *Avian Dis.* 4:384–390, 1960.
6. Hitchner, S.B., and P.G. White. A comparison of embryo and bird infectivity using five strains of laryngotracheitis virus. *Poul. Sci.* 37:684–690, 1958.
7. Howes, D.W., et al. The assessment of a potency standard for infectious laryngotracheitis vaccine in dose-response experiments. *Proc. XII World's Poul. Cong.* (Sydney), pp. 344–348, 1962.
8. Hudson, C.B., and F.R. Beaudette. The susceptibility of pheasants and a pheasant bantam cross to the virus of infectious bronchitis. *Cornell Vet.* 22:70–74, 1932.
9. Kernohan, G. Infectious laryngotracheitis in pheasants. *J. Am. Vet. Med. Ass.* 78:553–555, 1931.
10. May, H.G., and R.P. Tittsler. Tracheolaryngitis in poultry. *J. Am. Vet. Med. Ass.* 67:229–231, 1925.
11. Seddon, H.R. A detailed review of appearance and spread of ILT to certain physical and chemical factors. *J. Infec. Dis.* 56:210–223, 1935.
12. Winterfield, R.W. Susceptibility of turkeys to infectious laryngotracheitis. *Avian Dis.* 12:191–201, 1968.

Duck Plague Virus

Duck plague (DP) is a disease that infects only birds of the genus *Ansirinae*, and it is known to occur in the Netherlands, Belgium, India, China, and the United States.[8] Species affected include many of the common types of ducks, geese, swans, and wild waterfowl. The disease is also known as duck virus enteritis. The effects of duck plague have been most severe on large duck farms, where the disease may kill 90% of the flock in only 3–4 weeks. It is an acute or peracute disease lasting about 1–3 days. The first signs of the disease are apparent about 4–7 days after infection: the ducks are listless, moving only with difficulty; there is a sticky discharge from nostrils and eyes; the ducks experience total inappetence but increased thirst; and there is watery diarrhea with fouling around the cloaca.[2] Gross changes seen at autopsy include petechiae throughout the body, which is most marked on the heart, serous membranes, and mucosa of the esophagus. There also are hemorrhages of the ovary, peritonitis, and diptherial esophagitis and cloacitis. Microscopic lesions occur in all organs but are most frequent in lymphoid tissues.[9] Often inclusion bodies are seen in nuclei of cells in which the core wall is disrupted and indistinct. Under the electron microscope, duck plague virus particles have a dense core surrounded by an envelope, and, when in the nuclei of cells, the virion has a diameter of 91 nm and a core diameter of 48 nm; in the cytoplasm, the virus has a diameter of 181 nm and a core diameter of 75 nm. There also are smaller particles in the nuclei of cells that measure 32 nm in diameter.[3] When subjected to DNase for 2 hours, the core of the virus is digested. The virus is inactivated in about 10 minutes at 56°C and in 2 hours at 50°C.

Specimens

Virus can be recovered from blood, liver, spleen, and kidneys by inoculation of cell cultures and embryonating duck eggs.

Laboratory Procedures

Cultures. Inoculating tissue suspensions from field cases onto the CAM of embryonating duck eggs results in the death of the embryos about 5 days later. Primary isolation of the virus cannot be done in embryonating chicken eggs, but the virus will grow on the chick's CAM after about 12 duck egg passages. Duck embryonating eggs are used for producing the virulent strain of the virus and yield the highest concentrations at 144 hours when injected via the CAM route, and at 144 and 168 hours in the YS. After 20 passages in chicken eggs, the virus no longer is pathogenic for ducks. Chicken embryos used for the attenuated strain yield the highest titers when injected via the CAM. Concentration is highest in amnioallantoic fluid about 96 hours after inoculation and in the CAM at 144 hours.[1]

Duck plague virus can be adapted to grow well in tissue cultures of duck embryo fibroblasts.[6] Cultures inoculated with infectious material show typical herpes CPE and inclusion bodies in 3–4 days. To detect small quantities of virus, it may be necessary to inoculate a susceptible duck and reproduce the disease.

Animal inoculation. Laboratory animals other than ducks are not used.

Immunology and serology. The VN and PR tests are used to identify or assess serum antibodies or virus. The AD and FA tests also may be used. The serum antibody level is not a reliable indicator of resistance to reinfection.[7] Duck plague virus is not neutralized by serum from ducks infected with Newcastle disease, fowl plague, or duck hepatitis. The PR test may be used for this differentiation.

Vaccine made from the CAM of embryonating chicken eggs (attenuated strain) is effective against the virulent strain of duck plague virus. It will not revert to the virulent strain after passages in duck embryos. Injected IM, 1 ml of the suspension (one embryo CAM in 15 ml broth) protects against a dose of 1000 times the minimum lethal dose (MLD). The importance of an interference phenomenon has been demonstrated, in that the vaccine is effective when given 4 hours after introduction of the virus. Therefore, if an outbreak of duck plague should occur, ducks not showing signs often can still be protected by giving them the vaccine.[5] The presence of interferon in these circumstances has not been demonstrated although it is suspected.

References

1. Breese, S.S., Jr., and A.H. Dardiri. Electron microscopic characterization of duck plague virus. *Virology* 34:160–169, 1968.
2. Butterfield, W.K., F.A. Ata, and A.H. Dardiri. Duck plague virus distribution in embryonating chicken and duck eggs. *Avian Dis.* 13:198–202, 1969.
3. Dardiri, A.H., and W.R. Hess. A plague assay for duck plague virus. *Can. J. Comp. Med.* 32:505–510, 1968.
4. Dardiri, A.H., W.R. Hess, S.S. Breese, Jr., and H.R. Seibold. Characterization of a duck virus from a disease outbreak in the United States. *Abstr. Proc. 39th Northeastern Conf. Avian Dis.* (State University of New York, Stony Brook), 1967.
5. Jansen, J. Duck plague. *Brit. Vet. J.* 117:349–356, 1961.
6. Jansen, J. The interference phenomenon in the development of resistance against duck plague. *J. Comp. Path. Ther.* 74:3–7, 1964.
7. Jansen, J. Duck plague. *J. Am. Vet. Med. Ass.* 152:1009–1016, 1968.
8. Kunst, H. Isolation of duck plague virus in tissue cultures. *Tijdschr. Diergeneesk.* 92:713–714, 1967.
9. Leibovitz, L. Gross and histopathologic changes of duck plague (duck virus enteritis). *Am. J. Vet. Res.* 32:275–290, 1971.

Swine Cytomegalovirus

Swine cytomegalovirus (SCMV) infections are caused by a type B herpesvirus, and severe infections of young swine are often referred to as inclusion body rhinitis or cytomegalic inclusion disease. Piglets up to 4 weeks of age are most severely affected, and suffer increased nasal discharge, sneezing, and labored breathing, which may progress to death within 3 weeks.[2] When introduced into a noninfected herd, morbidity of all ages is almost 100%, although in herds where the disease has become established, only newborn animals are severely affected.[2]

Gross lesions seen at necropsy of swine with SCMV include petechiation of kidneys and edema of varying extent in the subcutis, which frequently involves the muscle tissues, hydrothorax, and interstitial pulmonary edema. In some cases, myocardial petechiation, fibrinous pericarditis, and hemorrhagic or necrohemorrhagic enteritis are observed.[6]

Microscopic changes are best observed in the mixed glands of the nasal mucosa. Cells in early stages of infection exhibit a swollen nucleus containing conspicuous intranuclear inclusion bodies. Eventually, the glands and ducts undergo necrosis and, unless secondary bacterial infection occurs, healing by granulation tissue and fibrosis results. Massive lymphoid infiltration of the propria is seen, forming larger and more numerous nodules than those found in the normal turbinate.[3]

The agent of SCMV is an ether-sensitive virus that induces greatly enlarged cells with characteristically large basophilic intranuclear inclusion bodies. Electron microscopy indicates that the cytomegalic state of affected cells is due to distension of the endoplasmic reticulum and Golgi apparatus and swelling of mitochondria. The inclusion body itself is composed of dense granular chromatin and 70–100 nm membrane-bound particles. Double-membraned particles measuring 100–150 nm are frequently seen in the distended endoplasmic reticulum and Golgi, as well as in the extracellular space. Single-membraned particles, resembling those in the nuclei inclusion bodies, are seen free in the cytoplasm and are believed to acquire the second membrane by budding into the endoplasmic reticulum.[4]

Specimens

Turbinate and nasal mucosal tissue from infected pigs 2–4 weeks old yield the greatest amount of virus. An electron microscopic study of the nasal mucosa of piglets from a natural outbreak disclosed that the SCMV particles are numerous, easily located, and arranged in crystalline arrays both in the nucleus and cytoplasm of the infected cells.[7] Thus specimens should be taken for electron microscopy, FA test, and histologic examination, as well as for viral isolation.

Laboratory Procedures

Cultures. A 1:20 suspension of pooled nasal mucosa and turbinate tissue prepared in PBS should be lightly centrifuged and passed through a 0.45 μm filter under positive pressure.[6] Swine cytomegalovirus can then be propagated in pig lung cell cultures.[5] The cell cultures should be inoculated with 0.1 ml of the ground turbinate and nasal mucosa filtrate, and serial passages made by transferring 0.1 ml of pooled cells and fluids to fresh pig lung cultures.[6] The CPE are usually first observed 17 days after inoculation of primary cultures. Initially, small foci of clear, refractile, but enlarged cells that retain their normal polygonal shape are observed. The foci appear to be slightly raised above the level of the surrounding cell sheet. The enlarged cells slowly become rounded or spindle shaped, very refractile, and detached from the glass. The CPE is progressive from the center to the periphery of the foci and involves only a small portion of the total cell sheet.

Inclusion bodies can be seen in stained cultures (May-Grünwald-Giemsa or MGG stain) as small, irregularly-shaped, granular pink-to-violet masses in the nuclei of cells in the early stages of infection. Some bodies may be surrounded by a clear zone. As CPE progresses, the inclusions become larger, stain a deep purple, and displace the nucleoli peripherally. Eventually, margination of chromatin and condensation of the inclusion bodies are evident, and some cells show enlarged, deformed nucleoli. At this point, the inclusion becomes very dense and is surrounded by a clear halo. The cytoplasm appears dense, especially adjacent to the nucleus, and is often filled with clear vacuoles. In the terminal stages of cell degeneration, the affected cells round up and become very dark and opaque.[6] Cell cultures prepared from kidneys, testes, and salivary gland tissues of infected animals also develop intranuclear inclusion bodies typical of the disease.[1]

Animal inoculation. Apparently only pigs are susceptible.

Immunology and serology. The VN and FA tests are used.

References

1. Booth, J.C., R.F. Goodwin, and P. Whittlestone. Inclusion body rhinitis of pigs: Attempts to grow the causal agent in tissue culture. *Res. Vet. Sci.* 8:338–345, 1967.
2. Cameron-Stephen, I.D. Inclusion body rhinitis of swine: Clinical aspects. *Austral. Vet. J.* 37:87–91, 1961.
3. Done, J.T. An inclusion-body rhinitis of pigs. *Vet. Rec.* 67:525–527, 1955.
4. Duncan, J.R., F.K. Ramsey, and W.P. Switzer. Electron microscopy of cytomegalic inclusion disease of swine. *Am. J. Vet. Res.* 26:939–947, 1965.
5. Hinz, R.W., and J.T. Syverton. Mammalian cell cultures for study of influenza virus. *Proc. Soc. Exp. Biol. Med.* 101:19, 1959.
6. L'Ecuyer, C., and A.H. Cornei. Propagation of porcine cytomegalic inclusion disease virus in cell cultures: Preliminary report. *Can. J. Comp. Med. Vet. Sci.* 30:321–326, 1966.
7. Valicek, L., B.I. Smid, and J. Mensik. Electron microscopy of porcine cytomegalovirus: Viral cystalline arrays and viral forms in the nasal mucosa of piglets. *Arch. ges. Virusforsch.* 41:344–353, 1973.

Guinea Pig Cytomegalovirus (GPCMV)

Cytomegalovirus in the salivary glands of guinea pigs causes enlargement of the duct cells and produces typical large intranuclear inclusions. Infection acquired naturally is chronic, and infected animals exhibit no overt clinical disease.[1] Electron microscopy reveals three distinct spherical forms of the virus in the nuclei and two distinct cytoplasmic forms. The virus particles appear to leave the nucleus as single particles or in clusters; extracellular virus appears to be similar to one of the two cytoplasmic forms.[2]

Salivary glands infected with GPCMV typically exhibit markedly enlarged duct cells that protrude into the lumen. These cells contain large acidophilic intranuclear inclusions and smaller basophilic cytoplasmic granules or bodies usually seen on the lumenal side of the cell nucleus. Cytoplasmic inclusions are not found in cells devoid of intranuclear inclusions and have not as yet been demonstrated in cell cultures.[2] Both cytoplasmic and intranuclear inclusions are Feulgen positive.

GPCMV primarily infects duct-cell epithelial cells of the serous parts of salivary glands, although occasionally the mucous portions are also involved. Frequently, varying degrees of mononuclear cell infiltration are observed around the infected ducts.[2]

Specimens

The submaxillary salivary glands of infected guinea pigs are the best sources of virus. Virus has also been isolated from spontaneously degenerating cell cultures prepared from infected salivary glands.[1]

Laboratory Procedures

Cultures. The submaxillary glands of guinea pigs are aseptically removed, ground, and diluted 1:10 by weight in Hanks' solution. After centrifugation, the supernatant fluid is further diluted 1:10 and filtered through a 0.45 μm filter under positive pressure. GPCMV can be cultivated in guinea-pig-embryo skin and muscle cells grown in Eagle's basal medium with 15% guinea pig serum. The cultures are maintained in Eagle's basal medium with 5% horse serum.[1] In cell cultures, GPCMV produces multiple foci of round retractile cells that spread peripherally in a slow progressive manner. Infected cells develop large acidophilic intranuclear inclusions surrounded by a clear halo.

Animal inoculation. The disease can be reproduced in guinea pigs by subcutaneously inoculating 0.2 ml of a 10% suspension of infected salivary glands.[3]

Immunology and serology. Although the CPE of GPCMV and human CMV in fibroblast cultures are similar, serologic studies have shown that GPCMV is not antigenically related to either human or murine CMV.[1]

Because most commercially available complement contains antibodies against the GPCMV antigen, it can be used as positive reference sera in the CF test. Only serum from young guinea pigs shown to be free of GPCMV antibodies can be used as a source of complement. Antigen for the CF test consists of tissue culture cells showing CPE that are ground in a Ten Broeck grinder and suspended in the cell culture fluid. CF antibody–free guinea pigs inoculated with GPCMV develop CF antibody titers of 1:64 within 3 weeks. Titers of 1:128 or greater are found in guinea pigs hyperimmunized with submaxillary gland suspensions.[1]

References
1. Hartley, J.W., W.P. Rowe, and R.J. Huebner. Serial propagation of the guinea pig salivary gland virus in tissue culture. *Proc. Soc. Exp. Biol. Med.* 96:281–285, 1957.
2. Middilkamp, J.N., G. Patrizi, and C.A. Reed. Light and electron microscopic studies of the guinea pig cytomegalovirus. *J. Ultrastruct. Res.* 18:85–86, 1967.
3. Smith, M.G. Propagation of salivary gland virus of the mouse in tissue cultures. *Proc. Soc. Exp. Biol. Med.* 86:435–441, 1954.

Pigeon Herpesvirus

Pigeon herpesvirus (PHV) disease was originally described in 1945 in U.S. Army pigeons being trained in the South and having contact with replacements from the United Kingdom.[5] It has since been described in Denmark and the United Kingdom, where it is probably widespread. Young pigeons are most susceptible and, in endemic areas, the disease recurs annually in young stock. Young chickens are not susceptible. The disease is characterized by several nonspecific signs varying in severity and is easily confused with pigeonpox and infectious laryngotracheitis. Affected birds are listless, sit perched and huddled together, and exhibit inappetence and frequently a mild conjunctivitis. In some pigeons, small diphtheroid patches are found in the mouth or pharynx.

The virus is an enveloped icosahedron with a nucleocapsid diameter of 100 nm. The virions are ether sensitive and labile at pH 4. Replication is inhibited by halogenated deoxyuridines and infectivity is destroyed in 30 minutes at 56°C. However, PHV is more stable at lower temperatures than other members of the group. The virus produces typical herpesvirus intranuclear inclusions and in cell culture produces CPE like that of cytomegaloviruses.[3]

In naturally infected pigeons the tissues primarily affected are the liver, kidneys, and the upper respiratory tract, but the effects may be more widespread. The most common lesion is a local necrotizing hepatitis, the severity of which is subject to much variation. The bile ducts contain cellular debris and the capsule of the liver is covered with fibrin containing many heterophils and small numbers of macrophages. Multiple foci of cream-colored necrosis are found in the renal cortex of some birds; these areas of necrosis are seen to be tubules when examined microscopically. Although serous conjunctivitis is seen in most infected birds and mild serous rhinitis is also common, overt lesions of the respiratory system occur infrequently. A diphtheritic membrane coating on the laryngeal mucosa or small ulcers coated with adherent caseous material may be present on the larynx and pharynx of some.

Intranuclear inclusions are readily seen in hepatic cells throughout the organ but are most numerous at the periphery of the smaller necrotic foci. These inclusion bodies vary from pale eosinophilia to intense basophilia upon staining.

Specimens

Liver, spleen, throat swabs, larynx, trachea, and lungs are the most desirable specimens for isolating the virus.

Laboratory Procedures

Cultures. The tissues are triturated in a mortar and pestle in BSS to yield a 10% suspension by volume. The supernatant fluid is harvested, treated with antibiotics, and inoculated into 12-day-old embryonating chicken eggs by dropping 0.2 ml of the inoculum onto the CAM. The eggs are incubated at 39.5°C and examined after 4 days. For further passage, a 10% suspension of the membranes from the first passage is used. At least three serial passages should be made before the sample is regarded negative. Optimum yields of virus are obtained from CAM inoculated eggs after 2 days incubation. Other inoculation sites are unreliable and show decreased virus yield.[2]

Pooled extracts of affected tissues inoculated onto the CAM of embryonating chicken eggs will produce discrete pocks on or before the fourth day. Embryonic death with associated small foci of embryonic hepatic necrosis occurs on about the fifth day. Pock numbers increase with further passaging. Pigeon herpesvirus is cytopathogenic in cell cultures of whole chick embryo, chick embryo kidney, chick embryo liver, chicken kidney, and pigeon kidney, but apparently will not grow in mammalian cells. Antiserum to PHV prepared in rabbits neutralizes PHV but not ILT in whole chicken embryo cell cultures.[1]

Animal inoculation. Pigeons must be used to study the disease. Antiserums may be prepared in rabbits.

Immunology and serology. The outbreaks of PHV described in the United States, Denmark, and the United Kingdom were most likely caused by the same or closely related viruses. The indirect FA test has been used to demonstrate the presence of the virus in the liver and pancreas. Specific viral antigen is found in the nuclei of pancreatic ascinar cells, especially, and in hepatic cells, either on the nucleic margin or uniformly throughout the nucleus.[4]

Little has been reported on immunity to PHV infections. Recovered birds have not been studied nor reported as having been re-exposed to the virus. The disease can be distinguished from ILT and pigeonpox infections, the two diseases with which it is most readily confused, by pathologic means. In embryonating chicken eggs, PHV causes pocks to appear on the CAM and there is early necrosis of the ectoderm, which soon invades the mesoderm, while ILT affects only ectoderm and causes the development of syncytia, in contrast to PHV and pigeonpox.

References
1. Cornwell, H.J.C., and A.R. Weir. A herpesvirus infection of pigeons. *Vet. Rec.* 81:267–268, 1967.
2. Cornwell, H.J.C., and A.R. Weir. Herpesvirus infection of pigeons. III. Use of embryonated eggs for the growth and characterization of the virus. IV. Growth of the virus in tissue culture and comparison of its cytopathogenicity with that of the viruses of laryngotracheitis and pigeon-pox. *J. Comp. Path.* 80:509–515, 517–523, 1970.
3. Cornwell, H.J.C., and N.G. Wright. Herpesvirus infection of pigeons. I. Pathology and virus isolation. *J. Comp. Path.* 80:221–227, 1970.
4. Cornwell, H.J.C., N.G. Wright, and H.B. McCusker. Herpesvirus infection of pigeons. II. Experimental infections of pigeons and chicks. *J. Comp. Path.* 80:229–232, 1970.
5. Smadel, J.E., E.B. Jackson, and S.W. Harman. A new virus disease of pigeons. I. Recovery of the virus. *J. Exp. Med.* 81:385–398, 1945.

Cottontail Rabbit Herpesvirus

The disease produced by the cottontail rabbit herpesvirus (CRH) appears as a progressive chronic malignant lymphoma. Infected rabbits carry the virus for life.[3] CRH was first isolated from the kidneys of apparently healthy weanling cottontail rabbits (*Sylvilagus floridanus*) trapped in southern Wisconsin.[1] No other animals tested have been shown to be susceptible to the infection, including New Zealand white rabbits (*Oryctolagus cuniculus*), mice, hamsters, guinea pigs, and embryonating hens' eggs.

The disease is characterized by massive infiltration of immature lymphoid cells, accompanied by an overall leukocytosis and an elevated lymphocyte differential count. In long-term chronic infection the total white blood cell count reaches 12,000–15,000 as compared to the normal of 6000–8000, with the lymphocyte component comprising about 95% as compared to normal values of 50–60%. The disease develops 6–8 weeks after inoculation but infected animals frequently appear clinically healthy.[2]

Electron microscopy reveals the CRH capsid to be icosahedrally symmetrical with a diameter of approximately 90 nm. Its core is DNA as shown by acridine-orange staining and use of chemical inhibitors. CRH produces intranuclear inclusion bodies typical of the herpesvirus group. Although no distinct envelope is evident, CRH is ether sensitive as well as heat and acid labile, characteristics placing it in the herpesvirus group.

Specimens
While the original isolation of CRH was from cell cultures of infected cottontail rabbit kidneys, the specimen of choice is fresh whole blood. The serum fraction alone will not yield significant quantities of infective virus.[2]

Laboratory Procedures
Cultures. To isolate CRH, dilute 0.5 ml fresh defibrinated blood with 4.5 ml nutrient medium and inoculate onto monolayer cultures of diploid New Zealand white rabbit primary kidney cells. Leave the inoculum on the cells for 2 days, after which the cells can be washed and incubated with fresh medium for 14–21 days at 37°C. CPE typical of the herpesviruses occurs in 10–15 days. Serial passage reduces this time interval; after repeated passages and inoculation with a high concentration of virus, CPE can be seen in 3–6 days. In cell culture CRH produces a similar type of cell destruction in both cottontail and New Zealand white rabbit cells. Initially, focal areas of round distorted cells

are seen, followed in 1 or 2 days by the development of multinucleate syncytial masses containing 50 or more nuclei. Complete cell destruction occurs in 5–7 days. Infected cells show typical type A intranuclear inclusion bodies.

Optimal storage conditions for the virus are obtained by harvesting cultures into medium containing 30% glycerol and storage at −65°C.[3]

Animal inoculation. Antiserum can be prepared by infecting adult cottontail rabbits or by repeatedly inoculating CRH into New Zealand white rabbits. Serum should be collected 12–14 weeks after infection of cottontail rabbits and 1–2 weeks after the final inoculation of the New Zealand whites.

Immunology and serology. CRH does not cross-neutralize with *Herpesvirus hominis*, *H. tamarinus*, *H saimiri*, or *H. suis*, and it also is antigenically distinct from *H. cunicali* (virus III), which causes a similar latent infection in domestic rabbits (*Oryctolagus*). Apparently, once infected, rabbits carry the virus in their leukocytes for life. The strongly cell-associated nature of CRH has been studied and is the basis for classifying CRH in *Herpesvirus* subgroup B.[4]

References

1. Hinze, H.C. Isolation of a new herpesvirus from Cottontail rabbits. *Bact. Proc.*, pp. 149–150, 1968.
2. Hinze, H.C. Rabbit lymphoma induced by a new herpes virus. *Bact. Proc.*, pp. 157–160, 1969.
3. Hinze, H.C. New member of the herpesvirus group isolated from wild Cottontail rabbits. *Infec. Immunity* 3:350–354, 1971.
4. Ley, K.D., and D. Burger. Cell-associated nature of Cottontail rabbit herpesvirus *in vitro*. *Appl. Microbiol.* 19:549–550, 1970.

Channel Catfish Herpesvirus

A virus with characteristics of the herpes group was isolated from several epizootics of an acute hemorrhagic disease causing high mortality in populations of young channel catfish (*Ictalurus punctatus*).[1] Affected fry and fingerlings swim in spirals and hang vertically with their heads at the water surface. The onset of channel catfish virus disease (CCVD) usually follows some kind of stress. It ends with the death of affected fish within 6–15 days. Apparently only channel catfish are suceptible to the virus. Goldfish (*Carrasius auratus*), bluegills (*Lepomis macrochiris*), red ear sunfish (*L. microlopis*), and striped bass (*Morone saxatilis*) are refractory.

Gross pathologic changes observed in moribund and dead fish affected with CCVD include hemorrhages in fins, musculature, liver, kidneys, and spleen. The spleen is often pale red and enlarged. Abdominal ascites is a frequent finding. Exophthalmos on one or both sides of the fish may be present. The stomach may be distended with mucus. However, in many fish the only internal gross pathologic changes are in the kidneys, which are pale and enlarged.

Specimens

Channel catfish disease virus can be isolated from a pooled specimen of viscera, brain, and gills of affected fish on primary cell cultures of channel catfish ovary.

Herpesviruses

Laboratory Procedures

Cultures. Brain, gill, and visceral tissue collected from fish affected with CCVD should be ground with crushed glass in a cold mortar. The resulting paste is diluted with cold Hanks' BSS. Bacteria and debris are removed by passing the suspension through an 0.45 μm filter. The filtrate can then be used to inoculate cell cultures or experimental animals. It may be stored for short periods at −20°C, or at −70°C for up to 20 days.

Primary channel catfish ovary cell cultures are prepared using techniques reported in the literature.[2,3,5] Cells are grown in 85% Eagle's minimum essential medium, 15% fetal bovine serum, plus 100 units per ml penicillin and 100 μg per ml streptomycin. Cell cultures incubated at 27°C develop confluent monolayers in 3–5 days. CCDV will grow in these cells, producing extensive CPE after 2 days. The virus will also replicate in cell cultures derived from the brown bullhead (*Ictalurus nebulasus*), referred to in the literature sometimes as BB cultures. However, the virus will not produce CPE or demonstrable infectious virus in cell cultures derived from at least 14 other animal species, including rainbow trout gonad, fathead minnow, bluegill fry, bullfrog tongue, primary chicken embryo cells, rabbit kidney, rhesus monkey kidney, human embryo, human epidermoid carcinoma #2 (Hep-2), and HeLa.[4]

Early in infection the cell nuclei become basophilic, and by the end of the second hour margination of the chromatin and the beginnings of syncytial formation can be observed. By the fourth hour, intranuclear inclusions are evident in most cell nuclei. Inclusions differ somewhat from the classic Cowdry's type A inclusion, being quite granular and irregular in shape. In the later stages of infection nuclear disintegration can be seen, and basophilic condensations, presumably of nuclear origin, appear in the cytoplasm.

Virus particles in all stages of development can be seen in the nuclei of infected cells from the fourth hour after infection. Three distinct nuclear particles have been described and have been shown by electron microscopy to acquire envelopes by budding into cytoplasmic vacuoles or from the inner lamella of the nuclear membrane into the perinuclear cisterna. Extracellular virus particles are usually enveloped and measure approximately 175–200 nm in diameter. Negative staining techniques reveal the nucleocapsid symmetry to be icosahedral and to contain probably 162 capsomeres. These structural observations, as well as evidence that the virus is ether sensitive and contains DNA, suggest that CCVD is a member of the herpesvirus group.[4]

Animal inoculation. Only channel catfish are susceptible.

Immunology and serology. Very limited studies have been made.

References

1. Fijan, N.N., T.L. Wellborn, Jr., and J.P. Naftel. An acute viral disease of channel catfish. Technical Paper 43. Bureau of Sport Fisheries and Wildlife, U.S. Department of Interior, Fish, and Wildlife Service, 1970.
2. Kinst, L., and N. Fijan. Preparation of primary monolayer cell cultures of carp ovary. *Vet. Arch.* 36:228–236, 1966.
3. Wolf, K. Some recent developments and applications of fish cell and tissue culture. *Prog. Fish Culturist* 27:67–74, 1965.

4. Wolf, K., and R.W. Darlington. Channel catfish virus: A new herpesvirus of Ictalurid fish. *J. Virol.* 8:525–533, 1971.
5. Wolf, K., M.C. Quimby, E.A. Pyle, and R.P. Dexter. Preparation of monolayer cell cultures from tissues of some lower vertebrates. *Science* 132:1890–1891, 1960.

Simian Herpesviruses

The simian herpesviruses consist of a group of at least four distinct serotypes, all of which possess the biologic, chemical, and physical properties generally attributed to the herpesvirus family. Each serotype has its own natural host in which fatal infections rarely occur. Cross-infections among simian species and between simian and humans do occur, and in some instances these result in fulminating fatal infections. Herpes simplex virus must be included or considered in any diagnostic procedure both because of its antigenic similarity to some members of the simian herpesvirus group and because it is infectious for some simian species.

The herpesvirus group may be divided into three subgroups: (1) the true herpesvirus as represented by herpes simplex, (2) the cytomegaloviruses, and (3) the varicella–herpes zoster group. Viruses representing all three groups have been recovered from species of the subhuman primates. This section deals mainly with the four "true herpesviruses" referred to above, but the researcher should be aware that other types of herpesviruses may be encountered in a monkey colony.

Cytomegaloviruses have been recovered from Asiatic, African, and New World simians generally as latent agents in cell cultures prepared from monkey tissues. One of these agents, simian *aethiops* no. 6 (SA6), has been isolated from the salivary glands of African green (vervet) monkeys.[12] No recognized clinical disease in monkeys has been ascribed to infection with these agents, nor is it known if they are infectious for humans. These simian cytomegaloviruses will propagate, however, in human cell cultures.

An agent called *Herpesvirus saimiri* (HVs) has been isolated from squirrel monkeys; it possesses some of the characteristics of both the true herpesviruses and the cytomegalovirus.[15] Growth of this agent is restricted to cells of several New World primates and of the African green monkey. No growth occurs in cells of Asiatic monkeys, humans, and many laboratory and domestic animals. Hamsters inoculated IM or IP were fatally infected. No disease was produced in squirrel monkeys following experimental infection, but both marmosets and owl monkeys developed a fatal disease with neoplastic features. Death occurred between 2 and 4 weeks postinfection. Histopathology was characterized by proliferation and invasion or replacement of organs and tissues by reticulum cells, i.e. reticulum cell sarcoma. Such changes were observed in the liver, kidney, adrenal gland, lymph nodes, spleen, lung, thymus, salivary gland, and Peyer's patches.

Two viruses, possibly identical, have been isolated from fatal exanthematous diseases in green and patas monkeys. The first of these was isolated from fatal infections in a recently colonized group of green monkeys and is referred to as LVV (Liverpool vervet virus).[1] The second was recovered under similar circumstances in a group of patas monkeys.[14] In both the natural and experimental disease in green monkeys the rash occurred first as macules that then progressed to papules and to vesicles. Death occurred 48 hours after onset. Histopathology consisted of disseminated focal necrosis with hemorrhage in the mucosa of the alimentary tract, bladder, uterus, lung parenchyma, liver, adrenal cortex, spleen, pancreas, visceral lymph nodes, and ovary. Infected cells contained intranuclear eosinophilic inclusion bodies, and electron microphotographs further revealed a particle with the physical properties of a herpesvirus. LVV was isolated and propagated in both green and rhesus monkey cell cultures but not in rabbit cells. Growth occurred in foci and the virus was cell associated as is seen with the varicella-zoster group. The virus recovered from patas monkeys had similar properties.

The four strictly simian herpesviruses to be considered in greater detail here are identified in Table 10.1.

Table 10.1. Four simian herpesviruses

Natural host	Virus	Other names
Macaques (*Macaca*)	B-virus	*Herpesvirus simiac*, herpes B
African green monkeys (*Cercopithecus*)	SA8	
Squirrel monkeys (*Saimiri*)	*Herpesvirus tamarinus*	Marmoset herpesvirus, *Herpesvirus platyrrhinae*
Spider monkeys (*Ateles*)	Spider monkey virus (SMV)	

Ecology and Primate Pathogenicity

B-virus. Natural infection with B-virus has been reported in four species of Asiatic macaques, namely *Macaca mulatta, M. irus, M. fuscata,* and *M. cyclopsis*.[3,4] All other Asiatic species should be considered as possibly being susceptible to B-virus until the facts are known. Natural B-virus infections have not been observed in either African or South American simians although the African green monkey (*Cercopithecus*) is susceptible to experimental infection. No clinical evidence of disease was noted, but virus was present in the throat and seroconversion occurred. The susceptibility of New World species to B-virus infection is as yet unknown. The susceptibility of humans to B-virus is probably very low, as judged by the few reported cases, but the virus is extremely virulent when accidental infection does occur.

B-virus produces clinically inapparent or minor disease in its natural host although the virus has been recovered from nearly every tissue or organ of rhesus monkeys. It may be excreted in the saliva, conjunctival fluids, or exudates, or in the urine. Virus has not been recovered, however, from stool or rectal swabs. Clinical disease, when it occurs, is generally limited to oral or skin lesions and to conjunctivitis.

B-virus infection may be more prevalent in colonies of captive rhesus monkeys than it is in the same species in the wild. In one study, sera obtained at time of capture revealed a 10% incidence of B-virus antibody.[11] Two weeks after capture, and following housing in gang cages, 70% of the same group of animals were found to be antibody positive. These observations plus others suggest that a high incidence of active infection might be expected in a recently trapped group of animals. The virus apparently becomes latent in some animals following primary infection, but recurrent active infection can be seen in a few animals at any time even in a well-conditioned colony. Evidence that this also occurs in the wild was presented recently in a report that described the persistence of B-virus infection for 30 years in an isolated but free-roaming colony of rhesus monkeys.[18]

SA8 virus. Little is known about this virus in the African green monkey, from which it was isolated, or in other primate species. Only two isolations have been reported and both of these were made from CNS tissues of green monkeys.[13] In one experimental study an African green monkey with low-level (1:4) neutralizing antibody was inoculated intradermally (ID) and onto scarified lip tissue with high-titered SA8 virus. Mild local lesions developed and persisted for about 1 week. Antibody titer rose to 1:2048 by 3 weeks postinfection. No other signs or symptoms of infection were observed. Although isolation of the virus from African green monkeys has been infrequent, antibody surveys suggest that infection with SA8 may be more common. In one study, 18 of 26 monkeys or a little over 70% were antibody positive. This incidence, however, may vary with different shipments of monkeys. No human infections with SA8 virus have been reported.

Herpesvirus tamarinus. This virus was first recovered from marmosets during an epidemic in a recently collected group of animals.[5] The infection in these animals was essentially 100% fatal. Subsequent study, however, of a number of New World species revealed that 80–100% of the squirrel monkeys (*Saimiri sciureus*) tested possessed high levels of neutralizing antibody to *H. tamarinus*.[6] Antibody was found in only an occasional animal of other species studied. The squirrel monkey therefore appears to be the natural host for this virus, which is carried as a latent infection. Cross-infection in marmosets or owl monkeys, however, generally results in fatal disease. The susceptibility of African or Asiatic species to this virus is unknown. One possible human infection with *H. tamarinus* has been reported, and this case was associated with squirrel monkeys. The patient suffered from encephalitis but recovered.[17]

H. tamarinus produces a generalized disease in marmosets that progresses to lethargy and death. Experimentally, marmosets have been infected by ID and IN inoculation and by gavage. Pathology varied with the different routes of infection. Rhinitis and pneumonitis followed IN inoculation and death occurred in 4–5 days. Local hemorrhagic lesions appeared within 2 days of intradermal inoculation and grew to 4–6 cm in diameter at the time of death 4–7 days postinoculation. Animals infected by gavage became lethargic and died between 12 and 14 days after infection. All animals at autopsy showed focal necrosis of the liver, spleen, and adrenals, while the intranasally inoculated animals revealed in addition an extreme necrotizing pneumonia. Focal necrosis was seen in the small intestine in the marmosets infected by gavage. Virus can be recovered from a large variety of tissues, including adrenals, kidneys, lung, liver, spleen, heart, thymus, and brain.

Spider monkey virus. SMV was originally isolated from a fatally infected, zoo-born and zoo-raised, 5-month-old black-handed spider monkey (*Ateles geoffroyi*).[10] Numerous crusty brownish-colored lesions were observed on the lips and nose, and large deep ulcerated areas were present on the tongue, palate, and gums. Death occurred within 24 hours. The virus was recovered from the brain and the lip lesions. This is the only reported isolation of this virus to date. A serologic survey of various New World primates suggested that the spider monkey was the natural host for this virus. High incidence and high levels of SMV antibody, however, were detected only in adult animals. Although the virus was recovered from a fatally infected animal, the infection must not be highly fatal in spider monkeys living in the wild, since most adult animals tested had antibody indicative of previous infection. The biologic and serologic properties of SMV are more closely related to *H. tamarinus* than to the herpesviruses of Old World simians. In laboratory experiments, SMV was found to be equally as virulent for marmosets as is *H. tamarinus*.

Herpes simplex virus. Herpes simplex virus has been recovered from cases of fatal encephalitis in laboratory gibbons,[2,19] owl monkeys,[16] and marmosets. Humans presumably were the source of infection in these instances. Attempts to experimentally infect rhesus monkeys with herpes simplex have failed, but this may have been due to cross-protection resulting from prior infection with B-virus. The susceptibility of African monkeys is as yet unknown.

Specimens

In the case of nonfatal infections, specimens should be obtained from visible lesions such as those seen on the skin, in the oral cavity, or in the conjunctiva. If possible, a portion of the scab should be raised to permit collection of the vesicular fluids, which are generally rich in viral content. Specimens can be obtained from the eye by swab; the swab should be rinsed and squeezed out in a small volume of BSS or other appropriate reagent. Throat and buccal swabs may also be useful when lesions are seen or suspected in these regions. At autopsy all tissues showing gross pathology should be collected, as well as brain and spinal cord tissues, even though gross lesions are not seen there. A 10% suspension should be prepared by triturating the tissue with an abrasive material (Alundum or sand) in BSS. All of these herpesviruses are relatively unstable; thus, if isolation attempts are not made immediately, the tissues or other specimens should be frozen at $-70°C$ until the assays are to be performed.

Laboratory Procedures

Cultures. Although various laboratory animals or embryonating eggs are susceptible to these viruses, tissue culture is the most sensitive and convenient tool available. Primary rabbit kidney cells, or a rabbit kidney cell strain such as LLC-RK$_1$, are the cultures of choice, since all the simian herpesviruses as well as herpes simplex will grow in these cells.[9] The viruses also will grow in African green monkey kidney cells or in a strain such as BS-C-1.[7] SMV, *H. tamarinus,* and herpes simplex will not grow in rhesus monkey kidney nor in a cell strain derived from this species, LLC-MK$_2$.[9] Human cells may be used, but SA8 will not grow in at least one strain, AV$_2$, derived from the amnion. Further, the sensitivity of human cells to B-virus is considerably lower than that of rabbit or monkey cells.

Tissue cultures should be inoculated with 0.1–0.5 ml of the prepared sample and also with a 1:10 and 1:100 dilution when possible. The overlay medium should contain approximately 5% bovine or horse serum, and the pH should be 7.4–7.6. These herpesviruses all grow best in the presence of serum and at an alkaline pH. Appropriate antibiotics also are necessary, especially when the specimen is obtained from local lesions. Cultures should be incubated at 35–37°C and observed for CPE for at least 2 weeks before discarding as negative. The CPE produced by these viruses in some cell systems is quite characteristic and is an aid in identifying the virus. The most striking CPE is produced by B-virus in monkey kidney cells where large multinucleated giant cells with spikelike processes are seen. In stained preparations the type A intranuclear inclusions will be seen in these cells. In rabbit kidney cells, however, B-virus CPE is characterized by a rounding up of the cells with little evidence of giant cell formation.[8] The CPE produced by the other viruses in these cells systems is either similar or intermediate to the two extremes described for B-virus. In most instances, however, giant cell formation is evident and the experienced observer should suspect a herpesvirus infection. All the viruses produce typical type A eosinophilic intranuclear inclusions in all cell types in which they will proliferate.

Animal inoculation. There is no single laboratory animal that is readily susceptible to all of these viruses. The rabbit is highly susceptible to B-virus by any route of inoculation. It is also susceptible to herpes simplex and *H. tamarinus* by the IC route and may develop local lesion following ID inoculation by any of the viruses. Rabbits so inoculated with SMV, SA8, or herpes simplex may develop a fatal encephalitis. Only herpes simplex and B-virus consistently produce a fatal infection following IP inoculation.

The mouse, either suckling or adult, is susceptible to *H. tamarinus,* SMV, and herpes simplex by the IC route of inoculation. The ATCC and the B-virus vaccine strains of B-virus do not infect mice, but some strains have been adapted to mice and produce fatal disease. Several strains isolated from human infections possess mouse virulence. Mouse virulence thus is not a stable characteristic. SA8 is avirulent for mice.

Guinea pigs develop local lesions following ID inoculation of all of these herpesviruses, but generalized infection and death is rarely observed. Herpes simplex, B-virus, and *H. tamarinus* will produce herpeticlike pocks on the CAM of inoculated embryonating chicken eggs. SMV and SA8 have not been studied in embryonating eggs.

Immunology and serology. Serologic techniques are of limited value in the diagnosis of infection by these simian herpesviruses, with the exception to be noted. There is a high incidence of homologous neutralizing antibody in the sera of the natural host species for each of the virus types. Thus a positive finding in a single serum sample taken during an acute episode or suspected infection is meaningless. Serial bleedings, however, showing seroconversion or a sharp rise in titer (fourfold or greater) provide presumptive evidence of infection. In situations where cross-infection results in severe or fatal disease, i.e. *H. tamarinus* or SMV in marmosets and owl monkeys or B-virus in humans, the finding of neutralizing antibodies in the sera or diseased animals has significance. Positive assays for herpes simplex antibody, however, in gibbons, marmosets, and owl monkeys in which it has produced fatal infection may or may not provide incriminating evidence, since it is not known at this time what the incidence of infection with herpes simplex virus is in these species. In any instance the assay technique of choice is the VN test.

Quantitative VN tests, or in some instances cross-neutralization tests, are necessary for virus identification. These viruses do not hemagglutinate, and although it is known that some do produce CF antigens, the specificity of CF tests with this group of viruses has not been determined. FA tests have been reported but the results have not been confirmed by VN tests. In performing the VN test, it is desirable to include antiserum prepared against all of the known simian herpesviruses plus herpes simplex antiserum because of the cross-reactions that occur.

Serum neutralization tests can be performed using a variety of techniques, but the one described here has proven most satisfactory. To obtain the maximum neutralizing titer of these antisera, it is necessary that a heat-labile factor (referred to as potentiating factor, PF, which may be complement) be present.[20] Some low-titered sera (1:32 or less) may show no titer after heat inactivation. Thus the sera should not be heat inactivated, or if they are heated, then 5% fresh normal guinea pig sera (final concentration) should be added to the serum-virus mixture as a source of PF. In practice, even if the sera are not heat inactivated, guinea pig serum is included in an attempt to standardize the level of PF from test to test. The techniques of the test are as follows: (1) The virus should be titrated in tissue culture (preferably rabbit cells) and a dilution selected that will assure a challenge dose of 30–300 $TCID_{50}$. This dilution should be prepared in culture medium to which 10% fresh normal guinea pig serum has been added. (2) Serial serum dilutions should be made either in culture medium or BSS and carried beyond the known homologous antibody titers of the sera. (3) Equal volumes of each serum dilution should be mixed with equal volumes of the challenge virus (0.6 ml plus 0.6 ml is frequently used) and incubated for 2 hours at room temperature. The virus control samples should be held in like manner. (4) Inoculate the mixture into susceptible tissue cultures (0.5 ml into each of two tube cultures) and add medium. (5) Make log 10 serial dilutions of the challenge virus and inoculate into tissue culture for $TCID_{50}$ determination. (6) Incubate in an appropriate tissue culture system at 35–37°C for 7 days and watch for CPE.

In order to interpret the results of the tests, the investigator must be aware of the likely cross-reactions. Although the extent of these cross-reactions may vary with individual pools of typing serum, the general pattern is as outlined in Table 10.2.

Table 10.2. Pattern of cross-reactions

	HSV	B-virus	SA8	H. tamarinus	SMV
HSV	1024	32	64	<8	<8
B-virus	4–8	64	32	<8	<8
SA8	4–8	16	256	<8	<8
H. tamarinus	<8	<8	<8	2048	16–64
SMV	<8	<8	<8	4–32	128

It is obvious that herpes simplex, B-virus, and SA8 form one group, and that *H. tamarinus* and SMV form another in respect to antigenic composition. B-virus and SA8 are both broader antigens than herpes simplex, since both of their antisera show a high degree of heterologous neutralization. Although B-virus and SA8 are closely related, a fourfold or greater difference in serum titers distinguishes the homologous from the heterologous virus. B-virus antiserum may quantitatively neutralize herpes simplex, and SA8 antiserum also will neutralize herpes simplex virus in fairly high dilutions. There is little or no reciprocal cross-neutralization, however, as hyperimmune herpes simplex antiserum either will not neutralize B-virus and SA8, or will do so only at dilutions of 1:4 or 1:8. SMV appears to be the broadest antigen of the other group, as most antiserum pools will show some neutralizing titer for *H. tamarinus*. Neutralization of

SMV by *H. tamarinus* antiserum, however, does not occur as frequently nor does it reach as high a titer.

Virus recovered by animal inoculation can also be identified by a tissue culture neutralization test, either by neutralization of virus contained in tissue suspension or more conveniently by first passing the virus in tissue culture before performing VN tests. It also is possible to do cross-protection tests by active immunization and challenge of susceptible animals, or by inoculation of preincubated serum-virus mixtures. Such tests, however, are time-consuming and expensive as compared to the TC neutralization test.

Tentative virus identification can be made based on clinical observations and upon the history of the infected animal. The species involved is of importance, because as noted above, each serotype not only has its own natural host but also may have the capacity to produce infection in other species. The severity and type of the infection, either in a natural host or in other susceptible species, may provide a clue as to the type of virus involved. A history of known exposure (or no exposure) to other species is of value in defining the possible agents involved. For example, a New World monkey that has never been exposed to Asiatic or African species most likely would not be infected with B-virus or SA8, but the researcher should consider *H. tamarinus,* SMV, and herpes simplex. An Asiatic macaque most likely would be infected with B-virus, and an African green monkey with SA8. The latter is susceptible to B-virus, but if there is no known exposure to rhesus or other macaques, then there is little reason to suspect B-virus infection.

When exposure to other species has occurred, it is more difficult to predict the likely etiology of a suspected herpesvirus infection due to our ignorance of the consequences of all possible cross-infections. It is not known, for example, if New World species are susceptible to B-virus, and if so, how severe a disease might result from such infection. Further, we do not know if African or Asiatic species can acquire infections with *H. tamarinus* or SMV through exposure to infected squirrel or spider monkeys or other New World species carrying these agents. In these situations caution must be exercised in making tentative diagnoses.

Once the virus has been isolated, its growth properties in tissue culture and its virulence for laboratory animals can serve as an aid to virus identification. The growth characteristics in a selected group of cell cultures will either tentatively identify the virus or reduce the number of possible types involved. Such a scheme is shown in Table 10.3.

Table 10.3. Scheme of virus identification

	pRK or LLC-RK$_1$	pRMK or LLC-MK$_2$	pAGMK or BS-C-1	pHA or AV$_2$
B-virus	+	+	+	+
SA8	+	+	+	0
H. tamarinus	+	0	+	+
SMV	+	0	+	+
HSV	+	0	+	+

Primary cell cultures: pRK, rabbit kidney; pRMK, rhesus monkey kidney; pAGMK, African green monkey kidney; pHA, human amnion.
Cell lines: LLC-RK$_1$, rabbit kidney, LLC-MK$_2$, rhesus monkey kidney; BS-C-1, green monkey kidney; AV$_2$, human amnion.

Inoculations of mice IC and rabbits IP will provide information as to the type of herpesvirus in an unknown sample. The results, based on the incidence of paralytic disease and death, can be compared to those in Table 10.4.

Table 10.4. Differential diagnosis of herpesviruses by animal inoculation

	B-virus	SA8	H. tamarinus	SMV	HSV
Mice, IC	±	0	+	+	+
Rabbits, IP	+	0	0	0	+

The problem of cross-infections has been emphasized, and it should be clear to all laboratories maintaining colonies of monkeys that isolation of species is necessary. This problem exists not only in respect to the possibility of cross-infection with herpesviruses, but with all other simian viruses, as well as many viruses common to man. Human contact should be limited, and where possible, separate caretakers should be employed for each species. Within a colony, separate cages enclosed on all sides but the front are preferred over gang cages. Isolation and quarantine of all new animals to the laboratory for a period of 6–8 weeks prior to use in experimental procedures is further recommended as a means of preventing epidemics within the colony, and as a safeguard against possible zoonoses.

References

1. Clarkson, M.J., E. Thorpe, and K. McCarthy. A virus disease of captive vervet monkeys (*Cercopithecus aethiops*) caused by a new herpesvirus. *Arch. ges. Virusforsch.* 22:219–234, 1967.
2. Emmons, R.W., and E.H. Lennette. Natural herpesvirus hominis infection of a gibbon (*Hylobates lar*). *Arch. ges. Virusforsch.* 31:215–218, 1970.
3. Endo, M., T. Kamimura, Y. Aoyama, T. Hayashida, T. Kinjo, Y. Ono, S. Kotera, K. Suzuki, Y. Tajima, and K. Ando. Etude du virus B au Japon. *Jap. J. Exp. Med.* 30:227–233, 385–392, 1960.
4. Hartley, E.G. Naturally-occurring B virus infection in cynomolgus monkeys. *Vet. Rec.* 76:555–557, 1964.
5. Holmes, A.W., R.G. Caldwell, R.E. Dedmon, and F. Deinhardt. Isolation and characterization of a new herpesvirus. *J. Immunol.* 92:603–610, 1964.
6. Holmes, A.W., J.A. Devine, E. Nowakowski, and F. Deinhardt. The epidemiology of a herpesvirus infection of New World monkeys. *J. Immunol.* 96:668–671, 1966.
7. Hopps, H.E., B.C. Bernheim, A. Nisalak, J. Hin Tjio, and J.E. Smadel. Biologic characteristics of a continuous kidney cell line derived from the African green monkey. *J. Immunol.* 91:416–424, 1963.
8. Hull, R.N. The simian viruses. In Virology Monographs no. 2, pp. 1–66. Springer-Verlag, New York, 1968.
9. Hull, R.N., W.R. Cherry, and O.J. Tritch. Growth characteristics of monkey kidney cell strains LLC-MK$_1$, LLC-MK$_2$, and LLC-MK$_2$ (NCTC-3196) and their utility in virus research. *J. Exp. Med.* 115:903–918, 1962.
10. Hull, R.N., A.C. Dwyer, A.W. Holmes, E. Nowakowski, F. Deinhardt, E.H. Lennette, and R.W. Emmons. Recovery and characterization of a new simian herpesvirus from a fatally infected spider monkey. *J. Nat. Cancer Inst.* 49:225–231, 1972.
11. Hull, R.N., and J.C. Nash. Immunization against B virus infection. I. Preparation of an experimental vaccine. *Am. J. Hyg.* 71:15–18, 1960.
12. Malherbe, H., and R. Harwin. Seven viruses isolated from vervet monkey. *Brit. J. Path.* 38:539–541, 1957.
13. Malherbe, H., and R. Harwin. Neurotropic virus in African monkeys. *Lancet* 2:530–534, 1958.
14. McCarthy, K., E. Thorpe, A.C. Laursen, C.S. Heymann, and A.J. Beale. Exanthematous disease in patas monkeys caused by a herpes virus. *Lancet* 2:856–857, 1968.
15. Melendez, L.V., M.D. Daniel, R.D. Hunt, and F.G. Garcia. An apparently new herpesvirus from primary kidney cultures of the squirrel monkey (*Saimiri sciureus*). *Lab. Anim. Care* 18:374–381, 1968.

16. Melendez, L.V., C. Espana, R.D. Hunt, M.D. Daniel, and F.G. Garcia. Natural herpes simplex infection in owl monkey (*Aotus trivirgatus*). *Lab. Anim. Care* 19:38–45, 1969.
17. Schrier, A.M. Editor's notes. *Primate Newsletter* 5(4):ii, 1966.
18. Shah, K.V. Comparison of three rhesus groups of antibody patterns to some viruses: Absence of active simian virus 40 transmission in the free-ranging rhesus of Cayo Santiago. *Am. J. Epidemiol.* 89:308–311, 1969.
19. Smith, P.C., T.M. Yuill, R.D. Buchanan, J.S. Stanton, and V. Chaicumpa. The gibbon (*Hylobates lar*): A new primate host for herpesvirus hominis. I. A natural epizootic in a laboratory colony. *J. Infec. Dis.* 120:292–297, 1969.
20. Stevens, D.A., T. Pincus, M.A.K. Burroughs, and B. Hampar. Serologic relationship of a simian herpesvirus (SA_8) and herpes simplex virus heterogeneity in the degree of reciprocal cross-reactivity shown by rabbit 7 S and 19 S antibodies. *J. Immunol.* 101:979–983, 1968.

11. Leukoviruses

The names thylaxovirus and oncornavirus have been proposed to include a group of viruses most of whose members are oncogenic. The criteria for this classification are: a loose saclike envelope, high water content, particle formation by budding from the cell membrane, and usually absence of CPE during rapid viral replication. The virus particles are spherical, 75–100 nm in diameter, and contain a core of single-stranded RNA. We propose to use the classification leukoviruses until some final agreement is reached on an appropriate name for the group. The avian leukosis-sarcoma viruses and the murine leukemia viruses will be discussed here.

Avian Leukosis-Sarcoma Viruses

The avian leukosis-sarcoma viruses possess several important characteristics in common. In size, structure, nucleic acid content, and susceptibility to lipid solvents and low pH, members of this group are indistinguishable from one another and resemble the myxoviruses, but no helical substructure has been demonstrated as yet. They all contain a characteristic group-specific antigen demonstrable by the CF test.[7,9]

In thin sections viewed under the electron microscope, avian leukosis-sarcoma viruses have an inner electron-dense nucleoid, an intermediate membrane, and an outer membrane. The viruses are sensitive to lipid solvents and highly resistant to UV irradiation.

Viruses of this group, whether isolated from birds with tumors or with inapparent infections, induce a spectrum of neoplasms (Table 11.1); however, under a given set of conditions, one particular response usually predominates. The type of neoplasm is influenced by the strain of virus (but not necessarily its serotypic subgroup), the dose of inoculum, the route of inoculation, the genetic source of the chicken, the sex and age at inoculation, and the previous history of the flock.

Serotype Division of the Leukosis-Sarcoma Viruses

Viruses of the avian leukosis-sarcoma group have been divided into seven subgroups, lettered A through G, on the basis of host range in genetically susceptible or resistant cells, interference spectrum, and viral envelope antigens.[12] A classification of the viruses most fully studied appears in Table 11.2. Chickens are the primary hosts for

Table 11.1. Neoplastic diseases produced by viruses of the leukosis-sarcoma group

Name	Synonyms	Target cells	Occurrence	Lesions
Lymphoid leukosis	Big liver disease, visceral lymphomatosis	Intrafollicular bursal lymphoid cells	Common	Lymphoid tumors of liver, spleen, bursa, and other visceral organs
Erythroblastosis	Erythroleukosis, erythromyelosis	Intravascular erythroblasts	Occasional	Proliferative—enlarged, cherry-red spleen and liver; aplastic anemia.
Myeloblastosis	Granuloblastosis, myeloid leukosis, leukomylosis	Extravascular myeloblasts	Rare	Enlarged grey liver and spleen, bone marrow firm and grey, myeloblastemia
Nephroblastoma	Renal adenocarcinoma, embryonal nephroma, Wilm's tumor	Embryonic kidney rests	Occasional	Tumors in kidney parenchyma or pedunculated; may be cystic, bone, etc.
Osteopetrosis	Marble bone, osteopetrotic lymphomatosis	Osteoblasts and periosteum	Occasional	Deposition of abnormal osseous tissue in long bones
Hemangioma	Endothelioma, hemangioendothelioma	Blood vessels including endothelial cells	Occasional	Cavernous—"blood blisters" in liver parenchyma; Capillary—solid masses
Sarcoma	Fibrosarcoma, myxofibrosarcoma	Fibroblasts	Occasional	Firm, fibrous, or myxomatous tumor in subcutis, etc.

viruses of this group; the subgroups F and G were isolated from pheasants. In addition, sarcoma viruses will produce tumors in many other avian and some mammalian species.

Host range and genetic resistance of cells. Cells resistant to growth of subgroup A or subgroup B viruses are termed C/A or C/B respectively. Cells susceptible to viruses of all known subgroups are termed C/O cells. Cellular resistance to leukosis-sarcoma viruses of subgroups A and B is governed by an independent pair of recessive alleles, a^r and b^r, for each subgroup. Stocks of virus and field isolates often contain representatives from more than one subgroup. It is quite possible that additional subgroups will be discovered.

Interference spectrum. The growth of the noncytopathic avian leukosis viruses in cells interferes with the CPE of other viruses belonging to the same subgroup, but not with viruses of different subgroups. This is the basis of the resistance-inducing factor (RIF) test.[8]

Envelope antigens. Virus neutralization and immunofluorescence of infected cells occur with avian sera prepared against envelope antigens of viruses of the same subgroup; however, within a subgroup, virus types can be distinguished by the degree of their neutralization by different antisera.

Disease Produced

In chickens, lymphoid leukosis is the most common neoplasm.[1,7] Other forms of the disease that are less frequently observed are listed in Table 11.1.

Lymphoid leukosis is a neoplasm of the bursa-dependent lymphoid system. The lymphoid cells of the bursa are considered to be the target cells, since removal of the bursa

Table 11.2. Classification of leukosis-sarcoma viruses

Virus strains	Virus subgroups and designations						
	A	B	C	D	E	F	G
Leukosis							
LL-erythro	RPL-12						
Rubin's LL	RIF-1	RIF-2					
Myeloblastosis str BAI-A	AMV-A	AMV-B					
Engelbreth-Holm erythro (Str R)			AEV				
Endogenous					RAV-0	RAV-61	GPV
Endothelioma							
MH-2			MH-2				
Nondefective sarcoma							
Schmidt-Ruppin	SR-RSV-A	SR-RSV-B		SR-RSV-D			
Carr-Zilber				CZ-RSV-D			
Prague	PR-RSV-A		PR-RSV-C				
B77			B77				
Defective sarcoma viruses (examples of each pseudotype)							
Bryan high-titer Rous	BH-RSV(RAV-1)	BH-RSV(RAV-2)	BH-RSV(RAV-7)	BH-RSV(RAV-50)			
Bryan standard Rous	BS-RSV(RAV-4)						
Fujinami	FSV(FAV-1)						
Harris		HA-RSV(RAV-6)					
Associated viruses							
Myeloblastosis-associated virus	MAV-1	MAV-2					
Leukosis-associated virus					RAV-60		
Rous-associated viruses							
High-titer Standard	RAV-1, RAV-3	RAV-2	RAV-2				
Harris	RAV-4, RAV-5	RAV-6					
Schmidt-Ruppin			RAV-49	RAV-50			
Carr-Zilber				CZAV			
Fujinami	FAV-1, FAV-2						

at any time prior to 4 months of age prevents the occurrence of lymphoid leukosis. Neoplastically transformed bursa follicles can be seen histologically before the tumor appears in other organs of the body. The viruses that cause lymphoid leukosis (LL) are almost ubiquitous; however, most strains that have been isolated from field cases are relatively nonpathogenic. The disease occurs mainly in chickens over 16 weeks of age. In the early stages, affected chickens show few signs of the disease, but later they lose weight and their abdomens are often enlarged. Large focal or diffuse tumors occur in the bursa of Fabricius, liver, spleen, and other visceral organs. The tumors are composed of masses of large uniform lymphoblasts.

Specimens

Plasma, serum, or tumor tissues are the best specimens for virus isolation, although virus can be isolated from most of the organs of the body and also from oral washings and feces. Leukosis viruses may be transmitted from parent to offspring through the egg.[2] The number of hens shedding virus by this route varies from flock to flock. When it is important to determine whether dams are shedding virus in their eggs, 10-day-old embryos should be used.

Chicks that hatch from infected eggs are viremic and usually remain so throughout their lives. They shed virus in their saliva and feces and act as a source of infection for other chicks. Chicks hatching from noninfected eggs usually possess maternal antibody from their dams, because most of the dams have antibody. Antibody is lost by 3–4 weeks of age, and shortly thereafter many chicks become infected with virus. Such chicks develop a transient viremia that occurs in most birds between the ninth and fifteenth weeks of age and is replaced by circulating antibody.

Tumors may contain large amounts of virus; however, sometimes no virus can be detected by any available method. All viruses of this group are very thermolabile and can only be preserved for long periods at temperatures below −60°C.

Laboratory Procedures
Leukosis Virsuses

The leukosis viruses, that is, those that induce lymphoid leukosis, erythroblastosis, and myeloblastosis, can be assayed by inoculation of chicks or embryos, the RIF test, COFAL test, NP test (Table 11.3), and FA test.[7] In addition, the adenosine triphosphatase of avian myeloblastosis virus and its ability to transform cultures of hematopoetic cells can be used under certain conditions for quantitative determinations.

In vivo assay. When leukosis viruses are inoculated via IAb or IV routes into day-old susceptible chicks, an adequate lymphoid leukosis response may be obtained in about 270 days.[1] The time required for quantitative assay can be shortened to 63 days by using the less sensitive erythroblastosis response and to 43 days by IV inoculation of embryos. Chicks inoculated as embryos hatch normally and later develop erythroblastosis. Avian myeloblastosis virus can also be assayed by chick or embryo inoculation.

RIF test. Leukosis viruses do not produce CPE in tissue culture except after prolonged passage. However, when sensitive cells (chick embryo fibroblasts) are infected with a leukosis virus, the cells become resistant to neoplastic transformation by a sarcoma virus

Table 11.3. Comparison of methods for assaying leukosis viruses

Methods	Requirements	Response measured	Subgroup determination	Time required (days)
In vivo				
Chick inoc. 1 day IAb	Lymphoid leukosis susceptible*	Lymphoid leukosis	Genetically resistant birds	270
Chick inoc. 1 day IAb	Erythroblastosis susceptible†	Erythroblastosis	Genetically resistant birds	63
Embryo inoc. 11 days IV	Erythroblastosis susceptible	Erythroblastosis	Genetically resistant birds	43
Cell cultures				
RIF Test	RSV pseudotypes, C/O cells‡	Resistance to formation of RSV foci in cell culture	Challenge virus	12§ + 6
COFAL test	Hamster antiserum, C/O cells, COFAL antigen-free cells	Complement fixation test	Genetically resistant cells	12 + 1
NP test	NP cells	RSV foci in cell culture or on CAM, or tumors in chicks	Genetically resistant cells or reverse RIF test	8 + 6
PM test	RSV pseudotypes, C/O, CE cells	RSV foci in cell culture or on CAM, or tumors in chicks	Genetically resistant cells or reverse RIF test	7 + 6

*Chickens susceptible to infection by the virus and susceptible to lymphoid leukosis tumor formation.
†Chickens susceptible to virus infection and to development of erythroblastosis (or myeloblastosis).
‡C/O means cells phenotypically susceptible to infection by viruses of all subgroups.
§Approximate number of days necessary to cultivate virus plus number of days to indicate presence of virus.

of the same subgroup.[8] Only viruses of the same subgroup interfere with one another in this way. The property of interference has been used extensively for assay of leukosis viruses by the RIF test and also in delineating the virus subgroups.[12] In the RIF test, chick embryo fibroblast cultures are inoculated with material suspected of containing a leukosis virus. Cells are subcultured at least three times at 3–4 day intervals, and at each passage a sample of the cells is tested for susceptibility to focus formation by Rous sarcoma viruses of different subgroups. Control cultures infected with known leukosis viruses and uninfected controls are always included. The presence of a lymphoid leukosis virus is indicated by a reduction of tenfold or greater in the number of foci produced by a standard stock of Rous sarcoma virus (RSV) when compared with the number of foci on sensitive control cells. Several different challenge viruses, one for each subgroup, must be used to ensure that all leukosis viruses are detected.

COFAL test. The CF test for avian leukosis viruses (COFAL test) is dependent upon a group-specific protein antigen of avian leukosis-sarcoma viruses.[9,10,11] The antigen is present in the supernatant fluids prepared from cells of infected cultures and in the virus particles themselves. The antigen is not present on the surface of the virus particles. When hamsters are infected with RSV (usually the Schmidt-Ruppin strain), a tumor develops and some hamsters produce sufficient or detectable antibody to the group-specific antigen. Rabbit antiserum prepared against the group-specific antigen and liberated from purified virus preparations with detergent can also be used. The mammalian antiserum is used in a CF test to detect the group-specific antigen produced in chick embryo fibroblast cultures by an infecting leukosis-sarcoma virus. A detailed description of current procedure follows:

1. Prepare secondary chick embryo fibroblast (CEF) cultures from virus-free embryos of known C/O phenotype that do not express the group-specific antigen.

2. Inoculate CEF cultures with test material suspected of containing LL virus and incubate at 35–37°C for 12–28 days to obtain maximum sensitivity. During this period, the CEF cells should be passed as often as necessary to maintain viability. Samples of cells from each passage can be examined in the CF test.

3. Positive controls: Inoculate additional CEF cultures with known LL virus material, using both a subgroup A virus and a subgroup B virus in separate cultures.

4. Negative controls: Use uninoculated CEF cultures.

5. At the end of the incubation period, place all CEF cultures in storage at −60°C or colder until needed in the CF test.

6. Just before use, thaw and refreeze all CEF cultures three times to disrupt intact cells and release the group-specific antigen. After centrifugation, the CEF preparations (test material, positive, and negative controls) become the antigens for the CF test.

7. The antiserum used in the CF test may be prepared in either hamsters or rabbits, using RSV. A standard antiserum for commercial vaccine manufacturers in the United States can be obtained from the Biologics Division at NADC. Four units of standard antiserum are used for each test. Commercial antiserums are also available.

8. Perform the microtiter CF test using either the 50 or 100% hemolytic endpoint technique to determine complement unitage. For the test, use either 5–50% or 2–100% hemolytic units of complement.

9. In the absence of anticomplementary activity, COFAL activity at the 1:4 dilution of the test material antigen is considered a positive test for LL viruses. COFAL activity at 1:2 dilution is considered a suspicious reaction. Occasionally, "normal" antigens may cause weak or false test reactions.

NP test. The nonproducer (NP) test requires NP cells that are transformed by a defective strain of RSV (Bryan high-titer strain) and that do not produce virus detectable in the usual tests on C/E cells (cells resistant to subgroup E viruses only).[10] Test samples are inoculated onto virus-free, genetically susceptible, chick fibroblast cultures that are subsequently co-cultivated with NP cells. Cultures infected with LLV can be identified because RSV is produced in large quantities by the NP cells activated by virus in the test sample. The RSV can be detected by assay in culture or in embryos. This test is highly sensitive but requires stocks of NP cells that are difficult to produce.

PM test. The phenotypic mixing (PM) test depends on the ability of a sarcoma virus (defective or nondefective) of one subgroup, when co-cultivated with a leukosis virus of another subgroup, to acquire the envelope host-range properties of the leukosis virus. Thus a subgroup E sarcoma virus will not form foci on C/E cells. However, when phenotypically mixed with a leukosis virus of subgroup A, it will infect and form foci on C/E cells. Thus, in the PM test, C/O cells (cells susceptible to infection with viruses of subgroups A through E), C/E cells, and stocks of RSV(O) are required.[4,6] A detailed description of the procedure follows:

1. Prepare secondary CEF cultures from virus-free embryos of known C/O phenotype in 35 mm diameter petri dishes.
2. Approximately 1 hour before infection on the monolayer, add DEAE dextran to the medium to a final concentration of 2 μg/ml.
3. Infect with about 10^3 plaque-forming units (PFU) of RSV(O) and incubate for 18–24 hours at 37°C.
4. Positive controls: Titrate known leukosis viruses (usually of subgroups A and B) to determine the sensitivity of the test.
5. Negative controls: Use cultures infected with RSV(O) to confirm the absence of a contaminating virus and the susceptibility of the cells.
6. Remove the supernatant fluid containing the DEAE dextran and residual RSV(O) inoculum and replace with fresh culture medium and 0.1–0.5 ml of the test material, or add one drop of heparinized whole blood directly to the supernatant medium.
7. Change the supernatant medium every second day and harvest it on the seventh day after inoculation with the sample.
8. Freeze and thaw once and centrifuge to remove cells and debris.
9. Assay for RSV by inoculating C/E cells as described above.

The presence of virus of subgroup A, B, C, or D in the test materials will result in a large number of RSV foci on the C/E cells. If the test materials lack virus, then no RSV foci will appear on the C/E cells.

Interpretation of RIF, COFAL, and PM tests. All three tests require a standard source of RIF-free chick embryos of known phenotypes for use in preparing cell cultures. For the PM test, C/O and C/E cells are necessary. Cells for use in the COFAL test must in addition be free of the genetically controlled antigen that reacts in the test. In the COFAL test, specific antiserum is a necessity; in the PM test, stocks of suitable sarcoma viruses are a prerequisite. None of the tests should be performed directly on cells obtained from embryos of unknown genetic origin, since the results may be confused by genetic resistance and genetically controlled nonspecific COFAL antigen.

The RIF and COFAL tests require several subcultures to propagate the virus sufficiently and therefore, involve considerably more work than the PM test. Also, the indicator systems are different in the three tests. In the RIF test, the number and appearance of Rous foci after challenge is highly dependent on the physiologic condition of the cells. Thus, when cell cultures are not in optimal condition, it is not possible to perform a RIF test. On the other hand, a cell extract is used in the COFAL test, and it can be stored frozen and tested on more than one occasion if necessary. Similarly, in the PM test, the supernatant fluid can be stored and tested for virus by either the cell culture, CAM, or chick inoculation techniques. The results are usually more clear-cut in the PM test than in the RIF or COFAL tests.

The subgroup of an infecting leukosis virus can be determined by any of these tests. In the interference test, only the Rous virus belonging to the same subgroup as the leukosis virus is interfered with. In the COFAL test, genetically resistant cells can be employed; thus a leukosis virus of subgroup A will not produce COFAL antigens in C/A cells. In the PM test, the supernate from the mixing phase, which contains Rous virus of the same subgroup as the leukosis virus, can be placed on genetically resistant cells or embryos, or used in a reverse RIF test with a known leukosis virus.

Fluorescent antibody tests. The direct and indirect FA tests have been used to detect viral antigen in chick embryo fibroblast cultures. When mammalian group-specific antisera are used, the test becomes analogous to the COFAL test. Avian sera are subgroup or even type specific.

Hematopoietic transformation. Avian myeloblastosis virus will infect cultures of avian hematopoietic tissue and induce focal transformation of the culture into myeloblasts. Assays are usually based on a quantal response in which individual cultures are scored as positive or negative.

Rous Sarcoma and Related Viruses

Rous sarcoma virus and many other sarcoma viruses produce tumors in a short time when inoculated SC, IM, IAb, or by contact with inoculated chickens, but SC inoculation into the wing web is most commonly used. On SC inoculation with high doses of virus, tumors are first palpable after about 3 days, and in susceptible chickens may grow rapidly, ulcerate, and metastasize. With low doses of virus, tumors may occur as late as 35 days after inoculation.

Rous sarcoma virus produces pocks on the CAM of susceptible embryos.[3] When the CAM of 11-day-old embryos are inoculated, pocks can be counted after an additional 8 days of incubation. Some strains of virus produce hemorrhages 7 days after IV inoculation into 11-day-old embryos. This has formed the basis of an assay procedure that, however, is not in general use because it takes so long to run.

In sensitive CEF cultures, sarcoma viruses produce foci of neoplastically transformed cells that can be seen microscopically after 4–5 days and grossly after about 10 days.[5] The foci consist of rounded refractile cells that become multilayered. The morphology of the transformed cells and the shape of the focus produced are characteristic of the infecting virus. Sarcoma viruses also activate NP cells, produce the group-specific CF antigen, and can be detected by the FA technique.

Serology. Serum or egg yolk is suitable for antibody determinations, but heparinized plasma should not be used when tests are made in cell culture.[10] Neutralization of an RSV pseudotype is an indication of current or past infection with a leukosis or sarcoma virus of the same or similar type. A virus of one subgroup will not be neutralized by antibodies provoked by a virus of a different subgroup. A 1:5 dilution of heat-inactivated serum (56°C for 30 minutes) is usually mixed with an equal quantity of a standard preparation of RSV of a known pseudotype, and after incubation the residual virus is quantitated by cell culture.

Immunity and challenges. The presence of antibody is evidence of infection but provides no indication of whether a particular bird will die of neoplasia. Thus serologic studies have very limited application in studies of immunity to the disease. Challenge of chickens, which are known to be genetically susceptible, with RSV or erythroblastosis virus under laboratory conditions can be used to test for immunity.

Among chickens, there are two levels of genetic resistance to leukosis viruses: resistance of cells to virus infection as described above, and resistance to the development of disease. In the latter case, chickens may become infected with the virus and produce antibody, but they do not develop neoplasms. Chickens can be challenged IC at 1 day of age to determine whether their cells are genetically susceptible to infection with RSV. Mortality occurs between day 7 and day 28 after inoculation. Genetic resistance to erythroblastosis can be examined by IV challenge of 12-day-old embryos or 14-day-old chickens with a laboratory-adapted strain of leukosis virus.

Diagnostic pathology. Birds with tumors caused by viruses of this group may have an anemia in the early stages and an anemia or leukemia in later stages. There is often a terminal dehydration. In leukemic cases, blood smears reveal cells characteristic of the disease, for example, erythroblasts in erythroblastosis, and so forth.

Birds with myeloblastosis, particularly the disease induced by the laboratory strain BAI strain A, have an increased adenosine triphosphatase activity in their plasma. Osteopetrotic birds have higher serum alkaline phosphatase levels than unaffected birds.

The pathology of each tumor condition has been described briefly above. In field outbreaks of lymphoid tumors the greatest difficulty is encountered in differentiating between lymphoid leukosis and Marek's disease. Marek's disease is a lymphoproliferative disease that affects the nerves and visceral organs, particularly the gonads, and is caused by a DNA virus belonging to the B subgroup of herpesviruses. The most important diagnostic features for differentiating between the diseases are included in Table 11.4. Impression smears of affected organs stained with methyl-green pyronin, acridine orange, or hematoxylin and Schorr's stain can be helpful in this differentiation.

Table 11.4. Comparison of pathologic differences between lymphoid leukosis and Marek's disease

Signs and lesions	Lymphoid leukosis	Marek's disease
Clinical signs		
Age of onset	>16 weeks of age	>4 weeks of age
Paralysis	Absent	Usually present
Gross lesions		
Peripheral nerve and ganglia involvement	Absent	Usually present
Bursa of Fabricius	Nodular tumor	Diffuse enlargement or atrophy
Skin and muscle tumors	Usually absent	May be present
Microscopic lesions		
Peripheral nerve infiltration	Absent	Usually present
Cuffing in white matter of cerebellum	Absent	Usually present
Skin infiltration with follicular patterns of lymphoid cells	Absent	Often present
Cell proliferation in bursa of Fabricius	Intrafollicular	Interfollicular
Cytology of lymphoid cells	Uniform "blast" cells	Pleomorphic mature and immature cells

References

1. Burmester, B.R., C.O. Prickett, and T.C. Belding. A filtrable agent producing lymphoid tumors and osteopetrosis in chickens. *Cancer Res.* 6:189–196, 1946.
2. Cottral, G.E., B.R. Burmester, and N.F. Waters. Egg transmission of avian lymphomatosis. *Poul. Sci.* 33:1174–1184, 1954.
3. Dougherty, R.M., and P.J. Simons. The sensitivity of Rous sarcoma virus. *Virology* 18:559–566, 1962.
4. Graf, T. A simple technique for the detection and classification of latent avian RNA tumor viruses. *Zeitschrift Naturforsch.* 27:223–226, 1972.

5. Manaker, R.A., and V. Groupe. Discrete foci of altered chicken embryo cells associated with Rous sarcoma virus in tissue culture. *Virology* 2:838–840, 1956.
6. Okazaki, W., H.G. Purchase, and B.R. Burmester. Phenotypic mixing test to detect and assay avian leukosis viruses. *Avian Dis.* 19:311–317, 1975.
7. Purchase, H.G., and B.R. Burmester. The leukosis/sarcoma group. In *Diseases of Poultry*, M.S. Hofstad, B.W. Calnek, C.F. Helmboldt, W.M. Reid, and H.W. Yoder, Jr. (eds.), pp. 502–568. 6th ed. Iowa State University Press, Ames, 1972.
8. Rubin, H. A virus in chick embryos which induces resistance *in vitro* to infection with RSV. *Proc. Nat. Acad. Sci.* 46:1105–1119, 1960.
9. Sarma, P.S., H.C. Turner, and R.J. Huebner. An avian leukosis group-specific complement fixation reaction: Application for the detection and assay of non-cytopathogenic leukosis viruses. *Virology* 23:313–321, 1964.
10. Solomon, J.J., P.A. Long, and W. Okazaki. Procedures for the *in vitro* assay of viruses and antibody of avian lymphoid leukosis and Marek's disease. ARS Agriculture Handbook no. 404, p. 18. U.S. Government Printing Office, Washington, 1971.
11. USDA, APHIS, Veterinary Services, Biologies Laboratories. *Supplemental Assay Method for Detecting Lymphoid Leukosis Biocontamination by the COFA Test*. Ames, Iowa, 1973.
12. Vogt, P.K., and R. Ishizaki. Criteria for the classification of avian tumor viruses. In *Viruses Inducing Cancer: Implications for Therapy*, W.J. Burdett (ed), pp. 71–90. University of Utah Press, Salt Lake City, 1966.

Murine Leukemia Viruses

The murine leukemia viruses (MuLV) are associated with various types of leukemia: lymphoid, myeloid, erythroid, hemocytoblastic, and reticulum cell. However, the type of hematologic disease each virus induces is not constant; it may vary under different conditions of inoculation or in different hosts. The viruses are found not only in leukemic tissues but also in the tissues of many normal-appearing mice and mouse embryos, especially AK strain mice, which have a high incidence of natural leukemia. This shows that MuLV are transmitted vertically from parent to offspring,[17] similar to the egg transmission of avian leukosis. Lateral transmission of the viruses also occurs. Mice with latent infections of MuLV may develop clinical leukemia following inoculation with various materials or after irradiation (Table 11.5). The main importance of murine leukemia is that it offers a relatively inexpensive model system for the study of a mammalian neoplastic disease.

There have been over 25 isolations of MuLV by almost as many different investigators. All of the MuLV are spherical, about 85–100 nm in diameter, contain a single-stranded RNA core, and are enclosed in a loose saclike envelope.

Another virus, called spleen focus-forming virus (SFFV), initiates the development of macroscopic foci of transformed hemopoietic cells in the spleens of susceptible adult mice within 9 days of IV infection. SFFV is a helper-dependent virus, found in both the Friend and Rauscher virus complexes. The MuLV in these complexes are called LLV-F, or Friend helper, and LLV-R, or Rauscher helper, respectively. SFFV is probably responsible, at least in part, for the rapid induction of erythroleukemia that is characteristic of "Friend disease" and "Rauscher disease," but it is not certain whether other viruses also contribute to this syndrome. Only in certain Friend virus preparations is the host range of SFFV naturally restricted so that other MuLV can substitute for its natural helper virus, LLV-F.[8] By studying the neutralization kinetics of these SFFV (MuLV) pseudotypes in the presence of murine-typing antisera, researchers have made a preliminary classification of some MuLV isolates based on their virus-bound envelope antigens (Table 11.6).[9]

Table 11.5. Partial list of murine leukemia viruses*

Inoculum or treatment of animal from which virus was isolated	Main type of leukemia	Reference
Spontaneous leukemias in Ak and C58 mice; normal Ak embryos	Lymphoid	17
Transplantable tumors		
Sarcoma 1 (ascitic)	Myeloid	15
Sarcoma 36 (solid)	Lymphoid	27
Ehrlich carcinoma	Erythroleukemia†	12
Ehrlich ascites	Reticulum cell	38
Schwartz leukemia	Erythroleukemia‡	31
Plasma cell #70429	Lymphoid	28
Irradiation-induced leukemia		
X-ray–induced	Lymphoid	22
^{32}P-induced	Lymphoid	19
Chemically induced leukemia		
DMBA-induced	Lymphoid	43
Hormone-induced leukemia		
Diethylstilbestrol-induced	Lymphoid	21
Leukemias induced by other viruses		
Vaccinia virus	Hemocytoblastic	23
WM1 virus	Erythroleukemia	30
Friend virus nucleoprotein	Lymphoid	32
Friend virus (low dose)	Lymphoid	36
Leukemia arising in mice inoculated with material from human leukemia	Lymphoid	7

*Space permits listing only half of the independent isolates of murine leukemia viruses; these were selected because of their frequency of use or their usefulness as examples.

†Polycythemia was later observed with certain Friend virus strains.

‡Lymphoid leukemias were observed in rats and in some mice given low doses of virus.

Table 11.6. Classification of murine leukemia viruses

Type and subtype*	Isolate
1	Gross
2	
A	LLV-F (Friend helper)
B	Moloney
C	LLV-R (Rauscher helper)
3	Buffett (334C)

*There is little or no cross-reactivity between subtypes A and B, but they both cross-react with subtype C.

Virus Titration Techniques

MuLV are usually quantified by measurement of their viral infectivity in vivo. However, most bioassay procedures for these viruses have serious drawbacks—chiefly their consumption of large numbers of mice (to offset irregular responses of individual mice) and their long duration (for endpoint dilutions of virus to induced leukemia). Consequently, many attempts have been made to detect these viruses by other means, but only recently have certain modifications in assay procedures simplified the problem of virus titration, and these will be emphasized here.

Virus may be prepared from the plasma or from enlarged leukemic organs (spleen, thymus, or lymph nodes) of infected mice. In some cases rats may be used to supply larger volumes of plasma for subsequent virus purification, although rat passage may alter the infective or antigenic behavior of the virus. Most routine work is carried out with cell-free filtrates of homogenized leukemic tissues. The homogenates (10–20% W/V), once cleared of coarse cellular debris by centrifugation (2400 $\times g$ for 20 minutes), should be heavily irradiated or passed through filter candles or Millipore-type filters whenever the action of cells must be ruled out.[18,27] For storage, samples of undiluted virus should be sealed in glass ampules and kept at very low temperatures, preferably that of liquid nitrogen ($-196°C$) if undiminished infectivity is required months later.

Prior to assay, thawed virus suspensions should be diluted into ice-cold medium, usually a simple diluent such as physiological saline (0.15 M), buffered at neutrality, or citrate buffer (0.05 M, pH 6.4). If required, thermal stability can be improved with the use of protein-rich diluent, such as Eagle's BSS supplemented with 15% calf serum. Serial dilutions of virus can then be inoculated into groups of 10–20 mice, the number of recipients depending on the assay method. Newborn mice (preferably less than 24 hours old) should be given IP injections; 0.1 ml via a 27–30-gauge needle can be inserted through the thigh muscle to prevent leakage of virus. Young adult mice may be inoculated IP or IV for titrations of virus stocks that contain SFFV; the latter route of inoculation provides virus titers about 10 times higher than the former. After a little practice, the lateral tail veins of mice (previously warmed under a flood lamp) can be penetrated quite easily with a 27-gauge needle; 0.5 ml volumes are delivered accurately with a glass tuberculin syringe.

It should be emphasized that the results of mouse leukemia virus titration may be modified by several factors, including (1) the passage history of the virus preparation, (2) the quantity of infective virus in the inoculum, (3) the route of inoculation, and (4) the age and genotype of the recipient. It is most important that these factors be considered in any comparison between virus titration data.

Quantal response assays. The potency of any MuLV preparation can be determined by observing the highest dilution of virus capable of eliciting a quantal (all-or-none) response in 50% of inoculated mice. The 50% endpoint for either physical signs of leukemia (ED_{50}) or death (LD_{50}) is usually estimated by the R & M method.

For titration of MuLV preparations that do not contain SFFV, quantal response assays are frequently chosen. Inoculated mice that survive the neonatal period are examined regularly for evidence of leukemia during the next 5–6 months. SFFV-containing virus preparations can also be titrated in a quantal response assay, such as one based on the incidence of spleens weighing more than 0.5 g at 21 days postinoculation (DPI). However, any quantal assay method suffers from a considerable amount of variation in host response to inoculations of a virus that has been diluted beyond the 50% endpoint.

Graded response assays. Certain measurable variables of the host response to MuLV infection can be correlated with the infecting dose of virus. For MuLV in general, this variable may be survival time or the time required for the development of leukemia or the time required for the production of specific cytotoxic antibodies.[20,27] For SFFV-containing virus preparations, the variable measured is usually spleen weight, although thrombocytopenia has also been employed. The chief advantage of these methods is that each mouse provides a quantitative value rather than a yes-or-no response; hence graded response data are often more reliable than quantal data. However, the interpretation of results can be more complicated than with quantal or enumerative assays, for virus potency is usually expressed in terms relative to a standard virus pool or in terms of a quantal or enumerative assay that has been standardized for the graded response assay. Two exceptions to this are the helper assays for MuLV, based on the ability of these viruses to provide a helper function—either for murine sarcoma virus–induced focus formation in mouse embryo fibroblasts in vitro[11] or for SFFV-induced spleen focus formation in vivo.[41] With these assays constant amounts of murine sarcoma virus or SFFV, used as the indicator virus, are added to serial dilutions of helper MuLV. After 5 or 9 days, respectively, the increase in focus formation over that observed with indicator virus alone, called helper activity and expressed in Δ focus-forming units per ml, is proportional to the dose of MuLV. Extrapolation of this linear relationship to the theoretical helper activity of undiluted MuLV will give its titer, expressed in helper units per ml.

Enumerative response assays. Virus assays based on the formation of discrete lesions or foci of infection provide a degree of precision not obtainable by other titration procedures. Such assays have been difficult to develop for MuLV, because while MuLV replicate in murine cells in vivo and in tissue culture, they do not normally produce CPE. Virus preparations that contain SFFV, though, can be titrated readily in vivo because of its remarkable capacity to induce focal lesions of leukemic cells in the splenic red pulp of susceptible mice within 9 days of infection.[5]

Other MuLV stocks that are free of detectable SFFV can also induce enumerative responses, but these can only be demonstrated with special techniques in cell culture. Examples include a focus assay for Gross MuLV that is based on the detection by immunofluorescence microscopy of focal areas of infected cells that synthesize specific antigen,[44] and a new line of murine sarcoma virus–transformed cells that, after superinfection with MuLV, responds with the formation of typical murine sarcoma virus–type foci in proportion to the concentration of MuLV used for superinfection.[6] But the most frequently used enumerative response assay for MuLV is a plaque (rather than a focus) assay, based upon syncytium formation between Rous sarcoma virus–infected rat tumor (XC) cells and MuLV-infected cells.[35]

With all of these assay methods the mean number of foci or plaques per spleen or culture dish is directly proportional (for susceptible cells) to the amount of virus in the inoculum. The product of the mean lesion count times the virus dilution factor will give an estimate of the virus titer in focus- or plaque-forming units per unit volume. This titer estimate should be constant through all dilutions for which enumeration of lesions is accurate, and the dose-response relationship is said to be "one-hit," implying that the development of one lesion was initiated by a single infectious entity in the virus preparation. However, the titration of MuLV stocks in certain partially resistant hosts may result in diminishing titer estimates with increasing dilutions of virus. These "two-hit" or "multiple-hit" dose-response relationships usually imply that more than one infectious entity was required to initiate the development of a given lesion. Occasionally such data will provide evidence of a helper-dependent relationship between two viruses, as between SFFV and its natural helper virus, LLV-F, in the Friend virus complex.[40]

Cell Transplantation Techniques

In 1914, Little developed the genetic theory of transplantation: inheritance of susceptibility or resistance to transplants occurs according to Mendelian laws and depends upon the matching of histocompatibility genes between donor and recipient. This concept is central to the development of assays for MuLV-transformed cells, to the analysis of MuLV-induced cellular antigens, and to an understanding of transplantation immunity.

To transplant leukemic cells, either tissue fragments or, for better quantitation, cell suspension may be used. The latter are prepared according to the form of the leukemia employed. For example, ascitic leukemias are ready-made cell suspensions. Splenic leukemias are dissociated easily by repeated injections of medium under the splenic capsule. Other leukemias, however, growing as subcutaneous tumors or in lymph nodes or thymus, must be thoroughly chopped with fine scissors and either passed through a fine wire-mesh screen or repeatedly forced through a syringe. Cell clumps are removed by allowing them to settle out of suspension or by filtration through several layers of gauze. Finally, a dye such as erythrocin or trypan blue is added to a diluted aliquot of the suspension and the cells are counted in a hemocytometer. The concentration of unstained (presumably living) cells is used to determine the amount of diluent required so that the inoculum contains a prescribed number of cells.

Quantal and graded response methods. The capacity of leukemic cells to multiply in a given host system is frequently expressed as the fraction of mice (out of the total number inoculated) that develop progressively growing tumors. However, this fraction approaches unity over a wide dose range for lines that require only a few cells to generate a successful take. While this is rare for virus-induced leukemias, more reliable data can be obtained by determining the least number of cells required to cause 50% of recipients to develop leukemia. Once this value is defined by the R & M method for the cell-host system under study, the potency of the cell preparation for transferring leukemia will be most simply expressed by the number of cells to be transplanted.

Occasionally, advantage is taken of graded host responses in order to estimate the number of cells with growth potential. Survival time of injected mice has been used with apparent success with certain transplantable murine leukemia lines, and spleen weight may also be a valid variable if the cells are injected IV.

Spleen colony method. The enumerative assay method for leukemia cells resembles in several ways the enumerative type of assay for leukemia virus, but only superficially. Because spleen foci are lesions of virus-transformed host cells, foci do not develop in lethally irradiated mice;[5] in contrast, spleen tumor colonies are transplants of donor cells and develop with the same frequency in irradiated or unirradiated hosts.[3]

The main resemblance between the two assay methods is the technique employed. A suspension of leukemia cells is usually washed at least once in medium and diluted so that 10^2–10^6 cells in 0.5 ml are inoculated into the tail vein of normal young adult mice of the same strain as the donor. Nine or ten days later the injected animals are killed and their spleens are removed and placed in Bouin's fixative. Spleen colonies are counted in much the same way as spleen foci, except that colonies are larger (1–6 mm in diameter) and protrude more from the splenic substance.

The number of spleen colonies generated by the inoculation of "spontaneous" Ak lymphoma cells into Ak mice is directly proportional to the number of cells injected. However, with Gross virus–induced lymphomas in C3H/Bi mice, the number of colonies per spleen tends to reach a plateau as the number of inoculated cells increases.[4] This phenomenon is considered to have an immunologic basis, because the dose-response relationship becomes linear again if the cells are inoculated into C3H mice previously made tolerant by injections of Gross virus shortly after birth.

Recently the spleen colony method was modified to assay Friend virus–induced leukemia cells.[42] To prevent foci from developing among the colonies, the titer of SFFV in the cell suspensions is diminished by washing the cells three times in medium. In addition, the cells, recovered from an inbred mouse strain that is susceptible to SFFV, are injected into first generation hybrids between the susceptible strain and a resistant strain (such as C57BL). Such hybrids, though resistant to SFFV, are fully susceptible (according to the laws of transplantation) to parental cell grafts.

Transplantation immunity. Resistance to transplants of virus-induced leukemias can be elicited in adult mice by several forms of immunization. These include (1) inoculation of virus, (2) injection of leukemic cells that have been rendered incapable of transferring leukemia by dilution past the threshold dose for a successful graft, (3) irradiation, or (4) recovery of cells from a histo-incompatible strain. Preparations that contain SFFV should also be treated with Formalin (1:500, 24 hours) to remove viral infectivity prior to immunization.[39] One injection of antigen may be sufficient to demonstrate significant immunity, but a schedule of two or three injections spaced at 1–3-week intervals provides better results. The degree of immunity is usually tested 4–10 days after the last injection of antigen. Groups of mice are given equal numbers or graded doses of leukemia cells, and quantal or enumerative host responses are determined as previously described.

Serologic Techniques

Group-specific antigens are common to all MuLV and are thought to exist chiefly within the nucleoid of the virion. Subgroup-specific antigens may be either G (Gross) or FMR (Friend-Moloney-Rauscher) in specificity; they occur on the cell membrane and also in soluble form in the plasma of leukemic mice. Type-specific antigens may take any of at least five forms, although there is some cross-reactivity among three of them

(Table 11.6). They exist on the viral envelope and on portions of the cell membrane involved in budding.[2]

The techniques described here are limited to those that usually detect only one of the three types of antigen. Techniques that may detect more than one type of antigen are based on serologic reactions such as CF, FA, and HI tests.

Group-specific antigens. Because mice have a very limited capacity (if any) to produce antibodies against MuLV group–specific (gs) antigens, sera are usually harvested from rats bearing MuLV-induced tumors. Another requirement for the detection of these antigens is their release from MuLV virions by disruption of the outer envelope with multiple cycles of freezing and thawing or with mild ether extraction. Under these conditions the soluble internal gs antigens will combine with antibody and form immunoprecipitation lines in the AD test.

A major gs antigen, called gs1, is common to Gross, Friend, Moloney, and Rauscher viruses,[16] but does not cross-react with leukemia viruses of other species. In contrast, another antigen, gs3, is shared with leukemia viruses of cats, rats, and hamsters, but not chickens.[13]

Subgroup-specific (cellular) antigens. Cells are thought to be destroyed immunologically when a critical concentration of complement is bound to antigen-antibody complexes at the surface.[26] Presumably, therefore, a cytotoxic test reflects the presence of cell-bound antigens only.[14] Certainly the cytotoxic test detects the subgroup-specific antigens of the G and FMR categories, but there remains some uncertainty whether it can also detect viral envelope antigens at the cell membrane during the budding process.[29]

The cytotoxic test has been modified for testing relatively dilute cell suspensions and is carried out as follows: obtain suspensions of viable cells from enlarged leukemic organs (usually spleen) and dilute to a concentration of 10^7 per ml. Incubate equal volumes (0.1 ml) of cells, diluted antiserum, and guinea pig serum, diluted one-third as a source of complement, for 45 minutes at 37°C. Percentage of viability is then determined microscopically from the ratio of unstained cells to total cells after the addition of trypan blue. (The latter is kept as a 0.2% stock solution; immediately before use, dilute 4 parts of this with 1 part of 4.25% saline.) In every test, controls must be included in which the cells are incubated with either guinea pig serum or antiserum; no more than 10% dead cells should be observed by the end of the test.

The cytotoxic test can be used to detect many other antigens on murine leukemias, including the soluble FMR antigen that has been adsorbed onto indicator EL4 leukemic cells.[3] The G soluble antigen will also adsorb onto these cells, but its detection requires the FA test.[1] These subgroup-specific antigens are probably not components of the virion envelope, because envelope antigens are type specific (Table 11.6).

Antigens. Several techniques have been used to study MuLV envelope antigens, such as virus agglutination or the immunoelectroadsorption technique, but the best technique is virus neutralization, which is quantitative, reliable, and simple, especially if an enumerative response virus assay is used. Neutralization experiments may be designed in either of two ways: keep the antiserum concentration constant and estimate the amount of virus neutralized,[10] or keep the virus concentration constant and determine the dilution of antiserum required to neutralize 50% of the virus activity. The former method is especially effective for discriminating between closely related viruses if the kinetics of virus neutralization are followed, which is only practical if a focus or plaque assay for MuLV is available.[5]

Briefly, the VN method is as follows: prewarm diluted serum and virus separately, and at time zero combine the two in a test tube and incubate in a 37°C water bath. At 10–15-minute intervals for up to an hour thereafter, remove a sample from the reaction tube, dilute appropriately in ice-cold saline, and immediately assay for viral infectivity. The fractional virus survival for each period of incubation is calculated by dividing the corresponding residual virus titer by the original virus titer at the beginning of the experiment (or better, by the titer of virus incubated under the same conditions with normal serum). Antiserum potencies are expressed in terms of the inactivation constant, K, determined from the following equation: $K = (D/t) \log_e (V_o/V_t)$, where D is dilution of an-

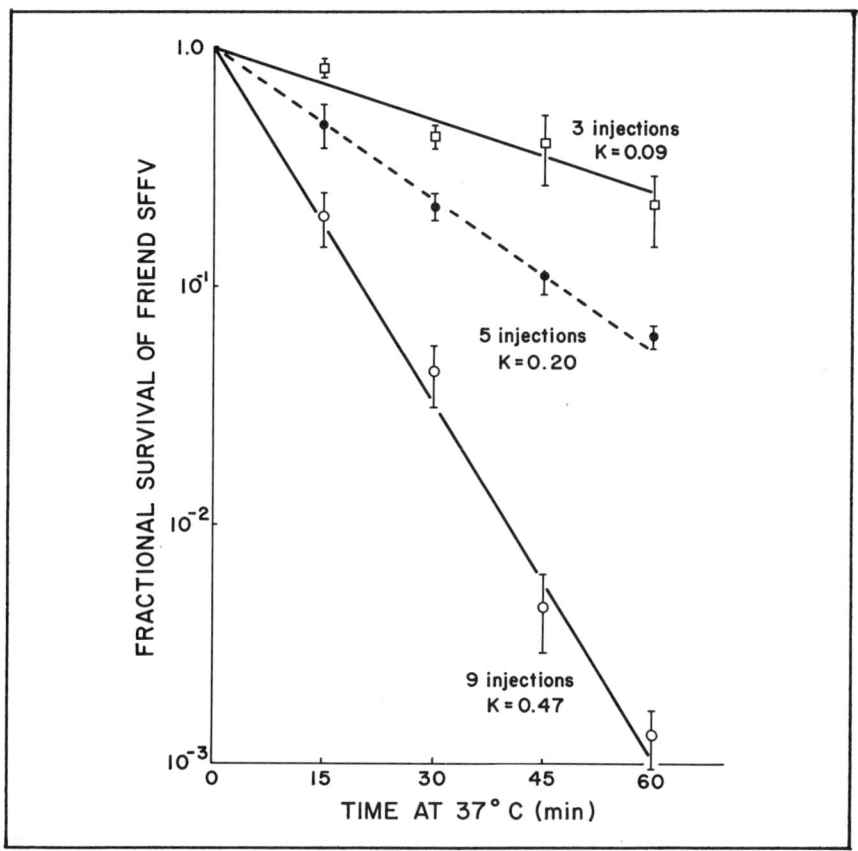

Figure 11.1. Neutralization kinetics of Friend spleen focus-forming virus (SFFV) by antisera of varying potency. C3H mice were injected at weekly intervals with 10^7 Formalin-treated leukemic cells induced by SFFV. Four days after the last injection, sera were recovered, diluted 1:4, and tested for SFFV-neutralizing activity. Standard errors are shown by vertical lines.

tiserum, V_o is virus titer at time zero, and V_t is virus titer at time t. Dilution of an antiserum reduces the slope of the curve but does not alter the value of K, nor, in the case of SFFV neutralization, does the presence of cellular debris.[39]

The neutralization curves of SFFV shown in Figure 11.1 demonstrate that with increasing numbers of immunizations (10^7 Formalin-treated SFFV-infected C3H leukemia cells) there is a corresponding increase in the potency (K value) of the antiserum recovered from C3H mice. Immunization of rabbits with normal C3H spleen cells, however, will result in antiserum with strong neutralizing activity for SFFV harvested from C3H mice (K > 0.8). Absorption with normal C3H spleen homogenates and normal liver powder will remove all of the neutralizing activity from this serum and most of the neutralizing activity of rabbit antiserum against SFFV-infected leukemia cells. These findings demonstrate the importance of complete absorption of antisera that have been recovered from a host different from that used for recovery of immunizing and target antigens since the virus apparently acquires some host-derived antigens during the budding process.

Absorption procedures are not required, of course, if antisera are produced in the same inbred mouse strain as the target antigen. Most mouse strains will respond to only three injections of Formalin-treated crude virus extracts, although 10–20 injections are recommended for potent antisera. It should be emphasized, however, that such antisera may contain antibodies against cellular as well as viral antigens; therefore, cross-reactivity even by virus neutralization would only indicate antigenic similarity between the leukemia used as immunizing antigen and the virus neutralized.

Additional Techniques

Morphology. Observations of gross pathologic changes in the size or shape of organs in virus-infected mice can be very useful, especially if they are made sequentially throughout the preleukemic period. In this way, leukemias have been classified according to the organ of origin: spleen, thymus, or intestinal lymph node.[33] Leukemias of splenic origin are further divided by observations at the cellular level into erythroid (Friend and Rauscher leukemias) and myeloid forms. Leukemias of thymic origin are lymphatic; those originating in intestinal lymph nodes begin as reticulum cell sarcomas.

Hematology. For routine hematologic procedures, blood samples may be collected in heparinized capillary tubes from the ophthalmic venous plexus by gentle pressure at the lateral canthus of the eye of anesthetized mice.[34] Counts of red or white blood cells per cu mm are made by dilution in Gower's solution or white cell count diluting fluid (respectively) in appropriate pipettes and by observation in a Neubauer counting chamber. In various strains of mice over 2 months of age, normal values range from 8–11 million RBC per cu mm and 5–12 thousand WBC per cu mm.[37] Hematocrit levels (ratio of packed red blood cell volume of total blood volume), which vary from 39–51% in normal mice, are now usually determined by the microhematocrit technique.[24]

Of the more specialized hematologic procedures for studying MuLV, the measurement of erythropoietic activity in the spleen by its uptake of radioactive ^{59}Fe has been especially useful as a sensitive indicator of infection with viruses that induce erythroleukemia.[25] At a given time after infection mice are injected intravenously with 1 μCi of

^{59}FeCl$_3$ diluted in saline. Twenty-four hours later the mice are killed and the radioactivity of each spleen is measured in a well-type scintillation counter. In mice infected with large doses of SFFV only 7 days previously, the percentage of injected ^{59}Fe taken up by the spleen is five to six times that of uninfected controls. Much lower virus doses can be detected by increasing the latent period before measuring the ^{59}Fe uptake.

References

1. Aoki, T., E.A. Boyse, and L.J. Old. Wild-type Gross leukemia virus. I. Soluble antigen (GSA) in the plasma and tissues of infected mice. *J. Nat. Cancer Inst.* 41:89–96, 1968.
2. Aoki, T., E.A. Boyse, L.J. Old, E. deHarven, U. Hämmerling, and H.A. Wood. G (Gross) and H-2 cell surface antigens: Location on Gross leukemia cells by electron microscopy with visually labeled antibody. *Proc. Nat. Acad. Sci.* 65:569–576, 1970.
3. Aoki, T., L.J. Old, and E.A. Boyse. Serological analysis of leukemia antigens of the mouse. National Cancer Institute Monograph, vol. 22, pp. 449–457, 1966.
4. Axelrad, A.A. Antigenic behaviour of lymphoma cell populations in mice as revealed by the spleen colony method. *Prog. Exp. Tumor Res.* 6:30–83, 1965.
5. Axelrad, A.A., and R.A. Steeves. Assay for Friend leukemia virus: Rapid quantitative method based on enumeration of macroscopic spleen foci in mice. *Virology* 24:513–518, 1964.
6. Bassin, R.H., N. Tuttle, and P.J. Fischinger. Isolation of murine sarcoma virus–transformed mouse cells which are negative for leukemia virus from agar suspension cultures. *Internat. J. Cancer* 6:95–107, 1970.
7. Buffett, R.F., J.T. Grace, Jr., and E.A. Mirand. Properties of a lymphoid leukemia agent isolated from Ha/ICR Swiss mice. *Proc. Am. Ass. Cancer Res.* 4:8, 1963.
8. Eckner, R.J., and R.A. Steeves. Defective Friend spleen focus-forming virus: Pseudotype neutralization by helper-specific antisera. *Nature—New Biology* 229:241–243, 1971.
9. Eckner, R.J., and R.A. Steeves. Classification of the murine leukemia viruses: Pseudotype neutralization by specific antisera. *Proc. Am. Ass. Cancer Res.* 12:57, 1971.
10. Fink, M.A., and F.J. Rauscher. Immune reactions to a murine leukemia virus. I. Induction of immunity to infection with virus in the natural host. *J. Nat. Cancer Inst.* 32:1075–1082, 1964.
11. Fischinger, P.J., and T.E. O'Connor. Tissue culture assay of helper activity of murine leukemia virus for murine sarcoma virus. *J. Nat. Cancer Inst.* 40:1199–1212, 1968.
12. Friend, C. Cell-free transmission in adult Swiss mice of a disease having the character of a leukemia. *J. Exp. Med.* 105:307–318, 1957.
13. Geering, G., T. Aoki, and L.J. Old. Shared viral antigen of mammalian leukemia viruses. *Nature* 226:265–266, 1970.
14. Gorer, P.A., and P. O'Gorman. The cytotoxic activity of isoantibodies in mice. *Transplant. Bull.* 3:142–143, 1956.
15. Graffi, A. Chloroleukemia of mice. *Ann. N.Y. Acad. Sci.* 68:540–558, 1957.
16. Gregoriades, A., and L.J. Old. Isolation and some characteristics of a group-specific antigen of the murine leukemia viruses. *Virology* 37:189–202, 1969.
17. Gross, L. "Spontaneous" leukemia developing in C3H mice following inoculation, in infancy, with Ak leukemic extracts or Ak embryos. *Proc. Soc. Exp. Biol. Med.* 76:27–32, 1951.
18. Gross, L. How many different viruses causing leukemia in mice? *Acta Haemat.* 32:44–62, 1964.
19. Holmberg, E.A.D., C. Vasquez, C. Dosne de Pasqualini, A. Pavlovsky, and S.L. Rabasa. Acellular passage of ^{32}P-induced leukemia: An electron microscopic study. *Cancer Res.* 27:198–204, 1967.
20. Klein, E., and G. Klein. Mouse antibody production test for the assay of the Moloney virus. *Nature* 204:339–342, 1964.
21. Kunii, A., H. Takemoto, and J. Furth. Leukemogenic filterable agent from estrogen-induced thymic lymphoma in RF mice. *Proc. Soc. Exp. Biol. Med.* 119:1211–1215, 1965.
22. Lieberman, M., and H.S. Kaplan. Leukemogenic activity of filtrates from radiation-induced lymphoid tumors in mice. *Science* 130:387–388, 1959.
23. Mazurenko, N.P. Induction of leukoses in mice with infectious viruses and the significance of the latter in the etiology of disease. *Problems Oncology* 6:873–882, 1960.
24. McGovern, J.J., A.R. Jones, and A.G. Steinburg. The hematocrit of capillary blood. *New Eng. J. Med.* 253:308–312, 1955.
25. Mirand, E.A., T.C. Prentice, J.G. Hoffman, and J.T. Grace, Jr. Effect of Friend virus in Swiss and DBA/1 mice on ^{59}Fe uptake. *Proc. Soc. Exp. Biol. Med.* 106:423–426, 1961.

26. Möller, E., and G. Möller. Quantitative studies of the sensitivity of normal and neoplastic mouse cells to the cytotoxic action of isoantibodies. *J. Exp. Med.* 115:527–553, 1962.
27. Moloney, J.B. Biological studies on a lymphoid-leukemia virus extracted from sarcoma 37. I. Origin and introductory investigations. *J. Nat. Cancer Inst.* 24:933–951, 1960.
28. Moloney, J.B. The murine leukemias. *Fed. Proc.* 21:19–31, 1962.
29. Old, L.J., and E.A. Boyse. Antigens of tumors and leukemias induced by viruses. *Fed. Proc.* 24:1009–1017, 1965.
30. Pope, J.H. The isolation of a mouse leukemia virus resembling Friend virus. *Austral. J. Exp. Biol.* 40:263–276, 1962.
31. Rauscher, J.B. A virus-induced disease of mice characterized by erythrocytopoiesis and lymphoid leukemia. *J. Nat. Cancer Inst.* 29:515–543, 1962.
32. Rich, M.A., J. Geldner, L.W. Johns, M. Kalocsky, P. Meyers, E.L. Rothstein, R. Siegler, and J. Gershoa-Cohen. Studies on murine leukemia-nucleic acids. *Trans. N.Y. Acad. Sci.* 25:580–589, 1963.
33. Rich, M.A., and R. Siegler. Virus leukemia in the mouse. *Ann. Rev. Microbiol.* 21:529–572, 1967.
34. Riley, V. Adaptation of orbital bleeding technic to rapid serial blood studies. *Proc. Soc. Exp. Biol. Med.* 104:751–754, 1960.
35. Rowe, W.P., W.E. Pugh, and J.W. Hartley. Plaque assay techniques for murine leukemia viruses. *Virology* 42:1136–1139, 1970.
36. Rowson, K.E.K., and I.B. Parr. A new virus of minimal pathogenicity associated with Friend virus. I. Isolation by end-point dilution. *Internat. J. Cancer* 5:96–102, 1970.
37. Russell, E.S., E.F. Neufeld, and C.T. Higgins. Comparison of normal blood picture of young adults from 18 inbred strains of mice. *Proc. Soc. Exp. Biol. Med.* 78:761–766, 1951.
38. Stansly, P.G., and H.D. Soule. Experiments on the transplantation and cell-free transmission of a reticulum cell sarcoma in BALB/c mice. *Proc. Am. Ass. Cancer Res.* 3:270, 1961.
39. Steeves, R.A., and A.A. Axelrad. Neutralization kinetics of Friend and Rauscher leukemia viruses studied with the spleen focus assay method. *Internat. J. Cancer* 2:235–244, 1967.
40. Steeves, R.A., and R.J. Eckner. Host-induced changes in infectivity of Friend spleen focus-forming virus. *J. Nat. Cancer Inst.* 44:587–594, 1970.
41. Steeves, R.A., R.J. Eckner, E.A. Mirand, and R.L. Priore. Rapid assay of murine leukemia virus helper activity for Friend spleen focus-forming virus. *J. Nat. Cancer Inst.* 46:1219–1228, 1971.
42. Thomson, S., and A.A. Axelrad. A quantitative spleen colony assay method for tumor cells induced by Friend leukemia virus infection in mice. *Cancer Res.* 28:2105–2114, 1968.
43. Toth, B. Development of malignant lymphomas by cell-free filtrates prepared from a chemically induced mouse lymphoma. *Proc. Soc. Exp. Biol. Med.* 112:873–875, 1963.
44. Woods, W.A., J. Massicot, and M.A. Chirigos. An immunofluorescent focus assay for Gross leukemia virus. *Proc. Soc. Exp. Biol. Med.* 135:772–777, 1970.

12. Orbiviruses

The name orbiviruses implies that circles or rings may be seen on the surface of the virion formed by the capsomeres. The International Committee on Taxonomy of Viruses has placed the orbiviruses under the family Reoviridae. A former name for the viruses was diplornaviruses, which indicated that they contained double-stranded (DS) RNA. The four diseases that will be discussed here are bluetongue, African horsesickness, Ibaraki disease, and epizootic hemorrhagic disease of deer.

Bluetongue Virus

Bluetongue (BT) is a noncontagious viral disease primarily of sheep, although cattle and other ruminants may undergo inapparent infection and occasionally clinical infection. The virus is vector transmitted and the disease therefore is seasonal in nature. The incubation period is 7–10 days.

Bluetongue was observed first in South Africa, after the importation of European breeds of sheep in 1905.[3,21] The disease became widespread throughout much of the African continent before appearing in other parts of the world, including Cyprus (1924), Turkey (1944), Israel (1951), Portugal and Spain (1956), Pakistan (1960), India (1964), and Australia (1977).[18,38] The disease was suspected in Texas in 1949 and was subsequently confirmed in California (1954) by isolation and identification of the virus.[24] It has since spread to most western and some midwestern states in which extensive sheep raising is carried on.[6]

The BT virus is transmitted by biting arthropods. Thus far, however, only species of the genus *Culicoides* have been incriminated.[8,30] On the basis of studies of *C. variipennis,* culicoides appear to be biologic rather than mechanical vectors.[12] In Africa, *C. pallidipennis* is the vector of BT.[38]

There are strong indications that epizootics of BT are initiated by virus transmitted from a reservoir host or hosts.[19] Cattle appear to be a likely source of virus, as inapparent infection occurs in these animals under natural conditions.[6,9] When cattle are experimentally inoculated they become viremic, but the infection is asymptomatic. Also, goats and white-tailed deer in the United States[36] and blesbuck in Africa[27] have been experimentally infected. Naturally occurring BT has been reported in bighorn sheep[32] and the virus has been isolated from wild rodents in Africa.[18] Serologic surveys have revealed evidence of infection in elk, antelope, Barbary sheep, moose, and three species of deer.[40] However, the role played by these species in the epizootiology of BT is unknown.

The lesions associated with BT infection in sheep vary greatly in severity, although they are more pronounced in the naturally occurring disease than in that produced experimentally. They include hyperemia and necrosis of the epithelial surfaces of the buccal cavity, dental pad, and occasionally the esophagus and rumen, in addition to coronitis and hemorrhagic streaking of the periople. Subcutaneous tissues of the neck, ventral thorax, and intermandibular space are infiltrated with a yellowish edematous fluid. Edema also may be present in the tissues of the gastrointestinal tract, heart, and lungs. Of considerable diagnostic significance are the petechial and ecchymotic hemorrhages frequently observed in the heart and the suffusion hemorrhages at the base of the pulmonary artery.[39] Microscopic findings are in keeping with the gross pathologic changes and consist essentially of degenerative and necrotic changes in the digestive tract, skeletal musculature, and myocardium. There is no evidence of inclusion bodies due to bluetongue infection.[26]

The mortality rate from BT is relatively low in the United States, rarely exceeding 5–10% of the infected animals. Death due to the virus occurs shortly after the acute stage of the disease, whereas that occurring later is usually due to pneumonia resulting from secondary bacterial infection. Ewes vaccinated with modified live virus vaccine between the fourth and eighth weeks of gestation may give birth to stillborn or living but deformed lambs as a consequence of in utero infection.[34] Presumably, naturally occurring BT causes the same syndrome.

Although BT was first reported (1934) to cause clinical disease in cattle,[3] signs and lesions in cattle are rarely seen.[38] However, the virus is known to invade the fetuses of subclinically infected cattle, causing hydranencephaly and cerebral hypoplasia in the offspring.[25] The frequency with which the virus has been recovered from clinically normal cattle, and the failure of the virus to produce signs of illness in cattle after experimental inoculation, raises doubts concerning the etiologic role of the virus in those rare instances when it is isolated from cattle with clinical signs of disease. Clinical signs similar to those of BT in sheep are seen in cattle with BVD-MD.

In epizootic areas of Africa where BT has existed for many years, the cattle population has acquired immunity as a consequence of repeated inapparent infection, and this immunity is passively transferred to the offspring. It is reinforced by repeated, naturally occurring, inapparent infection; consequently, clinical evidence of the disease in African cattle rarely if ever occurs.[18] Likewise, clinical evidence of BT in U.S. cattle rarely occurs. However, in the United States, BT in sheep is relatively mild as compared to that which occurs elsewhere. In countries where BT suddenly appeared (e.g. Israel, Spain, and Portugal), many cattle had clinical infections and some died.[18]

The BT virus has a diameter of 54 nm and the RNA is double stranded.[42] The protein coat has 32 capsomeres arranged in a 5:3:2 symmetry.[37] The virion does not have a true envelope.[10,37] The virus is inactivated by heating at 60°C for 30 minutes and by pH of 6 or less; it is stable in the alkaline range.[18] In blood with anticoagulant and preservative, the virus remains infectious for years at 4°C.[16]

Specimens

Blood provides the best material for viral isolation.[38] It is readily available and when taken at the acute stage of the infection contains almost as much virus as does splenic tissue. Spleen is the tissue of choice from animals dead of the disease, although other organs that contain considerable blood are also satisfactory. However, antibody is usually beginning to appear by the time of death, so the likelihood of isolating virus is greatly decreased.[38]

The stage at which the blood is obtained largely determines the success of isolation attempts. In experimentally inoculated sheep and presumably in those undergoing naturally occurring infection, the virus attains maximal levels prior to the febrile rise and before neutralizing antibodies appear, which is about day 9 after inoculation.[23] As the infection is usually not detected until clinical signs or death occur, viral isolation can be expedited by subinoculating blood or splenic tissue from affected sheep into a clinically normal sheep and subsequently drawing blood samples from this animal at the appropriate times for viral isolation. Blood should be treated with an anticoagulant solution such as oxalate, carbolic acid, and glycerol (OCG).[38]

Laboratory Procedures

Cultures. Bluetongue virus can be propagated in a number of host systems including sheep, chicken embryos,[1] cell cultures,[17] suckling mice,[41] and suckling hamsters.[7] However, not all are equally suitable for isolation of the virus.

Intravascular inoculation of 11–12-day-old chicken embryos provides a highly sensitive method for isolation of BT virus and is now the preferred method for isolating the virus from field specimens.[13,14] This method is also useful for VN tests.[15] Special equipment is not required and the technical details can be readily mastered. In contrast to the situation with YS inoculation, embryo deaths occur on the initial passage of virus-containing material and the titers obtained are 2–3 log units higher. Viral typing can also be carried out by IV inoculation; by this method, isolation and identification of BT virus can be accomplished within 10 days.[15] Chicken embryos inoculated with BT virus via any route must be incubated at 33.6°C and not at 37°C.[1]

Low-passage (1–5) cultures of ovine adult or fetal kidney, or ovine fetal lymph node, lung, or testicle cells in either lactalbumin-Earle's (LE) or Hanks' medium containing 3% fetal calf serum, are most satisfactory for either viral isolation or serologic investigation. Corresponding cultures of bovine fetal kidney and lymph node cells in the same mediums are also satisfactory. Line cell cultures of ovine or bovine fetal kidney or bovine lymph node likewise support viral multiplication, although the titers are lower than those in low-passage cultures of the same cells. Multiplication of the virus has also been reported in cultures of HeLa, Chang liver, McCoy synovial, and Henle's intestinal cells,[11] although in lower titer than in either bovine or ovine cells. Eagle's MEM is the medium of choice for these cells.

Ovine or bovine tissue cell monolayers in roller tubes inoculated when 3–5 days old give optimal yield of virus after 96 hours of incubation at 33.6–37°C. This temperature range is in contrast to the narrow range (33.6–34°C) required for multiplication of the virus in chicken embryos.[1] Incubation of cell cultures beyond 96 hours causes a decrease in the viral titer.

All isolates of BT virus recovered to date produce CPE in cell cultures. These changes appear in ovine or bovine cells from 24 to 36 hours after inoculation of cell culture–adapted virus and from 4 to 8 days in the case of specimen materials containing the virus.[18]

Animal inoculation. In addition to sheep, suckling mice and suckling hamsters can be used as laboratory animals.[5]

Immunology and serology. Bluetongue virus exists in a multiplicity of antigenic types, all of which share a common group antigen or antigens.[28] Currently there are 20 types of BTV that have been identified on a worldwide basis; 15 occur in Africa, 4 in the United States, 1 in Cyprus, 1 in Pakistan. The reference strains for 17 of the types of BTV are (1) Biggarsberg, (2) Urvheid, (3) Cyprus, (4) Theiler, (5) Massop, (6) Strathene, (7) Utrecht, (8) Camp, (9) University Farm, (10) Portugal (BT-8 California), (11) Neslpoort (BT-Station, Texas), (12) Blyenesport, (13) Westlands (BT-67-41B, Idaho), (14) Kolwani, (15) 133/60, (16) Pakistan, and (17) Newtype (BT-62-45S, Wyoming).[2,20] Thus the United States has types 10, 11, 13, and 17.[2] Portugal and Spain apparently have succeeded in eradicating BT.[38] Type 20 is Australia (CSIRO 19).

Either BT virus or antibodies may be detected with CF, VN, AD or FA tests. The CF test is group specific and is used for routine diagnosis.[35] A modification of the so-called "standard" CF test, as used in South Africa, is used in Canada and the United States. Both test procedures use antigen prepared from mouse brain after extraction with acetone-ether or, in the case of the standard test, virus propagated in eggs or cell culture.[18] The modified procedure differs from the standard in that the serums are inactivated at 60°C for 30 minutes instead of 53°C for 90 minutes, and are then incubated in the presence of antigen at 9°C for 18 hours rather than at 37°C for 90 minutes. Also, the guinea pig complement is supplemented in the modified test by addition of normal unheated calf serum free of BT antibodies in a concentration of 5%. The modified procedure is more sensitive than the standard test, giving titers three to eight times higher, and it can detect antibody in cattle serum, whereas the standard procedure cannot.[4] Complement-fixing antibodies can be detected in serums by day 14 postinoculation[33] and they persist for approximately 16 weeks.[4]

The VN test is probably the most widely used for diagnostic purposes, largely because of its relative simplicity, although it is a type-specific test. Indicator systems include chicken embryos inoculated IV, low-passage ovine or bovine renal cell cultures or cell lines such as McCoy cells, and baby mice or hamster cells. As the titer of stored BT virus does not remain stable, freshly prepared culture must be used as test antigen. The test procedure consists of titrating the virus in the presence of a constant dilution of the test and control serums. The cell cultures are incubated at 37°C after inoculation. Titers are expressed in terms of the NI.[31]

The AD test uses a group-specific soluble antigen derived by dialysis and low-speed centrifugation of BT virus culture in lamb kidney cells. Positive reactions may be obtained with serums from sheep as early as 14 days after infection and with some for as long as 3 years.[22] The direct FA technique may be used to detect BT virus; the indirect method is used for serums to detect group-specific antibodies.[29]

Reference laboratories. ADR Laboratory, Denver, Colo.; NADC; for wildlife ruminants only, Department of Veterinary Science, University of Wisconsin, Madison; for the WHO world reference laboratory for typing exotic strains of BT virus, Veterinary Research Institute, Onderstepoort, South Africa.

References

1. Alexander, R.A. The propagation of bluetongue virus in the developing chick embryo with particular reference to the temperature of incubation. *Onderstepoort J. Vet. Sci.* 22:7–26, 1947.
2. Barber, T.L., and M.M. Jochim. Serotyping bluetongue and epizootic hemorrhagic disease virus strains. *Am. Ass. Vet. Lab. Diagnosticians 18th Ann. Proc.,* pp. 149–162, 1975.
3. Bekker, J.G., G. DeKoch, and J.B. Quinlan. The occurrrence and identification of bluetongue in cattle—the so-called pseudo foot and mouth disease in South Africa. *Onderstepoort J. Vet. Sci. Anim. Ind.* 2:393–507, 1934.
4. Boulanger, P., G.M. Ruckerbauer, G.L. Bannister, D.P. Gray, and A. Girard. Studies on bluetongue. III. Comparison of two complement-fixation methods. *Can. J. Comp. Med. Vet. Sci.* 31:166–170, 1967.
5. Bowne, J.G. Bluetongue disease. In *Advances in Veterinary Science and Comparative Medicine,* C.A. Brandly and E.L. Jungherr (eds.), vol. 15, pp. 1–46. Academic Press, New York, 1971.
6. Bowne, J.G., A.J. Luedke, N.M. Foster, and M.M. Jochim. Current aspects of bluetongue in cattle. *J. Am. Vet. Med. Ass.* 148:1177–1180, 1966.
7. Cabasso, V.J., G.I. Roberts, J.M. Douglas, R. Zorzi, M.R. Stebbins, and H.R. Cox. Bluetongue. I. Propagation of bluetongue virus of sheep in suckling hamsters. *Proc. Soc. Exp. Biol.* 88:678–681, 1955.
8. DuToit, R.M. The transmission of bluetongue and horsesickness by *Culicoides. Onderstepoort J. Vet. Sci.* 19:7–16, 1944.
9. DuToit, R.M. Bluetongue—recent advances in research: The role played by bovines in the transmission of bluetongue in sheep. *J. S. African Vet. Med. Ass.* 33:483–490, 1962.
10. Els, H.J., and D.W. Verwoerd. Morphology of bluetongue virus. *Virology* 38:213–219, 1969.
11. Fernandes, M.V. Isolation and propagation of bluetongue virus in tissue culture. *Am. J. Vet. Res.* 20:398–408, 1959.
12. Foster, N.M., R.H. Jones, and B.R. McCrory. Preliminary investigations on insect transmission of bluetongue virus in sheep. *Am. J. Vet. Res.* 24:1195–1200, 1963.
13. Foster, N.M., and A.J. Luedke. Direct assay for bluetongue virus by intravascular inoculation of embryonating chicken eggs. *Am. J. Vet. Res.* 29:749–753, 1968.
14. Goldsmit, L., and E. Barzilae. Isolation and propagation of a bluetongue virus strain in embryonating chicken eggs by the intravenous route of inoculation (preliminary report). *Refuah Vet.* 22:279–285, 1965.
15. Goldsmit, L., and E. Barzilae. An improved method for the isolation and identification of bluetongue virus by intravenous inoculation of embryonating chicken eggs. *J. Comp. Path.* 78:477–487, 1968.
16. Haig, D.A. Bluetongue. *Proc. 14th Internat. Vet. Cong.* (Madrid) 1:215–225, 1959.
17. Haig, D.A., D.G. McKercher, and R.A. Alexander. The cytopathogenic action of bluetongue virus on tissue culture and its application to the detection of antibody in the serum of sheep. *Onderstepoort J. Vet. Res.* 27:171–177, 1956.
18. Howell, P.G. Bluetongue In *Emerging Diseases of Animals.* FAO Agricultural Studies no. 61, pp. 111–153, 1963.
19. Howell, P.G. Some aspects of the epizootiology of bluetongue. *Bull. Off. Internat. Epiz.* 66:341–352, 1966.
20. Howell, P.G. The antigenic classification and distribution of naturally occurring strains of bluetongue virus. *J. S. African Vet. Med. Ass.* 41:215–223, 1970.
21. Hutcheson, D. Fever or epizootic catarrh. *Rep. Coll. Vet. Surg.* 1880:12, 1881.
22. Jochim, M.M., and T.L. Chow. Immunodiffusion of bluetongue virus. *Am. J. Vet. Res.* 30:33–41, 1969.
23. Klontz, G.W., S.E. Svehag, and J.R. Gorham. A study of the agar diffusion technic of precipitating antibody directed against bluetongue virus and its relation to homotypic neutralizing antibody. *Arch. ges. Virusforsch.* 12:259–268, 1962.

24. McKercher, D.G., B. McGowan, and J.K. Saito, Isolation, identification and typing of the bluetongue virus and a preliminary report on the serodiagnosis of the disease. *Proc. Am. Vet. Med. Ass.* 91:167–177, 1954.
25. McKercher, D.G., J.K. Saito, and K.V. Singh. Serologic evidence of an etiologic role for bluetongue virus in hydranencephaly of calves. *J. Am. Vet. Med. Ass.* 156:1044–1047, 1970.
26. Moulton, J.E. Pathology of bluetongue of sheep. *J. Am. Vet. Med. Ass.* 138:493–498, 1961.
27. Neitz, W.O. The Blesbuck (Damaliscus albifrons) as a carrier of heartwater and bluetongue. *J. S. African Vet. Med. Ass.* 4:24–26, 1933.
28. Neitz, W.O. Immunological studies on bluetongue in sheep. *Onderstepoort J. Vet. Sci.* 23:93–135, 1948.
29. Pini, A., H. Ohder, A.P. Whiteland, and L.T. Lund. Studies on the fluorescent and neutralizing antibodies to bluetongue virus in sheep. *Arch. ges. Virusforsch.* 25:129–136, 1968.
30. Price, D.A., and W.T. Hardy. Isolation of bluetongue virus from Texas sheep: *Culicoides* shown to be a vector. *J. Am. Vet. Med. Ass.* 124:255–258, 1954.
31. Reed, L.J., and H. Muench. Simple method of estimating fifty percent endpoints. *Am. J. Hyg.* 27:493–497, 1938.
32. Robinson, R.M., T.L. Hailey, C.W. Livingston, and J.W. Thomas. Bluetongue in desert bighorn sheep. *J. Wildlife Mgmt.* 31:165–168, 1967.
33. Ruckerbauer, G.M., D.P. Gray, A. Girard, G.L. Bannister, and P. Boulanger. Studies on bluetongue. V. Detection of the virus in infected materials by immunofluorescence. *Can. J. Comp. Med. Vet. Sci.* 31:175–181, 1967.
34. Schultz, G., and P.D. DeLay. Losses in newborn lambs associated with bluetongue vaccination of pregnant ewes. *J. Am. Vet. Med. Ass.* 127:224–226, 1955.
35. Shone, D.K., D.A. Haig, and D.G. McKercher. The use of tissue culture propagated bluetongue virus for complement fixation studies on sheep sera. *Onderstepoort. J. Vet. Res.* 27:179–182, 1956.
36. Stair, E.L., R.M. Robinson, and L.P. Jones. Spontaneous bluetongue in Texas white-tailed deer. *Path. Vet.* 5:164–173, 1968.
37. Studdert, M.J., J. Bangborn, and R.B. Addison. Bluetongue virus structure. *Virology* 29:509–511, 1966.
38. Symposium on Bluetongue. Adelaide, South Australia, May 1974. *Austral. Vet. J.* 51:165–232, 1975.
39. Thomas, A.D., and W.O. Neitz. Further observations on the pathology of bluetongue in sheep. *Onderstepoort J. Vet. Sci.* 22:27–40, 1947.
40. Trainer, D.O., and M.M. Jochim. Serologic evidence of bluetongue in wild ruminants of North America. *Am. J. Vet. Res.* 30:2007–2011, 1969.
41. Van den Ende, M., A. Linder, and V.R. Kaschula. Experiments with the Cyprus strain of bluetongue virus: Multiplication in the central nervous system of mice, and complement fixation. *J. Hyg.* 52:155–164, 1954.
42. Verwoerd, D.W. Purification and characterization of bluetongue virus. *Virology* 38:203–212, 1969.

African Horsesickness Virus

African horsesickness virus (AHSV) causes an infection of solipeds characterized by edema and hemorrhage of the heart, lungs, and digestive organs. The clinical feature most often seen is swelling (from edema) of the neck and supraorbital tissues. A high mortality rate often occurs and the infected animals either die within 2 weeks or gradually recover.

The disease (types 1–8) has in the past mainly been confined to South, East, and Central Africa. However, recently AHSV type 9 has emerged and spread across North Africa and most of the Middle East, and has been found in Pakistan, India, Afghanistan, Turkey, Cyprus, and Spain.[4]

The incubation period of AHSV is from 1 to 2 weeks. Viremia occurs during the febrile stage. Fever, irregular respiration, and swelling of supraorbital, pharyngeal, jugular, axillary, scapular, abdominal, and scrotal areas are the main clinical signs. The mildest form of AHS is called horsesickness fever; usually only a febrile reaction is noted. This form is only seen with partially resistant animals.

For descriptive purposes the lesions of AHS have been divided into three types: cardiac, pulmonary, and mixed.[29] In the cardiac form the edema and hemorrhage involve the tissues of the heart and may extend from the supraorbital fat down the neck, forelegs, chest, and abdomen to the scrotum. In the pulmonary form the main findings are pulmonary edema, hydrothorax, and enlargement of the bronchial and mediastinal lymph glands. The mixed form combines features of both the cardiac and pulmonary forms and is the type most often seen in field cases. In all forms congestion of the liver and glandular fundus of the stomach are commonly found.[15] Some of the clinical signs and lesions of acute AHS resemble those of equine infectious arteritis, equine infectious anemia, trypanosomiasis, and anthrax. The differential diagnosis involves assessment of epizootic information, history, seasonal prevalence, arthropod presence, postmortem lesions of several animals, and hemograms. In enzootic areas it is necessary to consider in addition the locality, prevalence data, vaccination program, and the possibility of an infection by a new type of AHS virus.

For many years *Culicoides* sp. have been accepted as the major vectors of AHSV,[7] and *Aedes aegypti* also has been implicated.[26] Recent studies with *Culicoides, Aedes,* and *Culex* have failed to support the earlier work regarding survival of AHSV in these arthropods.[32] However, AHSV can be propagated in a mosquito TC cell line.[18] Also, field evidence on the occurrence of the disease during the mosquito season and in areas where mosquitos are abundant supports the original view of arthropod transmission.

AHSV has been listed as an unclassified arbovirus.[7] However, new evidence indicates that AHSV is very similar to bluetongue virus (BT)[19] and that both viruses may be classified as orbiviruses under the family Reoviridae.

AHSV and BT differ from the classical arboviruses in morphology, mode of replication, and resistance to lipid solvents.[12,19,30] AHSV and BT both have double-stranded RNA genomes.[19,31] The RNA of AHSV has been resolved into five components by sucrose gradient sedimentation analysis and into six segments in four size groups by polyacrylamide gel electrophoresis.[19] In thin sections the outer envelope of the AHS virion has a diameter of about 71 nm while the core is about 36 nm. Purified AHSV (without the envelope) has an icosahedral shape and is about 55 nm in diameter and probably consists of 32 capsomeres.[19]

AHSV is relatively resistant to various chemicals.[21] The virus is stable between pH 6.2 and 10 but is rapidly inactivated in acid solutions lower than pH 6. Neurotropic strains are destroyed at 60°C within 15 minutes. However, virus in tissue culture medium will withstand heating at 50°C for at least 3 hours and at 37°C for as long as 37 days.[21,25] When the virus is frozen and held at −35°C, a decrease in infectivity occurs.[30] It is more stable at −20 or −50°C.[13,23]

Specimens

Heparinized, oxalated, or defibrinated blood, or samples of the spleen, kidneys, or lymph nodes, may be used for tests during the early clinical stage. The specimens (particularly blood) should be refrigerated but not frozen unless the temperature can be maintained at −50°C or lower. The organ samples also can be preserved in buffered glycerol.

Laboratory Procedures

Cultures. Initially the field specimen should be inoculated IC, using suckling mice 3–5 days old. The incubation period may vary from 4 to 20 days. Mouse brain tissue should be harvested for additional passages after which the virus can be readily adapted to adult mice, guinea pigs, chick embryos, or tissue cultures.[1,3,8] AHSV will replicate well in Vero, MS, and baby hamster kidney (BHK) cell lines and in primary BHK cells.[18,24] These tissue culture cells also can be used for initial virus isolation. Not all types of AHSV produce clear CPE on the first passage but they usually do on subsequent passages. The Vero and MS cell cultures can also be used for the plaque technique.[11,20] Recently, a mosquito TC cell line has been developed for propagating AHSV.[18] In infected TC cells, multiple inclusion bodies are produced in the cytoplasm near the nucleus and can be demonstrated by FA technique. Virus titrations are usually made in mice or tissue cultures.

Animal inoculation. Horses and ponies are very susceptible, mules and donkeys are less susceptible, and zebras are highly resistant. Angora goats and sheep are occasionally infected and the virus may replicate in dogs that are fed large quantities of meat and organs from infected horses or are inoculated with AHSV.[2,6,28,29] Mice, ferrets, guinea pigs, and rats also can be infected by inoculation.[1,2] Human AHSV infections have not been reported.

Immunology and serology. There are nine types of AHSV (Table 12.1). Animals recovered from infection or vaccinated with one type of AHSV are susceptible to infection with any other type.[12,17] The nine types are readily differentiated by VN tests in mice or tissue culture.[10] The HI test can be used but has some drawbacks.[27] With VN tests many cross-reactions between types occur, particularly with types 6 and 9. AHS infection, but not the virus type, may be detected by CF, AD, and FA tests.[6,9,16,20] Two antigenic components common among all nine types were demonstrated by AD tests.

Table 12.1. Prototype strains representing established antigenic types of African horsesickness virus[12,22]

Types	Prototype strains
1	A501
2	OD
3	L
4	Vryheid
5	VH
6	114
7	Karen
8	18/60
9	S2

These strains are either tissue-culture or (neurotropic) mouse adapted. They are used as vaccine strains and to produce type-specific antiserums for tests. Strains 18/60 and S2 were attenuated at the Razi Institute, Teheran, Iran. The others were developed at the Onderstepoort Veterinary Research Laboratory in South Africa. Other virulent strains are used for challenge of immunity.

The early AHSV antibodies, which are detected by CF tests, usually appear within a week after the onset of fever, reach a peak level by the second week, continue at a high level for about a month, and then decline rapidly. In some infected animals neutralizing antibodies appear early and rapidly increase in titer, but more often they appear late and do not reach their peak titer until the second month after infection, and they may persist for years.

Attenuated live virus vaccines are mainly used;[6] however, killed virus vaccines also have had some successful trials.[22] In the southern parts of Africa, vaccine strains attenuated by mouse brain passage are used. Often the vaccines are polyvalent (7 types). In the Near East, Spain, and North Africa the vaccine strains used were attenuated by mouse brain passage and then passed in tissue culture. Some strains have been attenuated only by tissue culture passage and have given good results;[25] generally, these vaccines were monovalent (type 9).

Early in the Middle East outbreak of AHS, the polyvalent mouse brain vaccine containing types 1–7 conferred immunity to type 9 in most vaccinated horses.[13] In contrast, AHS was often observed in South Africa among horses reportedly vaccinated with polyvalent vaccines.[14]

Foals are usually vaccinated at about 7 months. The colostral antibodies they ingest from nursing their AHS-immunized mothers protest them for about 6 months.[5] Annual vaccinations are usually given to older animals before the mosquito season begins. The duration of immunity is quite variable. In experimental vaccine trials the immunity is challenged about a month after vaccination.

Reference laboratory. PIADC.

References

1. Alexander, R.A. Preliminary note on the infection of white mice and guinea-pigs with the virus of horsesickness. *J. S. African Vet. Med. Ass.* 4:1–9, 1933.
2. Alexander, R.A. Studies on neurotropic virus of horsesickness. I. Neurotropic fixation. *Onderstepoort J. Vet. Sci. Anim. Ind.* 4:291–322, 1935.
3. Alexander, R.A. Studies on the neurotropic virus of horsesickness. VI. Propagation in the developing chick embryo. *Onderstepoort J. Vet. Sci.* 11:9–19, 1938.
4. Alexander, R.A. The 1941 epizootic of horsesickness in the Middle East. *Onderstepoort J. Vet. Sci.* 23:77–92, 1948.
5. Alexander, R.A., and J.H. Mason. Studies on the neurotropic virus of horsesickness. VII. Transmitted immunity. *Onderstepoort J. Vet. Sci.* 16:19–32, 1941.
6. Dardiri, A.H., and Y. Ozawa. Immune and serologic response of dogs to neurotropic and viscerotropic African horsesickness viruses. *J. Am. Vet. Med. Ass.* 155:400–407, 1969.
7. DuToit, R.M. The transmission of bluetongue and horsesickness by Culicoides. *Onderstepoort J. Vet. Sci.* 19:7–16, 1944.
8. Goldsmit, L. Growth characteristics of six neurotropic and one viscerotropic African horsesickness virus strains in fertilized eggs. *Am. J. Vet. Res.* 28:19–24, 1967.
9. Hazrati, A., B. Mastan, and S. Bahrami. The study of African horsesickness virus by the agar double-diffusion precipitation test. I. Standardization of the technique. *Arch. Insti. Razi* 20:49–66, 1968.
10. Hazrati, A., and Y. Ozawa. Quantitative studies on the neutralization reaction between African horsesickness virus and antiserum. *Arch. ges. Virusforsch.* 25:83–92, 1968.
11. Hopkins, I.G., A. Hazrati, and Y. Ozawa. Development of plaque techniques for titration and neutralization tests with African horsesickness virus. *Am. J. Vet. Res.* 27:96–105, 1966.
12. Howell, P.G. The isolation and identification of further antigenic types of African horsesickness virus. *Onderstepoort J. Vet. Res.* 29:139–149, 1962.

13. Howell, P.G. African horsesickness. In *Emerging Diseases of Animals*. FAO Publication no. 61, pp. 73–108, 1963.
14. Howell, P.G. Observations on the occurrence of African horsesickness among immunized horses. *Onderstepoort J. Vet. Res.* 30:3–10, 1963.
15. Maurer, F.D., and R.M. McCully. African horsesickness—with emphasis on pathology. *Am. J. Vet. Res.* 24:235–266, 1963.
16. McIntosh, B.M. Complement fixation with horsesickness viruses. *Onderstepoort J. Vet. Res.* 27:165–169, 1956.
17. McIntosh, B.M. Immunological types of horsesickness virus and their significance in immunization. *Onderstepoort J. Vet. Res.* 27:465–538, 1958.
18. Mirchamsy, H. Propagation of African horsesickness virus in a mosquito cell line. *3d Internat. Conf. Equine Infect. Dis.* (Paris), 1972.
19. Oellermann, R.A., H.J. Els, and B.J. Erasmus. Characterization of African horsesickness virus. *Arch. ges. Virusforsch.* 29:163–174, 1970.
20. Ozawa, Y. Studies on the replication of African horsesickness virus in two different cell line cultures. *Arch. ges. Virusforsch.* 21:155–169, 1967.
21. Ozawa, Y. Studies on the properties of African horsesickness virus. *Jap. J. Med. Sci. Biol.* 21:27–39, 1968.
22. Ozawa, Y., and S. Bahrami. African horsesickness killed virus tissue culture vaccine. *Can. J. Comp. Med. Vet. Sci.* 30:311–314, 1966.
23. Ozawa, Y., and S. Bahrami. Effects of freezing on African horsesickness virus. *Arch. ges. Virusforsch.* 25:201–210, 1968.
24. Ozawa, Y., and A. Hazrati. Growth of African horsesickness virus in monkey kidney cell cultures. *Am. J. Vet. Res.* 25:505–511, 1964.
25. Ozawa, Y., A. Hazrati, and N. Erol. African horsesickness virus tissue culture vaccine. *Am. J. Vet. Res.* 26:154–168, 1965.
26. Ozawa, Y., F. Shad-Del, G. Nakata, and S. Navai. Transmission of African horsesickness by means of mosquito bites and replication of the virus in *Aedes aegypti*. *Proc. 1st Internat. Conf. Equine Infec. Dis.* (Stresa, Italy), pp. 196–207, 1966.
27. Pavri, K.M. Haemagglutination and haemagglutination-inhibition with African horsesickness virus. *Nature* 189:249–250, 1961.
28. Pilo-Moron, E., J. Vincent, and P. Sureau. Type 9 virus of African horsesickness in Algeria and identification of the strains isolated in 1965–1966. *Rev. Elevage Med. Vet. Pays Trop.* 20:5–20, 1967.
29. Theiler, A. *African Horsesickness: A System of Bacteriology in Relation to Medicine*, no. 7, pp. 362–375. H.M. Stationary Office, London, 1930.
30. Theiler, M. Action of sodium desoxycholate on arthropodborne viruses. *Proc. Soc. Exp. Biol.* 96:380–382, 1957.
31. Verwoerd, D.W. Purification and characterization of bluetongue virus. *Virology* 38:203–212, 1969.
32. Wetzel, H., E.M. Nevill, and B.J. Erasmus. Studies on the transmission of African horsesickness. *Onderstepoort J. Vet. Res.* 37:165–168, 1970.

Ibaraki Disease Virus

Ibaraki disease (ID) is a noncontagious viral infection that affects cattle clinically in a way that is similar to the manner in which bluetongue affects sheep.[1] Outbreaks of ID occurred in Japan in 1959 and 1960, but only during the late summer and fall, mostly south of 37° N latitude, and not at high altitudes, which suggests an anthropod vector. Serologic surveys demonstrated antibodies for ID in serums from cattle on Taiwan and Bali Island, Indonesia. However, the virus has only been isolated in Japan, and is named for the prefecture where this occurred.

The ID virus contains DS RNA, has 32 capsomeres, and does not have an envelope; the virion diameter is about 55 nm.[2] Thus it is morphologically similar to bluetongue virus.

ID causes a severe disease in cattle with a mortality rate of about 10%, but it does not cause clinical disease in sheep. In contrast, bluetongue is often a fatal disease in sheep and an almost inapparent disease in cattle. There is no known serologic relationship between ID and BT.

ID is characterized by fever, stomatitis, and difficulty in swallowing. The mucous membranes, skin, musculature, and vascular system are all involved in the disease. Degeneration of striated muscular tissue is observed in the esophagus, larynx, pharynx, tongue, and skeletal muscles.

Specimens

As in bluetongue, blood is the specimen of choice for virus isolation. The spleen also may be used.

Laboratory Procedures

Cultures. Primary bovine cell cultures are used. The CPE is usually seen in 3–7 days. Embryonating chicken eggs also can be used for viral studies.

Animal inoculation. Calf inoculation is a more sensitive method for viral isolation than cell cultures. It also helps rule out the presence of Bluetongue. The incubation period in calves is about 4–12 days. Suckling mice also can be used.

Immunology and serology. A vaccine has been used in Japan to control the disease. It is an egg-passaged, attenuated, live-virus, lyophilized vaccine. Either ID virus or antibodies may be detected with CF, VN, AD, or FA tests.

References

1. Inaba, Y. Ibaraki Disease and its relationship to Bluetongue. *Austral. Vet. J.* 51:178–185, 1975.
2. Ito, Y., Y. Tanaka, Y. Inaba, and T. Omori. Electron microscopy of Ibaraki virus. *Arch. ges. Virusforsch.* 40:29–46, 1973.

Epizootic Hemorrhagic Disease Virus of Deer

Epizootic hemorrhagic disease of deer (EHD) is a noncontagious viral disease that affects certain species of deer. The white-tailed deer (*Odocoileus virginianus*) is the host in the United States.[5,7] As in BTV, the EHD virus is transmitted by the midge, *Culicoides variipennis,* as a biologic vector.[1,3] EHD has been reported in the United States since 1955,[5] in Alberta, Canada, only in 1962 and not since,[3] and in Nigeria in 1974.[4]

Clinical EHD is rarely observed in natural outbreaks because most deer are found dead, often close to water.[3] The incubation period in experimental EHD infection is 4–12 days, and clinical signs and lesions are similar to those of BT infection of deer.[3,7] Both EHD and BT viruses have been isolated from a single deer in the southeastern United States[6] and from a herd of cattle in Colorado;[1] the cattle did not show clinical signs or lesions of infection. The EHD virus does not produce clinical disease in sheep or maintain itself in sheep,[3] and not all genera of deer are susceptible (unpublished transmission studies of E.P.J. Gibbs, Animal Virus Research Institute, Pirbright, Woking, Surrey, England).

The EHD and BT viruses have similar morphology and contain double-stranded RNA.[2] The regularly used serologic tests fail to show croos-reactivity between EHD and BT preparations; however, low-level cross-reactivity may be demonstrated with special CF techniques.[3] A plaque neutralization test is used to differentiate the serologic types of EHD and BT viruses.[1] Two serologic types of EHD have been proposed for U.S. viral isolates: type 1, strain New Jersey, and type 2, strain Alberta (Canada).[1] The Nigerian EHD viral isolates were of three distinct serotypes.[4]

References
1. Barber, T.L., and M.M. Jochim. Serotyping Bluetongue and epizootic hemorrhagic disease virus strains. *Am. Ass. Vet. Lab. Diagnosticians 18th Ann. Proc.*, pp. 149–162, 1975.
2. Borden, E.C., R.E. Shope, and F.A. Murphy. Physicochemical and morphological relationships of some arthropod-borne viruses to Bluetongue virus—a new taxonomic group: Physicochemical and serological studies. *J. Gen. Virol.* 13:261–271, 1971.
3. Frank, J.F., and N.G. Willis. Bluetongue-like disease of deer. *Austral. Vet. J.* 51:174–177, 1975.
4. Moore, D.L. Bluetongue and related viruses in Ibidan, Nigeria: Serologic comparison of Bluetongue, epizootic hemorrhagic disease of deer, and Abadina (Palyam) viral isolates. *Am. J. Vet. Res.* 35:1109–1113, 1974.
5. Shope, R.E., L.G. MacNamara, and R. Mangold. A virus-induced epizootic hemorrhagic disease of the Virginia white-tailed deer (*Odocoileus virginianus*). *J. Exp. Med.* 3:155–170, 1960.
6. Thomas, F.C., N. Willis, and G. Ruckerbauer. Identification of viruses involved in the 1971 outbreak of hemorrhagic disease in southeastern United States white-tailed deer. *J. Wildlife Dis.* 10:187–189, 1974.
7. Trainer, D.O., and L.H. Karstad. Epizootic hemorrhagic disease. In *Infectious Diseases of Wild Mammals*, J.W. Davis, L.H. Karstad, and D.O. Trainer (eds.), pp. 50–54. Iowa State University Press, Ames, 1970.

13. Orthomyxoviruses

The term myxoviruses (Greek, *myxo,* "mucus"), originally given to those viruses found to react with mucoproteins having N-acetylneuraminic acid determinants and found to agglutinate erythrocytes, has recently been changed to orthomyxoviruses.[10] This group comprises the influenza viruses of humans, swine, birds, and horses. Diseases caused by the influenza viruses usually but not always involve and are limited to the respiratory tract. Marked antigenic changes have occurred among some of the influenza viruses since they were first isolated. There has been considerable speculation about an extra-human reservoir of influenza viruses that infects humans, especially since the "Asian" influenza epidemic of 1957. Investigations to establish the exact relationship between human and animal influenza viruses have shown that there are several interspecies antigenic bridges among the influenza-A viruses.[1,6] The A_2/Hong Kong/68 influenza virus, originally isolated from human beings, also was isolated from pigs in Taiwan.[3]

The influenza viruses are 80–120 nm in diameter and have helical symmetry. They contain RNA and are ether sensitive and pH labile. Disruption of the particle by lipid solvents uncovers an inner helical component, the nucleocapsid, that has an approximate diameter of 9 nm.

The influenza viruses possess three principal antigenic components: the ribonucleoprotein (RNP) or "S" (soluble) antigen, and the surface antigens, hemagglutinin and neuraminidase. The RNP antigen can be assayed by the CF or AD tests and is used for the classification of influenza viruses into types A, B, and C. The hemagglutinin and neuraminidase antigens are strain specific, and they are used to determine antigenic differences among viruses of the same type by the CF, HI, VN, neuraminidase inhibition, and AD tests. There also are host component antigens on the virion.

The type A influenza viruses contain a number of subtypes, some of which are further divided into antigenic variants (Table 13.1). These subdivisions have been determined by assays of the surface antigens.

In human epidemics, three type A antigenic groups of influenza virus have been recognized: subtypes A_0, A_1, and A_2. In swine, only one serologic influenza-A type is known. Two subtypes of influenza-A virus have been detected in equines: A/Equine-1

Table 13.1. Methods for isolation and identification of influenza virus infections

Species affected	Preferred specimens	Chicken* embryos	Tissue† culture	Animals and lesions	Identification of virus Type	Identification of virus Subtype	Reference strain
Porcine	Washings or swabs of nasal passages, lung, trachea	9–11 days amnionic or allantoic sac	Monkey kidney, fetal swine trachea	Mice, ferrets; pneumonia	CF, AD	CF	A/Swine/1976/31
Equine	Washings or swabs of nasal passages	Same as above	Monkey kidney, calf kidney, horse kidney	Same as above	CF, AD	CF	A/Equine-1/Prague/1/56 A/Equine-2/Miami/1/63
Avian	Washings or swabs of nasal passages, conjunctiva, trachea, air sacs, lung, cloaca	Same as above	Chicken kidney, CEF, monkey kidney	Chicks, poults, ducklings; resp. signs, death	CF, AD	CF	A1/Turk/Eng/63 A2/Virus-N/49 A3/Duck/Eng/56 A4/Duck/Czech/56 A5/Chicken/Scot/59 A6/Turk/Ontario/3724/63 A7/Duck/Ukraine/63 A8/Turk/Ontario/618/67

*Preferred host. Most virus strains will adapt to growing in the allantoic cavity following three amnionic passages. Temperature of incubation of 35°C is preferable.
†Primary isolation of virus varies greatly with cells used and virus strains encountered.[3]

and A/Equine-2. Over 100 strains of influenza-A virus have been recovered from different species of birds. Recently, the avian isolates have been classified into eight serologic groups. Fowl plague virus (FPV) is designated A1, the N-virus (which does not produce clinical disease in chickens but is lethal for embryos) is A2, and the various other avian influenza viruses are designated A3 through A8 (Table 13.1). Reference strains for the major influenza virus groups in animals are also shown in Table 13.1. The subtypes cannot be strictly species delineated, the interspecies antigenic bridges of various proportions have been described.[5]

The antigenic differences among the influenza-B viruses are not as extensive as those of the type A viruses, and sufficient information is not available to establish subtypes. Antigenic differences among the type C influenza viruses have also not been great enough to establish subtypes.

In swine and horses, influenza is primarily a respiratory disease.[2,4,8,9,11] The morbidity is high but the mortality is generally low. Numerous subtypes and strains of the type A influenza virus have been recovered from the avian species. Influenza-A infections in poultry may range from subclinical to acute or chronic respiratory infections with little or no mortality; while in other instances, the disease (e.g. fowl plague) may be a highly acute, rapidly spreading septicemic infection resulting in mortalities approaching 100%.

Only type A influenza viruses have been isolated from avian, porcine, and equine species under natural conditions. The virus that was responsible for influenza in human beings during the 1918–1919 pandemic was clearly related to the swine influenza virus, based on retrospective serologic studies. Types B and C influenza viruses occur naturally only in humans. Because the general sequence of human influenza outbreaks is known for the past 50 years or more from serologic studies, it is possible to approximate a person's age in decades by assessing the serologic response of his or her serum to the various human influenza viruses.

Specimens

Frequency of isolation of the influenza viruses in all species is greatest during the very early stages of the acute phase of the disease or onset of clinical symptoms. Viremia is usually transient and is dependent upon the species of animal and strain of virus encountered.

Nasal swabs from swine and horses are generally adequate but swabs from the deeper nasal passages are preferable. In poultry, tracheal swabs, lung and sinus exudates, or swabs from the cloaca are most desirable. Frequently, isolations can be made from repiratory tissues of recently expired animals.

Laboratory Procedures

Cultures. Primary isolations of the influenza viruses can be made in 9–11-day-old embryonating chicken eggs or in cell cultures. Numerous subcultured primary-cell and line-cell cultures have been used for virus isolations in various species, as listed in Table 13.1. After appropriate preparation, the sample should be inoculated into either the amnionic or allantoic cavities, the AmC route being the more sensitive. Both AlC and AmC inoculations may be done in the same egg to increase the possibility of growth of the virus. Growth of the virus may result in the death of the embryo in 2–8 days. Also, the embryonic fluids may hemagglutinate chicken or guinea pig red blood cells. In all instances the AmC and AlC fluids should be serially blind passed at least three times before the sample is considered negative.

Various tissue culture cells may be used for primary isolation of many of the influenza viruses (Table 13.1); however, cytopathic effects may not always be seen.

Animal inoculation. See Table 13.1.

Immunology and serology. The standard HI, HAdI, CF, VN, and AD test procedures should be employed for identification of the agent and for serologic diagnosis of influenza infections.

The HI test is conducted using allantoic and/or amnionic fluid as antigen, chicken or guinea pig RBC, and known antisera prepared against specific influenza viruses to detect specific inhibition. Swine isolates should be tested with antisera prepared against any of the swine influenza viruses isolated during the past 10 years. Equine isolates should be tested against antisera prepared against A/Equine-1 and A/Equine-2 viruses. Since these viruses are serologically distinct, antisera of both subtypes must be used. Isolations made from avian species should also be tested against known antisera prepared against viruses of the paramyxovirus group (NDV, PI Yucaipa, and Turkey/Wisc/68). In all cases, avian isolates should be handled with caution in countries in which fowl plague is exotic until this disease is definitely eliminated as a diagnostic possibility.

Most orthomyxoviruses grow in tissue culture systems and exhibit hemadsorption. Although the HAdI is less sensitive than the HI test, it is useful in some instances, particularly during a known epizootic, to identify an isolate.

Nonspecific inhibitors may interfere with either the HI or HAdI tests, and sera from heterologous species should be treated by absorption and RDE before use.

The CF (and/or the AD) test is preferable to use when there appears to be a major shift in antigenic composition in a specific type of influenza virus or if nonavid strains are encountered that react poorly in the HI test. However, antisera prepared against the soluble antigenic component of influenza A, B, and C must be available. It should be remembered that most sera from the avian species are anticomplementary, that swine sera are procomplementary, and that difficulties with individual horse and mule sera must be taken into consideration.

Testing for all possible influenza and parainfluenza viruses is laborious and expensive unless there is sufficient evidence to narrow the possibility to one or two types. This is particularly important with the many isolates from the avian species. Detection procedures can be considerably narrowed by using the AD test, using the soluble antigen prepared against influenza-A,[7] and conducting the HI or HAdI tests with the known viruses of the paramyxovirus group (ND and PI Yucaipa viruses). Keep in mind that new antigenic variants which would not be detected by the HI test may appear.

Laboratories not familiar with identification techniques and not having the necessary influenza reference sera on hand should have the final identification conducted elsewhere.

Reference laboratories. World Influenza Center, National Institute for Medical Research, London; WHO Influenza Center for the Americas, CDC; for fowl plague, Plum Island Animal Disease Center (PIADC), Greenport, N.Y.

WHO Recommendation for Designating Influenza Viruses

Human influenza viruses. Type-subtype/place of origin/serial/year of isolation. Example: A2/Singapore/305/57.

Animal influenza viruses. Type/species of origin–subtype if any/place of origin/serial/year of isolation. Examples: A/Equine-1/Prague/1/56, A/Equine-2/Miami/1/63, A/Swine/Wisconsin/3/66, A/Pheasant/Italy/647/66.

References

1. Easterday, B., W.G. Laver, H.G. Pereira, and G.C. Schild. Antigenic composition of recombinant virus strains produced from human and avian influenza-A viruses. *J. Gen. Virol.* 5:83–91, 1969.
2. Francis, J., and H.F. Maassab. Influenza viruses. In *Viral and Rickettsial Infections of Man,* F.L. Horsfall and I. Tamm (eds.). 4th ed. Lippincott, Philadelphia, 1965.
3. Kundin, W.D. Hong Kong A_2 influenza virus infection among swine during a human epidemic in Taiwan. *Nature* 228:857, 1970.
4. Lief, F.S., and D. Cohen. Equine influenza: Studies of the virus and of antibody patterns in convalescent, interepidemic and postvaccination sera. *Am. J. Epidemiol.* 82:225–227, 1965.
5. McQueen, J.L., J.H. Steele, and R.Q. Robinson. Influenza in animals. In *Advances in Veterinary Science,* C.A. Brandly and C.E. Cornelius (eds.), vol. 12, pp. 285–336. Academic Press, New York, 1968.
6. Pereira, H.G., B. Tumova, and R.G. Webster. Antigenic relationship between influenza-A viruses of human and avian origins. *Nature* 215:982–983, 1967.
7. Samadieh, B., and R.A. Bankowski. Identification of influenza-A viruses by immunodiffusion. *Am. J. Vet. Res.* 32:479–484, 1971.
8. Scholtens, R.G., and J.H. Steele. U.S. epizootic of equine influenza, 1963: Epizootiology. *Public Health Rep.* 79:393–398, 1964.
9. Shope, R.E. Swine influenza. In *Diseases of Swine,* H.W. Dunne (ed.). 2d ed. Iowa State University Press, Ames, 1964.
10. Wildy, P. *Classification and Nomenclature of Viruses.* Monographs in Virology, vol. 5, pp. 1–81. S. Karger, New York, 1971.
11. Wilson, J.C., J.T. Bryans, and E.R. Doll. Recovery of influenza virus from horses in the equine epizootic of 1963. *Am. J. Vet. Res.* 26:1466–1468, 1965.

14. Papovaviruses

The term papova is derived from the first two letters of the common names of three viruses in the group: *pa*pilloma, *po*lyoma, and *va*cuolating.[33] The papovavirus group includes the papilloma viruses of human, rabbit, dog, deer, and bovine (subgroup A), as well as polyoma virus of rodents, K virus of mice, and rabbit vacuolating and simian vacuolating viruses (subgroup B). Although each papovavirus is antigenically distinct,[27] and all those studied differ in the base composition of their nucleic acids,[5] the members of the group have a number of characteristics in common. All are double-stranded DNA viruses that multiply in the nuclei of their host cells. The principal viruses in the group are oncogenic, particularly when given to young or newborn animals. Nucleic acid extracted from the viruses is also oncogenic.[9] Subacute, latent, and chronic infections are common. The sizes of the viruses are reported to be 45–50 nm[27] but some of the papilloma viruses are slightly larger, 55 nm in diameter.[5] The mature virus particles appear to be icosahedrons with 5:4:3 cubic symmetry. Filamentous forms of some of the viruses have been observed. In early studies the number of capsomeres was considered to be 42, but in recent years the number 72 has been more widely accepted. Smaller particles of the polyoma virus have also been observed—a particle 38 nm in diameter with 32 capsomeres, and a particle 22 nm in diameter with 12 capsomeres. The viruses are resistant to ether and therefore do not contain essential lipids. All remain viable under a variety of conditions that would destroy many other viruses.

The papovaviruses and the diseases that they induce are shown in Table 14.1. Some of the viruses not only have a narrow host range but also have specific tissue affinity. The rabbit oral papilloma virus, for example, produces disease only when injected into the oral mucosa of rabbits, but this tissue is not susceptible to the oncogenic activity of the Shope papilloma virus. Likewise, the oral mucosa of dogs but not the skin of dogs is susceptible to the canine papilloma virus. Simian virus 40 (SV40) infects rhesus monkeys, its natural host, and other monkeys such as patas, cynomolgus, and cercopithecus, but it is oncogenic only when injected into newborn hamsters.

Table 14.1. Diseases induced by papoviruses

Virus	Host	Age when infected	Disease	Latent period
Human wart	Humans	Young	Skin or genital warts, laryngeal papillomas[3]	6 wk–8 mo
Rabbit oral papilloma	Domestic rabbits	All ages	Papillomas[32]	9–38 d
Shope rabbit papilloma	Wild and domestic rabbits	All ages	Papillomas[24] Revert to carcinomas	6–12 d 9 mo
Rabbit vacuolating	Wild and domestic rabbits		None[21]	
Bovine papilloma	Cattle	Young	Papillomas[6]	1–3 mo
	Horses	Young	Fibrous nodules, sarcomas[29]	12–27 d
	Hamsters	2–52 wk	Connective tissue tumors[36]	100 d
	Mice		Connective tissue tumors[1]	
Deer fibroma	Deer	Young	Fibromas[38]	7 wk
Goat papilloma	Goat	Adult	Papillomas[7]	
Chamois papilloma	Chamois or Alpine goat	Adult	Papillomas[26]	
Pig genital papilloma	Pigs	Young	Genital skin papillomas[31]	4–10 wk
Equine papilloma	Horses	Young	Papillomas[4]	2–3 mo
Canine papilloma	Dogs	Young	Papillomas[8]	30–35 d
Hamster papilloma	Hamsters	Young	Papillomas[18]	4–18 mo
		Newborn	Lymphomas, sarcomas	
	Rats	Newborn	Lymphomas, sarcomas	
Polyoma	Mice	Newborn	Over 20 histologically different tumors[39]	1–10 mo
	Hamsters	Newborn	Sarcomas, hemangiomas[16]	21 d–7 mo
	Rats	Newborn	Sarcomas, hemangiomas[15]	56 d–4½ mo
	Rabbits	Newborn	Fibromas[14]	13–64 d
	Guinea pigs	Newborn	Sarcomas[12]	11–960 d
	Ferrets	Newborn	Sarcomas[20]	152–176 d
	Mastomys	Newborn	Sarcomas[34]	32–172 d
K	Mice	<10 d old	Fetal pneumonia[25]	9–12 d
SV40	Rhesus monkeys	Newborn	None[11]	
	Hamsters	Newborn	Sarcomas[11]	82–200 d

Specimens

Tumors are the specimens of choice for isolation of all the oncogenic papovaviruses. Of the known papilloma viruses, the hamster papilloma virus is the only one that can be propagated in cell cultures and the bovine papilloma virus is the only one that can be propagated in embryonating chicken eggs. In papillomas afflicting natural hosts, mature virus is usually plentiful in the nondividing keratinized portion but not in the proliferating basal layers.[28] In papillomas induced by the Shope rabbit papilloma virus in domestic rabbits or in the epidermoid carcinomas, which evolve from papillomas either in the domestic or in the natural host, mature virus may be sparse or absent.

Unlike the papillomas, mature virus is present only in small quantities in tumors induced by either the polyoma virus or SV40. The concentration of virus can be increased by culture of the tumor material in susceptible cell cultures.[10]

The rabbit vacuolating virus is present in some Shope rabbit papillomas and in some rabbit tumors induced by dimethyl-benzanthracene.[35] The virus is nonpathogenic but it can be propagated in cell cultures.

The K virus does not induce tumors but it is plentiful in the lungs, liver, spleen, and kidneys of infected mice, particularly if the mice are infected when less than 10 days of age.[25]

Laboratory Procedures

Cultures (Table 14.2). Crude extracts of the keratinized portion of papillomas—ground, diluted with saline solution, centrifuged, and either filtered or not filtered—usually contain sufficient virus to infect other susceptible animals. Virus in the tumor extracts can be concentrated or purified by methanol precipitation,[17] fluorocarbon treatment,[31] high-speed centrifugation, or cesium chloride, sucrose, or glycerol density-gradient centrifugation.[5]

Nucleic acid extracted from Shope rabbit papillomas or carcinomas, whether or not they contain mature virus, can induce tumors in rabbits.[22] Likewise, tumors can be induced in mice or hamsters by nucleic acid extracted from polyoma virus–induced tumors or from the polyoma virus, and tumors can be induced in hamsters by nucleic acid derived from SV40.

The rabbit vacuolating virus grows in rabbit kidney monolayers with cytopathic changes occurring and has titers of 10^5–10^7.[21]

Hamster papilloma virus grows in hamster embryo cell cultures without cytopathic changes. The virus was first recovered by incubating normal-appearing hamster embryo

Table 14.2. Papovavirus cultivation

	In animals				In embryonating eggs
Virus	Route of inoculation	Host	Tissue	In cell culture	
Human wart	Skin	Usually children	Wart[3]	No[27]	
Rabbit oral papilloma	Oral mucous membranes	Domestic rabbits	Papillomas[32]		
Shope rabbit papilloma	Skin	Cottontail rabbits	Papillomas[37]	No[21]	
Rabbit vacuo-lating virus				Rabbit kidney[21]	
Bovine papilloma	Skin, vagina, and urinary tissue	Calves, young cattle	Papillomas[6]	No[21]	CAM[30]
Deer fibroma	Skin	Deer	Fibromas[38]		
Goat papilloma	Skin	Goats	Papillomas[7]		
Chamois papilloma	Skin	Rabbits	Papillomas[26]		
Pig genital papilloma	Genital skin	Pigs	Papillomas[31]		
Equine papilloma	Skin	Young horses	Papillomas[4]		
Canine papilloma	Oral mucous membranes and neighboring skin	Young dogs	Papillomas[8]	No[2]	
Hamster papilloma				Hamster embryo[18]	
Polyoma				Mouse embryo or kidney[39,16]	No
K	IC, IP	Mice 10 d old	Liver, spleen, kidney[25]		
SV40				*Cercopithecus* monkey kidney[40]	

cultures 1–6 weeks, then injecting the culture fluid into newborn hamsters. Four to eighteen months later, papillomas developed in more than 20% of the hamsters. Different neoplasms appeared when centrifuged or filtered extracts of the papillomas were injected into newborn hamsters or rats: in some studies more than half the animals developed abdominal lymphomas and reticulum cell sarcomas that started in the liver and spleen.[18]

Tumors induced by polyoma virus and SV40 contain little infectious virus. Both viruses grow well but slowly in appropriate cell cultures, with characteristic cytopathic changes. The cultures of choice for the polyoma virus are mouse embryo or mouse kidney cells; for SV40, cercopithecus monkey kidney cells. Maximum cytopathic titers for both viruses are obtained 14–28 days following inoculation.

The cytopathic changes induced by the two viruses are different. Mouse embryo cultures infected with the polyoma virus first show foci of small dark shrunken cells. Degeneration continues until the entire cell sheet is involved and most of the cells fall off the glass. SV40-infected *Cercopithecus* monkey kidney cell cultures develop small patches of cells with multiple small vacuoles in the cytoplasm. Cell destruction continues until all cell morphology is erased and only patches of brown amorphous material remain on the glass.

There have been no reports of attempts to grow K virus in cell cultures. The virus is widespread in the tissues of infected mice. Extracts of pooled lungs, liver, spleen, and kidneys from infected mice titrated by the IC route in mice less than 10 days of age gave titers of 10^5.

Virus identification. All the papovaviruses have properties in common. The sizes vary from 45 to 55 nm and the particles, as seen in the electron microscope, are naked spheres without a surrounding membrane. When examined by fluorescent microscopy after staining with acridine orange, the greenish coloration characteristic of DNA viruses is noted in the nuclei. All the viruses are resistant to the action of ethyl ether and have slow growth cycles.[27]

Different criteria are necessary to identify the individual papovaviruses. The host, the site of tumor formation, and the length of the latent period for tumor development are indicative of some of the viruses. The human wart virus is species specific. Shope papilloma virus induces papillomas in the skin of rabbits but not in the oral mucosa, the site of tumors induced by the rabbit oral papilloma virus. Rabbits bearing Shope papillomas are susceptible to the rabbit oral papilloma virus and rabbits bearing oral papillomas are susceptible to the induction of papillomas by the Shope rabbit papilloma virus. The rabbit vacuolating virus differs from the other rabbit papovaviruses by being nonpathogenic, and it can be distinguished by its capacity to grow in rabbit kidney cell cultures with characteristic cytopathic changes.[21]

The bovine papilloma virus has a wider host range than other papilloma viruses. It induces fibrous nodules in horses and a variety of connective tissue tumors in hamsters and C3H strain mice. Although the tumors regress, the disease is of economic importance because of damage to the hides.

Deer are the only animals known to be susceptible to the deer fibroma virus. Little is known about the goat or chamois papilloma viruses. The bovine papilloma virus may be the etiologic agent in these species, or the etiologic agent may not belong to the papovavirus group. The pig genital papilloma also needs further study to determine if it actually is a papovavirus.

The equine and the canine papilloma viruses are highly species specific and the latter has specific tissue affinity; tumors appear only in the oral mucous membranes and nearby skin areas. The hamster papilloma differs from other papilloma viruses by its capacity to grow in cultures of hamster embryo and to produce tumors when injected into newborn rats.

The polyoma virus induces any of over 20 histologically different tumors (leukemias and lymphomas are the notable exceptions). The tumors may arise at almost any site. The most common sites in many strains of mice are the parotid glands, but in A strain mice, bone tumors are commonly seen. Sarcomas or hemangiomas are induced in a variety of tissues in hamsters, rats, guinea pigs, and ferrets. Rabbits are the only animals whose polyoma virus–induced tumors regress. Following inoculation of newborn rabbits with virus, multiple small hard nodules, some filled with amber or reddish fluid, appear on the skin. The nodules disappear after 3–4 months.

Virus can be isolated in mouse embryo or mouse kidney cell cultures from most of the polyoma virus–induced tumors; the cytopathogenic changes in the cultures are characteristic.

The K virus of mice is pathogenic for mice less than 10 days of age but it is nononcogenic. It differs histologically from other viruses in that endothelial swelling is an outstanding feature.

Rhesus monkeys are often carriers of SV40 and the virus can be recovered by culturing their kidney tissue for 2–3 weeks. Fluid from such cultures may be used to infect cercopithecus monkey kidney cell cultures or to infect newborn hamsters. The virus is cytopathic for cercopithecus monkey kidney cells and it induces sarcomas at the site of inoculation in hamsters inoculated SC, IP, or IM. Hamsters injected IC may develop ependymonas.[11]

Most of the papovaviruses are readily identifiable serologically by standard methods. Many are identifiable by tests carried out in vivo or in vitro, depending upon the virus involved. Three of the viruses produce HA. The rabbit vacuolating virus causes HA of guinea pig erythrocytes at either 4 or 20°C, but only after treatment of the virus in the culture fluids with RDE followed by heating at 56°C for 30 minutes. The polyoma virus causes HA with erythrocytes at 4°C from a variety of animal species, e.g. guinea pig, chick, mouse, human type O, but erythrocytes from guinea pigs are usually used. The virus, particularly when present in animal tissues, is often combined with nonspecific inhibitors. These inhibitors can be removed by heating at 56°C for 30 minutes or at 37°C for 2 hours, or by treatment with fluorocarbon or RDE.

The K virus agglutinates only sheep erythrocytes and HA takes place at 4°C, room temperature, or 37°C. Clearer patterns are generally seen at 4°C. Elution of the virus from the erythrocytes does not occur at any of the three temperatures.

Most of the papovaviruses that have been tested are capable of fixing complement or of reacting in FA tests.[23,28] These tests may reveal the presence of either virus or virus-induced cellular antigens. Positive CF antigens have not been demonstrated in hamster tumors induced by the bovine papilloma virus. The AD test has seldom been used in studies of the papovaviruses.[42]

Cell transformation in vitro. Some of the papovaviruses that fail to grow in cell cultures nevertheless have the capacity to transform such cultures. The Shope rabbit papilloma virus, for example, transforms cell cultures prepared from wild cottontail rabbits, domestic rabbits, and rats.[19] The bovine papilloma virus transforms bovine kidney cells, fetal cells from several mouse strains, and hamster embryo cells. The polyoma virus transforms cells from animal species such as cattle, mice, rats, or hamsters.[3] SV40 is of considerable interest because it can transform human buccal mucosa and kidney cells as well as cells from other animals. The K virus has been shown to transform mouse lung cells.[41]

Immunity and challenge. Animals that have papillomas which regress are usually immune to reinfection with the homologous virus. Polyoma virus–induced tumors, except in the rabbit, and SV40 induced–tumors do not regress. Most offspring of adult hamsters immunized by inoculation of live virus are resistant to challenge with the virus used to immunize the mother. Many hamsters born to unimmunized mothers and infected with SV40 when newborn do not develop tumors if repeatedly inoculated with large doses of the virus twice weekly starting approximately 20–25 days after the initial infecting dose of virus.[13]

The rabbit vacuolating virus infects rabbits but causes no known disease. The K virus is nonpathogenic for adult mice. Reports are not available regarding immunity in the offspring or immunized mice.

Diagnostic pathology. Histologically, tumors induced by the papovaviruses do not differ sufficiently from tumors induced by certain chemicals or other viruses to be conclusively diagnostic. Only the K virus, which causes ballooning of the nuclei and endothelial swelling when fixed in Zenker's solution and stained by H & E, is histologically different from the changes caused by other pneumonitis viruses with which it might be confused.

Clinical signs of disease are generally a rare indication of infection with a papovavirus. Many susceptible animals have low-grade infections that can only be diagnosed on the basis of serologic procedures, long incubation of cell cultures prepared from or inoculated with suspected virus-containing fluids or tissue extracts, or inoculation of susceptible animals with such materials.

References

1. Boiron, M., J.P. Levy, M. Thomas, J.C. Friedmann, and J. Bernard. Some properties of bovine papilloma virus. *Nature* 201:423–424, 1964.
2. Chambers, V.C., and C.A. Evans. Canine oral papillomatosis. I. Virus assay and observations on various stages of the experimental infection. *Cancer Res.* 19:1188–1195, 1959.
3. Ciuffo, G. Innesto positivo con filtrate di verruca vulgare. *Gior. Ital. Mal. Ven. Pelle.* 42:12–17, 1907.
4. Cook, R.H., and C. Olson, Jr. Experimental transmission of cutaneous papilloma of the horse. *Am. J. Path.* 27:1087–1097, 1951.
5. Crawford, L.V., and E.M. Crawford. A comparative study of polyoma and papilloma viruses. *Virology* 21:258–263, 1963.
6. Creech, G.T. Experimental studies of the etiology of common warts in cattle. *J. Ag. Res.* 39:723–727, 1929.

7. Davis, C.L., and H.E. Kemper. Common warts (papillomata) in goats. *J. Am. Vet. Med. Ass.* 88:175–179, 1936.
8. DeMonbreun, W.A., and E.W. Goodpasture. Infectious oral papillomatosis of dogs. *Am. J. Path.* 8:43–56, 1932.
9. Di Mayorca, G.A., B.E. Eddy, S.E. Stewart, W.S. Hunter, C. Friend, and A. Bendich. Isolation of infectious deoxyribonucleic acid from SE polyoma-infected tissue cultures. *Proc. Nat. Acad. Sci.* 45:1805–1808, 1959.
10. Eddy, B.E. Comparison of properties of two viruses—SV40 and polyoma virus—oncogenic for hamsters. *Perspectives Virol.* 3:138–158, 1963.
11. Eddy, B.E. Simian virus 40 (SV40): An oncogenic virus. *Prog. Exp. Tumor Res.* 4:1–26, 1964.
12. Eddy, B.E., G.S. Borman, R.L. Kirschstein, and R.H. Touchette. Neoplasms in guinea pigs infected with SE polyoma virus. *J. Infec. Dis.* 107:361–368, 1960.
13. Eddy, B.E., G.E. Grubbs, and R.D. Young. Tumor immunity in hamsters infected with adenovirus type 12 or simian virus 40. *Proc. Soc. Exp. Biol. Med.* 117:575–579, 1964.
14. Eddy, B.E., S.E. Stewart, R.L. Kirschstein, and R.D. Young. Induction of subcutaneous nodules in rabbits with the SE polyoma virus. *Nature* 183:766–767, 1959.
15. Eddy, B.E., S.E. Stewart, M.F. Stanton, and J.M. Marcotte. Induction of tumors in rats by tissue culture preparations of the SE polyoma virus. *J. Nat. Cancer Inst.* 22:161–171, 1959.
16. Eddy, B.E., S.E. Stewart, R. Young, and G.B. Mider. Neoplasms in hamsters induced by mouse tumor agent passed in tissue culture. *J. Nat. Cancer Inst.* 20:747–761, 1958.
17. Fischer, R.G. Methyl alcohol precipitation of the rabbit papilloma virus. *Proc. Soc. Exp. Biol. Med.* 72:323–325, 1949.
18. Graffi, A., T. Schramm, I. Graffi, D. Bierwolf, and E. Bender. Virus-associated skin tumors of the Syrian hamster: Preliminary note. *J. Nat. Cancer Inst.* 40:867–873, 1968.
19. Greene, H.S.N. The induction of the Shope papilloma in homologous transplants of embryonic rat skin. *Cancer Res.* 13:681–683, 1953.
20. Harris, R.J.C., F.C. Chesterman, and G. Negroni. Induction of tumors in newborn ferrets with Mill Hill polyoma virus. *Lancet* 1:788–791, 1961.
21. Hartley, J.W., and W.P. Rowe. New papova virus contaminating Shope papilloma. *Science* 143:258–260, 1964.
22. Ito, Y., and C.A. Evans. Induction of tumors in domestic rabbits with nucleic acid preparations from partially purified Shope papilloma virus and from extracts of the papillomas of domestic and cottontail rabbits. *J. Exp. Med.* 114:485–500, 1961.
23. Kidd, J.G. A complement-fixation reaction involving the rabbit papilloma virus (Shope). *Proc. Soc. Exp. Biol. Med.* 35:612–614, 1937.
24. Kidd, J.G., and P. Rous. A transplantable rabbit carcinoma originating in a virus-induced papilloma and containing the virus in marked or altered form. *J. Exp. Med.* 71:813–837, 1940.
25. Kilham, L., and H.W. Murphy. A pneumotropic virus isolated from C3H mice carrying the Bittner milk agent. *Proc. Soc. Exp. Biol. Med.* 82:133–137, 1953.
26. Kumer, Von L. Ueber die papillomatose der gemsen. *Wien. Klin. Wochenschr.* 48:890–891, 1935.
27. Melnick, J.L. Papova virus group. *Science* 135:1128–1130, 1962.
28. Noyes, W.F., and R.C. Mellors. Fluorescent antibody detection of the antigens of the Shope papilloma virus in papillomas of the wild and domestic rabbit. *J. Exp. Med.* 106:555–562, 1957.
29. Olson, C., and R.H. Cook. Cutaneous sarcoma-like lesions of the horse caused by the agent of bovine papilloma. *Proc. Soc. Exp. Biol. Med.* 77:281–284, 1951.
30. Olson, C., D. Segre, and L.V. Skidmore. Further observations on immunity to bovine cutaneous papillomatosis. *Am. J. Vet. Res.* 21:233–242, 1960.
31. Parish, W.E. A transmissible genital papilloma of the pig resembling condyloma acuminatum of man. *J. Path. Bact.* 8:331–345, 1961.
32. Parsons, R.J., and J.G. Kidd. A virus causing oral papillomatosis in rabbits. *Proc. Soc. Exp. Biol. Med.* 35:441–443, 1936.
33. Provisional Committee for Nomenclature of Viruses (PCNV). Proposals and recommendations. *Ann. L'Inst. Pasteur* 109:625–637, 1965.
34. Rabson, A.S., W.J. Branigan, and F.Y. Legallais. Production of tumors in Rattus (Mastomys) natalensis by polyoma virus. *Nature* 187:423–425, 1960.
35. Rashad, A.L., and C.A. Evans. A difference in sites of DNA synthesis in virus-induced (Shope) and in chemically induced epidermal tumors of rabbit skin. *Cancer Res.* 27:1639–1647, 1967.

36. Robl, M.G., and C. Olson. Oncogenic action of bovine papilloma virus in hamsters. *Cancer Res.* 28:1596–1604, 1968.
37. Shope, R.E., and E.W. Hurst. Infectious papillomatosis of rabbits with a note on the histopathology. *J. Exp. Med.* 58:605–624, 1933.
38. Shope, R.E., R. Mangold, L.G. MacNamara, and K.R. Dumbell. An infectious cutaneous fibroma of the Virginia white-tailed deer (Odocoileus virginianus). *J. Exp. Med.* 108:797–802, 1958.
39. Stewart, S.E., B.E. Eddy, and N. Borgese. Neoplasms in mice inoculated with a tumor agent carried in tissue culture. *J. Nat. Cancer Inst.* 20:1223–1243, 1958.
40. Sweet, B.H., and M.R. Hilleman. Detection of a "non-detectable" simian virus (vacuolating agent) present in rhesus and cynomologous monkey kidney cell culture material: A preliminary report. *Internat. Conf. Live Poliovirus Vaccines* (Washington) 2:6–7, 1960.
41. Takemoto, K., and P. Fabisch. Transformation of mouse cells by K-papovavirus. *Virology* 40:135–143, 1970.
42. Watson, D.H., G.L. LeBouvier, J.A. Tomlinson, and D.G.A. Walkey. Electron microscopy of antigen precipitates extracted from gel diffusion plates. *Immunology* 10:305–308, 1966.

15. Paramyxoviruses

The paramyxovirus group contains a number of distinct viruses that cause diseases in mammalian and avian species (Table 15.1). These viruses are roughly spherical, are heterogeneous in size, and have a particle diameter range of 125–250 nm. They are ether sensitive and contain lipoproteins. Not all members of the group have viral neuraminidase. The intact viral particle has a well-defined outer envelope covered with short projections. The virion contains single-stranded RNA that is about 17–18 nm in width. The viral replication takes place in the cell cytoplasm and perhaps in the nucleus also.

Unlike the orthomyxoviruses, some paramyxoviruses can hemolyze certain types of

Table 15.1. Properties of paramyxoviruses

Virus	Synonyms	Major host	Host range	Neuraminidase	HAd	HA
Mumps		Humans		+	+	+
Newcastle disease	Pneumo-encephalitis	Chickens, turkeys	Most birds	+	+	+
Yucaipa	None	Turkeys, chickens	Turkeys, chickens	+	+	+
Parainfluenza-1	Sendai, influenza-D, hemadsorption virus 2, HA-2[5]	Humans	Mice, guinea pigs	+	+	+
Parainfluenza-2	Croup-associated (CA) virus, DA virus[2]	Humans	Dogs	+	+	+
Parainfluenza-3	Shipping fever, SF-4, PI-3	Humans, cattle	Humans, cattle, buffalo, horses, sheep, guinea pigs, monkeys, swine, hamsters	+	+	+
Parainfluenza-4		Humans		+	+	+
Simian myxovirus	SV5, SA virus, DA virus, simian parainfluenza	Rhesus and cynomolgus monkeys	Dogs, humans		+	+
Measles		Humans	Monkeys	−	−	+
Distemper		Dogs	Wolf, coyote, mink, fox, ferret, weasel, skunk	−	−	−
Rinderpest		Cattle, buffalo	Order Artiodactyla, mice, rabbits, hamsters, chickens	−	−	−

erythrocytes and others can cause cell fusion under certain conditions. Some have common antigens that are not shared by the influenza viruses. Three serologically related viruses, those of measles, distemper, and rinderpest, have been tentatively allocated to the paramyxovirus group on the basis of the morphology of the virion.

Although the paramyxoviruses are a relatively homogeneous group, pathogenically they differ widely. Some cause localized infections of the respiratory tract and several produce generalized diseases. Among the latter, some are characteristically associated with skin rashes (measles) or CNS involvement (distemper and Newcastle disease). The more important veterinary paramyxoviruses are those of parainfluenza-3 (shipping fever), Newcastle disease, canine distemper, rinderpest, and peste des petits ruminants. In addition to the paramyxovirus diseases listed in Table 15.1, there are other viruses that ultimately may be included in the group, e.g. parainfluenza-5 of dogs,[1] pneumonia of mice,[4] and respiratory syncytial virus.[3]

References

1. Binn, L.N. A review of viruses recovered from dogs. *J. Am. Vet. Med. Ass.* 156:1672–1677, 1970.
2. Chanock, R.M. Association of a new type of cytopathogenic myxovirus with infantile croup. *J. Exp. Med.* 104:555–576, 1956.
3. Chanock, R.M., R.H. Parrott, K. Cook, B.E. Andrews, J.A. Bell, T. Reichelderfer, A.Z. Sapikian, F.M. Mastrota, and R.J. Huebner. Newly recognized myxoviruses from children with respiratory disease. *New Eng. J. Med.* 258:207–213, 1958.
4. Chu, C.M., J.K. Liang, and C.C. Wen. A study of a new mouse virus. I. Discovery of the virus. *Scientia Sinica* 6:1065–1080, 1957.
5. Johnson, K.M., R.M. Chanock, M.K. Cook, and R.J. Huebner. Studies on a new human hemadsorption virus. I. Isolation properties and characterization. *Am. J. Hyg.* 71:81–92, 1960.

Parainfluenza-3 Virus

Parainfluenza-3 virus plays an important role in respiratory disease of cattle. The virus has been isolated from humans, cattle, water buffalo, horses, and monkeys. Guinea pigs, hamsters, sheep, and swine are susceptible to experimental infection. Serologic evidence of infection has been found in humans,[1] cattle, horses, guinea pigs, swine, deer, and sheep.[2] Human and bovine strains of the virus that have been compared show a close relationship. Bovine strains have been isolated from cattle with and without signs of disease, suggesting that the virus may be harmless until conditions of stress precipitate the disease.

Severity of the disease varies from subclinical infection to severe fatal pneumonia. The apical, cardiac, and diaphragmatic lobes generally show small areas of consolidation. The severity of the lesions appears to depend on the presence of secondary bacteria, especially *Pasteurella multocida* and *P. hemolytica*. Histologic examination of involved areas reveals bronchiolitis and alveolitis. The bronchiolitis may extend into the bronchi, depending upon the severity and secondary involvement. There is also an infiltration with leukocytes and some edema, and multinucleated cells may be observed. Generally, acidophilic intracytoplasmic inclusions are found in alveolar macrophages and bronchiolar epithelial cells. Similar inclusions can be found in the nasal epithelium. In severely affected lungs there may be an extensive cellular infiltration with loss of alveolar structure and evidence of abscessation, emphysema, and/or edema.

Specimens

Parainfluenza-3 virus exerts its primary effect on the epithelial cells of the respiratory tract. It can generally be recovered from respiratory secretions, nasal scrapings, or tracheal or lung tissue. Optimally, nasal swabs should be obtained during the first 3–5 days following infection. Virus may be shed continuously or intermittently during the first 10 days of infection; thereafter, virus isolation becomes more difficult.

The nasal swabs should be placed in tissue culture fluid with penicillin, streptomycin, and an antifungal agent. The specimens should be chilled and inoculated promptly. When prolonged storage is unavoidable, the swab and tissue culture fluid should be quickly frozen and then stored, preferably at $-70°C$.

Laboratory Procedures

Cultures. Tissue culture methods are employed in the isolation and identification of the parainfluenza viruses. Primary bovine embryonic kidney cells (BEK) are most commonly used for making isolations from cattle. However, a variety of other cells are equally suitable, for example, kidney cells of bovine (BK), swine (SK), feline (FK), chicken embryo (CEK), and monkey (MK). Several cell lines also have been used, including MDBK and embryonic bovine tracheal (EBTr) cells. The cultures are used after monolayers are formed. Acceptable tissue culture media include Medium 199, Hanks' BSS plus 0.5% lactolbumin hydrolysate, Eagle's, Earle's, and others. The addition of serum is to be avoided where possible. The inoculated cultures are incubated at 35–37°C and observed for CPE under low-power microscope objective.

PI-3 produces good CPE in tissue culture after adaptation in most instances. The virus has also been reported to form plaques on BEK.

Some viral strains produce indefinite CPE, and sometimes CPE develops rather slowly; it is difficult to detect such stains or distinguish their effect from normal degenerative processes of the cell sheet. In these cases, the virus can be detected earlier by using the HAd technique. The cells can be tested for HAd using guinea pig erythrocytes on about the third day after inoculation, generally before CPE becomes evident. Positive HAd will be noted in infected cells when compared to uninoculated cell controls.

The virus can be further identified by demonstrating a specific HAdI with PI-3 antiserum. This procedure is rapid and simple. Some of the cells, with or without CPE, are washed and treated with antiserum. The erythrocytes are added after 15 minutes at room temperature. Lack of HAd is indicative of viral inhibition.

In some cases in which HA is used, parainfluenza virus will not produce HA until adapted to grow in vitro. Some virus isolates vary in HA activity with erythrocytes from different species. Generally, bovine or guinea pig erythrocytes are used in the HA test. Treatment of bovine erythrocytes with RDE results in a loss or reduction of HA titer.

Once the virus is isolated and shown to agglutinate erythrocytes, confirmatory identification can be achieved by the macro or micro HI test using specific anti-PI-3 serum.

Interferon activity has been reported in calf kidney cultures infected with some bovine strains of PI-3.

Animal inoculation. Guinea pigs, hamsters, pigs, or calves may be used as laboratory animals.

Paramyxoviruses

Immunology and serology. Serologic diagnosis of parainfluenza-3 infection commonly requires the use of paired sera. The HI and the VN tests are the two techniques most commonly used.

The HI test can be performed in tubes or in microtiter plates. The tube method usually gives a one- to twofold higher HA titer than the microtiter method. The antigen for the test is prepared by propagating PI-3 virus in cultures of primary BEK cells. The medium is harvested after the CPE of the virus is well marked and then the harvested fluid is stored frozen. (The antigen is supplied on request by Diagnostic Services, APHIS, NADC, Ames, Iowa.) The sera to be tested are treated with kaolin and inactivated at 56°C for 30 minutes. In addition, a RBC suspension is prepared from bovine blood.

HI titers as high as 1:40 have been observed in sera of cattle following a minimal exposure to PI-3 that did not produce clinical signs of disease. When cattle had a clinical response following infection, HI titers of 1:320, 1:640, and higher were found. Titers in the range of 1:10 to 1:40 indicate previous exposure to PI-3 virus but may not be related to a recent illness. Since the titers have been observed to increase about 2 weeks after infection, acute and convalescent serum samples should be tested. A fourfold increase or higher in HI titer is considered confirmation of a recent infection with PI-3 virus.

All serum samples for the VN test are inactivated for 30 minutes at 56°C. The test is carried out by using the constant virus–varying serum dilution technique as follows. A set of tubes is prepared to contain 0.4 ml volumes of twofold serially diluted (1:2 to 1:256) inactivated serum. To each tube is added an equal volume of a PI-3 virus suspension known to be cytopathic and to contain 100–500 $TCID_{50}$ per 0.1 ml. The serum-virus mixtures are incubated at room temperature for 1 hour. Each mixture is distributed in 0.2 ml quantities into at least 5 BK cell cultures.

At least two uninoculated TC tubes are used for controls. All the tubes are incubated at 35°C ± 1°C for 7 days. Interim readings are made at 3 or 4 days and the final readings at 6 or 7 days. The test is read by observing neutralization of CPE in TC tubes. An alternate method of reading the test is observing for HAdI of guinea pig RBC. If this system is used, the $TCID_{50}$ of the challenge virus must be determined by guinea pig erythrocyte HAd instead of CPE in order to dilute the virus properly.

As for cross-reactions, a common antigen has been demonstrated between the bovine and human strains of PI-3 virus. Among some bovine strains, there appear to be some differences in the AD test. Serologically, there is a difference between the human and bovine strains, the homologous strains showing a greater titer than the heterologous. The boine strains isolated from cattle in the United States, Sweden, Germany, and Japan are serologically identical.

The immunity to parainfluenza should be considered from at least two aspects—circulating antibody, and local immunity of the respiratory tract. It has been demonstrated that circulating antibody does result in protection of calves vaccinated with this agent. The part local immunity plays needs further definition. Vaccinated calves react with lower temperatures and less severe lung lesions when challenged with virus and *Pasteurella* organisms under stress. (The experimental reproduction of uncomplicated parainfluenza-3 infection with IN virus challenge is inconsistent.) After challenge, vaccinated cattle and sheep have less virus detectable in nasal swabs than unvaccinated controls. Maternal antibody will interfere with vaccination of young animals.

Acquired immunity to parainfluenza is not absolute. Infection can occur in the presence of circulating antibody; however, the presence of antibody has been shown to reduce the severity of the disease and the recovery of virus. Antibody titers following infection or the use of inactivated or attenuated vaccines do not completely correlate with the degree of protection.

References
1. Chanock, R.M., R.H. Parrott, K. Cook, B.E. Andres, J.A. Bell, T. Reichelderfer, A.Z. Sapikian, F.M. Mastrota, and R.J. Huebner. Newly recognized myxoviruses from children with respiratory disease. *New Eng. Med.* 258:207, 1958.
2. Gale, C. Bovine parainfluenza-3 immunization procedures. *J. Am. Vet. Med. Ass.* 152:871, 1968.

Newcastle Disease Virus

The synonyms for NDV are Ranikhet disease (named for a town in Uttar Pradesh, India), pseudofowl pest, pseudopoultry plague, Doyle's disease, avian pneumoencephalitis, respiratory nervous disorder, and avian fowl pest. Newcastle disease (ND) is a highly contagious viral disease, primarily of avian species.[7,9] In domestic and wild species, infection can vary from a subclinical to a highly fatal disease, with varied degrees of systemic or localized respiratory, nervous, or gastrointestinal involvement. There are many strains of the virus that vary considerably in pathogenesis and virulence. The strains of virus are grouped for convenience as velogenic (virulent), which produces severe disease, high mortality, and may produce viscerotropic lesions; mesogenic (less virulent), which produces moderate disease with little mortality, especially in older birds; and lentogenic (mild), which produces a mild infection principally of the upper respiratory tract.[8] An asymptomatic form of infection with a low morbidity has also been observed.[2]

Severity of the lesions varies considerably with the virulence and tropism of the ND virus involved.[12,13] Histologically the velogenic strains produce hyperemia, edema, hemorrhage, and other blood vascular changes in various organs. In blood vessels, hydropic degeneration, hyalinization of capillaries and arterioles, and development of hyaline thrombi followed by necrosis of the endothelial cells have been reported. Hemorrhagic necrotic lesions may be found in the intestine with the more virulent (velogenic) strains of the virus.

Identification of ND virus and diagnosis of the disease by gross or histopathologic lesions alone is not possible in view of the similarity of these lesions to those produced by other viruses. However, once an isolate has been made and identified as ND by serologic procedures, it may be classified as velogenic, mesogenic, or lentogenic on the basis of lesions produced in embryonating eggs, 1-day-old chicks, and 10-week-old chickens. A complete summary of the differentiation of these pathogenic types according to the reactions in experimental hosts may be seen on pages 71–74 of the report of the Poultry Disease Subcommittee on Animal Health.[16]

The ND virus is roughly spherical, enveloped, and notably pleomorphic, especially after exposure to high salt concentrations. It varies in size from 120 to 300 nm but is usually about 180 nm in diameter.[1,17,19] The envelope resembles that of influenza virus but the surface spikes or projections are not so prominent; they are about 8 nm long. Enclosed within the envelope is a coiled filament or nucleocapsid containing single-stranded RNA but no lipid. The inner component or tube is about 17–18 nm wide. The negatively stained preparations are consistent, with a helicle arrangement of the protein subunits. The virus is ether sensitive and pH labile.

Among the biologic properties of NDV is its ability to hemagglutinate RBC. The hemagglutinin is structurally identified with the projections on the envelope of the virus and has been chemically determined to be associated with the enzyme neuraminidase. The latter is associated with the release (elution) of the virus from the surface of RBC. The rate of elution may be complete in minutes or may take more than 12 hours, depending on the strain of the virus. Like other parainfluenza viruses, NDV possesses a hemolysin, but the degree of hemolytic activity differs among the strains. There is only one immunologic type of NDV; however, in vitro there is a considerable disparity in neutralization activity among the strains.

ND virus has been isolated from domestic chickens, turkeys, guinea fowl, and a great variety of other birds.[15] In humans the virus may cause a mild to severe conjunctivitis (usually unilateral), but a generalized form of the disease also has been authenticated.[14]

Specimens

The ND virus can be readily isolated from the respiratory tract of infected chickens during the first 3–5 days following infection. Generally the virus is recovered from respiratory secretions and the trachea and particularly from lung tissue.[10,11,16] Recovery of virus from one or more chickens of a flock that has the mild form of the disease does not necessarily mean that ND virus was the primary etiologic agent. In more severe and generalized forms of infection the virus is recovered readily from the spleen, blood, and cecal tonsils, and less frequently from the brain. Virus isolations from previously vaccinated or recovered birds that have become reinfected are more likely to be successful at a later date (day 6–14). When swabs of the trachea or cloaca are made from live specimens, these should be placed in a TC fluid containing penicillin, streptomycin, and antifungal agents for 4–24 hours at 4–9°C before inoculation into a suitable host.

Laboratory Procedures

Cultures. The embryonating chicken egg 9–11 days old is the most suitable host for isolation of ND virus.[4,16] The eggs should preferably be obtained from flocks known to be free from pathogenic organisms and lacking antibodies to ND virus. The suspected tissues should be inoculated into the allantoic chamber and incubated at 37–38°C. The inoculated eggs are candled once or twice daily for 5 days or until all or most of the embryos die. Embryonic deaths usually occur in 36–96 hours with the velogenic and mesogenic strains. Examination of the embryos will reveal generalized congestion or hemorrhages on the head and other parts of the body; the clear allantoic fluid contains the virus. The milder strains of the virus may not cause embryonic death. However, the allantoic and amniotic fluid should be examined for the ability to hemagglutinate chicken RBC. A sample should not be considered negative for the virus until at least three serial passages through embryos are made with embryo tissues suspended in allantoic and amniotic fluids.

The use of susceptible chickens for isolation and identification of ND virus may be necessary under certain circumstances. The birds can be inoculated by the respiratory route or IM to reproduce the disease. However, adequate isolation facilities should be available.

The ND virus can be propagated in primary cell cultures of avian origin and in some mammalian primary and cell lines,[3,4,16] but chicken embryo fibroblasts or chick embryo kidney cells are the preferred kinds of cell cultures. The highly susceptible chicken embryonating eggs, however, are more frequently employed because with cell cultures CPE may not always be seen, particularly with some strains of the virus and with lentogenic strains that do not produce plaques without the addition of magnesium ions and DEAE in the overlay medium, if this method is chosen.[6]

Animal inoculation. A definitive diagnosis of NDV can be accomplished by inoculating chickens or turkeys that have recovered from an infection suspected of being ND with a known virulent strain of ND virus. Susceptible controls should be inoculated simultaneously.

Immunology and serology. The HI, HAdI, and VN tests are employed for the identification of the agent and for serologic diagnosis of ND virus. Serologic examination may suffice to confirm suggestive history and signs in areas where ND is enzootic, but proof of new foci and characterization of the pathologic nature of the agent require recovery and identification of the virus.

In conducting the HI test, sera from suspected birds should be tested against 4 units of ND virus known to have good HA properties. The virus (in allantoic fluid) should have a titer of at least 10^6 infective doses to effectively induce HA.[8] In laboratories or countries in which infectious ND virus is prohibited or unacceptable, pools of infectious allantoic fluids can be inactivated with 0.1% Formalin, which destroys infectivity but retains the HA properties. The test is conducted with a series of doubling dilutions of serum in 0.25 ml quantities and 0.25 ml of a 0.5% RBC suspension, which is prepared from chicken blood. The reaction is allowed to stand for 30–35 minutes at room temperature (instead of 4°C overnight) or until HI is demonstrated in the positive control tubes. For identification of ND virus, the same test is conducted using infected allantoic fluids of embryos with a known anti-NDV serum. The HI test, which is simpler and faster than the VN test, cannot be used for evaluating the status of immunity; however, HI titer values of 1:20 or higher definitely indicate prior infection of the bird. HI antibodies do not persist as long as do VN antibodies following infection.

The HAd and HAdI tests are also useful in detecting the presence of a ND virus strain that does not produce distinctive CPE in cultures. Either chicken or guinea pig RBC may be used.

The constant serum–varying virus dilutions VN test is used. Serum samples from normal chickens having no previous contact with ND virus may neutralize as much as 100 infective units of virus. Therefore, neutralization of at least 100 LD_{50} is necessary for diagnosis. With chickens infected 10–20 days previously, the sera may neutralize 10^3–10^6 infective units of virus. Although all strains of Newcastle disease virus studied are immunologically cross-protective, differences in the neutralization capacity of antibodies produced by the various strains of virus have been demonstrated.[5,18]

Immunity to Newcastle disease should be considered from several aspects. Circulating antibody (HI or VN) in vaccinated chickens or turkeys does not always result in protection against infection of the respiratory tract or a drop in egg production in the absence of CNS signs or mortality following experimental challenge or field exposure. Also, parental antibody in chicks hatched from immune dams (first 4 weeks) interferes with vaccination.

References

1. Bang, F.B. Newcastle virus: Conversion of spherical form to filamentous forms. *Proc. Soc. Exp. Biol. Med.* 64:135, 1947.
2. Bankowski, R.A. A study of asymptomatic Newcastle disease in a breeding flock. *Res. Vet. Sci.* 2:193–201, 1961.
3. Bankowski, R.A. Cytopathogenicity of Newcastle disease virus. In *Newcastle Disease Virus: An Evolving Pathogen,* R.P. Hanson (ed.), pp. 231–246. University of Wisconsin Press, Madison, 1964.
4. Bankowski, R.A., H. Izawa, and J. Hyde. Tissue culture—a diagnostic tool—with particular reference to Newcastle disease and vesicular exanthema viruses. *Proc. Ann. Mtg. U.S. Livestock Sanitary Ass.* 63:377–388, 1959.
5. Bankowski, R.A., and T. Kinjo. Tissue culture systems with Newcastle disease virus and relationship of antigenicity to immunogenicity among strains. *Avian Dis.* 9:157–170, 1965.
6. Barahona, H.H., and R.P. Hanson. Plaque enhancement of Newcastle disease virus (lentogenic strains) by magnesium and diethylaminoethyl dextran. *Avian Dis.* 12:151–158, 1968.
7. Beach, J.R. The status of avian pneumoencephalitis and Newcastle disease in the United States. *J. Am. Vet. Med. Ass.* 108:372–376, 1946.
8. Hanson, R.P. Newcastle disease. In *Diseases of Poultry,* M.S. Hofstad et al. (eds.), pp. 619–656. 6th ed. Iowa State University Press, 1964.
9. Hanson, R.P. (ed.) *Newcastle Disease Virus: An Evolving Pathogen.* University of Wisconsin Press, Madison, 1964.
10. Hanson, R.P., J. Spalatin, and E.M. Dickinson. Criteria for determining the validity of a virus isolation. *Avian Dis.* 11:509–514, 1967.
11. Hofstad, M.S. A quantitative study of Newcastle disease virus in tissues of infected chickens. *Am. J. Vet. Res.* 12:334–339, 1951.
12. Jungherr, E.L. Pathogenicity of Newcastle disease virus for the chicken. In *Newcastle Disease Virus: An Evolving Pathogen,* R.P. Hanson (ed.), pp. 257–272. University of Wisconsin Press, Madison, 1964.
13. Jungherr, E.L, E.E. Tyzzer, C.A. Brandly, and H.E. Moses. The comparative pathology of fowl plague and Newcastle disease. *Am. J. Vet. Res.* 7:250–258, 1946.
14. Lippman, O. Human conjunctivitis due to the Newcastle disease virus of fowls. *Am. J. Ophthalmol.* 35:1021–1028, 1952.
15. Palmer, S.F., and D.O. Trainer. Newscastle disease. In *Infectious and Parasitic Diseases of Wild Birds,* J.W. Davis et al. (eds.). Iowa State University Press, Ames, 1971.
16. Poultry Disease Subcommittee on Animal Health. *Methods for the Examination of Poultry Biologics.* 3d ed. (rev.). Agricultural Board, NRC, Washington, 1971.
17. Rott, R. Antigenicity of Newcastle disease virus. In *Newcastle Disease Virus: An Evolving Pathogen,* R.P. Hanson (ed.), pp. 133–146. Univeristy of Wisconsin Press, Madison, 1964.
18. Upton, E., R.P. Hanson, and C.A. Brandly. Antigenic differences among strains of Newcastle disease virus. *Proc. Soc. Exp. Biol. Med.* 84:691, 1953.
19. Waterson, A.P., and J.G. Cruickshank. The effect of ether on Newcastle disease virus: A morphological study of eight strains. *Zeitschrift Naturforsch.,* ser. B, 18:114–118, 1963.

Canine Distemper Virus

Canine distemper (CD) in dogs is an acute or subacute, contagious, febrile viral disease with about a 50% mortality rate. Catarrhal or mucopurulent ocular and nasal discharge, pneumonia, diarrhea that is sometimes hemorrhagic, and in some cases nervous manifestations and hyperkeratosis of foot pads are the signs most commonly seen, singly or in combination, in dogs with CD. Retention of deciduous teeth in dogs after CD infection is often noted. Biphasic temperature elevation and leukemia in the acute phase of the disease are typical.[13] Most dogs with CD encephalitis have scattered focal areas of retinal degeneration.

The only consistent gross change in uncomplicated CD is reduction in size of the thymus in young animals, which is frequently almost absent.[1,16] Pneumonia and/or enteritis may be present but these are secondary to virus infection. Intracytoplasmic eosinophilic inclusion bodies in surface epithelium, lymphatic cells, or brain cells are pathognomonic; inclusion bodies in glial cells are often intranuclear. Demyelination is usually seen in cases of subacute CD encephalitis. Distribution of viral antigen, which can be stained with FA, corresponds with that of inclusion bodies. (The most viral antigen can be seen in impression smears or frozen sections.) The FA technique appears superior to H & E staining; however, eosinophilic inclusion bodies are detectable longer than viral antigen.

There is only one known serotype of CDV. The virus is closely related to the viruses of measles and rinderpest and has been placed in the measles, rinderpest, distemper (MRD) group of the paramyxoviruses. CD virus particles vary greatly in size and shape. Most particles are spherical and between 150 and 300 nm in diameter. Intact particles show an outer membrane of 5–8.5 nm thickness. Projections of 5–13 nm in length arise from the outer membrane. In partially disrupted particles the helix or nucleocapsid can be seen to have a width of 15–18 nm and a center hole approximately 5 nm in diameter.[15,26] The viral core is RNA.[30] The mean buoyant density of the infectious virion is 1.231 g/ml in cesium chloride.[29] The virus is easily inactivated by light, heat, and ether. The viral half-life was found to be 120 minutes at 21°C, 60 minutes at 37°C, 10 minutes at 45°C, and 2–3 minutes at 56°C,[34] but the virus can be maintained for several years at −70°C or in a lyophilized form. It is inactivated above pH 9 and below pH 4.5.[6] The HA and HI tests cannot be used.

Specimens

Virus isolation from CD-infected dogs depends on the form of the disease. In the early viremic phase after the first rise in temperature, when lymphatic tissue is mostly affected, buffy-coat cells and lymphatic tissues are best for virus isolation. Dogs with acute CD usually shed virus in all body excretions. Nasal, pharyngeal, and conjunctival swabs as well as feces and urine contain virus. Dogs that die from acute CD usually have little or no neutralizing antibody and virus can readily be isolated from lymphatic tissues (thymus, spleen, lymph nodes), lungs, intestine, or urinary bladder. If encephalitic signs are present, the cerebellum is a good source for virus isolation. However, in subacute or chronic CD, when neutralizing antibody is present in serum, and in cases of late encephalitis when neutralizing antibody also is present in the cerebrospinal fluid (CSF), virus isolation becomes more difficult.[1,3,14] Direct tissue culture cultivation of kidney or brain cells usually results in virus isolation. Virus isolation from washed buffy-coat cells sometimes can be achieved. For other species use the same specimen techniques as for dogs.

Laboratory Procedures

Cultures. CDV has been adapted to many cell culture systems. Isolation of virulent virus in a variety of cell culture systems has been reported, including kidney and lung cells from dogs and ferrets.[33,36] However, virus growth is often slow, virus isolation cannot always be achieved in these cultures, and CPE sometimes occurs only weeks after inoculation. The best method for isolation of virulent distemper virus appears to be in macrophage cultures from dogs[3] or ferrets.[31] Dog lung macrophages from distemper-susceptible dogs or from pups with maternal antibody are susceptible to CDV. Macrophages from dogs with active immunity to CDV are not susceptible. Macrophages are prepared from lungs of susceptible young pups in the following manner: (1) Mince lungs with scissors and stir pieces in tissue culture medium for approximately 1 hour at 25°C for release of alveolar macrophages. (2) Harvest released cells, wash, and suspend 1:150 in Medium 199 (or Hanks' BSS base) at pH 7 plus 20% fetal calf serum. All lots of calf serum should be tested for virus inhibition and support of macrophage growth before large-scale use. (3) Place suspension in flat-bottomed tubes or bottles, incubate at 36°C overnight, and allow cells to attach. (4) Change culture fluid but use the same medium. Care should be taken to adjust to about pH 7. (5) Inoculate material for virus isolation. Tissue suspensions should be inoculated in serial dilutions from 10% to 1% because undiluted material is often toxic to macrophages. Incubate at 37°C. (6) Observe cultures daily for round multinucleated giant-cell formations, which appear from 2 to 5 days after virus inoculation. Giant cells tend to detach, and not all cells form giant cells. (7) Identification of CDV can be made by neutralization of CPE with reference CDV antiserum or by the FA test. Features of a paramyxovirus can be demonstrated by electorn microscopy.

Animal inoculation. Many different species in the order Carnivora are susceptible to CDV (Table 15.2). The mortality rate varies greatly between species. Ferrets are most susceptible, with a mortality rate of close to 100%; they die within 8–14 DPI by any route of inoculation. The CDV has also been adapted to grow in embryonating chicken eggs, mice, and hamsters.[8,9,22,27]

Table 15.2. Natural host range of canine distemper (suborder Fissipeda)*

Family	Examples
Felidae	Cat, *lion*, tiger, etc.
Viverridae	Civet, fossa, mongoose, meerkat, linsang, *binturong* (questionable)
Hyaenidae	Hyena
Canidae	*Dog, dingo, fox, coyote, wolf,* jackal
Procyonidae	*Kinkajou, coati, bassariscus, raccoon, panda*
Mustelidae	*Weasel, ferret, mink, skunk, badger, stoat, marten, otter*
Ursidae	Bear

*The animal names in italic have all been reported as susceptible to infection with CD. Those in roman have not been adequately tested.

Immunology and serology. The VN test against CDV has been the method of choice for testing immunity in dogs, and for many years the growth inhibition of egg-adapted CDV in embryonating chicken eggs has been the most commonly used technique. At a symposium on CDV, a Committee on Standard Reagents and Test Procedures made recommendations for the standardization of this test.[12] Recommendations were based principally on the statistical evaluation of tests proposed by Robson et al.[32] The recommended test procedure follows: (1) The dilution of serum to be tested should not be greater than fourfold in saline. (2) Add equal volumes of serum and virus using between 100 and 1000 EID_{50} virus. Lederle CDV embryo-adapted strain (ATCC VR-128) at about the fortieth passage is recommended. In calculating the concentration of virus used in the test, the dilution factor of the serum should be taken into consideration. (3) Incubate virus-serum mixtures 2 hours at 25°C. (4) Inoculate 0.2 ml of each dilution on CAM, using the Gorham technique.[19] For each dilution, inoculate at least five embryonating chicken eggs that are about 8 or 9 days old. (5) Conduct an accompanying virus titration using 0.2 ml virus inoculum. Substitute diluent for serum. (Some laboratories use 0.1 ml inoculum.) Use five embryos per dilution and sufficient dilutions to establish that the test dose falls within the specified range of EID_{50}. (6) The CAM are usually examined after 7 days incubation at 35–37°C. Thickened whitish plaques on the membranes indicate presence of virus. A CAM should not be considered positive for CDV lesions unless two or more white plaques are found on the area where the infectious material was deposited.

Various tissue culture systems may be used for CDV VN tests. The tissue culture–adapted Rockborn strain[33] has been used in dog kidney cell cultures in several laboratories; however, this test system does not appear to be as sensitive as the chicken embryo system. Plaque reduction tests in tissue culture have been described and are useful.[21]

More recently, Vero cells[35] have appeared promising for use in VN tests. The tests can be made in Vero cells in microplates with egg-adapted CDV in the following manner. Use tissue culture microplates holding 96 flat-bottomed wells for 0.4 ml each, micropipettes dispensing 0.05 ml per drop, platinum Takatay loops (Linbro Co., New Haven, Conn.) holding 0.025 ml each, the Vero cell line, and the Onderstepoort egg-adapted virus that is adapted to Vero cells and human epidermoid carcinoma no. 2 (Hep-2) cells. Stock virus is grown in Hep-2 cells and harvests are made 3 days after inoculation when virus titers in Vero cells should be between 4 and 4.5 $\log_{10}$ per ml. Hep-2 cells yield higher virus titers for stock virus. Vero cells are better suited for neutralization tests. For the CDV control antiserum, use MEM with 0.5% lactalbumin hydrolysate, antibiotics, and 6% lamb serum as the preferred medium, although Medium 199 and 10% fetal calf serum will also work. Then (1) Place 0.5 ml TC medium into each well. (2) Make threefold serum dilutions with Takatay loops, four rows for each serum sample, eight dilutions per row. (3) Drop 0.05 ml of dilute CDV containing approximately 30 $TCID_{50}$ of stock virus into each well. Titrate virus without serum in threefold dilutions. (4) Incubate serum-virus mixtures for 2 hours at 25°C. (5) Add 0.05 ml TC medium containing approximately 12,000 Vero cells per drop to each well. (6) Cover microplates with one layer of sterile gauze and a plastic lid. (7) Incubate microplates at 35–36°C in a 5% CO_2 incubator. (8) Determine endpoints by staining 3 days after inoculation. Cells should be fixed in methanol for 10–20 minutes; plates should be air dried for 20 minutes, then stained with a freshly diluted Giemsa stain: 10 in water for approximately 20 minutes. Cells are then washed and drained. (9) Determine endpoints by the presence of giant cells and calculation by the S-K method. A well with one or more giant cells is considered positive.

Before techniques for the VN test were developed, the CF test was frequently used for CD antibody determination. CF antibody develops 3–4 weeks after initial CD infection; however, it disappears after several weeks.[24] It may appear again after re-exposure. CF antibody in serum indicates a recent infection. The most commonly used antigen source in this test has been 5% saline suspension of spleen and lymph nodes from dogs with acute CD, but the CAM from infected embryonating chicken eggs, or infected cell cultures, may also be used. The CF antigen is heat labile. Incubation for 30 minutes at 60°C destroys the antigen. For CF tests, incubation periods from 30 minutes at 37°C to 18 hours at 6°C have been used.

FA,[25] AD,[26] and measles HI tests[37] have been used in qualitative but not quantitative tests for the detection of CDV antibody. The best method for production of hyperimmune serum in dogs for these tests is the Laidlaw-Dunkin method: parenteral inoculation of Formalin-inactivated CDV followed 2 weeks later by IN inoculation of virulent virus. Serum should be harvested 10–14 days after the last inoculation.

Cross-reactions between CDV, measles, and rinderpest virus have been found.[23] CDV induces high levels of CDV antibody and usually low levels of rinderpest antibody but no measles antibody in various species. Dogs inoculated with measles or rinderpest virus become protected against later CDV challenge.

Acute CD in dogs without neutralizing antibody can be diagnosed by FA staining of buffy-coat, conjunctival, or vaginal cells. These tests usually fail in dogs with subacute or chronic CD, when neutralizing antibody is present. Frozen sections of foot-pad biopsies can be used in these cases for FA staining.

Dogs with CD encephalitis have increased amounts of protein and cells in the CSF. Presence of neutralizing antibody in CSF is pathognomonic. Dogs, after CD vaccination or after early recovery from CD, have high serum antibody levels but no antibody in their CSF. Dogs with subacute or chronic CD encephalitis have antibody in serum and CSF.Immunity in ferrets can be determined by observing clinical signs and mortality after challenge with virulent virus. The clinical criteria are valid in dogs only after IC challenge with virulent virus, e.g. the Snyder Hill strain. Immunity in dogs after IV, IN, or aerosol challenge can be determined by presence or absence of virus in spleen or thymus 5 days after challenge. The virus isolation method appears to be more sensitive than the FA method for this purpose.[4]

References

1. Appel, M.J.G. Pathogenesis of canine distemper. *Am. J. Vet. Res.* 30:1167–1182, 1969.
2. Appel, M.J.G., and J.H. Gillespie. Canine distemper virus. In Virology Monographs no. 11, pp. 1–96. Springer-Verlag, Vienna, New York, 1972.
3. Appel, M.J.G., and O.R. Jones. Use of aveolar macrophages for cultivation of canine distemper virus. *Proc. Soc. Exp. Biol. Med.* 126:571–574, 1967.

4. Baker, J.A. Measles vaccine for protection of dogs against canine distemper. *J. Am. Vet. Med. Ass.* 156:1743–1746, 1970.
5. Benson, T.F. The protection of susceptible puppies for ten days against canine distemper using quantitative amounts of antibodies. M.S. thesis, Cornell University, Ithaca, N.Y., 1960.
6. Bindrich, H. Untersuchengen über dis pH-Resistenz des Virus der Hundestaupe. *Exp. Vet. Med.* 4:119–126, 1951.
7. Bindrich, H. Beitrag zum Wesen der Staupevirusinfektion des Hundes und zu ihrer Bakämpfung I, II. *Arch. Exp. Vet. Med.* 8:131–162, 263–315, 1954.
8. Cabasso, V., and H.R. Cox. Propagation of canine distemper virus on the chorio-allantoic membrane of embryonated hen eggs. *Proc. Soc. Exp. Biol. Med.* 71:246–250, 1949.
9. Cabasso, V.J., J.M. Douglas, M.R. Stebbins, and H.R. Cox. Propagation of canine distemper virus in suckling hamsters. *Proc. Soc. Exp. Biol. Med.* 88:199–202, 1955.
10. Canine distemper supplement. *J. Am. Vet. Med. Ass.* 149:599–718, 1966.
11. Canine infectious disease report: Proceedings of a symposium on immunity to selected canine infectious disease. *J. Am. Vet. Med. Ass.* 156:1655–1817, 1970.
12. Conclusions and recommendations of the panel of the symposium on canine distemper immunization. *J. Am. Vet. Med. Ass.* 148:1400–1404, 1966.
13. Cornwell, H.J.C., R.S.F. Campbell, J.T. Vantsis, and W. Penny. Studies in experimental canine distemper. I. Clinicopathological findings. *J. Comp. Path.* 75:3–17, 1965.
14. Cornwell, H.J.C., J.T. Vantsis, R.S.F. Campbell, and W. Penny. Studies in experimental canine distemper. II. Virology, inclusion body studies and hematology. *J. Comp. Path.* 75:19–34, 1965.
15. Cruickshank, J.G., A.P. Waterson, A.D. Kanarck, and D.M. Berry. The structure of canine distemper virus. *Res. Vet. Sci.* 3:485–486, 1962.
16. Gibson, J.P., R.A. Griesemer, and A. Koostner. Experimental distemper in the gnotobiotic dog. *Path. Vet.* 2:1–19, 1965.
17. Gillespie, J., J.A. Baker, J. Burgher, D. Robson, and B. Gilman. The immune response of dogs to distemper virus. *Cornell Vet.* 48:103–126, 1958.
18. Gillespie, J.H. The virus of canine distemper. In *Comparative Virology. Ann. N.Y. Acad. Sci.* 101:540–547, 1962.
19. Gorham, J.R. A simple technique for the inoculation of the chorioallantoic membrane of chicken embryos. *Am. J. Vet. Res.* 18:691–692, 1957.
20. Gorham, J.R. Canine distemper. In *Advances in Veterinary Science,* C.A. Brandly and E.L. Jungherr (eds.), vol. 6, pp. 287–351. Academic Press, New York, 1960.
21. Gourlay, J.A. A note on the use of plaque reduction to test serums for canine distemper antibodies. *Cornell Vet.* 60:613–616, 1970.
22. Haig, D.A. Preliminary note on the cultivation of Green's distemperoid virus in fertile hen eggs. *Onderstepoort J. Vet. Sci. Anim. Ind.* 23:149–155, 1948.
23. Imagawa, D.T. Relationships among measles, canine distemper, and rinderpest viruses. *Prog. Med. Virol.* 10:160–193, 1968.
24. Karzon, D.T., J.H. Gillespie, and R.H. Bessell. Use of cell culture–adapted canine distemper virus in the complement-fixation test. *Am. J. Vet. Res.* 22:1069–1073, 1961.
25. Lium, C., and D.L. Coffin. Studies on canine distemper infection by means of fluorescein-labeled antibody. I. The pathogenesis, pathology, and diagnosis of the disease in experimentally infected ferrets. *Virology* 3:115–131, 1957.
26. Mansi, W. Slide gel diffusion precipitin test. *Nature* 181:1289–1290, 1958.
27. Morse, H.G., T.L. Chow, and C.A. Brandly. Propagation of a strain of egg-adapted distemper virus in suckling mice. *Proc. Soc. Exp. Biol. Med.* 84:10–12, 1953.
28. Norrby, E., B. Friding, G. Rockborn, and S. Gard. The ultrastructure of canine distemper virus. *Arch. ges. Virusforsch.* 13:335–344, 1963.
29. Phillips, L.A., and R.H. Bussell. Buoyant density of canine distemper virus. *Arch. ges. Virusforsch.* 41:310–318, 1973.
30. Phillips, L.A., and R.H. Bussell. The nucleic acid of canine distemper virus: Effects of 6-azauridine and actinomycin D on viral replication, and the incorporation of uridine into virions. *Am. J. Vet. Res.* 35:821–824, 1974.
31. Poste, G. The growth and cytopathogenicity of virulent and attenuated strains of canine distemper virus in dog and ferret macrophages. *J. Comp. Path.* 81:49–54, 1971.
32. Robson, D.S., B.P. Hildreth, G.F. Atkinson, L.E. Carmichael, F.D. Barnes, B. Pakkala, and J.A. Baker. Standardization of quantitative serological tests. *Proc. U.S. Livestock Sanitary Ass.* 65:74–78, 1961.

33. Rockborn, G. Canine distemper virus in tissue culture. *Arch. ges. Virusforsch* 8:485–491, 1958.
34. Russell, R.H., and D.T. Karson. Canine distemper virus in chick embryo cell culture: Plaque assay, growth, and stability. *Virology* 18:589–600, 1962.
35. Shishido, A., K. Yamanouchi, M. Hikita, T. Sato, A. Fukuda, and F. Kobune. Development of a cell culture system susceptible to measles, canine distemper, and rinderpest viruses. *Arch. ges. Virusforsch.* 22:364–380, 1967.
36. Vantsis, J.T. Preliminary note on the propagation of canine distemper virus in different tissue culture systems. *Vet. Rec.* 71:99–100, 1959.
37. Waterson, A.P., R. Rott, and G. Ruckle-Enders. The components of measles virus and their relationship to rinderpest and distemper. *Zeitschrift Naturforsch.*, ser. B, 18:377–384, 1963.

Rinderpest Virus

Rinderpest is an acute, sometimes subacute, febrile disease of ruminants and pigs, and it is characterized by severe congestion, hemorrhage, and erosion of the mucus membrane of the alimentary tract. Inapparent infections can occur but the disease is usually accompanied by severe diarrhea.

The recorded history of rinderpest dates back to before and during the early centuries of the Christian era. In the second half of the fourth century it was recognized as a distinct clinical entity. Outbreaks in Europe frequently came from the East and were believed to have originated in the area of the Caspian Sea and the adjacent steppes. Outbreaks of rinderpest invariably followed in the wake of major military campaigns.

With the exception of parts of Turkey, Europe has been reported to be free of the disease since 1930, largely due to slaughter and to strict enforcement of control measures. However, rinderpest has continued to be a problem in Africa, the Middle East, and Asia. Australia and North and South America have remained free of the disease except for one outbreak of short duration, in Brazil in 1921.

The rinderpest virus (RV) is classified as a paramyxovirus. It has a similar morphology and is immunologically related to the viruses of human measles and canine distemper forming the MRD group of viruses.[1,2,12] RV has a diameter of about 250–450 nm and a RNA core.

Clinically, rinderpest is characterized by pyrexia with ocular and nasal discharges, followed 2–4 days later by a necrotic stomatitis and, usually somewhat later still, by diarrhea.[4,7,13] The mortality rate varies considerably from well over 90% with highly susceptible breeds of cattle to possibly 10–20% in enzootic areas with more resistant breeds of cattle. In many areas where vaccines have been used, the clinical signs and lesions are quite mild and difficult to detect. The virus may be spread by the secretions and excretions of infected animals for a period of about 2–3 weeks after onset of the disease. Persistent carriers appear to be quite rare. The other diseases that could be confused with rinderpest are BVD-MD, FMD, vesicular stomatitis (VS), MCF, IBR, and anthrax.

Specimens

Blood with anticoagulant should be collected with aseptic precautions, preferably into a saline solution contributing a final 0.5% of EDTA (versene). The optimal time for taking blood and other tissues for virus isolation is during the early febrile (prodromal) phase, that is, the 3–4 days before specific clinical signs are easily detected. In the case of an outbreak, several such animals should be selected and sampled. Superficial lymph node material can also be obtained by biopsy.

At postmortem examination, the best materials for diagnosis are spleen and lymph nodes, particularly the mesenterics. A little buffered saline with an antibiotic mixture should be added to the storage bottles to control any contaminants; putrefaction rapidly destroys both virus infectivity and soluble antigens. If only late cases of the disease are available, that is, animals with advanced mouth lesions and/or dehydration, it may be better to take palatal tonsil or lung tissue for virus recovery.[6] All these materials should be stored immediately on ice. Tissues for virus isolation should be frozen rapidly at temperatures of about −70°C or below if they are to be stored.

Laboratory Procedures

Cultures. Japanese workers have described a method of isolation that consists of preparing buffy-coat cultures with coverslips from viremic animals. The infected cultures develop a particular type of syncytium, with intracytoplasmic and intranuclear inclusions demonstrable in stained preparations.[15]

For virus isolation in cell cultures, crude leukocyte fractions should be prepared from 10–20 ml of blood or 5% suspension of spleen of lymph nodes prepared by homogenizing the tissues in cell culture medium with 5–10% antibody-free serum. Tissue suspensions should be lightly centrifuged but should not be filtered prior to inoculation into cell cultures. The cultures of choice are primary 7–10-day-old monolayers of calf or bovine fetal kidney cells, using 0.2 ml amounts per tube or culture flask. Tissue culture tubes, which can be rolled and which show a zone of continuous cell proliferation at the periphery, are desirable. Following cell culture inoculation, the excess or unattached part of the inoculum should be removed by washing within 24 hours; thereafter the medium is replaced every 2–3 days. MEM plus 10% fetal calf serum is the preferred medium.

The CPE, normally detectable first at the periphery of the cell sheets, occurs after as little as 3 days, but small quantities of some field strains of virus do not produce recognizable changes for 10–12 days. The most important feature is the production of stellate cells or syncytia in which both cytoplasmic and intranuclear inclusions are demonstrable. The cytopathic effects of the agent can be neutralized specifically by high-titer convalescent or hyperimmune sera, which can be included if desired in the medium for a proportion of the original cultures as a means of rapid viral identification.

Animal inoculation. The most sensitive method for the detection of rinderpest virus is probably the parenteral inoculation of blood or tissue suspensions in large quantities into susceptible cattle of sensitive breeds, which should be maintained in strict isolation. The use of sheep, goats, or pigs may be justified when outbreaks occur that involve these species. In each case, the animals should develop the characteristic pyrexia and other clinical signs while immunized animals remain unaffected; the incubation period varies from 3–4 up to about 10 days depending on the strain and virus dosage.

The most important hosts of rinderpest are cattle (*Bos taurus* and *B. indicus*) and water buffaloes, but sheep, goats, yaks, domestic swine, and camels also can be naturally infected. A very large proportion of, if not all, wild ungulates (Order Artiodactyla) are susceptible. In the laboratory, RV can be adapted to growth in rabbits, mice, golden hamsters, and susliks, as well as embryonating chicken eggs.

Immunology and serology. All strains of RV are of a single immunologic type. A battery of serologic tests is available for the diagnosis of rinderpest.[13,14] The most generally useful is the AD test, which employs hyperimmune serum diffusing against soluble antigens from fragments of tissue or concentrated lymph node extracts. The tests should not be conducted if the rooms have a high ambient temperature. Positive results in the form of one or two precipitation zones can be expected within a minimum of 12 hours when using tissue from animals killed on the fourth to sixth days of pyrexia. All suspect antigens should of course be tested with suitable controls and should give a line of identity with a known positive preparation. The test may fail very early or very late in the clinical course of the disease and may fail with putrefied materials.

Complement-fixing antigens can be demonstrated in the lymph nodes of cattle and other animals, and also in chicken embryo spleens, infected cell cultures, and so forth. The antigen(s) can be boiled for 30 minutes,[5] is stable to acetone-ether extraction,[1] but can also be prepared as a simple saline extract of lymph nodes clarified by centrifugation. The antiserum is prepared by hyperimmunization of cattle or rabbits and the optimal dilution for diagnostic use should be established previously. Best results are given when the antigen-antibody mixtures, with about 5 units of complement, are allowed to react overnight in the cold.

Provost et al.[10] suggested a test based on the fact that rinderpest-immune sera inhibit the HA of measles virus. If the inhibiting antibody was first removed from the serum by reaction with a suspect antigen then measles HA occurred and the antigen was presumed to be that of rinderpest virus. The quantitative aspects of this test have not been defined,[10] however, and no hemagglutinin has been unequivocally demonstrated for rinderpest virus.[11]

Rinderpest virus strains can be readily identified by VN tests with convalescent or hyperimmune sera. One hour at 37°C or 18–24 hours at 4°C are suitable reaction times. Antisera are titrated using dilutions of serum and a constant 50–500 $TCID_{50}$ of virus in a cell culture system or an estimated 20–200 rabbit ID_{50} in rabbits. Constant serum tests have also been used to calculate a neutralization index. The critical level for the latter, that is, a level indicating significant activity, is a depression of about 2 $\log_{10}$ units. In a cell culture system, any complete neutralization of the test dose of virus is regarded as significant, while in the rabbit system the serum should be inhibitory at a dilution of 1:10.

VN tests can also be carried out in embryonating eggs, using embryo mortality or the development of complement-fixing antigens as criteria of infection. Similarly, a neurotropic mouse-adapted strain can be used for the same purpose but the sensitivity and accuracy of such tests have not been established.[3]

Hemagglutination inhibition tests, using measles virus hemagglutinin, have been applied to the detection of rinderpest antibodies but their sensitivity is inferior to that of VN tests. Complement-fixing antibodies appear irregularly in the sera of recovered or vaccinated cattle and are also short lived; their detection, while useful in diagnosis on a herd basis, is not suitable for epidemiologic surveys.[5]

A single successful exposure to infection with a living RV preparation, whatever its level of virulence, probably confers lifelong resistance to natural or parenteral challenge with any virulent strain. Limited multiplication of the challenge virus may occur in some clinically resistant animals, especially in the upper respiratory tract and associated lymphoid tissues of cattle or other species. Inactivated or killed virus vaccines, with or without adjuvants, are effective in producing a temporary resistance to challenge but reinfection may be frequent on exposure to virulent strains.

Immunity to rinderpest is normally proved by the parenteral inoculation of 10^4 or more $TCID_{50}$ of a strain that induces severe clinical reactions and a high proportion of deaths in the particular species—for cattle a suspension of virulent bovine spleen is commonly injected SC. The development of significant levels of VN antibody is reliable evidence of resistance to challenge, although a very small porportion of animals resistant to challenge may have no detectable circulating antibody.

Reference laboratories. Rinderpest is a reportable disease in all countries; the veterinary authorities must be notified immediately of suspected outbreaks. Reference laboratories for confirmation of a diagnosis of rinderpest exist in many countries where the disease is enzootic. In North America, PIADC and Grosse Isle Laboratories, Canada, are charged with this function. In Africa, reference laboratories exist at Dakar, Senegal; Farcha, Chad; and Muguga, Kenya. Similarly, diagnostic facilities are available in Asia at the Central Veterinary Research Institute, Mukteswar, Uttar Pradesh, India, and the National Institute of Animal Health, Tokyo, Japan.

References

1. Boulanger, P. Application of the complement-fixation test to the demonstration of rinderpest virus in the tissues of infected cattle using rabbit antiserum. *Can. J. Comp. Med.* 21:379–388, 1957.
2. Connaissances acquises récemment sur la peste bovine et son virus. *Rev. Elevage Med. Vet. Pays Trop.* 19:365–413, 1966.
3. Imagawa, D.J. Propagation of rinderpest virus in suckling mice and its comparison to murine adapted strains of measles and distemper. *Arch. ges. Virusforsch.* 17:203–215, 1965.
4. Jacotot, H., and P. Mornet. *La peste bovine.* L'Expansion, Paris, 1967.
5. Nakamura, J. *Complement-Fixation Reaction in Rinderpest Study: Guide for Technique and Application.* International Office of Epizootics, Paris, 1958.
6. Plowright, W. Studies on the pathogenesis of rinderpest in experimental cattle. II. Proliferation of the virus in different tissues following intranasal infection. *J. Hyg.* 62:267–281, 1964.
7. Plowright, W. Rinderpest. *Vet. Rec.* 77:1431–1438, 1965.
8. Plowright, W. Rinderpest virus. In Virology Monographs no. 3, pp. 27–110. Springer-Verlag, New York, 1968.
9. Plowright, W., and R.D. Ferris. Studies with rinderpest virus in tissue culture: A technique for the detection and titration of virulent virus in cattle tissues. *Res. Vet. Sci.* 3:94–103, 1962.
10. Provost, A., K. Bögel, and C. Borredon. Une nouvelle sérologie rapide d'identification du virus bovipestique. *Compte rendu Acad. sci.* 259:684–686, 1964.
11. Provost, A., and C. Borredon. Quelques recherches fondamentales sur le virus bovipestique. *Rev. Elevage Med. Vet. Pays Trop.* 21:33–48, 1968.
12. Scott, G.R. Rinderpest. In *Advances in Veterinary Science,* C.A. Brandly and E.L. Jungherr (eds.), vol. 9, pp. 113–224. Academic Press, New York, 1964.
13. Scott, G.R. *Diagnosis of Rinderpest.* F.A.O. Agricultural Studies no. 71. United Nations, Rome, 1967.
14. Scott, G.R., and R.D. Brown. Rinderpest diagnosis with special reference to the agar-gel double diffusion test. *Bull. Epiz. Dis. Afr.* 9:83–125, 1961.
15. Tokuda, G., K. Fukusho, T. Morimoto, and M. Watanabe. Studies on rinderpest virus in bovine leukocyte culture. *Nat. Inst. Anim. Health Q.* 3:55–63, 189–200, 1962.

Peste des Petits Ruminants Virus

Peste des petits ruminants (PPR), also known as pseudorinderpest of small ruminants, and kata (Nigerian name), is an acute or subacute virus disease of goats and sheep. The acute form is characterized by necrotic stomatitis and intestinal and lymphoid tissue syndromes that resemble those of rinderpest in cattle. The virus is closely related antigenically and immunologically to RV. Cattle are not clinically affected. The incubation period may range from 2 to 15 days. Goats are more susceptible than sheep and mortality rates in goats may range from 10 to 90%.

The acute form is accompanied by a sudden rise of temperature to 40–41°C. The affected animals appear ill and are restless. They have a dull coat, dry muzzle, depressed appetite, congested mucous membrane, and serous nasal discharge. Ulceration in the buccal cavity sometimes occurs. However, involvement may be limited to severe congestion of the laryngopharyngeal mucous membranes. The disease course is relatively short, about 8–10 days, usually resulting in death.

In the subacute form of the disease, which is the form usually seen in experimentally infected animals, clinical signs of disease are not evident until about the sixth day, when fever and a serous nasal discharge may be found. The fever reaches its peak after 2 or 3 more days and then falls after about a week with the onset of diarrhea. In fatal cases, diarrhea becomes progressively more severe, followed by dehydration, emaciation, and prostration. At about days 7–9 after inoculation, superficial erosions of the lip and buccal mucosa may be observed. Similar ulcerations or erosions may be found in females on the labial surface of the vulva. The sites of predilection for ulcerations are the lips, gums, buccal papillae, and the ventral surface of the tongue. Most goats die 6–12 days after the rise in temperature, but some may linger on for 3 weeks after onset of illness. The most frequent complications are secondary bacterial infections resulting in pneumonia and bronchopneumonia. *Pasteurella* and *Mycoplasma* organisms are frequently recovered from such cases. Infection with PPR may activate latent intestinal coccidial infection as well as hematophagous parasites. Abortions occur frequently.

Animals that die following an acute form of PPR do not exhibit lesions other than congestion of the mucous membranes. In some cases, there may be secondary bronchopneumonia. Lesions in frank clinical cases resemble those of RV infection in cattle but tend to be less intense. Pulmonary involvement is more frequent than in RV infections.

On histologic examination the necrosis of the mucosa of the oral cavity is marked by the presence of intranuclear and intracytoplasmic inclusion bodies and of occasional syncytia in the stratified epithelium, as in rinderpest. Intranuclear inclusion bodies also are found in the reticuloendothelial cells close to the sinus and germinal centers of the lymph nodes. Diseases such as bluetongue, coccidiosis, Nairobi sheep disease, contagious ecthyma, pox, and plant and mineral poisoning may cause clinical gross pathologic manifestations similar to those of PPR.

PPR has been confined mostly to the area of West Africa from Senegal to Nigeria. PPR has been reported since 1942; in Nigeria, kata was first recognized in 1965.[2] Various studies, including cross-immunity and serologic tests, indicate that PPR and kata are similar if not identical diseases.[2]

The PPR virus is similar to RV in its physical, chemical, and general antigenic properties. The viral particles are spherical in shape and have a diameter of about 250–450 nm. They contain an RNA core.

Specimens

Blood, spleen, and mesenteric lymph node specimens from affected animals should be taken for virus isolation. Recovered animals should be selected as serum donors for antibody detection tests.

Laboratory Procedures

Cultures. The PPR virus may be isolated by using cell cultures such as ovine embryo kidney cells. The virus induces the formation of large eosinophilic inclusion bodies within multinucleated giant cells.

Animal inoculation. Goats and sheep may be used for virus isolation. Cattle inoculated with PPR virus do not develop clinical signs or lesions of infection but do develop antibodies and resist challenge with RV.

Immunology and serology. The VN, CF, and AD tests may be used with PPR virus, as with RV. Cell culture RV vaccine has proved effective in the immunization of susceptible goats against natural or experimental exposure to PPR virus. Attenuated live-virus vaccines also are effective in protecting sheep and goats from natural exposure to PPR virus for about a year.

Reference laboratories. PPR is a reportable disease. See rinderpest for the reference laboratories.

References

1. Mornet, P., J. Orue, Y. Gilbert, G. Thiery, and M. Sow. La peste des petits ruminants en Afrique occidentale française: Ses rapports avec la peste bovine. *Rev. Elevage Med. Vet. Pays Trop.* 9:313–342, 1956.
2. Rowland, A.C., and P. Bourdin. The histological relationship between peste des petits ruminants and Kata in West Africa. *Rev. Elevage Med. Vet. Pays Trop.* 23:301–*307, 1970*

16. Parvoviruses

Parvoviruses ("parvo," small) are nonenveloped DNA-containing viruses whose particles have diameters of from 18 to 24 nm and are of cubic structure. They have icosahedral symmetry and probably have 32 capsomeres, each 2–4 nm in diameter. The buoyant density of parvoviruses ranges from 1.39 to 1.45 g/ml in cesium chloride gradients.

Many of these viruses contain single-stranded linear DNA. With some viruses (adeno-associated viruses, AAV; densonucleosis virus) the single strands are complementary and come together after extraction in vitro to form a double strand. The molecular weight of the DNA is between 1.2×10^6 and 1.8×10^6 daltons.

Parvoviruses are extremely stable in different environmental conditions. They resist lipid solvents, heat, and acid (pH 3) treatment, and can be stored at 4°C for years without significant loss in titer.

Most parvoviruses contain HA activity that is associated with the protein coat. However, when the viral particles disintegrate, a low density of HA activity of 1.31–1.32 g/ml is observed. The hemagglutinin usually is active with RBC from guinea pigs, human type O, rhesus monkeys, hamsters, rats, and mice. Some of the parvoviruses from domestic animals, however, show different HA patterns.

The growth of parvoviruses largely depends upon the physiological state of the cell. There is a preference for actively multiplying cells, and AAV needs a helper virus. Most if not all of the parvoviruses are highly host specific and usually multiply only in the original host or in cell cultures derived therefrom.

The parvoviruses are divided into three subgroups: subgroup A, viruses that replicate normally; subgroup B, viruses that replicate only in the presence of adeno- or herpesviruses, which serve as helper viruses; and subgroup C, parvoviruses from insects.

The viruses presently classified in subgroup A include as type species rat virus,[6] feline panleukopenia virus (FPLV), the H viruses,[18] minute virus of mice,[2] porcine parvovirus, bovine parvovirus, and parvoviruses II, III, and IV isolated from human cell lines.[5] Recently, a canine parvovirus was described that may be a member.[1]

Subgroup B includes all AAV. Five serotypes are suspected; they were isolated in association with other viruses from humans, monkeys, and recently from cattle.

An insect virus, the densonucleosis virus from *Galleria melonella*, is the most important parvovirus of subgroup C. (This virus is not described here.)

The term picodnavirus was previously used for this group as an analogy to the small RNA-containing picornaviruses, which are similar in morphology.

Rodent Parvoviruses

This group includes rat virus or Kilham's rat virus (RV), hamster osteolytic H virus (H-1 virus), and minute virus of mice (MVM). Each of these viruses is a distinct serotype. They do not cross-react in HI, CF, or VN tests.[3] They do seem to share one or more common antigens when subjected to the FA test, but they do not share common antigens with other parvoviruses (Table 16.1).

Table 16.1. Serologic relationships among subgroup A parvoviruses from different species, based on HI, VN, CF, and FA tests

Viruses	Specific antisera for designated viruses						
	RV	H-1	MVM	FPV	PPV	BPV	MVC
Rat virus (RV)	+	0^+	0^+	0	0	0	0
Hamster osteolytic virus 1 (H-1)	0^+	+	0^+	0	0	0	0
Minute virus of mice (MVM)	0^+	0^+	+	0	0	0	0
Feline panleukopenia virus (FPLV)	0	0	0	+	0	0	0
Porcine parvovirus (PPV)	0	0	0	0	+	0	0
Bovine parvovirus (BPV)	0	0	0	0	0	+	0
Canine parvovirus (MVC)	0	0	0	0	0	0	+

0^+, positive cross-reaction in FA test only.

Rat virus and H-1 viruses are prevalent in domestic and wild rats. There have been no indications that rat virus has other natural hosts besides rats.[3] Experimentally, rat virus is pathogenic for suckling hamsters (*Cricetus aureatus*)[6] and suckling multimammate mice (*Rattus [Mastomys] natalensis*).[20] One strain of rat virus has also been adapted to mice, although mice are normally resistant to infection.[7] Antibody to H-1 virus is found frequently in rats and the virus has been isolated from uninoculated rat organ cell cultures,[7,8] as well as from kidneys, livers, and lungs of normal rats.[3] H-1 virus is also suspected of being of human origin, because the virus has been isolated from human tumor material and the antibody has been found in laboratory personnel who had contact with the virus.[3,20] A viremia can be detected in humans and rhesus monkeys when they are inoculated experimentally with H-1 virus.[19,21]

Experimentally, H-1 virus produces clinical disease in newborn hamsters and mice. Natural hosts for MVM are mice and perhaps rats.[2,9,14] Antibody to MVM can frequently be found in rat sera; however, the specificity of this antibody is still doubtful. MVM produces an acute disease when given experimentally to newborn hamsters.

During the course of experimental disease various areas of the bodies of infected animals show pathologic changes. In the brain the external germinal layer of the cerebellum may be partially or totally destroyed and the Purkinje cells are scattered. This destruction usually leads to cerebellar hypoplasia. Tooth dysplasia may be present due to injury to the odontoblastic tissue. Runting and mongoloidism may also occur due to disturbance of growth as a result of widespread injury to immature tissues, along with defective repair of these tissues. In organs with rapidly multiplying cells, like the cerebellar germinal layer, the subependymal plate in the brain, and the hepatic parenchyma, typical intranuclear inclusion bodies are present.[11]

Specimens

During an acute disease, usually after experimental infection, rat virus, H-1, and MVM viruses can be isolated from almost all tissues, with highest titers in kidneys, liver, lung, blood, and large intestine. Feces and urine also contain virus, but the titer is lower than in the organs. High titers of virus occur from approximately 3 to 10 days after infection; however, virus may persist for long periods (especially in the gut, urine, and feces), even in the presence of circulating antibodies. In experimental subclinical or latent infections, rodent parvoviruses proliferate to high titers in the brain, where they can easily be isolated.[9]

Natural and spontaneous infection in normal rodents is generally latent and virus isolation can be difficult, although most colonies of mice or rats are infected. The presence of carcinogenic agents, tumors, or leukemia are inducing factors that allow virus isolation.[14]

Laboratory Procedures

Cultures. There are two kinds of virus isolation via tissue culture. Either rat embryo cell cultures (RECC) are inoculated with organ suspensions and the material is serially passaged, or cell cultures are prepared directly from organs of infected animals. In the first, secondary RECC should be inoculated with 10% organ suspensions and incubated for 10–14 days. In view of the affinity of Rat virus, H-1, and MVM for the dividing cell, RECC should be inoculated 24 hours after seeding when still subconfluent. Two to three blind passages may be necessary for CPE to develop. Cytologic changes are similar for all rodent parvoviruses. Large intranuclear inclusion bodies are apparent in stained cultures (MGG or H & E). Nucleoli are always preserved.

The CPE does not always lead to complete destruction of the cell sheet, and sometimes CPE does not occur in spite of the presence of virus. The antibody production test can then be employed for virus demonstration. Generally RECC are more sensitive for virus growth than are other cell cultures from rodents.[15] When RECC are used, blind passages of noninfected controls of all cell batches should be carried out, because vertical transmission can occur and result in latent infection of cultures.

A more successful method for isolating rodent parvoviruses is the preparation of cell cultures directly from organs of infected animals, although this method is more difficult. Kidneys, lung, testis, and brain are the best sources for cell preparation. The cultures should be subcultivated at least twice; if no CPE develops, the antibody production tests can be used for demonstration of virus.

Animal inoculation. The natural infection of rats with rat virus is generally subclinical. Only the hemorrhagic encephalopathy strain produces a lethal encephalopathy in young rats under natural condition.[4] Experimentally, rat virus can produce an acute fatal disease in neonatal rats if given in large quantities.[7,13] Death occurs approximately 8 days after infection. Small doses of virus induce dwarfism, mongoloidism, dental defects, and cerebellar hypoplasia. Similar changes are observed after infection of rats with H-1 virus.[13]

A more marked pathogenicity is seen when rat virus and H-1 are given to newborn hamsters. Animals inoculated up to 4–6 days after birth develop a fatal disease, which is manifested by hemorrhage of the gut, liver congestion, and anoxia 4–6 days postinfection. Death occurs soon after onset of clinical signs. Sometimes the animals also show deformities, when they survive. Newborn hamsters less than 24 hours old are especially sensitive to minute virus doses. H-1 and rat virus also produce dwarfism and runting in neonatal mice.[12]

Minute virus of mice does not produce a clinical disease in the natural hosts—mice and possibly rats. It is, however, pathogenic for neonatal hamsters and to a lesser extent for neonatal mice and rats when infected experimentally. Neonatal hamsters usually die from MVM infections within 6 days; in older suckling hamsters, mongoloidism, dwarfism, and peridontal disease occur.[9] In mice, only subclinical signs develop, accompanied by runting and growth retardation. A special target for the virus is the cerebellum, but no ataxia can be observed. Rats do not show symptoms after infection with MVM; however, subclinical infections are reported.[9]

All rodent parvoviruses can be transmitted vertically from mother to fetus, which may result in embryonic death or brain damage (cerebellar hypoplasia). Transplacental infection always occurs in association with maternal viremia.[11] Fetal infections can be induced experimentally between 24 hours and several days after infection of pregnant females. Primary isolation of all rodent parvoviruses can be achieved by IC or IP inoculation of neonatal hamsters (not older than 24 hours) with infected material. Signs of illness are generally absent on first passage, but blind passage of liver, spleen, or kidney suspension 7–10 days postinfection usually results in clinical signs and death as described earlier. Intranuclear inclusion bodies are prevalent in many tissues on histopathologic examination.[7]

Immunology and serology. The antibody production test (APT) is a relatively simple method for detection of rodent parvoviruses.[17] The APT can be used to titrate the amount of virus in a specimen or to isolate and identify a virus by the inoculation of the animals with tissue culture harvests or organ suspensions.[15,16] The entire procedure has to be performed under axenic conditions. Usually three to four animals are used per sample or dilution and they are inoculated under a light ether anesthesia with 0.5 ml IP and 0.05 ml IN. About 28 days later the animal's serum is tested for antibody by HI to rodent parvoviruses. Tests in mice are termed MAP tests, in rats RAP tests, and in hamsters HAP tests. Conditions essential in the test are use of animals from antibody-negative colonies, inclusion of adequate sham-inoculated controls, and isolation of the inoculated test animals to prevent cross-infection between test groups.

The FA method can only be used to differentiate between rodent parvoviruses and parvoviruses of other species. Differentiation between the rodent parvoviruses cannot be carried out, since they seem to share common antigens demonstrable by FA techniques only.[3]

All rodent parvoviruses contain a hemagglutinin that reacts with RBC from a number of animal species. Best results are obtained with RBC from guinea pigs, hamsters, human type O, and rhesus monkeys. The HA reaction is not pH or temperature dependent; however, best results are obtained after incubation at room temperature.

Titration of virus can be done in tubes or in microplates by preparing twofold dilutions of virus suspensions in saline or Bacto-HA buffer (pH 7.2–7.3), and then adding equal volumes of 0.5% guinea pig RBC suspended in buffered saline containing 0.25% of bovine serum albumin (BSA) to each dilution. (In microplates 1% RBC is used.) For tube tests use 0.2 ml amounts of all reagents; for microplates use 0.05 ml of virus dilution and buffer and 0.025 ml of RBC. Final readings are made in approximately 45–60 minutes at room temperature, when patterns have formed. H-1 and rat virus are read by the regular button method; MVM is read by the "tear drop" method.

HI tests can be carried out in tubes with 0.2 ml amounts of all reagents or using the microtiter technique with 0.025 ml amounts. Serial twofold serum dilutions are prepared in buffered saline after inactivation at 56°C for 30 minutes. Treatment of sera with equal amounts of RDE may be advisable to remove nonspecific activity.[17] About 8 HA units of antigen are added to each serum dilution and the mixture is incubated for 30–60 minutes at room temperature. An equal amount (0.2 ml or 0.025 ml) of 0.5% (tube test) or 1% (microtest) RBC in buffered saline containing 0.25% BSA is added to the serum-antigen mixture. After thorough mixing the test is incubated at room temperature for 1 hour and read, when patterns have formed. H-1 and rat virus are read by the regular button method, MVM is read by the tear-drop method.[14] Titers of 1:20 and higher are regarded as positive in RDE-treated sera. Known positive and negative sera should be included in the test for comparison.

The standard VN test can be used with the following modifications. Secondary RECC can be employed for all rodent parvoviruses. About 1000 $TCID_{50}$ in 0.1 ml are mixed with an equal amount of serum dilution and incubated at 37°C for 1.5–2 hours, and then 0.2 ml are inoculated into three to four tubes with RECC. Tubes are rocked for 1 hour and then fed with medium. Cell cultures are examined for CPE from day 5 to day 14 postinfection.[3]

CF antigens are prepared by infecting confluent monolayers of RECC with the appropriate virus, and cultures are harvested when approximately 50% of the cells show CPE.[3] Uninoculated cultures are handled in a similar manner as controls. The cells are suspended in 0.05 volume of the culture fluids, mixed with an equal volume of undiluted RDE, incubated overnight at 37°C, and then heated at 56°C for 30 minutes. The CF test is then carried out either in tubes or in microplates according to the Laboratory Branch Task Force Standardized Method,[10] employing 3 units of complement and 4 units of CF antigen. The serum-antigen-complement mixtures are incubated overnight at 4°C and then the hemolytic system is added. CF antibody titers of 1:10 or higher are considered positive. With each test, known positive and negative control sera should be used for comparison.

Animals that have been infected with either H-1, rat virus, or MVM after birth develop antibodies, which are long lasting. Such animals are immune to reinfection.

References

1. Binn, L.N., E.C. Lazar, G.A. Eddy, and M. Kajima. Recovery and characterization of a minute virus of canines. *Infec. Immunity* 1:503, 1970.
2. Crawford, L.V. A minute virus of mice. *Virology* 29:605, 1966.
3. Cross, S.S., and J.C. Parker. Some antigenic relationships of the murine parvoviruses: Minute virus of mice, rat virus, and H-1 virus. *Proc. Soc. Exp. Biol. Med.* 139:105, 1972.
4. Eidadah, A.H., N. Nathanson, K.O. Smith, R.A. Squire, G.W. Santos, and E.C. Melby. Viral hemorrhagic encephalopathy of rats. *Science* 156:392, 1967.
5. Hallauer, C., G. Kronauer, and G. Siegl. Parvoviruses as contaminants of permanent human cell lines. I. Virus isolations from 1960–1970. *Arch. ges. Virusforsch.* 35:80, 1971.
6. Kilham, L. Rat virus (RV) infection in hamsters. *Proc. Soc. Exp. Biol. Med.* 106:825, 1961.
7. Kilham, L. Viruses of laboratory and wild rats. In *Viruses of Laboratory Rodents*. National Cancer Institute Monograph no. 20, p. 117, Washington, 1966.
8. Kilham, L., and G. Margolis. Transplacental infection of rats and hamsters induced by oral and parenteral inoculations of H-1 and rat viruses. *Teratology* 2:111, 1969.
9. Kilham, L., and G. Margolis. Pathogenicity of minute virus of mice (MVM) for rats, mice, and hamsters. *Proc. Soc. Exp. Biol. Med.* 133:1447, 1970.
10. Laboratory Branch Task Force. *Standardized Diagnostic Complement Fixation Method and Adaptation to Micro Test*, H.L. Casey (ed.). Public Health Monograph no. 74. U.S. Government Printing Office, Washington, 1965.
11. Margolis, G., and L. Kilham. Parvovirus infections, vascular endothelium, and hemorrhagic encephalopathy. *Lab. Invest.* 22:478, 1970.
12. Matsuo, Y., and H.J. Spencer. Studies on the infectivity of rat virus (RV) in BALB/c mice. *Proc. Soc. Exp. Biol. Med.* 130:294, 1968.
13. Moore, A.E., and A.D. Nicastri. Lethal infection and pathological findings in A × C rats inoculated with H virus and RV. *J. Nat. Cancer Inst.* 35:937, 1965.
14. Parker, J.C., M.J. Collins, S.S. Cross, and W.P. Rowe. Minute virus of mice. II. Prevalence, epidemiology, and occurrence as a contaminant of transplanted tumors. *J. Nat. Cancer Inst.* 45:305, 1970.
15. Parker, J.C., S.S. Cross, M.J. Collins, and W.P. Rowe. Minute virus of mice. I. Procedures for quantitation and detection. *J. Nat. Cancer Inst.* 45:297, 1970.
16. Parker, J.C., R.W. Tennant, T.G. Ward, and W.P. Rowe. Virus studies with germfree mice. I. Preparation of serologic diagnostic reagents and survey of germfree and monocontaminated mice for indigenous murine viruses. *J. Nat. Cancer Inst.* 34:371, 1965.
17. Rowe, W.P., J.W. Hartley, and J.D. Estes. Studies of mouse polyoma virus infection. I. Procedures for quantitation and detection of virus. *J. Exp. Med.* 109:379, 1959.
18. Toolan, H.W. Studies on the H-viruses. *Proc. Am. Ass. Cancer Res.* 5:64, 1964.
19. Toolan, H.W. Susceptibility of the rhesus monkey (Macacca mulatta) to H-1 virus. *Nature* 209:833, 1966.
20. Toolan, H.W. The picodnaviruses: H, RV, and AAV. *Rev. Exp. Rath.* 6:136, 1968.
21. Toolan, H.W., E.L. Saunders, C.M. Southam, A.E. Moore, and A.G. Levin. H-1 virus viremia in the human. *Proc. Soc. Exp. Biol. Med.* 119:711, 1965.

Feline Panleukopenia Virus

Feline panleukopenia (FPL) is also known as infectious feline enteritis, cat distemper, infectious aleukocytosis, infectious feline agranylocytosis, infectious gastroenteritis, feline ataxia, feline cerebellar hypoplasia, and mink enteritis. All domestic and wild species of the family Felidae appear susceptible to FPL,[3,5,27] as well as mink and members of the raccoon family (raccoon, ringtail, and coati-mundi).[2,3,27] All FPL and mink enteritis isolates tested by serum neutralization procedures have been of one serotype.[8,11,24] There is no known cross-reaction between FPL virus and other small-DNA viruses (parvoviruses) such as Kilham's rat virus or H-1 virus.

In utero infection results in abortion, mummification of the fetus, stillbirth, neonatal death, or ataxia.[16,17,21] Typically, one or more kittens of a litter without previous history of illness will show varying degrees of symmetrical ataxia at 2–3 weeks of age. The surviving kittens are strong, alert, and in good condition. The affected kittens exhibit posterior ataxia and a rolling gait when attempting to walk, and also show a trembling of the head. If the kitten can eat, it will survive with persistent ataxia. Affected mink are anorexic and have abnormal enteric discharges containing mucus, blood streaks, or intestinal casts. Mortality varies between 10 and 80%.[2,23]

Three different types of diseases are seen. In weaned kittens or older susceptible cats, the disease varies from subclinical to an acute, often fatal, disease within 24 hours of the first signs. Typically, the affected cat will show depression, dehydration, vomition, and diarrhea. The most consistent finding is a mild to severe leukopenia. The reduction in circulating leukocytes, usually observed about 4 days postinoculation, may be gradual and reach 4000–6000 per cu mm, or the reduction may be precipitious, going from normal to less than 1000 per cu mm in less than 24 hours. Bone marrow smears usually reveal a severe reduction in leukopoietic cells.

The pathology observed in FPL is directly related to the affinity of the virus for cells in active mitosis. Hence, in postweaning kittens and adult susceptible cats, lesions are usually restricted to the intestinal epithelium and the reticuloendothelial system.

In the neonatal kitten, where the external granular layer of the cerebellum undergoes rapid mitosis, it is the primary tissue damaged, although virus and lesions are found in many other tissues.[4]

On autopsy, lesions are often not observed. The wall of the small intestine is thickened and edematous, especially the distal ileum, with petechial hemorrhages on the serosal and mucosal surfaces. The intestinal contents are scant and fluid. The mesenteric lymph nodes are edematous and often hemorrhagic. The thymus often appears edematous and even gelatinous after depletion of cellular elements, especially in young kittens. The bone marrow is more fluid and typically cannot be "shelled out." Leukocytes are absent in lesions and large vessels and greatly reduced in lymph nodes, thymus, spleen, and bone marrow. The epithelium of the small intestine, especially the base of the crypts of the ileum, show ballooned cells with desquamation of the epithelium and cell debris in the lumen.[7]

Eosinophilic intranuclear inclusions, with a wide halo and margination of chromatin and nucleoli, are present in the epithelium and mucosa of the small intestine. Inclusions are present in most tissues of neonatally infected cats, especially in the external granular layer of the cerebellum and subependymal cells of the ventricles;[17] they are more distinct when an acid fixative such as Bouin's or Zenker's is used. There is excellent correlation between the location of intranuclear inclusions in stained sections and FA-stained sections.

In kittens and ataxia, the external granular layer of the cerebellum is greatly reduced and the Purkinje cells are scattered.[16] The gross and histopathologic findings in mink are essentially the same as in the cat.[2,24]

FPL virus contains DNA; it resists ether, chloroform, heat, acid, phenol, and trypsin, but can be inactivated with Formalin.[8] Electron microscopy has shown that the size is 20–25 nm.[12,24] The specific gravity is 1.33.[12,24] Cytochemical studies indicate that FPL virus is probably single stranded.[12,24]

Specimens

During the acute disease, virus can be isolated from all tissues, blood, and excreta for 3–4 days until neutralizing antibodies appear in the blood (7 days after experimental inoculation). Spleen, small intestine, and thymus are the best tissues for isolation of virus from dead animals, while blood and feces should be used from living animals.

A carrier state may persist in recovered cats. Virus can be isolated from feces for several weeks in occasional cats, and from kidneys of kittens that have shown ataxia for several weeks.[16] Mink shed virus in their feces for at least 1 year after infection.[1]

Laboratory Procedures

Cultures. Cell cultures of feline kidney origin are preferred for the isolation and cultivation of FPL virus. Since the virus has a selective affinity for the mitotic cell, cultures should be inoculated early in their growth cycle.[9,13,16,24] Best results are obtained when secondary feline kidney cells are inoculated with virus material 2–3 hours after cells have been dispensed in tubes or flasks, or by mixing virus with cells before dispensing into containers. Maximum CPE is obtained at 37°C in 4–5 days, after which most cultures appear to recover unless a high multiplicity of virus was inoculated (Table 16.2).

Table 16.2. Effect of feline panleukopenia virus on feline kidney cell cultures

CPE	No. of inclusions per 125× field	Destruction of cell sheet	Approximate $TCID_{50}$ inoculated
+	<1	None	1–10
++	1–5	None	10–100
+++	>5	None to slight	100–1000
++++	Numerous	Partial	1000–10,000
+++++	Numerous	Complete	>10,000

Identification of the virus may be done in one of several ways. The CPE in unstained cultures appears as a transitory degenerative type and can easily be mistaken for nonspecific degeneration except in excellent cultures inoculated with high concentrations of virus.[24] The metabolic inhibition (MI) test can be used with the more cytopathic strains of the virus. Direct FA tests using Leighton tube coverslip cultures can be used for virus detection. A fluorescence of the entire nucleus is seen in infected cells.[18,24] For identification of the virus in cell cultures, the preferred method is the staining of Leighton tube coverslip cultures with MGG stain. A dark-red, Cowdry type-A intranuclear inclusion body is observed in infected cells.[24] H & E stain can also be used.[7,9] Frozen tissue sections from infected animals, examined by FA technique, can be used for rapid diagnosis of FPL.[27]

A direct correlation exists between the amount of virus inoculated into recently transferred secondary feline kidney tissue cultures and the resulting CPE, as outlined in Table 16.2.[24]

Animal inoculation. Susceptible cats may be challenged by oral, intragastric, cutaneous, SC, IP, IV, IN, or IC routes of inoculation.[17,25] Little if any difference in incubation period or clinical disease is observed by the different routes. Newborn ferrets inoculated intracerebrally can be used for assay of FPL virus.[17,22] Subclinical or mild infections occur frequently in susceptible cats with some strains of virus and in gnotobiotic cats with virulent virus.[22] To date, quantitative serology has not been used to evaluate the immune response in mink; studies have relied upon oral challenge of tissue suspensions from infected mink.

Most laboratory animals have been shown to be resistant to FPL infection, including the mouse, guinea pig, rabbit, ground squirrel, dog, rhesus monkey, hamster, canary, hedgehog, rat, and mongoose.[6,15,25] Neonatal ferret is the only animal known to be susceptible to FPL other than those previously mentioned.[17]

Immunology and serology. The VN test is the most suitable serologic technique for FPL.[24] Serum dilutions should be prepared and mixed with an equal volume of stock virus (100–300 $TCID_{50}$ per 0.1 ml). Aliquots of the serum-virus mixtures (0.2 ml) can be inoculated into secondary feline kidney cells in Leighton tube coverslip cultures 2–3 hours after transfer. Crandell cat cell line can also be used. After 4 days incubation at 37°C, the coverslips should be stained and examined for intranuclear inclusions as outlined under virus isolation. The coverslips can also be used for FA tests. The MI test can also be used, as can the direct examination of unstained cultures if the cultures are good; nonspecific degeneration often makes it difficult to arrive at an endpoint with these methods. The CF test has also been used by employing a purified mink enteritis isolate antigen.[14] FPL virus apparently does not hemmagglutinate erythrocytes as do some of the other parvoviruses.[21]

Neutralizing antibodies begin to appear in the serum of cats about 7 days after experimental inoculation, or about 3 days after clinical signs appear. Serum antibody titers between 1000 and 10,000 usually occur 14 days after experimental inoculation. Vaccination with modified live-virus (MLV) vaccines produce titers of between 1000 and 5000. Inactivated vaccines of feline or mink tissue origin produce titers between 10 and 200 following a single vaccination. A second vaccination may increase the titer.

Female cats that are immune to FPL transfer passive immunity to their offspring via the colostrum, which interferes with vaccination and protects the kittens against challenge with virulent virus. Serum antibody titers of the kittens are equal to that of the queen 24–48 hours postpartum, then gradually decline with an antibody half-life of approximately 9.5 days. Maternal immunity titers greater than 30 usually protect kittens against challenge with 1000–3000 $TCID_{50}$ of virulent virus, and serologic conversion does not occur. MLV vaccines will overcome maternal serum titers of 10 or less, while any demonstrable titer is sufficient to interfere with inactivated vaccines.

References

1. Bouillant, A., and R.P. Hanson. Epizootiology of mink enteritis. III. Carrier state in mink. *Can. J. Comp. Med. Vet. Sci.* 29:183–189, 1965.
2. Burger, D. The relationship of mink virus enteritis to feline panleukopenia virus. M.S. thesis, Washington State University, Pullman, 1961.
3. Cockburn, A. Infectious enteritis in the Zoological Gardens, Regent's Park. *Vet. J.* 103:261–262, 1947.
4. Csiza, C.K., A. de La Hunta, F.W. Scott, and J.H. Gillespie. Pathogenesis of feline panleukopenia in susceptible newborn kittens. *Infec. Immunity* 3:833–846, 1971.
5. Gorham, J.R., G.R. Hartsough, N. Sato, and S. Lust. Studies on cell culture adapted feline panleukopenia virus: Virus neutralization and antigenic extinction. *Vet. Med. Small Anim. Clin.* 61:35–40, 1966.
6. Goss, L.J. Species susceptibility to the viruses of Carré and feline enteritis. *Am. J. Vet. Res.* 9:65–68, 1948.

7. Hamman, W.D., and J.F. Enders. A virus disease of cats principally characterized by aleukocytosis, enteric lesions and the presence of intranuclear inclusion bodies. *J. Exp. Med.* 69:327–352, 1939.
8. Johnson, R.H. Feline panleukopenia. I. Identification of a virus associated with the syndrome. *Res. Vet. Sci.* 6:466–471, 1965.
9. Johnson, R.H. Feline panleukopenia virus. III. Some properties compared to a feline herpes virus. *Res. Vet. Sci.* 7:112–115, 1966.
10. Johnson, R.H. Feline panleukopenia virus. IV. Methods for obtaining reproducible *in vitro* results. *Res. Vet. Sci.* 8:256–264, 1967.
11. Johnson, R.H. Feline panleukopenia virus: *In vitro* comparison of strains with a mink enteritis virus. *J. Small Anim. Prac.* 8:319–324, 1967.
12. Johnson, R.H., and J.G. Cruickshank. Problem in classification of feline panleukopenia virus. *Nature* 212:622–623, 1966.
13. Johnson, R.H., G. Margolis, and L. Kilham. Identity of feline ataxia virus with feline panleukopenia virus. *Nature* 214:175–177, 1967.
14. Kääriäinen, L., J. Kangas, S. Keränen, M. Nyholm, and P. Weckström. Studies on mink enteritis virus. *Arch. ges. Virusforsch.* 19:197–209, 1966.
15. Kikuth, W., R. Gönnert, and M. Schweickert. Infektiöse aleukozytose der katzen. *Zentralblatt Bakt.* 146:1–17, 1940.
16. Kilham, L., and G. Margolis. Viral etiology of spontaneous ataxia of cats. *Am. J. Path.* 48:991–1011, 1966.
17. Kilham, L., G. Margolis, and E.D. Colby. Congenital infections of cats and ferrets by feline panleukopenia virus manifested by cerebellar hypoplasia. *Lab. Invest.* 17:465–480, 1967.
18. King, D.A., and D.L. Croghan. Immunofluorescence of feline panleukopenia virus in cell culture: Determination of immunological status of felines by serum neutralization. *Can. J. Comp. Med. Vet.* 29:85–89, 1965.
19. Lust, S.J., J.R. Gorham, and N. Sato. Occurrence of intranuclear inclusions in cell cultures infected with infectius feline enteritis virus. *Am. J. Vet. Res.* 26:1163–1166, 1965.
20. Margolis, G., and L. Kilham. Rat virus, an agent with an affinity for the dividing cell. In *Slow, Latent, and Temperate Virus Infections*. National Institute of Neurological Diseases and Blindness Monograph no. 2, pp. 361–367, 1966.
21. Margolis, G., and L. Kilham. In pursuit of an ataxic hamster, or virus-induced cerebellar hypoplasia. In *The Central Nervous System*. International Academy of Pathology Monograph no. 9, pp. 157–183. Williams and Wilkins, Baltimore, 1968.
22. Rohovsky, M.W., and R.A. Griesemer. Experimental feline infectious enteritis in the germfree cat. *Path. Vet.* 4:391–410, 1967.
23. Schofield, F.W. Virus enteritis in mink. *N. Am. Vet.* 30:651–654, 1949.
24. Scott, F.W. Feline panleukopenia. Ph.D. thesis, Cornell University, Ithaca, N.Y., 1968.
25. Syverton, J.T., J.S. Lawrence, R.J. Ackart, W.S. Adams, D.M. Erwin, A.L. Haskings, Jr., R.H. Saunders, Jr., M.B. Stringfellow, and R.M. Wetrich. The virus of infectious feline agranulocytosis. I. Characters of the virus: Pathogenicity. *J. Exp. Med.* 77:41–56, 1943.
26. Torres, S. Infectious feline gastroenteritis in wild cats. *N. Am. Vet.* 22:297–299, 1941.
27. Tuomi, J., and J. Kangas. A fluorescent antibody technique for studies of mink virus enteritis. *Arch. ges. Virusforsch.* 13:430–434, 1963.
28. Waller, E. Infectious gastro-enteritis in raccoons. *J. Am. Vet. Med. Ass.* 96:266–268, 1940.

Porcine Parvovirus

All isolates of porcine parvovirus (PPV) that have been reported belong to one serotype, and no antigenic relationships to other known parvoviruses have been found. Only swine are known to be susceptible to PPV. Recently, a virus that had similar properties and was serologically indistinguishable from PPV was isolated from a variety of established human cell lines as a contaminant.[7] the origin of these contaminations in human cell lines is unknown; the human being does not seem to be a natural host because no antibodies were found in 182 human sera from individuals of all ages, including sera from laboratory personnel working with PPV. In addition, the swine isolate G10/1 could not be adapted to growth in human cell lines.[12]

Swine do not develop a clinical disease whether infected neonatally or at older ages.[5] The virus readily passes the placenta and infects fetuses in pregnant sows. Virus can be recovered from aborted and stillborn piglets, and it has been suggested that PPV infections in pigs occur in connection with developing infertility in swine herds.[4] Experimentally, it has also been shown that PPV infects fetuses transplacentally; however, no significant effects were observed in any of these animals.[5,10] Only infection at the time of artificial insemination resulted in greater losses than normally would be expected.[5] Experimental in utero infection of porcine fetuses at various stages of gestation resulted in death and mummification of inoculated fetuses at up to 64 days of gestation, whereas controls in the other horn of the uterus within the same animal remained normal. Fetuses infected later in pregnancy developed antibodies in utero and were born apparently normal. It is obvious from these preliminary data that pathologic changes resulting in death and mummification can occur when PPV infection is induced early in pregnancy and that these changes are dependent upon the virus dose.[3]

Specimens

PPV has been isolated from aborted and stillborn piglets, mummified fetuses, and vaginal mucus and semen of pigs, as well as from testis and kidneys[4,12] of healthy piglets. Primary monolayer cultures from infected healthy piglets often harbor PPV,[9,12] and several strains of porcine adeno- and hog cholera viruses were shown to be contaminated with PPV, although not all reported PPV contaminations were eventually characterized as parvoviruses.[8]

In experimentally infected fetuses all organs contain large amounts of virus, and PPV can easily be isolated from kidneys, lung, liver, intestines, brain, testis, and lymph nodes of dead or mummified fetuses.[3]

Laboratory Procedures

Cultures. As in rodent parvovirus infections, two methods of virus isolation have been shown to be successful in tissue culture: the inoculation of cell cultures with organ suspensions, and the preparation of cell cultures directly from organs of infected animals.

Primary piglet kidney cell cultures or permanent porcine cell lines are most suitable for virus isolation. Because PPV has an affinity for the dividing cell similar to other parvoviruses, cultures must be subconfluent at the time of inoculation.[2] The primary cell cultures very often harbor latent PPV infections, so blind passages of noninfected controls of all cell batches must be carried out.[1] The SK cell line is very sensitive to growth of PPV,[11] but the porcine kidney (PK-15) cell line does not always yield satisfactory and reliable results.

PPV produces CPE 24–72 hours after infection, which appears as diffuse granulation, rounding up of cells, detachment, and lysis of the cell sheet.[12] If no CPE occurs, blind passages may be necessary for detection of virus. Infectivity titers obtained depend upon the cell system used and range from 10^5 to $10^{6.5}$ TCID$_{50}$ per 0.2 ml. HA titers go up to 1:1024. Intranuclear inclusion bodies can be detected from 16 to 36 hours after infection.[12]

Better results are obtained, however, when tissues of infected pigs are cultured as monolayers some time after infection. Best chances for virus isolation are reported from animals with high antibody titers. Virus persists at least 6–9 weeks after infection.[10] Isolation of virus from animals with longer periods of infection is usually not successful. Kidneys, testicles, and lungs are the tissues that most readily yield virus.

Animal inoculation. PPV shows no pathogenicity when inoculated IP in newborn hamsters or rats.[12]

Immunology and serology. The FA test can be used. This method will yield reliable results in tissue culture. The FA-positive nuclei are demonstrable between 8 and 36 hours postinoculation.

PPV possesses a hemagglutinin that is active with RBC from the guinea pig, human type O, rhesus monkey, mouse, rat, cat, and chicken, but no HA is observed with RBC from hamster, rabbit, dog, sheep, pig, horse, or goose. Optimal results are obtained with guinea pig (GP) RBC. Titration of virus can be done in tubes (0.2 ml amounts) or microplates (0.025 ml amounts) by preparing twofold dilutions of virus suspensions in saline or Bacto-HA buffer (pH 7.2–7.3), and adding equal volumes of 0.5% RBC in saline and 0.25% BSA to each dilution. In microplates 1% RBC are used.[1] Final readings are made in approximately 4–6 hours at 4°C, when patterns are formed. The regular button method is used. Incubation at room temperature gives somewhat less reliable results.

HI tests can be carried out in tubes or microplates as described under HA. Serial twofold serum dilutions are prepared in buffered saline after inactivation at 56°C for 30 minutes. Treatment of the sera for removal of nonspecific inhibitors is not necessary.[6,12] Isoagglutinins are removed by absorption of the sera with 50% GP RBC. About 8 units of HA antigen are added to the serum dilutions and the mixture is incubated for 60 minutes at room temperature. An equal amount of 0.5–1% GP RBC suspension is added. After mixing, the test materials are incubated at 4°C for 4–6 hours and read when patterns have formed by the regular button method. Titers of 1:8 or higher are regarded as positive.

Standard methods are used for the VN test with the following modifications. SK cells are employed.[11] About 1000 TCID$_{50}$ of PPV in 0.1 ml is mixed with an equal amount of inactivated serum dilution and incubated at room temperature for 2 hours. Then 0.2 ml is inoculated into three or four cell culture tubes, used 24 hours after seeding with 1×10^5 cells per ml. Tubes are rocked for 1 hour and then fed with medium. Cell cultures are incubated in roller drums at 37°C and examined for CPE from day 5 to day 10 postinfection with one fluid change at day 6.

Infected and contact pigs develop high (1:1024 to 1:4000) HI antibody titers against PPV.[1,12] Reinfection does not result in a rise of titer.[10]

In fetal infections later than 64 days of pregnancy, antibodies develop in utero. When infection occurs earlier than 33 days of pregnancy, a tolerance state is seen.[10] Antibodies develop rapidly after infection; usually within 7 days titers of 1:256 are present.[1,11] Fetal mummification is sometimes seen in PPV infections.[13] PPV is widely spread; it occurs in more than 50% of the pigs in Germany,[1] Great Britain,[4] the United States, and probably many other countries.

References
1. Bachmann, P.A. Vorkommen und Verbreitung von Picodna (Parvo)-Viren beim Schwein. *Zentrallblatt Veterinärmedizin*, ser. B, 16:341–345, 1969.
2. Bachmann, P.A. Porcine parvovirus infection *in vitro:* A study model for the replication of parvoviruses. I. Replication at different temperatures. *Proc. Soc. Exp. Biol. Med.* 140:1369–1374, 1972.
3. Bachmann, P.A., B.E. Sheffy, and J.T. Vaughn. Experimental *in utero* infection of fetal pigs with a porcine parvovirus (PPV). *Infec. Immunity* 12:455, 1975.
4. Cartwright, S.F., and R.A. Huck. Viruses isolated in association with herd infertility, abortions and stillbirths in pigs. *Vet. Rec.* 81:196–197, 1967.
5. Cartwright, S.F., M. Lucas, and R.A. Huck. A small hemagglutinating porcine DNA virus. II. Biological and serological studies. *J. Comp. Path.* 81:145, 1971.
6. Darbyshire, J.H., and D.H. Roberts. Some respiratory virus and mycoplasma infections of animals. *J. Clin. Path.* 21(suppl. 2): 61, 1968.
7. Hallauer, C., G. Kronauer, and G. Siegl. Parvoviruses as contaminants of permanent human cell lines. I. Virus isolations from 1960–1970. *Arch. ges. Virusforsch.* 35:80, 1971.
8. Horzinek, M., M. Mussgay, J. Maess, and K. Petzoldt. Nachweis dreier Virusarten (Schweinepest-, Adeno-, Picodna-Virus) in einem als cytopathogen bezeichneten Schweinepestvirusstamm. *Arch. ges. Virusforsch.* 21:98, 1967.
9. Huygelen, C., and J. Peetermans. Isolation of a hemagglutinating picornavirus from primary swine kidney cell cultures. *Arch. ges. Virusforsch.* 20:260, 1967.
10. Johnson, R.H., and D.F. Collings. Transplacental infection of piglets with a porcine parvovirus. *Res. Vet. Sci.* 12:570, 1971.
11. Kasza, L., J.A. Shadduck, and G.J. Christofinis. Establishment of viral susceptibility, and biological characteristics of a swine kidney cell line SK-6. *Res. Vet. Sci.* 13:46, 1972.
12. Mayr, A., P.A. Bachmann, G. Siegl, H. Mahnel, and B.E. Sheffy. Characterization of a small porcine DNA virus. *Arch. ges. Virusforsch.* 25:38, 1968.
13. Mengeling, W.L., R.C. Cutlip, R.A. Wilson, J.B. Parks, and R.F. Marshall. Fetal mummification associated with porcine parvovirus infection. *J. Am. Vet. Med. Ass.* 166:993–995, 1975.

Bovine Parvovirus

Bovine parvovirus (BPV) is also known as hemadsorbing enteric (HADEN) virus. All known isolates belong to the same serotype. There is no antigenic relationship to the recently isolated AAV X_7, which is associated with bovine adenovirus type 1, nor to other known parvoviruses.[2,3] Cattle are the only species known to be susceptible to BPV.

Mild clinical symptoms develop in calves inoculated with BPV strain HADEN; after *per os* infection, calves show diarrhea.[6] Clinical signs of the natural infection are unknown, although a large percentage of animals in the United States and in Europe contain antibodies. The virus can pass the placenta and infect the fetus, as shown by the demonstration of homologous antibodies in precolostrum newborn calves and by isolation of BPV from stocks of fetal calf serum.[4]

Specimens

Bovine parvovirus has been isolated from feces and from nasal swabs.[1,6] Possible sources of virus are fetal tissues and blood.

Laboratory Procedures

Cultures. Virus isolation can be carried out in primary or secondary cell cultures prepared from BEK or from bovine testis.[2,5] BPV does not seem to be as dependent upon the dividing cell as are other parvoviruses. BPV produces a CPE 3–4 days after infection that starts with a diffuse granulation and rounding up of cells and results in complete lysis of the cell sheet. Eosinophilic nuclear inclusion bodies develop 18–24 hours after infection in cell cultures.

Infectivity titers range from $10^{4.5}$ to $10^{5.5}$ TCID$_{50}$ per 0.1 ml, and HA activity goes up to titers of 1:4000. BPV can also be demonstrated by FA techniques. The nuclei of infected cells fluoresce brightly.

Animal inoculation. Only cattle are susceptible to BPV.

Immunology and serology. Standard methods similar to those used for porcine parvovirus are used for VN tests. Bovine testicular cell cultures are employed and examination of cultures for CPE is made from 5 to 12 days postinoculation.

Bovine parvovirus possesses a hemagglutinin that reacts with RBC from guinea pigs, human type O, and dogs, whereas negative results are obtained with rabbit, rat, mouse, chicken, cat, sheep, and bovine RBC. The reaction is independent of pH changes between 5 and 8.[2] Titrations of virus can be done using GP RBC as described for the porcine parvovirus. The test materials are incubated at room temperature for 1 hour before reading.

HI tests are carried out as described for the porcine parvovirus. Guinea pig RBC should be used and the reaction incubated at room temperature for 1 hour before reading by the regular button method. Titers of 1:20 and higher are regarded as positive. Sera have to be treated with 25% kaolin and should be adsorbed with 50% GP RBC before use to remove nonspecific inhibitors and isoagglutinins.

Infected and contact cattle develop antibodies but may still have a mild diarrhea when challenged with BPV. BPV antibodies are also present in precolostrum calves and in fetal calf serum.[3]

References

1. Abinanti, F.R., and M.S. Warfield. Recovery of a hemadsorbing virus (HADEN) from the gastrointestinal tract of calves. *Virology* 14:288, 1961.
2. Bachmann, P.A. Properties of a bovine parvovirus. *Zentralblatt Veterinärmedizin,* ser. B, 18:80, 1971.
3. Luchsinger, E., R. Strobbe, G. Wellemans, D. Dekegel, and S. Sprecher-Goldberger. Hemagglutinating adenoassociated virus (AAV) in association with bovine adeno-virus type 1. *Arch. ges. Virusforsch.* 31:390, 1970.
4. Molander, C.W., A.J. Kniazeff, C.W. Boone, A. Paley, and D.T. Imagawa. Isolation and characterization of viruses from fetal calf serum. *In vitro* 7:168, 1971.
5. Spahn, G.J., S.B. Mohanty, and F.M. Hetrick. Characteristics of hemadsorbing enteric (HADEN) virus. *Can. J. Microbiol.* 12:653, 1966.
6. Spahn, G.J., S.B. Mohanty, and F.M. Hetrick. Experimental infection of calves with hemadsorbing enteric (HADEN) virus. *Cornell Vet.* 56:377, 1966.

Adeno-Associated Viruses

Five serotypes of adeno-associated viruses (AAV) have been reported. Four serotypes (AAV 1, 2, 3, 4) are from humans and monkeys; the new AAV 5 was isolated from bovine adenovirus stocks.[11] The AAV type 2 and 3 show a cross-reaction in CF and FA tests.[7] AAV have no common antigens with subgroup A and C parvoviruses. The AAV isolated from humans and monkeys were found only in association with adenovirus infection. The AAV isolated from bovine adenovirus stocks is prevalent in cattle and humans.[11] No other species are known to be susceptible, no pathologic effects are known to be caused by AAV, and the natural history is unknown.[7]

Specimens

Isolations have been made from anal and throat swabs from people with adenovirus infections. Most isolations have been as contaminants of human, simian, canine, and bovine adenovirus stocks.[2,6,7,11]

Laboratory Procedures

Cultures. Monkey kidney, human embryo kidney, canine kidney, and bovine embryo kidney or testicle cell cultures can be used for isolation and propagation of AAV if the culture is first infected with an adenovirus helper. Adenoviruses types 7 and 12 are reported to be the best helper viruses[6,13] but numerous adenoviruses can be used, including SV15,[10] infectious canine hepatitis,[8,10] mouse adenovirus,[10] and bovine adenovirus,[11] as long as the appropriate cell system is employed. Cultures are preinfected with adenovirus 1 hour before inoculation of AAV, at a virus-cell multiplicity of 1 to 3.[3,4] At maximum adenovirus CPE (about 4–5 days), tubes are frozen and thawed, and then the fluid is tested for AAV antigen by the CF test using guinea pig antiserum against the different serotypes of AAV.[2,8] Cultures inoculated with AAV without adenovirus helper should be observed for CPE to eliminate other causes of CPE, since AAV alone will not induce the appearance of CPE in cell cultures.[7] AAV-infected cultures can also be identified by electron microscopy and by VN and FA tests.

Either the usual negative staining procedure can be used for purified virus suspensions, or the following method can be employed. Cultures infected with AAV (titers of at least 10^7 per ml) are clarified with fluorocarbon (Freon 113) for 1 minute in a mixer. A drop of this treated specimen is placed on a square of 2% agar, dialyze-dried at room temperature, covered with 0.25% parlodion in amyl acetate, and allowed to drain. The agar blocks are placed in 0.75% phosphotungstic acid. After stripping the collodian film and virus from the agar, the floating film is picked up on a grid, dried, and examined under the electron microscope. Particles can be examined and counted, giving a quantitative estimate of the particle concentration in the infected culture.

Animal inoculation. AAV replicates only in specific hosts.

Immunology and serology. Clean AAV preparations are required for serologic tests and for immunization of animals for the production of AAV type-specific antisera. Two techniques are used to prepare adenovirus-free AAV. One is isopycnic density-gradient centrifugation in CsCl.[7,8] This works because the adenoviruses have a density of about 1.35 g/ml, whereas the various AAV band at 1.385–1.44 g/ml. After double banding is carried out at 35,000 rpm for 48 hours each time, these AAV preparations will be free of adenovirus antigens.[7] The second technique is a combination of filtration through Millipore membranes (50 nm pore size), which retain the adenovirus particles, and differential centrifugation under conditions that pellet the AAV virions and allow the soluble antigen to remain in the supernatant fluid.[1]

For the FA test, antiserum to purified AAV can be prepared in either guinea pigs or rabbits by mixing the antigen with Freund's adjuvant and inoculating it into the foot pad of the animals. Then Leighton tube coverslip cultures are coinfected with adenovirus and AAV. After 1–3 days incubation, coverslips are removed and stained with specific AAV conjugate and examined for intranuclear fluorescence.[4,10,13]

AAV type 4 has a strong HA activity for human type O and to a lesser extent for monkey, sheep, and guinea pig RBC. The reaction gives optimal results when performed in the cold (4°C).[9] Similarly, AAV type 5 isolated from bovine adenovirus stocks shows a strong temperature-dependent HA activity. The same titers are obtained with human type O, guinea pig, and mouse RBC, while sheep and horse RBC are less sensitive. The titers are different at different temperatures with different blood cells; however, optimal results are obtained at 4°C.[11]

CF tests are widely used for detection of antigen or antibody in work with AAV. CF antigen is produced by purification in density gradients, and CF tests are carried out using 4–8 units of antigen according to standard methods previously mentioned.[8,12]

The VN test is based on the use of a FA technique to assay neutralizing antibodies for the AAV types.[3,4] A fluorescent focus reduction test has been described in which separate preparations of AAV serotypes that contained 10^6 TCID$_{50}$ per 0.1 ml are mixed with equal amounts of a 1:5 serum dilution and then incubated at room temperature for 45 minutes. Then 0.2 ml of the virus-serum mixture is inoculated on cell cultures that had been infected 4 hours earlier with adenovirus type 7 (free from AAV) at the multiplicity of three infectious particles per cell. Coverslips are fixed in acetone 24–30 hours after adenovirus infection. The number of infected cells is then determined by FA staining and plotted against numbers in control cultures with normal guinea pig serum. The reduction of fluorescent foci is used as a measure of neutralizing antibody.[2,7]

Another VN test, which has been used extensively, is similar to the standard test. Fluids from cultures infected with adenovirus and AAV are heated at 56°C for 15 minutes to eliminate infectious adenovirus. The standard VN test is run, using reference AAV antiserum and 100–1000 TCID$_{50}$ per 0.1 ml of AAV. The virus-serum mixtures are inoculated into cell cultures pre- or coinfected with adenovirus after incubation at room temperature for 45 minutes. Endpoints are determined by CF tests after harvesting the cultures, when the adenovirus CPE progresses to a 4+ reaction.

For AAV types 4 and 5, HI tests can be performed. Human type O RBC are used and the test is kept at 4°C before reading. A plaque inhibition test has also been described;[5] cultures infected with AAV have a reduction in the yield of adenovirus due to a reduction in the number of cells infected with adenovirus. However, large amounts of AAV are necessary for the test. After incubation of virus-serum mixtures for 1 hour at room temperature the mixtures are inoculated into cultures and the cultures are immediately challenged with 100 plaque-forming units (PFU) of adenovirus. After adsorption for 2 hours, the cell cultures are overlaid with agar and incubated for 7–9 days at 36°C. A 90% plaque reduction is taken as the endpoint.

Seroconversion occurs in children after AAV infection.[2] Antibodies against the various AAV have been detected in people,[2,14] monkeys,[2] and against type 5 in cattle.[11]

References

1. Atchison, R.W., B.C. Casto, and W. McD. Hammon. Adenovirus-associated defective virus particles. *Science* 194:754, 1965.
2. Blacklow, N.R., M.D. Hoggan, and W.P. Rowe. Isolation of adenovirus-associated viruses from man. *Proc. Nat. Acad. Sci.* 58:1410, 1967.
3. Blacklow, N.R., M.D. Hoggan, and W.P. Rowe. Immunofluorescent studies of the potentiation of an adenovirus-associated virus by adenovirus 7. *J. Exp. Med.* 125:755, 1967.
4. Blacklow, N.R., M.D. Hoggan, and W.P. Rowe. Serologic evidence for human infection with adeno-associated viruses. *J. Nat. Cancer Inst.* 40:319, 1968.
5. Casto, B.C., J.A. Armstrong, R.W. Atchison, and W.McD. Hammon. Studies on the relationship between adeno-associated virus type 1 (AAV-1) and adenovirus. II. Inhibition of adenovirus plaques by AAV: Its nature and specificity. *Virology* 33:452, 1967.
6. Domoto, K., and R. Yanagawy. Properties of a small virus associated with infectious canine hepatitis virus. *Jap. J. Vet. Res.* 17:32, 1969.
7. Hoggan, M.D. Adenovirus associated viruses. *Prog. Med. Virol.* 12:211, 1970.
8. Hoggan, M.D., N.R. Blacklow, and W.P. Rowe. Studies of small DNA viruses found in various adenovirus preparations: Physical, biological, and immunological characteristics. *Proc. Nat. Acad. Sci.* 55:1467, 1966.
9. Ito, M., and H.D. Mayor. Hemagglutinin of type 4 adeno-associated satellite virus. *J. Immunol.* 100:61, 1968.
10. Ito, M., J.L. Melnick, and H.D. Mayor. An immunofluorescence assay for studying replication of adeno-satellite virus. *J. Gen. Virol.* 1:199, 1967.
11. Luchsinger, E., R. Strobbe, G. Wellemans, D. Dekegel, and S. Sprecher-Goldberger. Hemagglutinating adeno-associated virus (AAV) in association with bovine adeno-virus type 1. *Arch. ges. Virusforsch.* 31:390, 1970.
12. Parks, W.D., J.L. Melnick, R. Rongey, and H.D. Mayor. Physical assay and growth cycle studies of a defective adeno-satellite virus. *J. Virol.* 1:171, 1967.
13. Smith, K.O., and J.F. Thiel. Adeno-associated virus studies employing a fluorescent focus assay technique. *Proc. Soc. Exp. Biol. Med.* 125:887, 1967.
14. Sprecher-Goldberger, S., D. Dekegel, J. Otten, and L. Thiry. Incidence of antibodies to adenovirus-associated viruses in patients with tumors or other disease. *Arch. ges. Virusforsch.* 30:16, 1970.

17. Picornaviruses

The name of this group means small RNA viruses. The group includes two very well known disease agents, foot-and-mouth disease virus (FMD) of cloven-hooved animals and poliovirus of humans. The main characteristics of the picornaviruses are (1) a single-stranded RNA core, (2) a diameter ranging from 20 to 40 nm, (3) the absence of essential lipids as shown by resistance to ether and other organic solvents, (4) the absence of an envelope, and (5) replication in the cell cytoplasm. Most of the picornaviruses so far examined have a small number of capsomeres, approximately 30–40, arranged in a fairly regular 5, 3, 2 icosahedral symmetry.

The picornaviruses are divided into three groups: rhinoviruses, enteroviruses, and caliciviruses. Members of each of the three groups are generally isolated from definite areas of the body, such as rhinoviruses from the upper respiratory tract, throat, and mouth, and enteroviruses from the intestinal tract. In addition, each of these groups has specific biochemical and biophysical properties that set them apart. Most of the rhinoviruses are inactivated at pH 3 and some at pH 5, they have a buoyant density (in CsCl) of 1.38–1.43 g/ml, and they can readily multiply in cell cultures at lower than customary temperatures. The enteroviruses are not inactivated at pH 3, are stabilized by the presence of certain cations, such as Mg^{++}, when subjected to thermal inactivation at 50°C for 60 minutes, and have a buoyant density of 1.34–1.35 g/ml. The caliciviruses are unstable at pH 3, have variable stability at pH 5, and have a buoyant density of 1.37–1.38 g/ml.

In the current classification, Picornaviridae is the family name for the group. The rhinoviruses include FMDV and human and equine viruses. The enteroviruses include human polio, coxsackie, and ECHO viruses, bovine, porcine, simian, and avian enteroviruses, and the viruses of swine vesicular disease, Teschen disease, Talfan, avian encephalomyelitis, and duck hepatitis. The caliciviruses include vesicular exanthema of swine and the feline picornaviruses, which are mostly respiratory or conjunctival isolates.

Foot-and-Mouth Disease Virus

Foot-and-mouth disease (FMD) is a contagious viral infection primarily of cattle, swine, sheep, and goats, but also of other cloven-footed domestic and wild animals. It is characterized by vesicular lesions and subsequently by erosions of the epithelium of the mouth, nares, muzzle, feet, teats, udder, and rumen pillars.[2,3,4,7] It also may cause focal degeneration of cardiac and skeletal muscle tissues. Except for the rumen and muscle lesions, FMD produces signs and lesions that are clinically indistinguishable from those of vesicular stomatitis (VS), vesicular exanthema of swine (VES) (including the marine mammal viruses), and swine vesicular disease (SVD).[3,8] The susceptibility of various hosts to these four diseases is given in Table 17.1.

Table 17.1. Susceptibility of various hosts to foot-and-mouth disease (FMD), vesicular stomatitis (VS), vesicular exanthema of swine (VES), and swine vesicular disease (SVD)

	FMD*	VS	VES†	SVD
Cattle	S	S‡	R	R
Swine	S	S	S	S
Sheep	S	S	R	E
Horses	R	S	E	R
Guinea pigs	S	S	R	S
Mice (newborn)	S	S	R	S
Humans	S	S	R	S

S, susceptible; R, resistant; E, experimental transmission only.
*The susceptibility of Australian marsupials and other fauna to FMD has been reported.[12]
†The recently isolated marine mammal viruses (San Miguel sea lion virus) have chemical and physical characteristics similar to VES virus and have a similar host range (see reference 13 under VES virus).
‡IM inoculation of VS virus in cattle gives negative results.

Although a high mortality rate does not occur often, FMD is of major concern to disease-control veterinarians of most countries because of its rapid spread; the resulting loss of milk, meat, and other animal products; the expense of eradication or vaccination programs; and the restrictions in international trade. The disease is enzootic in Africa, Asia, Europe, and South America. The continents of Australia and North America (from Panama north) do not have FMD. Likewise, Greenland, Iceland, Ireland, Japan, New Zealand, Norway, and most of the smaller islands of Oceania and the Caribbean are free of FMD.

Outbreaks of vesicular diseases should be reported promptly. Rapid laboratory confirmatory diagnosis and initiation of strict control measures are essential. In the United States there are trained foreign-animal-disease diagnosticians in various regions who are available to help in the event of an outbreak. By direction of the proper federal and state officials, appropriate field specimens can be sent by courier for diagnosis to PIADC.

The main mode of spread of FMD is via respiratory aerosols. The usual primary site of infection and initial viral replication is in the cells of the mucous membrane of the throat.[3,9,11,13] Less frequently the virus establishes the initial infection through abrasions in the mucous membranes or skin as a result of contact with contaminated materials.[3] When susceptible animals are in direct contact with infected animals that are in the clinical stage of the disease, transmission of FMD readily occurs and recognizable clinical signs may be seen in the exposed animals within 3–5 days, but longer incubation periods have been reported.[13] The peak period of transmission usually is at the time the vesicles rupture.[3,13] Pigs fed garbage contaminated with FMD virus may show signs of infection in 1–3 days. Artificially exposed animals may develop signs as early as 12 hours after inoculation; however, the usual interval is 24–48 hours.[3]

Carrier studies have shown that the oesophageal-pharyngeal (OP) fluids and respiratory aerosols from FMD-infected animals can contain virus before, during, and after appearance of clinical signs and lesions of the disease.[3,9,13] Thus normal-appearing animals that have recovered from infection, or were vaccinated for FMD and then exposed to the virus, may harbor the virus in their throat areas for variable periods of time (from 6 to as long as 24 months in cattle, about 4–6 months in sheep and goats, but only during the clinical stage of the disease in pigs).[9,13] It has been experimentally demonstrated that when humans inhale the respiratory aerosols of FMD-infected animals they can harbor the virus in the throat area as a subclinical infection for at least 24 hours, and during this time they may transmit the virus to other people or to animals via their respiratory aerosols.[11] This temporary infection in humans has rarely become a clinical entity. When clinical FMD has occurred in humans, vesicles have been found on the hands, feet, or in the mouth; however, recovery usually has been rapid. Thus FMD has not been considered a public health problem.[2,4]

The FMD virus is composed of a single-stranded RNA core (the infectious part) within a protein coat (the antigenic part), which consists of 32 capsomeres forming a symmetrical icosahedral capsid with a diameter of about 23 nm.[1] The virus has a molecular weight of about 6.9×10^6 daltons of which about 31% is RNA.[1] The intact virion has a sedimentation coefficient of 140 S. Two other antigenic particles have been described: 12 S, which may be a portion of the protein coat of degraded virus, and 75 S, an empty virion without an RNA core.[1,5] In addition, there is a virus infection–associated (VIA) antigen found in the host cells that may be a part of the virus or may be FMD-virus RNA polymerase.[5] In the AD test with specific FMD sera, the antigens of 140 S, 12 S, and VIA each form a distinct precipitin band.[5]

The FMD virus differs from most of the other picornaviruses (except rhinoviruses) by being more labile to pH changes.[1] Strong bases (e.g. sodium hydroxide) and organic acids (e.g. acetic acid) in 2% solutions are commonly used as disinfectants for FMD virus. The RNA of FMD virus may survive boiling under certain conditions.[1] The intact virion is more susceptible to heat because of rapid denaturization of the protein capsid above 43°C. However, when protected by tissue materials, FMD virus preparations may retain some infectivity even after heating to 85°C for as long as 4 hours.[1]

Specimens

Oral, nasal, or podal lesions may be used but they should be fresh and representative.[3] The following specimens may be taken from each of two or three animals: (1) vesicular fluid (all that is obtainable), (2) vesicular lesion epithelial coverings (5g), (3) flaps of epithelial tissue still attached to the edges of the lesions (5g) (old necrotic fibrinous material that is difficult to remove is undesirable), (4) blood with anticoagulant added (5 ml) (viremia ends about 4 or 5 days after onset of disease), (5) OP fluid obtained with a cup probang from cattle, sheep, or goats but not from pigs (about 5 ml before dilution; the OP fluid samples should be diluted immediately with an equal volume of cell-culture supporting fluid, e.g. HLH, and shaken vigorously for about a minute), (6) blood for serum samples (about 10 ml of serum), (7) from dead animals, a sample of lymph node, thyroid, adrenal, kidney, or heart (about 10 g). Samples of lesion epithelium, OP fluid, and serum should always be taken; the others are optional. With the exception of serum samples, it is important that all samples be promptly frozen and that they arrive at the laboratory in that state.[3]

Laboratory Procedures

The field specimens, i.e. vesicular fluid or lesions, should be prepared for use as the antigen in CF tests with known reference sera for the four vesicular diseases. If the samples contain sufficient virus and it happens to be one of the four vesicular diseases, a differential interpretation can be made. Because a battery of sera is used in the case of FMD and VS, the virus type also will be known. Additional tests are required for VES and SVD and to determine subtypes of FMD or VS.[3,6,8] In addition, some of the lesion tissues, OP fluids, blood with anticoagulant, and organ tissues should be used to inoculate animals of the same species as the source of the samples for reproduction of the disease and virus isolation. Newborn mice and tissue cultures should also be inoculated. All viral isolates can then be subjected to CF tests for identification.

Cultures. For initial isolation of FMD virus, primary swine and bovine kidney and bovine thyroid cell cultures should be used. Baby hamster kidney cell lines are used for virus production but not initial isolation. FMD virus produces CPE and, with various techniques, good plaque formation. Viral titrations can be made with either the CPE or PFU techniques.

Animal inoculation. In addition to the natural hosts of FMD (cattle, swine, sheep, etc.), newborn and suckling mice and guinea pigs are used as laboratory animals. The virus causes paralysis and death of young mice and foot pad lesions in guinea pigs. Viral titrations can be made in suckling mice, guinea pig foot pads, or the tongues of cattle.

Immunology and serology. One of the complicating factors about FMD is that seven immunologically distinct types have evolved, all of which produce similar signs and lesions.[3] Animals that recover from infection with one type of FMD are susceptible to infection with any of the other types.[3] The types of FMD have been designated as O, A, C, SAT-1, SAT-2, SAT-3, and Asia-1. The geographic distribution of the types is given in Table 17.2. Within the seven types of FMD, 63 subtypes have been designated by CF tests (Table 17.2). The subtypes are of importance primarily for the selection of viral strains to be used in vaccine production.[6] The seven types of FMD viruses are readily differentiated by CF, VN, direct FA, AD, and cross-immunity tests.[3,5,10]

Serum samples from convalescent animals can be used to differentiate between the vesicular diseases in VN, AD, or FA tests. When using sera from the suspected field animals, previous FMD infection (but not virus type) may be detected by AD tests using the VIA antigen or by indirect FA reactions.[3,5] The early FMD viral antibodies, which form soon after infection, begin to decline in about 14 days and are practically lost within 30 days. Their S-rate is 19 S. They react in the VN test but not in the CF test.

Table 17.2. Geographic distribution of types of foot-and-mouth disease virus and the number of subtypes for each type

Geographic distribution	Types	No. of subtypes*
Europe, South America, Africa, Asia, Near East	A	31
Europe, South America, Africa, Asia, Near East	O	10
Europe, South America, Africa, Asia, Near East	C	5
Africa and Near East	SAT-1†	7
Africa only	SAT-2	3
Africa only	SAT-3	4
Asia and Near East	Asia-1	3

*Each geographic area has its own group of subtypes (that is to say, Europe does not have all 31 type A subtypes).
†SAT, *Southern* African Territories (not *South*).

The late FMD virus antibodies, 7 S, may be detected in 10–14 days, reach a significant level in 28 days, and may persist for 12 or more months. The late antibodies are FMD virus type–specific in the CF, VN, and AD tests.[5]

Animals recovered from FMD infection resist reinfection with the same virus type for only about a year.[3] Resistance engendered by a good FMD vaccine wanes rapidly after 4–6 months; therefore, vaccinations must be repeated at intervals. Only inactivated viral vaccines are authorized in most FMD endemic areas and generally they are trivalent. In countries free of FMD, vaccination is prohibited and, if an outbreak occurs, attempts would be made to eradicate the disease by the "stamping-out" method of quarantine, slaughter, and so forth. Vaccination might be considered but only as a temporary adjunct to eventual eradication.

References

1. Bachrach, H.L. Foot and mouth disease. In *Annual Review of Microbiology*, C.E. Clifton (ed.), vol. 22, pp. 201–244. Annual Reviews, Palo Alto, Calif., 1968.
2. Callis, J.J., M.S. Shahan, and P.D. McKercher. Foot and mouth disease. In *Diseases of Swine*, H.W. Dunne (ed.). 3d ed. Iowa State University Press, Ames, 1970.
3. Cottral, G.E. Diagnosis of bovine vesicular diseases. *J. Am. Vet. Med. Ass.* 161:1293–1298, 1972.
4. Cottral, G.E., M.S. Shahan, and H.R. Seibold. Foot and mouth disease. In *Bovine Medicine and Surgery*, W.J. Gibbons, E.J. Catcott, and J.F. Smithcors (eds.), pp. 47–52. American Veterinary Publications, Wheaton, Ill., 1970.
5. Cowan, K.M. Immunochemical studies of foot and mouth disesse. IV. Preparation and evaluation of antisera specific for virus, virus protein subunit, and the virus-infection-associated antigen. *J. Immunol.* 101:1183–1191, 1968.
6. Davie, J. A complement fixation technique for the quantitative measurement of antigenic differences between strains of virus of foot and mouth disease. *J. Hyg.* 62:401–411, 1964.
7. Graham, A.M. Foot and mouth disease. *Vet. Rec.* 71:383–387, 1959.
8. Graves, J.H., and P.D. McKercher. Swine vesicular disease. In *Proc. 77th Ann. Mg. U.S. Anim. Health Ass.*, pp. 155–159, 1973.
9. McVicar, J.W., and P. Sutmoller. Sheep and goats as foot and mouth disease carriers. In *Proc. 72d Ann. Mtg. U.S. Livestock Sanitary Ass.*, pp. 400–406, 1969.
10. Mohanty, G.C., and G.E. Cottral. Foot and mouth disease virus: Rapid assay using the fluorescent antibody technique. *Arch. ges. Virusforsch.* 32:348–358, 1970.
11. Sellers, R.F., K.A.J. Herniman, and J.A. Mann. Transfer of foot and mouth disease virus in the nose of man from infected to non-infected animals. *Vet. Rec.* 89:447–449, 1971.
12. Snowdon, W.A. The susceptibility of some Australian fauna to infection with foot-and-mouth disease virus. *Austral. J. Exp. Biol. Med. Sci.* 46:667–687, 1968.

13. Sutmoller, P., J.W. McVicar, and G.E. Cottral. The epizootiological importance of foot-and-mouth disease carriers. I. Experimentally produced foot-and-mouth disease carriers in susceptible and immune cattle. *Arch. ges. Virusforsch.* 23:228–235, 1968.

Swine Vesicular Disease Virus

Swine vesicular disease (SVD) is a contagious viral infection of swine. It is characterized by vesicular lesions and subsequently by erosions of the epithelium of the mouth, nares, snout, and feet. The clinical lesions and signs of pigs suffering from SVD are indistinguishable from those caused by FMD, VS, and VES.

Although a high mortality rate does not occur, SVD is of major concern to disease control veterinarians of most countries because of its rapid spread and its close similarity to FMD. The disease has occurred in Italy, France, Poland, Austria, England, Scotland, Wales, Hong Kong, and Japan.

Outbreaks of SVD should be reported promptly, as described for FMD.

The primary mode of transmission is by contact of susceptible pigs with the excretions of infected pigs. The virus is much more resistant to disinfectants and environmental conditions than FMD virus, and during the attempted eradication of the disease from Great Britain in 1973, infection of susceptible animals used to restock decontaminated premises proved a problem. During the same campaign it was found that trucks that had carried infected pigs and had been decontaminated by standard FMD procedures were a major source of subsequent spread of the disease.

A major means of spread of the disease is the feeding of garbage or swill that contains contaminated materials. Because the virus is acid stable, a low pH of garbage or swill does not cause virus destruction.

The only known species susceptible to infection with SVD are swine, infant mice, and humans.

Swine vesicular disease virus (SVDV) is a member of the enterovirus group of picornaviruses. Its structure consists of single-stranded RNA (the infectious part) within a protein coat (the antigenic part). Its size is between 28 and 32 nm. It is acid stable and not adversely affected by organic solvents such as ether.

While separate virus isolations have been made in Italy,[4] Hong Kong,[3] England,[1] Poland, and Austria, all seem to be closely related serologically. Serologic strain differences have not been verified.

Swine vesicular disease virus is closely related to the human enterovirus Coxsackie B-5.[2] Human infection has been reported in laboratory workers and most human sera will show some neutralization of SVDV. Caution should be taken in handling highly virus-contaminated materials and unnecessary human contact with diseased pigs should be avoided.

Specimens

Oral, nasal, or podal lesions may be used but they should be fresh and representative. The following specimens may be taken from each of two or three animals: (1) vesicular fluid (all that is obtainable), (2) vesicular lesion epithelial coverings (5g), (3) flaps of epithelial tissue still attached to the edges of the lesion (5g) (old necrotic fibrinous material that is difficult to remove is undesirable), (4) blood with anticoagulant added (5ml) (viremia ends about 4 or 5 days after onset of disease), (5) blood for serum samples (about 10 ml of serum). Samples of lesion epithelium and serum should always be taken; the others are optional. With the exception of serum samples, it is important that all other samples be promptly frozen and that they arrive at the laboratory in that state.

Laboratory Procedures

The field specimens, i.e. vesicular fluid or lesions, should be prepared as the antigen for CF tests with known reference sera for the four vesicular diseases. If the samples contain sufficient virus and it happens to be one of the four vesicular diseases, a differential interpretation can be made. Because a battery of sera is used in the case of FMD and VS, the virus type also will be known. In addition, some of the lesion tissues should be used to inoculate animals of the same species as the source of the samples for reproduction of the disease and virus isolation. Newborn mice and tissue cultures should also be inoculated. All viral isolates can then be subjected to CF tests for identification.

Cultures. For initial isolation of SVD virus, primary swine or pig kidney cell lines should be used. SVD virus produces CPE and, with various techniques, good plaque formation. Virus titrations can be made with either the CPE or PFU techniques.

Animal inoculation. In addition to the natural hosts of SVD (swine), newborn mice are used as laboratory animals. The virus causes paralysis and death of the young mice in 48–96 hours, particularly after intracerebral inoculation. Virus titrations can be made in newborn mice.

Immunology and serology. Serum samples from convalescent animals can be used to differentiate the vesicular diseases in VN, AD, or FA tests. Serum from SVD convalescent swine will neutralize Coxsackie B-5 virus and react in the precipitin test in agar diffusion.

Animals recovered from SVD are resistant to reinfection. Experimental vaccines have been prepared but have not been used under field conditions.

For tables on differential diagnosis see the section on FMD.

References

1. Brooksby, J.B. Swine vesicular disease: A statement from Pirbright. *Vet. Rec.* 91:681–682, 1972.
2. Graves, J.H. Serological relationship of swine vesicular disease virus to Coxackie B-5 virus. *Nature* 245:314, 1973.
3. Mowat, G.N., J.H. Darbyshire, and J.F. Huntley. Differentiation of a vesicular disease of pigs in Hong Kong from foot and mouth disease. *Vet. Rec.* 90:618–621, 1972.
4. Nardelli, L., E. Lodetti, G. Bualandi, R. Burrows, D. Goodridge, F. Brown, and B. Cartwright. A foot and mouth disease syndrome in pigs caused by an enterovirus. *Nature* 219:1275–1276, 1968.

Equine Rhinovirus

Horses naturally or experimentally infected with equine rhinovirus have fever, anorexia, and nasal discharge.[4] There are at least two serotypes of the virus. In Canada, where both serotypes are found, most horses by 2 years of age have had one serotype and by 5 years have had both serotypes.[3] Serum antibodies are long lasting. The viruses have been isolated from equine feces, respiratory fluids, and in one case from an aborted foal.[1,2,4,6] Viremia occurs, and some horses excrete the virus in their feces for long periods of time. Antibodies have been detected in persons associated with horses, and pharyngitis and viremia was observed in a human volunteer who was experimentally infected with equine rhinovirus.[5] The viruses grow in equine, human, and monkey cell cultures.

References

1. Böhm, H.O. Über die isolierung und charakterisierung eines Picornavirus vom Pferd. *Zentralblatt Veterinärmedizin*, ser. B, 11:240–250, 1964.
2. Ditchfield, J., and L.W. MacPherson. The properties and classification of two new rhinoviruses recovered from horses in Toronto, Canada. *Cornell Vet.* 55:181–189, 1965.
3. Ditchfield, W.J.B. Rhinoviruses and parainfluenza viruses of horses. *J. Am. Vet. Med. Ass.* 155:384–387, 1969.
4. Plummer, G. An equine respiratory virus with enterovirus properties. *Nature* 195:519–520, 1962.
5. Plummer, G. An equine respiratory enterovirus: Some biological and physical properties. *Arch. ges. Virusforsch.* 12:694–700, 1963.
6. Plummer, G., and J.B. Kerry. Studies on an equine respiratory virus. *Vet. Rec.* 74:967–970, 1962.

Porcine Enteroviruses

The porcine enteroviruses, which have worldwide distribution, are picornaviruses that have an RNA core, are ether resistant, and are relatively stable at room temperatures, at pH 3, and with trypsin. They have icosahedral symmetry with no envelope and a particle diameter of 15–30 nm.

There are few diagnostic lesions or signs associated with enteroviruses other than the Teschen or Talfan infections. Occasionally, the more common enteroviruses produce convulsions, tremors, and even paralysis. Stillbirth, mummification, embryonic death, and infertility are frequently associated with enteroviruses, giving rise to the term SMEDI viruses. Teschen disease, the most virulent of the enteroviruses, is characterized by involvement of the CNS, with tremors, nystagmus, convulsions, paralysis, and death. Paralyzed animals may not recover, but others less affected may return to normal. Histologically, the CNS lesions involve mostly the gray matter, with perivascular cuffing, a degeneration of neurons, and neuronophagic and nodular cell formations. Most commonly the dorsal root ganglia are affected. Meningitis may be present. Other enteroviruses, though less virulent than Teschen disease, may produce mild lesions of the disease. Talfan disease, also known as benign enzootic paresis, porcine polioen-

Table 17.3. North American enteroviral strains suitable as type strains

Serologic groups	North American type strains*	SMEDI groups	WHO type strains*
1	PS34 (f)	C	Teschen, Talfan (b)
2	O3 (b)		T80 (b)
3	O2 (b)	B	O2 (b)
4	PS36 (f)	G	PS36 (f)
5			F26 (i)
6	PS37 (f)	E	PS37 (f)
7	WR2 (i)	F	F43 (i)
8†	PS27 (f)	A	PS27 (f)

*(b), brain; (f), fetus; (i), intestine.
†Subgroups of group 8: a, SMEDI D (PS32); b, ECPO1; c, PS30.

cephalomyelitis, and Ontario disease, usually affects young pigs and the mortality rate rarely exceeds 10%. The main clinical signs are fever and ataxia, generally of the hind legs; the unsteady gait may persist for many months. There is economic loss from the slower growth rate of affected pigs. The disease, which is caused by a group 3 virus (Table 17.3), also causes posterior paralysis. Histologic lesions of the CNS similar to those in Teschen disease are usually present if there are any clinical signs.

Specimens

The virus is most commonly isolated from rectal feces or from the contents of the gastrointestinal tract. Many of the virus types are capable of establishing a viremia and can be isolated from the brain, tonsil, or liver. At times it is possible to isolate the virus from stillborn pigs or pigs dying shortly after birth, but isolation is usually more successful if the pig lives until birth. Intrauterine infection established early in pregnancy usually does not persist until birth. Viruses isolated from tissues are likely to be more pathogenic than those isolated from feces and less likely to be contaminated with other viruses.

Little has been done to determine the period during which the virus will persist in the digestive tract. Limited results suggest that the virus persists as long as 2 months in the infected nonpregnant animal and as long as 3 months in the pregnant sow. Some evidence exists that the virus persists intermittently in carriers.

Laboratory Procedures

Cultures. The viruses grow well on primary swine kidney cells. Isolates usually grow quite well on PK-15 cell line, but isolation is more difficult to achieve using PK-15 cell line than using primary cultures. The viruses cause two types of CPE and most will form plaques readily.

Animal inoculation. The pig is the primary host but transmission to other animals has not been adequately explored.

Immunology and serology. Pigs infected with enteroviruses appear to have excellent immunity. Although experiments on the duration of immunity have not been done, sows recovering from enterovirus-induced infection, which is characterized by reproductive problems, will have normal litters at the next farrowing even though the infection may be evident in other sows not previously affected. Currently there is no vaccine for the disease.

Detection of antibodies to specific enteroviruses in fetuses at more than 70 days of gestation is an effective means of diagnosing infection where reproductive problems are encountered.

Currently there appear to be eight major serologic groups (Table 17.3). At least one of these (group 8), through use of the VN test, will probably be subgrouped later because of weak intragroup serologic relationships. Group 8 contains all strains with type II CPE and has the greatest intragroup serologic variation. Three possible subgroups are suggested.

The first five groups in Table 17.3 have been demonstrated to be pathogenic, causing polioencephalomyelitis or reproductive failure. The prototype enterovirus is the virus of

Teschen disease, which causes a classical polioencephalomyelitis with moderate to high morbidity in susceptible pigs. Many of the viruses (serogroups 1, 2, 3, and 8) are known to produce some degree of mild to moderate polioencephalomyelitis in susceptible young pigs. Groups 1, 3, 4, 6, 7, and 8 have been associated with reproductive disease and referred to as SMEDI viruses. Some of the viruses in group 3 have been shown to be immunogenically related to the Teschen-Talfan viruses. The group numbers have been assigned by the WHO International Subcommittee on Porcine Enteroviruses. Serotype strains of viruses usable in the United States and WHO reference serum serotypes are also indicated.

The FA techniques may be used. The HA test has not been adequately explored although apparently a few strains cause HA. The VN test in cell cultures is the serologic method of choice for virus identification. The test should be conducted using primary SK cells. The constant virus–varying serum dilutions test is recommended, using 100 $TCID_{50}$ (0.5 ml) with twofold dilutions of serum (0.5 ml). The serum-virus mixtures should be incubated at 37°C for 1 hour before seeding on cultures. Fetal calf serum should be used in the TC medium. The test should be read when one or more virus control cultures with 100 $TCID_{50}$ of virus develops clear-cut CPE.

References

1. Alexander, T.J.L., and A.O. Betts. Further studies on porcine enteroviruses isolated at Cambridge. II. Serological grouping. *Res. Vet. Sci.* 8:330, 1967.
2. Betts, A.O. Studies on enteroviruses of the pig. I. The recovery in tissue culture or two related strains of a polioencephalomyelitis virus from the tonsils of "normal" pigs. *Res. Vet. Sci.* 1:57, 1960.
3. Bohl, E.H., K.V. Singh, B.B. Hancock, and L. Kasza. Studies on five porcine enteroviruses. *Am. J. Vet. Res.* 21:99, 1960.
4. Cartwright, S.F., and R.A. Huck. Viruses isolated in association with herd infertility, abortions, and stillbirths in pigs. *Vet. Rec.* 81:196, 1967.
5. Dunne, H.W., D.C. Kradel, C.D. Clark, G.R. Bubash, and E. Ammerman. Porcine enteroviruses: A serologic comparison of thirty-eight Pennsylvania isolates with other reported North American strains, Teschen, Talfan, and T80 serums—A progress report. *Am. J. Vet. Res.* 28:557, 1967.
6. Dunne, H.W., J.T. Wang, and E.H. Ammerman. Classification of North American porcine enteroviruses: A comparison with European and Japanese strains. *Infec. Immunity* 4:619–631, 1971.
7. Dunne, H.W., J.T. Wang, C.D. Clark, J.F. Hokanson, T. Morimoto, and G.R. Bubash. The effects of *in utero* viral infection on embryonic, fetal, and neonatal survival: A comparison of SMEDI (porcine picorna) viruses with hog cholera vaccinal virus. *Can. J. Comp. Vet. Med. Sci.* 33:245, 1969.
8. Greig, A.S., G.L. Bannister, D. Mitchell, and A.H. Corner. Studies on the pathogenic porcine enteroviruses. II. Isolation of virus in tissue culture from brain and feces of clinical cases. *Can. J. Comp. Vet. Med. Sci.* 25:142, 1961.
9. Harding, J.D.J., J.T. Done, and G.F. Kershaw. A transmissible polioencephalomyelitis of pigs (Talfan disease). *Vet. Rec.* 69:2, 1957.
10. Izawa, H., R.A. Bankowski, and J.A. Howarth. Porcine enteroviruses. I. Properties of three isolates from swine with diarrhea and one from apparently normal swine. *Am. J. Vet. Res.* 23:1131, 1962.
11. Kasza, L., and A. Adler. Biologic and immunologic characterization of six swine enterovirus isolates. *Am. J. Vet. Res.* 26:625, 1965.
12. Lamont, P.H., and A.O. Betts. Studies on enteroviruses of the pig. IV. The isolation in tissue culture of a possible enteric cytopathogenic swine orphan (ECSO) virus (V13) from the feces of a pig. *Res. Vet. Sci.* 1:152, 1960.
13. McConnell, S., R.O. Spertzel, and J.N. Shively. Isolation, characterization, and serologic comparison of selected porcine enteroviruses by plaque reduction test. *Am. J. Vet. Res.* 29:245, 1968.
14. Morimoto, T., G. Tokuda, T. Omori, K. Fukusho, and M. Watanabe. Cytopathic agents isolated from the feces and the intestinal contents of pigs. I. Their isolation and serological classification. *Nat. Inst. Anim. Health Q.* 2:59, 1962.

15. Thorsen, J., and L.W. Macpherson. A study of porcine enteroviruses isolated from swine in the Toronto area. I. Isolation and serological grouping of viruses. *Can. J. Comp. Med. Vet. Sci.* 30:308, 1966.
16. Trefny, L. A serious disease of pigs in the Teschen area. *Zverol. obzor* 23:235, 1930.
17. Yamanouchi, K., R.A. Bankowski, and J.A. Howarth. Physical and biological properties of the CHICO strain of porcine enterovirus. *J. Infec. Dis.* 115:345, 1966.

Bovine Enteroviruses

Bovine enterovirus (BEV), bovine enteric viruses, and enteric cytopathic bovine orphan (ECBO) viruses are all synonyms. These viruses have been isolated from clinically normal cattle[4,9] as well as cattle suffering from mucosal disease,[1] reproductive disorders,[2] respiratory disease,[7] and enteritis accompanied by fever and nasal exudate.[8] However, the exact relationship of the bovine enteroviruses to any disease process is yet to be established.[5] Currently, more than 60 strains have been isolated in a dozen countries throughout the world.

Specimens

Rectal swabs and fresh stool samples are the most common specimens for virus isolation.

Laboratory Procedures

Cultures. Primary bovine embryonic kidney cell cultures have commonly been used for growth of BEV. However, the viruses also will replicate with the production of CPE in cell cultures of calf testicle, embryonic lamb kidney, human kidney, rhesus monkey testes and kidney, rabbit kidney, established bovine kidney cell lines, and diploid embryonic bovine trachea. For initial isolation, primary, secondary or tertiary embryonic calf kidney or calf testicle cell cultures appear to be the cells of choice.

Suspensions of specimens are prepared with trypticase soy broth or one of several other stabilizing solutions to which has been added 200–500 μg of streptomycin and 200–500 units of penicillin per ml. A neomycin-polymycin solution can be used but may cause mild toxic effects on some cells. The mixture is centrifuged for clarification at $10,000 \times g$ for 15 minutes. The supernatant fluid is inoculated onto medium-free cell monolayers in the quantity of 0.2 ml per tissue culture tube and allowed to adsorb to the cells for 30 minutes at 37°C. Maintenance medium with serum that is free of specific antibodies is added to the cultures and the tubes are returned to the incubator. Roller tubes appear to enhance the appearance of CPE. Most BEV strains readily produce plaques when the diploid or established bovine cell lines such as MDBK cells are used.

The CPE elicited by BEV is similar to that of other enteroviruses, consisting of rounding of cells, some of them clumping and then floating free from the cell sheet. Complete destruction of the cell sheet may occur within 24 hours but the average is between 3 and 4 days. To confirm identification as an enterovirus, the isolates should be subjected to the following tests: (1) exposure to chloroform at room temperature for 10 minutes, (2) exposure to pH 3 at room temperature for 3 hours, (3) exposure to 1 M $MgCl_2$ for 1 hour at 50°C, (4) filtration with a 50-nm-pore-size filter, showing less than 50 nm size particles. Enteroviruses show little loss in infectivity by these procedures.[3,10,11]

Animal inoculation. Hyperimmune serum for identification of BEV is produced most easily in roosters or goats. The presence of an inhibitor or a naturally occurring cross-reacting antibody in rabbit serum precludes the use of this animal for antiserum production.[6] Immunization schedules in general consist of two injections per week of virus-containing tissue culture fluid. The first injection of about 1×10^6 infectious units is given IV, followed 3 days later by a similar amount IM. About 7–10 days following the tenth injection the animals are bled for antiserum. An alternate and very satisfactory method consists of a small dose injected IM, followed 2 weeks later by 100 ml or more IV or IP. The animals are bled 10–14 days after the last inoculation. The latter procedure reduces the amount of cross-reactions that occur as well as lowering the number of anticell antibodies.

The use of laboratory animals or calves is of little value in identification or differentiation of enteroviruses. Virus instilled intranasally into clinically healthy cattle produces a slight and gradual temperature rise following an incubation period of 4 days.[9,12] Experimental inoculation of certain other strains produce diarrhea in calves but with no significant temperature change and minimal systemic host response.[12] The LC-R4 strain of BEV has been shown to be pathogenic when injected IP into suckling mice.[4]

Immunology and serology. A VN test employing plaque reduction has been shown to be more sensitive than tube neutralization and is the method of choice. However, either method can be used. One hundred $TCID_{50}$ or 100 plaque-forming units of virus with variable amounts of serum is the technique most likely to yield satisfactory results. Serum-virus mixtures should be incubated at 37°C for 30 minutes prior to inoculation of the tissue culture.

References

1. Darbyshire, J.H. The isolation, separation and identification of two viruses from a case of bovine mucosal disease. *J. Comp. Path. Ther.* 73:309–318, 1963.
2. Huck, R.A., and S.F. Cartwright. Isolation and classification of viruses from cattle during outbreaks of mucosal or respiratory disease and from herds with reproductive disorders. *J. Comp. Path.* 74:346–364, 1964.
3. Ketler, A., V.V. Hamparian, and M.R. Hilleman. Characterization and classification of ECHO 28-rhinovirus-coryzavirus agents. *Proc. Soc. Exp. Biol. Med.* 110:821–831, 1962.
4. LaPlaca, M., M. Portolani, and C. Lamieri. The basis for classification of bovine enteroviruses: Antigenic characters studied with chicken immune sera, and rhesus monkey erythrocytes agglutinating activity. *Arch. ges Virusforsch.* 17:98–115, 1964.
5. McFerran, J.B. Bovine enteroviruses. *Ann. N.Y. Acad. Sci.* 101:436–443, 1962.
6. Moll, T. Abortion and stillbirth of guinea pigs resulting from experimental exposure to bovine enteric viruses. *Am. J. Vet. Res.* 25:1757–1762, 1964.
7. Moll, T., and A.D. Davis. Isolation and characterization of cytopathogenic enteroviruses from cattle with respiratory disease. *Am. J. Vet. Res.* 20:27–32, 1959.
8. Moll, T., and A.V. Finlayson. Isolation of cytopathogenic viral agent from feces of cattle. *Science* 126:401–402, 1959.
9. Niederman, R.A., R.E. Luginbuhl, and C.F. Helmboldt. The separation and characterization of two enteric cytopathic bovine viruses isolated from a sample of bovine feces. *Cornell Vet.* 53:550–559, 1963.
10. Polson, A., and A. Kipps. Physio-chemical investigation of an enteric cytopathogenic bovine orphan virus, ECBO SA. I. *Arch. ges. Virusforsch.* 17:488–494, 1965.
11. Rovozzo, G.C., R.E. Luginbuhl, and C.F. Helmboldt. Bovine enteric cytopathogenic viruses. I. Characteristics of three prototype strains. *Cornell Vet.* 55:121–130, 1965.
12. Van der Maaten, M.J., and R.A. Packer. Isolation and characterization of bovine enteric viruses. *Am. J. Vet. Res.* 28:677–684, 1967.

Simian Enteroviruses

Viruses with the properties of the human enteroviruses have been readily isolated from the gastrointestinal tract of a wide variety of nonhuman primates.[8,10,14] Table 17.4 lists the currently recognized prototype strains of simian enteroviruses and the primate species from which they were originally isolated. In some instances strains of the SV group have been isolated from more than one species of Asian monkeys[1,5,7] but there is little evidence that these viruses are indigenous to African or New World monkeys. In addition, a large number of enterovirus strains, including some human enteroviruses, have been isolated from captive chimpanzees and a few isolates have been made from marmosets.[2,14]

Table 17.4. Prototype simian enteroviruses

Virus	Prototype strain	Species of origin	References
SV2	2382	*Macaca mulatta*	8
SV6	1631	*M. mulatta*	8
SV16	2450 SD	*M. mulatta*	9
SV18	2481 B2	*M. mulatta*	9
SV19	P2	*M. mulatta*	7, 9
SV26	3163	*M. mulatta*	9
SV28*		*M. mulatta*	4
SV35	A7987	*M. mulatta*	9
SV42	P1	*Macaca irus*	5
SV43	P12	*M. irus*	7
SV44	P13	*M. mulatta*	7
SV45	P14	*M. irus*	5
SV46	P15	*Macaca* sp.	5
SV47	P16	*M. irus*	5
SV49	P19	*M. mulatta*	5
SA4		*Cercopithecus aethiops*	11
SA5	B165	*C. aethiops*	11
A13	A13	*Papio doguera*	4

*SV4 is now considered to be a prime strain of SV28.

SV28 and SA4 (Table 17.4) possess all the chemical and physical properties of the enteroviruses but until recently they were listed as unclassified picornaviruses because they have not been isolated from the gastrointestinal tract. In contrast to the other viruses, these viruses have been frequently isolated as latent tissue culture contaminants.[8] It was originally believed that these viruses belonged in the reovirus group,[13] but this has been shown to be untrue because of the lack of serologic relationship between the simian reoviruses and SV28 or SA4. It was recently demonstrated that SV28 and SA4 are related to the simian enteroviruses. While antibody for SV28 and SA4 is frequently found in monkey sera, no evidence exists that they produce disease in monkeys.

The simian picornavirus group is large and isolates can easily be made from a captive primate group, but there is little evidence to suggest that they are of great importance in colony health. Identification of a specific serotype can be a difficult, time-consuming task that may provide information of little diagnostic value. Until more definitive studies are done on their pathogenicity they are primarily of academic interest.

Specimens

Although enterovirus isolations are frequently made from throat swabs, stool samples or rectal swabs are the specimens of choice. A particular virus can be isolated repeatedly over a period of weeks. In other instances a sporadic isolation pattern is observed.[6]

The enteroviruses are rather stable and have survived in rectal swab material shipped from India to the United States in 50% glycerol at ambient temperatures. Molar magnesium chloride also can be used to stabilize specimens containing these viruses.

Laboratory Procedures

Cultures. The enteroviruses are most readily isolated in primary kidney cell cultures of the primate species yielding the fecal specimen. In general, primary rhesus kidney cell cultures are the single most useful cell system but they do not support the growth of a number of the chimpanzee isolates and are of doubtful value in working with New World species. Established cell lines of simian tissues such as the LLC-MK_2, LLC-MK_4, BS-C-1, Vero, and MA 104 are useful in studying the simian enteroviruses but are generally much less sensitive than primary cell cultures. A chimpanzee liver culture has been useful in working with the chimpanzee enteroviruses.[3] In all instances typical enterovirus CPE is observed in infected cultures but the damage to the cell sheet may vary with the virus strain. This can be related to plaque morphology, a useful characteristic for separating these viruses into groups prior to serotyping.[5] Two of the prototype simian enteroviruses, SV19 and SV44, when inoculated IM are capable of producing lesions in suckling mice resembling those of the group B Coxsackie viruses, but the ease with which SV19 and SV44 are isolated in tissue culture makes TC the best method for their isolation.[7]

With the exception of the chimpanzee isolates, none of the simian enteroviruses will grow in cell cultures of human origin. This is further evidence that the simian viruses are unique and not the result of infection from a human source. The ability of chimpanzee enteroviruses to grow on human diploid cells may indicate a human source of virus infection or emphasize the close relationship of chimpanzees to humans.[14] The antigenic distinctness of the chimpanzee isolates indicates the latter may be more likely. Within the group of viruses listed in Table 17.4 there is considerable variation in the growth spectrum on a variety of Old and New World monkey species primary kidney cell cultures.[5] However, all these agents will grow on primary rhesus monkey kidney cell cultures.

In vitro studies have demonstrated that infected cells stained with H & E show typical enterovirus cytopathology. In these cells an eosinophilic mass develops in the cytoplasm causing the nucleus to be pushed to one side with indentation.[5]

Animal inoculation. No specific attempts have been made to immunize monkeys with simian enteroviruses for protection against disease. Antisera have been prepared in rhesus and cynomolgus monkeys using SV2, SV16, SV18, SV19, SV26, and SV35 by the IV or IM routes, with and without Freud's adjuvant. In no instance was evidence of disease noted. SV2, SV16, SV19, and SV35 produced highly specific antisera, whereas SV18 elicited no response and SV26 produced antibodies to itself as well as SV19, SV35, and SV44.

The large number of serotypes, lack of conclusive data for pathogenicity, and varied antibody response of the animals make active immunization with the simian enteroviruses impractical. Further, despite the fact that circulating antibody occurs in naturally infected animals, there seems to be no relationship between this antibody and virus excretion.[6]

In studies where monkeys were experimentally inoculated by the IC route with SV6, SV26, or SV35, a focal lesion was observed at the site of inoculation. This lesion was characterized by destruction of the choroid plexus and surrounding epithelial cells.[9,12] In one instance lesions were found in the lumbar segment of the spinal cord of a monkey inoculated with SV6. No histopathologic changes have been observed with SV16, SV18, and SV19. No histopathology studies have been carried out on gastrointestinal tract tissues of naturally or artificially infected monkeys.

Despite the fact that enteroviruses are frequently isolated from monkeys with intestinal disease, no causal relationship can definitely be assigned to these agents because the same viruses are isolated just as frequently from apparently healthy monkeys. In addition, limited studies with experimental infections of captive monkeys have been uniformly negative. Experimental infection of animals born in captivity is required for understanding the role these viruses play in simian disease. This would rule out the possibility of prior exposure and resultant immunity in animals used in such studies.

Immunology and serology. The method of choice for identifying serotypes of the simian enteroviruses is the VN test, but the poor antigenicity of these viruses and the cross-reactions frequently observed present problems that are difficult to overcome.[5] For this reason care must be taken in the preparation and testing of antisera to be certain that typing sera are sufficiently specific. Minimal immunization as well as homologous and heterologous cross-neutralization testing of each serum is necessary before use.

Of all the simian enteroviruses, only SV2 agglutinates rhesus RBC with regularity. The HI test is therefore of little value in identifying the current prototype viruses. The CF test has not been extensively employed for typing these viruses. Difficulties in obtaining purified antigens and specific antisera limit the use of this test for diagnostic purposes.

Identification of specific serotypes by the serum neutralization test is complicated by the fact that the simian enteroviruses are rather poor antigens, and production of antisera by extensive immunizing schedules frequently has resulted in cross-reacting sera.[5] Cross-reactions can be minimized by immunizing with less antigen, but this generally results in antisera with low homologous antibody titers.[8] There is some evidence that viral antigens purified by cesium chloride density-gradient centrifugation are more antigenic and can be used to produce highly specific antisera. The limited studies done on the simian enteroviruses have failed to demonstrate an antigenic relationship to any of the human enteroviruses.[7,12,14]

The WHO has designated the Southwest Foundation for Research and Education, San Antonio, Texas, as a Collaborating Laboratory in Comparative Medicine: Simian Viruses.[10] Support for this laboratory is received from NIH. Its purpose is to provide a diagnostic facility, source of materials, and information for simian viruses of all types as an aid to qualified users of nonhuman primates and investigators engaged in the study of simian viruses.

References

1. Bhatt, P.N., M.K. Goverdhan, M.F. Schaffer, C.D. Brandt, and J.F. Fox. Viral infections of monkeys in their natural habitat in Southern India. I. Some properties of cytopathic agents isolated from bonnet and laugur monkeys. *Am. J. Trop. Med. Hyg.* 15:551–560, 1966.
2. Deinhardt, F., A.W. Holmes, J. Devine, and J. Deinhardt. Marmosets as laboratory animals. IV. The microbiology of laboratory kept marmosets. *Lab. Anim. Care* 17:48–70, 1967.
3. Douglas, J.D., P.J. Vasington, and J.K. Noel. Viral spectrum of an established chimpanzee liver cell line. *Proc. Soc. Exp. Biol. Med.* 121:824–829, 1966.
4. Fuentes-Marins, R., A.R. Rodriquez, S.S. Kalter. A. Hellman, and R.A. Crandell. Isolation of enteroviruses from the "normal" baboon (*Papio doguera*). *J. Bact.* 85:1045–1050, 1963.
5. Heberling, R.L., and F.S. Cheever. Some characteristics of the simian enteroviruses. *Am. J. Epidemiol.* 81:106–123, 1965.
6. Heberling, R.L., and F.S. Cheever. A longitudinal study of simian enterovirus excretion. *Am. J. Epidemiol.* 83:470–480, 1966.
7. Hoffert, W.R., M.E. Bates, and F.S. Cheever. Studies of enteric viruses of simian origin. *Am. J. Hyg.* 68:15–30, 1958.
8. Hull, R.N. The simian viruses. In Virology Monographs no. 2, pp. 1–66. Springer-Verlag, New York, 1968.
9. Hull, R.N., J.R. Minner, and C.C. Mascoli. New viral agents recovered from tissue cultures of monkey kidney cells. III. Recovery of additional agents both from cultures of monkey tissues and directly from tissues and excreta. *Am. J. Hyg.* 68:31–44, 1968.
10. Kalter, S.S., and R.L. Heberling. The study of simian viruses. *WHO Chron.* 23:112–117, 1969.
11. Malherbe, H., R. Harwin, and M. Ulrich. The cytopathic effects of vervet monkey viruses. *S. Afr. Med. J.* 37:407–411, 1963.
12. McMillen, J., F. Macasaet, M. Lenahan, P. Kamitsuka, and H.A. Wenner. Lack of serologic relationship between several group A coxsackie and simian viruses. *Am. J. Epidemiol.* 88:126–131, 1968.
13. Rosen, L. Reoviruses in animals other than man. *Ann. N.Y. Acad. Sci.* 101:461–465, 1962.
14. Soike, K.F., F. Coulston, P. Day, R. Deibel, and H. Plager. Viruses of the alimentary tract of chimpanzees. *Exp. Mol. Path.* 7:259–303, 1967.

Vesicular Exanthema of Swine Virus

The disease, caused by the vesicular exanthema of swine (VES) virus is an acute, highly infectious and febrile disease of swine characterized by the formation of vesicles on the snout, mucous membranes of the mouth, soles of the feet, between the toes, and on the coronary band and dewclaws.

Clinically, VES is indistinguishable from FMD, VS, and SVD.[8] The mortality is usually less than 5% and the disease is self-limiting with recovery in about 1–2 weeks. Except for its occurrence in the Port of Honolulu[12] and in Iceland,[12] VES has never been reported as a natural infection in any part of the world other than the United States. The disease was eradicated from the United States in 1959, mainly because of a program of compulsory cooking of garbage before feeding to swine.

Recently, viruses were isolated from sea lions (San Miguel sea lion virus), fur seals, and gray whales in California that shared common physical and chemical characteristics with VES viruses.[13] In addition, neutralizing antibodies to one of these viruses have been found in feral pigs on the Channel Islands off Santa Barbara, California. These findings lend some credence to the conjecture that swine in California originally contracted VES as a result of being fed meat scraps from marine mammals.

Specimens

Oral, nasal, or podal lesions may be used, but they should be fresh and representative. The following specimens may be taken from each of two or three animals: (1) vesicular fluid (all that is obtainable), (2) vesicular lesion epithelial coverings (5 g). (3) flaps of epithelial tissue still attached to the edges of the lesion (5 g) (old necrotic fibrinous material that is difficult to remove is undesirable), (4) blood with anticoagulant added (5 ml) (viremia ends about 4 or 5 days after onset of disease), (5) blood for serum samples (about 10 ml of serum). Samples of lesion epithelium and serum should always be taken. With the exception of serum samples, it is important that all other samples be promptly frozen and that they arrive at the laboratory in that condition.

VES virus ordinarily retains its infectivity for long periods of time when stored in pieces of material or fluids from vesicles suspended in 50% glycerol in phosphate buffer (pH 7.4) at near freezing or lower temperatures.[1] Immunotype 101-43 virus, for example, was found to be infectious after storage at 4°C for over 10 years. However, marked differences in stability among the 13 known serotypes have been found. Serotypes I-34, G-55, and I-55 were found to be considerably more labile on storage.[1]

Laboratory Procedures

Cultures. All known serotypes of VES multiply and produce CPE in monolayers of swine kidney, lung, liver, testicle, and embryo cells,[6] but primary pig kidney cells and pig kidney line cells are most desirable. The virus does not produce consistent CPE in cell cultures prepared from other hosts. All serotypes of VES do not propagate readily in tissue culture on first passage using field specimens but the virus can be readily adapted to swine kidney culture.[1] Cytopathology in pig kidney cell cultures is produced in 48–72 hours under routine conditions. The appearance is similar to all other picornaviruses, with rounding and destruction of cells. Plaque formation occurs with methycellulose overlay.[1]

Animal inoculation. The virus is very host specific and under natural conditions has been confirmed only from swine. Horses vary in their susceptibility to inoculation with the various strains when inoculated in the tongue epithelium.[1,5] Dogs, hamsters, and guinea pigs were found to be irregularly and mildly affected on some occasions. Repeated attempts to initiate infection in cattle, calves, sheep, goats, mice, rats, rabbits, hedgehogs, adult chickens, and chicken embryos have failed.[1,5] Human cases of infection have not been reported.

Immunology and serology. There are 13 known immunologically distinct types of the virus as determined by complement fixation, virus neutralization, and cross-immunity tests (Table 17.5).[1,5]

The plurality of immunologic types and the ease with which VES virus mutates complicate diagnosis of this disease and make typing of serotypes difficult. The VN, AD, and CF tests can be employed for identifying the virus and its serotype.[1,3,5]

Neutralization antibodies can be detected in serum of swine as early as 10–12 days

Table 17.5. History, source, and identification of immunologic types of vesicular exanthema virus*

Types	Source and year of isolation	Reference
Crawford A†	San Diego, 1933	7
1. Crawford B (1-34)†	San Jose, 1934	7
Crawford C†‡	California, 1934	7
Crawford D†·§	California, 1934	7
2. 101-43†	San Francisco, 1943	6
1940-42 A	San Francisco, 1943	11
1940-42 B	San Francisco, 1943	11
1940-42 C	San Francisco, 1943	11
3. A-48†	Fontana, Calif., 1948	11
4. B-51	Davis, Calif., 1951	1
5. C-52	San Francisco, 1952	1
6. D-53	Riverside, Calif., 1953	2
7. E-54	Alameda, Calif., 1954	1
8. F-55	San Mateo, Calif., 1955	4
9. G-55	San Mateo, 1955	4
10. H-54‖	San Mateo, 1955	1
11. I-55	San Mateo, 1955	1
12. J-56	New Jersey, 1956	9
13. K-56	New Jersey, 1956	9

*There are 13 types of VESV currently available; they are numbered in this table. Those not numbered are of historical interest but are unavailable, as the viruses were not preserved.
†Samples of virus collected by J. Traum and submitted to laboratories where they were identified.
‡Mild for pigs, produced lesions in horses.
§Extremely virulent for hogs but not for horses.
‖Type was not established within the same year, causing discrepancy in sequence.

after infection. The titer reaches a peak between 21 and 28 days as measured by the VN, CF, and AD procedures.[5] Only convalescent sera retain their type specificity. Hyperimmune serums are not type specific and can react with heterologous VEV antigens. By using VN tests in cell culture, a clear differentiation can be made among types 1-34, 101-43, and A-48 through I-55.[1,5] A low level of cross-neutralization may occur between types K-56 and C-52, between J-56 and types E-54 and C-52, and between I-55 hyperimmune serum and type G-55 virus.[4] For this reason cross-immunity studies to show immunologic differences between serotype may be necessary. There is no cross-neutralization between anti-VES serums and viruses of FMD and VS.[3,5]

All serotypes of VES have a common CF antigenic component that is readily detected and the virus can be differentiated from the FMD and VS viruses by the CF procedures.[3,11] Complement (C') must be used sparingly in the antigen-antibody reaction and the procomplementary activity of swine serum must be recognized.[1]

The AD technique using borate buffer of pH 8.6 and ionic strength of 0.05 can be employed for the detection of VES virus using convalescent type-specific antiserums. Some cross-reactions similar to those found in the CF test can be expected.[1]

Information on the persistance of immunity to the various immunogenic types of VES is meager. However, studies of swine recovered from experimentally induced infection with serotypes A-48, B-51, and C-52 indicate that an immunity of less than a year can be expected.[1] Similarly, limited studies indicate that immune serum may have some prophylactic value providing it is administered within 24 hours after exposure.[9,10] Neither method is of practical value because of the multiplicity of serotypes and the progressive mutation of the virus under field conditions.

Differentiation and identification of a serotype of VES was formerly determined by cross-immunity challenge. The suspected virus was inoculated into swine IV or ID on the snout, using swine recently recovered from experimentally induced infection with the known serotypes.[1]

References

1. Bankowski, R.A. Vesicular exanthema. In *Advances in Veterinary Science*, C.A. Brandly and E.L. Jungherr (eds.), vol. 10, pp. 23–64. Academic Press, New York, 1965.
2. Bankowski, R.A., H.B. Keith, E.E. Stuart, and M. Kummer. Recovery of the fourth immunological type of vesicular exanthema virus in California. *J. Am. Vet. Med. Ass.* 125:383–384, 1954.
3. Bankowski, R.A., and M. Kummer. Vesicular stomatitis fixation. *Am. J. Vet. Res.* 16:374–376, 1955.
4. Bankowski, R.A., A.G. Perkins, E.E. Stuart, and M. Kummer. Recovery of new immunological types of vesicular exanthema virus. *Proc. U.S. Livestock Sanitary Assoc.* 60:302–320, 1956.
5. Barber, T.L., W.M. Moulton, and S.S. Stone. The identification and typing of vesicular exanthema by complement fixation and agar diffusion tests. *Proc. U.S. Livestock Sanitary Assoc.* 64:317–323, 1960.
6. Brooksby, J.B. Etude expérimentale de l'exanthème vésiculeux. *Bull. Off. Internat. Epiz.* 42:368–377, 1954.
7. Crawford, A.B. Experimental vesicular exanthema of swine. *J. Am. Vet. Med. Ass.* 90:380–395, 1937.
8. Graves, J.H., and P.D. McKercher. Swine vesicular disease. *Proc. U.S. Anim. Health Ass.* 77:155–159, 1974.
9. Holbrook, A.A., J.N. Geleta, and S.R. Hopkins. Two new immunological types of vesicular exanthema virus. *Proc. U.S. Livestock Sanitary Ass.* 63:332–339, 1959.
10. Madin, S.H. Preliminary studies on the prophylactic and therapeutic values of type "B" vesicular exanthema serum. *J. Am. Vet. Med. Ass.* 129:368–370, 1956.
11. Madin, S.H., and J. Traum. Experimental studies with vesicular exanthema of swine. *Vet. Med.* 48:395–400, 1953.
12. Madin, S.H., and J. Traum. Vesicular exanthema of swine. *Bact. Rev.* 19:6–19, 1955.
13. Smith, A.W., S.H. Madin, and T.G. Akers. Pinnipeds as a possible natural reservoir for a virus disease of domestic swine. In *Proceedings of the 10th Conference on the Biology of Sonar and Diving Mammals*. Stanford Research Institute, Menlo Park, Calif., 1973.

Feline Picorna Respiratory Viruses

The feline picorna respiratory (FPR) viruses appear to be limited to the Felidae. The domestic cat is the primary host but there is serologic evidence that the wild and larger cats are also susceptible.[5,6] Following a 1 or 2 day incubation period there is a febrile response and serous nasal and lacrimal discharge, which later may become mucopurulent. There is also a reddening of the nasal mucosa and conjunctiva and anorexia. The infection is usually limited to the upper respiratory areas but viral interstitial pneumonia is produced with certain strains and may cause a mortality of up to 30%. Ulcerative glossitis and stomatitis may occur as sequelae.[10] Secondary pneumonia occurs but generally can be controlled with proper supportive therapy. FPRV is widespread throughout the world. More than 50 isolations have been made and there are several different serotypes of the virus.[10] The viral isolates must be differentiated from herpes virus in cats.

The FPR viruses are about 36 nm in diameter and have a single-stranded RNA core.[1,11,13] They are replicated in the cytoplasm and some have been seen to form large crystalline arrays.[10] They are ether resistant and stable at pH 4.8 but labile at pH 2.8.[2,4,5,7,8] They are inactivated at 50°C for 30 minutes and are not stabilized in molar solutions of either $MgCl_2$ or $MgSO_4$.[4,5,10] The isolates that have been tested were found not to be sensitive to guanidine-HC1.[10] This chemical, which prevents the formation of viral RNA polymerase in cells infected with some picornaviruses, has been used for subdividing certain picornaviruses into groups that share common properties.[10]

Specimens

The FPR viruses have been isolated from the oral, pharyngeal, nasal, and conjunctival membranes, from rectal swabs, visceral organs, and occasionally from urine.[2,5,6] Virus can be isolated from approximately 2 days prior to the onset of clinical signs and for the duration of the illness. When the discharge becomes more purulent, virus isolation becomes more difficult. However, virus may still be isolated from swabs of the tonsillar area for as long as a year after infection.

Laboratory Procedures

Cultures. Primary feline kidney cell cultures are preferred for initial isolation; it is possible to differentiate between the various feline respiratory viruses on the basis of their distinctive CPE in these feline cell cultures. The supporting medium of choice is MEM fortified with 2% calf, fetal calf, or lamb serum. Infection is characterized by rapidly progressive CPE without the formation of inclusions. Infected cells develop fibrillar cytoplasmic processes and then round up and leave the glass.[7] Herpesvirus infection induces the formation of multinucleate giant cells, and Cowdry type-A intranuclear inclusions are observable in stained preparations of infected cultures.[6] Feline reovirus infection causes a slowly progressive cytopathic degeneration. Infected cells contain paranuclear cytoplasmic viral inclusions.[12]

A fetal diploid line of feline tongue cells (Fc_3Tg) also may be used for initial isolation of FPRV. The distinctive fibrillar cytoplasmic processes are a pronounced feature of the CPE observed with FPRV in this cell line and also with the Crandell feline kidney (CRFK) cell line. Infection of cell cultures with about 100 $TCID_{50}$ of virus is usually followed by CPE within 18–24 hours. Infected cells assume a neuronal appearance before rounding up completely and leaving the glass surface. The TC plaque technique also may be used.

Animal inoculation. Since the FPR viruses appear to be limited to the Felidae, only domestic cats are used for viral transmission studies. Goats may be used to produce specific antisera for the various viral strains.

Immunology and serology. The VN and FA techniques are used for serologic characterization. The constant virus–variable serum technique is commonly used for the VN test.[2] With this test it is apparent that there are distinct strain differences in FPRV, but there is some cross-reactivity between strains.[3,10] The FPR viruses thus far tested all share a common antigen, which is reactive in the FA test.[9] Thus a single fluorescent conjugated serum may be used with any of the FPRV isolates. The National Cancer Institute (NCI) has some reference antisera available to investigators for study of FPRV.

References

1. Almeida, J.D., A.P. Waterson, J. Prydie, and E.W.L. Fletcher. The structure of a feline picornavirus and its relevance to cubic viruses in general. *Arch. ges Virusforsch.* 25:205, 1968.

2. Bartholomew, P.T., and J.H. Gillespie. Feline viruses. I. Characterization of four isolates and their effects on young kittens. *Cornell Vet.* 58:248, 1968.
3. Bittle, J.L., C.J. York, J.W. Newberne, and M. Martin. Serologic relationship of new feline cytopathogenic viruses. *Am. J. Vet. Res.* 21:547, 1960.
4. Bürki, F. Picornaviruses of cats. *Arch. ges. Virusforsch.* 15:690, 1965.
5. Crandell, R.A. A description of eight feline picornaviruses and an attempt to classify them. *Proc. Soc. Exp. Biol. Med.* 126:240, 1967.
6. Crandell, R.A., and E.W. Despeaux. Cytopathology of feline viral rhinotracheitis virus in cultures of feline renal cells. *Proc. Soc. Exp. Biol. Med.* 101:494, 1959.
7. Fastier, L.B. A new feline virus isolated in tissue culture. *Am. J. Vet. Res.* 18:382, 1957.
8. Florio, R.M., M. Bertrand, M. Lapras, C. Papageorgiou, L. Valette, and J. Vicaria. De l'étiologie des principales maladies virales félines: Etude systématique des virus infectant le chat dans la region lyonnaise. *Rev. Med. Vet.* 117:97, 1966.
9. Gillespie, J.H., A. Judkins, and D.E. Kahn. Feline viruses. XIII. The use of the immunofluorescence test for detection of feline picornaviruses. *Cornell Vet.* 61:172–179, 1971.
10. Kahn, D.E., and J.H. Gillespie. Feline viruses. X. Characterization of a newly-isolated picornavirus causing interstitial pneumonia and ulcerative stomatitis in the domestic cat. *Cornell Vet.* 60:669–683, 1970.
11. McEwan, P.J., and J.A.R. Miles. An electron microscopic study of viruses associated with upper respiratory tract infections of cats. *Proc. Univ. Otago Med. School* 45:21, 1967.
12. Scott, F.W., D.E. Kahn, and J.H. Gillespie. Feline viruses. VIII. The isolation, characterization, and pathogenic effects in the domestic cat of a feline reovirus. *Am. J. Vet. Res.* 31:11, 1969.
13. Zwillenberg, L.O., and F. Bürki. On the capsid structure of some small feline and bovine RNA viruses. *Arch. ges. Virusforsch.* 19:373, 1966.

Encephalomyocarditis Virus

Encephalomyocarditis (EMC) is an often latent virus infection primarily of wild rats and to a lesser extent of other rodents; the virus has been isolated from various types of wild rats, mice, hamsters, mongooses, raccoons, and squirrels.[15,17,18,33] The virus also has been found as the cause of disease in swine and in a few calves.[11,12,22] Occasionally, EMC virus has been isolated from humans and other primates (rhesus and aotus monkeys, chimpanzees, and a mandrill baboon).[11,15,19,25,31] Serologic surveys have shown that EMC antibodies are present in a significant number of *Rattus norvegicus* and *R. alexandrinus* in certain areas of the United States (e.g. Mississippi 87%, Texas 30%),[35] in *R. kyjabius* and *R. coucha* in Uganda,[34] in *Mus booduga* (gray) in India,[14] and in 22% of water rats (*Hydromys chrysogaster*) and 5–10% of other types of rats in Queensland (*R. rattus, R. sordidus conatus, R. norvegicus,* and *Melomys lutillus littoralis*).[23,24] HI EMC antibodies were found in 2.1% of 1000 cattle sera tested in Queensland.[30] EMC antibodies also were found in sera from pigs, horses, mice, and bandicoots (*Isoodon macrourus*), but not in sera from dogs, cats, and kangaroos.[24,29]

Surveys for EMC antibodies in human sera have been made in the United States, Germany, Sweden, Mexico, and Australia.[16,24,34] These surveys showed that less than 3% of healthy people had EMC antibodies, but from individuals with signs of CNS disease the incidence was 12–16%.[34] There is some evidence that EMC appears in localized outbreaks in groups of humans (for example, the epidemic of "3-day fever" among U.S. troops in Manila in 1945–1946).[13,34] Human infections with EMC virus have been associated with a variety of clinical signs, varying from a mild febrile illness to a severe encephalomyelitis, but no deaths have been reported and myocarditis has not been observed.[34]

Apart from sudden death, EMC virus infection in pigs presents no consistent or reliable identifying clinical signs.[1,11] The clinical signs that have been reported in pigs include depression, inappetance, trembling, staggering, paralysis, vomiting, and dyspnea.[1] In experimental infection of pigs, viremia lasts for only about 2 days, while virus persists in heart and other tissues for a further 3–5 days.[20] The main heart lesion seen in pigs that have EMC is myocardial pallor, which may be diffuse or occur in focal areas 2–10 mm in diameter.[1] The right ventricle is more often and more severely involved than the left, especially the subepicardial muscle.[1] Histologically, lesions are most severe in the conus arteriosus, where extensive myocardial necrosis produces the pallor seen grossly.[1] EMC lesions of the heart atria are rarely seen.[1]

Skeletal muscle lesions are found in some outbreaks.[28] The myocardial lesions seen both grossly and microscopically in pigs with EMC very closely resemble those seen in pigs with FMD.[1] Other pig diseases that may present somewhat similar gross lesions are edema disease, vitamin E–selenium deficiency, hog cholera, and mulberry heart disease.[1] Gross myocarditis is seen infrequently in some outbreaks of EMC.[12] Encephalomyelitis rarely occurs in pigs with EMC, except when the virus is inoculated IC.[11,37]

In experimentally infected rats and mice, both encephalitis and myocarditis are features of EMC.[34] Also, a disease syndrome resembling diabetes mellitus, with severe necrotizing lesions of the pancreatic islets, hyperglycemia, decreased glucose tolerance, and glycosuria, developed in certain inbred lines of mice that survived the initial EMC infection.[2,9,21,38] Such diabetic signs and lesions were minimal in the C3H strain of mice.[6]

Mice inoculated IP with EMC virus usually die within 4–7 days.[1,34] Death may be sudden due to heart involvement or after signs of CNS illness, including short hopping locomotion with humped back, convulsive periods, and flaccid posterior paralysis.[1] Mice and hamsters of all ages are very susceptible to experimental EMC virus infection, while the resistance of albino rats to EMC increases with age.[17,34] The disease is fatal for about 10–50% of guinea pigs, but it is not fatal for rabbits and usually not for rhesus monkeys.[34]

Transmission of EMC virus by contact has been demonstrated in cotton rats, but experiments with swine were unsuccessful.[20,34] However transmission by feeding infectious material was demonstrated in swine and albino mice; it is presumed that pigs contract EMC from eating infected rats and mice or feed contaminated with their feces.[7,11,17,20,34] Intranasal exposure of swine also resulted in transmission of EMC.[20] Transmission by arthropods has not been proven, although the Mengo strain of the virus has been isolated from mosquitoes (*Taeniorrhynchus fuscopennatus*) in Uganda.[34]

EMC virus was first isolated in New York in 1940 from cotton rats that were being used for the passage of the Yale-SK polio virus, so the new isolate was at first named the Columbia-SK virus.[16,34] Subsequently, similar viruses were isolated in Florida, Uganda, the Netherlands, Germany, Columbia, Panama, and Australia, and they were variously designated as MM, EMC, Mengo, AK, Li 32, F, Ortlieg, S.V.M., and Innisfail.[23,34] They all are now recognized as strains of EMC virus.[10,36] The first isolation of EMC virus from primates was made from a chimpanzee at an animal farm near Dania, Florida, in 1945,[11,15,34] and from swine in Panama in 1958.[22]

The EMC virus is classified as a picornavirus under the cardiovirus group.[27] It has an icosahedral shape, a diameter of about 30 nm, and a molecular weight of about 8.5×10^6 daltons, of which about 30% is single-stranded RNA.[4,27] The virus has a buoyant density in CsCl of 1.33 g/ml, is stable at pH 3 and pH 8, but has been reported to be unstable at pH 6.[27] The virus may be stored at -30 to $-70°C$ as homogenized brain tissue from infected mice or as a cell culture harvest.[1,37] EMC virus does not respond well to lyophilization.[20]

Specimens

The specimens for EMC virus isolation from swine are: heart ventricle, liver, spleen, kidney, pancreas, brain, blood, and feces (2–5 g each).[20] For rodents or other animals exhibiting CNS signs, the brain may be the more important specimen, but samples from the heart, pancreas, and kidney also should be taken.[3,9] Titers of 10^8 TCID$_{50}$ per gram have been found in heart specimens from pigs with EMC infection.[20]

Laboratory Procedures

Cultures. Fetal mouse fibroblast (FMF) or swine embryo kidney (SEK) cell cultures are recommended.[1,5,26] However, EMC virus will grow and produce CPE within 2–4 days in a wide variety of cell cultures, including HeLa cells.[8] The virus also may be propagated via the CAM route in embryonating eggs, causing embryo death in 72–96 hours without pathognomonic lesions.[34]

Animal inoculation. SPF strains of laboratory mice or hamsters should be used for initial virus isolation or titrations, and the stock should be screened for latent EMC virus infection and antibodies. The animals can be inoculated via various routes, with preference for the IP or IC routes.[1,34] Rabbits can be given a single EMC virus inoculation via the IM route and bled 14 days later to produce antiserum.[1]

Immunology and serology. Standard VN, CF, FA, AD, and cross-protection tests can be used to identify the virus.[34] The VN test can be conducted in mice or cell cultures using either constant virus–variable serum dilutions or constant serum–variable virus dilutions. The HI technique is also used with EMC virus.[8,32] Agglutination of sheep RBC occurs at 4°C and the virus is eluted from the cells at temperatures above 20°C.[34]

References

1. Acland, H.M., and I.R. Littlejohns. Encephalomyocarditis virus infection of pigs. I. An outbreak in New South Wales. *Austral. Vet. J.* 51:409–415, 1975.
2. Boucher, D.W., and A.L. Notkins. Virus-induced diabetes mellitus. I. Hyperglycemia and hypoinsulinemia in mice infected with encephalomyocarditis virus. *J. Exp. Med.* 137:1226–1239, 1973.
3. Burch, G.E., C.Y. Tsui, and J.M. Harb. The early renal lesions of mice infected with encephalomyocarditis virus. *Lab. Invest.* 26:163–172, 1972.
4. Burness, A.T.H., A.D. Vizoso, and F.W. Clothier. Encephalomyocarditis virus and its ribonucleic acid: Sedimentation characteristics. *Nature* 197:1177–1178, 1963.
5. Chang, T.W., and L. Weinstein. Characteristics of growth of encephalomyocarditis virus in cultures of mouse muscle. *Proc. Soc. Exp. Biol. Med.* 102:181–183, 1959.
6. Craighead, J.E., and D.A. Higgins. Genetic influences affecting the occurrence of a diabetes mellitus-like disease in mice infected with the encephalomyocarditis virus. *J. Exp. Med.* 139:414–426, 1974.

7. Craighead, J.E., P.H. Peralta, T.G. Murnane, and A. Shelokov. Oral infection of swine with encephalomyocarditis virus. *J. Infec. Dis.* 112:205–212, 1963.
8. Craighead, J.E., and A. Shelokov. Encephalomyocarditis virus hemagglutination inhibition test using antigens prepared in HeLa cell cultures. *Proc. Soc. Exp. Biol. Med.* 108:823–826, 1961.
9. Craighead, J.E., and J. Steinke. Diabetes mellitus-like syndrome in mice infected with encephalomyocarditis virus. *Am. J. Path.* 63:119–129, 1971.
10. Dick, G.W.A. The relationship of Mengo encephalomyelitis, encephalomyocarditis, Columbia-SK and M.M. viruses. *J. Immunol.* 62:375–386, 1949.
11. Gainer, J.H. Encephalomyocarditis virus infections in Florida, 1960–1966. *J. Am. Vet. Med. Ass.* 151:421–425, 1967.
12. Gainer, J.H., J.R. Sandefur, and W.J. Bigler. High mortality in a swine herd infected with the encephalomyocarditis virus: An accompanying epizootiological survey. *Cornell Vet.* 58:31–47, 1968.
13. Gajdusek, C. Encephalomyocarditis infection in childhood. *Pediatrics* 16:819–834, 1955.
14. Ghosh, S.N., and P.K. Rajagopalan. Encephalomyocarditis virus activity in *Mus booduga* (Gray) in Barur Village (1961–1962), Sagar KFD area, Mysore State, India. *Indian J. Med. Res.* 61:989–991, 1973.
15. Helwig, F.C., and E.C.H. Schmidt. A filter-passing agent producing interstitial myocarditis in anthropoid apes and small animals. *Science* 102:31–33, 1945.
16. Jungeblut, C.W., and G. Bautista. Antibodies against Columbia-SK in Mexican sera. *Am. J. Trop. Med.* 3:466–474, 1954.
17. Kilham, L., P. Mason, and J.N.P. Davies. Pathogenesis of fatal encephalomyocarditis (EMC) virus infections in albino rats. *Proc. Soc. Exp. Biol. Med.* 90:383–387, 1955.
18. Kilham, L., P. Mason, and J.N.P. Davies. Host-virus relations in encephalomyocarditis (EMC) virus infections. II. Myocarditis in mongooses. *Am. J. Trop. Med.* 5:655–663, 1956.
19. Kissling, R.E., J.M. Vanella, and M. Schaeffer. Recent isolations of encephalomyocarditis virus. *Proc. Soc. Exp. Biol. Med.* 91:148–150, 1956.
20. Littlejohns, I.R., and H.M. Acland. Encephalomyocarditis virus infection of pigs. II. Experimental disease. *Austral. Vet. J.* 51:416–422, 1975.
21. Müntefering, H., W.H.K. Schmidt, and W. Korber. Zur virusgenese des diabetes mellitus bei der weissen Maus. *Deutsche Med. Wochenschrift* 16:693–697, 1971.
22. Murnane, T.G., J.E. Craighead, H. Mondragon, and A. Skelekov. A fatal disease of swine due to encephalomyocarditis virus. *Science* 131:498–499, 1960.
23. Pope, J.H. A virus of the encephalomyocarditis group from a water-rat, *Hydromys chrysogaster*, in north Queensland. *Austral. J. Exp. Biol. Med. Sci.* 37:117–124, 1959.
24. Pope, J.H., and W. Scott. A survey for antibodies to encephalomyocarditis virus in man and animals. *Austral. J. Exp. Biol. Med. Sci.* 38:447–450, 1960.
25. Roca-Garcia, M., and C. Sanmartin-Barberi. The isolation of encephalomyocarditis virus from Aotus monkeys. *Am. J. Trop. Med. Hyg.* 6:840–852, 1957.
26. Rouhandeh, H., R.R. Chronister, and M.L. Brinkman. Propagation of encephalomyocarditis virus in swine embryo kidney cells. *Proc. Soc. Exp. Biol. Med.* 116:610–612, 1964.
27. Rueckert, R.R. Picornaviral architecture. In *Comparative Virology*, K. Maramorosch and E. Kurstak (eds.), pp. 255–306. Academic Press, New York, 1971.
28. Southerland, R.J., G.W. Horner, R. Hunter, and B.H. Fyfe. An outbreak of encephalomyocarditis in pigs. *New Zealand Vet. J.* 25:225, 1977.
29. Spradbrow, P.B. Antibodies to reoviruses, parainfluenza 3 virus, encephalomyocarditis virus and infectious bovine rhinotracheitis virus in porcine serums. *Austral. Vet. J.* 44:320–322, 1968.
30. Spradbrow, P.B., and Y.S. Chung. Haemagglutination-inhibition antibodies to encephalomyocarditis virus in Queensland cattle. *Austral. Vet. J.* 46:126–128, 1970.
31. Verlinde, J.D., and H.A.E. van Tongeren. Human infection with viruses of the Columbia-SK group. *Arch. ges. Virusforsch.* 5:217–227, 1953.
32. Vivell, O., and R. Mauer. Untersuchungen über die Hämagglutination von Viren der Parapoliomyelitisgruppe (Enzephalomyocarditisgruppe). *Zeitschrift Immunitatsforsch.* 109:246–261, 1952.
33. Vizoso, A.D., M.R. Vizoso, and R. Hay. Isolation of a virus resembling encephalomyocarditis from a red squirrel. *Nature* 201:849–850, 1964.
34. Warren, J. Encephalomyocarditis viruses. In *Viral and Rickettsial Infections of Man*, F.L. Horsfall, Jr., and I. Tamm (eds.), pp. 562–568. 4th ed. Lippincott, Philadelphia, 1965.
35. Warren, J., S.B. Russ, and H. Jeffries. Neutralizing antibody against viruses of the encephalomyocarditis group in the sera of wild rats. *Proc. Soc. Exp. Biol. Med.* 71:376–378, 1949.

36. Warren, J., J.E. Smadel, and S.B. Russ. The family relationship of encephalomyocarditis, Columbia-SK, M.M., and Mengo encephalomyelitis viruses. *J. Immunol.* 62:387–398, 1949.
37. Watt, D.A., and P.B. Spradbrow. Experimental encephalomyocarditis virus infection of pigs. *Austral. Vet. J.* 50:316–319, 1974.
38. Wellmann, K.F., D. Amsterdam, P. Brancato, and B.W. Wolk. Fine structure of pancreatic islets of mice infected with the M variant of the encephalomyocarditis virus. *Diabetologia* 8:349–357, 1972.

18. Poxviruses

Members of the Poxviridae family have certain features in common: they are of large size, have a complex morphology, are antigenically complex, and contain double-stranded DNA of high molecular weight. They have a predilection for infecting epidermal cells, their site of replication is in the cell cytoplasm, and they all produce cytoplasmic inclusion bodies of type B. The phenomenon of nongenetic reactivation of denatured poxvirus occurs with all members of the family and does not occur with any other known viruses.

Most diseases due to poxviruses are associated with lesions of the skin and can be observed as localized pocks or as generalized rashes. There are, however, some poxvirus infections in which gross dermal lesions are not seen.

The poxviruses have been divided into genera and subgroups on the basis of host range, serologic reaction, and morphology of the virion (Table 18.1).

Orthopoxviruses (Variola-Vaccinia Subgroup)

This genus of poxviruses includes the important viruses of vaccinia, cowpox, variola, and alastrim. Although distinct, they resemble each other in their biologic properties and their ability to cross-protect. The less important members of this genus are rabbitpox, monkeypox, and ectromelia. Some of the important properties of members of the genus are that they (1) are relatively resistant to ethyl ether and sodium deoxycholate, (2) are readily inactivated at 56–60°C for 20–30 minutes, (3) are sensitive to pH 3 and to chloroform, (4) possess an ability to uncoat a heated poxvirus and then reactivate it, (5) induce the synthesis of thymidine kinase, and (6) exhibit growth suppression by chemicals such as bromodexoyuridine, a DNA inhibitor.[1,6,20]

Specimens

Virus may be isolated from vesicular fluid and from lesion crusts. From dead animals, the liver and spleen are suitable for viral isolation. With mousepox, the majority of successful viral isolations are made from the intestinal tract mucosa or from the epidermis in the tail region.

Table 18.1. Poxviridae genera, strains, and major characteristics

Genera and subgroups*	Strain	Size (nm)	Inclusion bodies Nucleus	Cytoplasm A	Cytoplasm B	Ether sensitivity
Orthopoxvirus (Variola-Vaccinia)	Vaccinia	250 × 300	−	+	+	R
	Cowpox	250 × 300	+	+	+	
	Variola	250 × 300		−	+	
	Alastrim	250 × 300		−	+	
	Rabbitpox	250 × 300	−	−	+	
	Monkeypox	250 × 300	+	−	+	
	Ectromelia	250 × 300			+	
Parapoxvirus (Orf)	Orf	157 × 263	−	−	+	MR
	Bovine pseudopox	160 × 260	−	−	+	
	Bovine papular stomatitis		+	−	+	
	Sealpox	196 × 352	+	−	+	
Capripoxvirus (Sheeppox)	Sheeppox	115 × 194	(NV)+	−	+	S
	Goatpox			−	+	R
	Bovine lumpy skin disease	300 × 350			+	S
Avipoxvirus (Avianpox)	Fowlpox	284 × 332	+		+	R
	Turkeypox					R
	Canarypox	263 × 311		+	+	R
	Pigeonpox				+	
Leporipoxvirus (Myxoma)	Myxoma (Brazil)	250 × 300	(NV)		+	S
	Myxoma (Calif.)	250 × 300	(NV)		+	
	Rabbit fibroma	250 × 300	−	+	+	S
	Squirrel fibroma	250 × 300			+	
	Hare fibroma					
(Molluscum)	Molluscum contagiosum	226 × 302	+		+	S
	Yaba pox	250 × 280	−	−	+	
	Yaba-like pox	125 × 310	+		+	
	Tana pox				+	S
(Swinepox)	Swinepox	250 × 300	(NV)+	−	+	S

NV, nuclear vacuolation; R, resistant; MR, moderately resistant; S, susceptible.

*The International Committee on Taxonomy of Viruses has assigned generic names to cover most of the Poxviridae family. Formerly, the genera listed here were called subgenera A to E, respectively, and earlier they were designated by the subgroup names, as listed in parentheses.

Laboratory Procedures

Cultures. The inoculation of embryonating chicken eggs of 10–12 days incubation is quite frequently used for initial viral isolation. Usually the artificial air cell technique is used and the inoculum dose of 0.1–0.2 ml is deposited on the CAM. For initial viral isolations, the eggs are incubated at 35–37°C. After a virus has been found, eggs inoculated with a subsequent viral passage may be incubated at various incubator settings from 37.5 to 41.5°C to determine the ceiling temperature of the viral isolate.[5] These results, the pock morphology on the CAM, and the viral lethality for the embryo help to differentiate the various viruses in the genus[5] (Table 18.2). On the CAM, variola virus produces more lesions sooner than does alastrium virus, a fact which helps to differentiate these two otherwise quite similar-reacting viruses. All of the viruses of this genus will produce some pocks on the CAM within 72 hours.

Table 18.2. Orthopoxvirus growth characteristics on the CAM of embryonating chicken eggs

Viruses	Pock morphology	Lethality for embryo	Ceiling temperature °C*
Vaccinia	Large, ulcerated, red to white, flat	+	40.5–41
Rabbitpox	Large, ulcerated, red to gray	+	40.5–41.5
Cowpox	Large, ulcerated, ring-shaped, red to white	±	40
Mousepox	Minute, white	±	39
Monkeypox	Small, white	±	39
Variola	Small, not ulcerated, white	–	38.5
Alastrim	Small, not ulcerated, white	–	37.5

*Ceiling temperature is the maximum temperature at which lesions are produced and is a constant characteristic of each of the viruses.[5]

The cell system of choice to study CPE and plaque characteristics of this genus is the chicken embryo fibroblast. The CEF cell cultures are prepared from embryos 9–11 days old. The head and feet of the embryos are discarded and the remaining bodies of the embryos are minced with scissors. After this point, the technique is similar to that described for primary monolayer cultures in Chapter 4.

Many other kinds of cell cultures may be used and, with the exception of alastrim virus, the other viruses of the genus have a broad range of cell cultures that they will attack. Cell cultures inoculated with poxviruses have a CPE characterized by the appearance of small foci of rounded up cells that degenerate, giving rise to a clear area surrounded by swollen rounded-up cells. Sometimes there is syncytial formation and cytoplasmic streaming. Vaccinia virus CPE is rapid, and the entire cell sheet may be destroyed in 3 or 4 days. The changes seen with other members of the genus are similar; however, the time sequence of cell destruction varies with the virus type.[16,17,18] Intracytoplasmic inclusion bodies produced by the poxviruses are distinct and characteristic of the virus group.[4,12,13,21] The inclusions may be found after staining coverslip cell culture preparations with the MGG or H & E stains.[7,9] With the MGG stain, the Feulgen-positive DNA of the virus stains red-purple and the ribonucleoprotein of the cytoplasm stains blue. With H & E stain, the inclusions and nuclei are blue and the cytoplasm is light red.

Plaque formation is seen without an agar overlay in cell cultures inoculated with vaccinia, cowpox, variola, and alastrim viruses.[18] With an agar overlay, all viruses of the genus may produce plaques, with the poorest results from variola and alastrim viruses.[18] As with CAM pock formation, there is a characteristic ceiling temperature of incubation for the production of CPE and plaques in cell cultures by the viruses of this genus[5,8] (Table 18.3).

Animal inoculation. Guinea pigs, rabbits, hamsters, mice, and occasionally other animal species have been used for viral isolations. Although less suitable for virus isolation, these species of animals are useful for virus differentiation. Vaccinia virus is readily passaged serially in rabbits from infected skin lesions whereas variola and alastrim viruses are passaged only with difficulty, if at all. For many years vaccinia virus has

Table 18.3. Orthopoxvirus growth characteristics on cell cultures[8,11,12,16,17,18]

Viruses	Cell culture range	CPE	Plaques formed		Critical temperature °C	
			Without agar	With agar	CPE	Plaques
Vaccinia	Broad	+	+	+	40	40
Rabbitpox	Broad	+		+		
Cowpox	Broad	+	+	+	40	40
Mousepox	Broad	+		+		38
Monkeypox	Broad	+	+			
Variola	Broad	±	+	±	38.5	38
Alastrim	Narrow	+	−	±	37.5	37.5

been grown on the shaved abdominal skin of calves and then harvested to make smallpox vaccine. Many laboratories still use this production method.

Immunology and serology. In general, the viruses of this genus contain several antigens: a soluble lipid protein, LS antigen; a nucleoprotein, NP antigen; and a lipoprotein hemagglutinin, HA antigen.[4] There is sharing of antigens within the genus, which makes serologic differentiation difficult.[23] For this reason, a combination of techniques is often necessary before a definite viral identification can be made. For the detection of antibody in serum or for serologic identification of an unknown viral isolate, the HI and VN tests are the methods of choice.[23]

Not all chickens produce RBC that are suitable for use in the HA or HI tests.[14] The following is a simple test for suitability of RBC. Collect the RBC in Alsever's solution (1:5) and store at 4°C. To use, wash the RBC three times with 0.85% saline solution and then prepare them as a 0.5% suspension. Mix 0.25 ml of the RBC suspension with 0.5 ml of a 1:10,000 dilution of cardiolipin microflocculation antigen. Shake and incubate for 60 minutes at room temperature. RBC that agglutinate are suitable for the HA or HI tests. Turkey RBC are more often suitable than are chicken RBC. Hemagglutination is best demonstrated using virus from CAM pocks, and the HA can be inhibited with specific antisera in the standard HI test.

The VN test may be used in both of its forms, either the constant virus or constant serum dilutions. The test may be conducted in cell cultures by plaque inhibition, on the CAM by pock inhibition, or as animal protection tests.

The FA test is useful for rapid diagnosis of poxvirus infection and differentiation from other disease agents.[15,19] The test may be conducted with smears of clinical specimens, infected CAM, or cell cultures on coverslips.

The AD test is also used to identify poxviruses. The CF, HAd, and HAdI tests are workable but are not frequently used.

The viruses of the *Orthopoxvirus* genus will all give some degree of cross-protection. One of the earliest recorded examples was Jenner's observation regarding the immunity of milkmaids to infection with smallpox. In general, very good vaccines may be prepared from these viruses. The worldwide use of vaccinia virus to protect against variola infection has reduced this once dreaded scourge to an infrequently occurring disease.

Reactivation test. Admittance of a virus to the poxviridae family is in part dependent upon the virus passing the reactivation test.[6] Vaccinia virus is the test agent. Vaccinia virus of known titer and ability to produce pock lesions on the CAM is inactivated by heating at 55°C for 2 hours. The inactivated vaccinia virus is then mixed with equal volumes of the virus under test. This mixture is inoculated on the CAM of embryonating chicken eggs, and positive and negative controls are inoculated into other eggs. If the inactivated vaccinia virus is reactivated and produces its typical pock lesions, the test virus is classified as a poxvirus.[10] When the vaccinia virus is heated, as in this test, an enzyme necessary for release of the DNA core from the protein coat is inactivated. Thus the DNA, which was not harmed by the heat, is trapped in the coat and can not start replication. The missing enzyme is supplied by the other poxvirus and then the vaccinia virus DNA is released from its coat and is free to start replication.[10]

Host Range of the Orthopoxviruses

Vaccinia. Vaccinia virus is considered to be a laboratory phenomenon that does not occur naturally. Its origin and early passage history have been lost. Attempts to rederive vaccinia virus from variola, cowpox, and alastrim viruses have not been successful.[2] However, hybrids derived from mixtures of variola and cowpox viruses do in many cases closely resemble vaccinia. Vaccinia and variola inclusion bodies are quite similar, and vaccinia resembles cowpox in having a broad experimental host range.[4] Thus the suggestion that vaccinia originated as a hybrid of variola and cowpox deserves serious consideration.[2] Vaccinia virus will infect a wide variety of species including humans, monkeys, cattle, horses, swine, sheep, chickens, cats, rabbits, rats, mice, guinea pigs, and ground squirrels.[1,11]

Rabbitpox. This is another laboratory phenomena. Rabbitpox has not been reported in wild rabbits; it only occurs in domestic rabbits.[2] It has been suggested that rabbitpox virus may be a variant of neurovaccinia virus.[2] The Utrecht strain of the virus causes minimal reactions in mice, guinea pigs, cattle, and chickens.

Cowpox. Cowpox is a natural occurring disease of cattle and can be contracted from cattle by humans as an occupational disease. Experimentally, cowpox virus readily infects a wide variety of animals. The virus has been studied in rabbits, mice, guinea pigs, and monkeys. Reports of natural infection of horses with cowpox have not been verified.

Mousepox. Mousepox is usually found only in the laboratory mouse but has been detected occasionally in wild mice in close association with laboratories. Under natural conditions mousepox has a restricted host range, but the virus is reported to infect rats, rabbits, guinea pigs, and cotton rats.[1] Serial transmission of the virus occurs only in mice.

Monkeypox. Monkeypox has been reported under natural conditions in the subhuman primates and in the giant anteater, *Myrmecophaga tridactyla*,[7] and appears to have a limited host range under natural conditions.[20,22]

Variola. Variola virus has a much more restricted host range than the other members of the vaccinia subgroup. Monkeys are the only animals other than humans that are known to be infected by variola virus under natural conditions.[3]

Alastrim. Alastrim virus has a host range similar to that of variola, has a low virulence for animals, and multiplies to a lower titer on the CAM of the chicken embryo.[12] Alastrim infects monkeys under natural conditions.[1]

References

1. Andrewes, C. Poxviruses. In *Viruses of Vertebrates*, C. Andrewes and H.G. Pereira (eds.), pp. 373–414. 3d ed. Williams and Wilkins, Baltimore, 1972.
2. Bedson, H.S., and K.R. Dumbell. Smallpox and vaccinia. *Brit. Med. Bull.* 23:119–123, 1967.
3. Bleyer, J.C. On the occurrence of variola among monkeys of the genera, Mycetes and Cebus, in the wake of a pox epidemic on the tributaries of the Alto Uruquay in the jungles of southern Brazil. *Medizinische Wochenschrift* 69:1009–1010, 1922.
4. Downie, A.W., and K.R. Dumbell. Poxviruses. *Ann. Rev. Microbiol.* 10:237–252, 1956.
5. Dumbell, K.R., and H.S. Bedson. The use of ceiling temperature and reactivation in the isolation of poxvirus hybrids. *J. Hyg.* 62:133–140, 1964.
6. Fenner, G., and B.M. Comben. Genetic studies with mammalian poxviruses. I. Demonstration of recombination between two strains of vaccinia virus. *Virology* 5:530–548, 1958.
7. Gispen, R., J.D. Verlinde, and P. Zwart. Histopathological and virological studies on monkeypox. *Arch. ges. Virusforsch.* 21:205–216, 1967.
8. Gurvich, E.B. Effect of different temperatures on viruses of the smallpox group in tissue cultures. *Voprosy Virusologii* 9:116–118, 1964.
9. Ichihashi, Y., and S. Matsumoto. Studies on the nature of marchal bodies (A-type inclusion) during Ectromelia virus infection. *Virology* 29:264–275, 1966.
10. Joklik, W.K., G.M. Woodroofe, I.H. Holmes, and F. Fenner. The reactivation of poxviruses. I. Demonstration of the phenomenon and techniques of assay. *Virology* 11:168–184, 1960.
11. Kantoch, M., and B. Kuczkowska. Studies on the differentiation of variola and vaccinia viruses. *Arch. Immunol. Ther. Exp.* 14:339–349, 1966.
12. Kato, S., J. Hara, M. Ogawa, H. Miyamoto, and J. Kamahora. Inclusion markers of cowpox virus and alastrium virus. *Biken's J.* 6:233–235, 1963.
13. Kato, S., M. Takahashi, S. Kameyama, and J. Kamahora. A study on the morphological and cytoimmunological relationship between the inclusions of variola, cowpox, rabbitpox, vaccinia (variola origin) and vaccinia IHD and a consideration of the term "Guarnieri Body." *Biken's J.* 2:353–363, 1959.
14. Kempe, C.H., and L. St. Vincent. Variola and vaccinia viruses. *Diagnostic Procedures for Viral and Rickettsial Diseases*, E.H. Lennette and N.J. Schmidt (eds.), pp. 665–692. 3d ed. American Public Health Association, New York, 1964.
15. Kirsch, D. and R. Kissling. The use of immunofluorescence in rapid presumptive diagnosis of variola. *Bull. WHO* 29:126–128, 1963.
16. Marennikova, S.S., E.B. Gurvish, and M.A. Yumasheva. Laboratory diagnosis of smallpox and similar viral diseases by means of tissue culture methods: Differentiation of smallpox virus from varicella, vaccinia, cowpox and herpes viruses. *Acta Virol.* 8:135–142, 1964.
17. McConnell, S., R.O. Spertzel, D.L. Huxsoll, L.H. Elliott, and R.H. Yager. Plaque morphology of monkeypox virus as an aid to strain identification. *J. Bact.* 87:238–239, 1964.
18. Mika, L.A., and J.B. Prisch. Differentiation of variola from other members of the poxvirus group by the plaque technique. *J. Bact.* 80:861–864, 1960.
19. Murray, H.G.S., and M.B. Belf. The diagnosis of smallpox by immunofluorescence. *Lancet* 1:847–848, 1963.
20. Rouhandch, H., R. Engler, M.T.A. Gouad, and L.L. Sells. Properties of monkeypox virus. *Arch. ges. Virusforsch.* 20:363–373, 1967.
21. Sauer, R.M., J.E. Prier, R.S. Buchanan, A.A. Creamer, and H.C. Fegley. Studies on a pox disease of monkeys. I. Pathology. *Am. J. Vet. Res.* 21:377–380, 1960.
22. Von Magnus, P., E.K. Andersen, K.B. Petersen, and A. Brich-Andersen. A pox-like disease in Cynomolgus monkeys. *Acta Path. Microbiol. Scand.* 46:156–176, 1949.
23. Woodroofe, G.M., and F. Fenner. Serological relationships within the poxvirus group: An antigen common to all members of the group. *Virology* 16:334–341, 1962.

Parapoxviruses (Orf Subgroup)

The genus *Parapoxvirus* presents a different morphology from other poxviruses, as demonstrated by electron microscopy. The virion is oval to cylindrical in shape with a conspicious cross-pattern made up of tubular fibrils. The virions are approximately 150–260 nm in size.[6,7,8,9] Thus far, only Orf virus, bovine papular stomatitis virus, pseudocowpox virus, and sealpox virus have been shown morphologically to belong to this genus.[2,11,12] Classification within the genus (Orf subgroup) is based on the animal species from which the virus is isolated rather than on other characteristics of the virus.[5]

Specimens

The viruses of this genus have been isolated from lesion scabs and fluids, skin scrapings, blood, lymph, milk, and nasal and pharyngeal washings and swabs.

Laboratory Procedures

Cultures. The viruses of this genus do not readily produce lesions on the CAM of embryonating chicken eggs. Likewise, they do not readily infect suckling mice. Thus, negative results with these systems are useful for differentiating these viruses from many of the other poxviruses and other viral families (Table 18.4).[1]

Table 18.4. Diagnostic features of parapoxviruses

Viruses	Isolation in cell cultures	Lesions on CAM	Cytoplasmic inclusions	Serology			Typical EM ovoid morphology	Laboratory animals	
				CF	HA-HAd	FA		Rabbits	Mice
Orf	+	−	+	+	−	+	+	±	−
BPS	+	−	+	+	−	+	+	−	−
Pseudocowpox	+	−	+	+	−	+	+	±	−
Sealpox	ND	ND	+	ND	ND	ND	+	ND	ND

Primary cell culture systems can be used for viral isolation of members of this genus. Cell cultures from the respective species involved in the disease in question may also be used. The viruses produce a typical poxvirus CPE.

Animal inoculation. The primary host species can be inoculated to reproduce the respective diseases, but other laboratory animals are not generally useful for laboratory tests.

Immunology and serology. The AD and FA tests are used for viral identification of members of this genus. By means of the FA test it was demonstrated that Orf, bovine papular stomatitis, and pseudocowpox viruses are related antigenically, but cross-reactions were not found with vaccinia virus.[4] The CF and VN tests have been used but success has been limited.

Other methods for viral identification. Electron microscopy is the method of choice for diagnosis of members of the *Parapoxvirus* genus. It is often possible to identify the virion in material taken from the lesion by a technique that can be completed in 3–4 hours. The electron microscope (EM) technique is as follows: (1) cut lesion material into small fragments, (2) suspend in 2 ml of 0.004 M McIlvaines buffer (pH 7.8), (3) sonicate at 4°C for 2.5 minutes at maximum setting, (4) centrifuge for 20 minutes at about 3000 rpm and discard debris, (5) centrifuge supernatant fluid at 20,000 rpm for 20 minutes ($32,000 \times g$), (6) remove supernatant fluid and discard, (7) suspend pellet in one drop of distilled H_2O, (8) on a waxed slide, deposit a drop of the suspended pellet and mix with a drop of 5% sodium phosphotungstate at about pH 6.5 (duplicate samples may be made), (9) transfer microdrops of the mixture to a carbon-coated nitrocellulose film on standard EM grids, (10) when the preparation is dry and is ready for placing in the EM, examine at a magnification of about 10,000×.

An even more rapid EM technique that may be used with many of the poxviruses, and with the capripoxviruses and avipoxviruses in particular, is as follows: (1) insert a needle into a lesion biopsy specimen and then touch a drop of distilled H_2O on a waxed slide with the point of the needle, (2) place a 400-mesh carbon-coated EM grid on the drop of specimen-contaminated water, (3) after 1 minute remove the grid and blot it, (4) stain 1 minute with a drop of phosphotungstic acid containing 0.4% sucrose (pH 7), (5) blot and air dry the grid, (6) examine under EM at magnifications of 20,000 and 40,000× for poxvirus virions.

The reactivation test (heated vaccinia virus) also may be conducted to verify that the isolate is a poxvirus. MGG and H & E stains may be used with smears of lesion material or preparations from cell cultures to demonstrate inclusion bodies. The acridine orange stain may be used to determine the nucleic acid of the virion since a DNA reaction indicates that the virus is a poxivirus.

Orf Virus

Synonyms for Orf disease are contagious pustular dermatitis, contagious ecthyma of sheep, and ovine pustular dermatitis. Orf is a viral disease of sheep and goats that has a worldwide distribution. The natural host range is restricted to sheep and goats, with humans and cattle as accidental hosts. In the naturally occurring disease, the oral mucosa is most commonly affected, although the virus may spread to other areas of the body.

Vesicular lesions appear 2–4 days after exposure and may spread rapidly to cover extensive areas of the face, lips, and buccal mucosa. Occasionally, lesions are found on teats and udders of ewes. After rupture of the vesicles, the lesions become encrusted and then heal after 2–3 weeks.

People in contact with Orf-infected animals may develop lesions on the fingers and hands. These lesions usually disappear within a matter of weeks unless secondary complications occur. Transmission from person to person has not been recorded.

Bovine Papular Stomatitis Virus

Bovine papular stomatitis (BPS) is characterized by proliferative lesions on the buccal mucosa, muzzle area, and margins of the lips.[10] It resembles early lesions of FMD and VS. Lesions are generally rounded areas that are slightly raised. The slow peripheral extension of the lesion forms concentric rings of different colors.[3]

The natural infection appears to be limited to cattle, with humans as accidental hosts. Significant levels of neutralizing antibodies apparently do not develop subsequent to infection with BPS virus although calves recovered from infection are immune to reinfection.

Pseudocowpox Virus

The synonyms are pseudopox, paravaccinia, milker's nodule, and spurious cowpox.[6] This disease, closely resembling cowpox, has long been recognized in cattle. It may vary in severity from one or two small scabs on a teat to extensive scabbing of teats and udders of several cows in the herd.

After an incubation period of 6–9 days, early lesions appear as dark red spots on the teats. The lesions may then develop into papules, which often erode, leaving a raw surface that scabs over and eventually heals. Secondary lesions may be found in adjacent areas 1–2 weeks after infection. The disease can be spread by milking machines. Sometimes lesions are found in the mouths of suckling calves.

In humans, a variety of clinical lesions can be seen, varying from a single nodule to multiple vesicles with enlargement of regional lymph glands.[2] The disease is generally characterized by nodular lesions of finger, hand, wrist, forearm, or face appearing about 1 week following exposure to an infected cow. The lesions begin as isolated papules or round areas 1–2 cm in diameter and have a reddish-brown color. The lesions regress, generally without treatment, in 2–5 weeks.

In individual animals, the lesions may persist for prolonged period of time and many animals may be reinfected on re-exposure to the virus. Animals recovered from cowpox or persons vaccinated with vaccinia virus are not protected against pseudocowpox infection.

Sealpox Virus

Sealpox disease occurs as a diffuse proliferative skin disease and may be accompanied by anorexia and respiratory distress. Skin papules and granulomas are common among pinnipeds, but the virus has only recently been identified. Viral morphology, as shown by electron microscopy, and cytoplasmic inclusion bodies in infected cells were the diagnostic criteria used.[11,12]

References

1. Castrucci, G., D.G. McKercher, V. Cilli, G. Arancia, and C. Nazionali. Characteristics of a paravaccinia virus from cattle. *Arch. ges. Virusforsch.* 29:315–330, 1970.
2. Friedman-Kien, A.E., W.P. Rowe, and W.G. Banfield. Milkers nodules: Isolation of a poxvirus from a human case. *Science* 140:1335–1336, 1963.
3. Griesemer, R.A., and C.R. Cole. Bovine papular stomatitis. I. Recognition in the United States. *J. Am. Vet. Med. Ass.* 137:404–410, 1960.
4. Lieberman, H. Serologic relationships between paravaccinia viruses. *Arch. Exp. Veterinärmed.* 20:1353–1354, 1966.
5. Morita, C., H. Izawa, and M. Soekawa. Isolation of a paravaccinia virus from a cow in Japan. *Jap. J. Vet. Sci.* 29:171–175, 1967.
6. Moscovici, C., E.P. Cohen, J. Sanders, and S.S. DeLong. Isolation of a viral agent from pseudo cowpox disease. *Science* 141:915–916, 1963.
7. Nagington, J. Electron microscopy in differential diagnosis of poxvirus infection. *Brit. Med. J.* 2:1499–1354, 1964.
8. Nagington, J., A.A. Newton, and R.W. Horne. The structure of Orf virus. *Virology* 23:461–472, 1964.
9. Peters, D., G. Muller, and D. Buttner. The fine structure of paravaccinia viruses. *Virology* 23:609–611, 1964.
10. Plowright, W., and R.D. Ferris, 1959. Papular stomatitis of cattle in Kenya and Nigeria. *Vet. Rec.* 71:718–722, 1959.

11. Wilson, T.M., N.F. Cherille, and L. Karstad. Seal pox. *Bull. Wildlife Dis. Ass.* 5:412–418, 1969.
12. Wilson, T.M., and P.R. Sweeney. Morphological studies on seal poxvirus. *J. Wildlife Dis.* 6:94–96, 1970.

Capripoxviruses (Sheeppox Subgroup)

This genus of poxviruses, *Capripoxvirus,* consisting of sheeppox virus, goatpox virus, and lumpy skin disease virus (Neethling strain), was formed on the basis of the cross-immunity among the three viruses and their failure to exhibit cross-immunity with viruses of the other genera of poxviruses.

The three viruses of the genus share common antigens in the AD test, cross-react in the CF test, and cross-protect either bilaterally or unilaterally.[2,3,5,9]

Cell culture techniques can be used to study these viruses. All three of them cause typical poxvirus CPE and form intracytoplasmic inclusion bodies. Their DNA content is readily demonstrated by the acridine orange staining procedure. For rapid EM techniques that can be used with capripoxviruses, see the laboratory procedures described for parapoxviruses.

Sheeppox Virus

The disease sheeppox has been known for centuries. At present, it is found only in the Mediterranean countries and the Near East. It may be seen as a severe generalized infection with a high mortality in young lambs, or as a milder, less severe pox infection in adults. Fever, lacrimation, nasal discharge, and skin lesions are the usual clinical signs and lesions. Typical lesions follow the classic pox cycle of erythema, papule, vesicle, pustuli with exudation, encrustation, and scab formation. When the scab dries and falls off, a pitted scar remains. The pox lesions also may occur on the pharyngeal mucous membrane. The lesions are generally large, often hemorrhagic, and are persistent.[2]

Sheeppox virus is readily isolated in cell cultures derived from the kidneys and testes of sheep, goats, and calves. The viral CPE develops within 4–6 days and tends to remain focal rather than generalized. Cytoplasmic inclusion bodies are readily seen in infected cells.[8] Morphologically, sheeppox virus resembles vaccinia virus but is smaller and more elongated. It is host specific and only sheep are naturally infected. Rabbits, hamsters, guinea pigs, and mice are resistant to the virus. Embryonating chicken eggs may be infected, but with difficulty. Sheeppox virus protects cattle against true lumpy skin disease[5] and goats against goatpox.[2] The disease clinically could be confused with Orf, bluetongue, photosensitization, or mycotic dermatitis.

Goatpox Virus

Goatpox is found in a few European countries but otherwise has a geographic distribution similar to sheeppox. The lesions are a pustulopapular type and are smaller and more transient than are the lesions of sheeppox. The disease could be confused with Orf or bluetongue.

The virus is readily grown in cell cultures of lamb and kid kidney and testes.[7] The CPE caused by the virus resembles that seen with other poxviruses, cytoplasmic inclusions are formed and the virus gives a typical DNA fluorescence with acridine orange stain. An AD test has been developed for the diagnosis of sheeppox and goatpox.[3]

Lumpy Skin Disease Virus

Lumpy skin disease, also known as *Knopvelsiekte,* is characterized by the development of cutaneous nodules and generalized lymphadenitis. The disease affects cattle and buffaloes and is confined to the African continent east and south of the Sahara. True lumpy skin disease is caused by the Neethling poxvirus (NPV).[1] The Allerton herpesvirus (AHV) is sometimes associated with NPV; by itself, however, it produces a milder skin disease that clinically may be confused with true lumpy skin disease.[1] AHV is also closely related to the bovine herpes mammillitis virus. In addition, other nonpathogenic orphan viruses are sometimes isolated from lumpy skin disease lesions or regional lymph nodes, either in pure culture or mixed with NPV.[1]

The incubation period for natural lumpy skin disease varies from 2 to 5 weeks. There is a diphasic fluctuating fever and skin eruptions coincide with the second temperature peak.[4] The animals are reluctant to move and have anorexia, increased salivation, and oculonasal discharge. The skin nodules are circumscribed, firm, raised, flat-topped intradermal swellings varying from 0.5 to 7 cm in diameter.[4] The hairs over the lumps stand erect thereby accentuating the lumpy appearance. There may be only two or three lumps, or there may be hundreds of lumps scattered over the body surface.[4] An important diagnostic sign is the obvious swelling of superficial lymph nodes.[4] Internal lesions are also found.[4]

In the milder AHV infection, skin lesions appear suddenly after a slight febrile reaction. The lesions are firm, round, raised nodules, with a depressed center in their otherwise flat surface. This is a differentiating feature between the AHV infection and the NPV infection. Also, the lymph nodes are not enlarged in AHV infection.

For specimens from live animals, several active skin lesions should be excised and a biopsy of an enlarged superficial lymph node should be made. From destroyed animals, specimens of lesions, enlarged lymph nodes, and internal lesions (if present) should be taken.

Virus isolation may be made in calf or lamb kidney or testis cell cultures. The CPE develops slowly similar to that of sheeppox virus. The virion morphology is similar to that of the vaccinia virus. There are Cowdrey type-A intranuclear inclusions with AHV, while NPV produces intracytoplasmic inclusions.[6] Rabbits can be infected with both NPV and AHV, but only AHV infects and kills suckling mice.

Cattle recovered from lumpy skin disease are resistant to reinfection. The disease can be prevented by vaccination with sheeppox virus.[5] When calves are naturally infected with NPV the mortality rate may be as high as 10%.

References

1. Alexander, R.A., W. Plowright, and D.A. Haig. Cytopathogenic agents associated with lumpy skin disease of cattle. *Bull. Epiz. Dis. Afr.* 5:489–492, 1957.
2. Bennett, S.C.J., E.S. Horgan, and M.A. Haseeb. The pox diseases of sheep and goats. *J. Comp. Path.* 54:131–160, 1944.
3. Bhambani, B.D., and D.K. Murty. An immuno-diffusion test for laboratory diagnosis of sheeppox and goatpox. *J. Comp. Path.* 73:349–358, 1963.
4. Burden, M.L., and J. Prydie. Lumpy skin disease of cattle in Kenya. *Nature* 183:949–950, 1959.
5. Capstick, P.B., and W. Coackley. Protection of cattle against lumpy skin disease. I. Trials with a vaccine against Neethling type infection. *Res. Vet. Sci.* 2:362–368, 1961.

6. Munz, E.K., and N.C. Owen. Electron microscopic studies on lumpy skin disease virus type "Neethling." *Onderstepoort J. Vet. Res.* 33:3–8, 1966.
7. Pandey, R., and I.P. Singh. Cytopathogenicity and neuralization of goatpox virus in cell culture. *Res. Vet. Sci.* 2:195–197, 1970.
8. Plowright, W., and R.D. Ferris. The growth and cytopathogenicity of sheeppox virus in tissue cultures. *Brit. J. Exp. Path.* 39:424–435, 1958.
9. Sharma, S.N., P.R. Nilakantan, and M.R. Ohanda. A preliminary note on pathogenicity and antigenicity of sheep and goatpox viruses. *Indian Vet. J.* 43:673–678, 1966.

Avipoxviruses (Avian Poxvirus Subgroup)

The avian poxviruses have long been described as one of two major subgroups of the poxviruses, the other being identified simply as mammalian poxviruses. In the early literature, the term fowlpox was applied to all pox diseases of birds, both domesticated gallinaceous and wild. They now have a generic name, *Avipoxvirus*.

This genus of poxviruses is comprised of a heterogenous group, with four major virus types recognized on the basis of cross-immunity and cross-protection tests. These four types are fowlpox virus, turkeypox virus, pigeonpox virus, and canarypox virus. In addition, three minor types are recognized—sparrowpox, starlingpox, and juncopox viruses. Comparative studies are needed to definitively position each of the virus types within the genus. Such studies have been hampered by the reported inability of many species of birds to produce high levels of antibody,[6] the migratory habits of many species of birds, which make it difficult to ascertain the source of infection, and the mechnical transmission of the poxviruses by hematophagous vectors, especially the mosquito.[7]

Excellent descriptions of the comparative pathogenesis of the major types of avian poxviruses have been published.[2] The disease is characterized by the appearance of nodular lesions on the unfeathered parts of the body or by an inflammatory response of the mucous membranes of the mouth and upper respiratory tract.

The morphology of the virion, as demonstrated by electron microscopy, is of the vaccinia subgroup type.[1] The virion is readily demonstrated with the electron microscope, which can be used as a simple, rapid diagnostic tool. (See the technique described under laboratory procedures for parapoxviruses.) All the known avian poxviruses share a common antigenicity as shown by the AD test and the CF test.[5,8]

The major avian poxvirus types may be differentiated by their growth characteristics in vivo and in vitro, and by comparative serologic procedures. A summary of these characteristics is presented in Table 18.5. Susceptibility of day-old chicken embryos inoculated IV and comparative VN studies in cell cultures are the best means of identifying the virus type.

Table 18.5. Differential characterization of the avipoxviruses

Virus	Growth on CAM	IV susceptibility of day-old chicks	Cross-reactions in VN test
Fowlpox	+	+	+
Turkeypox	+	+	−
Pigeonpox	+	−	−
Canarypox	+	−	+

Fowlpox Virus

Fowlpox has a worldwide distribution and has been observed in domesticated birds for many decades. The historical aspects of fowlpox are well documented and many excellent descriptions of this disease have been published.

The usual form of fowlpox is characterized by nodular lesions on the skin of the head or other unfeathered parts of the body. In this form, fowlpox disease can be diagnosed with a consistent degree of accuracy based on gross examination and the microscopic appearance of the cutaneous lesions.

Occasionally, the eyes and nasal sinuses are involved (roup) or involvement of the mucous membranes of the mouth and respiratory tract (fowl diphtheria) is encountered. Diagnosis of these forms of the disease is more difficult.

Tracheal fluids, materials from the eyes, mouth, or upper respiratory tract, and suspensions of skin nodules are excellent sources for virus isolation attempts. The viruses grow well on the CAM of 9–11-day-old embryonating chicken eggs, in cell cultures of chicken embryo kidney or fibroblasts, and in duck embryo fibroblast cells.[3] Typical pock lesions are produced on the CAM and a CPE is seen in cells under a fluid medium. Histochemical techniques such as acridine-orange and FA staining are excellent methods for virus identification.

The serologic methods of choice are the AD and VN tests in cell cultures. CF, indirect HA, HI, and FA techniques are also useful.

Fowlpox virus will infect many species of birds, but the definitive species range is undetermined. Host specificity studies reported by a number of investigators present a conflicting story,[4,6] which needs further clarification. Microscopically, the appearance of eosinophilic bodies (Bollinger bodies) in the cytoplasm of epithelial cells is a useful diagnostic marker.

References

1. Beaver, D.L., and W.J. Cheatham. Electron microscopy of junco pox. *Am. J. Path.* 42:23–39, 1963.
2. Cunningham, C.H. Avian pox. In *Diseases of Poultry,* M.S. Hofstad (ed.). 6th ed. Iowa State University Press, Ames, 1972.
3. Gelenczei, E.F., and H.N. Lasher. Comparative studies of cell-culture-propagated avian pox viruses in chickens and turkeys. *Avian Dis.* 12:142–150, 1968.
4. Irons, V. Cross-species transmission studies with different strains of bird-pox. *Am. J. Hyg.* 20:329–351, 1943.
5. Kato, K., T. Horiuchi, and H. Tsubahara. Isolation of sparrow pox virus and its serological properties. *Nat. Inst. Anim. Health Q.* 5:130–137, 1965.
6. Kirmse, P. Host specificity and pathogenicity of pox viruses from wild birds. *Bull. Wildlife Dis. Ass.* 5:376–386, 1969.
7. Kligler, I.J., and M. Ashner. Transmission of fowl pox by mosquitoes: Further observations. *Brit. J. Exp. Path.* 10:347–352, 1929.
8. Tsubahara, H., and K. Kato. Application of agar gel precipitin test to bird pox viruses. *Bull. Nat. Inst. Anim. Health* 41:43–54, 1961.

Leporipoxviruses (Myxoma Subgroup)

Many of the poxvirus infections of animals appear to be associated with benign localized tumors of the skin that are generally seen as single nodules. This is especially true with *Leporipoxvirus* infections. The genus includes two major antigenic types of

Table 18.6. Differential characteristics of leporipoxviruses

Virus	Susceptibility of newborn domestic rabbits	Primary rabbit kidney	Continuous rabbit kidney (RK-13)	Chick embryo fibroblasts
Myxoma (Brazil)	Very	CPE	CPE	Plaques*
Myxoma (Calif.)	Very	CPE	CPE	Plaques*
Rabbit fibroma	LLO†	CPE	CPE	Neg.‡
Squirrel fibroma	LLO	CPE	CPE	Neg.
Hare fibroma	LLO	CPE	Neg.	Neg.

*Plaques produced if DEAE (dextran) is added to overlay.
†LLO, localized lesion only.
‡Neg., negative reaction.

myxoma virus, Brazilian and Californian, and three distinct antigenic types of fibroma viruses, those of the rabbit, squirrel, and hare (Table 18.6).

Myxoma Virus

Either myxoma or myxomatosis are used as names for the disease produced by myxoma virus. Two antigenic variants of myxoma virus have been identified: the Brazilian myxoma virus that affects the tapetis (native rabbit) of South America, and the Californian myxoma virus of the sage brush rabbit. Morphologically the myxoma virion is indistinguishable from vaccinia. The virus is not ether resistant as are the more typical poxviruses. There is cross-protection and cross-neutralization between the myxoma viruses but no cross-immunity with vaccinia virus.[11]

Myxoma viruses produce a typical poxvirus CPE in monolayer cultures of cells derived from tissues of embryonic rabbits. These cellular changes are characterized by the formation of cytoplasmic inclusions and nuclear vacuolation. Cytopathic changes are best visualized using histochemical techniques, such as the acridine orange stain for nucleic acid identity and the MGG or H & E stains for evidence of cytoplasmic inclusions.

Plaques are produced under agar overlay in rabbit kidney and rabbit embryo fibroblasts, and in chicken embryo fibroblasts if DEAE (dextran) is added to the overlay.[11] Myxoma viruses also will replicate in human diploid cells, producing a typical poxvirus CPE.[2]

The embryonating chicken egg CAM is susceptible to the myxoma viruses, small pocks being produced in about 3 days. One-day-old mice are susceptible to the virus but older mice are not.

The FA, CF, VN, and AD tests are all useful for serologic identification of myxomatosis. The method of choice for virus isolation is ID inoculation of suspect material on the back of the domestic rabbit.[8]

Brazilian myxoma virus is widely distributed throughout South America. The disease was first described by Sanarelli in 1898 and the etiologic agent was called virus myxomatosum caniculi.[9] Under natural conditions the virus infects the tapetis, causing a benign disease characterized by localized skin tumors.[4]

In domestic rabbits, myxoma virus causes a generalized disease and is highly lethal. Local lesions develop in 3–5 days; the disease becomes generalized a few days later, evidenced by bilateral blepharoconjunctivitis with copious secretion. This is accompanied by swelling of the genital area, snout, and ears. A generalized papular rash develops and small tumors may develop over the body. The disease is usually fatal, death occurring between 8 and 15 days after exposure. Cage transmission occurs among domestic rabbits from virus shed in mucous secretions or by contact with infected cages or bedding. Under natural conditions, infection with myxoma virus is caused by mechanical transfer from infected rabbits by mosquitoes and rabbit fleas. Experimentally, the Brazilian myxoma virus will produce tumors and death in North American cottontail rabbits.[7]

Natural infection with Brazilian myxoma virus is found only with rabbits, *Sylvilagus braziliensis* and *Oryctolagus cuniculus,* and very rarely with hares, *Lepus europaeus* and *Lepus timidus.*[3] The Brazilian myxoma virus was deliberately introduced into Europe and Australia where it is now established in both areas as an enzootic disease. During the early period following introduction of the virus, epizootics in Europe and Australia resulted in the death of millions of rabbits.[3] However, in both cases, hares were rarely affected by myxoma and thrived very well.[3] Thus rabbits and hares have natural disease resistance differences. (While rabbits and hares may look alike, there are several biologic differences that justify placing them in different genera. The most obvious difference, to those who have raised both rabbits and hares, is explained in the following jingle: "Nude neonate rabbit heirs have nary hairs. / Au contraire, hasty hares have hairy heirs.")

Californian myxoma virus induces a disease in brush rabbits that is characterized by a mild localized fibroma. The virus is highly host specific, with only the brush rabbit and domestic rabbits yielding virus levels high enough for mosquito transmission.[8] In nature, maximum tumor growth is seen 7–10 days after infection; the tumors last for several weeks, scab over, and heal without scar formation.

As with the Brazilian strain, the Californian myxoma virus is extremely lethal for the domestic rabbit. The two strains are closely related antigenically with recovered animals having good immunity against reinfection with either virus.

Diagnosis is based on clinical appearance of infected animals. In vitro differentiation of the Californian (as with the Brazilian) myxoma virus is partially based on the small-sized pocks it produces on the CAM of embryonating chicken eggs. Similarly to other members of the genus, this strain grows well in cell culture and can easily be identified by the serologic procedures listed for the Brazilian biotype of myxoma virus.

Rabbit Fibroma Virus

Rabbit or Shope's fibromas occur naturally in feral rabbits in the eastern United States. First described by Shope in 1932, this disease is identical to that produced by the myxoma viruses.[10] This fibroma virus is closely related to myxoma viruses by immunologic tests, and cross-protection against the myxoma viruses is good.

Clinically, the only manifestation of disease in experimentally infected domestic rabbits is the appearance of tumors at the site of infection. This is a major departure from the myxoma viruses and is a useful diagnostic key.

The fibroma virus replicates on the CAM of embryonating chicken eggs and can be passaged on the membrane but produces no pock lesions. Neither does the virus produce plaques on monolayers of chicken embryo fibroblasts, although it replicates in this cell system. However, plaques are produced on monolayers of rabbit kidney cells and cytoplasmic inclusions are found in infected cells.[11]

The rabbit fibroma virus has a very limited host range and differs from the myxoma viruses in their ceiling temperature, that is, the fibroma virus does not grow at 40°C in cell culture, whereas myxoma virus will.[5] Like myxoma virus, the fibroma virus will multiply in the brain of newborn mice without producing symptoms of disease.[1]

Identification of the virus is based on morphologic characteristics or on serologic confirmation using standardized AD, CF, VN, or FA systems. Where electron microscopy is not available nor specific antiserum obtainable, the reactivation of an inactivated poxvirus is the diagnostic procedure of choice.

Squirrel Fibroma Virus

This virus causes multiple fibromatoses in young gray squirrels (*Sciurus carolinses*). Adult squirrels are relatively resistant. Geographic distribution is limited to the eastern United States and the virus is transmitted by blood-sucking vectors. Young woodchucks and domestic rabbits are susceptible to the virus.[6]

Immunologically (in cross-protection and plaque neutralization), squirrel fibroma virus is closely related to rabbit fibroma virus. The virus replicates in monolayer cell cultures of rabbit and squirrel kidneys and produces clear plaques on rabbit embryo fibroblasts but no visible lesions on CEF cells.[11]

Hare Fibroma Virus

The only indigenous member of the genus found in Europe, the hare fibroma virus causes a disease in the European hare (*Lepus* sp.) characterized by the formation of small localized fibromas. Immunologically and morphologically the virus qualifies for inclusion in the genus.[11]

Only newborn domestic rabbits are susceptible to the virus. Hare fibroma virus produces plaques on rabbit embryo fibroblasts, causes a CPE in rabbit kidney cells, and can be distinguished from the other members of the subgroup by its failure to cause CPE on monolayers of continuous rabbit kidney (RK-13) cells. Hare fibroma virus does not produce visible lesions on chicken embryo fibroblasts but will reactivate heat-inactivated poxviruses, a criterion for classification as a poxvirus.

References

1. Dalmat, H.T. Passage of Shope's rabbit fibroma virus through one day old mice. *Proc. Soc. Exp. Biol. Med.* 97:219–220, 1958.
2. DeFabritis, A., and D.D. Balducci. The cytopathic effects of tumor viruses in human diploid cells: Similarity with lesions of irradiated cells. *Oncologia* 19:391–400, 1965.
3. Fenner, F., and F.N. Ratcliffe. *Myxomatosis,* p. 379. Cambridge University Press, London, New York, 1965.
4. Fenner, F., and D.O. White. *Medical Virology.* Academic Press, New York, London, 1970.
5. Kilham, L. Relation of thermoresistance to virulence among fibroma and myxoma viruses. *Virology* 9:486–487, 1959.

6. Kilham, L., C.M. Herman, and E.R. Fisher. Naturally occurring fibromas of gray squirrels related to Shope's rabbit fibroma. *Proc. Soc. Exp. Biol. Med.* 82:298–301, 1953.
7. Regnery, D.C. The epidemic potential of Brazilian myxoma virus (Lausanne strain) for three species of North American (cottontails). *Am. J. Epidemiol.* 94:514–519, 1971.
8. Regnery, D.C., and I.D. Marshall. Studies in the epidemiology of myxomatosis in California. IV. The susceptibility of six Leporid species to Californian myxoma virus and the relative infectivity of their tumors for mosquitoes. *Am. J. Epidemiol.* 94:508–513, 1971.
9. Sanarelli, G. Das myxomatogene virus: Beitrag zum studium de krankheitserreger ausserhalb des sichtbaren (vorlaufige Mitteilung). *Zentralblatt Bakt.* 23:865–873, 1898.
10. Shope, R.E. A transmissible tumor-like condition in rabbits. *J. Exp. Med.* 56:793–802, 1932.
11. Woodroofe, G.M., and F. Fenner. Viruses of the myxomafibroma subgroup of the poxviruses. I. Plaque production in cultured cells, plaque-reduction tests, and cross-protection tests in rabbits. *Austral. J. Exp. Biol. Med. Sci.* 43:123–142, 1965.

Molluscum Contagiosum Subgroup

The molluscum contagiosum subgroup has not yet been assigned a genus name. Pox outbreaks attributed to this subgroup of poxviruses are few in number; in general, the infections appear to be associated with single or mutiple benign localized nodules of the skin. Members of this subgroup are molluscum contagiosum poxvirus, Yaba monkey tumor poxvirus, Yaba-like poxvirus, and tanapox virus.

Molluscum contagiosum is primarily a disease of humans, but a single episode of this disease has been reported in the chimpanzee.[1] The lesions of this disease resemble that of a common wart and the disease is a chronic proliferative process restricted to the skin epithelium. On rare occassions, mutiple discrete nodules may be seen. Humans and chimpanzees are the only species of animals naturally infected.

The disease can best be diagnosed using the technique described by Douglas.[1] Lesion exudate is placed on a glass slide and stained with Wright's stain. Microscopic examination will show large, blue, intracytoplasmic inclusion bodies typical of poxvirus infection. Alternate procedures include the use of acridine orange stain and electron microscopy.

Yabapox is a human disease that appears to be limited to Nigeria. The host range of the virus appears to be limited primarily to humans and experimentally to Asiatic monkeys, with most African and South American primates being resistant. The disease is characterized by the appearance of histiocytomas of a benign nature. The tumors are subcutaneous and nonencapsulated and lesions regress spontaneously.[3]

Yaba-like pox disease is primarily observed in the *Macaca* sp. of simians and is transmissible to humans. The lesions involve only the epidermis as in molluscum contagiosum, whereas Yaba tumors do not. Lesions may be single but are often multiple. They first appear as red, slightly elevated areas that rapidly progress to circular, circumscribed, raised nodules. In general, these lesions are not vesicular, purulent, or hemorrhagic. The disease is self-limiting and regression of the tumors begins as early as 10 days after infection.

Tanapox disease in humans is characterized by a short febrile illness with headache and prostration, and the disease is characterized by a single pocklike lesion on the body. The host range is limited to humans and monkeys. Apparently, this disease is a zoonosis transmitted from monkeys to humans, possibly by the mosquito as a mechanical vector.[2]

Yaba, Yaba-like, and tanapox viruses are serologically related. The Yaba antiserum cross-reacts strongly with Yaba-like virus by the FA technique but only weakly by the CF and VN tests. Yaba antiserum cross-reacts slightly with tanapoxvirus in the CF test but not in the VN test. Yaba-like and tanapoxviruses are closely related serologically and may be identical.

The viruses replicate in cell lines derived from human and subhuman primates. Primary rhesus monkey kidney cells, the continuous lines of *Cercopithecus* kidney, BS-C-1, and Vero are recommended. The adsorption period is relatively long (4–5 hours) and CPE may not be evident for 4–15 days. Coverslips of virus-infected cells stained by the acridine orange technique usually show the presence of virus at between 5 and 8 days.

Species specificity in vivo and in vitro are important in the differential diagnosis of poxviruses isolated from subhuman primates. Failure of these viruses to grow in rabbit

Table 18.7. Growth characteristics of molluscum contagiosum subgroup

Viruses	Tissue layer	Lethality to chick embryo	Growth on CAM	Microtumor in cell culture	Inclusions Cytoplasmic	Nuclear
Molluscum contagiosum	Epidermis	–	–	–	+	±
Yaba	Dermis	–	±	+	+	–
Yaba-like	Epidermis	–	–	–	+	+
Tana	Epidermis	–	–	?	+	?

kidney cell cultures readily distinguishes this subgroup of viruses from monkeypox and vaccinia viruses. The viruses of this subgroup are further differentiated by the properties shown in Table 18.7.

References
1. Douglas, J.D., K.N. Tanner, J.R. Prine, D.C. Van Riper, and S.K. Derwelis. Molluscum contagiosum in chimpanzees. *J. Am. Vet. Med. Ass.* 151:901–904, 1967.
2. Downie, A.W., C.H. Taylor-Robinson, A.E. Caunt, G.S. Nelson, P.E.C. Manson-Bahr, and T.C.N. Matthews. Tanapox: A new disease caused by a pox virus. *Brit. Med. J.* 1:363–368, 1971.
3. Yohn, D.S., V.A. Haerdiges, and J.T. Grace, Jr. Yaba tumor poxvirus synthesis *in vitro*. I. Cytopathological, histochemical, and immunofluorescent studies. *J. Bact.* 91:1977–1985, 1966.

Swinepox Subgroup

True swinepox occurs in most areas where pigs are raised. The subgroup at this time consists of only one virus biotype, which is an immunologically distinct member of the poxvirus group and has not been assigned a specific genus name. This disease must be differentiated from vaccinia virus infection of swine, which produces a similar clinical picture and is sometimes called pigpox.

In pigs free of biting arthropods, the virus usually produces a benign disease characterized by the appearance of pustular skin lesions on the ventral abdominal skin surface or in the inguinal and scrotal regions. Usually only localized pock lesions are seen in arthropod-free pigs. If hog lice or other biting arthropods are present, they disseminate the virus to other skin areas and multiple pock lesions will be seen. Mechanical transmission by the hog louse is frequently encountered in larger population of pigs reared in close contact.[6]

The best source of the virus for isolation and identification is from early skin lesions or from dried scabs. No lesions are produced on the CAM of embryonating chicken eggs or on the scarified skin of rabbits or guinea pigs. A localized skin reaction in the rabbit can be elicited with a high multiplicity of virus, but the virus is not serially transferred by passage of rabbit lesion material.[3]

The virus only infects in vitro the cells derived from swine, producing a nuclear vacuolation and cytoplasmic inclusions.[4] The CPE is evidenced generally only after serial passage of infected cells. Detection of viral antigen in first passage cell culture can readily be done by use of the FA technique.[2] This procedure is more rapid than adapting the virus to cells by passage in order to visualize the CPE of the virus.

Swine produce low levels of VN antibodies, limiting the usefulness of serologic procedures for diagnostic purposes. No cross-protection is seen between swinepox virus and vaccinia. Pigs recovered from swinepox are immune to reinfection.

The virion is ether sensitive and is morphologically similar to the virion of the vaccinia poxvirus subgroup but somewhat larger.[1,2] The virus is species specific and is readily transmitted experimentally to other susceptible pigs.[5,6]

Specific diagnosis depends on EM demonstration of the virion in skin lesions, the histopathologic demonstration in affected epidermal cells of characteristic cytoplasmic inclusion bodies and intranuclear vacuolation, or the demonstration of pathogenicity of the suspect material for young susceptible pigs and negative results with other animals.

References

1. Cheville, N.F. The cytopathology of swine pox in the skin of swine. *Am. J. Path.* 49:339–352, 1966.
2. Cheville, N.F. Immunofluorescent and morphologic studies on swinepox. *Path. Vet.* 3:556–564, 1966.
3. Datt, N.S. Comparative studies of pigpox and vaccinia viruses. I. Host range pathogenicity. *J. Comp. Path.* 74:62–69, 1964.
4. Kasza, L., E.H. Bohl, and D.O. Jones. Isolation and cultivation of swine pox virus in primary cell cultures of swine origin. *Am. J. Vet. Res.* 21:269–273, 1960.
5. Schwarte, L.H., and H.E. Biester. Pox in swine. *Am. J. Vet. Res.* 2:136–140, 1941.
6. Shope, R.D. Swine pox. *Arch. ges. Virusforsch.* 1:457–467, 1940.

19. Reoviruses

The name reovirus was originally proposed as a group name for a number of viruses previously classified as being identical with, or related to, ECHO type 10 virus, and in fact reovirus is an acronym for respiratory-enteric-orphan viruses. These viruses are approximately 60–70 nm in diameter and have icosahedral symmetry. They have no envelope, are ether resistant, contain double-stranded RNA arranged in a double-helical configuration, and are replicated in the cytoplasm of the cell. Three serotypes are known to exist and they infect humans and almost every species of animal so far examined. Although found in both the respiratory and enteric tract, they are as yet not causally associated with any disease.

Specimens

Reoviruses have been recovered from almost every conceivable type of specimen, but statistically, most isolates from living animals have come from fecal specimens. Specimens should be collected as early in the course of illness as possible, though reoviruses can be found in the feces of some individuals for weeks. Reoviruses have also been obtained from tissue grown in culture when suspensions of such tissue failed to yield virus by direct inoculation into TC.[2] Specimens should be stored in the frozen state at as low a temperature as possible. Reoviruses are generally considered relatively stable agents, but few data are available on their stability in clinical specimens.

Laboratory Procedures

Cultures. Mammalian reoviruses replicate and produce CPE in a remarkably wide variety of cell cultures, including cultures derived from domestic animals as well as those of primate origin. The type of cell culture that has been the most widely used for recovery of reoviruses from naturally infected animals is *Macaca* monkey kidney. In addition, KB (Karl Bis----) cells, HeLa cells, human fibroblasts, stable human amnion lines, primary human embryonic kidney, primary *Cercopithecus* kidney, BS-C-1 cells, and L-cells, among others, have been used in experimental studies.

Primary *Macaca* kidney cell cultures are satisfactory for routine isolation, but primary human embryonic kidney should be used in very critical work when the possibility of latent reovirus infection in the cells themselves must be excluded. Reovirus type 1 has been recovered frequently from simian kidney cell cultures maintained for long periods of time, suggesting that the virus was present in a latent state in the cells. However, latent reovirus infection has not been encountered when *Macaca* kidney cells are used as described below, nor have they been recovered from uninoculated human kidney cell cultures, even when the latter have been maintained for long periods of time.

Reoviruses can sometimes be isolated directly in newborn mice, although few isolates have been obtained in this way; cell cultures are believed to be more sensitive. A possible source of error in using mice is the presence of pre-existing reovirus type 3 infection in most colonies of laboratory mice.

Tube cultures of primary kidney cells are used when a confluent monolayer of cells has appeared. It is important that the cultures be washed free of serum before use, since it is likely that any mammalian serum present in the growth medium contains antibodies to one or more reovirus serotypes. Washing is accomplished by replacing the growth medium with three successive changes of 1 ml of Hanks' BSS containing 100 units of penicillin and 100 μg of streptomycin per ml. After the last change, 1 ml of Medium 199 or MEM with the same concentration of antibiotics is added as a maintenance medium.

The specimen is then inoculated into one or more culture tubes in 0.1 ml amounts. Tubes are incubated in the stationary position at 36–37°C and are observed microscopically every 2 or 3 days for 21 days. At the end of this time interval, 0.1 ml of the supernatant fluid of each tube is passed to a fresh culture tube that has been prepared in the same manner as the original tube. The passage tubes are incubated and observed in the same manner for 7 days. Maintenance fluid is not changed on either the original or the passage tube, and the isolation tubes are ordinarily kept for 21 days, even though the cell sheet may have degenerated before then.

The CPE typical of the reoviruses is often not seen in isolation tubes that are inoculated with relatively small amounts of virus. However, after 21 days even a very small amount of virus usually will have increased to the extent that typical CPE is seen in the passage tube. Even though the *Macaca* kidney cultures used in the isolation procedure could be maintained in better condition by periodic changing of the maintenance medium, such a procedure usually is not undertaken because of the increased risk of viral cross-contamination and because it is not necessary for the isolation of reoviruses.

Reoviruses usually can be distinguished from other viruses that are encountered in fecal specimens by the nature of their CPE in unstained *Macaca* kidney cultures. The cells become granular and do not slough off the glass as readily as do cells affected by most enteroviruses. Often they remain fastened to the glass by a single process and flutter in the medium as the tube is agitated during microscopic examination. The typical effect usually can be recognized with experience, but it is often confused with nonspecific cellular degeneration by inexperienced personnel. Of course, doubtful cases can be resolved by additional cell culture passages. One way to gain experience is to observe the effect of various dilutions of a known reovirus in *Macaca* kidney cultures of good quality.

Reoviruses can also be recognized by the cytoplasmic inclusions seen by conventional microscopy in stained preparations of infected cell cultures and by their intra- or extracellular morphology when examined with the electron microscope. Other characteristics of mammalian reoviruses that may assist in differentiating them from viruses of other groups are their (1) resistance to inactivation by ethyl ether, (2) size of 60–75 nm, (3) ability to agglutinate human RBC, (4) ability to produce CPE in cell cultures from a variety of animal species, (5) ability to multiply in a wide variety of animal hosts (some strains produce clinical disease in newborn mice), and (6) presence of a common CF antigen.

Animal inoculation. Type-specific immune sera can be prepared in guinea pigs, chickens, and geese.[1,10] Because the sera of guinea pigs frequently contain HI antibodies against one or more reovirus serotypes, preimmunization sera should be tested against antigens of each of the three serotypes before animals of this species are employed for immune serum production.

Guinea pigs can be immunized by instilling 0.1 ml of undiluted cell culture fluid into each nostril of an anesthetized animal. The virus titer of the fluid is not critical since reoviruses multiply in guinea pigs after intranasal inoculation. (Note that the infected guinea pigs can transmit their infection to animals housed in the same cage.) Animals should be exsanguinated as soon as a trial bleeding indicates that a sufficiently high titer of homotypic HI antibody (1:160) has appeared (usually 2–3 weeks after inoculation). The final serum also must be tested to determine if the animal has responded with only a type-specific reaction. Some animals develop heterotypic antibodies. An immune serum is considered satisfactory if it has a homotypic HI titer of at least 1:160 and heterotypic titers of less than 1:10. The preimmunization serum of each animal yielding a satisfactory immune serum should be preserved for reference purposes for use in the event that equivocal results are obtained in typing an isolate with the postimmunization serum. Considerable antigenic variation has been noted among strains of type 2; it may be necessary to prepare several immune sera for this serotype, using different strains as antigens.

Preimmunization sera of chickens and geese that are to be used for immune serum production should also be tested for HI antibodies against mammalian reoviruses, since there is one report of such antibodies in chickens.[17] Chickens can be immunized by a series of three IM inoculations of 1 ml of undiluted cell culture fluid given a week apart, followed by exsanguination 1 week after the last inoculation. Geese can be immunized by an initial inoculation of 10 ml of cell culture fluid IP and 5 ml IV, followed by 5 ml IP on day 15, 5 ml IV on day 27, 2 ml IM on day 40, and exsanguination on day 50. Domestic fowl apparently do not transmit mammalian reoviruses to each other and can be housed in the same cage. However, as with guinea pigs, postimmunization sera should be tested for homotypic and heterotypic antibodies and preimmunization sera should be preserved. Most mammalian species will respond with heterotypic antibodies when immunized with repeated parenteral inoculations of a single mammalian reovirus serotype.

Satisfactory immune sera can also be obtained by careful selection of sera from humans, cats, or cattle with naturally acquired antibodies.[10,16] Individual sera are tested against antigens of each of the three serotypes until some are found with the desired homotypic titers and the absence of heterotypic titers.

Immunology and serology. Mammalian reoviruses are usually identified as to serotype by HI techniques. All isolates so far described have the property of agglutinating human RBC, although this phenomenon is sometimes difficult to demonstrate with strains of type 3.

Human RBC are collected in Alsever's solution (glucose, 2.05 g; sodium citrate, 0.8 g; citric acid, 0.055 g; NaCl, 0.42 g/100 ml of distilled water; autoclave at 10 lb [68.9 kPa] pressure for 1 minute); add 10–20 ml of blood to 50 ml of the solution. The cells are then washed three times in dextrose-gelatin-Veronal (DGV) solution and can be stored as a 10% suspension in this solution for at least 1 week after collection. If the RBC are to be used less than 24 hours after collection, they can be washed and stored temporarily in 0.85% NaCl. Slightly higher titers have been reported when reoviruses are tested with human type A or AB rather than with type O RBC.

To minimize variation in the number of RBC employed in titrations of HA and in HI tests, the concentration of cells is standardized by means of a spectrophotometer. The standard value is determined by allowing 0.2 ml amounts of varying concentrations of human RBC in 0.85% NaCl to settle at room temperature in test tubes (12×75 mm) with hemispherical bottoms. The lowest concentration of cells producing a solid button of cells after complete sedimentation is chosen as the standard. The optical density of this test preparation is determined at a wave length of 490 nm on the spectrophotometer and thereafter all RBC suspensions are made at this value.

Supernatant fluid from infected tube cultures is tested for HA after the cell sheets have been completely destroyed by the virus and the cultures have been frozen and thawed once. Fluid from two or more culture tubes is usually pooled (before testing) in order to have enough hemagglutinin to complete the identification procedure. Serial twofold dilutions of the fluid are prepared in 0.85% NaCl in 12×75 mm test tubes. Dilutions should range from 1:2 to 1:1024 and each tube should contain 0.4 ml. The standard erythrocyte suspension is then added in 0.2 ml amounts. The tubes are shaken and the erythrocytes allowed to settle at room temperature. The highest dilution of cell culture fluid that shows a "one plus" pattern of sedimentation is taken as the endpoint, and this tube is considered to contain 1 unit of hemagglutinin.[3]

It is usually possible to demonstrate agglutination of human erythrocytes by strains of reovirus types 1 and 2 in any passage fluid from *Macaca* kidney cultures. However, strains of type 3 sometimes have low titers or give negative results when first tested. Thus far it has always been possible to obtain titers of hemagglutinin that are sufficiently high (20 units/ml) for purposes of identification of all strains of type 3 by testing additional passage levels. Hemagglutinin titers of type 3 strains are not necesssarily increased with continued cell culture passage. Rather it appears, for reasons unknown, that the multiplication of virus in one lot of cell cultures simply results in the production of a higher titer of hemagglutinin than does multiplication in another, grossly similar, lot of cultures.

HI tests for typing isolates are carried out as follows. First, the typing sera are absorbed with kaolin by mixing 1:5 dilution of serum in 0.85% NaCl with an equal volume of a 25% suspension of acid-washed kaolin in 0.85% NaCl (25 g of kaolin plus 100 ml of saline solution) and allowing the mixture to stand for 20 minutes at room temperature. The mixture is then centrifuged briefly to sediment the kaolin and the decanted supernatant fluid is considered as a 1:10 dilution of serum. After this treatment, the sera are adsorbed with human erythrocytes to remove any agglutinins for this type of cell that might be present. This is done by adding 0.1 ml of a 50% suspension of RBC to each 1 ml of the 1:10 dilution of serum and allowing the mixture to stand for 1 hour at approximately 4°C. The supernatant fluid is then decanted and is ready for use. The sera are not heat inactivated.

Since kaolin removes some antibody from serum, alternative methods of removing nonspecific serum inhibitors have been proposed.[9,14] However, these methods are more complicated and it has not been demonstrated that they offer any practical advantages.

The typing test is set by adding 0.2 ml amounts of hemagglutinin diluted in 0.85% NaCl so as to contain 20 units per ml (4 units per 0.2 ml) to 0.2 ml amounts of serial twofold dilutions of serum in 0.85% NaCl. Each serum is used from a dilution of 1:10 to, or beyond, its endpoint. The mixtures are shaken briefly and are then allowed to stand for 1 hour at room temperature before adding 0.2 ml amounts of the standard RBC suspension. The erythrocytes are allowed to settle at room temperature; the titer of a serum is that dilution which completely inhibits agglutination. The lowest dilution of each serum used is tested for the presence of RBC agglutinins by substituting 0.2 ml of saline solution for the antigen. An antigen titration is also included in the test.

An isolate is considered typed if it is inhibited at a titer of at least 1:40 by one of the typing antisera, and not inhibited at a dilution of 1:10 by the others. Because of the antigenic heterogeneity of type 2 strains, it sometimes may be necessary to prepare an antiserum against the isolated strain in order to demonstrate a relationship to this serotype.[4]

Relatively little information is currently available on the reoviruses of domestic fowl. These agents can be isolated either in chicken kidney cell cultures or in embryonating eggs. They are typed by VN tests since no hemagglutinins have yet been detected.

Most serology of mammalian reovirus infections has been done with the HI test. Not only is this procedure simpler in general than either the VN or the CF test, but the latter two procedures are also less satisfactory for diagnostic purposes in reovirus infections for the following reasons. In the VN test, a relatively large amount of test virus is required in order to attain a CPE before the tissue cultures degenerate spontaneously. Consequently, small amounts of antibody are difficult to detect. In the CF test it is often difficult or impossible to detect CF antibodies in convalescent sera. Thus both tests are less sensitive than the HI test. When CF antibodies are present, they apparently are group- rather than type-specific.

A microneutralization test for reoviruses has been described as somewhat more sensitive than the conventional tube VN test, but it does not appear to offer any particular advantage for diagnostic purposes.[15] A method for preparing relatively potent reovirus CF antigens also has been described, but the use of such antigens in diagnosis has not been reported.

It has been possible to demonstrate a fourfold or greater rise in homologous HI antibody in practically all natural or experimental reovirus infections that have been observed. A fourfold or greater rise is considered a positive result. Animals infected with reovirus type 3 almost invariably show only a homotypic HI response, whereas those infected with types 1 or 2 often develop heterotypic antibody also.[12,13] The heterotypic titers are usually, but not always, lower than the homotypic titers.

Reoviruses have an exceptionally wide host range. Aside from humans, they have been recovered from naturally infected wild and laboratory mice, dogs, cats, cattle, *Macaca* and *Cercopithecus* monkeys, chimpanzees, quokkas (an Australian marsupial), chickens, ducks, and turkeys.[11,16] In so far as they have been studied, all mammalian reoviruses of the same serotype, including those from humans, are indistinguishable from each other.[11] With one exception, all reoviruses recovered from birds are distinguishable from the mammalian serotypes. Reovirus type 3 (a mammalian serotype) was reportedly isolated from the blood of several species of wild birds, but because the isolations were made in suckling mice there is some question as to the validity of the findings.

HI tests for reovirus sera are carried out by a technique similar to that already described for typing reovirus isolates. The test antigens are prepared with representative or with homotypic strains in the same manner as described previously.

When available, paired sera are always run in the same test and are usually titrated in twofold dilutions from 1:10 through 1:320 against each of the three viral serotypes. Because of the antigenic heterogeneity of type 2 strains, it may be necessary to use more than one antigen of this type. An antigen prepared from a strain isolated from the animal is the most satisfactory in type 2 infections. This procedure has not been found necessary for types 1 or 3.

Hemagglutination-inhibition or neutralizing antibodies against reovirus types 1, 2, or 3 have been found in the sera of all species of terrestrial mammals (including marsupials) that have been examined, and it is probably safe to assume that all mammals are susceptible to infection with one or more of these agents. At present, relatively little is known of the host range of the reoviruses recovered from domestic fowl.

Because much uncertainty exists as to the etiologic role of reoviruses in the illnesses from which they have been recovered, very little can be said about supplementary diagnostic procedures. However, an interstitial pneumonitis has been observed in both natural and experimental infections in various mammals.[5,6,7,8,18] Upper respiratory disease in domestic acats may be caused by a reovirus, but differentiation must be made from picornavirus and herpesvirus infections, which produce similar clinical syndromes.

References

1. Behbehani, A.M., L.C. Foster, and H.A. Wenner. Preparation of type-specific antisera to reoviruses. *Appl. Microbiol.* 14:1051–1053, 1966.
2. Bell, T.M. Viruses associated with Burkitt's tumor. *Prog. Med. Virol.* 9:1–34, 1967.1
3. Canock, R.M., and A.B. Sabin. The hemagglutinin of St. Louis encephalitis virus. I. Recovery of stable hemagglutinin from the brain of infected mice. *J. Immunol.* 70:271–285, 1953.
4. Hartley, J.W., W.P. Rowe, and J.B. Austin. Subtype differentiation of reovirus type 2 strains by hemagglutination-inhibition with mouse antisera. *Virology* 16:94–96, 1962.

5. Joske, R.A., D.D. Keall, P.J. Leak, N.F. Stanley, and M.N.I. Walters. Hepatitis-encephalitis in humans with reovirus infection. *Arch. Internal Med.* 113:811–816, 1964.
6. Lamont, P.H. Some bovine respiratory viruses. *Proc. Roy. Soc. Med.* 59:50–51, 1966.
7. Lamont, P.H., J.H. Darbyshire, P.S. Dawson, A.R. Omar, and A.R. Jennings. Pathogenesis and pathology of infection in calves with strains of reovirus types 1 and 2. *J. Comp. Path.* 78:23–33, 1968.
8. Lou, T.Y., and H.A. Wenner. Natural and experimental infections of dogs with reovirus, type 1: Pathogenicity of the strain for other animals. *Am. J. Hyg.* 77:293–304, 1963.
9. Mann, J.J., R.D. Rossen, J.R. Lehrich, and J.A. Kasel. The effect of kaolin on immunoglobulins: An improved technique to remove the non-specific serum inhibitor of reovirus hemagglutination. *J. Immunol.* 98:1136–1142.
10. Rosen, L. Serologic grouping of reoviruses by hemagglutination-inhibition. *Am. J. Hyg.* 71:242–249, 1960.
11. Rosen, L. Reoviruses in animals other than man. *Ann. N.Y. Acad. Sci.* 101:461–465, 1962.
12. Rosen, L., F.R. Abinanti, and J.F. Hovis. Further observations on the natural infection of cattle with reoviruses. *Am. J. Hyg.* 77:38–48, 1963.
13. Rosen, L., J.F. Hovis, F.M. Mastrota, J.A. Bell, and R.J. Huebner. An outbreak of infection with a Type 1 reovirus among children in an institution. *Am. J. Hyg.* 71:266–274, 1960.
14. Schmidt, N.J., J. Dennis, and E.H. Lennette. Studies on filtrates from cultures of a psychrophilic *Pseudomonas sp.* which inactivate non-specific serum inhibitors for certain hemagglutinating viruses. *J. Immunol.* 93:140–147, 1964.
15. Schmidt, N.J., E.H. Lennette, and M.F. Hanahoe. Microneutralization test for the reoviruses: Application to detection and assay of antibodies in sera of laboratory animals. *Proc. Soc. Exp. Biol. Med.* 121:1268–1275, 1966.
16. Scott, F.W., D.E. Kahn, and J.H. Gillespie. Feline viruses. VIII. The isolation, characterization, and pathogenic effects in the domestic cat of a feline reovirus. *Am. J. Vet. Res.* 31:11–13, 1969.
17. Stanley, N.F., and P.J. Leak. The serologic epidemiology of reovirus infection with special reference to the Rottnest Island Quokka (*Setonix Brachyurus*). *Am. J. Hyg.* 78:82–88, 1963.
18. Tillotson, J.R., and A.M. Lerner. Reovirus Type 3 associated with fatal pneumonia. *New Eng. J. Med.* 276:1060–1063, 1967.

20. Rhabdoviruses

As the name implies, rhabdoviruses are rod shaped, with one end flat and the other rounded like a blunt bullet. All rhabdoviruses have an RNA core. This virus group contains some plant as well as animal viruses, but only three animal pathogens will be discussed: vesicular stomatitis virus, rabies virus, and ephemeral fever virus.

Vesicular Stomatitis Virus

The disease caused by vesicular stomatitis virus (VSV) is clinically indistinguishable from foot-and-mouth disease (FMD), vesicular exanthema of swine (VES), and swine vesicular disease (SVD).[1,4] The disease is characterized by a febrile response accompanied by the formation of vesicles on the mucous membranes of the mouth, the epithelium of the tongue, the interdigital area of the feet, the coronary band, and occasionally the teats and other areas of the body.

VSV is a member of the genus *Vesiculovirus*. Its particles are heterogeneous with respect to length. Infectivity is associated with the longer rods of approximately 185 nm.[5,9,10] Short rods, approximately 70 nm in length, have been found to be noninfectious but autointerfering.[5,6,10]

Infectivity of VSV may be sustained reasonably well at 4°C for about 30 days, for longer periods at $-20°C$, and indefinitely at -50 to $-70°C$.

The disease is usually self-limiting, with recovery in about two weeks. It is of extreme importance, however, because in cattle and swine it resembles FMD, and like FMD it can be economically disasterous. Suspected cases should immediately be brought to the attention of appropriate state and federal authorities.[1] Currently, the disease is present only in North, Central, and South America; past outbreaks in Europe have been eradicated.[8]

A wide variety of mammalian and avian species are experimentally susceptible. The most common naturally susceptible species are cattle, horses, and swine.[7] Humans are susceptible and should exercise caution when in contact with lesions and aerosols; particular care should be exercised where insect vectors are known to be present.[3] Recent experimental studies suggest that VSV may have originated as a plant virus and spread to animals via arthropods. In laboratory studies, VSV is important as an agent for the detection and titration of interferon.[8]

Specimens

The same specimens as reported for FMD should be taken from animals suspected of having VSV infection. Vesicular fluid and/or vesicle coverings are good sources of virus, and biopsy of the regional lymph nodes will usually yield virus. A transient viremia is often present within 24–72 hours following exposure. Information on a carrier state is speculative.

Laboratory Procedures

Cultures. Suspect material, following filtration or treatment with antibiotics, may be inoculated into 8–10-day-old embryonating eggs (any route), primary cell cultures of mammalian and/or avian origin, and certain cell lines such as BHK-21 (CCL-10) or MDBK (CCL-22) (available from ATCC). Embryonating eggs die 48–72 hours after viral inoculation and virus can be recovered from all fluids and tissues of the egg. Cytopathology is produced in 8–12 hours in any of the above cells under routine conditions. Plaque formation occurs under agar or Methocel.

Animal inoculation. Infection and disease can be obtained by ID inoculation into the foot pad of guinea pigs or by IC inoculation into mice. Titration of VSV may be made in the tongue epithelium of cattle. When cattle are inoculated IM clinical disease does not result.

Immunology and serology. There are two serologically distinct types: New Jersey and Indiana.[2] There are three subtypes of the Indiana type: (1) the classic subtype (Ft. Lupton), (2) the Cocal (Trinidad) subtype, and (3) the Alagoas (Brazil) subtype.[2] The New Jersey serotype is represented by only one virus. The reference virus strain for New Jersey is Hazlehurst (ATCC VR-159); for Indiana it is Indiana Lab (ATCC VR-158). Two additional viruses have been isolated; they have been shown to be morphologically similar and serologically related to VSV Indiana: Piry virus isolated from a marsupial in Brazil, 1967, and Chandipura virus isolated from a man in India, 1967, and also in Africa, 1973.[8]

The serologic test of choice is the VN test, using constant virus and varying amounts of antibody. The PR test also is reliable and simple.[1,2,8] The CF and mouse protection (MP) tests are also useful. Statistically significant reduction of 2–4 logs in virus titer, as compared to controls, is obtained with 21-day convalescent antisera.[2] Clear-cut serologic differentiation is found between the Indiana and New Jersey types. Certain cross-reactions, which sometimes may require further examination, are seen between various Cocal-like isolates and the Indiana classic reference strain. Other tests include metabolic inhibition and resin-agglutination inhibition.[8]

Despite the persistence (2 years) of demonstrable circulating antibody, cattle and swine are often susceptible to experimental reinfection for 2–6 months after recovery. Field data indicate that immunity can better resist natural exposure, presumably because of lower challenge levels. Experimental vaccines against VSV have been developed but are not often used.[7,8]

References

1. Cottral, G.E. Diagnosis of bovine vesicular diseases. *J. Am. Vet. Med. Ass.* 161:1293–1298, 1972.
2. Federer, K.E., R. Burrows, and J.B. Brooksley. Vesicular stomatitis virus: The relationship between some strains of the Indiana serotype. *Res. Vet. Sci.* 8:103–117, 1967.
3. Fields, B.N., and K. Hawkins. Human infection with the virus of vesicular stomatitis during an epizootic. *New Eng. J. Med.* 277:988–994, 1967.
4. Graves, J.H., and P.D. McKercher. Swine vesicular disease. *Proc. 77th Ann. Mtg. U.S. Anim. Health Ass.*, pp. 155–159, 1973.
5. Hackett, A.J. A possible morphologic basis for the autointerference phenomenon in vesicular stomatitis virus. *Virology* 24:51–59, 1964.
6. Hackett, A.J., F.L. Schaffer, and S.H. Madin. The separation of infectious and autointerfering particles in vesicular stomatitis preparations. *Virology* 31:114–119, 1967.
7. Hanson, R.P. The natural history of vesicular stomatitis. *Bact. Rev.* 16:179–204, 1952.
8. Hanson, R.P. Vesicular stomatitis. In *Diseases of Swine*, H.W. Dunne and A.D. Leman (eds.), pp. 308–324. 4th ed. Iowa State University Press, Ames, 1975.
9. Howatson, A.F., and G.F. Whitmore. The development and structure of vesicular stomatitis virus. *Virology* 16:466–478, 1962.
10. Huang, A.S., J.W. Greenwalt, and R.R. Wanger. Defective T particles of vesicular stomatitis virus. I. Preparation, morphology, and some biological properties. *Virology* 30:161–172, 1966.
11. Tesh, R.B., B.R. Chaniotos, and K.M. Johnson. Vesicular stomatitis virus (Indiana serotype): Transovarial transmission of Phlebotomine sandflies. *Science* 175:1477–1479, 1972.

Rabies Virus

Rabies is an acute infectious disease of the CNS to which all warm-blooded animals are susceptible. The virus replicates in the salivary glands, lungs, kidneys, pancreas, and mammary glands; it can maintain a cycle in wildlife without causing encephalitis.[3] The permanent hosts of rabies virus in the United States appear to be spotted skunks, weasels, and other members of the Mustelidae family.[3] The mongoose is the main host in Puerto Rico and the vampire bat is an important reservoir of the virus from Mexico to South America. The clinical disease with encephalitis is mainly seen in carnivorous or biting animals such as dogs, cats, foxes, wolves, and coyotes. The world areas that presently do not have rabies include Australia, New Zealand, New Guinea, the islands of Oceania, Sweden, Norway, Great Britain, Japan, Taiwan, Hong Kong, and Malaya.

At the present time, only one serotype of rabies is known. The virus, classified as a rhabdovirus (genus *Lyssavirus*),[6] is an ether-sensitive, acid-labile RNA virus with a helical nucleocapsid. Like other viruses of the same group, it is a rod-shaped organism with one hemispherical and one flat end, 80×200 nm, and a helix diameter of 10–20 nm. The surface of the virion is studded with protrusions 6–7 nm long.[3]

The most common natural transmission of rabies virus depends upon the virus being emitted in sufficient quantity from the salivary glands in vector animals, such as dogs, foxes, skunks, and bats, to allow for introduction of virus into a bite wound or open lesion. Transmission can also occur by ingestion of infected material, by intranasal and rectal instillation of virus suspensions, and by inhalation of contaminated air. The implication of nonbite transmission of the disease is of definite epidemiologic significance. The African shrew is a carrier of mokola virus, a new rabies-like virus.

Specimens

The brain usually provides the best source of rabies virus in an infected animal. In addition, the salivary glands often contain virus and are of special epidemiologic importance. Therefore, when decapitating an animal in the field, care should be taken to avoid damaging the brain and to include the submaxillary salivary glands with the head.

The head must be cooled promptly and kept cold. It should be delivered to the diagnostic laboratory by messenger service if possible. If such service is not available, the head should be placed in a tin or other suitable water-tight metal container. This container should in turn be put into a larger water-tight metal container and cracked ice packed between the inner and outer container.

The virus will survive in frozen specimens shipped in dry ice; however, quick microscopic examination may be delayed because of the thawing time. If it is necessary to freeze the material, the brain and salivary glands should be removed from the head, since frozen tissue specimens are easier to handle than frozen whole heads.

When it is not feasible to ship tissues in ice, a solution of 50% glycerol-saline can be used (equal parts glycerol to 0.9% NaCl solution). Rabies virus will be preserved during shipment and no refrigeration will be required. The portions of brain or salivary gland to be preserved in glycerol solution should be about the size of a mouse brain (300 mg), to give the laboratory worker enough material to work with. Pieces from the hippocampus, cerebellum, and cerebral cortex from each side of the brain should be included, as well as a portion of the medulla.

Glycerolated portions of brain must be washed thoroughly in saline to produce satisfactory impressions, since it is difficult to make the glycerolated specimens adhere to a slide. For this reason, it may be desirable to make impression slides of the pieces of nonglycerolated brain and to stain them with Sellers' stain; the slides can be packed in the same carton with the jar containing the glycerolated brain specimens.

Laboratory Procedures

Animal inoculation. Mice, especially the laboratory strains of white Swiss mice, are susceptible to intercerebral injection of rabies virus and are the animals of choice for rabies virus isolation.[6] Of the other common species of laboratory animals—hamsters, guinea pigs, and rabbits—the hamster is considered most susceptible. However, large quantities of rabies virus can be grown in rabbit brains, and these have been used to prepare rabies vaccines.

With the exception of the mouse inoculation, no specific animal test is used routinely for examination of rabies virus. A guinea pig potency test for evaluation of rabies vaccines is used by manufacturers of the products and by the Veterinary Biological Control Division of APHIS at NADC. Details for such a test can be obtained from that division. Rabbies vaccines have been fairly successful.[1,4,7,8,9]

Cultures. Laboratories that furnish rabies diagnostic services should be equipped to carry out mouse inoculation tests, since surveys have shown that even with the fluorescent rabies antibody (FRA) test, cases of rabies can be missed in direct microscopic examination of tissues. When microscopic examinations are negative or questionable, samples of the cerebral cortex, cerebellum, and hippocampus on each side of the brain, plus a sample from the brain stem, should be inoculated into mice. The procedure for virus isolation is as follows:

1. Portions of tissue (brain or salivary gland) are ground using either a chilled mortar

and pestle, a Ten Broeck grinder, or an electric blender, depending on the quantity of tissue to be triturated. Every precaution must be taken during this process to prevent creation of an aerosol of virus-laden material.

2. Diluent is added in the volume of four times the weight of tissues to make a 20% suspension. A commonly used diluent consists of 10% heat-inactivated animal serum (free of rabies antibodies) in physiological saline solution. Addition of 5000 units of penicillin and 500 μg of streptomycin per ml of diluent is often included to inhibit bacterial contamination.

3. The suspension is centrifuged for 5 minutes at 1000 rpm. An aliquot of this suspension should be diluted with an equal volume of diluent to make a 10% suspension for mouse inoculation. The remaining portion should be frozen at -40 to $-70°C$ for later reference if needed.

4. At least five 3–5-week-old mice under light anaesthesia should be inoculated intracerebrally with 0.03 ml amounts of suspension. Young mice are more sensitive to rabies infection than adult animals.

5. Mice are observed daily for at least 21 days. Deaths that occur within the first 48 hours after intracerebral inoculation are attributable to causes other than rabies virus (trauma, bacterial contamination, other viruses).

6. Mice showing signs of illness and paralysis may be rabid. Brains from these mice should be examined by the FRA test or Sellers' stain for rabies virus Negri bodies.

Rabies virus may be adapted to embryonating chicken eggs.[5,4,9] Baby hamster kidney cell cultures also are used to grow rabies virus, especially for use in serologic tests.[1]

Serologic identification of virus. The FRA test is a highly sensitive and specific test for detecting rabies virus in tissues and is the method of choice in initial examination of all rabies specimens. The direct method of FA staining is the one most commonly used in rabies diagnosis. The general procedure is as follows:

1. A longitudinal incision is made with sterile scissors into the dorsal surface of each cerebral hemisphere about 2 cm lateral to the longitudinal fissure on the midline of the brain. The incision is made from the occipital pole of the hemisphere and is extended forward 3–5 cm. The incision is made downward through the gray matter and then through the white matter until the lateral ventricle is reached. This will appear as a narrow space with a natural separation from the white matter of the cerebrum. The opening is widened by spreading the incised hemisphere, and Ammon's horn will be revealed as a semicylindrical white glistening body bulging laterally from the ventrical floor. It has a spiral contour and, on a cross-section, a characteristic rolled surface. A small cross-section of Ammon's horn is removed with the scissors and placed on a wooden spatula to make impression smears.

2. Small sections of the cerebral cortex and the cerebellum are removed and placed on wooden spatulas for impression smears.

3. The above procedures are then repeated for the opposite side of the brain so at least six slides are prepared from these three areas on each side of the brain.

4. When preparing smears from mouse brain, the entire brain is removed and placed on a wooden spatula. The anterior and posterior areas of the brain are cut off with a sharp scalpal. The center section is used for preparing the smears.

5. A microscope slide is touched very lightly to the brain cross-sections. Duplicate impression smears are made on the same microscope slide. The slide is allowed to dry for about 30 minutes.

6. The slide is dropped into a Coplin jar containing acetone at $-20°C$ and fixed for 4 hours. It is then removed from acetone and allowed to drain dry while still in the freezer.

7. Previously prepared slides fixed in the manner described can be stored in the freezer for 1 month or more to be used as known positive and negative controls.

8. Before staining with the fluorescent material, positive and negative control slides as well as test slides are removed from the freezer and allowed to warm to room temperature.

9. Areas of smear are surrounded with Vaseline-ether solution or Marktex pen to retain conjugate over the desired area during incubation.

10. Two equal portions of fluorescein-conjugated antirabies globulin are diluted; one with the recommended volume of dilution A, normal 20% mouse brain suspension (NMB), and the other with the recommended volume of dilution B, rabies 20% mouse brain suspension (RMB).

11. One smear of each slide is covered with a small drop of dilution A, the other with dilution B. The slides are then placed in a humid chamber (a plastic slide box with a wet blotter in the cover) at 37°C for 30 minutes.

12. The box lid is removed and the box of slides is immersed for 10 minutes in a pan of buffered saline. After the saline solution is poured off, a final rinse in distilled water will prevent formation of salt crystals during the drying. The smears are then drained dry.

13. Coverslips are mounted using glycerol mounting medium (90% glycerol buffered at pH 7).

To interpret the FRA test, examine the three slides with a UV microscope (see Chapter 5). The positive control slide consists of two impression smears of a known positive brain (e.g. mouse). First, examine the impression smear stained with dilution A containing antirabies fluorescein–conjugated globulin and NMB. This mixture should stain any rabies antigen in the impression. The green aggregates of staining appear as Negri bodies and/or as fine dustlike green fluorescing material.

Next, examine the impression covered with dilution B containing fluorescein-conjugated antirabies globulin and RMB (usually challenge virus standard, CVS). There should be an inhibition of green staining on this impression since the tagged antibody was absorbed by the RMB suspension. If any green staining is seen in this smear, the test is not conclusive and measures should be taken to determine the reason for the staining and to eliminate it.

The negative control slide consists of two impression smears of a known normal brain. Both impressions should be stained and read after the positive control slide. No green fluorescence should be observed.

As in the control slides, in the test slide the impression stained with dilution A is examined first; then the impression stained with dilution B is examined. If green fluorescence like that in the positive control slide is observed in the impression stained with dilution A and no green fluorescence is seen in the impression stained with dilution B, the test slide is positive. If no green fluorescence is seen in either impression, the slide is negative.

Direct microscopic examination for Negri bodies

1. Surfaces of the hippocampus, cerebral cortex, and cerebellum are cut and placed—with cut surface up—on clean blotting paper or a wooden tongue depressor.

2. A clean microscope slide is touched against the cut surface of the section and pressed gently downward. Just enough pressure is exerted to create a slight spread of the exposed surface of tissue against the slide. Three to four impressions can be made on one slide.

3. While still moist, the slide is covered with Sellers' stain (modified Lentz stain is also widely used), allowed to remain for a few seconds, rinsed with tap water, and dried at room temperature without blotting.

4. The slide is examined first under low power. Areas containing numerous large neurons to be examined for Negri bodies under immersion oil are selected.

The Negri body is usually rounded but can assume any shape. There is also great variation in size; generally, it is 0.24–27 μm in diameter. It characteristically stains acidophilic and is positioned in the cytoplasm within the neuron. However, the intracytoplasmic position of the Negri body can be expected with reasonable consistency only in fixed, cut histologic sections of the brain. In the tissue-impression techniques described above, normal structure is disturbed and Negri bodies often appear outside the neuron.

There is universal agreement that the Negri body is pathognomonic for rabbies. However, animal brains may contain other types of inclusion bodies that may be mistaken for Negri bodies. The acidophilic inclusion bodies of canine distemper or canine infectious hepatitis (fox encephalitis) are occasionally seen in the brains of dogs and foxes. Nonspecific acidophilic inclusion bodies are sometimes seen in the brains on nonrabid cats and laboratory white mice. The following outline is useful in the differentiation of Negri bodies and other inclusions occasionally seen:

Negri bodies	*Nonrabies inclusion bodies*
Presence of basophilic inner granules	Absence of internal structure
Heterogeneous matrix	Homogeneous matrix
Less refractive	More refractive
Magenta (heliotrope) tinge	Color more acidophilic (pinker)

Serologic diagnosis. The VN test is used for titration of antibodies in rabies hyperimmune serum that is to be used in the FRA test and for testing human or animal sera for antibodies to rabies. The CVS strain of fixed rabies virus is the standard reference virus; it is prepared as a 20% suspension of infected infant mouse brains. Both the constant serum–varying virus dilutions and the constant virus–varying serum dilutions tests are used. The serum-virus mixtures are incubated at 37°C for 1 hour. Infant mice inoculated IC are used as the test animals. The indirect FA test or the fluorescent focus inhibition test (FFIT) also can be used to test sera.

Stain formulas: Sellers' stock solutions. (1) Use 10 g of methylene blue (*Color Index,* no. 52015);[2] add enough methanol (absolute, acetone-free) to make 1000 ml. (2) Use 5 g basic fuchsin (*Color Index,* no. 42510);[2] add enough methanol (absolute, acetone-free) to make 500 ml.

Select dry dyes with a high content of methylene blue, preferably not less than 85%; for basic fuchsin, use preferably not less than 92%. While absolute, acetone-free methanol is recommended, CP methanol may be substituted if desired. The stock solutions are stored in screw-capped or ground glass–stoppered bottles.

For the staining solution, use 2 parts methylene blue (stock solution no. 1); 1 part basic fuchsin (stock solution no. 2). The solution is mixed thoroughly but not filtered. It is stored in screw-capped or ground glass–stoppered container. The mixed stain improves after standing for 24 hours and keeps indefinitely if protected from evaporation.

When the stock solutions have been accurately prepared, the above proportions will usually produce a stain that gives the desired color differentiation. However, it is well to make a trial stain. If the desired differentiation is not obtained, the stain can readily be adjusted. If the stroma is a bright red rather than rose-pink in the thinner areas, and the overall staining effect is reddish, the fuchsin is too dominant. Add methylene blue stock solution in measured amounts, checking with a trial stain after each addition until the desired color balance is obtained. When the methylene blue is too dominant, the Negri bodies are a deep muddy maroon color and the nerve cells stain too deeply. Adjustment may be made with the fuchsin stock solution in this case.

If the researcher wishes to use the modified Lentz rabies stain, the following solutions should be prepared: (1) methylene blue (saturated alcoholic)—2 g methylene blue plus 100 ml absolute ethanol; (2) basic fuchsin (saturated alcoholic)— 8.16 g basic fuchsin plus 100 ml absolute ethanol; (3) methyl alcohol with picric acid—0.25 g sodium carbonate (anhydrous) plus 0.5 g picric acid plus 500 ml methanol (absolute); mix the methanol and the Na_2CO_3, then add the picric acid (the sodium carbonate does not all dissolve); (4) stain (made fresh each time it is used)—9 drops methylene blue solution plus 2 drops basic fuchsin solution plus 30 ml *tap* water.

The procedure is as follows: (1) fix the slides in methyl alcohol with picric acid for 2 minutes, (2) air dry after fixing, (3) flood the slides with stain, (4) steam gently for 3 minutes, (5) rinse with tap water, (6) air dry and apply coverslip.

Negri bodies should stain magenta; RBC, salmon; nerve cells, blue.

References

1. Abelseth, M.K. An attenuated rabies vaccine for domestic animals produced in tissue culture. *Can. Vet. J.* 5:279–286, 1965.
2. *Color Index.* 4 vols. 2d ed. Society of Dyers and Colorists, Bradford, Yorkshire, Eng., and the American Association of Textile Chemists and Colorists, Lowell, Mass., 1956–1958.
3. Johnson, H.N. Rabies virus. In *Manual of Clinical Microbiology,* E.H. Lennette, E.H. Spaulding, and J. Truant (eds.), pp. 746–753. 2nd ed. American Society for Microbiology, Washington, 1974.
4. Koprowski, H,. J. Black and W.A. Johnson. Rabies in cattle. IV. Vaccination of cattle with high egg-passage chicken embryo-adapted rabies virus. *J. Am. Vet. Med. Ass.* 127:363–366, 1955.
5. Koprowski, H., and H.R. Cow. Studies on chick-embryo adapted rabies virus. I. Cultural characteristics and pathogenicity. *J. Immunol.* 60:533–544, 1948.
6. Lennette, E.H., and R.W. Emmons. The laboratory diagnosis of rabies: Review and prospective. In *Rabies,* Y. Nagano and F.M. Davenport (eds.), pp. 77–90. University Park Press, Baltimore, 1971.

7. Marx, M.B., and R.K. Sikes. Immunizing horses against rabies. *J. Am. Vet. Med. Ass.* 149:1159–1161, 1966.
8. Schmidt, R.C., and R.K. Sikes. Immunization of foxes with inactivated rabies vaccine. *Am. J. Vet. Res.* 29:1843–1847, 1968.
9. Starr, L.E., T.V. Clower, C.L. Bromley, and C.F. Routh. Antirabic immunization of cattle in Georgia using living virus vaccine of chick embryo origin. *Vet. Med.* 49:366–371, 1954.

Bovine Ephemeral Fever Virus

Bovine ephemeral fever (snyonyms: three-day sickness, bovine epizootic fever) is a noncontagious, arthropod-transmitted virus disease of cattle. It is characterized by fever (104–107°F, 40–41.7°C), anorexia, lacrimation, serous nasal discharge, drooling, depression, weakness, lameness, recumbency, and occasionally paresis. Clinical signs appear suddenly and regress in 3–5 days; spontaneous recovery is usual and rapid. Sequelae other than lameness are generally rare. A mortality rate of about 2% has been reported in purebred European-type cattle in Australia.[5] In milk cows there is cessation of lactation and, following recovery, milk production often fails to return to normal levels until the next lactation.[5] In fatal cases or in animals killed during the acute stage of the disease, the main lesions found include subcutaneous emphysema, edema of lymph nodes, and inflammation of nasal and ocular mucosa and joints.[2,5]

The disease was first described in South Africa in 1867.[2] Currently, the disease is seen in many parts of Africa, the Middle East, Pakistan, India, Indonesia, Australia, and Japan.[5] Ceratopogonid gnats have been incriminated as important vectors of the disease.[2]

The rod-shaped ephemeral fever virus (EFV) has dimensions of about 70×145 nm with an outer envelope of about 12 nm.[3] The virus is inactivated by ether, deoxycholate, high and low pH, or heat at 56°C for 10 minutes.[1] When stabilized with PBS plus 10% bovine serum, EFV may be stored for long periods at $-70°C$ or in the lyophilized state.[1] Infectivity declines rapidly at 4°C.[1]

Specimens

Animals in the acute stage of the disease should be selected for the collection of blood samples.[5] The virus is mainly associated with the buffy coat (leukocyte-platelet fraction) of blood.[5] Thus the blood should be collected in a sterile flask containing glass beads so it can be shaken for defibrination. The specimens may then be frozen for shipment.

Laboratory Procedures

Cultures. Samples of defibrinated blood are inoculated IC in newborn mice,[2,6] or cattle are inoculated IV, to reproduce the disease.[2] About 20% infected mouse brain or the buffy-coat fraction from infected cattle may be used as the source of viral antigen for serology.[6]

By the sixth or ninth serial passage IC in suckling mice, EFV becomes adapted to this host, causing paralysis and death within 2–4 days.[2,6] The mouse-adapted EFV is readily adapted to cell cultures within three or four passages.[1,2] In BHK-21 cell line and monkey kidney cell lines (MS and Vero), CPE develops in about 48–72 hours.[2] The plaque technique also may be used.

Animal inoculation. The EFV is very host specific, affecting only cattle under natural conditions. Experimentally, the disease was not transmitted when inoculated IV in horses, sheep, goats, dogs, rabbits, guinea pigs, rats, or adult mice.[5]

Immunology and serology. Neutralizing antibodies can be detected in serum of cattle by VN tests in suckling mice or cell cultures, or by the PR test in Vero cell cultures.[2,6]

Precipitating antibodies are demonstrable by the AD technique.[2] Buffy-coat fraction of whole blood from cattle during acute illness, 20% infected mouse brain, or 100–250× concentrated infected BHK or MS cell debris serve as suitable antigens for the precipitin test.[2] CF antibodies have been demonstrated using antigen prepared from infected bovine buffy coat or from infected mouse brain suspension.[5,6]

The existence of different serotypes has not been established. It has been reported that recovery from clinical disease confers solid immunity; however, instances of repeated attacks have been recorded in the field.[5] Multiple subcutaneous inoculations of mouse or cell culture–adapted EFV in oil adjuvant usually stimulate high titers of neutralizing antibody, and cattle thus inoculated are usually resistant to infection with virulent virus.[2,3]

Because bovine ephemeral fever is not present in the United States, suspected cases should be reported promptly to state and federal officials.

References

1. Heuschele, W.P. Bovine ephemeral fever. I. Characteristics of the causative virus. *Arch. ges. Virusforsch.* 30:195–202, 1970.
2. Heuschele, W.P., and D.C. Johnson. Bovine ephemeral fever. II. Response of cattle to attenuated and virulent virus. *Proc. 73d Ann. Mt. U.S. Anim. Health Ass.,* pp. 185–195, 1969.
3. Holmes, I.H., and R.L. Doherty. Morphology and development of bovine ephemeral fever virus. *J. Virol.* 5:91–96, 1970.
4. Lecatsas, G., A. Theodoridis, and B.J. Erasmus. Electron microscopic studies on bovine ephemeral fever virus. *Arch. ges. Virusforsch.* 28:390–398, 1969.
5. Mackerras, I.M., M.J. Mackerras, and F.M. Burnet. Experimental studies of ephemeral fever in Australian cattle. *CSIRO Bull.* 136, 1970.
6. Westhuizen, Van der, B. Studies on bovine ephemeral fever. I. Isolation and preliminary characterization of a virus from natural and experimentally produced cases of bovine ephemeral fever. *Onderstepoort J. Vet. Res.* 34:29–40, 1967.

21. Togaviruses

The envelope covering these viruses is reminiscent of the roman toga, hence the name togavirus. The togaviruses include the alphavirus group and the flavivirus group of the arboviruses. The alphaviruses to be discussed are the equine encephalomyelitis viruses: eastern, western, and Venezuelan types. Wesselsbron disease virus represents the flavivirus group. In addition, there are three viruses that have morphologic similarities to the togaviruses and they have been tentatively classified as such: hog cholera, bovine viral diarrhea–mucosal disease, and equine arteritis virus.

Equine Encephalomyelitis Viruses

There are three known serologic types of equine encephalomyelitis viruses (EEV): eastern equine encephalomyelitis (EEE), western equine encephalomyelitis (WEE), and Venezuelan equine encephalomyelitis (VEE) viruses.[2] The diseases caused by these viruses are enzootic over parts of North, Central, and South America. In 1971, VEE virus moved as far north as Texas, but prompt control measures and a vaccination campaign halted and pushed back the disease.[3,4] EEE and WEE are occasionally diagnosed in the United States in unvaccinated horses and in humans.[2]

Horses, donkeys, mules, and humans are susceptible to the clinical disease.[2,3] The viruses have been isolated from many species of birds and certain reptiles without clinical disease and they probably serve as reservoir hosts.[5] The principal vectors are mosquitoes of the genera *Culex* and *Aedes*.[2] EEE and WEE cause clinical encephalitis in humans, which is often fatal. VEE causes an influenzalike disease in humans.[2] Affected horses have fever, hypersensitivity to sound and touch, muscular tremors (especially of facial and shoulder muscles), incoordination of movements, depression, and sometimes penile erection. As the disease progresses the animal becomes somnolescent, then comatose until death. There are no characteristic gross lesions, but typical encephalomyelitis lesions are seen microscopically.

The three EEV have single-standard RNA cores, a nucleocapsid with cubic symmetry, and a lipid-containing envelope with prominent surface projections. EEE virus has a diameter of about 54 nm, a buoyant density in sucrose of 1.18 g/ml, and a molecular weight of 58×10^6 daltons.[1] VEE virus has a diameter of about 60–75 nm and a molecular weight of 6×10^7 daltons.[3] WEE virus has a diameter of about 45–48 nm.[2]

Specimens

From recently expired or destroyed moribund animals, cubed specimens (about 2 cm) may be cut from the cerebrum, medulla, pons, and cerebellum for viral isolation and histologic examination. During the viremic stage of the disease (acute), blood with anticoagulant may be taken for viral isolation.

Laboratory Procedures

Cultures. Embryonating chicken eggs inoculated on the CAM are often used for viral isolation. The embryo may die within 18–48 hours after inoculation and lesions (pocks) may be seen on the CAM.

Animal inoculation. Suckling mice, 2–5 days old, may be inoculated IC for viral isolation. Adult mice also may be used. The mice should show CNS disease clinical signs between 2 and 8 days after inoculation.

Immunology and serology. The three serologic types of EEV can be distinguished from each other in VN tests. However, they share antigenic determinants detectable by CF and HI tests. Good vaccines are available for all three EEV.

References
1. Fuscaldo, A.A., H.G. Halestad, and E.J. Hoffman. Biological, physical, and chemical properties of eastern equine encephalitis virus. I. Purification and physical properties. *J. Virol.* 7:233–240, 1971.
2. Hanson, R.P. Virology and epidemiology of eastern and western arboviral encephalomyelitis of horses. *Proc. 3d Internat. Conf. Equine Infec. Dis.* (Paris), pp. 100–114, 1972.
3. Johnson, K.M., and D.H. Marten. Venezuelan equine encephalitis. In *Advances in Veterinary Science and Comparative Medicine,* C.A. Brandly and C.E. Cornelius (eds.), vol. 18, pp. 79–116. Academic Press, New York, 1974.
4. McConnell, S. Venezuelan equine encephalomyelitis: Past, present and future. J. Am. Vet. Med. Ass. 161:1579–1583, 1972.
5. Thomas, L.H., and C.M. Eklund. Over wintering of western equine encephalomyelitis virus in experimentally infected garter snakes and transmission to mosquitoes. *Proc. Soc. Exp. Biol. Med.* 105:52–55, 1960.

Wesselsbron Disease Virus

Wesselsbron disease (WD) is a viral infection of sheep, cattle, and humans. It resembles Rift Valley fever (RVF) clinically. It was first noted in the Wesselsbron district of Orange Free State, Republic of South Africa.[3] Serologic surveys in Chad (northern Africa) revealed antibodies for WD in 43% of sheep and in 40 of 54 wild ruminants tested.[1]

The WD virus affects humans more readily but less severely than does RVF virus. The incubation period is about 3–4 days and the fever lasts about 24–48 hours. There is acute muscular pain, which may persist for about a month. Some patients have a body rash and some have hyperesthesia over scalp.[1]

In sheep, the disease may have mild, peracute, or chronic forms. The main clinical finding is abortion.[3] If aborted, the fetus usually is not infected; if retained, the fetus may become infected and die. It then may be absorbed or mummified. Some lambs are born showing signs of encephalitis. The mortality rate in lambs is usually about 25–30%. Affected sheep often are jaundiced. The lesions are similar to RVF, that is, they are disseminated small hemorrhages.

Specimens

Acute phase blood with anticoagulant, liver, spleen, and paired serum samples from acute and convalescent stages should be taken as specimens. Early embryos, but not full-term ones, should have samples taken of liver and brain.

Laboratory Procedures

Cultures. Lamb kidney cell cultures may be used, but mouse inoculation is preferred. The BHK-21 cell line is now being used for viral replication.[2]

Animal inoculation. Both day-old and adult mice should be inoculated, some IC and others IP. Adult mice will not show signs of infection following IP inoculation. WD virus causes fatal encephalitis, whereas RVF virus causes a fatal hepatitis in both suckling and adult mice in 3-5 days by both IC and IP routes.

Immunology and serology. The VN and CF tests are used. No serologic relationships between WD and RVF viruses have been established.

References

1. Kokernot, R.H., K.C. Smithburn, and E. Kluge. Neutralizing antibodies against arthropod-borne viruses in the sera of domestic quadrupeds ranging in Tongaland, Union of South Africa. *Ann. Trop. Med. Parasit.* 55:73-85, 1961.
2. Lecatsas, G., and K.E. Weiss. Formation of Wesselsbron virus in BHK 21 cells. *Arch. ges. Virusforsch.* 27:332-338, 1969.
3. Weiss, K.E., D.A. Haig, and R.A. Alexander. Wesselsbron virus: A virus not previously described, associated with abortion in domestic animals. *Onderstepoort J. Vet. Res.* 27:183-195, 1956.

Hog Cholera Virus

Hog cholera (HC) virus is known as swine fever virus in English-speaking countries of the world except Canada and the United States. In Germany, the disease is known as *Virusschweinepest* and in France, *peste du porc*.

Hog cholera is a highly contagious disease characterized in the acute form by multiple hemorrhages, necrosis, and infarctions of the internal organs with 90-100% mortality.[15] In the chronic form the clinical signs of depression, anorexia, pyrexia, and constipation followed by diarrhea are less severe and recovery sometimes occurs, particularly in older swine. In herds infected with low virulent strains of the virus only infant pig mortality is observed, along with abortions and stillbirths.[6] Affected pigs usually suffer severely from the invasion of secondary agents.

The histopathologic lesions are those of damage to the capillaries and the reticuloendothelial system. Significant brain lesions consisting of vascular and perivascular cuffing, microgliosis, infiltration of meninges and choroid plexus, capillary hemorrhages, and hyalinization of the vascular wall are found.[19,34,39] Sections through the medulla, cerebellum, midbrain, thalamus, and cerebral cortex should be examined. The neurons are not usually affected.

The signs and lesions of HC are similar to those of African swine fever, salmonellosis, erysipelas, and pasteurellosis. Differential diagnosis is an important consideration but the finding of other pathogens does not rule out the presence of HC virus.

The HC virus (genus *Pestivirus*) is about 53 nm in diameter, is pleomorphic but roughly spherical, and is covered by a compact nondistinctive membrane.[22] The virion has a lipid-containing RNA core[29] (see BVD-MD virus reference 27).

Specimens

The tissues of choice are spleen, tonsils, and lymph nodes (preferably mandibular) for virus isolation or detection of viral antigen by the FA tissue-section technique.[4,5,36,38,51,52] Specimens from at least 4–6 pigs should be collected. Although there are usually an ample number of dead pigs, it is desirable to euthanatize some pigs that have high rectal temperatures and, although visibly sick, are still able to move about. An extremely effective way of selecting pigs is to collect blood samples from 8–10 pigs, perform TWBC counts, and kill those for specimens whose TWBC counts are less than 10,000.[54]

In chronic HC the runt of the litter is a prime candidate for the persistent tolerant infection syndrome. Tissue specimens should also be collected from aborted fetuses and stillborn pigs. Many herds with chronic HC have severe infant pig losses and return trips may be necessary to get a good sampling of tissues.

Serum samples for VN tests should be collected from convalescent pigs, aborting sows, and sows giving birth to dead pigs and small litters.[5] If vaccination with live virus vaccine has been employed, antibody titers may be due to the vaccine virus. In herds infected with low virulent strains of HC, the diagnosis may be confirmed by finding ascending antibody titers in the breeding swine.

Laboratory Procedures

Cultures. Hog cholera virus may be propagated in pig kidney cell cultures. Since it is not cytopathogenic the virus is detected by staining the infected cells with a conjugate prepared from HC antiserum.[3,5,36,44,48,51,53] Specimen tissue suspension or heparinized blood is inoculated on coverslip cultures. After incubation the coverslips are removed, fixed, and stained with the conjugate (see Chapter 5). The HC infected cells have a bright green color when viewed by fluorescent microscopy, in contrast to the darker green or brown color of the uninfected cells.

Hog cholera viral antigen may be detected in tissue sections cut with a microtome cryostat, stained with HC conjugate, and examined by fluorescent microscopy.[16,20,31,43,45,49,55] Blocks of tissue approximately 10 mm square and 3 mm thick are cut from tonsil (cross-section), spleen, and mandibular lymph node and then frozen on microtome chucks with OCT compound (Ames Co., Elkhart, Ind.) or water so as to form a supporting matrix around the block. Frozen sections 8 μm thick are cut and mounted on glass slides directly from the microtome blade. The mounted sections are immediately immersed in acetone for 10 minutes and dried. The sections are flooded with HC conjugate and incubated in a moist chamber for 30 minutes. As controls, additional sections from each tissue are stained in the same manner with a mixture of equal parts of (1) normal swine serum and HC conjugate, and (2) HC antiserum and HC conjugate.[20] An alternative control is a duplicate section of each tissue stained with normal swine serum conjugate.[9]

The conjugate is decanted from the slides, the sections are rinsed in PBS, pH 7.2, and then immersed in PBS for 10 minutes. The sections are rinsed once with distilled water and coverslips are applied with buffered glycerol. The infected cells are bright green and are found singly or in clusters. In many specimens from acutely infected pigs all of the cells are infected and the entire section will fluoresce. The fluorescence of the viral antigen is most easily detected in the epithelial cells of the tonsil section. Fluorescence in the germinal centers may be confused with the nonspecific brightness of macrophages. In difficult cases careful examination of the control sections is necessary. The specific fluorescence is blocked in the section stained with the antiserum-conjugate mixture, while it is only slightly reduced in the section treated with the normal serum-conjugate mixture. If normal swine serum conjugate is employed as a control the section should be negative for specific fluorescence and should provide an indicator of the degree of brightness inherent in the specimen tissue.

When fluorescence is observed only in the germinal centers of the tonsil and the epithelial cells are negative for viral antigen, confirmatory fluorescing cells should be detected in spleen and lymph node sections from the same pig. Blocks of known HC infected tissue should be sectioned and examined with each group of specimens.

Hog cholera antigen may be detected in tissue impressions or smears[1,4,6] using the same procedure as with the FA tissue-section technique.

A variety of other techniques have been employed to confirm the presence of HC virus in specimen tissues, such as the AD technique[32,37,41] and the exaltation of Newcastle disease (END)[26,27,28] tests. However, these methods lack the speed and accuracy of the FA techniques.

Animal inoculation. The pig is the only animal that develops clinical signs of disease when exposed to HC virus although the virus will replicate in other animals when inoculated experimentally, such as the rabbit, sheep, goat, deer, and calf.[2,24,30] Hog cholera virus was passaged successfully in 4–10-day-old suckling mice by IP inoculation.[17] Passages were made at 24-hour intervals. Pigs exposed to inoculum from passage levels 21, 30, 39, and 50 developed signs of HC. Several species of mammalian cell cultures are also susceptible to infection with HC virus.

The most sensitive system for detecting HC virus is the inoculation of specimen material into the natural host, the pig.[8,35] Blood or tissue suspension is inoculated IM into one or two weanlings (18 kg body weight) and the pigs are maintained in strict isolation. Plastic cages with negative airflow that permit feeding and watering without opening the cage door are excellent for this purpose. The source herd should be free of HC and BVD infection as determined by VN tests, and negative preinoculation tests should be obtained on sera from the test pigs.[7]

As soon as anorexia is observed or at 7 DPI, blood samples are collected and cultured for HC virus. If the pigs sicken and die, tonsil, spleen, and mandibular lymph node are cultured for virus. If the pigs recover or remain healthy through 21 DPI, serum specimens are obtained for the VN test and inoculations of virulent HC virus are administered.

The trial is considered positive if HC virus is recovered from the blood or tissues or if the pigs develop VN titers and are immune to the challenge virus. The trial is negative if the pigs remain healthy, fail to develop VN titers, and are susceptible to a virulent strain of HC virus. When test pigs become sick or die and HC is not isolated, differential examinations should include bacterial and viral culture for other swine pathogens. Blood samples should be cultured for virus routinely even though signs of HC infection are not observed, in order to detect the immune tolerant type of HC infection frequently found with low virulent strains of HC virus.[6]

Occasionally field specimens will contain *Salmonella* or *Erysipelothrix* species in addition to HC virus. Then it is necessary to either pass the tissue suspension through a bacteria-retaining filter before inoculation or administer appropriate antibiotics to the test pigs.

The presence of HC virus may also be confirmed through the use of HC antiserum or vaccine. Specimen material is inoculated SC into two pigs, one of which is also given 0.5–1 ml of HC antiserum per 0.45 kg of body weight. If the specimen contains HC virus, the passively immunized pig will remain healthy while the unprotected pig will develop signs of HC. If a source herd of HC vaccinated pigs is available, a pig with active immunity may be substituted for the serum pig. In either of these procedures, if the pig receiving only the specimen does not develop signs of HC, then at 21 DPI both pigs should be inoculated with virulent HC virus. The vaccinated pig or the pig receiving serum should be protected against the challenge virus.

If the specimen contains a bacterial pathogen then the susceptible and the HC immune pig may both become sick. An even more confusing situation may result if the HC antiserum contains antibodies that protect the pig against bacterial pathogens. In this case an erroneous diagnosis may be made.

The precision of the trial may be enhanced by using increased numbers of pigs, employing an extra susceptible pig for contact exposure, and varying the protective dose of serum. As a differential diagnosis, the sickness and death of the immune pigs in the trial may indicate the presence of ASF virus. Pigs previously infected with BVD virus will become acutely ill when exposed to virulent HC virus but will often recover because there is a degree of cross-protection produced by the BVD immune response.[50]

Immunology and serology. Serum antibody against HC virus may be detected with a VN test using pig kidney cell cultures and the FA technique.[7,40] Employing a fourfold dilution scheme, $\log_{10}$ titers of 0.6–1.2 (1:4 to 1:16) are detected as early as 21 days after infection and peak titers of 1.8–3 (1:64 to 1:1024) are found at 5–6 weeks. Coverslip cell cultures of PK-15 or primary SK cells are prepared. Cultures are employed in the test 48–72 hours after seeding when the monolayers are at least 75% confluent.

A cell culture–adapted strain of HC virus, such as strain A, may be propagated in 250 ml plastic bottle cultures of PK-15 cells containing 25 ml of medium.[7,40] A virus inoculum of approximately 20,000 infective doses is inoculated into each culture flask and the cultures are incubated at 37°C for 4 days. The virus is harvested by freezing and thawing the cultures and then clarifying the fluid by centrifugation, 1400 RCF (relative centrifugal force) for 20 minutes at 4°C. A standard virus suspension is prepared that will produce 3000–3800 foci of infected cells on a coverslip when 0.1 ml is inoculated. This virus suspension may be stored without loss of titer at −84°C for 4 months.

Serum from a healthy specific pathogen–free (SPF) pig is used for a negative control and serum from a pig hyperimmunized against HC virus for a positive control. All sera are heat inactivated at 56°C for 30 minutes before testing.

A constant virus inoculum is titrated against varying serum dilutions. The standard virus suspension is prepared in Earle's medium containing 0.5% lactalbumin hydrolysate and 25 mg $MgCl_2 \cdot 6 H_2O$ (5.07 g/L). This medium is also used for diluting the sera. A fourfold dilution scheme is set up so that final dilutions of 1:4 through 1:1024 are obtained when 1.5 ml of each serum dilution is mixed with an equal volume of the virus suspension. The serum dilution–virus mixtures are agitated and incubated at 37°C for 1 hour.

After incubation, 0.2 ml of each serum dilution–virus mixture is inoculated onto each of two coverslip cell cultures. Controls on each set of tests are performed as follows: HC virus suspension and HC hyperimmune serum, HC virus suspension and normal swine serum, HC virus suspension and diluting fluid, and diluting fluid alone.

The cell cultures are incubated at 37°C for 18–24 hours and the coverslips are removed, fixed, stained with HC conjugate, and examined by fluorescent microscopy.

The number of foci of fluorescing cells on each coverslip is determined by obtaining an average number of foci per microscopic field and multiplying it by a conversion factor relating the area of the field to the area of the coverslip. The endpoint titer of a serum is the dilution that reduces the number of foci by at least 90% compared with the count obtained on the normal serum control. If less than 90% reduction of foci is found in the 1:4 dilution, the serum is classified as negative for HC antibodies.

Titers ranging from 1.8–3 (1:64 to 1:1024) are found following recovery from infection with a sublethal strain of HC virus or the administration of a modified live-virus vaccine.[7] In chronic HC infections where it is often difficult to isolate the virus, the serologic evidence of the infection can be determined by finding HC antibody titers in convalescent pigs. Hog cholera titers have been found to persist as long as 4 years after vaccination in a closed herd. Baby pigs nursing HC immune sows will have titers as high as their dams due to the ingestion of colostrum.

A significant source of confusion in interpreting low HC antibody titers is the inapparent BVD infection of pigs that are maintained in close contact with infected cattle.[50] Pigs with VN titers of 1.5–3 against BVD-MD virus will have cross-reacting titers of 0.6–1.2 against HC virus.

On the basis of experimental and field evidence there is only one serotype of HC virus. Pigs that recovered from infection with field isolates of HC virus had specific VN test titers[7,10] and resisted exposure to virulent challenge strain (Ames) HC virus. However, a strain of HC virus that produced a persistent infection in experimentally infected pigs was found to have different antigenic properties than the highly virulent Ames strain.[42]

Evidence has been developed that HC virus should be classified with the togaviruses.[11,21,22,23] This is also true of equine arteritis, rubella, and BVD-MD viruses.[29] An antigenic relationship between HC and BVD-MD viruses has been shown by CF,[18] AD,[12,13,33] and VN tests.[7,14,25,47,50] Pigs previously infected with BVD-MD virus were protected against fatal infection with virulent HC virus (Ames strain); however, marked clinical signs of HC were observed.[50]

References

1. Aiken, J.M., K.H. Hoopes, E.L. Stair, and M.B. Rhodes. Rapid diagnosis of hog cholera: A tissue impression fluorescent-antibody technique. *J. Am. Vet. Med. Ass.* 144:1395–13977, 1964.
2. Baker, J.A. Serial passage of hog cholera virus in rabbits. *Proc. Soc. Exp. Biol. Med.* 63:183–187, 1946.
3. Bool, P.H., and A.A. Ressang. Het onderzoek van pratijk-materiaal op de aawezigheid van varkenspestvirus met de IF-, ETV-, en END technieken. *Tijdschr. Diergeneesk.* 91:1164–1176, 1966.
4. Carbrey, E.A., H.A. McDaniel, W.C. Stewart, E.J. Henry, and J.I. Kresse. Comparison of frozen section and cell culture immunofluorescent techniques for the detection of hog cholera infection in experimentally infected pigs. *Proc. U.S. Anim. Health Ass.* 74:502–514, 1970.
5. Carbrey, E.A., W.C. Stewart, J.I. Kresse, and L.R. Lee. Technical aspects of tissue culture fluorescent antibody technique. *Proc. U.S. Livestock Sanitary Ass.* 69:487–500, 1965.
6. Carbrey, E.A., W.C. Stewart, J.I. Kresse, and L.R. Lee. The incidence and characteristics of strains of hog cholera virus causing fetal abnormalities, death and abortion in swine. In *Proceedings of the Symposium on Factors Producing Embryonic and Fetal Abnormalities, Death, and Abortion in Swine*. Chicago, October 2–3, 1967. U.S. Department of Agriculture, ARS 91–73, pp. 111–116, 1969.
7. Carbrey, E.A. W.C. Stewart, J.I. Kresse, and L.R. Lee. Confirmation of hog cholera diagnosis by a rapid serum-neutralization technique. *J. Am. Vet. Med. Ass.* 155:2201–2210, 1969.
8. Carbrey, E.A., W.C. Stewart, S.H. Young, and G.C. Richardson. Transmission of hog cholera by pregnant sows. *J. Am. Vet. Med. Ass.* 149:23–30, 1966.
9. Cherry, W.B., and T.R. Carski. *Fluorescent Antibody Techniques in the Diagnosis of Communicable Diseases*. Public Health Service Pub. no. 729. U.S. Government Printing Office, Washington, 1961.
10. Coggins, L., and B.E. Sheffy. A serological (neutralization) test for hog cholera. *Proc. U.S. Livestock Sanitary Ass.* 65:333–337, 1961.
11. Cunliffe, H.R., and P.A. Rebers. The purification and concentration of hog cholera virus. *Can. J. Comp. Med.* 32:486–492, 1968.
12. Darbyshire, J.H. A serological relationship between swine fever and mucosal disease of cattle. *Vet. Rec.* 72:331, 1960.
13. Darbyshire, J.H. Agar gel diffusion studies with a mucosal disease of cattle. II. A serological relationship between a mucosal disease and swine fever. *Res. Vet. Sci.* 3:125–128, 1962.
14. Dinter, Z. Relationship between bovine virus diarrhea and hog cholera virus. *Zentral Bakt.* 188:475–486, 1963.
15. Dunne, H.W. (ed.). *Disease of Swine*. 3d ed. Iowa State University Press, Ames, 1970.
16. Englerf, E., Urbaneck, D., and Olechnowitz, A.F. Immunhistologische untersuchungen bei schweinepest. I. Methode zun nachweis des schweinepestvirus in organmaterial experimentell infizierter schweine mit der direkten immunofluoreszenz unter verwendung der kontrastfarbung mit evans blue. *Arch. exp. Veterinärmed.* 24:481–501, 1970.
17. Goldman, G., and K.H. Pehl. Uber die vermehrung des schweinepest virus in der sauglingsmaus. *Arch. Exp. Veterinärmed.* 9:732–735, 1955.
18. Gutekunst, D.F., and W.A. Malmquist. Complement fixing and neutralizing antibody responses to bovine viral diarrhea and hog cholera antigens. *Can. J. Comp. Med. Vet. Sci.* 28:19–23, 1964.
19. Helmboldt, C.F., and E.L. Jungherr. The neuropathologic diagnosis of hog cholera. *Am. J. Vet. Res.* 11:41–49, 1950.
20. Henry, E.J., and H.A. McDaniel. Examination of specimens from suspected hog cholera cases by the fluorescent antibody tissue section and cell culture techniques. *Proc. U.S. Anim. Health Ass.* 74:664–667, 1970.
21. Horzinek, M. Characterization of hog cholera virus. II. Determination of sedimentation coefficient. *Arch. ges. Virusforsch.* 21:447–453, 1967.
22. Horzinek, M., J. Maess, and R. Laufs. Studies on the substructure of Togaviruses. II. Analysis of equine arteritis, rubella, bovine viral diarrhea, and hog cholera viruses. *Arch. ges. Virusforsch.* 33:306–318, 1971.
23. Horzinek, M., E. Reezko, and K. Petzoldt. On the morphology of hog cholera virus. *Arch. ges Virusforsch.* 21:475–478, 1967.
24. Koprowski, H., T.R. James, and H.R. Cox. Propagation of hog cholera virus in rabbits. *Proc. Soc. Exp. Biol. Med.* 63:178–183, 1946.
25. Kumagai, T., T. Morimoto, T. Shimizu, J. Sasahara, and M. Watanabe. Antigenic relationship between hog cholera virus and bovine viral diarrhea virus as revealed by cross neutralization. *Nat. Inst. Anim. Health Q.* 2:201–206, 1962.
26. Kumagai, T., T. Shimizu, S. Ikeda, and M. Matumota. A new *in vitro* method (END) for detection and

measurement of hog cholera virus and its antibody by means of effect of HC virus on Newcastle disease virus in swine tissue culture. I. Establishment of a standard procedure. *J. Immunol.* 87:245–268, 1961.
27. Kumagai, T., T. Shimizu, and M. Matumoto. Detection of hog cholera virus by its effect on Newcastle disease virus in swine tissue culture. *Science* 128:366, 1958.
28. Loan, R.W. Increased sensitivity of the END (exaltation of Newcastle disease virus) test for hog cholera virus. *Am. J. Vet. Res.* 26:1110–113, 1965.
29. Loan, R.W. Studies of the nucleic acid type and essential lipid content of hog cholera virus. *Am. J. Vet. Res.* 25:1366–1370, 1969.
30. Loan, R.W., and M.M. Storm. Propagation and transmission of hog cholera virus in non-porcine hosts. *Am. J. Vet. Res.* 29:807–811, 1968.
31. Maess, J., and B. Liess. Untersuchungen mit der immunofluoreszenzmethod zur laboratoriums diagnose der Europaischen Schweinepest. *Zentralblatt Veterinärmedizin,* ser. B, 13:660–670, 1966.
32. Mattheus, W., and K. Korn. Die prazipitationsreaktionen im agargel bei der europaischen schweinepest. *Zentralblatt Veterinärmedizin,* ser. B, 17:1010–1020, 1970.
33. Mattheus, W., and A. van Aert. Die beiziehung zwischen den immunpräzipitaten der europaischen schweinepest und der mucosal disease des rindes. *Arch. ges. Virusforsch.* 34:385–393, 1971.
34. McDaniel, H.A. Fozen brain sections as a diagnostic aid for hog cholera. *Proc. U.S. Livestock Sanitary Ass.* 68:479–487, 1964.
35. McNutt, S.H., H.W. Dunne, J.D. Ray, D.K. Sorenson, and J.P. Torrey. A standard method using animal inoculation for the detection of hog cholera virus. *Proc. U.S. Livestock Sanitary Ass.* 67:597–598, 1964.
36. Mengeling, W.L., and J.P. Torrey. Evaluation of the fluorescent antibody-cell culture test for hog cholera diagnosis. *Am. J. Vet. Res.* 127:1653–1659, 1967.
37. Molnar, I. Precipitation experiments with swine fever virus-containing material. *Acta Vet. Hung.* 4:247–251, 1954.
38. Nobuto, K., U. Sato, and M. Sawada. An instrument for harvesting tonsillar material for diagnosis of hog cholera. *Nat. Inst. Anim. Health.* 10:94–95, 1970.
39. Peckham, J.C., J.R. Cole, and A.R. Pursell. Fluorescent antibody and histopathologic procedures for hog cholera diagnosis. *J. Am. Vet. Med. Ass.* 157:1204–1207, 1970.
40. Phillips, C.E. *In vitro* potency tests for anti-hog cholera antibodies: a test for anti-hog cholera serums and a test for herd exposure. *Am. J. Vet. Res.* 29:1097–1102, 1968.
41. Pirtle, E.C. A soluble precipitating antigen (HCA) from hog choler virus propagated in tissue culture. I. preparation and characterization of the antigen. *Can. J. Comp. Med. Vet. Sci.* 28:193–196, 1964.
42. Pirtle, E.C., and W.L. Mengeling. Antigenic differences in two hog cholera virus strains. *Am. J. Vet. Res.* 32:1473–1477, 1971.
43. Robertson, A. G.L. Bannister, P. Boulanger, M. Appel, and D.P. Gray. Hog cholera. V. Demonstration of the antigen in swine tissues by the fluorescent antibody technique. *Can. J. Comp. Med. Vet. Sci.* 29:299–305, 1965.
44. Robertson, A., A.S. Grieg, M. Appel, A. Girard, G.L. Bannister, and P. Boulanger. Hog cholera. IV. detection of the virus in tissue culture preparations by the fluorescent antibody technique. *Can. J. Comp. Med. Vet. Sci.* 29:234–241, 1965.
45. Samol, S. Value of the immunofluroescence test in the laboratory diagnosis of swine fever. *Medycyna wet.* 26:69–72, 1970.
46. Sawada, M., U. Sato, T. Hanaki, T. Matsuno, and K. Nobuto. Studies on fluorescent antibody staining on tonsillar smear preparations (the FAST method) for rapid diagnosis of swine fever. *Rep. Nat. Vet. Assay Lab.* (Tokyo) 6:80–90, 1969.
47. Snowdon, W.A., and E.L. French. The bovine mucosal disease–swine fever virus complex in pigs. *Austral. Vet. J.* 44:179–184, 1968.
48. Solorzano, R.F., J.E. Thigpen, D.M. Bedell, and W.L. Schwartz. The diagnosis of hog cholera by a fluorescent antibody test. *J. Am. Vet. Med. Ass.* 149:31–34, 1966.
49. Stair, E.L., M.B. Rhodes, J.B. Aiken, N.R. Underdahl, and G.A. Young. A hog cholera virus–fluorescent antibody system: Its potential use in study of embryonic infection. *Proc. Soc. Exp. Biol. Med.* 113:656–660, 1963.
50. Stewart, W.C., E.A. Carbrey, E.W. Jenney, C.L. Brown, and J.I. Kresse. Bovine viral diarrhea infection in pigs. *J. Am. Vet. Med. Ass.* 159:1556–1563, 1971.
51. Stewart, W.C., J.I. Kresse, and E.A. Carbrey. Isolation of hog cholera virus from tonsil biopsies: Developmental studies and laboratory investigations. U.S. Department of Agriculture, ARS 91–99, pp. 10–16, 1971.

52. Teebken, D.L., J.M. Aiken, and M.J. Twiehaus. Differentiation of virulent attenuated and inactivated hog cholera viruses by fluorescent antibody test. *J. Am. Vet. Med. Ass.* 150:53–58, 1967.
53. Turner, L.W., chairman. Recommended minimum standards for the isolation and identification of hog cholera by the fluorescent antibody–cell culture technique. *Proc. U.S. Livestock Sanitary Ass.* 72:444–447, 1968.
54. Young, S.H. The use of supplemental tests in the diagnosis and eradication of hog cholera. *J. Am. Vet. Med. Ass.* 157:1855–1859, 1970.
55. Zimmerman, T. Zur diagnose der europaischen schweinepest mit der immunofluoreszenz-method. *Deutsche Tierarzt. Wochenschrift* 72:250–252, 1967.

Bovine Viral Diarrhea–Mucosal Disease Virus

Before it was determined that one virus caused both disease syndromes, bovine viral diarrhea (BVD) and mucosal disease (MD) were reported as two distinct diseases. Hence, the dual name for the virus and the disease complex, BVD-MD. The so-called mucosal disease complex is often seen as erosions of the bovine oral mucosa, and most clinically diagnosed mucosal disease is etiologically associated with the BVD-MD virus. However, similar clinical signs and lesions may occur in papular stomatitis, bluetongue, malignant catarrhal fever, rinderpest, infectious bovine rhinotracheitis, and foot-and-mouth disease (if seen only after FMD vesicles have ruptured and erosion has occurred).

Experimental or natural exposure of cattle to BVD-MD virus results in leukopenia, diphasic febrile response, and antibody production.[3,18,21] Unless these variables are monitored, the infection is usually inapparent.[3,24] In pregnant cattle, infection may be followed by fetal mummification,[24] abortion,[3,17] birth of weak calves,[23] or birth at term of calves with cerebellar or ocular defects.[17,30,32] Infrequently there is an acute disease with anorexia, persistent fever, nasal discharge, salivation, erosions of the oral mucosa, intractable diarrhea, terminal dehydration, and death. Chronic cases occur. Occasionally some cattle will have only mild diarrhea, cough, nasal discharge, and rapid respiration without pneumonia. Careful scrutiny frequently reveals oral lesions in otherwise normal-appearing herdmates of clinical cases.[17] The virus has been associated with fatal diarrhea in newborn calves.[18,21,23]

At necropsy examination the principal diagnostic changes occur in the alimentary tract, in the buccal cavity, on the tongue, in the esophagus, abomasum, rumen, small intestine, and colon. However, the lesions may be present in any part of the tract. Congestion and erosions of the mucosa may be found. The ulceration that occurs in the mucosa over Peyer's patches is characteristic of the disease. Often Peyer's patches are swollen to two to four times normal size. Edema and hemorrhages of lymph nodes associated with the tract frequently occur. Laminitis often may be seen in calves or yearlings.

The BVD-MD virus (genus *Pestivirus*) is 50–80 nm in diameter, is pleomorphic but roughly spherical, and is covered by a compact nondistinctive membrane. The virion has a lipid-containing RNA core. Thus the virus is structurally similar to rubella (RU) and HC viruses. However, unlike RU, some BVD-MD virus particles display a mottled appearance inside the outline of the outer membrane. Also, both BVD-MD and HC viruses have lower sedimentation and density values and lesser nucleocapsid diameters than RU virus.[14,28]

It is ether and chloroform sensitive. It has a sedimentation coefficient of about 80–90

S and a buoyant density of about 1.13–1.14 g/ml. It does not cause hemagglutination of RBC.[7,14]

Specimens

In acute cases, virus can be isolated from lesions, blood, urine, and nasal or ocular discharges.[3,4,21,27] At necropsy, spleen, mesenteric lymph nodes, or bone marrow are the specimens of choice.[3,4]

Laboratory Procedures

Cultures. The virus grows in many primary fetal bovine cell cultures including kidney, spleen, testicle, and trachea.[1,4,5,9,11] Stable cell lines of bocine kidney, trachea, turbinate, and testicle are commonly used.[4,19,29] Cytopathic changes vary slightly between virus strains and cell cultures and include rouding, stranding, cytoplasmic vacuolation, and eventual detachment of the cell sheet.[1,19] Noncytopathogenic strains are less commonly reported (probably because of difficulty in isolation rather than actual lower prevalence) and they must be identified by the FA test, by the induction of cellular resistance to known cytopathic strains, or by the use of Newcastle disease virus in the END test.[11,15,26] Organ cultures from infected animals have not been used extensively for viral isolation. However, anyone using cell cultures of bovine origin should be aware that such cultures should be checked by the FA or other tests mentioned above for the presence of BVD-MD virus.[29]

Animal inoculation. The ready availability of cell cultures makes calf inoculation impractical for primary isolation attempts. Gross lesions are not always produced by inoculation of susceptible cattle by various routes, but if monitored closely, other clinical signs and antibody production are usually observed.[3,19,24] Fetopathy may occur when susceptible pregnant cattle are inoculated.[17] Transmission studies using infective spleen material resulted in infection of rabbits, but not embryonating hens' eggs, guinea pigs, dogs, cats, goats, or mice.[3] The virus multiplies in experimentally inoculated pregnant sheep producing congenital anomalies and stimulating an antibody response.[31] Other studies with tissue culture–propagated virus demonstrated that some BVD-MD virus strains multiply in swine, inducing BVD-MD antibody production and protection against some strains of hog cholera.[2,25,27] The antigenic relationship between BVD-MD and hog cholera virus is demonstrable by animal inoculation and challenge,[2,4,25,27] by AD tests,[4,27] and by FA assay.[20,21,27] The two viruses may share a common soluble antigen.[6,12,13,28]

Immunology and serology. The strains of BVD-MD virus isolated thus far have been found to be identical by qualitative cross-VN tests in tissue culture[9,10,28] and by reciprocal cross-immunity tests in calves.[3,9,29] Quantitative strain differences (demonstrable in tissue cultures by differing magnitude of virus neutralization with homologous and heterologous antisera) are *not* sufficient to cause problems in virus identification or in serologic diagnostic procedures.[10,13,16] The VN test in primary Bk cell cultures in roller tubes is the procedure most commonly used. The strain of virus selected for the test must be as cytopathogenic as possible. The NADC strain is satisfactory. The test should consist of 100 TCID$_{50}$ of virus with twofold dilutions of serum, since antibody titers are generally low. Incubation at 37°C in a water bath for 30 minutes is the usual procedure, although overnight incubation at 4°C has been used.[4,5] The CF test may be used but has not been popular.[12,13]

The neutralization test is an indicator of immunity to challenge.[18,22] Massive challenge can overwhelm waning passive immunity. Neonates infected in utero have active immunity detectable in sera collected before nursing.[17,29,30]

References

1. Angulo, A.B., and M. Savan. In vitro study of bovine virus diarrhea virus: Interactions with some selected viruses. *Proc. U.S. Anim. Health Ass.* 73:551–559, 1969.
2. Atkinson, G.F., J.A. Baker, C. Campbell, L. Coggins, D. Nelson, D. Robson, B.E. Sheffy, W. Sippel, and S. Nelson. Bovine virus diarrhea (BVD) vaccine for protection of pigs against hog cholera. *Proc. U.S. Livestock Sanitary Ass.* 66:326–338, 1962.
3. Baker, J.A., C.J. York, J.H. Gillespie, and B. Grayson. Virus Diarrhea in cattle. *Am. J. Vet. Res.* 15:525–531, 1954.
4. Carbrey, E., Chairman, Committee for Recommended Standard Techniques for Diagnosing Bovine Respiratory Disease. Recommended standard laboratory techniques for diagnosing infectious bovine rhinotracheitis, bovine virus diarrhea, and shipping fever (parainfluenza-3). *Proc. U.S. Anim. Health Ass.* 75:629-648, 1971.
5. Coggins, L. Standardization of virus-neutralization test for bovine virus diarrhea. *Am. J. Vet. Res.* 25:103–107, 1964.
6. Coggins, L., and S. Seo. Serological comparison with rabbit antisera of hog cholera virus and bovine virus diarrhea virus. *Proc. Soc. Exp. Biol. Med.* 114:778–780, 1963.
7. Ditchfield, J., and F.W. Doane. The properties and classification of bovine viral diarrhea virus. *Can. J. comp. Med. Vet.* 28:148–152, 1964.
8. Fernelius, A.L. Noncytopathogenic bovine viral diarrhea viruses detected and titrated by immunofluorescence. *Can. J. Comp. Med. Vet. Sci.* 28:121–126, 1964.
9. Gillespie, J.H., J.A. Baker, and K. McEntree. A cytopathogenic strain of virus diarrhea virus. *Cornell Vet.* 40:73–79, 1960.
10. Gillespie, J.H., L. Coggins, J. Thompson, and J.A. Baker. Comparison by neutralization tests of strains of virus isolated from virus diarrhea and mucosal disease. *Cornell Vet.* 51:155–159, 1961.
11. Gillespie, J.H., S.H. Madin, and N.B. Darby, Jr., Cellular resistance in tissue culture, induced by noncytopathogenic strains, to a cytopathogenic strain of virus diarrhea virus of cattle. *Proc. Soc. Exp. Biol. Med.* 110:248–250, 1962.
12. Gutekunst, D.E., and W.A. Malmquist. Separation of a soluble antigen and infectious particles of bovine viral diarrhea viruses and their relationship to hog cholera. *Can. J. Comp. Med. Sci.* 27:121–123, 1963.
13. Gutekunst, D.E., and W.A. Malmquist. Complement-fixing and neutralizing antibody response to bovine viral diarrhea and hog cholera antigens. *Can. J. Comp. Med. Vet. Sci.* 28:19–23, 1964.
14. Horzinek, M., J. Maess, and R. Laufs. Studies on the substructure of togaviruses. II. Analysis of equine arteritis, rubella, bovine viral diarrhoea, and hog cholera. *Arch. ges. Virusforsch.* 33:306–318, 1971.
15. Inaba, Y., T. Omori, and T. Kumagai. Detection and measurement of non-cytopathogenic strains of virus diarrhea virus by END method. *Arch. ges. Virusforsch.* 13:425–427, 1963.
16. Kahrs, R.F. Determination of a 95 per cent dose for bovine virus diarrhea vaccine. *Am. J. Vet. Res.* 27:1551–1554, 1966.
17. Kahrs, R.F., F.W. Scott, and A. deLahunta. Congenital cerebellar hypoplasia and ocular defects in calves following bovine viral diarrhea–mucosal disease infection in pregnant cattle. *J. Am. Vet. Med. Ass.* 156:1443–1450, 1970.
18. Lambert, G., A.L. Fernelius, N.F. Cheville. Experimental bovine viral diarrhea in neonatal calves. *J. Am. Vet. Med. Ass.* 154:181–189, 1969.
19. Marcus, S.J., and T. Moll. Adaptation of bovine viral diarrhea virus to the Madin-Darby bovine kidney cell line. *Am. J. Vet. Res.* 29:817–819, 1967.
20. Mengeling, W.L., D.E. Gutekunst, and A.L. Fernelius. Demonstration of an antigenic relationship between bovine viral diarrhea and hog cholera viruses by immunofluorescence. *Can. J. Comp. Med. Vet. Sci.* 27:162–164, 1963.
21. Mills, J.H.L., and R.E. Luginbuhl. Distribution and persistence of mucosal disease virus in experimentally exposed calves. *Am. J. Vet. Res.* 29:1367–1375, 1968.

22. Robson, D.S., J.H. Gillespie, and J.A. Baker. The neutralization test as an indicator of immunity to virus diarrhea. *Cornell Vet.* 50:503–509, 1960.
23. Schipper, I.A., and D.F. Eveleth. Mucosal disease in calves. *Vet. Med.* 52:73–75, 1957.
24. Scott, F.W., R.F. Kahrs, and I.M. Parsonson. A mummified bovine fetus following experimental bovine viral diarrhea–mucosal disease in a pregnant cow. *J. Am. Vet. Med. Ass.* 156:876, 1970.
25. Sheffy, B.E., L. Coggins, and J.A. Baker. Relationship between hog cholera virus and virus diarrhea virus of cattle. *Proc. Soc. Exp. Biol. Med.* 109:349–352, 1962.
26. Smithies, L.K., and S.M. Robertson. The laboratory diagnosis of bovine virus diarrhea by fluorescent antibody. *Poc. U.S. Anim. Health Ass.* 73:539–549, 1969.
27. Snowdon, W.A., and E.L. French. The bovine mucosal disease–*swine fever virus complex in pigs*. *Austral. Vet. J.* 44:179–184, 1968.
28. Stott, E.J., J.D. Almeida, and K.J. O'Reilly. Characterization of mucosal disease virus as a togavirus by electronmicroscopy. *Microbios* 11:79–83, 1974.
29. Tyler, E., and F.K. Ramsey. Comparative pathologic, immunologic and clinical responses produced by selected agents of the bovine mucosal disease–virus diarrhea complex. *Am. J. Vet. Res.* 26:903–913, 1965.
30. Ward, G.M. Bovine cerebellar hypoplasia apparently caused by BVD-MD virus: A case report. *Cornell Vet.* 59:570–575, 1969.
31. Ward, G.M. Experimental infection of pregnant sheep with bovine viral diarrhea–mucosal disease virus. *Cornell Vet.* 61:179–191, 1971.
32. Ward, G.M., S.J. Roberts, K. McEntee, and J.H. Gillespie. A study of experimentally induced bovine viral diarrhea–mucosal disease in pregnant cows and their progeny. *Cornell Vet.* 59:525–538, 1969.

Equine Arteritis Virus

Equine arteritis virus (EAV) causes a severe disease of horses that is characterized clinically by anorexia, edema, and fever, and histologically by lesions of the vascular system particularly necrosis of the small arteries. It causes abortion in pregnant mares. EAV was first isolated in Ohio ("Bucyrus" prototype strain)[3] but its occurrence in the United States is infrequent. There is evidence for the existence of EAV in Austria, France, India, Italy, Sweden, Switzerland, and the United Kingdom.[7] Serologic evidence indicates that EAV subclinically infects a large proportion of standardbred but not thoroughbred horses in the United States.[7] The significance of subclinical EAV infection with regard to horse performance and sporadic abortion is not known. A carrier status for EAV is thought to exist but is not proved; however, EAV may persist for short periods of time in the kidneys and may be found in the urine. EAV is highly contagious and inhalation may be the major method of transmission. Transmission by arthropods or by coitus has not been demonstrated.

After an incubation period of 1–3 days, virulent EAV causes anorexia, fever, palpebral edema, conjunctivitis ("pink eye"), nasal catarrh, and edema of legs and abdomen. Photophobia, respiratory distress, restlessness, colic, weakness, diarrhea, and loss of weight also may be seen. Infected horses exhibit leukopenia. The acute stage of the disease varies from 3 to 7 days although some clinical signs may persist for longer periods. All age groups are susceptible but the disease is more severe in pregnant mares, foals, and highly parasitized horses. Experimental infection can be fatal but mortality is low in natural outbreaks.

Abortion has been recorded in up to 90% of susceptible pregnant mares, occurring from 10 to 33 days after exposure and usually during the period of clinical disease or early in convalescence. The fetus is infected by transplacental passage of the virus and usually is expelled without signs of impending abortion. Fetal death occurs before the onset of abortion, sometimes up to 4 days prior to expulsion. Thus autolyzed fetuses are common. Infrequently, there is a retained placenta and metritis. In contrast, equine rhinopneumonitis virus abortions occur most often in the ninth and tenth months and autolysis is uncommon. Except for abortion, which can occur up to 10 weeks after exposure, ERV infection of pregnant mares is usually asymptomatic.

Gross lesions due to EAV consist of hemorrhages and edema. Petechial hemorrhages occur in all serous membranes and in the lungs, mediastinal tissues, and gastric mucosa. The adrenals show larger hemorrhages. Hemorrhagic and edematous changes can occur in the heart, spleen, lung, kidney, the uterus in pregnant mares, conjunctiva, eyelids, the subcutis below the knees or hocks, the sheath, scrotum, and testicles. Serous cavities have large amounts of fluid containing protein and strands of fibrin. Lesions result from an acute panvasculitis.[2,8] Terminal lesions consist of massive necrosis of lymph nodes and the mucosa of the cecum. Chronic lesions, observed at about day 14 in clinically recovered horses, consist of extensive generalized arteritis and severe glomerulonephritis. Viral replication and lesions occur in most parts of the cardiovascular system. EAV infects pulmonary macrophages and spreads to the bronchial node. Replication occurs in macrophages and endothelium and secondarily in the medial cells, mesothelium, and epithelium of certain organs.

Histologic examination reveals necrosis of the musculature of small arteries with replacement by hyaline or fibrinoid material. Hemorrhage and edema is associated with veins and lymphatics. Arteries less than 0.3 mm are not affected. Vessels larger than 0.5 mm, veins, and lymphatics are distended. Large elastic arteries show little change apart from endothelial and intimal involvement. Arterial lesions may be irregularly distributed along the length of the vessel. The pathogenesis of the panvasculitis of EA as deduced by histologic, EM, and FA studies is as follows.[4] The EAV infects the endothelial cells, bringing about increased permeability and leukocyte infiltration of the vessels' intima. This leads to internal elastic lamina damage and disruption, which in turn allows penetration of leukocytes and virus into the media. The virus then infects the medial muscle cells. The destruction of the muscle cells and the influx of other cells and plasma finally results in fibrinoid necrosis.[4] The arteries become surrounded by lymphocytes and edema.

Thrombosis with infarction occurs in the intestinal tract and lung. Arterial lesions may be more common in the gut and adrenal glands but can occur in all organs with accompanying edema. By 10 days after experimental infection, lesions in veins and lymphatics have largely subsided but arterial necrosis is still at a peak. Arteries regenerate by about 2 months after infection.[8]

The aborted fetus is edematous and petechial hemorrhage may be seen in the respiratory mucosa and splenic capsule. Inclusion bodies are not observed (these are seen in ERV abortion). Specific arterial lesions are not seen in the aborted fetus or in those that die in utero.

EAV is an RNA virus, is ether sensitive, and is resistant to trypsin. The particle is roughly spherical, with an outer envelope. Particle size has been recorded as approximately 43 nm[1] or 55 nm[5] from electron microscopic studies. The inner core is approximately 35 nm. Spikes of 3–5 nm may be seen on the surface.

Specimens

For diagnosis, clinical observations must be complemented by laboratory examination to differentiate from other equine diseases exhibiting similar clinical signs. Specimens should include whole blood (heparinized or citrated) from acute cases, nasal swabs if there is discharge, the aborted fetus (if available), and serum from suspect cases. Fresh and Formalin-treated specimens of lung, spleen, and lymph nodes should be collected at postmortem. Specimens for virus isolation should be transported on ice. Histologic examination of lung, lymph node, and spleen of adult horses should reveal characteristic lesions after H & E staining.

Laboratory Procedures

Cultures. Preparations of whole blood and/or buffy coat, nasal swabs, aborted fetal tissue (especially spleen), adult lung, and spleen are inoculated into susceptible cell cultures. The virus replicates in equine cells (kidney, testis, dermis), LLC-MK$_2$, BS-C-1, and rabbit kidney cells; the CPE should appear in 3–5 days in positive specimens. Intracytoplasmic inclusions have been reported in infected cell cultures. EAV can be assayed by plaque formation in equine and other cell types.

Animal inoculation. Only horses seem to be affected by EAV and ponies are often used for experimental studies. Laboratory animals do not develop clinical signs or lesions, but rabbits, guinea pigs, hamsters, and mice can be used for production of antiserum.

Immunology and serology. EAV produces a solid and perhaps lifelong immunity. Horses experimentally infected by aerosol produce detectable serum neutralizing antibody by day 4, with constant titers by day 8. The CF, AD, and indirect FA tests can be used for serologic diagnosis.[2] The 50% endpoint plaque reduction test is a sensitive VN test.

An attenuated live-virus vaccine prepared in nonequine cell culture has given a high degree of immunogenicity with long-lasting protection (up to 3 years) against EAV.[6] Natural protection of foals by colostral antibodies may persist for 2–4 months.

References

1. Breese, S.S., and W.H. McCollum. Electron microscopic characterization of equine arteritis virus. *Proc. 2d Internat. Conf. Equine Infect. Dis.* (Paris, 1969), pp. 133–139. Karger, Basel, 1970.
2. Crawford, T.B., and J.B. Henson. Immunofluorescent, light-microscopic and immunologic studies of equine viral arteritis. *Proc. 3d Internat. Conf. Equine Infect. Dis.* (Paris, 1972), pp. 282–302. Karger, Basel, 1973.
3. Doll, E.R., J.T. Bryans, W.H. McCollum, and M.E.W. Crowe. Isolation of a filterable agent causing arteritis of horses and abortion by mares: Its differentiation from the equine abortion (influenza) virus. *Cornell Vet.* 47:3–41, 1957.
4. Henson, J.E., and T.E. Crawford. The pathogenesis of virus induced arterial disease: Aleutian disease and equine viral arteritis. *Adv. Cardiol.* 13:183–186, 1974.
5. Magnusson, P., B. Hyllseth, and H. Marusyk. Morphological studies on equine arteritis virus. *Arch. ges. Virusforsch.* 30:105–112, 1970.
6. McCollum, W.H. Vaccination for equine viral arteritis. *Proc. 2d Internat. Conf. Equine Infect. Dis.* (Paris, 1969), pp. 143–151. Karger, Basel, 1970.
7. McCollum, W.H., and J.T. Bryans. Serological identification of infection by equine arteritis virus in

horses of several countries. *Proc. 3d Internat. Conf. Equine Infect. Dis.* (Paris, 1972), pp. 256–263. Karger, Basel, 1973.
8. Prickett, M.E., W.H. McCollum, and J.T. Bryans. The gross and microscopic pathology observed in horses experimentally infected with the equine arteritis virus. *Proc. 3d Internat. Conf. Equine Infect. Dis.* (Paris, 1972), pp. 265–272. Karger, Basel, 1973.

22. Bunyamwera Group Viruses

The Bunyamwera is an uninhabited area within the Semliki Forest of western Uganda. A virus found in this area received the area name and later became the prototype virus for a group of arboviruses. The diseases to be discussed are Rift Valley fever and Akabane.

Rift Valley Fever Virus

Rift Valley fever (RVF) is a virus disease of ruminants, humans, and rodents, usually transmitted by mosquitoes.[2] It was first reported in the Rift Valley in Kenya in 1912, and it is now known to occur in Uganda, Southern Rhodesia (now Rhodesia), Mozambique, and South Africa.[1] *Arvicanthus,* the East African forest rat, may be the reservoir of infection.[1,2]

In the peracute form of the disease, the incubation period may be as short as 12 hours and may result in the death of lambs, calves, and kids within 24–36 hours. In the acute form of the disease the clinical signs are pyrexia, vomition, nasal discharge, dysentery, and muscular pain or weakness, as evidenced by unwillingness to move or a staggering gait. Pregnant ewes may abort and about 20% die. Other nonpregnant adult cattle and sheep may have only a transient fever, anorexia, muscle weakness, and a fall in milk yield.

Humans have an influenzalike reaction to RVF infection, with an incubation period of 2–6 days. There is a sudden onset of chills and fever, vomiting, epistaxis, "fullness" over the liver, muscle pains, and headache. Some patients have retinitis and temporary blindness. Usually, the disease runs its course within 2–3 days.[1]

In animals the lesions may be catarrhal gastroenteritis; subcutaneous hemorrhages, especially over shoulders and hindquarters; subcapsular hemorrhages in the spleen, liver, and kidneys; and hemorrhagic areas in the epicardium and endocardium. The spleen and lymph nodes may be enlarged.

The RVF virus contains single-stranded RNA, is enveloped, and has a diameter of about 70–94 nm. It is ether- and pH-sensitive and is inactivated at pasteurization temperatures. However, it survives very well in blood when stored at 4°C.

Specimens

A freshly aborted fetus is a good specimen for viral isolation. Blood with an anticoagulant taken during the acute phase, and liver, spleen, kidney, and brain specimens are also good sources of virus. Acute and convalescent paired serum samples are also desirable for serology.

Laboratory Procedures

Cultures. RVF will replicate in lamb, mouse, rat, or chick kidney cells. After 2–3 days incubation, CPE is detectable. If coverslip cultures are used and stained with H & E or other special stains, eosinophilic intranuclear inclusions can be seen.

Animal inoculation. The specimen material also should be inoculated IC into at least two litters of very young suckling mice and also into about 10 adult mice. RVF virus produces a fatal hepatitis in mice within 3–5 days. Liver specimens from such mice should be tested by inoculation into embryonating chicken eggs (8 days old) by the CAM or YS routes, and by smears for FA tests.

Immunology and serology. Serologic surveys have shown that many wild and domestic animals have antibodies for RVF, including buffalo, camel, many antelope, and goats.[2] The standard VN, CF, AD, and FA tests may be used. Vaccines for RVF are available for the protection of laboratory workers and animals.[1]

References

1. Easterday, B.C. Rift Valley fever. In *Advances in Veterinary Science,* C.A. Brandly and E.L. Jungherr (eds.), vol. 10, pp. 65–127. Academic Press, New York, 1965.
2. Henderson, B.E., A.W.R. McCrae, B.G. Kirya, Y. Ssenkubuge, and S.D.K. Sempala. Arbovirus epizootics involving man, mosquitoes, and vertebrates at Lunyo, Uganda, 1968. *Ann. Trop. Med. Parasit.* 66:343–355, 1972.

Akabane Virus

Akabane virus (named for a village in Japan) produces congenital defects in the offspring of nonimmune cattle, sheep, and goats characterized by hydranencephaly (HE), arthrogryposis (AG), micrencephaly (ME), or porencephaly. Infection can also lead to abortion. The disease occurs as epizootics and as sporadic isolated cases. In Japan during 1972–1973 there were 31,000 estimated cases of abortion, stillbirth, and congenital AG/HE in calves, much of which was associated with Akabane virus infection.[7,10] In Australia, from April to December 1974, about 5000 calves (excluding abortions) were lost with encephalomyelitis, AG, and HE.[1]

The virus has been isolated in Japan from the mosquitoes *Aedex vexans* and *Culex tritaeniorhynchus* and in Australia from the biting midge *Culicoides brevitarsis* on three occasions.[1,7] Outbreaks of congenital AG/HE associated with Akabane virus have occurred in central and western Japan,[7] in Australia in the Southeastern area of New South Wales,[1,4,5] and (on serologic evidence) in Israel.[8,11]

Pregnant, nonimmune animals become infected with Akabane virus, which is transmitted by arthropod vectors. The infected pregnant animals do not have a febrile response or show any other clinical signs of infection. Following IV inoculation of cattle with Akabane virus, viremia occurs from day 3 to day 6, with virus titers (assayed in mice) of about 10^2 LD$_{50}$ per ml of blood. Serum VN antibodies appear about day 7 to day 10 after infection, rapidly rising to titers of 1 in 32 to 1 in 512 by the fourth week after infection. A significant level of VN antibodies can be detected more than a year after infection. The virus infects the fetus at various stages of gestation to produce the different clinical entities of the disease.

In cattle, the disease results in congenitally acquired encephalomyelitis, arthrogryposis, hydranencephaly, various intermediate stages in these syndromes, and an increased number of abortions.[1,2,4,7,11] The following description of the lesions is based on the 1974 Australian outbreak. The lesions are grouped into several stages, probably approximating the gestational age of the fetus at the time of infection.[2] There is some overlap of lesions between the various stages. *Stage 1:* The calves have lesions of the CNS or elsewhere, but microscopically there is a universal nonsuppurative acute encephalomyelitis of varying intensity. *Stage 2:* The calves are either incoordinate or have flacid paralysis or mild arthrogryposis. Microscopically there is a mild to moderately severe active Wallerian-type degeneration of all levels of the spinal cord except the dorsal funiculi. *Stage 3:* The calves (June to September) have fixed flexion (arthrogryposis) or sometimes extension of one or more limbs, and occasionally have scoliosis. Microscopically there is a severe diffuse loss of myelinated fibers in the lateral and ventral funiculi of affected areas of the spinal cord, together with loss of ventral horn neurons and marked loss of nerves. *Stage 4:* Towards the end of the epizootic (July to October) and sometimes associated with lesions of arthrogryposis, the affected calves are able to walk quite well, but are blind, often have a slightly domed cranium, and are somewhat dejected. In the majority of such calves, both cerebral hemispheres are almost completely replaced by a fluid-filled cavity (hydranencephaly).

The disease also occurs in sheep and goats. In lambs, micrencephaly, arthrogryposis, hydranencephaly, and proencephaly are seen.[3,11] In kids, arthrogryposis and hydranencephaly may be observed.[11] Similar lesions are produced by congenital infections with bluetongue virus in cattle, sheep, and goats.

Akabane virus belongs to the serologic subgroup of arboviruses called the Simbu group. This group has been placed in the Bunyamwera group of viruses based on their weak serologic cross-reactions and on their morphologic similarity.[6] The virion density for these viruses is about 1.20 g/ml in CsCl and 1.18 g/ml in sucrose.[9,12] These viruses possess a glycoprotein-lipid envelope surrounding 3–4 pieces of single-stranded RNA, which is found as coiled helices of nucleoprotein.[12,13]

Specimens

The most important specimens for the diagnosis of this disease are the samples of serum from the mother and its affected offspring. Every attempt should be made to obtain a precolostrum serum sample from the affected neonate. In addition, tissue should be collected from an aborted fetus or stillborn affected animal for histologic and virologic examination. Samples of the brain and spinal cord should be preserved in 10% neutral Formalin for histologic examination. Samples from the cerebral remnants, cerebellum, spinal cord, heart, spleen, CSF, muscle, and placenta should be taken for virus isolation and sent immediately on wet ice to the laboratory.

Laboratory Procedures

Cultures. Either Vero or BHK-21 cell lines are used for virus production. Virus titrations are carried out in Vero cells, either by CPE or plaque techniques.

Animal inoculation. Tissues are made into a 10% suspension in nutrient broth containing antibiotics and clarified by low-speed centrifugation. A sample of the material is stored below $-10°C$ for confirmation of any virus isolation. The fresh material is inoculated IC into 1–2-day-old suckling mice (0.02 ml per mouse), using a litter of at least six suckling mice for each sample. Mice are observed daily for signs of nervous disease for 10 days. The brains from mice showing nervous signs or from mice 10 days after inoculation are harvested and a second passage is made for virus isolation. Virus isolates are identified by VN tests.

Immunology and serology. All isolates of Akabane virus found thus far appear to be serologically identical. The most common serologic test is VN performed in Vero cells. Tube cultures or microtiter trays are used with 100 $TCID_{50}$ or 12–25 $TCID_{50}$ doses of Akabane virus, respectively. The serum-virus mixtures are incubated at room temperature (20–25°C) for 1 hour.[1,7] The test is read 4 days postinoculation when 75–100% of the cell sheet is destroyed by the virus. CF, HI, and FA tests are not in use at present. The serologic test must differentiate Akabane from other teratogenic viruses, e.g. BT, BVD-MD, and PI-3. It is unlikely that virus will be recovered from an animal born with neutralizing antibodies to the virus.[2]

Recently, an extensive field survey was undertaken in Australia to define the limits of distribution of animals with VN antibodies against Akabane virus.[1] Most of the cattle in northern Australia, where the Australian vector, *Culicoides brevitarsis,* usually ranges, were found to have been exposed to the virus. The 1974 epizootic in southeastern New South Wales appears to have been associated with a southward extension of *C. brevitarsis,* due to favorable climatic conditions. Thus infected vectors brought the virus to pregnant animals in herds that had not been previously exposed to the virus. These herds produced up to 40% affected calves. In the areas where the epizootic was most severe, 80–100% of the animals tested had VN antibodies.[1] As there are only sporadic isolated cases of AG/HE calves in the endemic areas, it appears that animals are immune to reinfection. In Japan, recurrence of deformed calves from previously infected animals has not been observed.[7] Possibly the disease could be controlled by vaccination of young nonpregnant female animals in the epizootic areas. If a live vaccine is used, it should be administered only during periods when vectors are not active.

References

1. Della-Porta, A.J., M.D. Murray, and D.H. Cybinski. Congenital bovine epizootic arthrogryposis and hydranencephaly in Australia: Distribution of antibodies to Akabane virus in Australian cattle after the 1974 epizootic. *Austral. Vet. J.* 52:496–501, 1976.
2. Hartley, W.J., and W.G. deSaram. Pathology of Akabane disease in cattle. *Proc. 53d Ann. Conf. Austral. Vet. Ass.,* pp. 89–90, 1976.
3. Hartley, W.J., and K.G. Haughey. An outbreak of micrencephaly in lambs in New South Wales. *Austral. Vet. J.* 50:55–58, 1974.
4. Hartley, W.J., and R.A. Warner. Bovine congenital arthrygryposis in New South Wales. *Austral. Vet. J.* 50:185–188, 1974.
5. Hartley, W.J., R.A. Wanner, A.J. Della-Porta, and W.A. Snowdon. Serological evidence for the associa-

tion of Akabane virus with epizootic bovine congenital arthrogryposis and hydranencephaly syndromes in New South Wales. *Austral. Vet. J.* 51:103–104, 1975.
6. Holmes, I.M. Morphological similarity of Bunyamwera supergroup viruses. *Virology* 43:708–712, 1971.
7. Kurogi, H., Y. Inaba, Y. Goto, Y. Miura, H. Takahashi, K. Sato, T. Omori, and M. Matumato. Serologic evidence for etiologic role of Akabane virus in epizootic abortion-arthrogryposis-hydranencephaly in Japan, 1972–74. *Arch. Virol.* 47:71–83, 1975.
8. Markusfeld, O., and E. Mayer. An arthrogryposis and hydranencephaly syndrome in calves in Israel, 1969/70: Epidemiological and clinical aspects. *Refuah Vet.* 28:51–61, 1971.
9. McLerran, C.J., and R.B. Arlinghous. Structural components of the California encephalitis complex: La Cross virus. *Virology* 53:247–257, 1973.
10. Miura, Y., S. Hayashi, T. Ishihara, Y. Inaba, T. Omori, and M. Matumoto. Neutralizing antibody against Akabane virus in precolostral sera from calves with congenital arthrogryposis-hydranencephaly syndrome. *Arch. ges. Virusforsch.* 46:377–380, 1974.
11. Nobel, T.A., U. Klopper, and F. Neuman. Pathology of an arthrogryposis-hydranencephaly syndrome in domestic ruminants in Israel, 1969/70. *Refuah Vet.* 28:144–151, 1971.
12. Pettersson, R., L. Kaariainen, C.H. von Bonsdroff, and N. Oker-Blom. Structural components of Uukuneimi virus, a noncubical tick-borne arbovirus. *Virology* 46:721–729, 1971.
13. Saikku, P., C.H. von Bonsdorff, M. Brummer-Korvenkontvo, and A. Vaheri. Isolation of non-cubical ribonuceloprotein from Inkoo virus: A Bunyamwera supergroup arbovirus. *J. Gen. Virol.* 13:335–337, 1971.

23. Unclassified Viruses

The three unclassified viruses to be discussed are African swine fever (ASF), equine infectious anemia (EIA), and Borna disease (BD) viruses. ASF virus was for a time classified as an iridovirus; EIA and BD were classified as arboviruses. Their exact placement has never been settled.

African Swine Fever Virus

African swine fever (ASF) is a highly contagious, usually fatal disease of domestic swine. It is characterized by fever, cyanosis of skin, and extensive hemorrhages of lymph nodes, kidney, heart, and other internal organs. Animals surviving longer than 2–3 weeks develop chronic lesions such as fibrinous pericarditis, pneumonia, and enlargements over the leg joints. Clinically and pathologically, ASF resembles hog cholera, which is the prime suspect in a differential diagnosis in areas where hog cholera is present. In the acute disease, pigs generally sicken 5–7 days after exposure and death occurs in 10–15 days. Mortality is generally considered to approach 100%. With the less virulent ASF viruses, especially those modified in the laboratory, pigs may show febrile reactions for several weeks before dying, or may appear to recover then later react and die. The virus usually persists in surviving pigs but some pigs appear able to rid themselves of it completely. Inhibitors of virus growth can be found in the serum and tissues of surviving pigs.

In areas where ASF virus has become endemic in domestic swine, the milder forms of ASF are more common. Such cases may escape the accepted methods of disease control and, as carriers, are potential spreaders of ASF infection in domestic swine. The disease is present in parts of Africa, Spain, and Portugal.

Specimens

Primary isolations are made from spleen, lymph nodes, or blood of sick or dead pigs.[5] The Kenya (Hinde) isolate is suggested as a prototype because it has been studied most extensively and shares characteristics with other ASF isolates, including the nonhemadsorption property.[2]

Unclassified Viruses

Laboratory Procedures

Cultures. Swine bone marrow or buffy-coat cultures are the most sensitive in vitro systems available for the detection and propagation of ASF virus. These systems appear to be equally effective in the cultivation of ASF virus, but buffy coat is more convenient and does not require sacrificing the donor pig. Two distinct reactions are observed in these cultures when inoculated with ASF virus: HAd and cytolysis. HAd occurs from 10 hours after inoculation onward, depending on virus concentration, and is followed by cytolysis and detachment of infected leukocytes. Buffy-coat cultures usually contain sufficient erythrocytes to give the HAd reaction without addition of erythrocytes to the system. Slight agitation of cultures before microscopic examination facilitates the distinction between HAd and erythrocytes settled on the surface of leukocytes. Most infected cultures show HAd by the third or fourth day after inoculation and peak virus yields are obtained at this time if the inoculum contains a high titer of virus. Plaque techniques have not yet been perfected. Thus virus titers are determined by the tube dilution method using 50% HAd endpoints. Final readings on virus titrations are made after 6 days.

To prepare swine buffy-coat cultures: (1) Collect blood from a normal pig into a flask containing glass beads and defibrinate by shaking. (2) Filter blood through sterile gauze and centrifuge at 2000 rpm for 30 minutes. Aspirate serum and save. (3) Collect buffy-coat layer using a wide-mouth pipette and resuspend leukocytes in about three-quarters of the serum from which they separated. (4) Add antibiotics and dispense in 1 ml amounts into culture tubes. About 75 tube cultures can be obtained from 200 ml of blood. (5) Although cultures may be used immediately, better results are obtained if cultures are incubated at 37°C for at least 24 hours before use.[5]

Swine kidney cell cultures (primary or established cell lines) support the growth of ASF virus but usually require adaptation of the virus system before CPE is observed. Hess et al. have discussed methods of adaptation of the virus to SK cell culture.[6] The CPE occurs in 3–5 days once the virus is adapted and consists of a rounding of the cells, which become dislodged, leaving holes in the monolayer. Infection may also be confirmed by the addition of a 2.5% suspension of washed swine RBC to the culture. HAd occurs in cells in the vicinity of the CPE. Plaque techniques are still in developmental stages.

Animal inoculation. Although there are reports of successful propagation of ASF virus in rabbits or embryonating chicken eggs, neither appears to be a very satisfactory method of cultivation.[5] Domestic swine is the only species in which ASF virus is known to cause disease. Wild pigs such as the wart hog, bush pig, and giant forest hog have been shown to harbor the virus but with no apparent clinical signs or lesions.

Immunology and serology. HAd, HAdI, AD, CF, and FA tests are useful in the identification of ASF virus. All known isolates possess a common antigen as measured by the last three tests, whereas the HAdI test distinguishes between isolates of ASF virus. However, for practical purposes, the presence of HAd alone in swine buffy-coat cultures is useful in the differential diagnosis of ASF and hog cholera.

Common procedures for HAdI tests are not satisfactory for use with ASF virus presumably because ASF virus can overgrow the temporary inhibitory effect of antisera. However, by modifying the HAdI test to measure the capacity of an antiserum to block the attachment between erythrocytes and infected leukocytes, antibody can be detected. The technique is as follows: (1) Inoculate 3-day-old buffy-coat cultures with 0.1 ml amount of virus containing at least 10^5 HAd_{50}. (2) Incubate cultures for 24 hours or until a high percentage of leukocytes exhibit HAd. (3) Wash cultures with 2 ml of distilled water to hemolyze attached RBC. (4) Decant water and add 1 ml of a twofold dilution of antiserum (inactivated at 56°C for 30 minutes) to two tubes per dilution. Incubate at 37°C for 1 hour. As a HAd control use dilution media in place of antiserum. (5) Test for HAd by the addition of 0.1 ml of 2.5% suspension of washed swine RBC to each culture. Read after a further 30 minutes of incubation or when HAd is clearly evident in the control tube.

Complete inhibition of HAd by a known antiserum identifies the isolate as ASF virus. The serum titer is the highest dilution inhibiting HAd. The HAdI titer is not correlated with the immune status of the pig.

AD precipitation tests are useful in the detection of ASF antigen and ASF antibody. For ASF antigen detection, place small pieces of lymph node, liver, kidney, or spleen in wells cut in agar plates. Known ASF antiserum and antigen should be included in the test. Infected swine kidney tissue culture cell debris is the antigen commonly used as a control.[5] Precipitin lines specific for ASF appear between the positive sample and the ASF antiserum in 24–48 hours and merge with the lines between the control antigen and the antiserum. For detection of ASF antibody the procedure is similar except the precipitin lines form between the serum and the ASF antigen.[1,3]

The CF test is useful in the detection of ASF antibodies in swine serum. Antigen is prepared from culture fluids obtained from infected SK cell cultures. Dilute Formalin is used to eliminate the procomplementary activity of swine serum, and normal bovine serum is employed to enhance the detection of low antibody titers.[4] A modification of the standard direct CF test is the addition of 5% fresh unheated bovine serum to the guinea pig complement, to demonstrate ASF antigen or antibody.[1] Antigen is prepared from liver or spleen following an extraction with acetone-ether to remove the nonspecific activity of the tissues. Others have found that it is not always necessary to pretreat swine sera with Formalin, and the addition of bovine serum is used only to detect trace amounts of antibody.[6]

Precipitating and CF antibody are virus specific but not isolate specific. Presence of these antibodies appears to indicate only some previous exposure to the virus, and titers are not correlated with the immune status of the animal.

Standard FA techniques may be used to detect ASF antigen in SK and buffy-coat cell cultures infected with the virus.[1,7] Thus far, however, similar procedures have been unsatisfactory on frozen sections and tissue smears from pigs known to be infected with ASF virus. The test detects antigen common to all isolates of ASF virus. The technique for direct staining is as follows: (1) Remove coverslips from Leighton tubes containing infected cells. (2) Wash coverslip preparations in PBS, dry at room temperature, and fix in acetone for 10 minutes. (3) Dry at room temperature and overlay with fluorescein-labeled anti-ASF serum. Let react 30 minutes at 37°C in a petri dish containing a moist filter pad. (4) Wash in PBS, dry at room temperature, mount with buffered glycerol, and observe under a UV microscope.

The specificity of fluorescence is established by the following controls: (1) absence of fluorescence when tested with labeled normal serum, (2) inhibition of specific fluorescence by the addition of unlabeled anti-ASF serum to preparations before staining with labeled antiserum, (3) absence of fluorescence in uninfected cultures. Specific ASF fluorescence occurs in the form of granular or globular cytoplasmic inclusions juxtanuclear in position, which is also where the Giemsa-stained inclusions are seen in infected cell cultures. Fluorescent and Giemsa-stained inclusions are often ring shaped. Cells with inclusions generally have karyorrhexia of the nuclei.

Thus far, VN antibody has not been demonstrated consistently in survivor sera. Certain sera appear to inhibit growth of ASF virus but the effect is of a low degree and is often temporary.

Several isolates of ASF virus have been attenuated by passage in swine buffy-coat and bone-marrow cultures, generally after 70–100 passages. Such vaccines, however, have still retained a low degree of virulence and have not produced satisfactory immunity in the majority of pigs vaccinated. They have made possible the production of antisera against many of the isolates of ASF virus. Pigs may be effectively challenged with virulent ASF virus by almost any route, parenterally or orally. The dose of challenge virus does not appear to be a very important factor.

Reference laboratory. ASF is a reportable disease. In the United States, PIADC is the diagnostic laboratory.

References

1. Boulanger, P., G.L. Bannister, A.S. Greig, D.P. Gray, and G.M. Ruckerbauer. Diagnosis of African swine fever by immunofluorescence and other serological methods: *Bull. Off. Internat. Epiz.* 66:1–6, 1966.
2. Coggins, L. Segregation of a non-hemadsorbing African swine fever virus in tissue culture. *Cornell Vet.* 58:12–20, 1968.
3. Coggins, L., and W.P. Heuschele. Use of agar diffusion precipitation test in the diagnosis of African swine fever. *Am. J. Vet. Res.* 27:485–488, 1966.
4. Cowan, K.M. Immunological studies on African swine fever virus. II. Enhancing effect of normal bovine serum on the complement-fixation reaction. *Am. J. Vet. Res.* 24:756–760, 1963.
5. DeTray, D.E. African swine fever. In *Advances in Veterinary Science,* C.A. Brandly and E.L. Jungherr (eds.), vol. 8, pp. 299–309. Academic Press, New York, 1963.
6. Hess, W.R., B.F. Cox, W.P. Heuschele, and S.S. Stone. Propagation and modification of African swine fever virus in cell cultures. *Am. J. Vet. Res.* 26:141–145, 1965.
7. Heuschele, W.P., L. Coggins, and S.S. Stone. Fluorescent antibody studies on African swine fever virus. *Am. J. Vet. Res.* 27:477–480, 1966.

Equine Infectious Anemia Virus

Equine infectious anemia (EIA) is also known as swamp fever and equine relapsing fever. The primary hosts are animals of the Equidae family. The experimentally produced and the spontaneous cases of the disease vary considerably. There are three clinical types of the disease. In the first type, animals develop acute, severe disease with initiation of fever and clinical signs 8–10 days after experimental inoculation. These animals are continually febrile for weeks or months and often die within 3–8 weeks after the initial appearance of clinical signs. In the second type, animals develop clinical disease as evidenced by fever, depression, and anorexia, but recover from this and subsequently have periodic exacerbations of clinical disease interspersed with variable periods of clinical normalcy. The duration of the periodic clinical disease in these animals varies from 1 day to a week or more. The third type of the disease takes a chronic, relatively asymptomatic course. Animals with this type may develop acute disease for a short period and then become asymptomatic for months or years. Their brief periods of illness are widely spaced.

The packed cell volume and erythrocyte counts decline during the course of EIA. The rapidity of the decline is associated with and determined by the degree of clinical disease activity. The anemia is principally hemolytic although the hemolytic aspect is complicated by hyporesponsiveness in the bone marrow during febrile periods.[9] The hemolytic anemia appears to be immunologically mediated, as the RBC of diseased horses have been shown to be coated with complement and are Coombs positive.[10] The RBC have a decreased half life, which is often the only detectable alteration in horses with chronic asymptomatic EIA. The mechanisms by which the complement coats the RBC and causes decreased red cell survival and extravascular hemolysis is unknown. Probably, these events occur as a result of the presence of antibody directed against either the red cell itself or against EIA viral antigen that is in or on the erythrocytes. The quantity of antibody on the RBC appears to be small or of low affinity. Diseased horses also have deranged coagulation time so that surgical procedures such as biopsies must be approached with caution during active disease.

Examination of buffy-coat cells for the presence of iron reveals a variable number of circulating leukocytes that contain stainable iron. These cells, sideroleukocytes, are present in all horses with active clinical disease. The number of sideroleukocytes varies, but it is unusual to find more than three or four per 100,000 cells in normal horses. Sideroleukocytes are also seen in diseases such as equine piroplasmosis and in intoxication with hemolytic compounds such as phenothiazine. The total WBC count varies, but in some animals there is a decrease during pyrexic episodes. The decrease is usually found in the granulocytic series of cells, resulting in a relative lymphocytosis. Hypergammaglobulinemia with decreased albumin-globulin ratios also occurs. In horses with active disease, serum glutamic oxalacetic transaminase values are frequently elevated in those animals that develop hepatic changes. There are also decreases in haptoglobin values and indirect bilirubin, and plasma hemaglobin transiently increases during the active phases of EIA infection. Whether all or some of the clinical pathologic changes described above are seen in an individual horse will depend on the stage of disease activity at the time of examination.

The gross lesions observed in diseased horses include splenomegaly, lymphadenopathy, anemia, emaciation, edema, and accentuated hepatic lobular architecture. Microscopic lesions include lympholiferative changes with lymphocytic infiltrates, especially perivascular ones, in most organs and tissues. In addition, there is lymphoid and reticuloendothelial hyperplasia of the lymphoid tissues of the body. Liver cell necrosis occurs but is not a dominant feature of the disease and may be principally the result of anoxia. There is considerable periportal hepatic lymphoid infiltration and hyperplasia of the reticuloendothelial cells of the liver. Hemosiderin is prominent in the hepatic macrophages. The severity of the hepatic changes is related to clinical disease activity. Asymptomatic carriers that have not experienced an attack of disease for several months will often have no morphologic hepatic changes. Conversely, horses experiencing severe disease will have severe liver lesions. The hepatic changes are characteristic of EIA, although some researchers have suggested that similar-appearing lesions may be found in equine piroplasmosis. In addition, there is often generalized hemosiderosis with hemosiderin-laden cells detectable in the circulation as well as in a number of organs. A proliferative glomerulitis with increased glomerular cellularity and thickening of the glomerular tufts is also prominent. The glomerulitis appears to be the result of immune complex deposition since the glomerular capillaries contain granular deposits of complement (C'3) and IgG. Erythrophagocytosis can be found in lymphoid tissues, bone marrow, and liver. The principal microscopic changes upon which a diagnosis can be made are the hepatic changes associated with pyrexia, especially periodic pyrexia, and the presence of sideroleukocytes and anemia. Inclusion bodies have not been demonstrated and special stains are of little value.

Specimens

For virus isolation or transmission studies, whole peripheral blood, serum, and spleen have been most extensively used. Blood collected during the first fever episode appears to contain the highest concentration of virus, but comparative quantitative viral assays have not been carried out.

Experimentally infected horses become viremic 5–10 days after inoculation and the virus is continuously detectable in the circulation for many years and probably for the life of most animals. The lymphoid tissues and the blood probably contain the virus in the highest concentration, but sufficient experimental data is not available to completely evaluate this aspect. The virus is also present in the leukocytes and becomes detectable 5–8 days after inoculation. EIA virus is present in all tissues that have been tested as well as in urine, semen, and probably other excretions and secretions.

Laboratory Procedures

Cultures. Primary peripheral leukocyte cultures have been used for propagation of EIA virus;[4] this system has given favorable results in laboratories in Japan and the United States. Cultures must be maintained in good condition for 14–21 days in order to be useful in this technique. Because leukocyte cultures from most horses will not survive this long (21 days), selection of a suitable donor horse is of ultimate importance and depends upon trial and error. Because herpesvirus infection is very high in the general horse population, donor horses must also be screened for inapparent infection by such agents.

The leucocyte cultures are prepared in the following manner. Blood is collected from the jugular vein of the donor horse in citrate and allowed to stand at either room temperature or 4°C for approximately 1 hour. The rapid sedimentation rate of the erythrocytes allows the buffy-coat cells to be collected. The buffy-coat cells are washed twice in sterile Hanks' solution and resuspended in growth medium to a concentration of approximately 2×110^7 cells per ml. At the end of 24 hours the cultures are lightly centrifuged and the medium changed to 100% serum, Medium 199, or Hanks' solution enriched with 50–75% bovine or ovine serum. The serum donor is important since sera from some animals can be toxic to the cultures. Some laboratories use 40% newborn calf serum in Medium 199 as the initial culture medium. Incubation is stationary at 37°C.

The cultures are ready for inoculation after 24–72 hours. The inoculum should be left on the cultures for 1 hour at 37°C, then the cultures should be washed and new medium added.

Virus propagation in leukocyte cultures can be evaluated by observing three characteristics: cytopathic changes, production of CF antigen, and immunofluorescence. A CPE has been reported but the appearance of the change is similar to that occuring spontaneously in some cultures. Endpoints of infectivity cannot be determined accurately by CPE alone. The most specific method of evaluation appears to be the detection of CF antigen in cultures using a standard antiserum in the CF procedure described by Kono and Kobayashi.[6] Direct and indirect tests for immunofluorescence have been described using convalescent sera for preparation of the conjugates.[8,11]

Kono[5] used leukocyte cultures as the indicator system for infectivity and found that virus titers were highest in the serum during the initial febrile response, then declined, but tended to increase with each subsequent pyrexic episode; however, the levels of viremia did not reach that noted during the initial episodes.

Animal inoculation. Horses and related species are the only animals that have been conclusively proven to be susceptible to EIA virus. There have been reports of propagation in other animals, such as the rabbit, but these findings have not been verified.

The presence of EIA virus in affected horses has historically been demonstrated by inoculating susceptible horses with whole blood. The selection of susceptible recipient animals is accomplished by cross-transfusion tests, which are performed as follows. Approximately 100 ml of blood is collected from each of the animals to be checked and additional blood (50 ml) is collected and pooled. Each individual sample is then injected IV or SC into another horse. This is repeated until each animal has received 100 ml of whole blood from another horse. Each animal is then temperatured twice daily, and weekly sideroleukocyte counts and packed cell volume determinations are carried out. Preinoculation samples as well as postinoculation serum collected at 2-week intervals should be evaluated using the CF test. All animals are observed for 90 days. Hepatic biopsies can also be taken before and after inoculation. The pooled sample is injected into a known negative horse. If none of the horses exhibit changes in the variables described for EIA, they are considered free of EIA and can be used for horse inoculation.

In testing a horse for EIA, approximately 100 ml of blood is collected and injected IV or SC into a proven negative horse. The above described variables are checked for 90 days for changes associated with EIA. If they remain negative, the horse is considered negative for EIA.

Immunology and serology. No definitive information is available concerning serotypes of EIA. Kono and Kobayashi compared isolates of EIA virus from the United States, Japan, and Germany in the CF test and reported that they all share common CF antigens.[6] Incomplete evidence indicates there is no relationship to other known virus groups.

The CF test is conducted by the complement dilution method with the antigen prepared in infected leukocyte cultures.[6,7] In this test, a complement titer of 1.2 or higher is interpreted as an indicator of a positive serologic test for EIA, a titer of 0.75–1.19 as questionable, and one of less than 0.75 as negative. CF antibody responses have been demonstrated in both spontaneously and experimentally infected horses. The antibody response becomes detectable approximately 14–21 days after infection, persists for several weeks to over 2 months, then declines and becomes undetectable regardless of the clinical disease that the animal experiences thereafter. No cross-reacting CF antibodies have been noted when sera from animals infected with equine herpesviruses, including types I and II, equine influenza virus, and equine viral arteritis virus have been tested.

The VN test is conducted by standard methods, using leukocyte cultures for inoculation. The neutralization of CPE that is observed appears to be the result of antibodies; however, this has not been proven conclusively. This neutralization effect has been demonstrated in some but not all experimentally infected horses 20–30 days after inoculation and may be detectable for over 500 days. This test, however, has been only superficially investigated and additional research is needed before the significance of serum antibody titers can be evaluated.

For the AD test, spleen from an acutely ill pony or horse is used as antigen.[1,3] The animal must react severely and the spleen must be harvested 9–11 days after inoculation. Formation of a single line of identity with that of a reference control serum determines the specificity. EIA precipitating antibody generally appears between the second and third week following infection and seems to persist for the life of the animal. This test correlates well with data determined by the animal inoculation tests. By statistical analysis, the test is at least 95% accurate for the diagnosis of all forms of this infection.[2] The test should be employed to determine the negative status of any horse to be used in an animal inoculation test.

There is no evidence in either naturally or experimentally infected horses of immunity to EIA virus infection; hence the development of the carrier state. Humoral antibody responses have been demonstrated in infected horses, however; and the possibility of cellular immunity occurring must also be investigated. The evaluation of immunity by challenge procedures has not been effective. When infected horses have been reinoculated with EIA virus the results have varied; in some reports infected horses developed an exacerbation of clinical disease following challenge, while in other reports challenged horses remained normal.

References

1. Coggins, L., and N.L. Norcross. Immunodiffusion reaction in equine infectious anemia. *Cornell Vet.* 60:330, 1970.
2. Coggins, L., N.L. Norcross, and S.R. Nusbaum. Diagnosis of equine infectious anemia by immunodiffusion test. *Am. J. Vet. Res.* 33:11–18, 1972.
3. Coggins, L., and V. Patten. Immunodiffusion test for equine infectious anemia. *Proc. U.S. Anim. Health Assoc.* 74:568–571, 1970.
4. Kobayashi, K. Studies on the cultivation of equine infectious anemia virus *in vitro*. III. Propagation of the virus in leukocyte culture. *Virus* 11:249–256, 1961.
5. Kono, Y. Viremia and immunological responses in horses infected with equine infectious anemia virus. *Nat. Inst. Anim. Health Q.* 9:1–9, 1969.
6. Kono, Y., and K. Kobayashi. Complement fixation test of equine infectious anemia. I. Specificity of the test. *Nat. Inst. Anim. Health Q.* 6:194–203, 1966.

7. Kono, Y., and K. Kobayashi. Specificity of assay of equine infectious anemia virus in horse leukocyte culture. *Nat. Inst. Anim. Health Q.* 7:138–144, 1967.
8. McGuire, T.C., T.B. Crawford, and J.B. Henson. Immunofluorescent localization of equine infectious anemia virus in tissues. *Am. J. Path.* 62:283–292, 1971.
9. McGuire, T.C., J.B. Henson, and D. Burger. Complement (C'3) coated red blood cells following infection with the virus of equine infectious anemia. *J. Immunol.* 103:293–299, 1969.
10. McGuire, T.C., J.B. Henson, and S.E. Quist. Impaired bone marrow in equine infectious anemia. *Am. J. Vet. Res.* 30:2099–2104, 1969.
11. Ushimi, C., H. Nakajima, and S. Tanaka. Demonstration of equine infectious anemia viral antigen by immunofluorescence. Nat. Inst. Anim. Health Q. 10:90–91, 1970.

Borna Disease Virus

Borna disease (BD) is an infectious viral encephalomyelitis and meningitis of horses, sheep, and domestic rabbits. The disease is named after a village in Saxony, Germany, where a particularly severe outbreak occurred from 1894 to 1896.[4] BD is endemic in the West German states of Bavaria, Hesse, and Baden-Württemberg, and in the East German states of Thuringia and Saxony. The question of whether BD exists elsewhere in the world is unanswered; the disease may be present in Poland, Rumania, and the Soviet Union. In the enzootic areas, BD occurs throughout the year; thus arthropod vectors are not essential for transmission. Cattle may be inapparent carriers of the disease.[4]

The clinical signs of BD in horses include inappetence, constant chewing and grinding of teeth, priapism, head drooping, frequent lying down, unsteady gait, muscular contractions, colic, and frequent bending of neck to the side. Some cases resemble the EEV infections of the Americas. The mortality rate may be as high as 75–90%. The incubation period for experimental BD by IC inoculation of horses and sheep is 6–7 weeks.[2]

The clinical signs of BD in sheep include inappetence, unnatural stance, hyperexcitability alternating with lethargy and depression, and eventual paralysis. Some sheep may appear normal between attacks of sudden collapse, which may occur several times a day. Rabbits may show clinical signs similar to horses or sheep. An inability to lift the ears is often the first sign.[5]

No gross lesions are found. Microscopic lesions are found as inflammatory changes throughout the brain and spinal cord. The findings of lymphocytic infiltration, glial cell proliferation, and neuronal degeneration are considered diagnostic for BD. The midbrain is the most severely affected, involving the gray matter around the aqueduct and in the substantia nigra. Other sites include the caudate nucleus, Ammon's horn, the pyriform area, the medulla at the floor of the fourth ventricle, and the nuclei of cranial nerves V through X, generally excepting VII.[1,4] Gliosis is an early occurring, prominent feature of BD. Acidophilic intranuclear inclusion or JD (Joest-Degen) bodies are found in ganglion cells. The JD bodies vary from 0.1 to 3 μm in diameter and are considered pathognomonic for BD. FA reactions are found only in neurons and are concentrated in nuclei where JD bodies occur. Thus ganglia may be the primary site of virus replication.[5]

Electron microscopy has not yet demonstrated the BD virus ultrastructure, nor has the nucleic acid core been established. The virion is thought to have an envelope and the diameter may be greater than 85 nm.[3] The virus is considered to be quite resistant to usual environmental influences, for example, it can survive in tap water and in milk for over a month.

Specimens

The entire brain and portions of the spinal cord are needed for histopathologic examination, FA studies, and for inoculation of laboratory rabbits.

Laboratory Procedures

Cultures. Secondary lamb kidney cell cultures, with the slow-growing virus being carried along with passage of the cells, will support viral replication. However, animal inoculation, FA, or other tests must be used to detect the virus, which does not produce significant gross cytopathology.[4] Embryonating chicken eggs inoculated on the CAM also may be used for viral replication.

Animal inoculation. Rabbits inoculated IC are used for diagnostic and experimental studies. Laboratory rats and guinea pigs also can be used, but they are not as reliable as rabbits for BD studies.

Immunology and serology. As yet there is no reliable test for serum antibodies that can be used for diagnostic purposes. However, using laboratory antisera the BD virus may be detected with CF and FA tests.[6] Rabbits are used to produce antisera for BD. Vaccines have been developed that seem to provide protection for sheep but are less effective for horses.[4]

References

1. Anzil, A.P., and K. Blinzinger. Electron microscopic studies of rabbit central and peripheral nervous system in experimental Borna Disease. *Acta Neuropath.* 22:305–318, 1972.
2. Heinig, A. Experimental infection of horses and sheep with the virus of Borna Disease. *Arch. Exp. Vet. Med.* 18:753–766, 1964.
3. Mayer, A., and K. Danner. Production of Borna Disease in tissue culture. *Proc. Soc. Exp. Biol. Med.* 140:511–515, 1972.
4. Reichard, R.E., and R. Uskavitch. Borna disease: A literature review. U.S. Department of Agriculture, ARS-NE-56, pp. 1–25, 1975.
5. Shadduck, J.A., K. Danner, and E. Dahme. Fluorescent serological studies on the occurrence and localization of Borna virus antigen in the brains of experimentally infected rabbits. *Zentralblatt Veterinärmedizin* 17:453–459, 1970.
6. Von Sprockhoff, H. Experimental studies on Borna Disease: Soluble antigen and infection of young rabbits. *Zeitschrift Immunforsch. Exp. Ther.* 115:161–168, 1958.

24. Viruses of Chronic Degenerative Diseases

There are certain diseases of animals that can be categorized as chronic and degenerative and that have a virus etiology or are of presumed viral origin. Investigators in Iceland attached the label "slow viruses" to the etiologic agents of a group of such diseases of sheep.[5] However, all these qualities are not always applicable in the present concept of these diseases. In diseases where the causal agent is propagated in vitro, growth of the virus does not proceed any more slowly than with viruses causing acute diseases. Therefore, the term slow viruses does not now seem appropriate, as the slowness or chronicity of the infections may reflect the host's reaction to the infecting agent.

Basically, the diseases to be described in this section result from the continuous or intermittent presence of the causative agent over long periods and disease occurs after a latent period of weeks to years. The diseases are grouped on clinical criteria rather than on the basis of the qualities of the infecting agents. Such an approach seems appropriate in view of the paucity of information on the nature of some of these agents.

Visna and Maedi Viruses

Visna, meaning wasting, is a chronic demyelinating viral encephalitis of sheep with an extremely long incubation period.[6] Maedi, the Icelandic name for dyspnea, is a chronic progressive respiratory disease of sheep caused by a virus.[5] While these diseases are obviously dissimilar, they are presented together because the causative agents appear to be strains of the same virus.

Visna and maedi viruses are not only similar serologically but also share similar physical, chemical, and biologic properties. Electron microscopic studies have shown that virus particles are formed by budding at the surface of the host cells. The particles range in size from 60 to 90 nm, appear to be bounded by a single membrane, and contain a centrally located electron-dense core about 30–40 nm in diameter. All observations indicate that the virus particle contains RNA, and an RNA-dependent DNA polymerase has been demonstrated in visna virus, providing evidence of the similarity between visna and the avian and murine leukemia viruses.[8] Both visna and maedi viruses are ether sensitive, are inactivated at 56°C in 10 minutes, and are inactivated at a slow rate by UV light. They retain their infectivity for months at −60°C, almost as well at −20°C, and are viable for about 4 months at 4°C. The viruses are relatively stable in the range of pH 5.1–10 but are inactivated at pH 4.2.

The diseases, visna and maedi, have been economically important diseases of sheep in Iceland. Apparently, the diseases were introduced into Iceland by importation of sheep from Europe, but now they have been essentially eradicated. While no disease comparable to visna has been reported outside Iceland, the lung disease of sheep (*zwoegerziekte*) in the Netherlands and progressive pneumonia of sheep (Montana lung disease) in the United States have been shown by serologic cross-neutralization to be causally similar or related to maedi.[9]

Visna is usually insidious in its onset, beginning with slight ataxia and paresis, particularly in the hind legs. The paresis progresses slowly and usually ends in paraplegia or in total paralysis. The clinical disease can last from a few weeks to several months and appears to be invariably fatal. The clinical signs observed in experimentally transmitted cases of visna were apparently identical with the signs observed in natural cases. Transmission experiments have shown that the clinical stage of the disease is preceded by a subclinical period lasting from a few months up to several years.[6] During the subclinical period the main sign of the infection is an increase in the number of cells in the CSF, usually beginning 1 or 2 months after intracerebral inoculation. This is accompanied by an increase in the protein content of the CSF, particularly gamma globulins.

During this period virus may be found in the CSF, whole blood, and saliva, sometimes concurrently with a high concentration of VN antibodies in the serum.[2,3] Visna virus has also been recovered from various organs of sheep inoculated several months or even years earlier and not yet showing clinical signs. Sheep that become moribund following visna virus infection are consistently found to harbor the virus in various organs.

The primary lesion in the CNS is the appearance of meningeal and subependymal infiltration or proliferation of cells of the reticuloendothelial system, principally lymphocytes and microglia. Perivascular infiltrations of lymphocytes are common. Demyelination of the white matter of the CNS seems to occur secondarily. The gray matter is usually only slightly affected. Hyperplasia of the reticuloendothelial elements in the lungs, lymph nodes, and spleen of visna-infected sheep has also been noted. No changes have been observed in other organs.[6]

Maedi is a chronic respiratory disease, the early signs of which are characterized by dyspnea and a loss of condition, particularly under exertion. Both signs gradually become more distinct as the disease progresses. The respiration, even at rest, becomes extremely labored. The clinical disease usually lasts for 3–8 months or longer and usually ends in death.[5]

Epidemiologic studies, as well as transmission experiments with maedi, indicate a subclinical period of 2–3 years or more prior to the appearance of clinical signs. During this period, experimentally transmitted cases of maedi have developed leukocytosis beginning at least 1 year before the onset of clinical signs. The leukocyte count may or may not return to normal.[5] If the leukocyte count returns to normal the infection generally remains subclinical in nature.

Typical macroscopic changes are confined to the thoracic cavity. The weight of the lungs and of the tracheobronchial and mediastineal lymph nodes is increased up to four times that of the normal. The entire lungs are more or less uniformly thickened and when the thorax is opened they collapse much less than normal lungs. The color of the lungs is changed from pinkish-red to grayish-brown. The diaphragmatic lobes often seem to be more affected by the infection than the cardic and apical lobes.

On microscopic examination, the lungs show proliferation of the mesenchymal tissue with thickening of the alveolar septa. In advanced cases alveolar tissue is transformed into strands of mesenchymal cells separated by irregular spaces infiltrated with large mononuclear cells. The trachea and bronchi are normal. The enlarged lymph nodes show generalized hyperplasia and chronic inflammatory changes. Microscopic examination of lungs from sheep experimentally infected with maedi but killed before clinical signs appeared showed characteristic lesions consisting of perivascular and peribronchiolar infiltrations, mainly of lymphocytes, plasma cells, and monocytes.[5] The alveolar walls appear to be thicker than in normal lungs.

Specimens

Visna virus is readily recovered in cell cultures from brain material.[7] In experimentally infected sheep, the virus has been recovered from the choroid plexus, spleen, mediastinal lymph nodes, salivary glands, lungs, blood, and CSF, and in a few instances the kidney.

Maedi virus may be recovered from specimens of lung either by inoculation of suspensions of lung material or by explants of lung tissue.[7] The virus is also readily recovered from the spleen, mediastinal lymph nodes, and leukocytes, and less frequently from the choroid plexus and CSF. The virus has not been recovered from nasal or salivary secretions.[1] In experimentally infected sheep, virus was recovered from the above mentioned sources and also from the salivary gland and occasionally the kidney.[4]

Laboratory Procedures

Cultures. Visna and maedi viruses can be recovered from explants of choroid plexus and lung, respectively, as well as suspension of these and the previously mentioned organs onto cell cultures.[7] Preparation and inoculation of specimens onto choroid plexus or kidney cell cultures are similar to those used to recover other viruses.

Visna virus propagates readily on cell cultures derived from various organs of the sheep, other animals, and humans.[7] Most of the studies of the virus have been conducted in primary or serially propagated choroid plexus cells from sheep brain; however, the virus grows well in kidney and choroid plexus cells from calves.

Growth of maedi virus readily occurs in both primary and secondary cell cultures of sheep choroid plexus. No growth of the virus has been demonstrable in cultures of chick embryo cells. Growth in other types of cell cultures has not been studied.

Choroid plexus cell cultures are optimal to work with 3–8 weeks after primary harvesting. Tubes for subcultures are ready in 2–3 days. In the original research, both primary and secondary propagated cultures were grown in Medium 199 with 20% sheep serum and, following full growth, were maintained with the same medium plus 2% sheep serum. All serum should be previously checked for the presence of antibodies or inhibitors.

The growth of both viruses produces similar CPE in sheep choroid plexus cell cultures in about 4 days following inoculation. These changes include the formation of multinucleated giant cells, which in unstained cultures appear as large stellate cells with increased refractility. Other changes often observed are the formation of spindle-shaped cells with only one or very few nuclei, increased refractility, and the development of irregular processes extending from the cell. Similar changes occur in cultures of calf kidney and choroid plexus when inoculated with visna virus, but fewer and less distinct changes are produced in cell cultures of choroid plexus from human embryos, pigs, guinea pigs, dogs, and cats. No evidence of visna virus growth has been demonstrated in cultures of human amnion, chick embryo fiberblasts, HeLa, and L-cells.

Animal inoculation. When sheep are experimentally infected with visna virus, they develop pathognomonic CNS lesions, but, unlike in the naturally occurring disease, they also develop lung lesions similar to maedi.[3] When sheep are either naturally or experimentally infected with maedi virus, the characteristic lung lesions are found, but the sheep also may have CNS lesions that are indistinguishable from those seen in visna.[1,4] No other experimental animals have been successfully used.

Immunology and serology. Similar serologic procedures may be used for both visna and maedi viruses. The VN test may be accomplished by using standard methods; however, VN titers are greatly increased by incubating the serum and virus mixtures for a period of 3 hours at 37°C. CF antibodies are readily demonstrable. The standard CF test appears to be a more sensitive serologic method than the VN test for detecting early rises in antibody titer. No evidence of HA or HAd has been demonstrable with either virus.

Subclinical infection commonly occurs in maedi-infected flocks, as evidenced by widespread presence of circulating antibodies in members of the infected Icelandic flocks.[8,10] The percentage of sheep with antibodies was two to three times larger than the percentage showing macroscopic changes of maedi in the lung. Visna virus infection was eliminated from the Icelandic sheep much earlier; thus similar serologic data is not available for this disease. However, the presence of circulating antibodies does not confer immunity to infected sheep.[3] On the contrary, the evidence suggests that those sheep developing the highest levels of antibodies are more likely to succumb to the disease.[3] The long incubation period in which circulating antibodies can be found in the CSF concomitantly with virus raises the possibility that these diseases result from immune complexing. There are no reported attempts to immunize animals with these viruses.

References

1. Gudnadottir, M., G. Gislason, and P.A. Palsson. Studies on natural cases of maedi in search for diagnostic laboratory methods. *Res. Vet. Sci.* 9:65–67, 1968.
2. Gudnadottir, M., and P.A. Palsson. Successful transmission of visna by intrapulmonary inoculation. *J. Infec. Dis.* 115:217–225, 1965.
3. Gudnadottir, M., and P.A. Palsson. Host-virus interaction in visna infected sheep. *J. Immunol.* 95:1116–1120, 1966.
4. Gudnadottir, M., and P.A. Palsson. Transmission of maedi by inoculation of a virus grown in tissue cultures from maedi-affected lungs. *J. Infec. Dis.* 117:1–6, 1967.

5. Sigurdsson, B., P.A. Palsson, and A. Tryggvadottir. Transmission experiments with maedi. *J. Infec. Dis.* 93:116–175, 1953.
6. Sigurdsson, B., P.A. Palsson, and L. Van-Bogaert. Pathology of visna, transmissible demyelinating disease in sheep in Iceland. *Acta Neuropath.* 1:343–362, 1962.
7. Sigurdsson, B., H. Thormar, and P.A. Palsson. Cultivation of visna virus in tissue culture. *Arch. ges. Virusforsch.* 10:368–381, 1960.
8. Stone, L.B., E. Scolnich, K.K. Takemoto, and S.A. Aaronson. Visna virus: A slow virus with an RNA dependent DNA polymerase. *Nature* 229:257–258, 1971.
9. Thormar, H. A study of maedi virus, lung tumors in animals. In *Proceedings of the Third International Conference on Cancer,* L. Severi (ed.), pp. 393–401. Division of Cancer Research, University of Perugia, Italy, 1966.
10. Thormar, H., G. Gislason, and H. Helgadottir. A survey of neutralizing antibodies against maedi virus in sera from flocks of sheep affected with maedi and from healthy flocks. *J. Infec. Dis.* 116:41–47, 1966.

Transmissible Mink Encephalopathy Virus

Transmissible mink encephalopathy (TME) is a naturally occurring, subacute spongiform disease of mink.[2] It is a slowly progressive noninflammatory neuropathy that invariably terminates in death.

There are no serotypes known. The infecting agent has not been demonstrated by FA tests nor has any antibody been detected.[5] The naturally occurring disease is observed only in mink; however, it has been experimentally transmitted to golden hamsters and squirrel monkeys.[1,3] Naturally occurring and experimentally produced TME are clinically and pathologically indistinguishable. The incubation period following oral exposure is about 8 months. It is reduced to 5 months by IM inoculation, and further reduced to an average of 130 days by intracranial injection of a 10^{-1} dilution of a 10% brain suspension. The onset of disease is insidious and difficult to recognize unless one is well-acquainted with the behavioral characteristics of the individual mink affected. Some mink become very quiet and furtive while others become more excitable, active, and aggressive. Often, the first sign is anorexia. The mink gradually lose weight and become weakened, exhibiting locomotor disturbance beginning in the pelvic limbs. This is accompanied by roughened fur and a characteristic change in the posture of the tail, which is often arched up over the back in the manner of a squirrel. The neuropathy becomes more severe as it progresses: somnolence is more pronounced, and weakness to the point of incapacitation accompanies progressive disorientation.

Necropsies are characterized by a conspicuous absence of gross lesions. Consistent microscopic changes are only found in the brain; they include astrocytosis, neuronal degeneration, vacuolation of neurons, and spongiform degeneration of the gray matter. Neuronal vacuolation is less prominent than in scrapie. The lesions are most prominent in the hippocampus, hypothalamus, thalamus, and brain stem. Loss of Purkinje cells in the cerebellum is readily apparent. The astrocytosis is best observed if Cajal's gold sublimate stain for astrocytes is used. The other changes are adequately seen using H & E staining procedures.

Specimens

The specimen of choice is brain tissue. In mink exposed IM or orally, the spleen and liver also are suitable sources of the agent in the terminal phase of the disease.[4]

Laboratory Procedures

Cultures. Cell cultures of brains from mink with TME are prepared by trypsinization.[4] Brain material is minced and washed three times in saline, and the cells are dispersed by exposure to 0.25% trypsin at room temperature for 10 minutes. The cell suspension is mixed with 10 ml of calf serum and centrifuged for 10 minutes at $1200 \times g$ and the supernatant fluid is discarded. This process may be repeated if more cells are needed. The cell pellets are resuspended in complete Medium 199 containing 20% lamb serum to make a final concentration of 1:30 for planting. A confluent sheet of cells develops in approximately 3 weeks; subcultures develop in 72–96 hours.[4] Assay for infectivity is performed by intracerebral inoculation of mink. Cultures have titers of about 10^1 LD_{50} per 0.1 ml; whole cells, $10^{2.5}$; disrupted cells, $10^{3.5}$.

Animal inoculation. The most common test for TME in specimens from suspected mink involves the inoculation of normal young mink. The specimen, preferably brain, spleen, or liver, is homogenized in a tissue grinder and mixed with BSS to produce a 1:10 dilution by volume. The test mink are anesthetized with ether. A 0.75 inch (1.91 cm), 19-gauge needle is forced into the calvarium. A 2-inch (5.08 cm), 22-gauge needle is inserted into the lumen of the 19-gauge needle to deliver the inoculum into the cerebrum. Transmission of TME requires from 4 to 6 months, using a 10^{-1} dilution of the inoculum. Exposure by oral or IM routes results in incubation periods of 8–12 months.

Immunology and serology. No serologic tests are known. Recovery from the disease is not known. Whatever resistance exists appears to be natural or genetic.

References

1. Eckroade, R., G.M. Zurhein, R.F. Marsh, and R.P. Hanson. Transmissible mink encephalopathy: Experimental transmission to the squirrel monkey. *Science* 169:1088–1090, 1970.
2. Hartsough, G.R., and D. Burger. Encephalopathy of mink. I. Epizootiologic and clinical observations. *J. Infec. Dis.* 115:387–392, 1965.
3. Marsh, R.F., D. Burger, R. Eckroade, G.M. Zurhein, and R.P. Hanson. Preliminary report on the experimental host range of the transmissible encephalopathy agent. *J. Infec. Dis.* 120:713–719, 1969.
4. Marsh, R.F., D. Burger, and R.P. Hanson. Transmissible mink encephalopathy: Behavior of the disease agent in mink. *Am. J. Vet. Res.* 30:1637–1642, 1969.
5. Marsh, R.F., I.C. Pan, and R.P. Hanson. Failure to demonstrate specific antibody in transmissible mink encephalopathy. *Infec. Immunity* 2:727–730, 1970.

Scrapie Virus

Scrapie is a naturally occurring, relentlessly progressive, afebrile neuropathy of sheep and less often of goats. French-speaking people have called it *tremblent du mouton,* and in Iceland it is known as *rida.* Scrapie is considered to be one of the subacute spongiform virus encephalopathies along with TME and the human diseases, Kuru and Creutzfeldt-Jacob disease, which scrapie resembles in its pathologic features and biologic properties.[9] Scrapie has been recognized for more than 200 years and now is present on all the continents except Australia and South America.

No serotype is recognizable, as the agent has not been found to be antigenic.[2] Experimental infections have been established in mice,[3] rats,[4] hamsters,[11] mink,[8] and monkeys.[6] Efforts to infect pigeons, chickens, and rabbits have not been successful. Goats have been found to be highly susceptible to experimental inoculations; nearly 100% develop the disease, as opposed to 60% of sheep similarly exposed.[10] Vertical spread of the disease occurs; with considerably less facility lateral spread has been experimentally achieved among sheep, between sheep and goats, and among mice.

Scrapie is a disease of adult animals; it is virtually unknown naturally among sheep less than 2.5 years of age. There is no definable limit to the length of the incubation period. The subtle onset of the syndrome is deceptive in all species, whether natural or experimental infection is present. In the early stages the sheep is more excitable than usual and fine tremors of the head and neck may be observed. The most characteristic feature is an intense pruritus that usually beings at the rump and extends down the limbs, along the sides to the shoulders, and down the forelimbs, and concomitantly occurs in the mandibular and occipital areas. The sheep rubs against anything firm with subsequent loss of wool, which has become dull, separable, and brittle. During a spasm, the sheep lifts its head and with nodding motions makes viperlike extrusions of its tongue. The sheep in recumbancy will nibble vigorously at the short-wooled portions of the limbs, often denuding the surfaces that can be reached. With the gradual deepening of the neuropathy, locomotor disturbances become more pronounced. The gait is altered, especially at a trot or run. The limbs are characteristically overflexed and the pelvic limbs abducted. Emaciation and gradual weakness signal the terminal phase, although the appetite remains strong well into it. A convulsion often precedes the final agonal period.

There are no gross changes on which to base a diagnosis of scrapie in any species, whether naturally or experimentally affected. Microscopic changes of diagnostic importance are confined to the CNS. The most striking response to scrapie is astrocytosis of the hippocampus, diencephalon, cerebellar cortex, brain stem, and spinal cord. This may be observed best using Cajal's gold sublimate stain for astrocytes. There is also vacuolization of neurons, status spongiosus, and neuronal necrosis in all areas of the brain, but especially in the thalamus, hypothalamus, midbrain, and cerebellum. These changes may be observed by using H & E stain and by electron microscopy.

Several unusual qualities of the scrapie agent must be kept in mind. Attempts to release a viral-type agent from scrapie-affected brains have not been successful. Efforts to visualize it electron-microscopically have given essentially negative results. No marked changes from normal patterns of RNA and protein biosynthesis have been found. Although an increased rate of nuclear DNA synthesis has been found in the brain, the scrapie agent is cytoplasmically associated with organelles. The number of DNA-active nuclei reach a maximum long before any significant amount of the agent is present in the brain. Other remarkable properties are its resistance to heat, lack of antigenicity, resistance to Formalin, lack of inflammatory response to its presence, and bilateral symmetry of the lesions in the CNS. B-propriolactone reduces the activity in much less measure than it does for viruses that fit the criteria subscribed to by virologists.

Specimens

High concentrations of the agent have been demonstrated in the thalamus, midbrain, and brain stem of affected sheep. The brain, spleen, and thymus are excellent sources of the agent in mice.[5]

Laboratory Procedures

Cultures of infected tissues. Cell cultures of any part of the brain are prepared using 3-minute trypsinization periods with 0.25% trypsin. Overtrypsinization is to be carefully avoided. The number of cells that cling to the glass and eventually give rise to a monolayer culture through colonization is low. Ten days to two weeks are required for colonization to become clearly established. The character of the cultures, as compared with those from normal animals, is significant.[7] Cells originating from scrapie-infected tissue grow more readily and show wider variation in size and multinucleation than cells from normal tissue; polar orientation is also not as constant or orderly. In cell cultures established from mice 150 days after intracranial inoculation with 10% suspension of brain from an affected mouse, there are four times as many cells showing N-acetyl-b-d glucosaminidase (GAM) and b-glucuronidase (GUR) activity as in controls. At 120 days there is greater GAM activity than in controls but not greater GUR.[1]

Animal inoculation. The most common test for the presence of scrapie in specimens of suspected animals involves the inoculation of mice intracranially with a 10% suspension of brain. A portion of brain is frozen and triturated in that state and thoroughly mixed 1 part by volume with 9 parts of BSS. The suspension is centrifuged at moderate RCF for 30 minutes. The supernatant fluid is removed and filtered through an 0.045 μm filter prior to use. Transmission of scrapie from sheep to mice requires from 13 to 20 months. The second passage in mice requires from 5 to 7 months, and the third passage in mice may reach a steady state at 4–5 months of incubation. Strains of mice vary in their susceptibility.

Immunology and serology. No serologic tests are available.[2] Only rarely have there been reports of animals recovering from the disease; consequently, little is known of acquired immunity.

References

1. Buening, G.M., and D.P. Gustafson. Enzymatic changes in astrocytes of scrapie-affected mouse brains. *Am. J. Vet. Res.* 32:959–966, 1971.
2. Chandler, R.L. Attempts to demonstrate antibodies in scrapie disease. *Vet. Rec.* 71:58–59, 1959.
3. Chandler, R.L. Experimental scrapie in the mouse. *Res. Vet. Sci.* 4:276–285, 1963.
4. Chandler, R.L., and J. Fisher. Experimental transmission of scrapie to rats. *Lancet* 11:1165, 1963.
5. Ecklund, C.M., R.C. Kennedy, and W.J. Hadlow. Pathogenesis of scrapie virus infection in the mouse. *J. Infec. Dis.* 117:15–22, 1967.
6. Gibbs, C.J., Jr., and D.C. Gajdusek. Cell-virus interactions in slow infections of the nervous system. In *The Neurosciences,* F.O. Schmitt and F.G. Worden (eds.). Third Study Program. Paper no. 90, pp. 1025–1027. MIT Press, Cambridge, 1974.
7. Gustafson, D.P., and C.L. Kanitz. Evidence of the presence of scrapie in cell cultures of brain. In *Slow, Latent and Temperate Virus Infections.* National Institute for Neurological Diseases and Blindness Monograph no. 2, pp. 221–236, 1965.

8. Hanson, R.P., R.J. Eckroade, R.F. Marsh, G.M. Zurhein, C.L. Klanitz, and D.P. Gustafson. Susceptibility of mink to sheep scrapie. *Science* 172:859–861, 1971.
9. Lampert, P.W., D.C. Gajdusek, and C.J. Gibbs, Jr. Subacute spongiform virus encephalopathies: Scrapie, Kuru, and Creutzfeldt-Jacob disease—A Review. *Am. J. Path.* 68:626–646, 1972.

Sheep Pulmonary Adenomatosis (Jaagsiekte) "Virus"

Sheep pulmonary adenomatosis (SPA) is a distinct contagious lung tumor often occurring as a metastasizing adenocarcinoma.[3] The infectious agent that causes alveolar epithelial cell transformation by a progressive adenomatous process has not been elucidated, but available evidence incriminates a virus. The disease sometimes occurs with and can be confused with maedi.[1] The old name, Jaagsiekte, means driving sickness in Dutch, and was given because sick sheep in advanced stages of the disease had accelerated respiration as if they had been rapidly driven. When actually driven, they suddenly stopped, gasping for breath, and died soon afterward.[3] There are reports of SPA in goats, but other researchers have observed no transmission to goats or cattle when in contact with infected sheep.[3] With the exception of Australia and New Zealand, SPA has been reported as sporadic or enzootic in the major sheep-producing countries. The disease was eradicated from Iceland.

The incubation period usually varies from 4 to 8 months but may be as long as 2 years, depending upon host susceptibility. The course varies from 2 to 5 months. The chief clinical signs are progressive emaciation, overt respiratory distress, greatly increased respiratory rate, moist rales, discharge of mucinous watery fluid from lungs through the nostrils, and lack of fever. The adenomatous process appears to start from the anteroventral aspects of the diaphragmatic lung lobes and to progress dorsally and posteriorly. The affected zone of the lungs may have scattered, irregularly circumscribed, firm grayish-white nodules of varying size that eventually coalesce into a continuous glandlike tissue.

Histopathologic studies suggest that the initial change is a thickening of the interalveolar septa brought about by congestion, mononuclear cell invasion, and the presence of the epithelium of collapsed alveoli.[3] The adenomatous foci of transformed epithelial cells are first found in the thickened septa. The foci enlarge and coalesce to form larger nodules and eventually obliterate most of the normal lung tissue. With PAS staining, mucin may be demonstrated in cytoplasmic vacuoles in some of the adenomatous cells.[3] Metastatic foci are found mainly in the tracheobronchial and mediastinal lymph nodes.[2] When diagnosing SPA, only progressive interstitial pneumonia (maedi), chronic bronchopneumonia, and chronic verminous pneumonia need also be taken into consideration.

References
1. Marsh, H. Progressive pneumonia of sheep in the United States and its relation to diseases of the Jaagsiekte complex. In *Lung Tumors in Animals,* L. Severi (ed.), pp. 285–294. Division of Cancer Research, University of Perugia, Italy, 1966.
2. Nobel, T.A., F. Neumann, and U. Klopfer. Metastases in pulmonary adenomatosis of sheep. *Refuah Vet.* 25:57–62, 1968.
3. Wandera, J.G. Sheep pulmonary adenomatosis (Jaagsiekte). In *Advances in Veterinary Science and Comparative Medicine,* C.A. Brandly and E.L. Jungherr (eds.), vol. 15, pp. 251–283. Academic Press, New York, 1971.

PART THREE: BACTERIOLOGY

25. Enteric Organisms

Ewing defines the family Enterobacteriaceae as consisting of gram-negative, asporogenous, rod-shaped bacteria that grow well on artificial media.[6] Some species are atrichous, and nonmotile variants of motile species also occur. Motile forms are peritrichously flagellated. Nitrates are reduced to nitrites, and glucose is utilized fermentatively with the formation of acid or of acid and gas. The indophenol oxidase test is negative and alginate is not liquefied. Pectate is liquefied by members of only one genus (*Pectobacterium*). Many enteric organisms are potential hazards to laboratory personnel.

The family is divided into tribes, which in turn are divided into numerous genera and species. The tribes and genera are biochemically defined; species differentiation is based upon biochemical, serologic, and phage susceptibility characteristics. While researchers differ over the assignment of genera to tribes and in some cases over what constitutes a species, they agree on the characteristics that should be elucidated in the laboratory. Probably the two more common classification schemes are those of Kauffmann[16] and Ewing.[6] The classification proposed by Ewing is as follows:

Tribe I ESCHERICHIEAE
   Genus I *Escherichia*
   Genus II *Shigella*
Tribe II EDWARDSIELLEAE
   Genus I *Edwardsiella*
Tribe III SALMONELLEAE
   Genus I *Salmonella*
   Genus II *Arizona*
   Genus III *Citrobacter*

Tribe IV KLEBSIELLEAE
   Genus I *Klebsiella*
   Genus II *Enterobacter*
   Genus III *Pectobacterium*
   Genus IV *Serratia*
Tribe V PROTEEAE
   Genus I *Proteus*
   Genus II *Providencia*

All genera of the enterics are considered nonpathogens under ordinary circumstances. Nonetheless, they are discussed here because they regularly appear in the diagnostic bacteriology laboratory.

The material in this chapter will emphasize those genera (*Escherichia*, *Shigella*, *Salmonella*, *Arizona*, and *Klebsiella*) that are generally considered to be pathogenic or to have pathogenic species. Nonpathogenic members of the family will be mentioned at

Table 25.1. Differentiation of Enterobacteriaceae by biochemical tests

Test	Esch.	Shig.	Edwa.	Salm.	Ariz.	Citr.	Kleb.	Serr.	Pect. (25°C)	Enterobacter cloa.	aero.	hafn.	liqu.	Proteus vulg.	mira.	morg.	rett.	Providencia alca.	stua.
Indole	+	−+	+	−	−	−+	−	−	−+	−	−	−	+−	+	−	+	+	+	+
Methyl red	+	+	+	+	+	+	−	−	+−	−	−	+−	+−	+	+	+	+	+	+
Voges-Proskauer	−	−	−	−	−	−	+	+	−	+	+	+−	−+	−	−	−	−	−	−
Simmons' citrate	−	−	−	d	+	+	+	+	−+	+	+	(+)−	+	d	+(+)	−	+	+	+
H₂S (TSI)	−	−	+	+	+	+	−	−	d	−	−	−	−	−	−	−	−	−	−
Urease	−	−	−	−	−	dʷ	+	dʷ	dʷ	+−	−	+	d	+	+	+	+	+	+
KCN	−	−	−	−	−	+	+	+	+−	+	+	+	+	+	−	+	+	+	+
Motility	+−	−	+	+	+	+	−	+	+−	+	+	+	+	+	+	+	+	+	+
Gelatin (22°C)	−	−	−	−	+(+)	−	−	+	+(+)	−(+)	−(+)	−	d	+(+)	−	−	−	−	−
LYS-DC-ase	d	−	+	+	+(+)	−	+	+	−	−	+	+	+−	−	−	−	−	−	−
ARG-DH-ase	d	−(+)	−	+(+)	+(+)	d	−	−	+	+	+	−	+−	−	−	−	−	−	−
ORN-DC-ase	d	d	+	+	+	d	−	+	−	+	+	+	+	−	+	+	−	−	−
PHE-DA-ase	−	−	−	−	−	−	−	−	−	−	−	−	−	+	+	+	+	+	+
Malonate	−	−	−	−	+	d	+	−	+	+	+	−	−	−	−	−	−	−	−
Glucose gas	+	−	+	+	+	+	+	+−	+	+	+	−(+)	d	+	+	d	−	+	−
Lactose	+	−	−	−	d	d	+	−(+)	+	+(+)	+	d	d	+−	−	−	−	−	−
Sucrose	d	−	−	−	−	d	+	+	d	−+	+	−	+	+	d	−	d	d	d
Mannitol	+	+−	+	+	+	+	+	+	+	+	+	+	+	−	−	−	+−	+	−
Dulcitol	d	d	−	d	−	d	d	−	+	−	−	−	d	d	d	−	d	−	−
Salicin	d	−	−	−	+	d	+(+)	+	+	+(+)	+	d	d	d	−	d	d	−	−
Adonitol	−	−	−	−	−	−	+	d	−	−+	+	−	+	−	−	−	d	−	−
Inositol	−	−	−	d	−	d	+	d	+	d	+	−	d	−	−	−	+	+	d
Sorbitol	+	d	−	+	+	+	+	+	−	+	+	−	+	+	−	−	−	+	−
Arabinose	d	d	−	+	+	+	+	−	+(+)	+	+	+	+	−	−	−	−	−	−
Raffinose	d	d	−	−	−	d	+	−	+	−+	+	−	d	−	−	−	+−	−	−
Rhamnose	d	d	−	+	+	+	+	−	d	+	+	+	+	+	−	−	+	−	−

+, 90% or more positive in 1–2 days; −, 90% or more negative; +−, most strains positive; −+, most strains negative; +(+), positive or delayed positive; −(+), negative or delayed positive; (+)−, delayed positive or negative; d, different biochemical types; w, weakly positive reaction.

Enteric Organisms

Table 25.2. Biochemical reactions of Enterobacteriaceae at 37°C

Nitrate	Indole	MR	VP	Citrate	Phenylalanine deaminase	H_2S*	Motility	Tartrate	Gas in glucose†	Lactose‡	Sucrose	Salicin	Dulcitol	Tentative identification	Refer to Table
+	−	−	−	−	+	−	−	−	−	−	−	−	−	Proteus or Providencia	25.4
+	−	−	+	−	−	−	−	−	−	−	−	−	−	Klebsiella, Enterobacter, or Serratia	25.10
+	+	+	−	−	−	−	+	−	+	1§	−	−	−	E. coli	
+	+	+	−	−	−	−	−	−	+	−	−	+	−	E. coli	
+	+	+	−	−	−	−	−	−	+	−	−	−	−	Shigella flexneri; confirm serologically‖	25.3
+	1	+	−	−	−	−	−	−	−	−	−	−	−	Shigella; confirm serologically‖	25.3
+	−	+	−	−	−	−	−	−	−	−	−	−	+	Salmonella gallinarum	25.6
+	−	+	−	−	−	1	−	+	−	−	−	−	−	Salmonella pullorum	25.6
+	−	+	−	+	−	+	+	+	+	−	−	−	+	Salmonella or Citrobacter	25.8
+	−	+	−	+	−	+	+	−	+	−	−	−	−	Arizona (monophasic) or Citrobacter	25.8
+	−	+	−	+	−	+	+	+	+	−	−	−	−	Arizona (diphasic) or Citrobacter	25.8
+	−	+	−	+	−	+	+	+	+	+	−	−	+	Citrobacter or aberrant Salmonella	25.8
+	−	+	−	+	−	+	+	−	+	+	−	−	−	Citrobacter or Arizona	25.8
+	−	+	−	+	−	+	+	−	−	−	−	−	−	Aberrant Salmonella	25.8
+	−	+	−	+	−	+	−	−	+	−	−	−	−	Nonmotile Salmonella	25.8
+	+	+	−	+	−	+	+	−	+	1	−	−	−	Arizona	25.8
+	+	+	−	−	−	+	+	−	+	−	−	−	−	Edwardsiella tarda	25.8
+	−	+	−	−	−	+	+	−	+	−	−	−	−	Salmonella (citrate neg.)	25.8
+	−	+	−	−	−	−	+	−	+	−	−	−	−	Salmonella typhisuis	25.7, 25.8
+	−	+	−	+	−	−	+	−	+	−	−	−	−	Enterobacter hafnia or Salmonella	25.8

*Measured by blackening on TSI agar.
†All Enterobacteriaceae produce acid in glucose.
‡Lactose fermentation read in 1 day.
§1 means either + or −.
‖Shigellae are to be expected only in primates.

points where they are likely to be encountered in the procedures outlined, as will other organisms that are occasionally encountered in the enteric bacteriology laboratory. The chapter concludes with general comments and precautions on media preparation and use.

Tables 25.1 and 25.2 summarize the biochemical reactions and differentiation of the Enterobacteriaceae. Table 25.2 also provides cross-references to other tables listing the biochemical tests that will help complete the identification.

Escherichia

Escherichia coli, an inhabitant of the intestinal tract of many animals, aids in the digestive process but can cause disease when conditions are conducive. *Dorland's Medical Dictionary* defines colibacillosis as infection caused by *E. coli.*

In the neonatal animal, septicemia is produced when *E. coli* reaches the blood via the tonsils, umbilicus, lungs, or digestive tract. Toxemia is due to endotoxin, enterotoxin, neurotoxin, and some as yet unidentified toxin produced by *E. coli*. Septicemia, meningitis, and toxemia syndromes usually have a rapid fatal course with few previous clinical signs. In the enteric form, certain *E. coli* strains dominate the intestinal flora, produce an enterotoxin, and cause diarrhea. The diarrhea becomes progressively worse until the animal dies. In older animals, infection of the mammary gland (mastitis), reproductive tract, and urinary tract occurs. Diarrhea may be common but is not considered as serious in the newborn. Infections in poultry occur in the intestine (coli granuloma), air sacs (airsacculitis), ovary (salpingitis), and heart sac (pericarditis). Infection may kill embryos and chicks.[1,24]

Factors involved include unsanitary conditions, crowding, stress, cold, damp weather, poor nutrition, lack of antibody, lowered resistance of the host, and increased virulence of the agent. While a specific serotype of *E. coli* may be involved in an outbreak of colibacillosis, and while certain serotypes are pathogenic for one animal species but not another, individual host susceptibility does occur. This is observed in litters of pigs where a variety of serotypes are isolated from the litter and where a different serotype may predominate in each of the individual pigs that die. In a herd of cattle, individual calves may die from different *E. coli* serotypes.

Specimens

Collect fresh feces in sterile jars and add a preservative (buffered glycerol) if the specimen must be shipped. Freshly obtained fecal swabs can be streaked directly on agar plates. Sterile broth can then be added to the tube containing the swab for back-up tests. Fecal samples should be obtained at the first sign of diarrhea, before treatment, and several samples should be collected while the diarrhea persists. The samples should be cultured as soon as possible after collection.

Blood samples are usually negative for bacteria until the animal is in the terminal stage of disease. About 1 ml of blood may be drawn directly into 10 or 15 ml of broth medium.

Fluids must be removed aseptically immediately after the body cavity is opened. A heated spatula or small portable propane torch having a fine-flame tip can be used to sear the tissue surface, and fluids (heart blood, bile, urine, joints) can be withdrawn with a sterile syringe. Pieces of tissue should be placed in individual sterile jars. Both ends of a piece of intestine should be tied off to seal in contents before cutting. Sterile swabs can be used for thick fluids.

Laboratory Procedures

Direct examination of specimens for *E. coli*, especially in toxemia or septicemia, is usually of no value. The odor, consistency, and color of feces or intestinal contents varies. Smears, stained or unstained, would not necessarily add any useful information.

The use of conjugated *E. coli* antisera and the FA technique is practical for rapid screening where attention is focused on identification of a few specific serotypes. It is not practical for classification of a variety of *E. coli* serotypes. Because unheated cells are examined by FA, the reaction observed is due to K antigen-antibody, not to O antigen-antibody. Observation of the K reaction does not verify the presence of O antigen. If a K minus form is used to prepare an O antiserum for conjugate, O agglutination would occur with identical K minus forms in the specimen. Care must be exercised in the preparation and use of sera and the observation of results by FA. Confirmation of positive results and elimination of cross-reactions should be carried out by tube titer and the use of reciprocally cross-absorbed sera when required.

Cultures. Feces and fluids should be streaked directly to agar plates. Violet red bile

Enteric Organisms

(VRB) agar, MacConkey (MaC) agar, deoxycholate (Des, from the British spelling, desoxycholate) agar, or eosin methylene blue (EMB) agar may be used for this purpose. VRB is preferred for isolation of *E. coli*. Addition of a blood agar plate will help to identify hemolytic strains and increase the probability of isolating the fastidious *E. coli*. Smear a 2-3 cm strip on the agar surface with one sterile loop, then use another sterile loop to spread the inoculum over the plate so that isolated colonies will be obtained.

For necropsy specimens, sear the surface by flaming, then use sterile forceps and scissors to cut into, but not through, tissue. Enter the tissue with a sterile loop and streak plates as above. If there are only a few bacteria in the specimen, they will grow in the 2-3 cm strip. If large numbers are present, they will be adequately spread out to insure well-isolated colonies.

Differential reactions. Cultures of *E. coli* grow readily at 36°C with overnight incubation. Typical lactose-fermenting *E. coli* produce acid, with a characteristic change in the indicator in differential media. On EMB, black colonies with a metallic sheen are evident. On VRB, MaC, and Des, red colonies are produced. Where growth is crowded, colonies are small, pink to red, or even colorless. Well-isolated colonies can be entire or irregular, flat or raised, pink or deep red, and can have a solid color or a red center with transparent edge. Colonies of *E. coli* are rarely mucoid or watery. Slow lactose fermenters appear gray to colorless, the red color becoming apparent (VRB) in 2–7 days.

In addition to other gram-negative bacteria, more than one type of *E. coli* may be present on the differential medium. A well-isolated colony of each different colony type should be carefully pricked with a straight sterile needle for further identification. On VRB agar, transparent or gray colonies usually are *Salmonella, Proteus,* or *Pseudomonas.* Very thick, mucoid, white-edged to solid red colonies are characteristic of klebsiellae. After 48 hours, *Klebsiella* colonies are much larger and are viscous or watery.

Colonies of *Proteus* sp. sometimes spread in an even, thin film over the surface of the agar medium. If the plate is not carefully examined, mixed cultures may result from transferred proteus cells.

The above procedure should be applied to each specimen that is cultured. In the case of *E. coli,* multiple isolates of the same serotype from every specimen provide data that is of etiologic significance. Biochemical and serologic identification of as many colonies as possible provides information on the frequency of individual *E. coli* serotypes alone or in combination with other enteric bacteria.

Biochemical reactions of *E. coli* are listed in the tables on Enterobacteriaceae (Tables 25.1, 25.2). For preliminary tests, acid and gas in glucose, acid in lactose and mannitol, formation of indole, a positive methyl red (MR) test, a negative Voges-Proskauer (VP) test, no H_2S production in triple sugar iron (TSI agar), and no utilization of citrate (Simmons') are evidence of typical *E. coli*. However, slow lactose fermenters and anaerogenic strains do occur and can be identified by further biochemical and serologic tests (Table 25.3). The term paracolon should not be used since it only indicates a lack of intrest in confirming the genus and species.

Cellular morphology. *E. coli* bacteria are gram-negative rods. The rods may be short or long, single or paired, thin or fat, and occasionally bipolar. Pleomorphic forms occur. Flagella can be demonstrated on actively motile forms with Leifson's stain. Spores are

Table 25.3. Diagnostic features of *Shigella* and anaerogenic nonmotile *E. coli* (A-D organisms)[5]

	Motility	Indole	Gas in glucose	Salicin	Esculin	Mucate	Lysine
*Shigella**	–	1†	–	–	–	–	–
A-D group	–	+	–	1	1	1	1

*Confirm by agglutination tests with polyvalent antiserum.
†1means either + or –.

not produced. Capsules are associated with the mucoid strains having the A type of K antigen and can be demonstrated in conjunction with a specific K serum by use of an India ink slide preparation or in an unstained live suspension examined with a phase contrast microscope.

Animal inoculation. Animal inoculation is not required for isolation or identification but has been used for research purposes.

Immunology and serology. Serologic identification of *E. coli* cultures is based on their O (somatic), K (capsular) and, if motile, H (flagellar) antigens.[1,4] The O antigens are not inactivated by heat at 121°C for 2 hours. The three kinds of K antigens, L, B, and A, vary in sensitivity to heat and in their ability to mask or inhibit agglutination of unheated culture supension in O antisera. This inhibitory effect is inactivated by heat at 100°C for L and B, and at 121°C for A. When *E. coli* strains do not contain a K antigen (K minus, or K–) the inhibitory effect is absent. The H antigens are inactivated by heat at 100°C.

The antigenic differences in K antigens listed by Kauffmann include the assertion that heating at 121°C destroys the agglutinability of A and B antigens in their respective A and B antisera. This is observed in the tube agglutination method. Because the antibody binding remains intact, lines of identity are formed in the AD method. The L antigens are thermolabile; heating at 100°C for 1 hour destroys antigenicity, agglutinability, and antibody binding power.

An outline of the serologic methods is illustrated in Figure 25.1. A well-isolated colony is transferred to an agar slant that serves as a stock culture. Heated broth cultures are used for O antigens and unheated Formalinized cultures for H antigens. If the broth culture does not remain homogenous after heating (clumps or coarse precipitate), the culture is rough and further serologic tests are useless. The original stock culture can be plated on infusion agar and an attempt made to locate a smooth colony.

Actively motile forms can be obtained by passage of a culture through the semisolid Motility Test Medium of Ewing. Passage is facilitated by the use of glass tubing closed at the bottom with a rubber stopper or a screw cap.[10] The top of the medium is inoculated and the growth of flagellated forms recovered from the bottom. A screw cap provides better control of the semisolid medium when opened for transfer of growth. When motile forms stop short of the bottom, the medium can be easily removed until the line of growth is reached.

Since living or Formalinized antigen is used for preparation of K antiserum, O and H (if motile) antibodies are also produced in the serum. Growth from a dry agar slant is

Figure 25.1. Outline of serologic methods

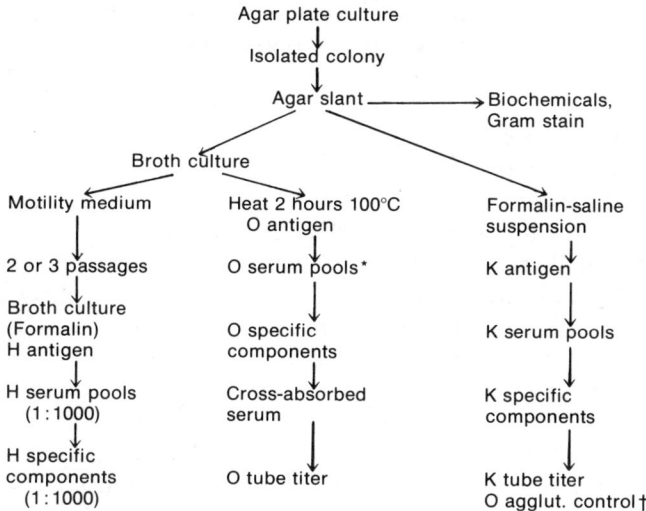

*If negative, repeat test with antigen heated at 121°C for 2 hours.
†K antigen tested with O serum of O group to which the strain belongs.

preferred for the K antigen, as flagellated forms (H) that interfere with K antigen identification are inhibited.

Antisera for *E. coli* are prepared in rabbits using standard strains. Extreme care must be used in handling *E. coli* standard strains and sera to eliminate contamination or misidentification. All serum prepared must be tested for purity, conformation to type, and known cross-reactions. Antisera from commercial sources should include a list of homologous and heterologous titers, and should be titered with standard strains and known cross-reactors before using. Serum can be mixed with an equal part of sterile glycerol as a preservative and stored at 5°C. Glycerol should not be used with serum prepared for FA studies.

Agglutination tests are carried out in 13 × 75 mm tubes, on slides, or by AD technique. The most rapid method, slide agglutination, requires a more concentrated serum (1:10 to 1:20) and more cross-reactions may occur. An advantage of the slide method is that serum pools and specific components, stored in small cartridge racks (Raymond Brass Mfg., Pittsburgh), take up less space and are ready for use at the touch of a button. Tube agglutination requires more time (3 days), but at the higher dilutions (1:500 to 1:1000), less serum is used and fewer cross-reactions occur. Typical O and K agglutination appears as precipitated particles that remain in suspension when the contents are shaken. A good K reaction is visible as a tighty precipitated pellicle or button that slips free when the tube is hit sharply; the titer rarely exceeds 1:320. A "cotton ball" or fluffy precipitate that goes back into suspension when shaken is typical of H agglutination. After the tube is shaken, the H agglutinate reoccurs promptly upon standing.

For the slide test, a modified Accu-Drop rectangular-pattern dispenser cartridge rack (Accu-Tech Corp., New York), cartridges, needles, and slides with 20 circles are required. A drop of each O pool serum (1:20) is placed on the slide using the dispenser, *E. coli* O antigen is added, this is mixed on a rotary shaker 8 minutes, and the reaction is recorded. Specific components (1:10) of positive pools are dropped on the slide and tested as above.

Reciprocally cross-absorbed serum (1:10) from small dropping vials are used to determine the probable O group. Tube titer agglutinations, 1:40–1:5120, are then used to confirm the O antigen group.

The slide method can be used for identification of O, K, and H antigens, with the time of shaking reduced to 4 minutes for H and K antigens.

For the tube test of O antigen, O antigen is added to the O pool serums at a final dilution of 1:100. The tubes are shaken and placed at 50°C overnight. O antigen is then added to tubes containing specific components (1:500) of positive pools and incubated at 50°C overnight. Tests with cross-absorbed sera are carried out on a slide, and serial dilutions are made in tubes as above.

For the tube test of K antigen, dilutions and procedure are the same as for O agglutination except the test is incubated at 37°C for 2 hours and refrigerated overnight. Cross-absorbed sera are usually not required. A tube titer agglutination of 1:40 to 1:320 is sufficient for K serum and 1:40 to 1:1280 for O serum control.

For the tube test of H antigen, H serum pools and H specific components are used at a dilution of 1:1000. Tubes of antigen plus antiserum are mixed, incubated at 50°C, and the results read at 15 minutes, 1 hour, and 2 hours. H agglutination is prompt, and the degree of reaction is read before the tubes are shaken.

A great deal of confusion exists in regard to the correct terms for reporting serologic classification of *E. coli* strains. The correct terms and their meanings follow:

O group 111 O antigen group 111 Serogroup 111 O111	The strain belongs to *E. coli* O group 111.
O antigen 111ab O antigen subgroup 111ab Serogroup 111ab O111ab	The O antigen of the strain has the sub–O group factor ab.
O111ab:K58(B4) OB group 111ab:K58(B) OK group 111ab:K58	The O and the K antigen of the strain is known. K58 is a B type of K antigen that in an earlier classification was number 4 (B4).
O111ab:K58:H12 Serotype 111ab:K58:H12 A serotype of O group 111 serotype	The O, K, and H antigens are known. The sub–O group factor ab completes the serotype formula.
O K H	The antigen in question has been examined but does not react with standard *E. coli* sera.

Phage typing of *E. coli* is not as widely used as serotyping and has been for the most part confined to individual studies. Thus the phage types reported in animal disease in one area cannot be compared with those found in another unless the phage types are exchanged. A comparison of human enteropathogenic *E. coli* serotypes of O111, O55, and O26 with a variety of *E. coli* phage types has indicated that a phage type exists for each *E. coli* serotype examined.[20]

Newborn calves, lambs, and pigs deprived of colostrum have been found susceptible to pathogenic *E. coli* serotypes administered orally. Colostrum-deprived animals apparently are more susceptible to *E. coli* serotypes that produce a septicemia. Newborn pigs given *E. coli* orally developed a fatal infection that their uninoculated littermates also acquired, even though all pigs were nursing the sow. *E. coli* strains, and the enterotoxin of the strains, produced a diarrhea in calves, pigs, and lambs that had received colostrum.[1,8,24]

Mice inoculated intraperitoneally with *E. coli* and hog gastric mucin were susceptible to 10 or less *E. coli* serotypes isolated from organs other than the intestine. The majority of serotypes from enteric sources required more than 10^5 *E. coli* to produce a LD_{50} with or without mucin.[1]

Embryonated chicken eggs and poultry of different ages are suscepitble to *E. coli* pathogenic for poultry but not to serotypes pathogenic for pigs. A difference in susceptibility of chicks was related to hatchery source.

The ligated intestinal loop method has been used to assess virulence of enteropathogenic *E. coli* serotypes and their toxins in rabbits, calves, pigs, and lambs.

E. coli produce endotoxin, enterotoxin, and neurotoxin. Endotoxins are produced by all gram-negative bacteria and have been studied by a variety of methods.[17,19] Live *E. coli* or their enterotoxin given orally produced diarrhea in neonatal animals and caused a positive intestinal loop reaction in calves, pigs, and lambs. The serotypes used for these enterotoxin studies were associated with enteritis or diarrhea. Studies on neurotoxin have not been extensively reported; neurotoxin is not clearly understood but may be involved in edema disease of swine.

Reference laboratory. Complete serologic classification, as well as a variety of *E. coli* antisera and serotypes, are available at cost from Paul J. Glantz, Pennsylvania State University, 105 Animal Industries Building, University Park, Pa. 16802. Diagnostic Services, Animal Health Division, NADC, offers assistance to qualified diagnostic laboratories throughout the United States. Consult the veterinarian in charge of your state.

Shigella[9,23]

Members of the genus *Shigella* are an important cause of gastrointestinal infection in primates. Several outbreaks of shigellosis can occur in any one colony of animals, and the disease is a major problem where monkeys are held and conditioned for shipment to laboratories. Poor sanitation contributes to the spread of the disease. Carrier animals transmit the disease by fecal contamination of food and drink. Infections may remain latent until stress conditions precipitate an acute attack.

The usual sign is diarrhea and the stools may contain blood or mucus. Rapid emaciation and death may result from acute infections. In these cases the mucosa of the large intestine is generally swollen and necrotic ulcers are usually found in the colon. In some cases, ulceration is slight and the lesions are those of catarrhal colitis. Adjacent lymph nodes are inflamed and the spleen is congested. The liver may or may not show gross pathologic change.

In animals with chronic infections, the size and variety of the lesions vary. Some form of colitis is invariably present and periodically the animals pass unformed stools.

Specimens

For rectal swabs, insert and rotate a cotton-tipped swab beyond the anal sphincter.

For fecal samples, collect recently passed feces in a sterile container. If immediate examination is not possible, a preservative should be used (e.g. 1 g feces to 10 ml of 30% glycerol in buffered 0.6% saline).

For necropsy specimens, collect all internal organs that show pathologic change. If the intestines appear normal, take the cecum.

Cultures. For rectal swabs, plates of xylose lysine deoxycholate (XLD) and salmonella-shigella (SS) agar should be streaked immediately after collecting the swab. The swab should then be submerged in 10 ml of gram-negative (GN) broth. Incubate these at 35–37°C. After 6 hours incubation, inoculate another set of plates using a loopful of the broth culture. Examine the plates after 18–24 hours incubation.

For fecal samples, fresh samples are suspended in saline (1 g per 3 ml saline). Inoculate media as above using a loopful of the fresh or preserved suspension for the plates and 2 ml of suspension in 10 ml of broth.

For necropsy specimens, culture organs or tissues other than the intestine by direct inoculation of any good, rich, solid culture medium that does not contain inhibitors. Incubate inoculated media at 35–37°C. Mince portions of the intestinal tract with sterile scissors. Add GN broth in a ratio of 1 part tissue to 10 parts of broth. Proceed as above.

Differential reactions. Shigellae grow well at 35–37°C. Colonies on XLD agar are pink, on SS agar are pale or colorless, and on MaC agar are colorless. Characteristic colonies are smooth and glistening and have an entire edge, but rough (R) forms do occur. Shigellae do not grow on brilliant green or bismuth sulfite agars.

Colonies suspected to be shigellae should be used to inoculate TSI agar. Cultures producing acid (yellow) butts and alkaline (red) slants and without evidence of H_2S may be shigellae. Additional evidence may be obtained by conducting an agglutination test with polyvalent shigella O antiserum. If no agglutination occurs, the culture should be boiled for 15 minutes to remove the envelope and capsules. Cultures agglutinating with the polyvalent antiserum may then be typed by serologic methods but they should also be confirmed biochemically using the following media: nitrate agar, tryptone water (for indole test), MR-VP medium, Simmons' citrate agar, phenylalanine agar, motility test medium, and fermentation broth media such as glucose, lactose, sucrose, and salicin. Refer to Tables 25.2 and 25.3 for interpretation of the reactions.

Salmonella and Arizona

Organisms in the genus *Salmonella* infect a very wide range of animals and humans. They are found in all domesticated mammals and birds and have been isolated from a wide variety of wild and captive mammals, birds, and reptiles. The importance of the organisms lies not only in their ability to cause disease in domestic livestock and poultry, often with large economic losses, but also in the fact that carrier animals and birds contribute to the contamination of human foods. Contaminated food is a major source of salmonellosis in humans. Direct infection of humans through contact with carrier animals, especially pets, is known to take place, but on the whole is secondary in importance.

Salmonellosis is primarily a disease of the very young, the old, and the debilitated. Mature adults succumb to infections when resistance is lowered by stress, virus disease, inadequate diet, or grossly unsanitary surroundings.

In birds the course of the disease may vary somewhat with species and breed infected and with the serotype causing the infection. In young birds there is a general picture of depression, weakness manifested by drooping wings and heads and staggering, loss of appetite, dehydration, and diarrhea with pasting around the vent. The birds tremble and huddle together as if chilly and, when the lungs are infected, breathing is labored. Heavy losses usually begin two or three days after hatching and begin to decline by the third or fourth week. The mortality rate varies from low to 100% and is affected by many factors including incubator and brooder management. The birds show generalized infection; internal organs are enlarged and may show streaks of hemorrhage or minute white spots. Yolk sacs may be dry and cheesy, intestines are inflamed and have cecal cores, and sometimes joints are swollen.

Acute infection is rare in adult birds. The chronic form of the disease is more commonly seen, with low death loss and no outward symptoms. In these birds the ovary may be infected and the organisms transmitted in the eggs. This type transmission results in poor fertility, low hatchability, and very early mortality starting at 1 day of age, with surviving chicks weak or deformed.

In fowl typhoid, caused by *Salmonella gallinarum,* there is heavy loss in all age groups from acute infection. Fowl typhoid is most common during the warm months.

Organisms in the genus *Arizona* are closely related to the salmonellae both biochemically and serologically. The first such organism was isolated from a reptile in Arizona and was named *Salmonella arizona* by Kauffmann. Most of the work on this group of organisms has been done by the late P.R. Edwards and co-workers.[5] Edwards concluded that the organisms were sufficiently different from salmonellae to warrant a separate serologic classification scheme.[21] Kauffmann, who now subdivides the genus *Salmonella* into four subgenera, includes the arizonae as subgenus III.[16] The seventh edition of *Bergey's Manual* classifies the organisms in the genus *Paracolobactrum*,[2] but those most knowledgeable about the group have not adopted the term. Ewing has proposed that organisms in the genus *Arizona* be designated *A. hinshawii,* in honor of W.R. Hinshaw, who has worked extensively with arizona infections in turkeys and reptiles.[7]

Accumulated evidence indicates that the arizonae recognize no host barriers. Clinical signs usually closely resemble those for salmonellosis. A notable exception to this is the eye infection of turkeys often caused by the serotype *Arizona* 7:1,7,8. Another serotype, *Arizona* 26:29–30, has been recognized as a cause of abortion in sheep. Cycles of infection among animals and between animals and humans appear to be very similar to those for salmonellae.

Specimens

For fecal samples, collect recently passed feces in a sterile container. If prompt examination is not possible, a preservative should be used.

For necropsy specimens, collect all internal organs that show pathologic change. Swollen joints or infected eyes should also be taken. Tissues of particular interest include the liver and gall bladder, spleen, abnormal ova, heart, pancreas, and intestines. Avian reactors to the blood tests for *S. pullorum, S. gallinarum,* and *S. typhimurium* should be handled following the procedures of the National Poultry and Turkey Improvement Plans and Auxilliary Provisions (*Code of Federal Regulations,* Title 9, part 147, subpart B, available from U.S. Government Printing Office, Washington).

Intestinal carriers of salmonellae cannot be diagnosed by serologic tests. Birds that have chronic infections with *S. pullorum* and *S. gallinarum* and turkeys that have chronic infections with *S. typhimurium* will react to serologic tests that have been developed for these organisms. Follow procedures of the National Poultry and Turkey Improvement Plans as above.

Cultures. Isolation of *S. choleraesuis* from swine intestines is difficult but can be done using selective enrichment broth media (tetrathionate or selenite F). Suspend 1 g of intestinal contents or feces in 3 ml of sterile saline. Mince intestines, add a small amount of saline, and macerate with a sterile glass rod. Streak one loopful onto a bismuth sulfite (BS) agar plate. With the remaining suspension, proceed as for all other animals.

For all other animals, add about 1 g of intestinal contents or feces to 10 ml of tetrathionate or selenite F broth. Mince with sterilized scissors regions of intestines that show lesions and add to selective enrichment broth in a ratio of 1 g of tissue to 10 ml of broth. Culture the gall bladder by cutting it and letting about 10 ml of the contents run into a flask or jar, then mince the emptied gall bladder and add it to the gall. Add selective enrichment broth in a 1:10 ratio. Incubate at 35–37°C for 18–24 hours.

Streak selective enrichment media onto brilliant green (BG), BS, and XLD agar plates. In streaking the plates of these differential media, use a generous loopful of inoculum and spread it out thoroughly, flaming the loop each time the plate is turned. The importance of obtaining well-isolated colonies cannot be overemphasized. Extra moments taken to streak a plate carefully are returned with interest at later stages. Incubate plates at 35–37°C for 24 hours (48 hours for BS agar). Return negative plates to the incubator for an additional 24 hours.

For necropsy specimens from acutely infected animals, use the common aseptic techniques: culture all internal organs that show pathologic changes, as well as fluid from swollen joints and eyes, by direct inoculation of any good rich solid culture medium that does not contain inhibitors. Incubate at 35–37°C. Treat intestines and gall bladder as previously described.

For necropsy specimens from animals with evidence of chronic infection, or where little pathologic change is seen, aseptically remove a plug about 1 cm square from the liver, spleen, and pancreas. Macerate the tissue and streak some directly onto plates of culture medium as above. Add 10 ml of any good rich broth (without inhibitors) to the remainder. Aseptically open the heart and culture one loopful of blood onto plates and put another loopful into broth. Put an abnormal ova into tubes of sterile broth and mash with a sterile glass rod. Incubate at 35–37°C. Treat intestines and gall bladder as above.

When broth shows growth, streak plates of any good rich noninhibitory culture medium and incubate at 35–37°C. If the plates show a highly mixed flora, subculture 0.5 ml of the broth culture in 10 ml of tetrathionate or selenite F broth. Hold all broth cultures and plates for 48 hours before discarding for lack of growth.

For milk, incubate at 35–37°C for 18–25 hours. Streak plates of BG or SS agar and of XLD agar. Also subculture 0.5 ml of incubated milk in 10 ml tetrathionate broth and incubate 18–24 hours, then streak plates of above agars.

For eggs, disinfect the outside of the egg and open it with aseptic precautions. Put contents (whether yolk and white, or dead embryo) into a sterile blender jar. Add noninhibitory broth in a ratio of 1 part egg to 10 parts of broth and blend. Transfer to sterile container. Incubate *a full 24 hours.*

For feed and feed ingredients, follow the procedures recommended by USDA (*Recommended Procedure for the Isolation of Salmonella Organisms from Animal Feeds and Feed Ingredients,* ARS 91-68), if the material is being examined for USDA purposes. Otherwise, weigh 25 g into a sterile jar, add 225 ml sterile lactose broth and 1.5 ml of Tergitol no. 7, and stir. Incubate a full 24 hours. Subculture 0.5 ml in 10 ml tetrathionate broth and incubate overnight. Streak onto brilliant green sulfa (BGS) and XLD agars. Incubate for 24 hours. Return negative plates to the incubator for an additional 24 hours.

For other materials, treat material that is expected to be grossly contaminated as in paragraph 3a of *Recommended Procedure;* if the material has been dessicated or frozen and is likely to be contaminated with unwanted organisms, treat as in paragraph 3f; if salmonellae or arizonae are likely to be present in pure culture but in small numbers, treat as in the paragraph on intestines, and so forth.

Differential reactions. Salmonellae and arizonae grow well at 35–37°C. Typical colony appearance on nutrient agar varies from translucent to moist and opaque. The consistency of the colonies usually is butyrous and the edge is entire; however, rough and mucoid colonies are encountered. Encapsulated strains are stringy when touched with a platinum wire. Size on nutrient agar (24-hour incubation) varies from less than 0.5 mm (*S. typhisuis*) to 4 mm (*Enterobacter* sp.). Some *Proteus* sp. will swarm over the entire surface.

On BG or BGS agar, salmonellae and slow lactose-fermenting arizonae are pink, translucent, smooth, and glistening with an entire edge. Size varies from less than 1 mm to 33 mm in 24 hours. The surrounding medium is red. If the colony is in a crowded area of the plate, it may be tan in color. Plates must be examined in 18–24 hours and again in 48 hours. Rapid lactose-fermenting arizonae, *E. coli, Enterbacter* sp., and *Klebsiella* sp. produce yellow or yellowish-green colonies. *Proteus* sp. may give yellow or red colonies or they may swarm.

On BS agar, *Salmonella* and *Arizona* colonies are black or brown with the surrounding agar having a blackened appearance and a metallic sheen. This appearance is not manifested until the plates have incubated for 48 hours. Colonies of salmonellae that fail to produce H_2S will appear green.

On SS agar, colonies of the genera *Salmonella*, *Arizona* (slow lactose-fermenting types), *Shigella*, and *Proteus* are pale. *Proteus* colonies tend to be stringy when touched with a needle; they do not swarm. *E. coli*, *Enterobacter* sp., and rapid lactose-fermenting arizonae are deep pink.

On XLD agar, in 24 hours *Salmonella* colonies in pure culture are pink with a black center and the surrounding medium is pink. However, in mixed cultures they usually are yellow with a very black center in 24 hours; by 48 hours the periphery of the colony may have turned pink. H_2S negative strains may resemble shigellae (pink). *Proteus* colonies are yellow and develop a grayish center. (For other diagnostic features of *Proteus*, see Table 25.4.)

Table 25.4. Diagnostic features of *Proteus* and *Providencia*[5]

	Indole	Methyl red	Voges-Proskauer	Citrate	H_2S	Phenylalanine deaminase	Urease	Gas from glucose
Prot. vulgaris	+	+	−	d*	+	+	+	1†
Prot. mirabilis	−	+	1	+	+	+	+	+
Prot. morganii	+	+	−	−	−	+	+	d
Prot. rettgeri	+	+	−	+	−	+	+	1
Prov. alcaligaciens	+	+	−	+	−	+	−	d
Prov. stuartii	+	+	−	+	−	+	−	−

*d means different reactions: +, delayed +, −.
†1 means either + or −.

To identify Enterobacteriaceae species isolated on noninhibitory media in the shortest time, inoculate a number of media simultaneously. Pick a colony and inoculate about 2 ml of veal infusion broth. Incubate at 35–37°C until growth becomes visible and then use the broth to inoculate the following media: nitrate agar, tryptone water (for indole test), MR-VP medium, Simmons' citrate agar (inoculate lightly), phenylalanine agar, TSI agar, motility medium, tartrate agar of Jordan and Harmon, and fermentation broth media such as glucose, lactose, sucrose, salicin, and dulcitol.

Incubate these cultures at 37°C for 24 hours. Test for nitrate reduction and phenylalanine diamination and record the appearance of the other media. Reincubate for another 24 hours. Test for indole formation and MR and VP reactions. Note any changes in the other media since the 24-hour reading. Refer to Tables 25.1 and 25.2 for interpretation of results.

If one is looking specifically for salmonellae or arizonae, cultures should be screened by inoculating slants of TSI and lysine iron (LI) agars (Table 25.5). When picking colonies from selective media, care should be taken to touch only the center of the selected colony. Contaminating organisms may remain viable on the selective media even though they do not colonize. Inoculate both agar slants with one pick. Incubate the slants at 37°C for 18–24 hours. LI agar reactions must be read after a single day's incubation.

Enteric Organisms

Table 25.5. Screening cultures from selective plating media specifically for salmonellae or arizonae

| LI agar | | | | | | TSI agar | | | | | | Interpretation |
| Butt | | Slant | | H$_2$S | | Butt | | Slant | | H$_2$S | | |
Purple	Yellow	Purple	Reddish	Present	Absent	Red	Yellow	Red	Yellow	Present	Absent	
+		+		+			+	+		+		*Salm.* or *Ariz.*
+		+		+			+	+ (either)	+ (either)		+*	Plate on noninhib. agar and see Table 25.1
+		+			+		+	+		+		See Table 25.1
+		+			+		+		+	+		Not *Salm.* or *Ariz.*
	+	+†			+		+		+	+		Not *Salm.* or *Ariz.*
	+	+†			+		+	+			+	Possibly *Shigella* or *S. typhisuis* ‡
	+	+†		+			+	+		+		Not *Salm.* or *Ariz.*
	+	+†		+			+		+	+		Not *Salm.* or *Ariz.*
	+		+				+	+ (either)	+ (either)	+		Not *Salm.* or *Ariz.*
	+		+ (either)				+	+ (either)	+§	+		Not *Salm.* or *Ariz.*
+ (either)	+ (either)						+		+			Not *Salm.* or *Ariz.*

*Cultures sometimes fail to have visible evidence of H$_2$S on TSI agar when much acid is produced from carbohydrates. At such times LI agar may indicate H$_2$S while TSI agar does not.

†The slant of lysine-negative cultures is often unchanged (light purple) while the butt is yellow, but sometimes both butt and slant are yellow.

‡If from primate, test with *Shigella* polyvalent serum. If from swine, test with *Salmonella* polyvalent serum. Otherwise, discard.

§Also has swarming growth.

Refer to Table 25.5 for an interpretation of the results and a suggestion on how to proceed.

Organisms that produce blackening along the stab line and purple throughout the media in LI agar, as well as those that produce red slants, yellow butts, and blackening (H$_2$S) in TSI agar, are almost certainly either salmonellae or tardy lactose-fermenting arizonae. If *Salmonella* grouping antiserums are available or if the tests are negative, the organism should be further characterized biochemically by inoculating the media listed above.

Occasionally salmonellae are encountered that do not produce H$_2$S in these media but are otherwise typical; they should be examined further. Biochemical tests should be done, and certain rapid tests can be used to advantage at this point. A positive test for indole on PathoTec-I paper strips (available from General Diagnostics Division, Warner-Chilcott, Morris Plains, N.J.) will screen out some cultures. Indole is not produced in abundance on TSI agar so the test will be weaker than a test done with growth from tryptose agar. Growth on LI agar is unsuitable for the indole test. In situations where *S. gallinarum* is expected, it will save time to test growth from the slant with *Salmonella* O group D (9,12) antiserum. Cultures giving agglutination should be subjected to the biochemical tests required to differentiate *S. gallinarum* and *S. pullorum* (Table 25.6).

S. paratyphi A and *S. typhisuis* are both lysine and H$_2$S negative. Do not expect the

Table 25.6. Diagnostic features of *Salmonella pullorum* and *S. gallinarum*

Salmonella	O antigens	Motility	Glucose	Maltose	Dulcitol	Tartrate	Citrate	H_2S	Growth characteristics
pullorum	1,9,12	–	AG*	–	–	–	–	weak +	Sparse
gallinarum	1,9,12	–	A	A	A	+	–	–	Moderate
gallinarum var. duisberg	1,9,12	–	A	slow A	A	–	+ in 2–3 days	–	Moderate

*Some strains, acid only. AG means acid and gas production, A means acid only.

former in cultures from animals. The latter is rare in swine. It grows sparcely and slowly and may be very difficult to isolate on differential plating media (Tables 25.7, 25.8).

Any organism that blackens TSI agar, even though the slant may be yellow and have a purple reaction throughout the LI agar in 24 hours, may be a rapid lactose-fermenting member of the genus *Arizona* or an aberrant *Salmonella* (Table 25.9). It should be plated on noninhibitory agar to assure a pure culture and then be identified by biochemical tests.

Cellular morphology. The salmonellae and arizonae are gram-negative nonsporogenic rods. They are usually motile, with peritrichous flagella, but nonmotile forms do occur.

Serology. Since procedures used to serotype salmonellae by means of the Kauffmann-White schema are described in detail in *Identification of Enterobacteriaceae*, the reader is referred to that book.[4] Actually, most laboratories will not find it feasible to attempt serotyping, but they can benefit by using antisera to assign the O antigens of a culture to one of the salmonella O groups. Antisera for this purpose are available from commercial companies or can be made by injecting rabbits.

Most of the cultures of the genus *Salmonella* that are encountered will have O antigens that can be identified by using only a few antisera. There are group B (4,5,12 and 4,12,27), group C_1 (6,7), group C_2 (8), group D (9,12), group E_1 (3,10), group E_2 (3,15), and group E_4 (1,3,19). If group F (11), group G (13,22 and 1,13,23), group H (6,14,24 and 1,6,14,25), group I (16), and group K (18) are added, then 98% of all the *Salmonella* cultures encountered in animals at the present time can be grouped. *Salmonella* O18 corresponds to Arizona O7 and will thus agglutinate *Arizona* 7:1,2,6 and *Arizona* 7:1,7,8, the most common *Arizona* serotypes.

The recommendations of the manufacturers must be followed when using commercial antisera. Some of these antisera have been partially adsorbed to remove natural cross-agglutination patterns, although information on the extent of the adsorption is not revealed.

Table 25.7. Diagnostic features of *Salmonella typhisuis* and *S. choleraesuis*

	O antigens	H antigens	H_2S	Citrate	Tartrate	Lysine	Trehalose	Arabinose
S. choleraesuis	6,7	1,5	–	–	+	+	–	–
S. choleraesuis var. kunzendorf	6,7	1,5	+	+	Usually +	+	–	–
S. typhisuis*	6,7	1,5	–	–	–	–	+	+

*Very sparse growth.

Table 25.8. *Salmonella* sp. and similar organisms

	Moeller's decarboxylase reactions*						Other characteristics
	Urease	KCN	Lysine	Arginine	Ornithine	Malonate	
Salmonella subgenus 1†	−	−	+	−	+	−	
Salmonella subgenus II†	−	−	+	−	+	+	
Salmonella subgenus III (*Arizona*)†	−	−	+	−	+	+	See Table 25.9
Salmonella subgenus IV†	−	+	+	−	+	−	
S. typhisuis	−	−	−	−	+	−	Sparse growth of *Salmonella* O6,7
Citrobacter freundii	weak +	+	−	−	1‡	−	"Rotten cabbage" odor
Edwardsiella tarda	−	−	+	−	+	−	Indole produced
Enterobacter hafnia§	−	+	+	−	+	1	

*Read in 2 days.
†Terminology of Kauffmann.[16]
‡1 means either + or −.
§See also Table 25.4.

Usually grouping is done with a saline suspension of the organism taken from an agar slant (the TSI agar slant is satisfactory for this purpose). Seven drops of the suspension, *equal in size,* are put down on a glass plate or slide. About 2–3 cm below them the seven O grouping antisera (B–E_4) are placed. Serum drops should be the *same size* as the culture suspension. After all the sera are placed, each serum is connected to a drop of culture suspension and mixed with a wire inoculating needle with an up-and-down motion; then the plate is tilted backward and forward to hasten the mixing of serum and antigen. Record as positive the agglutination that appears first and is strongest. Minor agglutination should be ignored. Agglutination tests done in this manner allow approximately the same time for each serum-antigen interaction and they do not dry out as fast as when spread out in a circle.

If there is no reaction in the first seven antiserums, try any additional O antisera available. If all are negative, and the culture's biochemical reactions are those of the genus *Salmonella,* the culture probably has one of the more unusual O antigens.

Cultures that agglutinated in O grouping antiserum may next be tested for H (flagellar) agglutination. The extent of the work done at this stage will depend on the use in-

Table 25.9. Abbreviated diagnostic features of *Salmonella* and *Arizona*

	Dulcitol	Malonate	Jordan's tartrate	Lactose	ONPG
Salmonella	+	−	+	−	−
Arizona	−	+	−	+	+

tended for the information. The presence of H antigen can be detected by simply using polyvalent H antiserum with a tryptose broth culture that has been diluted with saline containing 0.5% Formalin; for some purposes this step is sufficient. When epidemiologic studies are being carried out, however, the H antigens *must* be studied in a detailed manner. Also, it is strongly urged that all cultures from sick or from carrier animals be further examined.

Antiserum for identification of individual H antigens is available from commercial companies or can be made by injecting rabbits. Those wishing to attempt such identification should study the Edwards and Ewing book,[4] as well as the manufacturer's literature.

A somewhat simpler procedure was described by Spicer.[25] It uses sets of pooled antisera, and individual H antigens are recognized by their patterns of agglutination in the pools. Such pooled antisera are available commercially, and since the serum pools have been altered from Spicer's original suggestion, again the manufacturer's literature must be followed.

A unique feature of *Salmonella* flagellar antigens is phase variation; that is, a culture may have two quite different H antigens. One antigen may be present at a time or both may be present simultaneously. By use of an appropriate antiserum and a soft agar medium, it is possible to switch the phases at will. This is an integral part of serotyping, but it is not recommended for those using Spicer's pooled antisera.

The true usefulness of Spicer's serum pools is in reducing the number of cultures from a common source that need be submitted to a serotyping center. For example, if several cultures from a single animal or from one flock all belong to the same O group and all give identical reactions in the pooled sera, then only one representative culture need be serotyped.

Reference laboratories. The Animal Health Division, ARS, has facilities for serotyping salmonella and arizona cultures in several locations. In order to have a culture serotyped, the sender is requested to do a reasonable number of biochemical tests to assure that the culture is a *Salmonella* or an *Arizona*. It is also requested that O grouping and Spicer-Edwards H pool agglutination tests be attempted and that the results of this preliminary serology be submitted with the culture. A submission form must be completed for each culture submitted. A supply of these forms and the address of the appropriate serotyping laboratory can be obtained from the federal veterinarian in charge in each state.

Culture collection. A repository for salmonella cultures isolated from avian species is maintained at the Southeast Poultry Research Laboratory, ARS, Athens, Ga.

Klebsiella

Klebsiella strains are most commonly found in mastitis and in respiratory, genital, and intestinal infections in animals. Mastitis due to klebsiellae usually is very severe, difficult to treat, and often fatal. In newborn animals, klebsiellae may cause pneumonia or a severe enteritis with or without septicemia. Serologic typing has not produced evidence that one strain is more pathogenic than another. Under suitable conditions, each of the 72 known capsular types can be pathogenic.

Enteric Organisms

Laboratory Procedures

Cultures. Inoculate plates of VRB, MaC, and Des agar.

Differential reactions. Klebsiellae grow well at 37°C on most common media. They are aerobic and facultatively anaerobic. *Klebsiella* and *Enterobacter* colonies on VRB, MaC, and Des agar are thick, mucoid, watery, and pink to red in color. The viscid appearance is associated with the amount of capsular material present.

Preliminary tests should give the following reactions: acid and gas in glucose and lactose, citrate utilization, MR negative, H_2S negative, indole negative, and VP positive. A more complete pattern of biochemical reactions can be found in Table 25.1. Important differential reactions are listed in Table 25.10.

Cellular morphology and staining. *Klebsiella* and *Enterobacter* organisms are gram-negative rods 0.5 μm × 1–5 μm. In contrast to enterobacter strains, klebsiellae are nonmotile and frequently encapsulated.

Immunology and serology. *Klebsiella* strains are classified serologically by determination of the capsular antigens. Slide and tube agglutination, precipitin tests, and quellung reactions are used. Serologic identification includes testing the antigen with pooled serum and specific components of positive-reacting pools on a slide. An individual serum is then tested by quellung reaction to confirm that the reaction is capsular and not somatic. The quellung test is then used with serial dilutions of serum to determine titer

Table 25.10. Diagnostic features of *Enterobacter* sp. and related organisms[5]

	Klebsiella			Enterobacter					
	pneumonia	ozaenae	rhinoscleromatis	cloacae	aerogenes	hafnia 37°C	hafnia 22°C	liquifaciens 37°C	liquifaciens 22°C	Serratia marcescens
Capsule	+	+	+	−	−	−		−		−
Motility	−	−	−	+	+	+		+		+
Methyl red	−	+	+	−	−	1	−	1	1	−
Voges-Proskauer	+	−	−	+	+	1	+	1	1	+
Simmons' Citrate	+	1	−	+	+	1	1	1	+	+
Gelatin, 25°C, 2 days complete liquification	−	−	−	−	−	−		+		+
Urease	−	1	−	2	2	−		2		2
Gas from glucose	−	1	−	+	+	+		+		1
Lactose, 2 days	+	1	−	+	+	−		−		−
Adonitol, 2 days	1			1	+	−		−		−
Inositol, 2 days	+			−	+	−		1		−
Sorbitol, 2 days	+			+	+	−		+		+
Raffinose	+			+	+	−		−		−
Rhamnose	+			+	+	+		+		−
Arabinose	+			+	+	+		−		−
Malonate	+	−	+	1	1	1		−		−
Mucate	+	1	−	1	+	−		−		−
Lysine decarboxylase	+	1	−	−	+	+		1		+
Arginine dihydrolase	−			+	−	−		−		−
Orthin. decarboxylase	−			+	+	+		+		+

1, + or −; 2, weak or −.

of reaction. Because many relationships exist among the 72 different capsule types, cross-absorbed sera may be required. Although serologic typing of enterobacter is usually not done, a number of serologic studies of the *hafnia, cloacae,* and *aerogenes* groups have been reported.

Alcaligenes

Alcaligenes faecalis is not considered to be a pathogen since there is no clear-cut disease syndrome for which this organism is responsible. It is frequently encountered in clinical work, as are organisms classified in eight other genera that have the following in common: they are all gram-negative rods, are unpigmented, and fail to ferment carbohydrates. Such an organism may belong in any one of the nine genera: *Achromobacter, Alcaligenes, Bordetella, Comamonas, Herellea, Mima, Moraxella, Pseudomonas,* and *Bacterium.* (Some workers identify *Herellea vaginicola* with *Bacterium anitratum,* but the two are probably not identical.)

Although the published description of these organisms may lead one to believe that each species has varying sizes of organisms, actually size varies greatly with the age of the culture, the medium on which it is grown, and the length of time the organism has been cultivated on artificial media. Faced with the identification of a gram-negative nonfermenting rod, the first questions to be answered are: (1) Can the organism produce acid from carbohydrates by oxidation? (2) Is it motile? (3) If motile, what is the arrangement of the flagella?

Alcaligenes faecalis is to be found among the organisms that produce an alkaline reaction in Hugh and Leifson's oxidation-fermentation (OF) medium[31] containing glucose. *Achromobacter, Herellea vaginicola,*[3] *Bacterium anitratum,*[14] and many members of the genus *Pseudomonas* produce acid by oxidation in this medium.

Further, *A. faecalis* is motile by means of peritrichous flagella, a characteristic shared by *Bordetella bronchicanis* (*B. bronchiseptica*).[18] *Mima polymorpha*[3] and the genus *Moraxella* are nonmotile. *Comamonas terrigena* and members of the genus *Pseudomonas* have polar flagella.[11] Since many microbiologists avoid making flagella stains, it cannot be emphasized too strongly that there is no possible identification of an organism as *Alcaligenes faecalis* unless flagella stains have been made. Indeed, there is a polar flagellated organism known variously as *Pseudomonas alcaligenes,*[12] *Vibrio alcaligenes,* and *Vibrio percolans* that has nearly identical biochemical characteristics.[15]

Five other organisms in the genus *Alcaligenes* are described in *Bergey's Manual* and three of these are nonmotile.[2] Unfortunately the type cultures either do not exist today or, after years of being grown on artificial media, they no longer resemble the original descriptions. The modern tendency is to identify a gram-negative, nonpigmented, nonmotile rod that produces an alkaline reaction in Hugh and Leifson's medium containing glucose, and that grows well on nutrient agar, as *Mima polymorpha.*

Laboratory Procedures

Cultures. Agar colonies are opaque, entire, and unpigmented. Agar slant growth is white and glistening. Broth is turbid, has a thin pellicle and viscid sediment, and gives off ammonia.

Differential reactions. Gelatin is not liquefied; indole is not produced; urea is not hydrolized; nitrites may or may not be produced from nitrates.

Acid is not produced from carbohydrates in Hugh and Leifson's OF medium by fermentation or oxidation; an alkaline reaction is produced. Inoculate duplicate tubes of this medium containing glucose by stabbing to the depth of the column of medium. Seal one tube with a layer of sterile mineral oil or petrolatum. Incubate at 37°C for 18–24 hours. Fermentative organisms will produce acid (yellow color) in both tubes; oxidative organisms will produce no acid in the sealed tube but will produce acid in the open tube (yellow color at the top of the agar column). Organisms producing an alkaline reaction turn the medium from green to a deep blue.

Cellular morphology. The rods are approximately 0.5×1–2 μm, occur singly, in pairs, and in chains, are gram negative, are not acid fast, do not have spores, are normally not encapsulated, and are motile by means of peritrichous flagella.

Media

There are few glassware requirements for the media used in the identification of enteric organisms. Size of the tubes is relatively unimportant. If economy of material and space is important, 13×100 mm tubes can be used for all media and tests. If screw-capped tubes are used, the caps should be loosened during incubation.

In the preparation of media, it is very important that the directions for each different type be closely followed. Some media are not autoclaved but only heated to boiling or sterilized by filtration. Others must be autoclaved at 112 or 121°C and for the exact length of time stated on the label. Excessive temperature and time can cause a breakdown in components (sugars, alcohols). This may lead to false reactions when the media are inoculated.

CAUTION: Isolation of salmonellae from intestines, feces, and grossly contaminated materials requires culture media that contain selective inhibitors; that is, inhibitors that inhibit other enteric organisms while allowing salmonellae to grow. Laboratory workers must evaluate the dehydrated media they purchase and the brilliant green dye they use to assure that these will not unduly inhibit the organisms they hope to recover.

Different lots of brilliant green dye vary in their toxicity with respect to salmonellae.[22] Therefore, titrate this dye by making serial dilutions of it and inoculating lightly with an 18-hour culture of a *Salmonella*. This titration may be carried out in skim milk or tetrathionate broth (in ordinary broths the dye is very toxic at 1:100,000). An inoculum of exactly 0.1 ml per tube of a 10^{-6} dilution of *S. typhimurium* is usually satisfactory. Make a pour plate of the inoculum at the same time to check on the number of organisms in the inoculum; between 25 and 100 organisms is a desirable number.

Since evaluating dehydrated media is time consuming, it is desirable to purchase a year's supply at one time. Make plates of the medium and of tryptose or trypticase soy agar the day before they will be used and leave at room temperature so the surfaces will be dry.

Dilute 18–24-hour cultures of *S. typhimurium, S. gallinarum, S. pullorum,* and *S. choleraesuis* 10^{-5}, 10^{-6}, and 10^{-7} in sterile physiological saline or Butterfield's buffered diluent. For each dilution of each culture, use three plates with 0.1 ml on each. Spread the inoculum over the plate surface with bent glass rods shaped like hockey sticks. Incubate at 35°C for 2 days, then count the colonies. By using three dilutions, you will not miss the countable range. Record the ratio of colonies that develop on the test medium to the organisms on the noninhibitory medium and measure the size of the colonies on the two plates.

S. typhimurium is the least sensitive of the four organisms and any medium that does not give at least 75% recovery of this type is unsatisfactory.

References
1. Barnum, D.A., P.J. Glantz, and H.W. Moon. *Colibacillosis.* CIBA Veterinary Monograph, ser. 2, pp. 1–44, 1967.
2. Buchanan, R.E., and N.E. Gibbons (eds.). *Bergey's Manual of Determinative Bacteriology.* 8th ed. Williams and Wilkins, Baltimore, 1974.
3. DeBord, G.G. Descriptions of *Mimeae* tribe nov. with three genera and three species and two new species of *Neisseria* from conjunctivitis and vaginitis. *Iowa State Coll. J. Sci.* 16:471–480, 1942.
4. Edwards, P.R., and W.H. Ewing. *Identification of Enterobacteriaceae.* 2d ed. Burgess, Minneapolis, 1962.
5. Ewing, W.H. *Enterobacteriaceae Taxonomy and Nomenclature.* Communicable Disease Center, Atlanta, Ga., 1966.
6. Ewing, W.H. *Revised Definitions for the Family Enterobacteriaceae, Its Tribes and Genera.* Communicable Disease Center, Atlanta, Ga., 1967.
7. Ewing, W.H. *Arizona hinshawii* Comb. Nov. *Internat. J. Syst. Bact.* 19:1, 1969.
8. Gay, C.C. *Escherichia coli* and neonatal diseases of calves. *Bact. Rev.* 29:75–101, 1965.
9. Geiman, Q.M. Shigellosis, amebiasis, and simian malaria. *Lab. Anim. Care* 14:441–446, 1964.
10. Glantz, P.J. Simplified tube method for preparation of H antigens. *J. Bact.* 85:942–943, 1963.
11. Hugh, R. *Comamonas terrigena* comb. nov. with proposal for a neotype and request for an opinion. *Internat. J. Syst. Bact.* 12:33–35, 1962.
12. Hugh, R., and P. Ikari. The proposed neotype strain of *Pseudomonas alcaligenes* Monias 1928: Request for an opinion. *Internat. J. Syst. Bact.* 14:103–107, 1964.
13. Hugh, R., and E. Leifson. The taxonomic significance of fermentative vs oxidative metabolism of carbohydrates by various gram-negative bacteria. *J. Bact.* 66:24–26, 1953.
14. Hugh, R., and R. Reese. Designation of the type strain for *Bacterium anitratum* Schaub and Hauber. *Internat. J. Syst. Bact.* 17:245–254, 1967.
15. Hugh, R., and E. Ryschenkow. *Pseudomonas maltophilia,* an *Alcaligenes*-like species. *J. Gen. Microbiol.* 26:123–132, 1961.
16. Kauffmann, F. *The Bacteriology of Enterobacteriaceae.* Williams and Wilkins, Baltimore, 1966.
17. Landy, M., and W. Braun. *Bacterial Endotoxins.* Institute of Microbiology, Rutgers University, New Brunswick, N.J., 1964.
18. Leifson, E., and R. Hugh. A new type of polar monotrichous flagellation. *J. Gen. Microbiol.* 10:68–70, 1954.
19. Mesrobeanu, F., I. Mesrobeanu, and N. Mitrica. The neurotoxins of gram-negative bacteria: The thermolabile endotoxin. *Ann. N.Y. Acad. Sci.* 133:685–699, 1966.
20. Nicolle, P., L. LeMinor, S. LeMinor, and R. Buttiaux. Relation entre la sensibilite aux bacteriophages des *E.coli* des gastroenterites infantiles et leurs caracteres antigeniques et biochemiques. *Compte Rendu Acad. sci.* 239:462–464, 1954.
21. Peluffo, C.A., P.R. Edwards, and D.W. Bruner. A group of coliform bacilli serologically related to the genus *Salmonella. J. Infec. Dis.* 70:185–192, 1942.
22. Read, R.B., Jr., and A.L. Reyes. Variation in plating efficiency of *Salmonella* on eight lots of brilliant green agar. *Appl. Microbiol.* 16:746–748, 1968.
23. Ruch, T.C. *Diseases of Laboratory Primates.* Saunders, Philadelphia, 1959.
24. Sojka, W.J. *Escherichia coli in Domestic Animals and Poultry.* Commonwealth Agriculture Bureau, Farnham Royal, Eng., 1965.
25. Spicer, C.C. A quick method of identifying *Salmonella* H antigens. *J. Clin. Path.* 9:378–379, 1956.

26. Mima

The genus *Mima* was proposed by DeBord in 1942.[6] In spite of considerable attention, the appropriate designation and taxonomic position of this group is not yet settled.[3,4,5,7,13] Possibly *Mima polymorpha* var. *oxidans* will be grouped with the *Moraxella* while the oxidase-negative *Mima polymorpha* will be assigned to the *Achromobacter* or to the *Acinetobacter*.

These organisms were so named because of their mimicry of the *Neisseria* and their pleomorphism. They have been found as "normal" inhabitants of human skin and mucous membrane.[9] They also have been found in the blood and CNS.[7,11] Their role varies from that of normal flora to that of saprophytes, secondary invaders, or even primary pathogens.[2,7,8] The *Mima* have also been found in water, soil, and dairy products.[4,10] Further studies will determine their proper status in disease processes, and their relative importance as pathogens.[1]

Specimens

Any body fluid, tissue, feces, or soil may be collected and prepared as an inoculum without special treatment.

Laboratory Procedures

Cultures. The *Mima* grow satisfactorily on ordinary 5% blood agar. Human, rabbit, and cattle blood have been used. Primary isolation has been obtained on trypticase-soy agar (TSA) and on EMB agar. The *Mima* grow aerobically under normal atmospheric conditions at temperatures from 20–37°C.

After 24-hour incubation, colonies on blood agar are circular, convex, entire, smooth, opaque, grayish-white, and glistening. Consistency may vary from butyrous to mucoid or viscid. On EMB agar the colonies are blue or bluish-purple. In liquid media, the growth tends to be diffuse near the surface and usually there is a viscid sediment.

Differential reactions. On EMB agar, *Mima polymorpha* (*Achromobacter lwoffii*) colonies appear bluish or bluish-purple; they produce an alkaline reaction on TSI agar. They are MR negative, VP negative, citrate variable, indole negative, do not reduce nitates, and are oxidase negative and catalase positive. The *Mima* do not ferment carbohydrates in infusion base, but more sensitive procedures may demonstrate variation in this characteristic.[8] With *Mima polymorpha* var. *oxidans* (*Moraxella duplex*), the reactions are similar, except that the organism produces an oxidase-positive reation.

Cellular morphology. The degree of pleomorphism shown may be related to the medium used and to the time spent on the culture medium. Freshly isolated cultures on solid mediums tend to be predominantly diplococci or short diplobacilli. In liquid media both forms may be seen along with short chains or filaments. The *Mima* are gram-negative but show a modified bipolar appearance and a tendency to retain the gram-positive stain. DeBord described the dimensions as: the rod forms, 0.5–0.7×1–3 μm; and the cocci forms, 0.5–0.7 μm in diameter.[7] A capsule can be demonstrated.

Animal inoculation. Mima may be lethal for mice and guinea pigs by the IP route, but insufficient information is available to recommend this as a diagnostic criterion.

Immunology and serology. These aspects of identification have not been adequately worked out but some heterogeneity has been observed.[12] Phage susceptibility has not been reported. Toxins have not been demonstrated.

References

1. Alami, S.Y., and H.D. Riley, Jr. Infections caused by Mimeae with special reference to *Mima polymorpha*: A review. *Am. J. Med. Sci.* 252:537–544, 1966.
2. Ballard, S., M.A. Griffith, and G. Controni. The morphology and biochemical reactions of the *Moraxella-Mineae* group. *Am. J. Med. Tech.* 30:263–269, 1964.
3. Baumann, P., M. Doudoroff, and R.Y. Stanier. Study of the *Moraxella* group. I. Genus *Moraxella* and the *Neisseria catarrhalis* group. *J. Bact.* 95:58–73, 1968.
4. Baumann, P., M. Doudoroff, and R.Y. Stanier. A study of the *Moraxella* group. II. Oxidative-negative species (genus *Acinetobacter*). *J. Bact.* 95:1520–1541, 1968.
5. Controni, G., S. Ballard, and M.A. Griffith. A review of the literature on classification of the *Mima-Moraxella*. *Am. J. Med. Tech.* 30:257–262, 1964.
6. DeBord, G.C. Descriptions of Mimeae Trib. Nov. with three genera and three species and two new species of Neisseria from conjunctivitis and vaginitis. *Iowa State Coll. J. Sci.* 16:471–480, 1942.
7. Gilardi, G.L. *Achromobacter* and *Moraxella* (Tribe Mimeae): Review and new studies. *Am. J. Med. Tech.* 33:200–220, 1967.
8. Gilardi, G.L. Morphological and biochemical differentiation of Achromobacter and Moraxella (DeBord's Tribe Mimeae). *Appl. Microbiol.* 16:33–38, 1968.
9. Irving, W.R., and W. Herrick. The bacteria Mim-Herellea: Isolation and clinical significance in a general hospital. *Am. J. Clin. Path.* 47:729–733, 1967.
10. Koburger, J.A. Isolation of *Mima polymorpha* from dairy products. *J. Dairy Sci.* 47:646, 1964.
11. Lewis, J.F., T. Marshburn, H.P. Singletary, and S. O'Brien. Fatal meningitis due to *Moraxella duplex*: Report of a case with Waterhouse-Friderichsen Syndrome. *S. Med. J.* 61:539–541, 1968.
12. Nelson, J.D., and S. Shelton. Cultural, biochemical, and immunological properties of *Mima, Herellea,* and *Flavobacterium* species. *Appl. Microbiol.* 13:801–807, 1965.
13. Pickett, M.J., and C.R. Manclark. Tribe Mimeae: An illegitimate epithet. *Am. J. Clin. Path.* 43:161–165, 1965.

27. Pseudomonas

Seven species of pseudomonads have been isolated as primary or opportunistic pathogens in animals and humans: *Pseudomonas aeruginosa, P. fluorescens, P. pseudomallei* (etiologic agent of melioidosis), *P. mallei* (etiologic agent of glanders), *P. cepacia, P. maltophilia,* and *P. putrefaciens.* Six species of questionable pathogenicity include *P. putida, P. stutzeri, P. alcaligenes, P. pseudoalcaligenes, P. acidovorans,* and *P. diminuta.* The classification of *P. pseudomallei* and *P. mallei* has been the subject of considerable controversy for many years. They have at times been placed in *P. feifferella, Malleomyces, Actinobacillus,* and *Loefferella,* but recent characterizations of these organisms support their current assignment to the genus *Pseudomonas.*[10,11]

P. aeruginosa, an opportunistic pathogen, has been associated with necrotic pneumonitis, rhinitis, and enteritis in swine, septicemia and scours in calves, mastitis and abortion in cows, enteritis in chickens and turkeys, abortion in horses, pneumonia in mink, enteritis in chinchillas, and numerous infections in humans. The organism is commonly found in soil, water, and the excreta of animals and humans. Therefore, it is readily available for invasion of untreated wounds. It is found in dermal abscesses in a wide variety of animals and is a serious contaminant of the broken or burned skin of humans. The organism may cause death if effective antibiotics are not administered early in the infection.

P. fluorescens is a natural inhabitant of soil and water, but it has been recovered from necrotic lesions in reptiles and from the blood of lizards and snakes with fatal septicemia. The organism recovered in these cases was formerly called *P. reptilivora* but now is considered to be identical with *P. fluorescens. P. fluorescens* was judged responsible for one case of septicemia in humans, but generally this organism, and the closely related *P. putida,* do not appear to be of clinical significance in humans.

P. pseudomallei causes a fatal natural disease (melioidosis) of rodents, swine, sheep, and goats. The disease also occurs in incidental hosts such as humans, dogs, cats, horses, and cattle. Sometimes called "false glanders," the disease affects the nasal membranes, subcutaneous tissues, muscles, joints, and vital organs. The organism causes purulent discharges from ulcerated mucosa, pustular eruptions, severe polyarthritis, and multiple abscesses in the lungs, liver, and spleen. The disease is most common in Southeast Asia where the organism is found in soil and water.

P. mallei causes a fatal disease (glanders) of horses, cats, and, rarely, humans. The organism produces extensive nodule formation and necrosis in lymph glands, lungs, skin, and nasal membranes of infected animals.[7] Septicemia results in death. The disease once was worldwide but has been largely eliminated in developed countries.

P. cepacia (*P. multivorans*) is recovered from soil, water, and clinical materials from humans, and is phytopathogenic. Nutritional and genetic studies have shown that *P. cepacia* is related to the animal pathogens *P. pseudomallei* and *P. mallei*.[2] In humans it has been responsible for urinary tract infections, pneumonitis, endocarditis, and postoperative wound infections.

P. maltophilia is widespread in nature and has been recovered from soil, water, milk, animal, and human sources. With the exception of *P. aeruginosa*, it is the most frequently isolated pseudomonad from human clinical sources. Isolates from urine have been implicated in epididymitis, periurethral abscess, and urinary tract infections. Pseudomonads have been judged responsible for wound infections, including infection of an ankle injury, gangrene of the foot, gun-shot wound, and postoperative joint infections. *P. maltophilia* has been isolated in association with a wide variety of infections of the upper and lower respiratory tract, including pneumonia, empyema, sinusitis, and otitis.

P. putrefaciens is recovered from soil, water, milk, and fresh and frozen cod fillets, is the cause of putrid deterioration of butter, and is responsible for spoilage in haddock fillets and poultry. The organism has been judged to be responsible for chronic otitis media in humans and has been recovered from leg ulcers, sputum, and urine with apparently no etiologic relationship.

P. stutzeri is widely distributed in soil and water and has been frequently isolated from a variety of clinical specimens. Assessing a pathogenic role to *P. stutzeri* is difficult since the organism lives as a saprophyte in the human body.[8] It may cause serious infection if the general defense mechanisms of the patient have been weakened, but it is probably only occasionally an opportunistic pathogen.

P. alcaligenes, P. pseudoalcaligenes, P. acidovorans, and *P. diminuta* are found in soil and water and have been recovered from a variety of human specimens but probably are only rarely opportunistic pathogens.[1]

Specimens

All of the above pseudomonads can be isolated readily from exudate-containing lesions caused by the organism. The exudate or lesion-bearing tissue should be removed from the diseased animal and kept refrigerated until bacteriological examination can be made. Preferably, the exudate should be transferred and streaked directly on bacteriological media. Precautions should be taken in handling exudates of diseased animals so that infective material does not gain access to cuts or abrasions in the skin of the examiner. Because of the strong proteolytic activities of some of these species, they may cause ulcerative lesions on the skin or mucous membranes, which in turn may be contaminated with many other organisms. Direct staining of exudates is of little diagnostic value except to ascertain the Gram reaction of the predominant organism. Notation of the color of the exudate may be of diagnostic assistance since most strains of *P.*

aeruginosa produce a blue-green soluble pigment that gives the exudate a characteristic "blue pus" appearance.

Laboratory Procedures

Cultures. The above organisms may be isolated directly from lesion exudates by plating on peptone agar plus 5% defibrinated sheep or rabbit blood and incubating the inoculated plate aerobically at 37°C. Growth of *P. mallei* is favored by the addition of glycerol to a final concentration of 1%, but it is not essential. Addition of thionine to a final concentration of 0.04% inhibits growth of some contaminants but does not interfere with growth of *P. mallei*. Because ulcerative lesions often contain numerous organisms other than the etiologic agent, lesion exudates should be streaked on certain selective as well as nonselective media. *P. aeruginosa,* for example, grows well on SS, EMB, and MaC agar, while many other bacterial contaminants do not.

Differential reactions. Pseudomonads are gram-negative, aerobic, nonsporeforming bacilli with monotrichous or multitrichous flagella in the motile forms. They grow well on ordinary peptone medium, are usually oxidase positive, and either do not attack carbohydrates or attack them oxidatively with the production of acid but no gas. Indole, methyl red, and acetylmethylcarbinol tests are negative. They can be identified according to the morphologic and biochemical characteristics listed below and in Table 27.1.

The fluorescent group, *P. aeruginosa, P. fluorescens,* and *P. putida,* have several features in common, including the presence of the arginine-dihydrolase system, oxidase-positive activity, and the production of fluorescent pigment. Not all strains of *P. aeruginosa* produce pyocyanine and these strains must be identified by other means. Uniform characteristics for identification of apyocyanogenic strains of *P. aeruginosa* include the presence of monotrichous flagella, growth at 42°C, and inability to produce acid from disaccharides. *P. fluorescens* and *P. putida* can be differentiated from *P. aeruginosa* because the former are multitrichous, do not grow at 42°C, and are characterized by variable acid production from disaccharides.[9] *P. fluorescens* and *P. putida* can be differentiated by gelatin liquefaction and the egg yolk (lecithinase) reaction, characteristics possessed by the former but not the latter species.

The principal characteristics of the pseudomallei group, *P. pseudomallei, P. mallei,* and *P. cepacia,* include the presence of multitrichous flagella in the motile species, variable oxidase activity, and resistance to antibiotics of the polymyxin group. The color of growth of the species in this group is highly variable ranging from gray to yellow. The colony morphology of *P. pseudomallei* is variable, ranging from smooth to wrinkled in structure. *P. mallei* is nonmotile and can be further differentiated from *P. pseudomallei* on the basis of acid production from xylose. *P. cepacia* can be distinguished from *P. mallei* and *P. pseudomallei* on the basis of denitrification and arginine dihydrolase and lysine decarboxylase activity.

The alcaligenes group, *P. alcaligenes, P. pseudoalcaligenes,* is monotrichous, grows at 42°C, generally fails to accumulate intracellular fat, and assimilates pelargonate but not norleucine. Acid production from fructose and other carbohydrates distinguishes *P. pseudoalcaligenes* from *P. alcaligenes. P. acidovorans,* which is similar to the alca-

Table 27.1. Characteristics of *Pseudomonas* species

Test	aeru.	fluo.	puti.	pseudomall.	mall.	cepa.	acid.	alca.	pseudoalca.	stut.	putr.	malt.	dimi.
Flagella no.	1	>1	>1	>1	NM	>1	>1	1	1	1	1	>1	1
Fluorescein	+	+	+	−	−	−	−	−	−	−	−	−	−
Pyocyanin	V	−	−	−	−	−	−	−	−	−	−	−	−
Brown color	−	−	−	−	NT	−	−	−	V	−	−	+	+
Wrinkled col.	−	−	−	+M	−M	−	−	−	−	+	−	−	−
SS agar	+	+	+	−	NT	−	V	−	V	+	+	−	−
NaCl 6.5%	−	−	−	−	NT	−	−	−	−	+	+	−	−
NaCl 2.5%	+	+	+	−	NT	+	−	V	+	+	+	+	+
pH 5.6	+	+	+	+	NT	+	+	+	+	−	−	+	+
42°C	+	−	−	+	V	V	−	+	+	+	+	V	+
H₂S (KIA)	−	−	−	−	−	−	−	−	−	−	+	−	−
Nitrite	V	−	−	+M	V	V	+	+	+	V	+	V	−
N₂ gas	V	−	−	+	V	−	−	−	−	+	−	−	−
Glucose	+	+	+	+	+	+	+w	−	+w	+	+d	+	−
Fructose	+M	+M	+M	+	+	+	+	−	+	+	Vd	+M	−
Mannose	+M	+	+	+	+	+	−	−	V	+M	−	+M	−
Rhamnose	V	V	V	+M	−	−	−	−	−	V	Vd	−	−
Xylose	+M	+	+	+	−	+	−	−	V	+	−	V	−
Lactose	−	−M	−M	+	+	+	−	−	−	−	Vd	+M	−
Sucrose	−	V	−M	+M	−	+M	−	−	−	−	−	+M	−
Maltose	−	V	V	+	+	+	−	−	−	+	−	+	−
Mannitol	V	V	V	+	V	+	+	−	−	+M	−	−	−
Oxidase	+	+	+	V	V	V	+	+	+	+	+	−M	+
Arg-DH-ase	+	+	+	+	+	−	−	−	−	−	−	−	−
LYS-DC-ase	−	−	−	−	−	+	−	−	−	−	−	−	−
ORN-DC-ase	−	−	−	−	−	−	−	−	−	−	+	−	−
PHE-DA-ase	−	−	−	−	NT	−	−	+M	V	V	−	−	−
Aesculin	−	−	−	V	NT	+M	−	V	−	−	−	+	−
Lipase	V	+M	−M	+M	+	+	−M	−	−	+M	+	+	−
Starch	−	−	−	V	V	−	−	−	−	+M	−	−	−
DNase	−M	−	−	−	NT	−	−	−	−	−M	+	+	+
Lecithinase	−M	+	−	+	NT	+M	−	−	−	−M	+	+	−
Gelatinase	V	+	−	+	+	V	−	−M	−	−M	+	+	+
Intracell. fat	−	−	−	+	+	+	+	−	V	−	−	−	+
Polymyxin res.	−	−	−	+	NT	+	−	−	−	−	−	−	+
ONPG	−	−	−	−	NT	+	−	−	−	−	−	+	−
BMM	+	+	+	+	+	+	+	+	+	+	+	−	−
Assimilations													
D-glucose	+	+	+	+	+	+	−	−	+	+	−	+	−
D-fructose	V	+M	+M	+	V	+	+	−	+	+M	−	V	−
Maltose	−	−	−	+	V	−	−	−	−	+M	−	+	−
D-trehalose	−	+	−	+	+	+	−	−	−	−	−	+	−
D-mannitol	V	+	−M	+	+	+	+	−	−	V	−	−	−
Acetate	+	+	+	+	+	+	+	+	+	+	+	+	+
Pelargonate	+	+	+	+	−	+	−	+	+	+	−	−	−
Citrate	+	+	+	+	V	+	+	+	+M	+	−	+	−
β-alanine	+	+	+	+	+M	+	+	+	+	−	−	−	−
DL-norleucine	−	−	−	−	−	−	+	−	−	−	−	−	−

NM, nonmotile; V, variable; NT, not tested; +M, most strains positive; −M, most strains negative; +w, weak positive; +d, delayed positive; Vd, variable—delayed when positive. Nearly all reactions are read after 24–48 hours incubation at 37°C. Method details are given in *Manual of Clinical Microbiology*[6] and in the paper by Stanier et al.[11]

Pseudomonas

Figure 27.1. Identification of some gram-negative nonfermentative rods

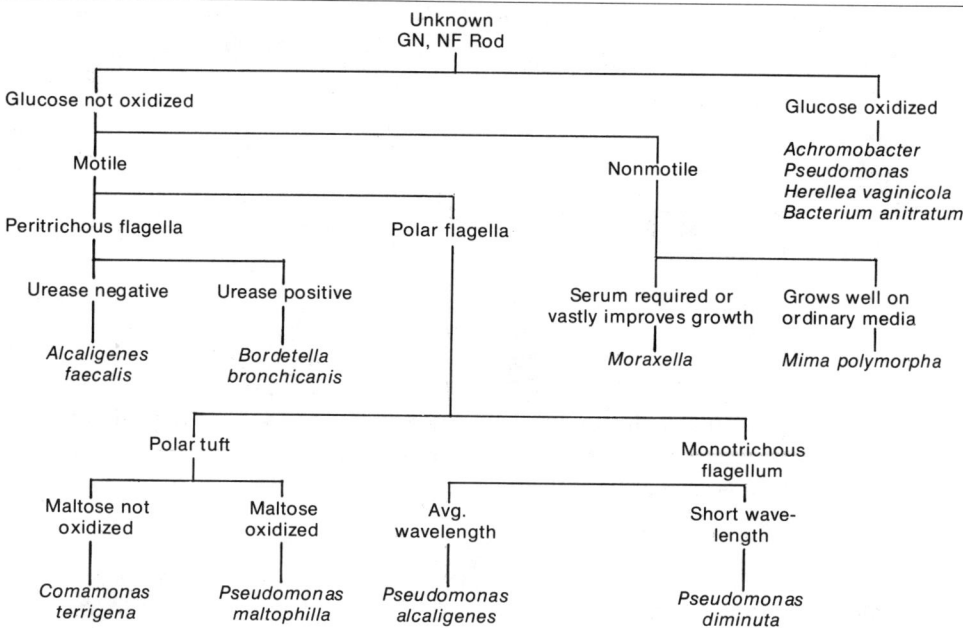

ligenes group, is multitrichous, accumulates intracellular fat, fails to grow at 42°C, and assimilates norleucine but not pelargonate.

P. stutzeri can be identified on the basis of its colony morphology and its production of nitrogen gas. The strains are diphasic, consisting of both rough and smooth colonial forms, yellow or light brown in color. Other distinctive features include starch hydrolysis, growth on 6.5% NaCl, and inability to grow at pH 5.6.

P. putrefaciens is characterized by the production of hydrogen sulfide from Kligler's iron agar (KIA) and a tan pigment. It produces decarboxylase for ornithine, is deoxyribonuclease positive, grows on 6.5% NaCl, and fails to grow at pH 5.6.

P. maltophilia and *P. diminuta* will not grow on the basal mineral medium unless supplemented with growth factors. *P. maltophilia* requires methionine and *P. diminuta* requires pantothenate, biotin, and cyanocobalamin.[6] *P. maltophilia* is multitrichous, is generally oxidase negative, produces decarboxylase for lysine, and is ortho-nitrophenol-beta-d-galactopyranoside (ONPG) positive. *P. diminuta* is monotrichous, accumulates intracellular fat, is oxidase positive, and fails to produce acid from carbohydrates (Fig. 27.1).

Animal inoculation. The various species of hosts naturally infected by pseudomonads are listed at the beginning of this chapter. The species of laboratory animals that can be experimentally infected are listed in Table 27.2.

Immunology and serology. Serology or skin sensitivity tests have not been used routinely for the diagnosis of diseases caused by pseudomonads except in the case of *P. mallei* infections. In this disease, the infected animal first develops antibodies that can

Table 27.2. Laboratory animals susceptible to pseudomonad infection

Host	Pseudomonas			
	aeruginosa	fluorescens	pseudomallei	mallei
Rat	+	−	+	+
Mouse	+	−	+	−
Rabbit	+	−	+	+
Guinea pig	+	−	+	+

+, septicemia, death after IP or IM inoculation; −, very mild or no disease.

be detected by CF, agglutination, or precipitin methods (although cross-reactions occur with antibodies produced against *P. pseudomallei*). Second, the animals become allergic to products of bacterial breakdown during infection, and skin sensitivity to these products can be detected by the mallein test. The test may be administered cutaneously, subcutaneously, or ophthalmically (dropped onto the inner eyelid). Swelling, hyperemia, congestion, or mucopurulent discharge at the site of inoculation and hyperthermia occur in animals that have been sensitized to *P. mallei*. Mallein is an extract of *P. mallei* cells or a culture filtrate.

Epidemiologic studies of *P. aeruginosa* have assumed an important role because this organism is of the greatest concern in nosocomial infections, replacing the *Staphylococcus* problem of a decade ago. One method of subdividing *P. aeruginosa* for epidemiologic purposes has been serotyping, but this method has limited use since most strains fall into a relatively few serologic types. An antigen schema based on challenge protection in mice, as distinguished from serologic reactions in vitro, was recently formulated; seven groups of cross-protective homogeneity were defined.

Phage and pyocin susceptibility. In addition to serotyping, pyocin typing and phage typing have been used for epidemiologic studies.[5] However, these methods are limited because of frequent changes in the phage lysis pattern, and because most strains of *P. aeruginosa* fall into a few pyocin types, as is the case with serotypes.[3] A method has been developed to circumvent these limitations; the relationship between unknown strains is established by identifying *P. aeruginosa* through both the production of and sensitivity to pyocin and phage.[4] In this procedure, the pyocin and phage are liberated from the unknown strains, the lysates are then tested against 27 indicator strains, and the zones of clearing are differentiated into pyocin or phage action.[12,13] Then 24 standard pyocin-phage lysates are applied to each unknown and the sensitivity patterns recorded. Thus the 51 operational characteristics establish the identity or dissimilarity of the unknown strains.

P. aeruginosa has been shown to produce a thermostable exotoxin, but it has limited toxicity for experimental animals. The pseudomonads probably contain endotoxins of the general gram-negative bacterial type, but they have not been studied sufficiently to ascertain their role in the causation or prevention of disease by the use of antitoxin.

Reference laboratories. Department of Microbiology, School of Medicine, George Washington University, Washington; Bacteriology Division, Hospital for Joint Diseases and Medical Center, New York.

References

1. Ballard, R.W., M. Doudoroff, and R.Y. Stanier. Taxonomy of the aerobic pseudomonads: *Pseudomonas diminuta* and *P. vesiculare*. *J. Gen. Microbiol.* 53:349–361, 1968.
2. Ballard, R.W., N.J. Palleroni, M. Doudoroff, R.Y. Stanier, and M. Mandel. Taxonomy of the aerobic pseudomonads: *Pseudomonas cepacia, P. marginata, P. alliicola,* and *P. caryophylli*. *J. Gen. Microbiol.* 60:199–214, 1970.
3. Farmer, J.J., and L.G. Herman. Epidemiological fingerprinting of *Pseudomonas aeruginosa* by the production of and sensitivity to pyocin and bacteriophage. *Appl. Microbiol.* 18:760–765, 1969.
4. Fisher, M.W., H.B. Devlin, and F.J. Gnabsik. New immunotype schema for *Pseudomonas aeruginosa* based on protective antigens. *J. Bact.* 98:835–836, 1969.
5. Gillies, R.R., and J.R.W. Govan. Typing of *Pseudomonas pyocyanea* by pyocyine production. *J. Path. Bact.* 91:339–345, 1966.
6. Hugh, R. Pseudomonas and aeromonas. In *Manual of Clinical Microbiology,* J.E. Blair, E.H. Lemnette, and J.P. Truant (eds.) pp. 175–190. American Society for Microbiology, Bethesda, Md., 1970.
7. Merchant, I.A., and R.A. Packer. The genera *Pseudomonas, Aeromonas,* and *Alcaligenes,* pp. 251–254. The genus *Malleomyces,* pp. 364–369. In *Veterinary Bacteriology and Virology,* Merchant and Packer (eds.). 7th ed. Iowa State University Press, Ames, 1967.
8. Palleroni, N.J., M. Doudoroff, and R.Y. Stanier. Taxonomy of the aerobic pseudomonads: The properties of the *Pseudomonas stutzeri* group. *J. Gen. Microbiol.* 60:215–231, 1970.
9. Pickett, M.J., and M.M. Pederson. Characterization of saccharolytic and nonfermentative bacteria associated with man. *Can. J. Microbiol.* 16:351–362, 1970.
10. Redfearn, M.S., N.J. Palleroni, and R.Y. Stanier. A comparative study of *Pseudomonas pseudomallei* and *Bacillus mallei*. *J. Gen. Microbiol.* 43:293–313, 1966.
11. Stanier, R.Y., N.J. Palleroni, and M. Doudoroff. The aerobic pseudomonads: A taxonomic study. *J. Gen. Microbiol.* 43:159–271, 1966.
12. Sutter, V.L., V. Hurst, and J. Fennell. A standardized system for phage typing *Pseudomonas aeruginosa*. *Health Lab. Sci.* 2:7–16, 1965.
13. Verder, E., and J. Evans. A proposed antigenic schema for the identification of strains of *Pseudomonas aeruginosa*. *J. Infec. Dis.* 109:183–193, 1961.

28. Staphylococcus

Staphylococci are frequently found in a wide variety of suppurative lesions in humans and animals. They can occasionally be recovered from the apparently healthy skin, mucous membranes, and the environment of humans and animals. They can also be found in milk, meat, and other food products. Of the two species of *Staphylococcus*, *S. aureus* is definitely pathogenic, whereas *S. epidermidis* has generally little or no pathogenicity. In veterinary medicine, staphylococci present problems as causative microorganisms in mastitis of cattle, sheep, and other animals, staphylococcic mastitis of cows being of particular importance. The staphylococci are associated with pyodermitis of dogs. They are often the cause of abscesses, generalized pyogenic lesions, and even fatal septicemias in all domestic animals including poultry. In addition, some strains of *S. aureus* elaborate enterotoxins that cause food poisoning in humans. However, in spite of this wide spectrum of pathogenicity, staphylococci have some degree of host specificity; certain staphylococcic strains infect predominantly humans, others mainly cattle, others dogs, and so forth.

Specimens

The samples should be collected as aseptically as possible, avoiding exposure to other contaminating microorganisms. Samples can be taken with sterile syringes or milked directly into sterile tubes. Milk samples from individual quarters should be collected after the udder has been thoroughly cleansed with a disposable towel soaked in a 200-ppm chlorine or other disinfectant solution and after each teat, particularly the area around the teat opening, has been rubbed with 70% alcohol on a separate piece of cotton.[6] The first streams of milk should be discarded into a strip-cup, because they may contain contaminating bacteria. In the strip-cup, abnormal milk can also be more readily recognized. Then 5–10 ml of milk should be drawn into sterile screw-capped vials.

Staphylococci from infections of animals can also be pathogenic for humans. Therefore, care should be taken in handling specimens.

Laboratory Procedures

In many cases of suspected staphylococcic infections a direct microscopic examination of the specimen is desirable. Although it cannot provide a final diagnosis, it may reveal the staphylococci, the cells of inflammation, and the association of the staphylococci with the cells. The latter could indicate the etiologic role of the staphylococci in the disease process.

For the direct microscopic examination, thinly spread films of specimen are dried in the air without heating. They are stained, preferably with the Kopeloff and Beerman modification of the Gram stain.[20] For staining smears of pure cultures, on the other hand, the Hucker modification of the Gram stain should be applied.[20] The findings of the direct microscopic examination should be confirmed by the isolation and identification of the staphylococci.

Cultures. Other than aseptic collection, most specimens of suspected staphylococcic infections do not require special preparation for culturing. Tissues may have to be ground in a blender. Usually, it is best to culture the specimens directly without delay. If this is not possible, keep them refrigerated or even frozen until they can be cultured. This reduces the chance of overgrowth by contaminating bacteria, which might occur at room temperature. Milk samples from individual quarters of cows can also be preincubated overnight at 37°C, provided they have been taken aseptically. During preincubation of the milk the staphylococci can multiply and become more easily detectable upon culture. However, this should not be done if the number of staphylococci in the original sample is to be estimated, or if the sample is presumed to be contaminated.

Staphylococci can be readily cultivated in a variety of laboratory media. In synthetic media they require amino acids as a source of nitrogen and vitamins for growth. The conventional media, based mostly on blood, meat digests (tryptic digest, peptones), and meat or yeast extracts, are still much more suitable for diagnostic bacteriology, and they are more easily prepared, are less expensive, and are more reliable in supporting initiation of growth by small inocula. For optimal growth of staphylococci adjust media to about pH 7.2.

Blood agar is the medium of choice for the isolation of staphylococci from infected animals. It readily supports staphylococcic growth and reveals hemolysins. Ovine blood agar gives somewhat clearer hemolytic reactions than bovine blood agar, although both can be used (and defibrinated), or the researcher can take blood from a donor animal that does not have detectable concentrations of staphylococcic antitoxins in its blood.[6] If the status of the donor is not known the red blood cells can be washed by repeated centrifugation in sterile 0.14 M NaCl at about $1500 \times g$ for 15 minutes to remove the antibodies. The washed red blood cell suspension, or the whole blood, is incorporated at a final concentration of 5% into a previously autoclaved base medium cooled in a water bath to 48°C. Suitable blood agar base media are available in dehydrated form from several manufacturing companies (e.g. Difco Lab., Detroit; Baltimore Biological Lab.; Albimi Lab., Brooklyn).

Selective media should be used for the isolation of staphylococci from specimens that are likely to contain large numbers of other bacteria, e.g. bulk milk, skin swabs, some food samples, feces, and so forth.

Staphylococci (*S. aureus* and *S. epidermidis*) grow vigorously in media containing up to 10% NaCl.[8,13] Most of the other bacteria are inhibited at these salt concentrations. Some of the commercially available media are the mannitol salt agar of Chapman,[13]

Staphylococcus medium 110,[14] and Chapman-Stone medium[15] (see Appendix A for formulas for the last two media). All of these media also indicate oxidation of mannitol, and the latter two show liquefaction of gelatin.

An enrichment broth for staphylococci can be prepared by the addition of NaCl at a final concentration of 7.5% to a nutritionally rich medium such as heart infusion or brain-heart infusion broth.

Staphylococci, like corynebacteria, are not inhibited on tellurite-glycine media and form jet black colonies. The tellurite-glycine media of Zebovitz et al. (see Appendix A for formula)[43] and of Baird-Parker[2] are commonly used. They are also commercially available.

Incorporation of polymyxin B into a nutrient agar at a concentration of 75 μg per ml medium also provides for selective growth of *S. aureus*. *S. epidermidis* is slightly, and most of the gram-negative bacteria are strongly, inhibited by the antibiotic.[26]

Staphylococci grow best aerobically. They also grow in an atmosphere of CO_2, which may enhance production of toxins, and even under anaerobic conditions. The optimum temperature of incubation is 37°C, although growth occurs between 10 and 42°C.

There is abundant growth in nutritionally adequate broth and agar media within 24 hours at 37°C. On agar media the colonies reach diameters of 2–3 mm. They are round, convex, opaque, and glistening. On blood agar, hemolysis is mostly seen with *S. aureus* and rarely with *S. epidermidis*. Staphylococcic cultures form golden pigment, others produce yellow or grayish-white colonies.

Differential reactions. All staphylococci are strongly catalase positive and utilize glucose anaerobically. *S. aureus* ferments mannitol and is coagulase positive. *S. epidermidis* does not ferment mannitol and is coagulase negative.

Fermentation of mannitol must be tested under anaerobic conditions.[7]

Coagulase production is the most reliable single criterion for the tentative identification of *S. aureus*. Coagulase is an enzymelike substance that mediates the conversion of fibrinogen into fibrin. This reaction can be demonstrated in a tube, slide, or plate test.[21]

The tube test can be conducted with citrated rabbit (or human) plasma, diluted 1:4 with sterile 0.14 M NaCl or broth. It can also be conducted with a fibrinogen-plasma solution, particularly when many cultures are to be tested. The fibrinogen-plasma solution consists of 2% (W/V) bovine fibrinogen (Armour Lab., Kankakee, Ill.) and 3% rabbit plasma in sterile 0.14 M NaCl. Usually 0.3 ml of the 18–24-hour staphylococcic broth culture in question, or in exceptional cases a loopful of the staphylococci from an agar colony, are mixed with 0.5 ml of either the diluted rabbit plasma or the fibrinogen-plasma solution in an agglutination tube. The test is read after 3 hours at 75°C. Formation of a coagulum indicates a positive coagulase reaction.

The slide test is a more rapid procedure giving essentially the same results as the tube test.[9,21] A loopful of staphylococci from a colony is first suspended in a drop of sterile 0.14 M NaCl on a slide. The suspension should be uniformly dense. Autoagglutinating or granular mixtures cannot be tested. A drop of fresh citrated rabbit plasma is placed near the staphylococcic suspension. Then, with a sterile loop, the suspension is induced to flow into the plasma. Coagulation of the plasma within 15 seconds at room temperature indicates a positive reaction.

The plate test reveals coagulase production of individual colonies. The staphylococci are grown on a fibrinogen agar medium. As the colonies develop coagulase diffuses into the fibrinogen medium, where it mediates the conversion into fibrin. Thus coagulase-positive staphylococcic colonies are surrounded by opaque zones of fibrin. The fibrinogen media can be prepared simply by spreading citrated rabbit plasma or a bovine fibrinogen solution over the surface of certain solidified agar media.[23] Selective media, such as the tellurite-glycine agar can also be used. The fibrinogen media are, therefore, useful for the isolation and presumptive identification of S. aureus in one step.

Besides their ability to ferment mannitol and to produce coagulase, many, but not all, S. aureus cultures and a few S. epidermidis cultures are hemolytic. Presently the alpha- beta-, and delta-hemolysins are recognized. After incubation at 37°C on sheep blood agar the alpha-hemolysin gives a zone of complete hemolysis, the beta-hemolysin a zone of hemolytic discoloration (partial hemolysis) and the delta-hemolysin a relatively narrow zone of complete hemolysis. A more specific differentiation of the hemolysins can be achieved by a variety of other procedures.[1,23] Their value for routine diagnosis, however, is limited, because the hemolytic pattern of staphylococci is not sufficiently constant.

A number of additional enzymes and toxins are frequently produced by S. aureus and only rarely, if at all, by S. epidermidis. A study of these substances may be helpful for diagnosis and for elucidation of staphylococcic pathogenicity.

Nuclease is formed by most S. aureus strains. It can be readily detected in an agar medium containing 2 mg DNA per ml medium.[27] After growth of the staphylococci for 48 hours at 37°C on the DNA agar, the plates are flooded with 1 N HCl. Nuclease-positive colonies are surrounded by zones of clearing.

Egg yolk opacity factor is produced by a number of S. aureus strains, particularly by those from abscesses. It can be demonstrated in egg yolk medium (see Appendix A).[28] Egg yolk factor–positive staphylococci produce a marked turbidity in the medium after incubation at 37°C for 24 hours.

Fibrinolysin activity is usually assayed on a fibrin agar.[34] For quantitative determinations a fibrinogen-plasma-coagulase solution can be used. Many staphylococcic cultures from dogs and human beings and a few from cattle are fibrinolytic.

Phosphatase can be tested in one of the phenolphthalein-diphosphate media.[21] However, a considerable number of S. epidermidis strains elaborate this enzyme also.

Leukocidic substances are likely to be important virulence factors in staphylococcic infections. Although much work has already been done, the leukocidic substances, particularly of S. aureus strains from animals, are still not completely known. The Panton-Valentine (P-V) leukocidin can be demonstrated microscopically[29] with human and rabbit leukocytes or by a color test.[42] The leukolysin is probably identical with delta-hemolysin and can be detected with human and rabbit leucocytes and also with leukocytes from other animal species.[29] The Neisser-Wechsberg leukocidin may be identical with the alpha-hemolysin and is demonstrable with rabbit leukocytes.[42]

The public health significance of staphylococcic mastitis of cows revolves around the potential of the staphylococcic strains involved to produce enterotoxin. One investigator reports that of the strains isolated from mastitic cows less than 10% of the total examined were enterotoxigenic.[11] However, dried milk products have been involved in food poisoning outbreaks.

The enterotoxins are proteins produced by the staphylococci in many foods and are one cause of food poisoning in man. Four enterotoxins, designated A, B, C, and D, have been identified.[4,12] but only three have been purified and their specific antibodies prepared in quantity. The purified enterotoxins are sensitive to heat but the crude toxins, e.g. enterotoxin A (which is the one most frequently involved in food poisoning), can withstand pasteurization and boiling for several minutes.[3,25]

The detection of enterotoxin and enterotoxin-producing staphylococci presents a difficult problem because there is no practical sensitive test that can be used to detect all the enterotoxins. Methods based on the use of specific antibodies have made it unnecessary to use animals except when testing for unidentified enterotoxins. For this work the animals most frequently employed are cats and monkeys.[4,11] The most reliable bioassay for an enterotoxin is feeding it to young rhesus monkeys, because the enterotoxins are the only substances produced by staphylococci that cause emesis in these animals. The cost of both the monkeys and their upkeep, and the fact that they do become resistant to the enterotoxins, limits their use. Next to monkeys, cats are the most reliable animal, although they are subject to nonspecific reactions and are relatively insensitive to enterotoxin C.[3] Because the enterotoxin is injected IV in cats, substances that may provoke symptoms similar to those cause by enterotoxin must be inactivated by digestion with trypsin or pancreatin.[10,24]

Of the methods based on the enterotoxin-antienterotoxin precipitation reaction, the microslide technique has been used most widely.[10,33] With this method, it is possible to detect as little as 0.1 μg of enterotoxin per ml of solution and to compare unknown samples directly with known enterotoxins.[11] The single gel-diffusion tube method has been adapted for quantitative measurement of the enterotoxins. Passive hemagglutination and reversed passive hemagglutination are sensitive methods for detection of enterotoxin, but as yet they have not been widely adopted.[38] As little as 0.0015 μg of enterotoxin per ml can be detected by the latter method. Procedures for the detection of enterotoxin in food extracts make use of the microslide, the Oakley double gel-diffusion tube, and the reversed passive hemagglutination methods.[33,38]

Subdivision of *Staphylococcus aureus* into three subspecies—*hominis, bovis,* and *canis*—has been proposed. The subdivision is based on (1) phage typing, (2) coagulase activity in bovine and human plasmas, (3) the crystal-violet test, (4) types of hemolysins, (5) production of fibrinolysin, and (6) pigment formation. Further differentiation of strains is also useful for epizootiological investigations and for studies on pathogenicity.

In the crystal-violet test, a nutrient medium containing crystal violet at a concentration of 1:100,000 is inoculated with the staphylococci in circular spots of about 6 mm diameter.[35] After incubation for 24 hours at 37°C, staphylococci from cattle form mostly yellow, those from human predominantly violet, and those from dogs mainly white macrocolonies. This test is particularly useful if the source of the staphylococci is to be determined.

Staphylococci frequently yield drug-resistant mutants. Consequently, with the extensive use of antibiotics the antibiotic resistance of staphylococci has greatly increased.

Therefore, whenever feasible, antibiotic sensitivity tests should be conducted for the most effective therapy. The results of these tests can also characterize staphylococcic strains in epizootiological and other research studies. For routine testing, the disc method can be used. The staphylococci in question are heavily seeded on a nutrient agar (preferably blood agar). Then the antibiotic discs are applied. (They are commercially available.) The concentrations of the antibiotics in the discs relate somewhat to the levels in the patient. The plates are incubated at 37°C overnight. Growth of the staphylococci directly around the discs indicates resistance and inhibition of growth susceptibility to the respective antibiotics. The sum of these reactions is the antibiogram of a certain staphylococcic strain. It indicates to the clinician which antibiotics may be and which will not be effective in treatment.

Phage typing provides useful markers for the differentiation of many (coagulase-positive) *S. aureus* strains.[5] *S. epidermidis*, on the other hand, is not susceptible to the typing phages.

With a series of internationally standardized phages ("human" phage set),[41] about 65–95% of the *S. aureus* cultures from humans and approximately 40–75% of those from cattle can by typed.[19,39] The typability of *S. aureus* cultures from cattle can be increased to more than 90% with a specifically selected set of "bovine" phages.[36] The bovine phage set has been developed mainly by Davidson.[22] It has less phages in groups I and II and more phages in groups IV and M than the human set.[41] Recently, the bovine phage set has been further modified.[37] Staphylococci from dogs are usually not typable with either the human or the bovine set.[18,19] However, phages have been isolated that could be used for typing canine staphylococci.[18]

With their respective staphylococcic propagating strains, some phages can be best produced in a liquid medium (broth) and others on the surface of a solid medium.[5] Propagation in broth is the simpler method and is recommended for the production of most typing phages. Propagation on a solid medium may yield somewhat higher titers. The latter methods can be applied to all phages. After propagation, the remaining staphylococci are removed from the lysate by centrifugation and subsequent filtration.[5,41]

Tenfold dilution of each lysate, prepared with separate pipettes, are titrated on agar plates inoculated with the respective propagating strain. The dilution that gives a nearly confluent lysis is the routine test dilution (RTD).[5]

The lytic activity of each phage preparation is tested on its propagating strain and a set of standard test strains.[5] This is done to characterize the typing phages and to detect any possible mutations or modifications of the phages during propagation.

The phages must be titrated and characterized by their lytic spectra before they are applied in order to obtain comparable results. Staphylococci from humans should be typed with the human set, those from cattle with the bovine set, and those from dogs with the "canine" set of phages. If the source of the staphylococci is not known, it could possibly be estimated by the crystal-violet test and bovine plasma coagulation.[35]

Cellular morphology. Staphylococci are spheres, approximately 0.7–1 μm in diameter. They occur frequently in irregular clusters, particularly in tissues, but also singly, in pairs, and in short chains. They are gram-positive, nonmotile, and not acid fast. They do not form spores or flagella and usually have no capsules.

Animal inoculation. Because staphylococci can be isolated readily on a number of conventional and selective culture media, there appears to be no need to use animals or embryonating eggs for the isolation of staphylocci in routine diagnosis.

Immunology and serology. Serologic characterization of staphylococci has been studied extensively. Agglutination with specifically adsorbed antisera appears to be most promising.[14] It is particularly useful as an adjunct to phage typing, because serology and lysotopy give independent results.[16,36,39] With the system of adsorbed antisera, *S. aureus* cultures from humans,[30] cattle,[31] dogs,[32] and possibly from other animals can be typed. However, the antigens are still ill-defined and may overlap. Blocking antigens may interfere with agglutination. Preparation of the specific antisera and the typing itself are time consuming and often difficult. Furthermore, reproducibility of serologic typing results is not always satisfactory. For these reasons, serotyping in its present form cannot be recommended as a routine procedure in epizootiological studies and other research on *S. aureus*. Nevertheless, in selected cases, serotyping may yield valuable results.

Immunology of *S. aureus* has been stimulated mainly by the difficulties in the control of staphylococcal infections. Antibiotics and other modern therapeutics have not always been effective. Most of these drugs are eliminated from the infected animals within several days. Antibodies, on the other hand, may persist for several weeks or even months.

Vaccination is of value as an additional control measure.[40] It may reduce the incidence and severity of clinically apparent staphylococcosis.[16,40] The protection against infection, on the other hand, appears to be strain specific.[16] This may indicate the use of autogenous vaccines in particularly troublesome cases and herd problems. The preparation of an autogenous vaccine presents no particular problems, but it requires a careful selection of the vaccine strain or strains. For this, the causative staphylococci have to be differentiated with some of the above-mentioned procedures. Then the vaccine has to be tested for its safety. Its effectiveness, however, cannot be predicted, because the immunogenicity of individual staphylococcic strains varies greatly. Therefore, for most field cases a proven commercial antistaphylococcic vaccine may be preferable. It can be used to supplement other control measures.

Pathogenicity in experimental animals. Experimental animals are relatively resistant to infection with *S. aureus*. Quite large inocula are required to produce lethal disease.[17] Rabbits inoculated IV with 10^9–10^{10} staphylococci usually die within 24 hours. Mice are killed within 24 hours after IP infection with 5×10^8 to 5×10^9 or IV injection with 10^8–10^9 staphylococci. Other experimental animals, such as guinea pigs, are no more suitable for studies on *S. aureus* than mice and rabbits. The disease in experimental animals including chick embryos cannot be related accurately to that produced by the same staphylococci in a particular species of domestic animals. In addition, characterization of individual staphylococcic strains by their pathogenicity in certain experimental animals is not sufficiently precise and therefore usually not justifiable.

References

1. Adamczyk, B., and C. Blaurock. Aum Nachweis spezifischer Staphylokokkenhämolysine. *Zeitschrift ges. Hyg.* 9:456–471, 1963.

2. Baird-Parker, A.C. An improved diagnostic and selective medium for isolating coagulase-positive staphylococci. *J. Appl. Bact.* 25:12–19, 1962.
3. Bergdoll, M.S. The staphylococcal enterotoxins. In *Biochemistry of Some Foodborne Microbial Toxins*, R.I. Mateles and C.N. Wogan (eds.), pp. 1–25. M.I.T. Press, Cambridge, 1967.
4. Bergdoll, M.S., O.R. Borja, and R.M. Avena. Identification of a new enterotoxin as enterotoxin C. *J. Bact.* 90:1481–1485, 1963.
5. Blair, J.E., and R.R.O. Williams. Phage typing of staphylococci. *Bull. WHO* 24:771–734, 1961.
6. Blobel, H., and D.T. Berman. Vaccination of dairy cattle against staphylococcic mastitis. *Am J. Vet. Res.* 23:7–14, 1962.
7. Brown, R.W., O. Sandvik, R.K. Scharer, and D.L. Rose. Differentiation of strains of *Staphylococcus epidermidis* isolated from bovine udders. *J. Gen. Microbiol.* 47:273–287, 1967.
8. Buchanan, R.E., and N.E. Gibbons (eds.). *Bergey's Manual of Determinative Bacteriology*. 8th ed. Williams & Wilkins, Baltimore, 1974.
9. Cadness-Graves, B., R. Williams, C.J. Harper, and A.A. Miles. Slide test for coagulase-positive staphylococci. *Lancet* 1:736–738, 1943.
10. Casman, E.P., and R.W. Bennett. Culture medium for the production of staphylococcal enterotoxin A. *J. Bact.* 86:18–23, 1963.
11. Casman, E.P., R.W. Bennett, A.E. Dorsey, and J.A. Issa. Identification of a fourth staphylococcal enterotoxin, enterotoxin D. *J. Bact.* 94:1875–1882, 1967.
12. Casman, E.P., H.S. Bergdoll, and J. Robinson. Designation of staphylococcal enterotoxins. *J. Bact.* 85:715–716, 1963.
13. Chapman, G.H. The significance of sodium chloride in studies of staphylococci. *J. Bact.* 50:201–203, 1945.
14. Chapman, G.H. A single culture medium for selective isolation of plasma-coagulating staphylococci and for improved testing of chromogenesis, plasma-coagulation, mannitol permentation, and the stone reaction. *J. Bact.* 51:409–410, 1946.
15. Chapman, G.H. An improved Stone's medium for the isolation and testing of food poisoning *Staphylococci*. *Food Res.* 13:100–105, 1948.
16. Cohen, J.O., and P.B. Smith. Serological typing of staphylococcus aureus. II. Typing of slide agglutination and comparison with phage typing. *J. Bact.* 88:1364–1371, 1964.
17. Cohn, Z.A. Determinants of infection in the peritoneal cavity. I. Response to and fate of *Staphylococcus aureus* and *Staphylococcus albus* in the mouse. *Yale J. Biol. Med.* 35:12–28, 1962.
18. Coles, E.H. *Staphylococcus* aureus of canine origin. I. Bacteriophage typing and antibiotic sensitivity of cultures isolated from diseased dogs. *Am. J. Vet. Res.* 101:803–807, 1963.
19. Coles, E.H., and A. Eisenstart. Staphylococcic phages. II. The use of human typing phages and adapted human typing phages in the typing of *Staphylococcus aureus* of animal origin. *J. Vet. Res.* 20:835–837, 1959.
20. Conn, H.J. Staining methods. In *Manual of Microbiological Methods*, Conn (ed.), pp. 10–36. Society of American Bacteriologists. McGraw-Hill, New York, 1957.
21. Cruickshank, R. *Medical Microbiology*. 11th ed. E. & S. Livingstone, Edinburgh, 1965.
22. Davidson, I. A set of bacteriophages for typing bovine staphylocci. *Res. Vet Sci.* 20:396–407, 1961.
23. Deneke, A., and H. Blobel. Fibrinogen media for studies on staphylocci. *J. Bact.* 83:533–537, 1962.
24. Denny, C.B., and C.W. Bohrer. Improved cat test for enterotoxin. *J. Bact.* 86:347–348, 1963.
25. Denny, C.B., P.L. Tau, and C.W. Bohrer. Heat inactivation of staphylococcal enterotoxin A. *J. Food Sci.* 31:762–767, 1966.
26. Elek, S.D. *Staphylococcus pyogenes and Its Relation to Disease*. E. & S. Livingstone, Edinburgh, 1959.
27. Fusillo, M.H., and D.L. Weiss. Qualitative estimation of staphylococcal deoxyribonuclease. *J. Bact.* 78:520–522, 1959.
28. Gillespie, W.A., and V.G. Alder. Production of opacity in egg-yolk media by coagulase-positive staphylococci. *J. Path. Bact.* 64:187–200, 1952.
29. Gladstone, G.P., and W.B. Von Heyningen. Staphylococcal leucocidins. *Brit. J. Exp. Path.* 38:123–137, 1957.
30. Grün, L. Die serologische Differenzierung von Staphylokokken. *Zeitschrift ges. Hyg.* 146:129–141, 1959.
31. Hahn, G., and H. Blobel. Serologische Typisierung der Staphylokokken vom Rind. *Zentralblatt Veterinärmedizin* 15:794–801, 1968.
32. Hahn, G., and H. Blobel. Serologische Typisierung der Staphylokokken vom Hund. *Zentralblatt Veterinärmedizin* 15:979–983, 1968.

33. Hall, R.E., Angelotti, R., and K.H. Leuis. Detection of staphylococcal enterotoxin in food. *Health Lab. Sci.* 2:179–191, 1965.
34. Hentschel, G., and H. Blobel. Untersuchung über Staphylokokken-fibrinolysin. *Zentralblatt Bakt.* 296:193–201, 1968.
35. Meyer, W. Differenzierungaschema für standortvarianten von *Staphylococcus aureus*. *Zentralblatt Bakt.* 201:464–481, 1966.
36. Nakagawa, M. Studies on bacteriophage typing of staphylococci isolated from bovine milk. *Jap. J. Vet. Res.* 8:331–342, 1960.
37. Renin, W., and H. Blobel. Typisierung "boviner" Staphylokokken. *Zentralblatt Bakt.* 205:390–318, 1967.
38. Silverman, S.J., A.R. Knott, and M. Howard. Rapid, sensitive assay for staphylococcal enterotoxin and a comparison of serological methods. *Appl. Microbiol.* 16:1019–1023, 1968.
39. Slanetz, L.W., and C.H. Bartley. Bacteriophage and serological typing of staphylococci from bovine mastitis. *J. Infec. Dis.* 110:238–245, 1962.
40. Slanetz, L.W., C.H. Bartley, and F.E. Allen. Vaccination of dairy cattle against staphylococcis mastitis. *Am. J. Vet. Res.* 24:923–932, 1963.
41. Wentworth, B.B. Bacteriophage typing of the staphylococci. *Bact. Rev.* 27:253–272, 1963.
42. Woodin, A.M. Fractionation of a leucocidin from *Staphylococcus aureus*. *Biochem. J.* 73:225–237, 1959.
43. Zebovitz, E., J.B. Evans, and C.F. Niven. Tellurite-glycine agar: A selective plating medium for the quantitative detection of coagulase-positive staphylococci. *J. Bact.* 70:686–690, 1955.

29. Streptococcus

The genus *Streptococcus* contains numerous species of bacteria that have spherical or ovoid cells which tend to form chains and to stain gram-positive. Streptococci are widely distributed in nature. Saprophytic species, such as *Streptococcus lactis,* occur as contaminants of raw milk and in the fermentation of plant juices. Most members of the viridans and enterococcus groups, represented by *Str. equinus* and *Str. faecalis* respectively, are a part of the normal flora of the mucous membranes (especially those of the oral cavity and gut) of warm-blooded animals including humans. These kinds of streptococci are parasitic but normally do not cause disease. However, when a portal of entry is provided due to disrupting or devitalizing of mucous membranes, sporadic cases of disease (e.g. peritonitis) may occur. Other species of streptococci have emerged as important pathogens of humans and animals, and a high percentage of these pathogens are beta-hemolytic. The pathogenic streptococci are not considered part of the normal microflora of animals, but small numbers of one or more species of them may occur as inapparent infections. Postconvalescent carriage of pathogenic streptococci, especially in the nasopharynx, is common.

The infected host animal is the basic source of streptococci for infecting other animals. Newborn animals tend to acquire streptococci of the normal flora variety within the first hours of their lives by direct contact with their dams or indirectly by contact with the contaminated environment. Animals with active streptococcal infections or postconvalescent carriers are the basic sources of pathogenic streptococci. These pathogens may be shed in nasal exudates and aerosols. Exudates of wounds or abscesses and secretions such as milk (in cases of streptococcal mastitis) are also sources of pathogenic streptococci.

The species of pathogenic streptococci show considerable variation in host range and anatomic sites of preference for colonizing and causing disease. *Streptococcus zooepidemicus* and *Str. equisimilis* affect many species of animals and may cause either septicemia or localized purulent infections, with or without abscessation, in one or more of many different anatomic sites. *Streptococcus pyogenes* is almost entirely a pathogen of humans. It commonly causes disease of the pharynx but also affects many other anatomic sites as well. It may occasionally be transferred from humans to dairy cows and cause mastitis. *Streptococcus equi* and Lancefield's group E *Streptococcus* sp. (*Str. suis*) are important pathogens of equines and swine respectively. Each of these two species has a marked predilection for localizing and causing disease in the pharyngeal region of their hosts. The mastitis group of streptococci, *Str. agalactiae, Str. dysgalactiae,* and *Str. uberis,* are serious pathogens of the mammary gland of dairy cows but are of little significance elsewhere. Horses, swine, cattle, and dogs are commonly infected by streptococci, while domestic fowl, cats, and sheep tend to be less frequently affected. Pharyngitis of horses and dogs is largely limited to young animals. Urinary tract infections tend to occur in young and aged animals. Contagious streptococcic lymphadenitis of swine apparently affects susceptible swine of various ages.

Specimens

Tissues collected in the field for transport to the laboratory should be placed in watertight containers and refrigerated (not frozen) en route. If possible, exudates from abscesses of live animals should be aseptically aspirated from unopened lesions that have healthy overlying skin. (*Proteus* sp. and other contaminants readily invade the contents of abscesses through necrotic skin.) Material from swabs can be transferred to sterile strips of filter paper simply by rolling the freshly taken swab on the paper, which can be mailed in a sterile vial or strong plastic bag. Sterile filter paper strips can be prepared in the laboratory.

Streptococcal infections induce mucopurulent exudate on mucous membranes. Purulent exudates, usually not malodorous and of variable viscosity, are associated with various pyogenic infections such as abscesses, arthritis, and metritis. Mastitic milk may contain clots or flakes of exudate depending on the stage of development of the infection. Hyperemia and subcapsular hemorrhage of the visceral organs are indications of streptococcal septicemia. In valvular endocarditis, verrucae, ulceration, and fibrin plaques may occur.

Thin smears of mastitic milk, defatted by flooding the dried slides with xylol and then fixed in alcohol, can be stained with methylene blue for microscopy of bacterial cell morphology. Direct smears of throat or vaginal swabs, fixed by gentle heat or methanol and Gram stained, are also of diagnostic value. Thick exudates should be diluted with sterile water prior to preparation of smears.

Laboratory Procedures

Cultures. Dried exudate on a cotton swab or filter paper strip can be rehydrated with enough sterile brain-heart infusion broth to yield up to 0.5 ml of expressed fluid. Routine incubation of this material at 37°C for 2–6 hours prior to culturing will increase the percentage of isolations of streptococci. One inoculating loopful of this material is an adequate quantity for dilution streaking of a blood agar plate. Aseptically drawn milk samples may be cultured at once, but the samples should routinely be incubated at 37°C overnight and cultured again.

Blood agar medium provides the nutrients required for growth and gives information on hemolytic patterns. Blood agar base medium plus 5% sterile sheep blood is satisfactory. Some laboratories routinely use cattle blood (antibiotic free). An ordinary streak-dilution inoculation is generally satisfactory, although a pour plate may be used.

Sodium azide–crystal violet (SA-CV) blood agar medium is satisfactory for isolating streptococci from mixtures containing enterobacteria and staphylococci.[6] Viscous thioglycollate medium is excellent for growing streptococci. Brain-heart infusion (BHI) broth is a good liquid growth medium. The addition of a few drops of sterile blood serum may be necessary to obtain growth in certain sugar broth media; the serum should first be dialyzed to remove the native glucose. (See Appendix A for media formulas.)

Incubate in saturated humidity at 37°C. Initial growth is generally enhanced by routine use of the candle jar. At least 48 hours of incubation is usually essential for hemolytic patterns to adequately develop.

Differential reactions. Colonies on blood agar tend to be punctiform. The hemolytic pattern may not be well-developed at 24 hours of incubation. At 48–72 hours of incubation, colonies are approximately 1 mm in diameter and are generally glossy or smooth with opaque centers and clear margins. Occasional mucoid strains with confluent streaklines of growth are seen. Colony profiles may be single or biconvex. Hemolytic patterns, alpha (greening), beta (complete clearing), or gamma (no change), are very significant in the identification process. Most streptococcal pathogens are beta-hemolytic.

Depending on the species of *Streptococcus* concerned and the concentration of crystal violet and sodium azide used, the growth rate of colonies and hemolytic patterns on the SA-CV agar may vary from those observed on blood agar. For this reason the colony characteristics and hemolytic patterns of all streptococci initially isolated on SA-CV blood agar should be compared with their reactions on blood agar.

In viscous thioglycollate medium, streptococci may grow as a layer of granular pellets but generally produce characteristic "comet" or "streamer" growth. In broth media such as BHI, the short-chain streptococci, e.g. *Str. uberis,* are relatively stable in suspension, the medium is turbid, and some closely packed sediment is seen. The long-chain streptococci, of which *Str. agalactiae* tends to be extreme, are less stable in suspension and settle out, forming a loose or flocculent sediment and a clear supernatant fluid. Streptococci do not form pellicles.

All streptococci depend on the lactic acid fermentation of carbohydrate material to obtain energy. Variation among different species of streptococci in the kinds of carbohydrate media fermented provides a useful diagnostic tool. The ability or inability to hydrolyze sodium hippurate is likewise useful. The beta-hemolytic group of streptococci does not grow at either test temperature of 10 or 45°C, at pH 9.6, in the presence of 6.5% NaCl, or in media containing 0.1% methylene blue, whereas members of the viridans, enterococcus, and lactic acid groups tolerate some if not all of these factors (Table 29.1).

Most kinds of streptococci except the viridans group have a polysaccharide C substance that enables the bacteriologist to place them in Lancefield's antigenic groups, which are designated by capital letters.[5] In the case of group A (*Str. pyogenes*) numerous serotypes occur within the group.

Any unknown microorganism having the cellular characteristics and growth require-

Table 29.1. Characteristics of selected species of streptococci

Streptococcus	Lancefield group	Hemolytic patterns*	Grows in 0.1% meth. blue	Grows at 10°C	Grows at 45°C	Grows in 6.5% NaCl	Grows in broth at pH 9.6	Sodium hippurate split
pyogenes	A	b	−	−	−	−	−	−
equisimilis	C	b	−	−	−	−	−	−
Group E (Str. suis)	E	b	−	−	−	−	−	−
agalactiae	B	m	−	−	−	−	−	+
dysgalactiae	C	m	−	−	−	−	−	−
uberis	X†	m	−	+	−	−	−	+
equinus	X†	a	−	−	+	−	−	−
faecalis	D	g	+	+	+	+	+	V‡
lactis	N	ag	+	+	−	−	−	V‡

*b, beta; m, may be either a, b, or g; a, alpha; g, gamma; ag, alpha or gamma.
†X, not indicated in literature cited.
‡V, variable, some strains positive, others negative.

ments listed above is considered to be a member of the genus *Streptococcus*. If the isolant is beta-hemolytic it is likely to be a pathogen. This degree of identification may suffice to indicate the regimen of therapy or other clinical measures to be undertaken, but more precise identification is generally needed to determine the medical significance of a streptococcal isolant.

The approved practice in human medical laboratories is to subject all isolants of beta-hemolytic streptococci to Lancefield's grouping test.[5] If a given isolant is group A–positive, the identification of *Str. pyogenes* is considered confirmed and the procedure for determining the serologic type is undertaken. In veterinary laboratories, serotypes within Lancefield's groups are of little concern, but the grouping test should be used routinely to increase the validity of the identification.

Essentially all of the pathogenic streptococci encountered in veterinary medicine, except *Str. uberis*, are members of certain Lancefield groups. Streptococci of groups B, C, and E are most frequently encountered; group C contains several species. Once it has been established that an unknown *Streptococcus* sp. is a member of group C, the species can be identified by the use of a small battery of carbohydrate differential broth media (Table 29.2). Group E appears to contain one pathogenic species (of swine) for which the name *Str. suis* has been proposed.[2] Groups L and M contain beta-hemolytic streptococci that appear to be pathogenic for dogs and swine. Group L isolants have been obtained from the skin and pharynx of humans. Group P isolants are beta-hemolytic and have been isolated from chicken and swine.

Table 29.2. Differentiation of beta-hemolytic streptococci of group C

Streptococcus	Lactose	Salicin	Sorbitol	Trehalose
canis	+	+	−	−
equi	−	+	−	−
equisimilis	V*	+†	−	+
zooepidemicus	+	+	+	−

*V, variable, some strains positive, others negative.
†Occasionally isolates of human origin are negative.

Since *Str. agalactiae* is the only species in group B, there is some doubt as to what additional identification procedures are justified once an unknown *Streptococcus* sp. is placed in this group. Traditionally, the Hotis test[4] or the use of the sodium hippurate test plus a battery of selected carbohydrate media have served as alternate or supplementary methods for identification of *Str. agalactiae*.

Streptococcus dysgalactiae is a member of group C, is variable (i.e. alpha, narrow beta, or not hemolytic) in its hemolytic pattern, has a carbohydrate fermentation pattern similar to *Str. equisimilis,* and does not hydrolyze sodium hippurate. It is negative on the Christie, Atkins, and Munch-Petersen (CAMP) test, while most isolants of both *Str. agalactiae* and *Str. uberis* are positive.[1] *Streptococcus uberis* is considered to be a member of the viridans group even though its hemolytic pattern is also variable. Typical of this group, however, *Str. uberis* is not susceptible to Lancefield's grouping test and has a wide growth temperature range. It is a short chain former, thus tending to maintain a stable suspension in broth media. It hydrolyzes sodium hippurate and ferments many kinds of carbohydrate broth media. It can be differentiated from *Str. agalactiae* and *Str. dysgalactiae* with a small battery of test media (Table 29.3). Definite identification of species of streptococci included in the enterococcus, lactic acid, and normal flora species of the viridans group is usually not necessary. Their ability to tolerate certain conditions not tolerated by the beta-hemolytic group of pathogens tends to categorize them. Furthermore, the enterococcus and lactic acid groups are members of Lancefield's groups D and N respectively.

Table 29.3. Differentiation of mastitis streptococci

*Streptococcus**	Sodium hippurate	Mannitol	Salicin	Sorbitol	Lancefield group
agalactiae	+	−	+†	−	B
dysgalactiae	−	−	−	−	C
uberis	+	+	+	+	X‡

*Hemolysis varies: gamma, alpha, or narrow beta.
†Occasional isolates are negative.
‡X, not indicated in literature cited.

Corynebacterium pyogenes is commonly encountered in the same environment as beta-hemolytic *Streptococcus* sp., especially in cattle and swine. *C. pyogenes* produces a small smooth colony and a narrow zone of complete hemolysis on blood agar. A gram-stained smear of a colony frequently reveals short gram-positive elements that on cursory examination may be mistaken for streptococci. It typically causes reduction, acid coagulation, and slow liquefaction of litmus milk. Colonies of *Erysipelothrix insidiosa* (rhusiopathiae) and *Listeria monocytogenes,* young colonies of *Staphylococcus aureus,* and colonies of *Hemophilus* sp. also resemble those of streptococci. Critical examination of Gram-stained cells plus attention to cellular arrangement in broth medium usually will enable the researcher to distinguish between these colonies.

Cellular morphology. The cells of beta-hemolytic streptococci tend to be nearly spherical but are flattened in the plane of cleavage where one cell abuts another. Cleavage tends to be incomplete and residual bits of cell wall material (intercellular bridges) loosely bind streptococci into chains. The bond is strongest between cells most recently formed, giving the impression on some stained smears of paired cocci in chains. Chaining tends to be less pronounced in exudates than in broth media. Cells of the viridan and enteric streptococci tend to be more ovoid. The cells of beta-hemolytic streptococci are approximately 0.5 μm in diameter. Streptococci do not have spores and essentially do not have flagella. Capsules may be present and can be demonstrated by either direct or indirect staining techniques. Streptococci stain gram-positive. Young (6 hour) broth cultures in a neutral pH medium should be used for Gram-staining. Old cultures or those from media containing acid tend to stain false gram-negative.

Formamide extraction or Lancefield's grouping antigen. Using centrifugation, sediment the streptococcal cells from 5 ml of an 18–24-hour BHI broth culture of the unknown *Streptococcus*. Remove the supernatant fluid as completely as possible and discard it. Add 0.1 ml of formamide, shake the tube, and place it in a mineral oil bath at 150–160°C for 15 minutes. Allow the tube to cool and then add 0.25 ml of acid alcohol. Sediment the precipitated bacterial debris by centrifugation. Pipette off the suernatant fluid into a small test tube and add 0.5 ml of acetone. Mix the contents of the tube by shaking, spin down the precipitate, and discard the supernatant fluid. The small precipitate contains the group "antigen". (The group-specific material is not a complete antigen because it does not stimulate antibody production following parenteral injection.) Add 1 ml of physiological salt solution and a drop of phenol red indicator to the precipitate and neutralize the material with sodium carbonate. The antigen is ready for use.

The formamide method of extraction is preferred in veterinary medicine because there is no need to preserve any protein type–specific antigens, as is the case in human medicine where *Str. pyogenes* is the main concern. The formamide method eliminates non-group-specific substances that may give cross-reactions in the precipitin test when using antisera prepared against whole cells. It is an efficient method requiring a minimal quantity of cells for extraction.[3] Streptococcal grouping diagnostic sera A through O and MG are available commercially. (*Streptococcus* MG is nonhemolytic and is associated with atypical pneumonia of humans.)

Reference laboratory. The streptococcus laboratory of CDC will accept occasional cultures of streptococci for serologic identification. Route these cultures through your state public health veterinarian.

References

1. Christie, R., N.E. Atkins, and E. Munch-Peterson. A note on a lytic phenomenon shown by group B streptococci. *Austral. J. Exp. Biol. Med. Sci.* 22:197–200, 1944.
2. Collier, J.R. Abscesses of swine. *J. Am. Vet. Med. Ass.* 146:344–347, 1965.
3. Fuller, A.T. The formamide method for extraction of polysaccharides from haemolytic streptococci. *Brit. J. Exp. Path.* 19:130–139, 1938.
4. Hotis, R.P., and W.T. Miller. A simple method for detecting mastitis streptococci in milk. *USDA Circular no. 400,* 1936.
5. Lancefield, R.C. A serological differentiation of human and other groups of hemolytic stretococci. *J. Exp. Med.* 57:571–595, 1933.
6. Packer, R.A. The use of sodium azide (NaN) and crystal violet in a selective medium for streptococci and *Erysipelothrix rhusiopathiae. J. Bact.* 46:343–349, 1943.

30. Brucella

Brucellosis is primarily a disease of sexually mature animals wherein the inciting organisms circulate systemically for variable lengths of time depending upon the host. The organisms then localize in reticuloendothelial tissue, reproductive organs, and less frequently bones and joints. The most dramatic clinical manifestation of brucellosis is abortion resulting from placentitis.

Following an abortion, the organisms are often cleared from the uterus and vagina within 30–40 days but they usually remain localized in reticulendothelial tissues, with the animal remaining chronically infected and excreting the organisms via the mammary gland for prolonged periods of time, or from the urogenital tract at subsequent parturitions, even for the rest of the animal's life.

The frequency with which clinical manifestations of brucellosis are apparent and the rate of infection in male animals depend upon the kind of animal, the species of infecting organism, and the degree of exposure. *B. abortus* occasionally localizes in the testicle and epididymis of bulls and an enlarged and indurated scrotum results. The orchitis is usually unilateral. The same is true of *B. melitensis* in rams and bucks. However, in chronically infected herds of swine and reindeer, males with orchitis, bursitis, arthritis, and spondylitis may be observed frequently.

Among the livestock populations within the United States, infection with *B. suis* is prevalent in swine and in Alaskan reindeer. However, the type of *B. suis* that affects reindeer is different from the types that affect swine. Infection with *B. abortus* is prevalent in cattle. With the possible exception of a few goats along the Texas-Mexico border, there has been no known infection with *B. melitensis* in goats and sheep in the United States. However, rams in the western and southwestern states have been infected with *B. ovis*. Clinical evidence of infection with *B. ovis* is not always apparent, although chronically infected animals may have palpable lesions of the epididymis. While this organism can cause abortion in ewes and neonatal lamb mortality, such events rarely occur under conditions of natural transmission.

An organism that is unquestionably a member of the genus *Brucella* has recently been incriminated as the cause of an infection of dogs, predominately beagles.[5] Clinical manifestations consist of abortion in the female and epididymitis and periorchitis in the male. The causative organism has been provisionally designated as *Brucella canis*.[5]

In addition to the hosts already mentioned, many other animals have been found either enzootically infected with brucellosis or susceptible to the disease: horses, yaks, bison, water buffalo, camels, llama, vicuna, alpaca, moose, elk, deer, hares, rabbits, foxes, ferrets, mink, chickens, and various species of rodents. The incidence of infection and species of organisms inciting the infections differ in various parts of the world according to the predominate kinds of animals used as livestock, to local husbandry practices, and to prevailing control and eradication measures.

Specimens

Brucella organisms are infectious for humans, and brucellosis (undulant fever) can be severe, disabling, or chronic. Therefore, the utmost care should be exercised in collecting specimens and in examining them in the laboratory. Containers that completely obviate any chance of leakage or breakage during transport must be used. Heavy plastic bags that can be securely sealed are excellent for collecting animal tissues.

The most useful specimen for the recovery of *Brucella* organisms is the aborted fetus. In the fetus, the stomach content is the material of choice, followed by lung and spleen specimens. If the fetus cannot be cultured, attempts should be made to recover the organisms from the fetal membranes and cotyledons. Both can be rich sources of *Brucella* organisms but they are frequently grossly contaminated.

Clean and disinfect the udder and teat orifices, discard the first two or three streams of milk, and collect into sterile containers 50–60 ml of milk from each quarter.

Culturing of the blood is a particularly rewarding technique for the recovery of *B. suis* from infected swine and *B. canis* from infected dogs, because the hosts frequently have prolonged periods of bacteremia, with or without apparent clinical manifestations. Aseptically draw 20–30 ml of blood from swine and place in flasks containing tryptose broth or in casteneda-style bottles. Blood from dogs is treated in the same manner except smaller quantities are required and part of the specimen may be placed directly on agar media.

Brucella organisms occasionally can be recovered from the semen of bulls, boars, and bucks. Culture of the semen is the method of choice to establish diagnosis of *B. ovis* epididymitis in live rams.[4]

B. melitensis has been retrieved by vaginal swabs from sheep and goats for periods of up to 45 days postabortion, *B. abortus* from cattle up to 101 weeks postabortion, and *B. suis* from swine up to 31 months postexposure. However, the majority of animals clear the organisms from their reproductive tract much more rapidly, and this may not be successful unless swabs are obtained within 2–4 weeks after abortion. Vaginal swabs following abortion or parturition in dogs is one of the methods of choice for recovery of *B. canis*.

Because *Brucella* organisms localize in reticuloendothelial tissues, the tissues of choice from the carcass are lymph nodes, particularly the supramammary, internal iliac, submaxillary, and retropharengeal. The spleen, uterus, testicles, male accessory genital organs, bone marrow, and lesions of bones and joints often are also rich sources of *Brucella* organisms. Placentas from animals that have aborted as a result of *Brucella* infections are usually thickened and leathery in consistency. The surface of the maternal cotyledons has granular yellowish necrotic areas and the rest of the chorion is opaque, with adherent brownish exudate. In infected sows, the uterine mucosa may be studded with pinpoint yellowish nodules.

Other lesions that may be grossly evident are enlargement of lymph nodes, enlarged and nodular spleen, abcesses in testes and epididymis, seminal vesiculitis, and enlargement of joints. Swine are more apt to develop abseses in internal organs than are other livestock.

There are, however, no observable lesions in the majority of infected animals. While typical lesions are suggestive of *Brucella* infection, especially if abortion has occurred in the individual or in other animals in the herd or flock, they are not diagnostic for brucellosis. However, a presumptive diagnosis can be made in the event that direct smears are positive.

Direct examination either by tinctorial or FA staining of tissue impression smears is particularly valuable on material that is apt to be contaminated, such as placental membranes, cotyledons, parts of partially destroyed fetuses, and smears made from vaginal swabs. Both methods of staining also can be used to establish a presumptive diagnosis on uncontaminated material. Because it is necessary to isolate the organism to determine species identity, and because it is usually desirable to know the species responsible for infection, an effort to isolate the organism should be made on all specimens irrespective of staining results. Koster's stain is recommended.

Laboratory Procedures

Cultures. Since it is not always possible to recover *Brucella* organisms from infected tissue or milk on direct culture, the researcher should preserve aliquots of the specimens by freezing. In the event of negative results, they can be recultured and also used for inoculating guinea pigs. Some skim milk should be saved for serology and the cream used for isolation attempts.

The problem of gross contamination of the fetal membranes can be partially overcome by washing the placenta in water, followed by several rinses in sterile saline, before culturing of the tissue is attempted. After washing, select areas with obvious lesions, mince with sterile instruments, and rub the cut surfaces of the tissue onto plates of selective media.[9]

Because *B. abortus,* biotype 2, and *B. ovis* require serum for growth, the media for initial isolation of *Brucella* organisms from all tissue and milk specimens should consist of a basal media to which serum and selected antibiotics are added.

Tryptose agar (Difco Lab., Detroit) is most frequently used as the basal medium, although Albimi *Brucella* agar or ABA (Albimi Lab., Brooklyn) and trypticase-soy agar (Baltimore Biological Lab.) support growth equally well. When it is necessary to use liquid media for isolation, as it is in culturing blood, broth made of any of the commercially available media is entirely satisfactory. About 20–30 ml of whole blood from cattle, swine, or sheep is added to 30–50 ml of citrated broth and mixed by gentle shaking. After 5–7 days incubation, subculture daily. Another popular method is to use a Casteneda-style blood culture bottle, which is simply serum-tryptose agar slanted in a Blake bottle with 15–20 ml of broth added after the agar media has solidified. Incubate the bottles in a standing position. All broth to be used for culturing blood should have sodium citrate added to a final concentration of 1% to prevent clotting. *B. ovis* and many biotypes of *B. abortus* require an atmosphere containing approximately 10% CO_2 to initiate growth on primary isolation. Thus all primary cultures from field specimens should be incubated in either CO_2 incubators or jars wherein the atmosphere can be controlled. On primary isolation, *Brucella* colonies may become visible in 72 hours but growth sufficient for recognition usually requires 4 or 5 days. However, cultures should not be discarded as negative for 14 days.

On serum-enriched media after 72–96 hours incubation, the colonies are small (pinpoint to pinhead in size), circular with smooth edges, convex, butyrous in consistency, and aged-ivory in color. As colonies age, they become larger in size (2–3 mm in diameter) and brownish in color but they remain translucent.

Organisms of the species *B. abortus, B. suis,* and *B. melitensis,* when freshly isolated from animal tissue, are usually of smooth colony morphology. In contrast, smooth colonies have not been found under any growth condition in the species *B. ovis* or *B. canis*.

Because serologic techniques are involved in ascertaining the generic identity of *B. abortus, B. suis,* and *B. melitensis,* and because colony morphology helps distinguish *B. ovis* and *B. canis,* the researcher should first determine the incidence of rough colony growth before proceeding with species identification.

Colony morphology can be determined by direct observation of the plates with oblique lighting, by staining the growth on the plates according to the method of White and Wilson,[14] and by testing individual colonies using the acriflavin test of Braun and Bonestell.[3]

Rough colonies are more granular in appearance, are more opaque than smooth colonies, and are reddish-yellow in color. Smooth colonies are green-blue in color. Rough colonies are drier than smooth colonies and sometimes are brittle in consistency rather than butyrous. For the inexperienced, more definite results can be obtained by staining the colonies and observing them under low magnification.

For the White and Wilson stain, allow plates to incubate 96 hours and choose a plate with well-separated colonies. Flood the plate with 1:2000 aqueous crystal violet solution, allow to stand for 15–20 seconds, decant excess stain into disinfectant, and then examine.[14] Smooth colonies show a central area of ivory surrounded by a zone of light blue, or the whole colony may be a pale blue. Rough colonies are a deep reddish-violet, crinkled in appearance, and very brittle in consistency.

If the isolate has been recovered from a blood culture and is on a slant, or if the diagnostician needs to determine the morphology of a single colony, the acriflavin agglutination test of Braun and Bonestell can be used.[3] For each daily use, prepare a fresh 1:1000 solution of neutral acriflavin in distilled water. Place one drop of the solution on a microscope slide with a loop. Then, in the drop, emulsify part of a colony or a small amount of growth from a slant. Smooth colonies remain in an even suspension; rough colonies clump, with the reaction resembling agglutination.

Cellular morphology. Organisms in the genus *Brucella* are small, nonmotile, nonsporing, gram-negative coccobacilli. They vary in size from 0.5×0.5 to 0.5×2 μm. Rough organisms stain irregularly and are more apt to show pleomorphism. The species cannot be distinguished morphologically. Capsules can sometimes be demonstrated with special stains on freshly isolated organisms, but this does not help in their generic or species identification. All members of this genus are aerobic, although some strains require 10% carbon dioxide added to the incubation atmosphere to initiate growth.

Differential reactions. For the tube agglutination test, proceed as follows: (1) prepare an antigen from smooth colonies of the unknown isolate by washing off the growth of a 48-hour slant in phenolized saline (approximately 10 ml), (2) inactivate the suspension by heating to 65°C for 1 hour, (3) with a spectrophotometer, adjust the cell density so it is equivalent to that of the NADC standard *Brucella abortus* antigen,[6] and (4) perform the standard tube agglutination test using known positive antiserum and known negative serum, and also using standard antigen on duplicate serum samples as controls. A positive result is persumptive evidence that the isolate is a member of the genus *Brucella*. Because *B. ovis* and *B. canis* are of nonsmooth colony morphology and therefore are autoagglutinable, this test cannot be used for their generic identification.

For FA staining make smears from suspensions of the unknown isolate and stain with fluorescein-conjugated anti-*Brucella* serum, using both positive and negative controls. No information is available on the stainability of *B. canis,* and the few strains of *B. ovis* that have been examined for FA staining have proved refractory. All other species show specific staining. A positive reaction is considered sufficient evidence that the isolate is a member of the genus *Brucella*.[12]

The following four methods are recommended for species and biotype identification: (1) the conventional biochemical methods as originally proposed by Huddleson,[7] which are (a) the need for added carbon dioxide to initiate growth on primary isolation, (b) hydrogen sulfide production, (c) bacteriostatic effect of basic fuchsin and thionin incorporated into the growth media; (2) agglutinability in monospecific antisera;[15] (3) lysis by *Brucella* bacteriophage; and (4) manometric determination of oxidative utilization of individual amino acid and carbohydrate substrates (Table 30.1).

All cultures of field strains should initially be incubated in carbon dioxide. After growth is established, make duplicate subcultures on slants, selecting serveral representative colonies (avoid picking just one colony). Incubate one subculture in an air atmosphere and place the other in an atmosphere containing 10% carbon dioxide. Carbon dioxide–dependent strains often lose this need after repeated subculture because of the occurrence of CO_2-independent mutants; therefore, this test should preferably be done on the first subculture and certainly before the strain has been subcultured repeatedly.

To measure hydrogen sulfide production, (1) prepare a saturated solution of neutral lead acetate in distilled water, then heat to boiling and cool; (2) dip filter paper in the solution and hang up to dry; (3) cut in strips; (4) inoculate the unknown isolate onto a slant of enriched media and insert the strip so only the top is showing, then secure with a cotton plug. Replace paper every 24 hours for four times and record results according to the amount of blackening that occurs at the bottom tip of the paper.

To show the bacteriostatic effect of basic fuchsin and thionin, (1) make up 0.1% aqueous stock solutions and dissolve by placing in flowing steam for 20–30 minutes; (2) while dye solutions are still warm, add desired amounts of dyes to melted basal media, enriched with serum if necessary, and pour into plates; (3) dyes are normally used in

Table 30.1. Differential characters of *Brucella* species and their biotypes

	Biotype	CO₂ required	H₂S produced	Growth on dyes* Thionin a	b	c	Basic fuchsin a	b	c	Agglut. by sera† A	M	Lysis by phage Tb at RTD	Metabolic test§ Glutamic acid	Ornithine	Ribose	Lysine	Most common reservoir
melitensis	1	−	−	−	+	+	+	+	+	−	+	−	+	−	−	−	Sheep, goats
	2	−	−	−	+	+	+	+	+	+	−	−	+	−	−	−	Sheep, goats
	3	−	−	−	+	+	+	+	+	+	+	−	+	−	−	−	Sheep, goats
abortus	1	+u‡	+	−	+	+	−	+	+	+	−	+	+	−	+	−	Cattle
	2	+	+	−	+	+	−	−	−	+	−	+	+	−	+	−	Cattle
	3	+u	+	+	+	+	−	+	+	+	−	+	+	−	+	−	Cattle
	4	+u	+	−	+	+	−	+	−	−	+	+	+	−	+	−	Cattle
	5	−	−	+	+	+	+	+	+	−	+	+	+	−	+	−	Cattle
	6	−	V‡	+	+	+	+	+	+	+	−	+	+	−	+	−	Cattle
	7	−	V	+	+	+	+	+	+	+	+	+	+	−	+	−	Cattle
	8	+	−	+	+	+	+	+	+	+	−	+	+	−	+	−	Cattle
	9	V	+	+	+	+	+	+	+	−	+	+	V	−	+	−	Cattle
suis	1	−	+	+	+	+	−	−	−	+	−	−	+	+	+	+	Pigs
	2	−	+	+	+	+	+	−	−	+	−	−	V	+	+	+	Hares, pigs
	3	−	−	+	+	+	+	+	+	+	−	−	+	+	+	+	Pigs
	4	−	−	+	+	+	+	+	−	+	+	−	+	+	V	+	Reindeer
neotomae	1	−	+	+	−	−	−	−	−	+	−	−	+	−	+	−	Desert wood rat
ovis	1	+	−	−	+	+	−	−	−	−	−	−	+	−	−	−	Sheep
canis	1	−	−	−	+	+	−	−	+	−	−	−	+	+	+	+	Dogs

*Concentrations of dyes (obtainable from National Analine Division, Allied Chemical & Dye Co., New York): a, 1:25,000; b, 1:50,000; c, 1:100,000.
†A, anti–*B. abortus* monospecific serum; M, anti–*B. melitensis* monospecific serum.
‡+u, usually positive; V, variable, some strains positive, others negative.
§Only 4 substrates for species differentiation are given in the table. We recommend that 12 substrates be used.

graded amounts, with the final concentrations of dye media being 1:25,000, 1:50,000, and 1:100,000. To 1000 ml of media, add 40 ml, 20 ml, and 10 ml, respectively, for each dye; (4) suspend the unknown isolate in saline and distribute the suspension over the surface of the dye plates with a glass rod or cotton swab. Include as controls an inoculated plate of medium that does not contain dyes, and sets of dye plates inoculated with strains of known species identity. Ideally, the control strains should be WHO reference strains.

The serotyping of *Brucella* strains can best be done by reference or research laboratories that have personnel experienced in preparing and standardizing the reagents and that use the technique frequently enough to maintain a fresh stock of standardized, absorbed, high-titer, monospecific antisera. Laboratories wishing to undertake preparation of their own absorbed sera should obtain from a reference laboratory samples of sera to use as a standard for titer comparison before using their sera on unknown isolates.[2]

The Tbilisi (Tb) strain of bacteriophage is the reference strain used for typing *Brucella* cultures. At the RTD, which is the highest dilution of phage causing complete lysis of susceptible strains of organisms, this phage lyses only members of the species *B. abortus*, and then only when they are of smooth or smooth-intermediate colony morphology. The WHO reference strain of *B. abortus*, strain 544, or *B. abortus*, strain 19, are used as propagating host organisms for this phage.[8]

To test a culture for its phage susceptibility, wash the growth off 24-hour slants of both the unknown isolate and the host strain of *B. abortus* and adjust each suspension to contain approximately 10^9 cells per ml. Soak a cotton swab in the cell suspensions and inoculate plates of enriched media by making an even streak across the plate with the swab. Then, with a fine tipped pipette, deposit a drop of phage on the streak. Incubate plates 24 hours. Vials containing the RTD of Tbilisi bacteriophage and cultures of *B. abortus*, strain 544, can be obtained from the FAO/WHO Brucellosis Center.

Since *Brucella* phage is easily propagated and can be stored at refrigerator temperatures for long periods without loss of titer, and since phage typing is especially useful in identifying *B. abortus*, laboratories that are more or less continuously engaged in the identification of *Brucella* strains should obtain a vial of concentrated phage for propagation and maintain their own stock of phage at the RTD.

The method described by Adams is entirely satisfactory for the propagation of *Brucella* phage.[1] Wash the growth off a 24-hour slant of *B. abortus*, strain 544, or *B. abortus*, strain 19, with sterile saline and adjust the cell concentration to contain approximately 10^8 cells per ml. Add 1 ml of this cell suspension and 1 ml of concentrated phage to 2 ml of semisolid agar that has previously been melted and allowed to cool to 45°C. Mix and distribute evenly over a plate of basal media. Incubate in carbon dioxide 24 hours. Harvest by adding 4–5 ml of broth to the plate, mixing the broth and the layer of semisolid agar with a glass rod, scraping this into a centrifuge tube, and after centrifugation filtering the supernatant fluid. Filtrate should have a high titer of phage and can be stored at 4°C as concentrated stock phage. To determine the RTD, make a saline suspension of a 24-hour slant of *B. abortus*, strain 544, or *B. abortus*, strain 19, and adjust cell concentration to approximately 10^9 cells per ml. Deposit approximately 0.5 ml on the surface of each of two plates of basal media. Distribute evenly over the surface with a glass rod and allow to thoroughly dry.

Withdraw 1 ml of the concentrated phage and make 10-fold dilutions with tryptose broth. With a fine-tipped pipette previously calibrated to deliver 50 drops per ml, deposit 1 drop of each phage dilution on each of the seeded plates, being careful to identify precisely the location of each dilution on the plates. Incubate 24 hours. The highest dilution that causes complete lysis is the RTD.

If the identity of a strain is still in doubt after all the other recommended tests have been done, the strain then should be sent to a reference laboratory for an examination of its oxidative metabolism. By using a Warburg respirometer and ascertaining the rate of utilization of amino acid and carbohydrate substrates by washed and resting (nonproliferating) cells, a researcher can identify each of the species of organism in this genus, as each has a pattern of utilization that is definitive.[10,11,13]

Animal inoculation. Guinea pigs can be used for isolating *B. abortus, B. suis,* or *B. melitensis* from contaminated specimens or from tissues and fluids that contain only a small number of organisms, because guinea pigs are highly susceptible to some strains of these organisms. The guinea pigs should weigh between 350 and 500 g.

Centrifuge macerated or ground tissue and inoculate 3–5 ml of the supernate IP using at least two guinea pigs for each tissue sample. If material is grossly contaminated, use SC or IM routes of inoculation, injecting smaller amounts on each of several successive days. Milk samples, prepared as previously described, usually can be injected IP in 5 ml amounts. However, if spoilage has occurred, use the IM route.

Obtain a sample of heart blood and necropsy half of the guinea pigs at 21 days after inoculation and half at 35–42 days. An agglutinin titer of 1:25 or greater indicates that the inoculum contained *Brucella* organisms.

At necropsy, aseptically remove and culture any organ or tissue with gross lesions and also remove and culture the spleen, liver, regional lymph nodes, and testicles whether gross lesions are present or not.

Immunology and serology. The preparation of reagents, testing procedures, and interpretation of test results on blood, milk, and semen have been carefully standardized and are documented in detail in a series of manuals prepared by NADC.[6] The directions presented in these manuals should be carefully adhered to in the testing of all herds and flocks of animals. Information on testing dog sera for antibodies to *B. canis* can also be obtained from NADC.

Reference laboratories. FAO/WHO Brucellosis Center, Ministry of Agriculture, Fisheries, and Food, Central Veterinary Laboratory, New Haw, Weybridge, Surrey, Great Britain; Animal Health Diagnostic Laboratory, NADC; Department of Veterinary Microbiology, School of Veterinary Medicine, University of California, Davis.

References

1. Adams, M.H. *Bacteriophages.* Interscience Publishers, New York, 1959.
2. Alton, G.G., L.M. Jones, and D.E. Pietz. *Laboratory Techniques in Brucellosis.* 2d ed. WHO Monograph Series no. 55. WHO, Geneva, 1975.
3. Braun, W., and A.E. Bonestell. Independent variation of characteristics in *Brucella abortus* variants and their detection. *Am. J. Vet. Res.* 8:386–390, 1947.

4. Buddle, M.B. Studies on *Brucella ovis* (NSP), a cause of genital disease in sheep in New Zealand and Australia. *J. Hyg.* 54:351–364, 1956.
5. Carmichael, L.E., and R.M. Kenny. Canine abortion caused by *Brucella canis*. *J. Am. Vet. Med. Ass.* 152:605–616, 1968.
6. Diagnostic Services, NADC, manuals as follows: *The Propagating of Brucella abortus 1119-3 for the Production of Brucella Antigens*, no. 65A; *The Production of Brucella abortus Standard Agglutination Test Antigens*, no. 65B; *The Production of Brucellosis Supplemental Test Antigens and Reagents*, no. 65C; *Standard Agglutination Test Procedures for the Diagnosis of Brucellosis*, no. 65D; *Supplemental Test Procedures for the Diagnosis of Brucellosis*, no. 65E; *Laboratory Procedures for Isolating, Identifying and Typing Brucella*, no. 65F.
7. Huddleson, I.F. Brucella. In *Bergey's Manual of Determinative Bacteriology*, pp. 404–406. 7th ed. Williams and Wilkins, Baltimore, 1957.
8. Joint FAO/WHO Expert Committee on Brucellosis. WHO Technical Report Series no. 289, pp. 9–17. WHO, Geneva, 1969.
9. Kuzdas, C.D., and E.V. Morse. A selective media for the isolation of brucellae from contaminated materials. *J. Bact.* 66:502–504, 1953.
10. Meyer, M.E. Metabolic characterization of the genus *Brucella*. IV. Correlation of oxidative metabolic patterns and susceptibility to brucella bacteriophage, type abortus, strain 3. *J. Bact.* 82:950–953, 1961.
11. Meyer, M.E. The epizootiology of brucellosis and its relationship to the identification of *Brucella* organisms. *Am. J. Vet. Res.* 105:553–557, 1964.
12. Meyer, M.E. Identification of *Brucella* by immunoflourescence. *Am. J. Vet. Res.* 117:424–429, 1966.
13. Meyer, M.E., and H.S. Cameron. Metabolic characterization of the genus *Brucella*. I. Statistical evaluation of the oxidative rates by which type I of each species can be identified. *J. Bact.* 82:387–395, 1961.
14. White, P.G., and J.B. Wilson. Differentiation of smooth and nonsmooth colonies of brucellae. *J. Bact.* 61:239–240, 1951.
15. Wilson, G.S. and A.A. Miles. The serological differentiation of smooth strains of the *Brucella* group. *Brit. J. Exp. Path.* 13:1–3, 1932.

31. Bordetella

Bordetella bronchiseptica is the only one of three species of the genus *Bordetella* that is known to affect domestic animals. *Bordetella pertussis* and *B. parapertussis* are commonly associated with whooping cough in humans.

B. bronchiseptica is a cause of inapparent to chronic infection of the respiratory tract of pigs, dogs, cats, rabbits, rats, mice, guinea pigs, turkeys, horses, and humans.[3,7,10,11,13] It also affects a number of wild animals such as raccoons, opposums, foxes, and skunks.[18] Latent infections can be activated by unfavorable conditions.[20] Only one-tenth of 1% of the clinical cases of whooping cough in humans are caused by *B. bronchiseptica*. A chronic pharyngitis sometimes occurs in animal caretakers caring for infected laboratory animals. *B. bronchiseptica* has no particular seasonal occurrence and is rather widespread in nature, as 28 of 80 SPF swine herds were found positive for the organism.[3] It was isolated from midwestern U.S. swine in 54% of the herds surveyed in 1963.[16] It has also been isolated in England, Canada, Norway, France, and Germany.

Four general types of lesions of the respiratory tract are elicited by infection with *B. bronchiseptica*. (1) Turbinate atrophy occurs in young pigs (4 weeks of age or less) infected with virulent strains of *B. bronchiseptica*. This atrophy is also known to occur in rabbits, cats, and some other laboratory animals. (2) A chronic fibrous bronchial pneumonia occurs in stressed animals infected with *B. bronchiseptica*. (3) A mucopurulent rhinitis and pharyngitis may accompany turbinate atrophy or may occur without occasioning turbinate stunting or hypoplasia. (4) Necrosis of the tracheal lining in some human infections produces a typical whooping cough lesion.

Common histopathologic lesions are hyperplasia, metaplasia and loss of cilia of the respiratory epithelium, submucosal fibroplasia, bone resorption, periarterial fibrosis, and peribronchial fibrosis.[1,2]

Specimens

The upper respiratory tract is the most likely source for recovering *B. bronchiseptica*. For isolation of the organism, nasal and tracheal mucus should be collected on sterile cotton-tipped applicator sticks. When collecting nasal samples from the live animal, a protective face mask should be worn to prevent inhalation of the organisms. Lung samples should be emulsified in tryptose phosphate broth before inoculation onto agar.

Laboratory Procedures

Cultures. Due to the variety of organisms usually present in the nasal cavity, the modified MacConkey's agar should be used. Colonies on this agar are grayish-tan in color and have a smooth surface with an irregular central area and an umbellate margin. They reach 2–3 mm in diameter after 48 hours incubation aerobically at 37°C. Old cultures have an odor similar to that of musty bread. Blood agar may also be used for isolation. The organism appears on horse and bovine blood agar as a white semitranslucent colony after 48 hours of incubation aerobically at 37°C. Beta-hemolysis may occur but is of little value in characterizing the organism. Animal inoculation is of no particular value in the isolation. The motility of *B. bronchiseptica,* due to peritrichous flagella, can be demonstrated by hanging-drop preparations of young broth or agar cultures, or by the Leifson staining method and by electron microscopy.

Cellular morphology. *B. bronchiseptica* is a gram-negative rod approximately $0.5-1 \times 1.5-4$ μm in size, occurring singly, in pairs, or occasionally in chains. It is nonsporeforming, nonencapsulated, and nonacid-fast.

Differential reactions. Isolates should alkalinize media containing glucose and lactose, hydrolyze urea within 24 hours and alkalinize litmus milk within 5 days. They should utilize citrate as the only source of carbon and be agglutinated by hyperimmune anti–*B. bronchiseptica* rabbit sera (Table 31.1).

Rapid plate agglutination tests employing hyperimmune rabbit sera against *B. bronchiseptica* can be used for identification of the typical colonies, in addition to the biochemical reactions.

The nutritional requirements of *B. bronchiseptica* have been partially defined by Ulrich and Needham.[19] *B. bronchiseptica* is extremely sensitive to sulfonamides and

Table 31.1. Media used to identify *B. bronchiseptica*

Test	Result
Colony morphology	Small, round, convex, smooth,* glistening, gray
Motility	Positive
Flagella	Peritrichous
Blood agar	No hemolysis
Urea	Positive
Lactose	Negative
Litmus milk	Alkaline
Glucose	Negative*
Maltose	Negative*
Gelatine	Not liquefied
Catalase	Positive
Indole	Negative
Phenylalanine deaminase	Negative
Niacin-free media	No growth
Agglutination with rabbit antisera	Positive in high titer

*There are rough variants that ferment glucose and maltose.
Slightly adapted from Richter and Kress, *Lab. Invest.* 16:187–210, 1967.

moderately sensitive to the antibiotics that are usually effective against gram-negative rods.[9]

The organism may be stored as frozen culture fluid or on agar slants or be lyophilized. It has been recovered from inoculated soil samples exposed to the sun for as long as 3 weeks after inoculation.

All three *Bordetella* species are considered to have common species-specific K (heat-labile) antigens and common O (heat-stable) antigens. *B. bronchiseptica* is believed to have 7 of the 14 heat-labile antigenic factors of the three *Bordetella* species.[5]

A preliminary report indicates that various strains of *B. bronchiseptica* can be typed according to phage susceptibility. *B. parapertussis* is sensitive to *B. bronchiseptica* phage. However, *B. pertussis, Alcaligenes faecalis,* and *Brucella* sp. appear to be insensitive to *B. bronchiseptica* phage.[14]

Filtrates of *B. bronchiseptica* contain a heat-labile toxin that is lethal to guinea pigs and causes dermal necrosis in rabbits.[6] Lipopolysaccharides (endotoxins) have been isolated from the three *Bordetella* sp.[4] *B. bronchiseptica* is toxic for mice and embryonating hens' eggs.[4] The chemical and biological properties of *Bordetella* sp. lipopolysaccharides are similar to those of other gram-negative bacteria.[12]

B. bronchiseptica has been shown to parasitize tissue culture cells and to undergo certain changes within the latter. The bacteria were readily cultured from cell cultures, and growth of the bacteria was not suppressed by the following antibiotics: penicillin, 100 units/ml; streptomycin, 100 µg/ml; tetracycline, 10 µg/ml; polymixin B, 10 µg/ml.[15]

Animal inoculation. Inoculation of 24-hour broth cultures of low passage isolates into 6–8-day-old embryonating hens' eggs via the YS route will cause death of the embryo in 24–48 hours. Such an embryo passage enhances the virulence of *B. bronchiseptica.* Inoculation of a *B. bronchiseptica* culture IP in the male guinea pig results in septic peritonitis and orchitis.

Immunology and serology. Both naturally and experimentally infected pigs have low or undetectable levels of circulating-agglutinating antibody for *B. bronchiseptica.*[17] High levels of circulating-agglutinating antibodies can be produced by injection of Formalinized bacterin. However, these pigs are not resistant to IN challenges by *B. bronchiseptica.* On the other hand, guinea pigs injected with Formalinized bacterin do not succumb to a pulmonary infection by *B. bronchiseptica.*[8]

At the present, serologic methods of diagnosis of *B. bronchiseptica* infection are of no value. Because the causative agent usually remains on the surface of the respiratory tract during the course of disease, direct cultural identification is the best diagnostic technique.

To prepare anti–*B. bronchiseptica* rabbit serum antigen, inoculate blood agar plates with a heavy suspension of *B. bronchiseptica* broth culture. After 48 hours incubation at 37°C, harvest bacteria into 0.85% salt solution containing 1:5000 Merthiolate. Sediment bacteria by centrifugation and wash bacteria two to three times in salt solution. Resuspend cells and standardize suspension to the desired density with the aid of a photometer.

To prepare the antisera, inject young adult white rabbits with graded doses of antigen increasing from 0.1 to 0.8 ml per kg of body weight, given at 3 day intervals over a 4–6 week period. When a satisfactory level of antibody titer has been reached, exsanguinate the rabbits. Inactivate antisera at 56°C for 30 minutes and preserve with Merthiolate 1:10,000. Dilute serum with approximately 20 volumes of 0.85% NaCl containing 1:10,000 Merthiolate prior to use. Rabbits with a preimmunization titer of 1:4 or greater for *B. bronchiseptica* should be rejected.

References

1. Duncan, J.R., F.K. Ramsey, and W.P. Switzer. Pathology of experimental *Bordetella bronchiseptica* infection in swine: Pneumonia. *Am. J. Vet. Res.* 27:467–472, 1966.
2. Duncan, J.R., R.F. Ross, W.P. Switzer, and F.K. Ramsey. Pathology of experimental *Bordetella bronchiseptica* infection of swine: Atrophic rhinitis. *Am. J. Vet. Res.* 27:457–466, 1966.
3. Dunn, J.W., M.J. Twiehaus, and L.C. Welch. Further studies and observations on atrophic rhinitis in the field. *Proc. U.S. Livestock Sanitary Ass.* 68:266–275, 1964.
4. Eldering, G. A study of the antigen properties of Hemophilus pertussis and related organisms. I. A factor obtained from *Br. bnronchiseptica*. *Am. J. Hyg.* 34:1–7, 1941.
5. Eldering, G., C. Hornbeck, and J. Baker. Serological study of *Bordetella pertussis* and related species. *J. Bact.* 74:133–136, 1957.
6. Evans, D.G., and H.B. Maitland. The toxin of *B. bronchiseptica* and the relation of the organism to *H. pertussis*. *J. Path. Bact.* 48:67–78, 1939.
7. Gallagher, G.L. Isolation of *Bordetella bronchiseptica* from horses. *Vet. Rec.* 77:632–633, 1965.
8. Ganaway, J.R., A.M. Allen, and C.W. McPherson. Prevention of acute *Bordetella bronchiseptica* pneumonia in a guinea pig colony. *Lab. Anim. Care* 15:156–162, 1965.
9. Hagen, K.W., Jr. Effect of antibiotic sulfonamide therapy on certain microorganisms in the nasal turbinates of domestic rabbits. *Lab. Anim. Care* 17:77–80, 1967.
10. Keegan, J.J. The pathology of epidemic pneumonia in mice and guinea pigs. *Arch. Internat. Med.* 26:570–593, 1920.
11. L'Ecuyer, C., E.D. Roberts, and W.P. Switzer. An outbreak of *Bordetella bronchiseptica* pneumonia in swine. *Vet. Med.* 56:420–424, 1961.
12. Maclennan, A.P. Specific lipopolysaccharides of Bordetella. *Biochem. J.* 74:398–409, 1960.
13. McGawen, J.P. Some observations on a laboratory epidemic, principally among dogs and cats, in which the animals affected presented the symptoms of the disease called "Distemper". *J. Path. Bact.* 15:372–426, 1911.
14. Rauch, H.C., and M.J. Pickett. *Bordetella bronchiseptica* bacteriophage. *Can. J. Microbiol.* 7:125–133, 1961.
15. Richter, G.W., and Y. Kress. Observations on commensal cultures of *Bordetella bronchiseptica* and rat hepatoma cells. *Lab. Invest.* 16:187–210, 1967.
16. Ross, R.F. Method of identification of certain etiologic agents of atrophic rhinitis. *Proc. U.S. Livestock Sanitary Ass.* 67:512–515, 1963.
17. Ross, R.F., W.P. Switzer, and J.R. Duncan. Comparison of pathogenicity of various isolates of *Bordetella bronchiseptica* in young pigs. *Can. J. Comp. Med. Vet. Sci.* 31:53–57, 1967.
18. Switzer, W.P., C.J. Mare, and E.D. Hubbard. Incidence of *Bordetella bronchiseptica* in wildlife and man in Iowa. *Am. J. Vet. Res.* 27:1134–1136, 1966.
19. Ulrich, J.A., and G.M. Needham. Differentiation of *Alcaligenes faecalis* from *Brucella bronchisepticus* by biochemical and nutritional methods. *J. Bact.* 65:210–215, 1953.
20. Winsser, J. A study of *Bordetella bronchiseptica*. *Proc. Anim. Care Panel* 10:87–104, 1960.

32. Haemophilus

The genus *Haemophilus* includes a group of gram-negative, nonmotile bacteria that are found in a variety of inflammatory conditions. Diseases associated with members of this group are swine influenza, polyserositis of swine, avian coryza, and possibly a pleuropneumonia of swine. Other conditions in which these organisms have been found to play a prominent, perhaps causative, role, include pneumonias of cattle, sheep, and swine, septicemia, meningitis, arthritis, cerebral abscess, metritis, abortion, vaginitis, and balanoposthitis. Except for coryza and influenza, which occur during the cool months of the year, *Haemophilus* infections may be encountered the year round. Because of their largely sporadic incidence, *Haemophilus* infections have not attracted widespread attention, but they have been found wherever they have been closely looked for. The organisms apparently occur also on normal mucous membranes.

Specimens
Specimens will vary widely according to disease manifestations. Since the organism is fastidious, speedy transfer to the laboratory is important. *Haemophilus* sp. has been recovered fairly consistently from deep-frozen tissues. As with other organisms, swabs should be used for collection and they should be shipped without delay in a suitable transport medium such as Stuart's. The organisms do not present a public health hazard.

Laboratory Procedures
Cultures. Since direct streaking onto solid media frequently fails to initiate growth, inoculation of a liquid medium, e.g. thioglycollate, should be routinely done. Into this medium, a piece of tissue, about 0.5 g, should be placed, or an equivalent amount of exudate or fluid. The large amount is intended not only to introduce an adequate inoculum but also to supply critical nutrients.

By the accepted definition, the *Haemophilus* species require one or both of two cofactors, one being nicotinamide riboside or another effective nicotinamide adenine dinucleotide (NAD) precursor (V factor), the other an iron porphyrin (X factor). Both are present in fresh blood, but, while X is stable, the V level rapidly declines below useful concentrations on storage. The same statement holds for chocolate agar (i.e. agar to which blood was added at 70–75°C), except that the V factor is more abundant in this medium. A convenient way of supplying both is in the form of a feeder culture streak growing simultaneously on the plate. Staphylococci are most commonly used for this purpose since they supply X and V needs consistently in adequate quantities.

All strains seem to benefit by being incubated in an atmosphere of about 10% CO_2. Some, especially the fowl coryza agent, *H. (para)gallinarum,* and the swine parasites, *H. suis* and *H. parasuis,* will often not grow without it. The optimum incubation temperature is 37°C.

On adequate blood agar, growth is apparent in 18–24 hours as translucent colonies less than a millimeter in size. On chocolate agar and in the vicinity of a feeder streak the colonies may reach much larger sizes and attain gray opalescence. As a rule growth is butyrous and easily removed. Older colonies may develop contoured edges and some degree of brittleness. In broth supplemented with the proper growth factors uniform turbidity is produced by most strains.

Differential reactions. All known strains show fermentative activity but the reactions are so variable and inconstant that little use is made of them for purposes of identification. All animal strains are indole negative and reduce nitrates to nitrites. The two most useful characteristics for assigning them to existing species are the cofactor requirements and the action on red blood cells. Cofactor requirements are determined by attempts to cultivate suspect isolates in proteose-peptone broth containing (1) no supplements, (2) 1 μg of NAD and 1 μg of hemin per ml, (3) 1 μg of NAD per ml only, (4) 1 μg of hemin per ml only. The broth may be further supplemented with serum to permit propagation of *H. suis, H. parasuis,* and *H. (para)gallinarum.*

Hemin is extremely insoluble in aqueous media, although the addition of crystalline hemin will allow sufficient amounts to dissolve. For quantitative additions, dissolve 50 mg in 1 ml of triethanolamine (Eastman Kodak, Rochester, N.Y.) and make aqueous dilutions of this. Another method calls for addition of 2.5 mg hemin to 1 ml 0.2 M KOH in 47.5% ethanol and dilution to 5 ml. Storage of NAD and hemin solutions should be at −20°C.[11]

Table 32.1 outlines a differentiation scheme for the genus *Haemophilus,* with special reference to animal isolates.

The V-requiring, X-independent types make up the vast majority of animal isolates. On very rare occasions strains requiring both X and V are encountered. To differentiate between the two types, the suspect organism may be inoculated heavily over the entire surface of a proteose-peptone agar plate. A single streak of a catalase-positive feeder (e.g. *Stapholocuccus aureus*) is drawn over one-half the diameter, and a similar streak of a catalase-negative feeder (e.g. *Streptococcus faecalis*) over the remainder. The X-independent *Haemophilus* will grow satellites along both streaks, the X-dependent only along the catalase-positive feeder streak.[8] In the absence of clear-cut results, serial passage on the test media may be advisable, because the first passage inoculum may have contained enough of a critical nutrient to allow limited growth even on a qualitatively inadequate medium.

Impregnated disks containing V, X, and both factors have been described[7] and are

Table 32.1. Differentiation of species in the genus *Haemophilus*[12]

	influenzae	suis	haemolyticus	parainfluenzae	parasuis	parahaemolyticus	haemoglobinophilus	influenzae-murium	gallinarum	paraphrophilus	paragallinarum	aphrophilus	ducreyi	ovis	putoriorum	citreus	piscium	aegyptius
X requirement	+	+	+	−	−	−	+	+	+	−	−	+	+	(+)	N	N	−*	+
V requirement	+	+	+	+	+	+	−	−	+	+	+	−	−	−	N	N	−*	+
Hemolysis	−	−	+	−	−	+	−	−	−	−	−	−	(+)	−	−	S	+	−
CO_2 requirement	−	−	−	−	−	−	−	−	+	+	+	+	+	−	−	−	−	−
Nitrites from nitrates	+	+	+	+	+	+	+	N	+	+	+	+	N	+	N	+	−	+
Indole	S	−	S	S	−	−	+	−	−	−	−	−	N	−	N	+	−	−
Catalase	+	+	+	+	+	+	+	−	N	+	−	(+)D	N	N	N	N	N	N
Beta-alanine utilization	−	−	N	+	+	+	N	N	N	N	+	N	N	N	N	N	N	N

( ), weak reaction or poor growth—in *H. ovis*, X requirement is demonstrable in freshly isolated cultures; N, not determined, not known; S, some (less than 90%) strains positive, some negative; D, delayed.

H. piscium requires diphosphothiamine or ATP.

Note: *H. influenzae, H. haemolyticus, H. aphrophilus, H. paraphrophilus, H. ducreyi,* and *H. aegyptius* have so far been reported from human sources only. *H. pleuropneumoniae,* described by Shope,[10] is bacteriologically indistinguishable from *H. parahaemolyticus*. A hemolytic equivalent of *H. paraphrophilus* has been described as *H. paraphrohaemolyticus*.

commercially available (Difco Lab., Detroit; Baltimore Biological Lab.). The kind containing both factors has inhibitors intended to restrain contaminants from human pharyngeal specimens. Unfortunately, they sometimes inhibit animal *Haemophilus* strains.

Although serologic types of *Haemophilus* species have been recognized, particularly for *H. suis-parasuis,* no typing reagents are in general use. There are no typing phages available for the identification of *Haemophilus* of animal origin. Soluble toxic fractions of uncertain chemical and immunologic character have been described for *H. influenzae*.[9,4] An endotoxin of the Boivin type has been isolated from *H. gallinarum*.[3]

Cellular morphology. Members of the genus *Haemophilus* are gram-negative coccobacilli and are typically of delicate appearance and occur singly or in short chains. The size of cellular elements is quite variable within a strain, between strains, and from species to species. All known forms are nonmotile and nonacid fast. Morphologic capsules are difficult to demonstrate in animal isolates, but serologic information points to the existence in some strains of *H. suis* of a readily extractable substance that may be analogous to capsular material.[2]

Animal inoculation. Most strains of *Haemophilus* will grow well in, and kill, embryonated hens' eggs. In view of the difficulties sometimes encountered in making recoveries on lifeless media directly from pathologic material, this detour may be justified provided an uncontaminated inoculum is available. Inoculation into the YS of 6-day embryos usually leads to death in 1–3 days. Mice are susceptible to large IP doses, probably due to their sensitivity to the endotoxin, rather than to true susceptibility to infection. Occasional strains prove pathogenic for mice by the IN route. Swine have been fatally infected by IP doses of *H. parahaemolyticus* and *H. parasuis,* and Shope set up lethal respiratory infections by IN instillation of a small number of *H. parahaemolyticus* (*H. pleuropneumoniae*) into swine.[10]

H. gallinarum cultures from field outbreaks of coryza readily reproduce the disease by nasal-cleft swabbing or intrasinal injection of previously unexposed chickens. Other avian species appear to be less susceptible.

Immunology and serology. Serologic tests are not currently employed in the diagnosis of *Haemophilus* infections. In contrast to the situation with human *H. influenzae*, the serology of animal *Haemophilus* has not reached the stage of direct typing of capsular swelling or fluorescent antibody tagging of bacteria in exudate. For demonstration of *Haemophilus* colonies in tissue, the Barbeito-Lopez stain has proved useful. It is non-specific, however, and does not substitute for isolation and cultural identification.

A group of gram-negative organisms resembling *Haemophilus* in many respects have in recent years been found to be associated with purulent and necrotizing infections of sheep and cattle. The most notorious of these is a meningoencephalitis of feedlot cattle.[5] Others, isolated from pneumonia of cattle and sheep, orchitis, epididymitis, arthritis, mastitis, meningitis, and septicemia of sheep, are bacteriologically similar. They differ from classic *Haemophilus* in that the cofactors V and X are not required. They resemble it morphologically, colonially, and in the satellite growth patterns they exhibit around feeder colonies on deficient media. Many strains will not grow or grow very sparingly on unsupplemented media. The demand for increased carbon dioxide may be quite strict. The first organism of this group that was isolated was called *Haemophilus agni,*[6] and the name *Haemophilus somnus* has been suggested for the cattle organism. At present the undefined nature of their accessory requirements excludes both organisms from the genus. The genus *Actinobacillus* has been suggested instead.[1]

These organisms are identified by their morphologic and colony similarity to nonhemolytic *Haemophilus,* their satellitism on tryptose agar, their unresponsiveness to NAD and hemin, and their CO_2 requirements. The cattle organism produces indole from suitable precursors.

References

1. Bailie, W.E., H.D. Anthony, and K.D. Weide. Infectious thromboembolic meningoencephalomyelitis (Sleeper Syndrome) in feedlot cattle. *J. Am. Vet. Med. Ass.* 148:162–166, 1966.
2. Bakos, K. *Studien über Haemophilus suis, mit besonderer Berücksichtigung der serologischen Differenzier ung seiner Stämme.* Academic Paper, Veterinärhögskolan, Stockholm. Appelberg, Uppsala, 1955.
3. Cundy, K.R. Isolation and characterization of an endotoxin from *Haemophilus gallinarum.* Ph.D. thesis, University of California, Davis. *Abstr. Bact. Proc.* 65:39–40, 1965.
4. Dubos, R.J. A soluble toxin produced by *Hemophilus influenzae. J. Bact.* 43:77–78, 1942.
5. Kennedy, P.C., E.L. Biberstein, J.A. Howarth, L.M. Frazier, and D.L. Dungworth. Infectious meningoencephalitis in cattle, caused by a Haemophilus-like organism. *Am. J. Vet. Res.* 21:403–409, 1960.
6. Kennedy, P.C., L.M. Frazier, G.H. Theilen, and E.L. Biberstein. A septicemic disease of lambs caused by *Hemophilus agni* (new species). *Am. J. Vet. Res.* 19:645–654, 1958.
7. Parker, R.H., and P.D. Hoeprich. Disc method for rapid identification of Haemophilus species. *Abstr. Bact. Proc.* 61:128, 1961.
8. Pickett, M.J., and M.A. Stewart. Identification of Hemophilic bacilli by means of the satellite phenomenon. *Am. J. Clin. Path.* 23:713–715, 1953.

9. Platt, A.E. Serological study of *Haemophilus influenzae:* Two serologically active protein fractions isolated from Pfeiffer's bacillus. *Austral. J. Exp. Biol. Med. Sci.* 17:19–24, 1939.
10. Shope, R.E. Porcine contagious pleuropneumonia. I. Experimental transmission, etiology, and pathology. *J. Exp. Med.* 119:357–368, 1964.
11. White, D.C. Respiratory systems in hemin-requiring *Haemophilus* species. *J. Bact.* 85:84–96, 1963.
12. Zinnemann, K., and E.L. Biberstein. The genus Haemophilus. In *Bergey's Manual of Determinative Bacteriology,* R.E. Buchanan and N.E. Gibbons (eds.). 8th ed. Williams and Wilkins, Baltimore, 1974.

33. Pasteurella, Yersinia, and Francisella

The species considered in this section are *Pasteurella multocida, P. haemolytica, P. pneumotropica, P. gallinarum, P. anatipestifer, Yersinia pestis, Y. pseudotuberculosis,* and *Francisella tularensis.* All were formerly classified in the genus *Pasteurella.* They are a group of loosely related, widely distributed, gram-negative bacteria that are primarily pathogens of mammals and birds. They may be the primary or secondary cause of disease. Clinical manifestations of infection vary from inapparent to those terminating in death.

The first four species are true *Pasteurella. P. anatipestifer* is currently included in this genus although it differs from the other species in major respects: it liquefies gelatin and does not ferment carbohydrates. Two closely related species, having properties that set them apart from the others, are now classified as *Yersinia pestis* and *Y. pseudotuberculosis.* The organism causing tularemia is also classified in a new genus, as *Francisella tularensis,* because it is markedly distinct in its cultural requirements and other characteristics. These last three species are included in this section, which is concerned mainly with the pasteurellae, for convenience, and because of their long historical association with this group.

Pasteurella multocida (P. septica)

This organism is the etiologic agent of fowl cholera,[19] an acute or chronic, highly infectious, septicemic disease of domestic and feral birds; snuffles, a disease (possibly secondary) of domestic rabbits, characterized by inflammation of the mucous membranes of the air passages, which may terminate with pneumonia or septicemia; hemorrhagic septicemia,[12] a septicemic disease causing high mortality in cattle, buffalo, swine, and other animals in Asia and Africa but seldom fatal in the United States; and shipping fever, a respiratory disease complex of livestock in which *P. multocida* or *haemolytica* are largely responsible for severe or terminal pneumonia. These organisms are often carried in the upper air passages of healthy animals and cause disease only when the host's resistance has been lowered, as with infection by parainfluenza-3 virus in the case of bovine shipping fever.

P. multocida is sometimes isolated from the respiratory tract, localized lesions, and blood of humans. The bite of a cat or dog is often the source of infection for humans.

The organism is usually transmitted by oral or nasal excretions from infected animals and ordinarily enters tissues through mucous membranes of the upper air passages but may gain entrance through the conjunctiva or cutaneous wounds. The virulence of *P. multocida* from one host species to another is its most variable characteristic. An isolate that produces acute septicemia in turkeys or in ducks may be avirulent for chickens, an isolate that severely affects cattle may be avirulent for turkeys, and so forth. Virulence also may be lost when the organism is subcultured on laboratory media. Thus the organism may cause an inapparent, an acute septicemic, an acute respiratory, or a chronic localized infection.

Specimens

Blood or mucus are the preferred specimens from live animals. Blood (1 ml) is aseptically collected and inoculated into 10 ml of trypticase-soy broth (TSB). Mucus is collected by inserting a cotton-tipped applicator (moistened with broth) into the nostrils, tonsil area, or along the gum line. At necropsy, bone marrow, liver, heart blood, sinus cavities, or localized lesions are preferred sources for specimens and can be collected on cotton swabs or with wire loops. The specimen is transferred to 5 ml of TSB, which can be incubated or frozen for later examination. A provisional diagnosis can be made by demonstrating bipolar organisms in blood smears or liver imprints using Wright's or other suitable stains. The FA technique can be used to identify the organisms in tissue,[17] but it is seldom used.

Laboratory Procedures

Cultures. The broth containing the specimen is incubated for 2 hours at 37°C and then streaked on a blood agar plate; however, blood specimens in broth should be incubated longer (16–24 hours) before plating. After the plate cultures have incubated for 18–24 hours, they are examined for colonies. A more definitive colony study can be made using plates of dextrose starch (Difco Lab., Detroit) containing 5% avian serum and MaC agar. These plates are examined with a stereomicroscope using obliquely transmitted light, which is obtained by directing a light beam up through the agar at an angle or by reflection from a mirror on the table.[19] Colonies on dextrose starch agar, when observed with obliquely transmitted light, are iridescent, sectored with variable iridescence, or blue with little or no iridescence. Older colonies usually are not iridescent. Colonies grown on blood agar are about 2 mm in diameter, smooth, entire, slightly convex, translucent, and butyrous. Older colonies are larger and often viscous.

Differential reactions. A selected isolated colony is inoculated onto a slant of stock culture agar (Difco), incubated 18–24 hours at 37°C, and then used for subculturing into differential test media. The sugars are prepared as 1% solutions in tubes of phenol red broth. The production of acid but no gas from glucose, sucrose, and mannitol (usually) is characteristic of *P. multocida;* lactose and maltose usually are negative. Indole is produced by most isolates of *P. multocida,* using Kovac's test and tubes of 2% tryptose (Difco) in 0.85% NaCl solution incubated 24–48 hours. No growth occurs on MaC agar, and blood is not hemolyzed. A summary of biochemical reactions of the pasteurellae, yersiniae, and francisellae is given in Table 33.1.

Pasteurella, Yersinia, and Francisella

Table 33.1. Biochemical and other reactions of *Pasteurella*, *Yersinia*, and *Francisella*

	multoc.	haemol.	gallin.	pneumo.	pestis	pseudo.	tulare.	anatip.
Arabinose	−u	V	−	V	+	+	−	−
Dextrin	−u	+	+	+	−	+	V	−
Dulcitol	−u	V	−	−	−	−	−	−
Fructose	+	+	+	+	+	+	V	−
Galactose	+	+	+	+	+	+	−	−
Glucose	+	+	+	+	+	+	+	−
Glycerol	V	+u	−	−u	V	+	V	−
Inositol	−	+u	V	−u	−	−	−	−
Lactose	−u	+u	−	+u	−u	−	−	−
Maltose	−u	+	+	+	V	+	+	−
Mannitol	+u	+	−	−	+	+	−	−
Mannose	+u	V	+	+u	+	+	+	−
Melibiose	X	X	X	X	−	+	X	X
Raffinose	−u	+	+	+u	−	−	−	−
Rhamnose	−u	V	−	−	−u	+	−	−
Salicin	−	V	−	−	V	+u	−	−
Sorbitol	+u	+	V	V	−	−	−	−
Sucrose	+	+	+	+	−u	V	−	−
Trehalose	V	V	+u	+	+	+	−	−
Xylose	V	+	−V	V	+u	+	−	−
Gelatin stab	−	−	−	−	−	−	−	+u
Hemolysis	−	+	−	−	−	−	−	−
H₂S	+u	+u	V	V	−	−u	+	−
Indole	+u	−	−	+	−	−	−	−
Litmus milk	−	Sac	−	−	Sac or −	Sal	− or Sac	*
MaC	−	+	−	−	−	+u	X	−
Motility	−	−	−	−	−	+	−	−
Nitrate red.	+	+	+	+	+	+	X	−
Urease	−	−	−	+	−	+	X	+

−u, usually negative reaction; +u, usually positive; V, variable; X, not known; Sac, slightly acid; Sal, slightly alkaline.
*Slowly becomes alkaline and casein is digested.

Cellular morphology. P. multocida cells are gram-negative, nonmotile, nonspore-forming rods that usually stain bipolarly. On primary isolation from an animal with septicemia, cells usually occur singularly and occasionally in pairs, and a capsule can be demonstrated with indirect India ink staining. In primary cultures from the respiratory tract of healthy animals, cells from iridescent colonies usually occur singularly, but sometimes they are mixed with filamentous forms and short chains. Under suboptimal growth conditions cells usually become pleomorphic. The long chains occur in gray colonies.

Animal inoculation. Animal inoculation is used when specimens may contain organisms that overgrow *P. multocida*. Rabbits, hamsters, or mice are injected IP with a 0.2 ml specimen of exudate, mucus, urine, or tissue suspended in TSB. Heart blood or liver should be cultured from animals that die within 24–48 hours. Usually a pure culture can be isolated by this technique. IM, IP, or IV inoculation of rabbits or mice with as few as 10 organisms often results in death. Instillation of the organisms in the nostrils of mice or rabbits often results in death within 18–48 hours. IM inoculation of guinea pigs produces necrosis at the site of injection, while IP inoculation usually results in death. Otherwise guinea pigs and rats are quite refractory to the organisms.

Immunology and serology. The antigens of *P. multocida* are many and complex. By combining the results of the indirect HA and the serum agglutination tests, researchers have found 12 serotypes.[5,16,20] The AD test is very effective for serotyping *P. multocida*;[11] 16 serotypes have been identified. There is a good correlation between the serologic reaction and the immune response in chickens and turkeys. The antisera for the AD test are prepared with *P. multocida* grown on dextrose starch agar, suspended in 0.85% NaCl solution containing 0.3% saturated solution of formaldehyde, and adjusted to a concentration corresponding to the density of 10× McFarland no. 1. An equal quantity of the cell suspension is emulsified with Bayol F mineral oil (Esso Standard Oil Co., Linden, N.J.) containing 3% Arlacel A (Atlas Powder Co., Wilmington, Del.). One ml of the antigen is injected SC in the neck of young mature male chickens. If the titer of the serum is satisfactory, the birds are exsanguinated 3 weeks after injection. Feed is removed from cages the night before. If the titer of the serum is too low, another injection is made IM and the birds are exsanguinated 2 or 3 weeks later. The serum is separated from the clot within 3 hours by centrifuging 1 hour at $1500 \times g$ and is preserved with 0.01% thimerosal and 0.06% phenol. Antigens are prepared with 18–24-hour growth from a heavily seeded culture plate. The cells are suspended in 1 ml of 8.5% NaCl, 0.02 M phosphate, and 0.3% saturated solution of formaldehyde, heated in a water bath at 100°C for 1 hour, and sedimented by centrifugation. The supernatant fluid is used as the antigen. The gel consists of 0.9% Special Noble agar (Difco) and 8.5% NaCl in distilled water. Five ml of melted agar is placed on 25 × 75 mm microscope slides; wells 4 mm in diameter and 6 mm from center to center are cut in the agar. Results are recorded after 24–48 hours at 37°C.

Pasteurella haemolytica

This organism is involved in the etiology of septicemia of lambs; mastitis of ewes and possibly of cattle; bovine shipping fever, causing pneumonia as a secondary invader in a manner similar to *P. multocida;* pneumonia of sheep, goats, and swine; and salpingitis of young hens. Human infections are infrequent. Some urease-positive isolates from respiratory infections were first considered to be variants and were classified as *P. haemolytica* var. *ureae;* they now are classified as a separate species, *P. ureae. P. haemolytica* is often isolated from the respiratory tract of healthy animals but the carrier rate is less than with *P. multocida*.

Specimens

Specimens similar to those of *P. multocida* can be used. In mastitis of ewes, the organism can be isolated from milk.

Laboratory Procedures

Cultures. The methods described for *P. multocida* are also applicable here. Colonies grown on agar are similar to those of *P. multocida,* though less mucoid and coalescent. A zone of hemolysis (beta) surrounding the colonies on blood agar is an aid in recognizing the organism; if hemolysis is not apparent, it often can be seen by scraping the colony off the agar, or by holding the culture for an additional period at 5°C. Some nonsmooth colonies are normally present and can easily be detected by flooding with

1:2000 aqueous crystal violet for 15 seconds. Nonsmooth colonies stain intensely purple and become brittle, while smooth colonies do not absorb dye and adhere to the agar. In liquid media, such as BHI broth, there is a diffuse cloudiness and sedimentation is formed by the organism.

Differential reactions. The most important reactions that differentiate *P. haemolytica* from *P. multocida* are growth on MaC agar, hemolysis on blood agar, and failure to produce indole.[27] Certain strains of *P. haemolytica* ferment arabinose (type A), while others ferment trehalose (type T).[25] Tests for arabinose fermentation should be conducted in the medium of Bosworth and Lovell.[25,27]

Cellular morphology. The cells are similar to those of *P. multocida* but they rarely form chains.

Animal inoculation. Because the organism has a low pathogenicity for laboratory animals, isolation by animal inoculation is not often used. The IP inoculation of about a 10^8 concentration of cells will kill a mouse or guinea pig within 48 hours; for a hamster a higher dose is required.[26] The organism is not pathogenic for rabbits.

Immunology and serology. With the indirect HA test, 12 serotypes are currently recognized.[2] The tube agglutination test may also be used. Antisera can be prepared by inoculating the live organisms into rabbits. Suspensions containing about 1.75×10^9 cells per ml are inoculated every 4 days in the amounts of 0.5, 1, 2, and finally 3 ml; rabbits are bled at 5 or 6 weeks.

Pasteurella pneumotropica

This organism, present in many mouse colonies, is a potential pulmonary pathogen of mice, particularly those used in experiments and exposed to other pathogens or stresses.[9] It also has been isolated from guinea pigs, hamsters, rats, and dogs.[14] A closely related organism differing only in its enzymatic activity also has been isolated from mice; the name *P. pneumotropica* var. *xylophil* was proposed.[13]

Specimens

The organism can be isolated from the lungs, eyes, uterus, kidneys, heart blood, or peritoneal fluid of infected animals.

Laboratory Procedures

Cultures. The procedures described for *P. multocida* are used. Colonies, when grown 24 hours at 37°C on blood agar, are about 1 mm in diameter, entire, convex, and grayish yellow.[14]

Differential reactions. Glucose, lactose, sucrose, maltose, and trehalose are fermented without producing gas.[3] Indole is produced, gelatin is not liquefied. There is no growth on MaC agar and no hemolysis on blood agar. Urea is hydrolyzed.

Cellular morphology. Cells are short, occasionally coccoid, about $0.4-1 \times 0.6-2$ μm. In old cultures, threadlike and swollen forms are often found.

Animal inoculation. Mice are susceptible when exposed IN but are quite resistant when exposed by other conventional routes. Rats, hamsters, guinea pigs, rabbits, and chickens are resistant to infection.

Immunology and serology. Agglutinating and CF antibodies are produced in experimentally infected mice, but carrier mice are often serologically negative.

Pasteurella gallinarum

This organism is often present in the respiratory tract of poultry and occasionally of cattle and sheep.[10] Pathogenicity is low, and the organism is best classified as a secondary invader. *P. gallinarum* has been identified in the United States, Australia, Japan, Nigeria, and Iran.

Specimens

Specimens are collected from the nasal cleft, sinuses, air sacs, trachea, and sometimes from the viscera of infected birds as described for *P. multocida*.[6] The FA technique can be used on smears of tissue or exudate.[19]

Laboratory Procedures

Cultures. The procedures described for *P. multocida* are used. Colonies, when grown 24 hours at 37°C on blood agar are 1–1.5 mm in diameter, smooth but often with concentric rings, entire, low convex, and translucent.

Differential reactions. Acid but no gas is produced from glucose, sucrose, and maltose (usually). Lactose is not fermented. Indole is not produced; there is no hemolysis on blood agar and no growth on MaC agar.

Cellular morphology. The cells are similar to those of *P. multocida*.

Animal inoculation. IM or IV inoculation of chickens may produce severe local necrosis but seldom death. YS inoculation of chicken embryos (10 days old) results in death within 24 hours. The other laboratory animals are resistant.

Immunology and serology. Agglutinins and precipitins can be detected in the serum of birds inoculated IM, but carrier birds are often serologically negative.

Pasteurella anatipestifer

P. anatipestifer infection has been called infectious serositis[7] and new duck disease.[4] It is an acute or chronic septicemic disease, usually in 1–8-week-old domestic ducklings.[23] The respiratory tract may also be infected. The organism has also been isolated from wild waterfowl, pheasants, turkeys, and quail. Signs are mild coughing and sneezing, ocular and nasal discharge, greenish diarrhea, ataxia, tremor of head and neck, and coma. Gross lesions are fibrinous pericarditis, fibrinous perihepatitis, fibrinous airsacculitis, caseous salpingitis, and arthritis.

Specimens

The brain, liver, lung, and trachea are the preferred tissues for specimens. The material for culture examination is collected as described for *P. multocida*. The FA test may be used on tissues.[18]

Laboratory Procedures

Cultures. P. anatipestifer is nutritionally fastidious. Chocolate agar (Difco) or its equivalent is preferred for primary isolation; for subculturing, TSA containing 5% defibrinated bovine blood may be used. On primary isolation, cultures should be incubated in a candle jar. Colonies grown at 37°C for 24 hours are about 1 mm in diameter, convex, transparent, glistening, and butyrous. Older colonies are larger and viscous.

Differential reactions. The organism does not ferment carbohydrates, and hydrogen sulfide and indole are not produced. Nitrates are not reduced and starch is not hydrolyzed. There is no growth on MaC agar and no hemolysis on blood agar. Gelatin is liquified, urease is usually produced, litmus milk may slowly become alkaline, and casein is digested (see Table 33.1).

Cellular morphology. Cells occur usually singly or in pairs, infrequently as filaments. They vary in size from $0.2–0.4 \times 1–5$ μm. A capsule can be demonstrated by the indirect India ink method. The cells are gram-negative, occasionally bipolar, nonmotile, nonsporeforming rods.

Animal inoculation. The organism is pathogenic for young ducklings when inoculated into the footpads or given by the IT or IV routes. Guinea pigs may die when inoculated IP. Chickens, pigeons, rabbits, and mice are resistant. Pathogenicity may be lost through subculturing. The YS of chicken embryos (10 days incubation) may be inoculated with 0.1 ml of prepared specimens. The embryos usually die within 24 hours, and the organisms can be isolated from the allantoic fluid.

Immunology and serology. Ducks that recover from infection are immune. In England, serotypes A–H have been differentiated by their agglutinogens.

Yersinia pestis (Pasteurella pestis)

This organism is the causative agent of plague (sylvatic), an infection primarily of wild rodents that is maintained as a continuous infection chain by an insect vector, the flea.[1] The principal animal hosts are ground squirrels, rats, prairie dogs, chipmunks, mice, and rabbits. Humans may become a victim of the bubonic form (the Black Death of historical reports) when bitten by an infected flea or by handling infected wild rodents. If the disease becomes generalized and the lungs are involved, human to human transmission may occur.

Specimens

Plague-suspect specimens may be obtained from rodents, other small animals, fleas, or humans. The preferred specimens from animals are lymph nodes, spleen, liver, and bone marrow. Fleas are pooled, washed in physiological saline solution, and ground to make a suspension. Blood or material from buboes would be taken from human patients. Smear examination of blood-stained sputum may be used to make a presumptive diagnosis of the pneumonic form of plague. Wayson's stain is preferred for use on tissue impression films. The FA technique may also be used for tissues; the bone marrow is preferred when decomposition of the cadaver is evident.[15]

Laboratory Procedures

Cultures. Blood agar or TSA may be used for the primary isolation. About 5 ml of a blood specimen is placed in 50 ml of trypticase soy broth so that subcultures can be made daily on agar to increase chances for isolation of the organism.[1] Cultures should be observed for 21 days. Incubation of some of the cultures in a candle jar may be valuable. *Y. pestis* grows slowly, but after 2 or 3 days colonies on blood agar are small, round, glistening, and colorless, resembling *E. coli*. On nutrient agar they are grayish-white and translucent. Broth cultures are turbid, or clear with flocculent sediment. Old cultures show a pellicle with streamers.

Differential reactions. Peptone water containing 1% carbohydrate and 1% Andrade's indicator is the recommended medium for fermentation tests, but the standard phenol red broth also is satisfactory. The tubes should be inoculated with heavy suspensions of the organisms. Often the fermentation tubes can be read in a few days, but an observation period of two weeks is recommended. The fermentation of carbohydrates and other biochemical tests for *Y. pestis* is given in Table 33.1.

Cellular morphology. The cells are small ($0.5-0.7 \times 1.5-1.75$ μm), short, plump rods, occurring singly, in pairs, or in short chains, with a marked pleomorphism in old cultures. In other features the cells are similar to those of *P. multocida*.

Animal inoculation. The cutaneous exposure of guinea pigs is useful when only heavily contaminated materials are available, such as putrified rodent organs.[1] The infected material is rubbed into the skin of the abdomen or medial surface of the thigh. Other more desirable specimens may be inoculated into the thigh or lower abdomen of rats or guinea pigs or into the abdomen of mice. Animals usually die within 4–5 days. IP inoculation will result in death of the animals within 24–36 hours, but this route should be restricted to specimens free of extraneous contaminants.

Immunology and serology. Antisera for plague agglutination tests are usually produced by immunizing rabbits. Avirulent organisms or heat- or Formalin-inactivated virulent cultures are inoculated IV for immunization. Rapid slide agglutination tests may be performed by placing loopfuls of bacterial suspensions (about 2×10^9 cells per ml) on a slide and mixing with a suitable dilution of the antiserum (final dilution about 1:100). Results can be read with a hand lens. *Y. pseudotuberculosis* cross-reacts with the antiserum of *Y. pestis* giving false positive test results.[24] However, preliminary absorption with *Y. pseudotuberculosis* organisms renders the serum specific for *Y. pestis*.

When it is important to confirm a diagnosis of plague in a human patient who has had antibiotic therapy, serum from the patient can be used in the agglutination test, but low titers of 1:3 or 1:4 may be found.

Precipitin tests done with soluble antigens from the tissues of animals dead from plague are used with some success, and HA tests with protein fractions of *Y. pestis* are useful since they are highly specific, even to the point of excluding *Y. pseudotuberculosis*. Except in laboratories specifically engaged in work on plague, however, antigens and antisera are usually not available.

Yersinia pseudotuberculosis (Pasteurella pseudotuberculosis)

This organism causes a natural disease in guinea pigs, rabbits, mice, pigeons, turkeys, canaries, and humans. It may be transmitted experimentally to wild rats, dogs, cats, monkeys, and horses. In epizootics, guinea pigs exhibit three clinical forms of the disease: septicemia, fatal in 24–48 hours; classic pseudotuberculosis, with emaciation, diarrhea, and death in 3–4 weeks; or lymphadenopathy of the cervical and thoracic nodes. Infection enters through skin or with contaminated feed and water. In human adults the disease may be a severe, often fatal, typhoidal form, or more often, especially in children, a benign form with symptoms of chronic appendicitis.

Another species, *Yersinia enterocolitica,* isolated from various sources including pseudotuberculosis in chinchillas and mesenteric lymphadenitis in humans, is related to but distinct from *Y. pseudotuberculosis.*

Specimens

Cultures may be obtained from the liver, lymph nodes, spleen, and blood (bacteremia occurs only during the early stages of the disease). The organism has been found in soil, dust, water, and milk. Because it is excreted by birds and rodents, recovery from fecal material is often possible.[22] The techniques are similar to those of *Y. pestis.* The FA test may be used, but cross-reactions with *Y. pestis* occur with some strains.[1]

Laboratory Procedures

Cultures. The organism grows well in ordinary peptone broth; growth at 22°C is diffuse, with some clumped masses and with occasional ring and pellicle formation. At 37°C in acid media, dissociation is accelerated. On plain agar the organism forms colonies that are smooth to slimy, granular, translucent, butyrous, grayish-yellow, and 0.5–1 mm in diameter. On blood agar, the colonies grow to 2–3 mm by the second day; at 37°C the colonies are thin, dry, and irregular. The organism is motile at room temperature but not at 37°C. Ordinarily the SIM (Difco) motility agar medium should be used instead of the hanging-drop suspension, but for fecal isolations the medium of Paterson and Cook is recommended.[22]

Differential reactions. Biochemical tests are carried out as outlined for *Y. pestis* (see Table 33.1).

Cellular morphology. The cells vary from coccal to ovoid; rods vary from 0.5×1.5–5 μm, with rounded ends. The cells do not take a bipolar stain as regularly as *Y. pestis.* Neither spores nor visible capsules are formed, although at 22°C an envelope may be seen in India ink preparations.

Animal inoculation. Guinea pigs, rabbits, mice, sparrows, and canaries are very susceptible. White laboratory rats are refractory. Isolation of the organism is usually done culturally rather than using animal inoculation. When guinea pigs are inoculated with the organisms SC they may die in 15–45 days. The necropsy findings include local abscesses, enlarged lymph nodes with caseous centers, and focal necrosis of the spleen, liver, lungs, and bone marrow. When ingested, the bacilli produce necrotic nodules in the ileum and cecum, with caseous necrosis of the mesenteric lymph nodes.

Immunology and serology. On the basis of agglutination reactions, *Y. pseudotuberculosis* strains have been divided into types I–V and subtypes IA and IB. Antisera prepared with these types generally agglutinate *Y. pseudotuberculosis* but not *Y. pestis*, while plague antiserum agglutinates both organisms.

Francisella tularensis (Pasteurella tularensis)

Tularemia is caused by this organism. It is primarily a disease of rabbits, rodents, and birds, and is transmitted by flies, fleas, lice, and ticks. Humans are accidental and terminal hosts, usually becoming infected by contaminating their hands or eyes with infected tissue, by the bite of arthropod vectors, by ingestion of contaminated food or water, or by inhalation. Tularemia is an acute febrile disease, often with pneumonic complications. *F. novicida* (*P. novicida*) is a closely related species isolated from water; it does not cause natural infection but will produce lesions similar to tularemia and will kill mice and guinea pigs when experimentally infected.[21]

Specimens

Lymph, blood, sputum, or localized lesions are the preferred specimens. The arthropod vectors also may be used as specimens for bacterial isolation.

Laboratory Procedures

Cultures. The organism will not grow on the regular laboratory media unless cystine or cysteine is added. Cultivation is most successful on cystine-glucose-blood agar slants incubated at 37°C in a candle jar. Primary growth from specimen material usually requires from 4 to 7 days. Subcultures on the same kind of agar grow in 2–3 days. In young cultures the colonies are very tiny; later, heavier growth of small, gray, transparent to translucent, mucoid colonies develop. Gelatinized egg yolk media also may be used. Liquid media of protein hydrolysates with extracts of blood cells support good growth.

Differential reactions. Biochemical tests should be carried out with media supplemented with cystine or cysteine. In addition to the tests shown in Table 33.1, tests for glutaminase, asparaginase, and citrullinase are often included. All strains of *F. tularensis* contain the first two enzymes, but only virulent strains degrade citrulline.

Cellular morphology. The organism is very pleomorphic, ranging from minute coccoid to bacillary forms, from $0.2–1 \times 1–3$ μm. The organism stains only faintly with the usual dyes but is definitely gram-negative and sometimes shows bipolar staining. It is nonmotile.

Animal inoculation. If isolation of the organism from humans is attempted, the most useful technique during the first week of illness is inoculation into guinea pigs. Blood from the patient should be diluted with an equal volume of 0.85% NaCl solution and 4–8 ml of the mixture inoculated IP into the animal. A single bacterium of a highly virulent strain can produce a fatal infection in a guinea pig, rabbit, hamster, or mouse. About 10 virulent organisms will produce a systemic infection in a monkey. Rats are quite resistant.

Immunology and serology. Direct agglutination, either using slide or tubes, will identify isolates of *F. tularensis*. If the tubes are placed on a reciprocal shaker for 5 minutes before incubating in a 50°C water bath, the agglutination test can be read in 4 hours.[9] The agglutination test is helpful in differentiating *F. tularensis* from *F. novicida*.[21]

References

1. Baltazard, M., D.H.D. Davis, R. Devignat, G. Girard, M.A. Gohar, L. Kartman, K.F. Meyer, M.T. Parker, R. Pollitzer, F.M. Prince, S.F. Quan, and P Wagle. Recommended laboratory methods for the diagnosis of plague. *Bull. WHO* 14:457–509, 1956.
2. Biberstein, E.L., M. Gills, and H. Knight. Serological types of *Pasteurella hemolytica*. *Cornell Vet.* 50:283–300, 1960.
3. Brenna, P.C., T.E. Fritz, and R.J. Flynn. *Pasteurella pneumotropica*: Cultural and biochemical characteristics, and its association with disease in laboratory animals. *Lab. Anim. Care* 15:307–312, 1965.
4. Bruner, D.W., and J. Fabricant. A strain of *Moraxella anatipestifer (Pfeifferella anatipestifer)* isolated from ducks. *Cornell Vet.* 44:461–464, 1954.
5. Carter, G.R. Studies on *Pasteurella multocida*. I. A hemagglutination test for the identification of serological types. *Am. J. Vet. Res.* 16:481–484, 1955.
6. Clark, D.S., and J.F. Godfrey. Atypical pasteurella infections in chickens. *Avian Dis.* 4:280–290, 1960.
7. Dougherty, E., 3rd, L.Z. Saunders, and E.H. Parsons. The pathology of infectious serositis of ducks. *Am. J. Path.* 31:475–480, 1955.
8. Engelfried, J.J., and F. Spear. Modified agglutination test for *Pasteurella tularensis*. *Appl. Microbiol.* 14:267–270, 1966.
9. Flynn, R.J., P.C. Brennan, and T.E. Fritz. Pathogen status of commercially produced laboratory mice. *Lab. Anim. Care* 15:440–447, 1965.
10. Hall, W.J., K.L. Heddleston, D.H. Legenhausen, and R.W. Hughes. Studies on pasteurellosis. I. A new species of *Pasteurella* encountered in chronic fowl cholera. *Am. J. Vet. Res.* 16:598–604, 1955.
11. Heddleston, K.L., J.E. Gallagher, and P.A. Rebers. Fowl cholera: gel diffusion precipitin test for serotyping *Pasteurella multocida* from avian species. *Avian Dis.* 16:925–936, 1972.
12. Heddleston, K.L., K.R. Rhoades, and P.A. Rebers. Experimental pasteurellosis: Comparative studies on *Pasteurella multocida* from Asia, Africa, and North America. *Am. J. Vet. Res.* 28:1003–1012, 1967.
13. Heyl, J.G. A study of *Pasteurella* strains from animal sources. *Antonie Van Leeuwenhoek* 29:79–83, 1963.
14. Jawetz, E. A pneumotropic *Pasteurella* of laboratory animals. I. Bacteriological and serological characteristics of the organism. *J. Infec. Dis.* 86:172–183, 1950.
15. Kartman, L. The role of rabbits in sylvatic plague epidemiology, with special attention to human cases in New Mexico and use of the fluorescent antibody technique for detection of pasteurella pestis in field specimens. *Zoonoses Res.* 1:1–27, 1960.
16. Little, P.A., and B.M. Lyon. Demonstration of serological types within the nonhemolytic pasteurella. *Am. J. Vet. Res.* 4:110–112, 1943.
17. Marshall, J.D. The use of immunofluorescence for the identification of members of the genus *Pasteurella* in chemically fixed tissues. Ph.D. thesis, University of Maryland, College Park, 1963.
18. Marshall, J.D., P.A. Hansen, and W.C. Eveland. Histobacteriology of the genus *Pasteurella*. I. *Pasteurella anatipestifer*. *Cornall Vet.* 51:24–33, 1961.
19. *Methods for the Examination of Poultry Biologics*. 3d ed. Pub. 705. National Academy of Sciences, Washington, 1971.
20. Namioka, S., and D.W. Bruner. Serological studies on *Pasteurella multocida*. IV. Type distribution of the organisms on the basis of their capsule and O groups. *Cornell Vet.* 53:41–53, 1963.
21. Owen, C.R., E.O. Buker, W.L. Jellison, D.B. Lackman, and J.F. Bell. Comparative studies on *Francisella tularensis* and *Francisella novicida*. *J. Bact.* 87:676–683, 1964.
22. Paterson, J.S., and R. Cook. A method for the recovery of *Pasteurella pseudotuberculosis* from feces. *J. Path. Bact.* 85:241–242, 1963.
23. Price, J. Studies of *Pasteurella anatipestifer* infections in white Pekin ducks. *Avian Dis.* 3:486–487, 1959.
24. Quan, S.F., W. Knapp, M.I. Goldenberg, B.W. Hudson, W.D. Lawton, T.H. Chen, and L. Kartman. Isolation of a strain of *Pasteurella pseudotuberculosis* from Alaska identified as *Pasteurella pestis*: An immunofluorescent false positive *Am. J. Trop. Med. Hyg.* 14:424–432, 1965.
25. Smith, G.R. The characteristics of two types of *Pasteurella haemolytica* associated with different pathological conditions in sheep. *J. Path. Bact.* 81:431–440, 1961.

26. Wessman, G.E. Susceptibility of mice, guinea pigs, and hamsters to challenge with *Pasteurella haemolytica* and its enhancement by microbial polysaccharides and related compounds. *J. Infec. Dis.* 117:421–428, 1967.
27. Wessman, G.E., and G. Hilker. Characterization of *Pasteurella hemolytica* isolated from the respiratory tract of cattle. *Can. J. Comp. Med.* 32:498–504, 1968.

34. Listeria

Listeria monocytogenes is a specific cause of meningoencephalitis, abortion, and neonatal death in humans, sheep, cattle, goats, swine, and other animals.[1,2,4] In the northern hemisphere the meningoencephalitic form of the disease is most apt to affect animals during the months of January through March. The disease in ruminants is frequently associated with the feeding of silage that contains the bacterium. Laboratories involved in rabies diagnosis sometimes encounter *L. monocytogenes* as the cause of CNS disorders rather than rabies virus. Infections occur in a wide range of domestic and feral hosts including at least 37 species of mammals and 17 species of birds.[1,2]

Specimens

When the clinical process includes encephalitis, the head of the animal should be sent to the laboratory for aseptic removal of the brain. When the process involves genital infections, a portion of the placenta and some cotyledons along with the fetus should be included. All specimens should be taken aseptically, chilled, and promptly transported. Protective gloves and clothing should be worn while handling these materials since the organism is pathogenic for humans. Blood samples should be taken from affected animals and from some of the apparently normal animals for serologic support of a diagnosis.

Gross lesions are not obvious in fatal encephalitis cases in adult animals such as ruminants, but foci of necrosis may be seen in the liver, lungs, and spleen of fetuses, newborn animals, and various adult monogastric animals. The liver, spleen, lung, and uterus should be examined histopathologically for small multiple foci of necrosis. In cases of encephalitis the lesions are concentrated in the brain stem and anterior cervical cord. Tissue imprints stained by the Gram's or Giemsa methods, or by the FA technique, can be helpful in making a presumptive diagnosis.

The organism may not replicate readily when isolated from fresh tissue. To assure good opportunity for isolation, a 1 cm cube of tissue should be removed aseptically and titrated in a tissue grinder.

Laboratory Procedures

Cultures. Ample portions of organ paste should be streaked on tryptose agar plates (Difco Lab., Detroit) or blood agar plates. The same media plus the inhibitor potassium tellurite (0.05%) may also be used. Broth media such as tryptose or BHI broth are useful if one is reasonably certain that the inoculum is free of contaminating organisms. At the time original cultures are prepared, the remainder of each tissue specimen should be set aside for reculture. The tissue paste is taken up in about 5 ml of tryptose broth, placed in tubes, and held in the refrigerator (4°C) for 6 weeks to 2 months. Plating at weekly intervals from samples held at 4°C will greatly increase positive isolations of *L. monocytogenes*.

Visible colonies ordinarily form on plating media within 24–48 hours at 37°C. Examine the plates daily for 5 days, since visible colonies form slowly on media containing inhibitors such as potassium tellurite. To demonstrate motility, inoculate tubes of motility agar (SIM, from Difco) and hold at 22°C, since few or no flagella are produced at 37°C.

The colonies that arise from tissue isolations are smooth and round and have entire borders. They appear translucent in transmitted light and glistening and watery in reflected light. The colonies are approximately 0.5–1.5 mm in diameter. Isolations are frequently made from materials that may be contaminated with other microorganisms. The use of streak plates offers the advantage of colony separation, and cultivation on blood agar may aid recognition by the development of clear zones of hemolysis around the *L. monocytogenes* colonies. Many diagnosticians use a clear medium such as tryptose agar and examine the plates with obliquely transmitted light. In addition, the colonies have a blue-green color that differentiates them from the colors of contaminating organisms. After 24 hours of incubation, broth cultures give rise to a uniformly turbid broth that is light to moderate in the amount of growth. Further incubation will produce sedimented masses of cells that are viscous in character.

Differential reactions. *L. monocytogenes* ferments several carbohydrates, with the production of acid but not gas. Characteristically there is fermentation in glucose, trehalose, and salicin in 24 hours of incubation at 37°C; these fermentations are useful in the differentiation of *L. monocytogenes* from *Erysipelothrix insidiosa*. The organism is relatively resistant to potassium tellurite, which makes the inhibitor useful when isolations are made from contaminated specimens. Potassium tellurite will permit the growth of *L. monocytogenes* in addition to enterococci, *Corynebacteria*, and a few other organisms. All bacterial colonies appear black if grown in the presence of potassium tellurite.

Cellular morphology. Virulent *L. monocytogenes* cells are characteristically small, gram-positive rods that show some V-shaped figures where cells have not separated following fission. Some palisading is observed. The rods are approximately 1–2 μm long by 0.5 μm wide. The organism is not acid fast, does not form spores, and is generally considered to be noncapsulated. Motility, by means of one to four peritrichous flagella, is apparent in cultures grown at reduced temperatures.

Animal inoculation. Listeria monocytogenes produces a characteristic keratoconjunctivitis when instilled in the eye of a rabbit or guinea pig. The Anton test may be performed by touching the conjunctiva with a cotton swab dipped in a broth culture. Purulent exudate appears within 24 hours and is well advanced at 48 hours, with developing opacity of the cornea.

Several species of laboratory animals can be used to determine the pathogenicity of this organism. However, the mouse is often used because of its high susceptibility and convenience. Four or five mice are inoculated SC with each of several doses of a 24-hour tryptose broth culture, starting at 0.5 ml and decreasing to 0.001 ml. Death usually occurs 3–10 days following inoculation, and necropsies should reveal the characteristic multiple necrotic foci in the liver and spleen. Mice receiving the lower doses commonly survive.

The organism is pathogenic to a wide spectrum of mammals and birds following inoculation by several routes. Rabbits and mice are the most commonly used laboratory species for diagnosis. Guinea pigs and rats are somewhat more resistant. The characteristic monocytosis associated with this infection is readily observed in laboratory rodents but is not a feature of the disease in ruminants.

Immunology and serology. Serotypes are determined by antigenic analysis of somatic and flagellar antigens. The species is usually divided into five serotypes, designated types 1, 2, 3, 4a, and 4b. Some investigators have reported additional types on the basis of more critical analysis of the antigens. Type 4b appears to be most common among isolates from ruminants in the United States, and type 1 is most common in Europe.

Serodiagnosis has been difficult to apply because nearly all "normal" human beings and ruminants have serum antibodies that are reactive with *L. monocytogenes*.[3] It is now known that these antibodies in "apparently normal" individuals are of the IgM immunoglobulin class. When animals are infected with the organism, they synthesize antibodies of the IgG immunoglobulin class. A somatic agglutination test for the latter antibodies can be performed by treating whole serum with 2-mercaptoethanol (0.1 M). The chemical depolymerizes the IgM molecules and thus permits testing for the 2-mercaptoethanol–resistant IgG molecules. The method is simple and readily adaptable to the routine procedures of the serologic laboratory.

Listeria monocytogenes is susceptible to bacteriophages, which makes phage typing a possible method for categorizing strains. The method has not received wide application, though, because the phage types fall into essentially the same categories as the serotypes and therefore give no additional information.

The pathogenesis of the disease suggests that toxicity plays a role in the process; however, a toxin has not yet been convincingly described or characterized.

Reference laboratories. Laboratories for serologic typing include the CDC and the Institute for Hygiene and Microbiology, University of Würzburg, Würzburg, W. Ger.

References

1. Gray, M.L., and A.H. Killinger. *Listeria monocytogenes* and listeric infections. *Bact. Rev.* 30:309–382, 1966.
2. Osebold, J.W. The diagnosis of listeriosis. *Ann. Proc. U.S. Livestock Sanitary Ass.* 63:394–398, 1959.
3. Osebold, J.W., and O. Aalund. Interpretation of serum agglutinating antibodies to listeria monocytogenes by immunoglobulin differentiation. *J. Infec. Dis.* 118:139–148, 1968.
4. Seeliger, H.P.R. *Listeriosis*. Hafner, New York, 1961.

35. Erysipelothrix

Erysipelothrix rhusiopathiae (insidiosa) is worldwide in distribution, affects a variety of animals, and has been associated also with marine and fresh water fish.[3,5] The organism has been isolated from a variety of ectoparasites, processed meat, decomposing animal carcasses, and sewage from slaughterhouses and streams. The tonsils of healthy-appearing pigs are a common reservoir of the organism. The effect of the disease on domestic pigs, turkeys, and sheep, and on captive animals in zoos and aquariums, is of major economic importance. Erysipelas in its acute form cannot readily be differentiated from other diseases characterized by signs of septicemia; however, urticarial lesions in pigs and porpoises are indicators of infection by *E. rhusiopathiae*. The chronic form of the disease is characteristically associated with arthritis. Animals of all ages can be affected, and the sudden appearance of the acute form seems to be related to stress, which in turn has been related to late summer temperatures or inadequate precautions during transportation. Outbreaks in turkeys have been related to infected wounds incurred in fighting among maturing males. Infection by *E. rhusiopathiae* is also an occupational hazard (erysipeloid) for persons processing fresh meat and fish and for veterinarians.

Specimens

Hemocultures from the living animal can be useful in establishing a herd diagnosis of erysipelas, but because hemocultures of one affected animal may not be positive every day, they should be made from several animals.

Tissues for bacteriological examination should include portions of the main body organs, representative lymph nodes, one or more intact articulations, and, when urticarial lesions are observed, a section of affected skin with its underlying tissue. Also, sterile cotton-tipped applicators in individual containers can be used to obtain inoculum during the necropsy. The omission of tissues can lead to the failure of a laboratory confirmation of the clinical diagnosis, because the organisms may be few in number or seemingly absent in one or more locations, and numerous and easily isolated in others.

Erysipelothrix can cause a painful wound infection, even by way of superficial abrasions of the skin. For this reason, the use of rubber gloves and disinfectants and sterilization of instruments is recommended.

Urticarial lesions of a square or rhomboid appearance are the only characteristic clinical findings that can be directly related to infection with *Erysipelothrix*. Other lesions that may be seen (or have been described) are those of septicemia, and they cannot be referred to as typical of the disease. The presence in pigs, however, of an enlarged pulpy spleen, enlarged edematous lymph nodes, and a history of lameness with enlargement of one or more articulations are suggestive of infection with *E. rhusiopathiae*.

Direct staining of whole blood, synovial fluid, and tissue impressions can be accomplished with the usual bacteriological stains, particularly crystal violet or methylene blue for demonstrating cellular morphology. This diagnostic approach, however, cannot be considered a reliable means of positively determining the identification of *E. rhusiopathiae*.

For specimens for histologic examination, collection of soft tissues can be made in a routine manner. Before examining an articulation, remove the entire articulation and immerse it in a Formalin solution (10%); after 24 hours, divide the articulation with a saw longitudinally on the medium line parallel to the long axis and return it to the fixing solution. Subsequent sectioning after decalcification allows a comprehensive examination of the articulation because the relationships of the anatomic structures are retained.

Laboratory Procedures

Cultures. Cultures at necropsy from soft body organs such as the liver, spleen, and lungs can be made quickly from the organs *in situ* by plunging a sterile cotton-tipped applicator into the tissues after first making an opening in the surface with the broken end of a sterile wood applicator. The surface of an agar slant or plate is streaked with the cotton-tipped applicator, which then is snapped off into a tube of broth. Firm organs such as heart and kidney can be cultured in the same manner after making an opening in them with a sterile scalpel. This method of culture is generally quite adequate if acute erysipelas is suspected, and inoculations can be completed quickly during necropsy, an advantage when many cultures must be made.

Specimens of the skin of pigs affected by erysipelas are often cultured, and this is best done after removing the specimen along with part of the subcutaneous fat. The underside of the specimen is seared and a well made by removing a section of tissue down to the epidermis; carefully avoid puncturing the relatively thin epidermis. By making numerous crisscross cuts into the dermis and scraping with a sterile scalpel, tissue fluid and debris can be made available for inoculation into media with a flamed wire loop. Care must be taken to prevent hot grease from entering the well, as the organisms may be killed.

Because *E. rhusiopathiae* often causes arthritis, the joints of swine and other animals are usually cultured. This can be accomplished quickly during necropsy by opening the joint capsule at a point where the joint can be cracked open and sampling the synovial fluid with a sterile cotton-tipped applicator. An alternate method is to penetrate the joint capsule with a sterile hypodermic needle and aspirate some of the synovial fluid into a sterile syringe. The material obtained then can be cultured.[5] In many cases, especially with chronic arthritis, the organism is difficult to detect. Therefore, it is advisable to culture joints as efficiently as possible. The following procedure is recommended: the joint is removed intact by sawing through the limb on either side of it. The entire specimen is clamped in a vise and the skin is removed with a scalpel. The surface is seared thoroughly with a flame and the joint capsule is opened aseptically. Cultures are made from the contents with a flamed wire loop or sterile cotton-tipped applicator. It is important to probe all parts of the joint and to enter all synovial sacs, because the organism may be localized in only a small area.

It may be necessary to examine decomposing animal tissues, tonsils of swine, intestinal lymphoid tissue, feces, urine, soil, and other materials that contain large numbers of other organisms. There are several useful methods for isolating *E. rhusiopathiae* from such sources. A sensitive method for the detection of the organism is through the use of *Erysipelothrix* selective broth (ESB),[8] consisting of tryptose broth with the addition of antibiotics, followed by subculture on Packer's medium,[4] consisting of tryptose agar with sodium azide, crystal violet, and serum.

Preparation and culture of specimens are recommended as follows: body tissues are prepared by mincing or chopping into small pieces with scalpel or scissors and are placed directly into ESB. Liquid specimens, such as urine, are centrifuged at $13,000–14,000 \times g$ or put through a bacteria-retaining filter to concentrate the flora. The sediment or residue is suspended in ESB. The entire filter element can be placed in the liquid medium if desired. A particulate specimen, such as feces or soil, is dispersed in 5–10 times its weight of 0.1 M phosphate buffer with a stirring motor or by hand mixing. The suspension is then mixed with an equal volume of ESB that contains all ingredients except buffer salts in double concentration, so that final culture preparation contains the proper concentrations of antibiotics.

Increasing the relative concentration of bacterial flora in fecal specimens is usually desirable to reduce the relative content of other organic matter. A method for this procedure is as follows: a quantity of feces up to 50 g is placed in 5 times its weight of buffered 1% peptone solution. The mixture is stirred thoroughly to break up the material into small particles. Excessive foaming should be avoided; therefore a blender or other high-speed stirrer is not suitable. A stirring motor with a propeller operated at about 1500 rpm is satisfactory. The suspension is centrifuged for 8–10 minutes at $1000 \times g$ to settle the larger particles. The cloudy supernatant fluid is decanted and centrifuged at $13,000–14,000 \times g$ to settle the bacterial flora. The sediment is suspended in a quantity of ESB about 10 times the weight of the original fecal sample.

If time is not an important factor, a simple and sensitive method for cultural detection of *E. rhusiopathiae* in tissue specimens is the extended refrigeration method. A tissue specimen is placed in a flask containing tryptose broth or beef infusion broth and held at 4–5°C for 4–5 weeks. Subcultures are then made onto Packer's medium. This method is quite satisfactory for detection of the organism in tonsils and intestinal lymphoid tissue of swine; however, it has not been found satisfactory for fecal specimens.

Examination for *E. rhusiopathiae* can be made by direct inoculation onto solid selective media, but the sensitivity of this method is less than with the use of enrichment culture. Direct culture, however, has the advantage of being much faster, and is satisfactory if the organism can be assumed to be present in sufficient numbers to offset the loss of sensitivity. The most commonly used solid medium for selective growth of *E. rhusiopathiae* is Packer's medium, with either whole blood or serum. The use of serum has the advantage of leaving the medium transparent for easy observation of colonies with transmitted light. Packer's medium is sometimes modified by lowering the concentration of the sodium azide or crystal violet, or by eliminating one of them.

Primary cultures can be made in tryptose agar containing whole blood or serum, tryptose broth containing serum, and beef infusion broth or agar. Primary cultures from contaminated materials can be made in ESB and subcultures made on Packer's medium.

Usually, incubation of liquid mediums for 18–24 hours at 37°C is sufficient; however, 48-hour incubation is recommended when ESB medium is used. Cultures on commonly used solid mediums can be examined after 24–48 hours incubation. Subcultures on Packer's medium (plates or slants) should be examined after 72 hours of incubation. When ESB is used for enrichment culture, growth of the organism usually will be confluent wherever the inoculum is spread on the agar surface, if the culture contains *E. rhusiopathiae*.

E. rhusiopathiae is a facultative anaerobe. Growth is relatively scanty in ordinary media and requires serum or other highly nutritive material in the medium for abundant growth. The optimal temperature for growth is 37°C at a pH of 7.4–7.8.

Growth in liquid media is fairly distinctive when observed in pure culture in beef infusion or tryptose broth. Growth is relatively slow and at 24 hours presents a scanty appearance (about 10^6 cells per ml) that was best described by Theobald Smith in 1885 as "a faint opalescence . . . which on shaking, was resolved for the moment into delicate rolling clouds." At 48 hours and later, a slight sediment is visible, which will spiral upward forming a tail when the tube is gently shaken in a circular motion. Growth is much heavier in broth enriched with serum, and a powdery sediment is usually present after 24 hours. There is no pellicle.

The organism is observed in smooth, rough, and intermediate colony forms. Dissociation to rough forms is most readily seen in older cultures when colonies are well isolated and are observed for several days. Smooth colonies are 0.7–1 mm in diameter at 48 hours, are circular and convex, and have entire edges and a smooth surface. Rough colonies are circular, usually slightly larger than smooth colonies, and have an irregular edge with a flattened rough surface. Intermediate colonies have characteristics of both smooth and rough forms and can assume a variety of appearances.

Colonies are typically bluish-gray in diffuse transmitted light at 24–48 hours, and become darker and more opaque as they age. Characteristic granulelike structures appear in the medium under the thickest part of a colony. These granules are nearly always present, except in some smooth forms. Colonies of *E. rhusiopathiae* can be easily overlooked because of their small size, especially when less than 24 hours old and mixed with faster-growing colonies of other organisms.

On blood agar, a very slight zone of hemolysis is usually seen around smooth colonies. The hemolysis is seldom complete, and usually a greenish color appears that is similar to alpha-hemolysis in streptococci.

On Packer's medium, growth consists of tiny (<1 mm), slightly convex, translucent colonies. When viewed under a dissecting microscope at 7–30 diameters with diffused transmitted light, they give an appearance of opaque or frosted glass, because they have a rough surface and do not accumulate crystal violet dye from the medium.

The growth of a stab culture of *E. rhusiopathiae* in nutrient gelatin is characteristic and provides a simple test for tentative identification. A tube of nutrient gelatin is stabbed with inoculum and incubated at 20°C for 3–5 days. It is important that the gelatin not be allowed to melt at any time. The growth radiates out from the stab in all directions with a filamentous appearance, resembling the bristles of a test tube brush; hence the commonly used term "test tube brush" growth. The organism does not liquefy gelatin.

Differential reactions. Erysipelothrix rhusiopathiae is catalase negative, does not produce indole, does not produce nitrites from nitrates, does not hydrolyze esculin, produces weak acid or no change in litmus milk, and most strains produce H_2S in TSI agar, a medium recommended by Vickers and Bierer.[6] The medium should not be more than 2 weeks old. The pattern of carbohydrate fermentation will vary according to the medium, indicator, and method of measuring acid production. White and Shuman[7] found that Andrade's base with 10% serum was the most dependable medium because it allowed the least variation in patterns. The typical pattern of acid production in the medium from 20 fermentable carbon compounds by *E. rhusiopathiae* is given in Table 35.1. If other media are used, the researcher should become familiar with the patterns of reactions of known strains in those media.

Table 35.1. Acid production by *E. rhusiopathiae* in 48 hours from fermentable carbon compounds in Andrade's base with 10% serum

Compound	Reaction	Compound	Reaction
Arabinose	−	Maltose	+
Dextrin	+	Mannitol	−
Dulcitol	−	Mannose	+*
Fructose	+	Raffinose	−
Galactose	+	Rhamnose	−
Glucose	+	Salicin	−
Glycerol	−	Sorbitol	−
Inositol	−	Sucrose	±†
Inulin	−	Trehalose	−
Lactose	+	Xylose	−

*Acid produced slowly (5–10 days).
†±, slight acid produced.

Cellular morphology. E. rhusiopathiae is gram-positive but easily decolorized, especially older cultures. The organism appears as a straight or curved slender rod, $0.2-0.4 \times 0.5-2.5$ μm, or as filamentous forms 4–15 μm in length. It is nonmotile, noncapsulated, and nonacid-fast, and does not form spores. The cellular morphology of *E. rhusiopathiae* depends on the type of colony. In smooth colonies the organism is a slender rod, often curved, occurring singly or in very short chains. The latter tend to be sharply curved or angular, suggesting the snapping division and palisade formation of diphtheroids. In rough colonies, long filamentous forms predominate. These may appear to be solid or in a definite chain. The filamentous forms resemble fungus mycelia, but without branching. Granules or beading are often seen, further suggesting diphtheroids.

A form intermediate between smooth and rough is seen most often, especially in isolates from sources other than acutely ill animals or from cultures several days old. The typical cell morphology consists of chains two to several cells in length and sharply curved, suggesting the letters C, S, and J. Considerable variation in morphology of the intermediate forms may be seen in the same field, from coccoid to filamentous.

Animal inoculation. Mice may be used for culture of *E. rhusiopathiae* from tissues and other specimens as follows: (1) direct SC inoculation of mice with material from the specimen; (2) a short period of incubation of the culture in a liquid medium, followed by inoculation onto scarified skin of the ears of mice; or (3) extended refrigeration in a liquid medium followed by inoculation of mice SC or onto scarified ears.

Inoculum is prepared by grinding the specimen in a mortar and pestle on a Ten Broeck grinder with a small amount of buffered 0.85% NaCl solution. Then 0.1–0.5 ml is injected SC into each of several mice (white Swiss, 16–20 g). When death occurs (ordinarily within 3–6 days), the heart blood is cultured.

The use of mice has the disadvantage of depending on the virulence of the strain of *E. rhusiopathiae* being sought. However, inoculation of mice via scarified skin instead of by SC injection has the advantage of eliminating many deaths caused by infection of the mouse by a contaminant, since most of the common contaminants do not possess the invasiveness of *E. rhusiopathiae* for scarified skin. Thus it is best to use this method for specimens that have a heavy population of other organisms.

Immunology and serology. The mouse protection test is commonly used for identification of *E. rhusiopathiae*. It is generally regarded as necessary for complete confirmation of identification, especially of newly isolated strains. The test is based on the protection of exposed mice with specific hyperimmune serum. The test requires, of course, that the strain in question be virulent for mice. Commercial equine hyperimmune anti-erysipelas serum is satisfactory for the test and is readily available from manufacturers of veterinary biologics. The procedure is as follows: each of a group of mice is inoculated with 0.1 ml of 24-hour broth culture by injection. The loose skin of the flank area is recommended. In the opposite flank, 0.3 ml of antiserum is injected. Another group of mice is inoculated with culture only. If the organism is *E. rhusiopathiae,* the mice receiving culture and antiserum should survive, and those receiving culture without antiserum should become ill and die within 6 days. It is advisable to conduct a parallel test with a known virulent strain of *E. rhusiopathiae* as a check on the antiserum. If the unknown is avirulent for mice, the serum of rabbits can be tested, after a series of IV inoculations, for the presence of specific agglutinins, using *E. rhusiopathiae* tube or plate antigen. A strong agglutination reaction will confirm the identification.

Serologic examination is now necessary for identification of *E. rhusiopathiae;* however, a precipitation test is used to identify serologic variants within the species. These variants are based on specific acid-soluble antigens, and most strains fall into one of two groups, A or B. In addition, several minor groups have been reported. Strains in which no antigen is detected are called N forms. A microagar double diffusion method is recommended. The procedure is as follows: in preparing the acid extract, a pure culture is grown at 37°C for 18–24 hours in beef infusion or tryptose broth with 10% serum. The cells are harvested by centrifugation and washed twice in 0.85% NaCl solution containing 0.01% thimerosal. Washed cells are resuspended in a volume of 0.03 N acetic acid that is equal to one-fortieth of the original culture volume, and they are then heated 45 minutes in a boiling water bath. The residue is then removed by centrifugation and discarded. The supernatant fluid is neutralized with 4% NaOH and centrifuged again to clarify it. The extract may be stored at 4°C. Agar diffusion slides are prepared using a 1% agar solution containing 0.03% $NaH_2PO_4 \cdot H_2O$, 0.06% Na_2HPO_4, and 0.01% thimerosal. Standard 25–75 mm microscope slides that have a frosted marking area on one end are preferable. A line is made with a wax pencil across each slide at the junction of the frosted and smooth portions, and 3 ml of melted agar is applied to the slide with a pipette. If done carefully, the liquid will not run off the edge or onto the marking area. The slides are left undisturbed until the agar hardens. These preparations can be stored for several days at 4°C in a container to retard dehydration.

Wells 3 mm in diameter and 3–5 mm apart are cut in the desired pattern, and agar within the wells is removed by aspiration with a micropipette. After the wells are charged with appropriate extracts and antisera, the slides are incubated overnight at room temperature in a covered petri dish. A piece of moistened cotton may be placed in the dish to prevent drying.

The FA test can be applied to *E. rhusiopathiae* and has been used for rapid tentative identification or confirmation of results of other tests. The test, however, is not essential for identification of the organism. The methods given by Cherry et al.[2] are applicable.

Brill and Politynska[1] have reported that two isolated phages were capable of lysing a number of strains of *E. rhusiopathiae*. On further investigation, they found no correlation between lysis and serologic type.

Pathogenicity is variable over a large number of animal species. Commonly available species such as mice, rabbits, and pigeons are susceptible to experimental infection. Pigs of all ages also are susceptible providing they have had no previous contact with the organism, or, when young pigs are employed, have had no colostrum from immune dams.

No toxin has been associated with *E. rhusiopathiae*.

Reference laboratories. NADC; ATCC.

References

1. Brill, J., and E. Politynska. The phages and lysogeny of *Erysipelothrix rhusiopathiae*. *Proc. Internat. Vet. Cong.* 16(2):511–512, 1959.
2. Cherry, W.B., M. Goldman, and T.R. Carski. *Fluorescent Antibody Techniques in the Diagnosis of Communicable Diseases*. Public Health Service Publication no. 729. U.S. Government Printing Office, Washington, 1961.
3. Clark, W.A., and H.P.R. Seeliger. Minutes of the international committee on nomenclature of bacteria, July 23–25, 1966, Moscow: Minute 16. *Internat. J. Syst. Bact.* 17(1):73–78, 1967.
4. Packer, R.A. The use of sodium azide (NaN_3) and crystal violet in a selective medium for streptococci and *Erysipelothrix rhusiopathiae*. *J. Bact.* 46:343–349, 1943.
5. Shuman, R.D., and G. Wellmann. Status of the species name *Erysipelothrix rhusiopathiae* with request for an opinion. *Internat. J. Syst. Bact.* 16(2):195–196, 1966.
6. Vickers, C.L., and B.W. Bierer. Triple sugar iron agar as an aid in the diagnosis of Erysipelas. *J. Am. Vet. Med. Ass.* 133:543–544, 1958.

7. White, T.G., and R.D. Shuman. Fermentation reactions of *Erysipelothrix rhusiopathiae*. *J. Bact.* 82:595–599, 1961.
8. Wood, R.L. A selective liquid medium utilizing antibiotics for the isolation of *Erysipelothrix insidiosa*. *Am. J. Vet. Res.* 26:1303–1308, 1965.

36. Bacillus

The genus *Bacillus* comprises a large group of gram-positive, aerobic, spore-forming rods that are abundant in soil and are commonly found as laboratory contaminants. Most of these species are not pathogenic for animals or humans, although some, such as *Bacillus subtilis,* can cause infection if given an opportunity, and *Bacillus cereus* can grow in food and may lead to food poisoning in humans. The pathogenic species is *Bacillus anthracis,* the causative organism of anthrax. The task of laboratories dealing with veterinary bacteriology is to differentiate this organism from saprophytic *Bacillus*. Identification is not difficult, but it is important because conclusive diagnosis of anthrax depends upon laboratory confirmation. The procedures for identification described in this chapter use techniques readily available to any bacteriology laboratory. Identification is made by a progression of tests in which a few fundamental characters are used first to suggest the presence of a *Bacillus,* and then additional tests are used to determine whether the organism is *B. anthracis*.

Anthrax can occur as an acute, subacute, or chronic disease. Cattle, horses, mules, sheep, and goats are most commonly affected, and in these animals the disease can be apoplectic, with death occurring suddenly in the absence of noticeable prodromal signs. Usually the disease progresses more slowly with signs developing within 24 hours. Animals manifest fever, depression, weakness, bloody discharges from body orifices, and edematous swellings of the body. Death may occur within 2–5 days, although some animals completely recover. Chronic anthrax occurs mostly in swine and is characterized by enlarged submaxillary, cervical, or mesenteric lymph nodes. Postmortem examinations of acute or subacute anthrax show edematous and hemorrhagic changes throughout the body, particularly in serous membranes. Lymph nodes are usually swollen, edematous, and hemorrhagic. The spleen is characteristically enlarged, dark, friable, and engorged with blood. Microscopic examination of smears of splenic tissue usually show large numbers of rod-shaped bacteria.

Anthrax is worldwide in distribution, with the highest incidence in animals occurring in Iran, Chile, and Central America.[11] The true incidence is difficult to establish because countries vary in their accuracy of reporting the disease. Endemic areas exist in the United States, particularly along the Gulf Coast, but sporadic outbreaks occur throughout the country. Many outbreaks of anthrax in the United States, Canada, and the western European countries stem from the use of animal feeds imported from countries in which anthrax is prevalent. The disease in animals usually occurs during the temperate time of year. Infection in humans occurs secondarily to the disease in animals, usually by the handling of infected carcasses or products such as hair, hides, or wool.

Specimens

All animals suspected of having anthrax should be handled only by a veterinarian, and postmortem examinations should be done with extreme caution to prevent infection of people and to limit contamination of the soil. Immediately after examination, infected carcasses must be cremated on the spot to prevent spread of anthrax bacteria to surrounding areas. Since virulent *B. anthracis* can be recovered from samples of soil stored for many years, careful adherence to these measures will help prevent future outbreaks.

Specimens for the laboratory should be collected as soon after death as possible. Usually, specimens collected from decomposed carcasses are of little value because *B. anthracis* may be destroyed or overgrown by putrefactive microorganisms. If animals have been treated with antibiotics prior to examination, anthrax bacteria may be impossible to isolate from specimens.

Specimens for laboratory examinations may include the following: (1) smears from blood or spleen made on clean glass slides; (2) sterile cotton swabs, gauze, or suture tape impregnated with splenic pulp and then placed in sterile sealed containers; and (3) a few milliliters of blood drawn aseptically with a sterile syringe and placed in a sterile sealed tube. The time-honored practice of submitting a severed ear to the laboratory is not satisfactory, although many isolations of *B. anthracis* have been made from the blood of such specimens. Rapid submission of specimens to the laboratory is most important for bacteriological diagnosis, since *B. anthracis* can be readily isolated from fresh materials that are not grossly contaminated with other microorganisms.

In cases of suspected anthrax in which the signs and pathology are not characteristic, samples are best taken from localized edematous areas or from lymph nodes, particularly those in the cervical region. These specimens are particularly important in chronic anthrax of swine, where it is difficult to isolate organisms from the blood. A diagnosis of anthrax cannot be made by gross examination. An enlarged dark spleen is suggestive, particularly if associated with edematous and hemorrhagic changes in other parts of the carcass, but positive diagnosis of anthrax can be made only by the laboratory after isolation and identification of virulent *B. anthracis* from a specimen.

In typical cases of anthrax, a presumptive diagnosis may sometimes be made by microscopic examination of stained smears from the blood or spleen, particularly if the specimen is fresh. However, it must be emphasized that this diagnosis is only presumptive, since many other bacilli microscopically resemble *B. anthracis*. Ordinary stains do not demonstrate the typical appearance of virulent anthrax bacteria when they are present in fresh specimens. Giemsa or Wright's stains can be used, but the simplest effective method is staining with polychrome methylene blue. When stained by the latter procedure, virulent encapsulated cells of *B. anthracis* appear as short chains of blue rods with square ends, surrounded by pink amorphous material that probably represents remnants of the capsule. This method was first described by McFadyean and still represents one of the best procedures for the presumptive diagnosis of anthrax.[9] Methods in which FA are used to identify *B. anthracis* are not specific and cannot yet be used for diagnosis.[5]

Tissue from the spleen or from lymph nodes can be taken for histologic examination, but since the etiologic diagnosis of anthrax depends upon isolation and identification of *B. anthracis,* these specimens are not essential.

Laboratory Procedures

Cultures. Fresh specimens collected from uncontaminated sources onto cotton swabs, gauze, or suture tape are wetted with a few milliliters of sterile nutrient broth and shaken for a few seconds, and then the broth is streaked with an inoculating loop on plates of blood agar and bicarbonate agar. Samples of blood can be streaked directly on the same two media. If specimens are heavily contaminated, they may be heated to 65°C for 5 minutes before streaking; this procedure should eliminate many contaminating bacteria that do not form spores. However, as a precautionary measure, the original specimen should also be streaked before heating, because anthrax bacteria that have not yet sporulated can be killed by heating.

Anthrax bacteria are difficult to isolate from sources such as bone meal, animal feeds, hair, hides, and wool that may be heavily contaminated with other microorganisms. An effective procedure is to cut about 10–20 g of the sample into small pieces, place the pieces in a sterile container, cover them with 2% aqueous phenol, and allow the mixture to stand with occasional shaking for about 30 minutes. Resuspend the material before streaking the suspension directly on blood agar and bicarbonate agar. This method enhances the likelihood of recovering *B. anthracis* because anthrax spores are quite resistant to phenol. Samples also can be heated as previously described, or they can be soaked in caustic agents such as KOH for about 20–30 minutes before streaking.

Blood agar may be prepared from any of the commercial brands of dehydrated media sold for this purpose. Bicarbonate agar plates must be freshly prepared. Selective media that permit growth of *B. anthracis* but inhibit growth of various other microorganisms are described in the literature but have not been widely used.[6,10] Cultures are incubated at temperatures between 25 and 37°C. Most important is incubation of bicarbonate agar plates both aerobically and in candle jars.

Colonies will appear on agar plates within 24 hours of incubation at 35–37°C. When incubated in air, isolated colonies on blood agar are nonhemolytic and have an irregular, ground-glass, hairlike appearance ("Medusa head" colony) that is characteristic of rough forms of bacteria. However, these dull, gray, flat colonies are not unique to the species because other saprophytic members of the genus have a similar colony morphology when grown aerobically. Most strains of *B. cereus* are hemolytic.

An important colony characteristic of virulent anthrax bacilli is their appearance on bicarbonate agar when the plates are incubated in the atmosphere of CO_2 provided by a candle jar. Under these conditions, virulent *B. anthracis* may be readily distinguished from avirulent strains and from *B. cereus* and *B. megaterium*. Colonies of *B. anthracis* are unique, being smooth, gray, mucoid, and glistening, with a brightly reflecting sur-

Table 36.1. Characteristics of some common species of bacillus

	Motility	Gelatin liquefaction	Starch hydrolysis	Hemolysis of sheep RBC	Milk peponization	Citrate use	Nitrate reduction	V-P reaction	Arabinose	Acid production from Glucose	Mannitol	Salicin
anthracis	−	+	+	−	−	+	+	+	−	+	−	−
brevis	+	+	−	X	V	V	−	−	−	+	+	X
cereus	+	+	+	+	+	+	+	+	−	+	−	V
circulans	+	+	+	X	acid	−	+	+	+	+	V	X
licheniformis	+	+	+	−	V	+	+	−	+	+	+	+
megaterium	+	+	+	X	V	+	+	−	+	+	+	V
mycoides	+	+	+	−	+	+	+	+	−	+	+	X
pumilus	+	+	−	X	+	+	−	+	+	+	−	X
sphaericus	+	+	−	X	−	−	−	−	−	−	−	X
subtilis	+	+	+	V	+	+	+	+	+	+	+	V

X, not indicated in literature cited; V, some strains positive, others negative.

face. In contrast, colonies of avirulent anthrax strains or of *B. cereus* are rough and show a dull gray surface that neither glistens nor reflects light. Colonies of *B. megaterium* are usually pale yellow with a dull surface. If bicarbonate agar plates are incubated in air, colonies of virulent and avirulent *B. anthracis, B. cereus,* and *B. megaterium* all appear rough, with a dull, gray, ground-glass surface that does not glisten or reflect light. Usually *B. megaterium* does not grow on bicarbonate agar plates incubated in air, and virulent anthrax strains often also fail to grow under these conditions. These striking morphologic differences have been neglected as a means to identify virulent strains of *B. anthracis*, although Burdon et al.[3] reported a perfect correlation between the capacity to form smooth colonies on bicarbonate agar plates incubated in CO_2 and the virulence of anthrax strains. Even inexperienced technicians can readily distinguish the colony differences.

Differential reactions. Table 36.1 lists several bacteriological characteristics of *B. anthracis*, as well as those of other species of *Bacillus* that are commonly encountered in the laboratory. A multitude of tests are required to differentiate all of these species. Fortunately, a few important characteristics can be selected that enable the laboratory to identify *B. anthracis*. Most investigators now agree that it is a separate and distinct species of *Bacillus*.[7]

Differentiation of *B. anthracis* from *B. cereus* or *B. megaterium* causes the most confusion. The three species can be readily differentiated by using four criteria from Table 36.1 plus two additional tests, and by animal pathogenicity. A list of these characteristics is given in Table 36.2. All the tests can be readily done by a laboratory doing routine diagnostic bacteriology.

The presence or absence of growth on agar containing pencillin is an important differentiating criterion, since virulent strains of *B. anthracis* are sensitive to penicillin.[1] This sensitivity is probably responsible for the "string of pearls" phenomenon.[8] To observe this phenomenon, anthrax bacteria are streaked on agar containing penicillin, and after a few hours of incubation the areas where growth might be expected are examined

Table 36.2. Characteristics that distinguish *B. anthracis*, smooth and rough, *B. cereus*, and *B. megaterium* (all cultures incubated at 35–37°C)

Tests	B. anthracis Smooth	B. anthracis Rough	B. cereus	B. megaterium
Motility in agar	−	−	+	+
Hemolysis on sheep's blood agar (24 hr)	−	−	+	−
Litmus milk peptonization (72 hr)	−	−	+	V
Salicin fermentation	−	−	+	−
Growth on penicillin agar	−	−	+	−
Growth on bicarbonate (0.7%) agar				
In air	R	R	R	NG
In a candle jar	S	R	R	SY
Death of mice				
Within 24–48 hr	+	−	−	−
Spleen smear, capsular stain of bacteria with polychrome methylene blue	+	−	−	−

V, variable, some strains positive, others negative; R, rough, dull, gray, flat colonies; S, smooth, mucoid, glistening, raised colonies; SY, smooth, yellow, dull, raised colonies; NG, no growth.

microscopically for the presence of large round cellular forms. According to Leise et al., even avirulent rough strains of *B. anthracis* that are resistant to penicillin can be characterized by the reaction.[8]

As mentioned, no one characteristic will differentiate strains of *B. anthracis* from other members of the genus. For instance, although there have been no reports of motile strains of *B. anthracis,* nonmotile strains of other species such as *B. cereus* or *B. megaterium* are found. Similarly, some strains of *B. cereus* are sensitive to penicillin. In particular, rough strains of *B. anthracis* may resemble *B. cereus.* Some rough strains are resistant to penicillin, others produce hemolysis, others effect peptonization of milk; and the colony morphology on agar media, including bicarbonate agar incubated under CO_2, is similar to that of *B. cereus.* However, a single rough strain will not exhibit all the characteristics of *B. cereus* and thus can be identified as a strain of *B. anthracis.*[4,8]

Cellular morphology. *B. anthracis* is a large gram-positive rod that usually occurs in short chains. The bacteria vary in size from 4.5 to 10 μm in width. Spores are formed aerobically but are not formed in vivo where the oxygen tension is lower. These spores usually are located centrally within the cell and do not exceed the diameter of the vegetative cell. The bacteria are not motile and do not possess flagella. When examined in smears from infected animals or from smooth colonies growing on bicarbonate agar in a candle jar, virulent anthrax bacilli are surrounded by a large capsule. However, the capsule is difficult to see in gram-stained preparations. Capsules are best demonstrated from in vitro cultures by examining wet India ink preparations.

Animal inoculation. Mice or guinea pigs are preferred for inoculation. The strain of mice is not important; mature hash mice of 15–20 g are as useful as purebred types.

Typical colonies grown on either blood agar or bicarbonate agar are emulsified in a few milliliters of saline. Mice are inculated SC in the thigh or abdominal region with 0.1 ml, or with 0.5 ml IP. Injection of virulent *B. anthracis* will usually cause death within 16–48 hours. If injected mice are not dead at the end of 72 hours, the suspected organism is probably not virulent *B. anthracis*. Death before 16 hours is also not usually due to anthrax.

All dead animals are autopsied. Smears are made from the spleen and blood, and heart blood is inoculated onto bicarbonate agar plates. Autopsies are carried out with caution, preferably in dissecting trays. Liberal use of disinfectants both on the carcass before it is opened and on the dissecting tray itself is advisable. A wise procedure is to place the animal's carcass on paper towels soaked with a disinfectant such as 1:1000 $HgCl_2$ or 5% phenol.

Animal inoculations are best carried out with suspensions of pure cultures, because contaminating organisms can limit the in vivo growth of *B. anthracis* or cause death of the injected animal earlier than anthrax infection. However, if the need arises, contaminated material or impure cultures can be inoculated into mice or guinea pigs by the scratch method, in which a few drops of material are rubbed into a previously scarified area of skin. Anthrax bacteria can usually penetrate the skin and establish an infection more readily than contaminating microorganisms. When this procedure is employed, the laboratory must be certain that virulent forms of *B. anthracis* are isolated and identified from injected animals that die.

Animal pathogenicity must be demonstrated before identifying a *Bacillus* as a virulent strain of *B. anthracis*. An important sequence to animal pathogenicity is recovery of typical virulent anthrax bacilli from heart blood and demonstration of capsules in vivo. For the latter, use impression smears made from the cut surface of the spleen and stained with polychrome methylene blue.

Immunology and serology. Although the species of *Bacillus* have a number of antigens, serologic procedures are not of value for differentiation. A complex group of toxic materials are produced by *B. anthracis* but they are not used for identification. Good commercial vaccines are available for control of anthrax.

Specific bacteriophages are available for *B. anthracis,* but as Wright points out, no one strain of bacteriophage will lyse all strains of *B. anthracis,*[13] and some phages may lyse only nonencapsulated strains. For identification, the gamma or W phages are used since these phages apparently are most specific.[2,8] However, none of the phages are as yet readily available, and for this reason, susceptibility to phage is not included in the procedure for identifying virulent *B. anthracis*. Lysis by bacteriophage is, rather, a confirmatory test that can be carried out in special laboratories.

Reference laboratory. Although the procedure outlined for identification of virulent *B. anthracis* will usually be sufficient for bacteriological confirmation and diagnosis of typical cases of anthrax, problems may arise from atypical cases. The CDC can be called upon for assistance.

One additional problem may occur: an anthrax disease that arises from infections with vaccine strains of *B. anthracis*. Because these strains are usually rough, they do not form smooth colonies on bicarbonate agar medium incubated in a candle jar, nor are they pathogenic for mice within the time period indicated in Table 36.2. However, these strains can usually be differentiated from *B. cereus* by the other criteria listed in that table. The question of whether a vaccine strain caused anthrax in an animal must then be decided by the veterinarian once a culture has been identified as a rough strain of *B. anthracis*.

References

1. Bennett, E.O., G.E. Peterson, and R.P. Williams. Penicillin sensitivity as compared with nucleic acid phosphorus content of virulent and avirulent strains of *Bacillus anthracis* and *Bacillus cereus*. *Antibiot. Chemother.* 9:115–120, 1959.
2. Brown, E.R., and W.B. Cherry. Specific identification of *Bacillus anthracis* by means of a variant bacteriophage. *J. Infec. Dis.* 96:34–39, 1955.
3. Burdon, K.L., E. Comstock, R.D. Wende, and B. Henry. Capsule formation in bicarbonate-containing medium as a test for the identity and virulence of anthrax bacilli. *Bact. Proc.* 55:106, 1955.
4. Burdon, K.L., and R.D. Wende. On the differentiation of anthrax bacilli from *Bacillus cereus*. *J. Infec. Dis.* 107:224–234, 1960.
5. Cherry, W.B., and E.M. Freeman. Staining bacterial smears with fluorescent antibody. *Zentralblatt Bakt.* 175:582–597, 1959.
6. Knisely, R.F. Selective medium for *Bacillus anthracis*. *J. Bact.* 92:784–786, 1966.
7. Lamanna, C. The anthrax question. *Fed. Proc.* 26:1491–1492, 1967.
8. Leise, J.M., C.H. Carter, H. Friedlander, and S.W. Freed. Criteria for the identification of *Bacillus anthracis*. *J. Bact.* 77:655–660, 1959.
9. McFadyean, J.A. A peculiar staining reaction of the blood of animals dead of anthrax. *J. Comp. Path. Ther.* 16:35–40, 1903.
10. Morris, E.J. A selective medium for *Bacillus anthracis*. *J. Gen. Bact.* 13:456–460, 1955.

11. Sterne, M. Distribution and economic importance of anthrax. *Fed. Proc.* 26:1493–1495, 1967.
12. Wilson, J.B., and K.E. Russell. Isolation of *Bacillus anthracis* from soil stored 60 years. *J. Bact.* 87:237–238, 1964.
13. Wright, G.C. The anthrax bacillus. *In Bacterial and Mycotic Infections of Man,* R.J. Dubos and J.G. Hirsch (eds.). 4th ed. Lippincott, Philadelphia, 1965.

37. Moraxella

The genus *Moraxella* has been found associated exclusively with the conjunctiva or the upper respiratory tract. Although the guinea pig has recently been recognized as a natural host, the principal hosts are humans and cattle. *Moraxella lacunata* (Morax-Axenfield bacillus) has been found only in humans. *Moraxella liquefaciens* (diplobacillus of Petit) produces central corneal ulcers in humans and has also been isolated from the conjunctivas of normal guinea pigs.[10] *Moraxella bovis* produces conjunctivitis and central corneal ulcers in cattle.[1,2,4,5,7] Under experimental conditions, conjunctival infection has been established in mice and sheep but corneal lesions occurred only in mice.

There has been considerable interest in the taxonomic aspects of this genus.[3] It is quite possible that the number of *Moraxella* species will be enlarged to include other similar types of organisms. Only one species, *Moraxella bovis,* appears to be of veterinary significance, and it is the cause of bovine infectious keratoconjunctivitis, in conjunction with certain environmental factors.[7] The disease is seen during the summer months in calves and older cattle. It appears in a cyclic pattern. After a particularly severe outbreak, a given herd may have several summers with only a few individual cases before the next severe epizootic occurs. The disease begins as a conjunctivitis that is recognized only by an increased vascular congestion and an increase in the tear pool. When the cornea becomes involved, there is a distinct lacrimation with tears overflowing the eyelid and running down the cheek. The corneal lesion begins as a minute ulcer that is usually central. The cornea surrounding the ulcer becomes edematous and, as a consequence of the edema, becomes translucent as the ulcer progressively enlarges. Severely affected corneas become completely opaque within 2–3 days and by 5–7 days vascularization commences at the limbus. By day 20, the vascular ring has progressed to the center of the cornea where it coalesces. Thereafter the vascularity diminishes into a dense central scar. Less frequently, corneal erosion occurs, which may result in panophthalmitis and functional loss of the eyeball.

Erosion of the margin of the eyelid occurs in some chronically infected eyes. These ulcers are usually moist, grayish, and quite variable in size and shape. They may involve one or both canthi as well as all or part of either or both lid margins; eventually they heal spontaneously after a few days or weeks duration.

The disease is recognized in most states of the United States and has been reported from several regions of the world (Australia, Great Britain, India). In the midwest region of the United States, at least, the disease is nearly universal in that most herds have the disease periodically, if not annually.

Specimens

Material for cultural examination is gathered on sterile cotton-tipped applicators. The swab is introduced into the conjunctival sac and rotated to collect lacrimal secretions as well as conjunctival secretions. Allow the swab to become saturated. Care should be taken to avoid the lid margins, which usually are contaminated. Swabs should be kept moist until cultures are made. Any suitable proteinaceous diluent will be satisfactory. Swabs may be preserved by freezing (in diluent) for long periods with only a slight reduction in viability.

The isolation of *M. bovis* from cattle eyes in relation to the time of appearance of overt signs of disease is quite variable. An incubation period of hours to more than 1 month has been seen. Some authors have reported isolation of *M. bovis* for periods of 1 year. Furthermore, not all infected eyes develop disease. For the foregoing reasons, then, both normal and diseased eyes should be examined.

Swab specimens are characteristically devoid of gross material. The lacrimal secretions are clear and free from pus. Occasionally, hair may be removed from the ventral conjunctival sac, particularly from beef-type animals. Smears may be made for Gram's or Wright's staining, but the results are equivocal. Histopathologic examination of the cornea usually shows only edema, epithelial discontinuity, and loss of stroma.

Laboratory Procedures

Cultures. The swab specimens of lacrimal and conjunctival fluids should be streaked directly on the culture medium. Considerable variation exists in the number and types of bacteria present in these specimens. The streaking should be carried out in such a way that maximum exposure of the swab is made on the surface of the medium while still obtaining discrete colony distribution.

The medium of choice is any blood agar base enriched with 5% defibrinated bovine blood.[9] Plates should be incubated aerobically for 24 hours at 37°C. An additional 24 hours at 22°C (room temperature) will facilitate the selection of hemolytic *M. bovis* colonies.

After 24 hours incubation at 37°C, *M. bovis* colonies, 1–3 mm in diameter, appear circular with an entire edge, convex to umbonate, glistening, translucent, grayish-white, and slightly indented into the medium. The colony texture is firm and adherent but tends to fracture when moved along the surface of the medium. The hemolytic zone, of the beta type, ranges from 0.5 to 1 mm in width. After an additional 24 hours at 22°C, the colonies increase to 3–4 mm in diameter and appear flat, and the hemolytic zone increases to 1–1.5 mm in width.

Nonhemolytic variants of *M. bovis* occur both in stock cultures and culture from cattle eyes. These variants are stable and are indistinguishable from *M. bovis* in all other respects.

The tendency toward rough colony formation is pronounced, and unless care is taken to select smooth colonies for transfer, the rough colonies rapidly become the predominant type.

Smooth colony growth in liquid medium is scant even after 48–72 hours incubation. Turbidity is slight but considerable coarse sediment develops. Selection of turbid growth for transfer results in a more turbid culture with correspondingly less sediment; at the same time the rough colony types become increasingly predominant.

Smooth colony growth scraped from the surface solid medium is difficult to suspend in most liquids. Uniform dispersion has been achieved in 10% magnesium chloride solution, thereby permitting viable cell counts.[8]

Cellular morphology. *M. bovis* cells are gram-negative, short ($0.5–1 \times 1.5–2$ μm), plump rods with rounded ends, and occur in pairs or in short chains. Older cultures show progressively more pleomorphism. The organism is nonacid-fast, nonsporeforming, and nonmotile. Capsules may be seen in recently isolated cultures.

Differential reactions. *M. bovis* and *M. liquefaciens* do not ferment or oxidize the usual carbohydrates and the media become slightly more alkaline. Both species are oxidase positive.

Gelatin is liquified slowly and growth in litmus milk is characteristic. After several days incubation, three distinct zones become discernible—an upper zone of clear dark blue liquid, a middle zone of lavender soft curd, and a bottom layer of pale lavender coagulated casein. Complete peptonization occurs after prolonged incubation. Nitrates are reduced by *Moraxella liquefaciens* but not by *Moraxella bovis*.

Use of conventional diagnostic immunologic and serologic tests or animal inoculation tests is not practical for routine purposes. No bacteriophage has been demonstrated. Genetic transformation studies and DNA base ratio determinations may yet prove to be of some value in taxonomic research but are not practical for diagnostic use.

A labile hemolytic toxin, associated with the viable cell, and a thermostable dermonecrotic toxin have been reported.[6] These toxins may be associated with the virulence of *M. bovis*.

References

1. Adinarayanan, N., and S.B. Singh. Infectious bovine keratitis with special reference to isolation of *Moraxella bovis*. Vet. Rec. 73:694–696, 1961.
2. Barner, R.D. A study of *Moraxella bovis* and its relation to bovine keratitis. Am. J. Vet. Res. 13:132–144, 1952.
3. Bovre, K. Transformation and DNA composition in taxonomy, with special reference to recent studies in Moraxella and Neisseria. Acta Path. Microbiol. Scand. 69:123–144, 1967.
4. Faul, W.B., and M.B. Hanksley. Infectious keratitis in cattle associated with *Moraxella bovis*. Vet. Rec. 66:311–312, 1954.
5. Gallagher, C.H. Investigations of the etiology of infectious ophthalmia of cattle. Austral. Vet. J. 30:61–68, 1954.
6. Henson, J.B., and L.C. Grumbles. Infectious bovine keratoconjunctivitis. III. Demonstration of toxins in *Moraxella* (Haemophilus) *bovis* cultures. Cornell Vet. 51:267–284, 1961.

7. Hughes, D.E., G.W. Pugh, Jr., and T.J. McDonald. Ultraviolet radiation and *Moraxella bovis* in the etiology of bovine infectious keratoconjunctivitis. *Am. J. Vet. Res.* 26:1331–1338, 1965.
8. Pugh, G.W., Jr., and D.E. Hughes. Inhibition of autoagglutination of *Moraxella bovis* by 10% magnesium chloride. *Appl. Microbiol.* 19:201–203, 1970.
9. Pugh, G.W., Jr., D.E. Hughes, and T.J. McDonald. The isolation and characterization of *Moraxella bovis*. *Am. J. Vet. Res.* 27:957–962, 1966.
10. Ryan, W.J. Moraxella commonly present on the conjunctiva of guinea pigs. *J. Gen. Microbiol.* 35:361–372, 1964.

38. Haemobartonella

Haemobartonella species are pathogenic microorganisms that parasitize erythrocytes of several vertebrate species and are probably naturally transmitted by arthropods.[2] Clinical disease, characterized by anemia, is usually not apparent unless the animal is splenectomized, except in the case of *Haemobartonella felis*.[1] Representative species are *Haemobartonella muris* of mice and rats, *Haemobartonella felis* of cats, *Haemobartonella bovis* of cattle, and *Haemobartonella canis*, which has been widely reported in dogs.[4] *Haemobartonella* organisms are susceptible to broad spectrum antibiotics such as tetracycline but not to penicillin.

Attempts have been made to culture the organism in embryonated eggs and in various blood-containing media but no successful cultivation has been reported. Animal inoculation is the only means by which the organism can be isolated. The organism can be recovered from whole blood obtained from acutely infected animals. Blood films stained by Romanowsky-type stains can be preserved as record specimens. Blood, other body fluids, or tissue homogenates of infected animals will cause infection in susceptible animals when inoculated by any parenteral route. This procedure results in either patent infection or a carrier state.

Microscopic examination of blood films stained by various histochemical methods reveals the pleomorphism of *Haemobartonella*. The organisms are slender rods with rounded ends, frequently showing granules or swellings at either one or both extremities and dumbbell, coccoid, or diplococcoid forms. They occur singly, in pairs, or in short chains of three or four elements and, when abundant, in parallel groupings. Rod-shaped organisms measure $0.1 \times 0.7–1.3$ μm while the coccoid forms measure $0.1–0.2$ μm in diameter. Eperythrozoa can be distinguished from haemobartonellae microscopically by their morphology.[3] Stained with Romanowsky dyes, eperythrozoa appear as rings, cocci, or short rods, 1–2 μm in their greatest dimension.

Preferred stains for light microscopy are those of the Romanowsky type. With Giemsa stain, various investigators reported (1) an intense red color, (2) a bluish tinge with distinct pink shade, or (3) a blue color with purple granules. With Wright's stain, the organism is bluish with reddish granules at the ends. With Schilling's methylene blue–eosin stain, the organism is a bright red color and the erythrocytes stain blue. The organism stains faintly with Manson's stain, pyrorin–methyl green, or fuchsin.

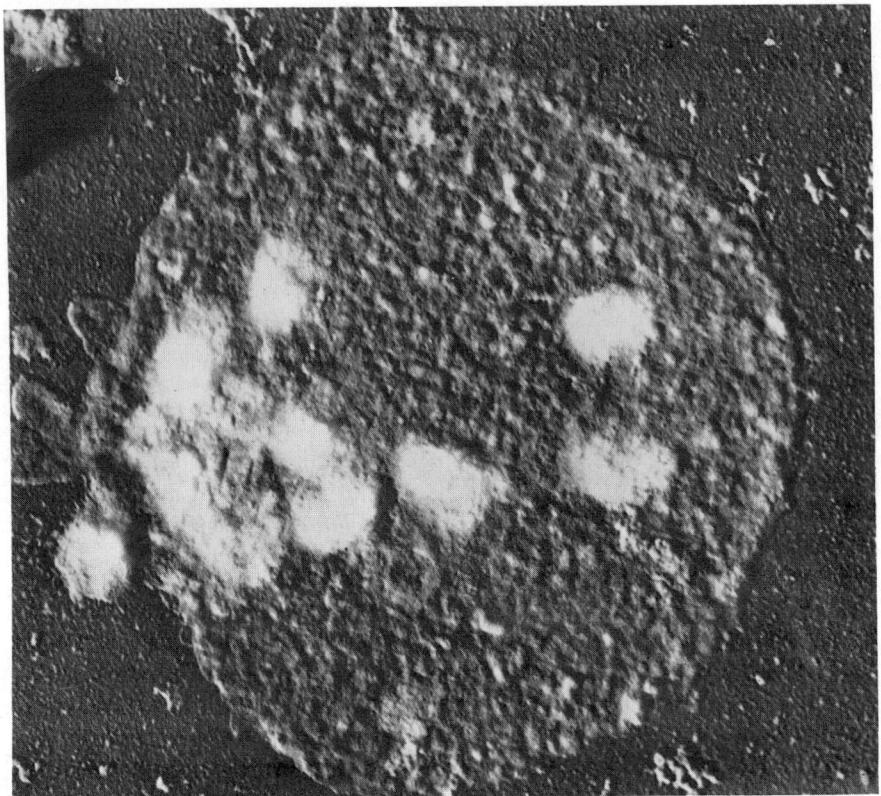

Figure 38.1. *Haemobartonella felis* on the erythrocytes of an infected cat. Electron micrograph, shadow cast preparation. × 40,000. (From Small and Ristic, *Am. J. Vet. Res.* 28:845–851, 1967.)

Living organisms can be stained with brilliant cresyl blue. They are gram-negative and can also be stained by acridine orange.

Electron microscopy of shadow cast preparations of infected erythrocytes reveals the parasites as coccoid and occurring singly, in pairs, and in groups of three or four.[3] They appear partially embedded in the erythrocyte membrane (Fig. 38.1). They have neither flagella nor cilia and appear to lack a rigid cell wall. In ultrathin sections, the organisms have two membranes and contain a dense granular material embedded in an electron-lucid granular substance. No true nucleus, organelles, or cell wall are observed. The results of enzyme treatment and histochemical staining indicate the presence of both RNA and DNA.

The organisms are nonfilterable with either the Seitz or Berkefeld N filter. They will survive for 3–6 days at 4°C and can be preserved by freezing at −65°C and lower in the presence of glycerol.

No case of true natural immunity in rats has been established. Acquired immunity occurs in (1) the latently infected rat; (2) the infected rat after splenectomy and recovery from the disease, the period of resistance corresponding to the duration of latency; and

(3) the nonsplenectomized, noncarrier rat following infection. Serum from *H. muris*–infected rats does not yield a positive Weil-Felix reaction. In the CF test, weak complement binding has been obtained with *Anaplasma marginale* and *Eperythrozoon coccoides* antigens. Agglutinins for trypsin-modified erythrocytes are present in the serum of acutely infected rats. The direct and indirect FA techniques have been applied to studies of *H. felis* and its antibodies, respectively. The experimental host range is restricted; however, an organism infective for one species of rodent may commonly infect other rodents.

References
1. Flint, J.C., M.H. Roepke, and R. Jense. Feline infectious anemia. I. Clinical aspects. *Am. J. Vet. Res.* 19:164–168, 1958.
2. Kreier, J.P, and M. Ristic, *Haemobartonellosis, Eperythrozoonosis, Grahamellosis and Ehrlichiosis in Infectious Blood Diseases of Man and Animals,* D. Weiman and M. Ristic (eds.), vol. 2, pp. 387–472. Academic Press, New York, London, 1968.
3. Small, E., and M. Ristic. Morphologic features of *Haemobartonella felis*. *Am. J. Vet. Res.* 28:845–851, 1967.
4. Weinman, D. Infectious anaemias due to Bartonella and related red blood cell parasites. *Trans. Am. Phil. Soc.* 33:308–312, 1944.

39. Actinobacillus

Microorganisms of the genus *Actinobacillus* generally show the following characteristics: they are gram-negative, nonmotile, medium-sized rods that vary in form from coccoid to long filamentous cells; they are catalase positive or negative, oxidase positive or negative, and facultatively anaerobic, and attack some carbohydrates fermentatively without gas production. Growth of these species is favored by cultivation on agar containing blood or serum. The genus contains five species: *lignieresi, equuli, actinomycetemcomitans, actinoides,* and *seminis*.

Actinobacillus lignieresi

Actinobacillus lignieresi is pathogenic for cattle, sheep, pigs, and humans. Actinobacillosis is distributed worldwide and is relatively common among cattle in the western hemisphere. The mortality, however, is not high and the majority of cases can be successfully treated with iodine. The symptoms and gross lesions of actinobacillosis in cattle resemble superficially those of actinomycosis, which is caused by *Actinomyces bovis*. Both diseases are characterized by granulomatous lesions and granules in the pus. The greatest dissimilarity of these two diseases is in their favored sites of localization. Actinomyces usually involves the bones of the head, especially the jaw bones, as a rarefying osteitis with formation of sinuses and is generally confined to the immediately surrounding soft tissues of the head and neck. Its most obvious manifestation is the hard, irregular enlargement resulting from the infection of the mandible or the maxilla, which gives the disease its common name, lumpy jaw. Actinobacillosis may involve the jaw of cattle, but more frequently the invasion is primarily of the tongue ("wooden tongue"), lymph nodes of the head, neck, and thorax, less frequently the lung, and rarely other organs.

In the early stages of infection in sheep, enlargement of the lymph nodes of the head occurs, and in the later stages, multiple abscesses form in the tissues of the head. Thickening of the skin occurs, accompanied by a discharge of pus, and spread of the infection to the region of the face is common.

It is generally believed that the entry of *A. lignieresi* into the animal is through wounds and abrasions of the skin, the mucous membranes of the oral cavity, and the rumen. Wherever the microorganisms locate, they act as an irritant giving rise to a low-grade inflammatory reaction of the granulomatous type. The predominating cells are large mononuclear phagocytes, lymphocytes, and fibroblasts. The colonies of actinobacilli assume the form of rosettes, which gradually become surrounded with large mononuclear phagocytes. In some cases the inflammation is a mixed granulomatous and suppurative type and the rosettes float in pus. Surrounding the zone of neutrophils is a mixture of lymphocytes and macrophages, and outside this is a capsule of fibroblasts. With continued growth of the organisms and the proliferation of connective tissues, large tumorlike masses form, which may be hard or soft, depending upon whether the predominant tissue form is leukocytic or granulated. In the central mass of the tumors are the colonies of organisms, which are formed into what are called sulfur granules.

Specimens

Samples of pus from lesions should be collected by aspiration with a sterile syringe and needle and placed in a sterile test tube. The specimen should be shipped to a laboratory immediately, or, if this is not possible, it should be refrigerated. Accompanying information should indicate whether the lesions were open or closed and the type of tissue that is involved. Precautions should be taken to avoid contamination of the hands, especially if cuts and abrasions are present; the organism is not generally considered a human pathogen, but many cases of actinobacillosis in humans have been reported.

The pus, which is usually thick, viscid, or gelatinous, and usually is greenish-yellow, should be examined macroscopically, the sample being placed in a glass petri dish and held over a dark surface and examined for characteristic sulfur granules. Although in actinomycotic pus the sulfur granules are visible to the unaided eye, in actinobacillosis the granules are in the form of thin whitish flakes, usually visible only with the aid of a hand lens or microscope. Microscopic examination of material that has been pressed or crushed to break granules reveals rayed formations of elongated club-shaped structures known as rosettes. Thin films of the exudate should be prepared and stained with Gram stain; the absence of gram-positive cells and the presence of short gram-negative rods with rounded ends are highly suggestive of actinobacillosis.[14]

In actinomycotic lesions, the rosettes are irregularly shaped, variable in size, and as a general rule considerably larger than the uniformly small formations in lesions of actinobacillosis. In addition, the individual clubs in the lesions of actinobacillosis are more slender and have more pointed ends than those in actinomycotic lesions. In old lesions, calcareous changes may occur in the rosette, and there is an extensive replacement of the granulomatous tissue by connective tissue, forming a tumorlike mass that may be mistaken for a fibroma.

Caution should be exercised in the interpretation of the "ray fungi" or rosettes because these appear also in botryomycosis (*Staphylococcus aureus*) and in coccidioidal granuloma (*Coccidioides immitis*).

Laboratory Procedures

Cultures. Pus or tissue from lesions of actinobacillosis is ground in saline, which breaks down the clubbed masses about the organisms. The compact rosettes contain very few organisms and heavy seeding of the medium with a well-triturated inoculum is necessary to obtain good growth.

Heart infusion agar containing 5–10% horse or rabbit blood is employed for the primary isolation of this organism from pus or tissues. Isolation of the organism from the ruminal contents or from the bovine tongue is facilitated by the use of a selective medium containing 1 μg oleandomycin and 200 units nystatin per ml. Growth is greatly improved by incubating in an atmosphere containing 10% CO_2.

Freshly isolated strains on blood or serum agar produce small, bluish-white, smooth colonies in 24 hours; they generally increase in size with further incubation. In nutrient broth, growth takes the form of small granules, which adhere to the walls of the tube or collect on the bottom, leaving the clear broth above. Following several transfers, the character of the growth changes. Growth in bulk is diffuse and a pellicle may be present.

There are three colony types: (1) fluorescent, 5–10 mm diameter, flat, rough surface, often with irregular edge; (2) granular, 2–4 mm diameter, bluish, raised, edge entire, translucent with fine internal granulation; (3) dwarf, 0.5–1 mm diameter, raised, gray, colorless, edge entire. The dwarf colonies occur only in freshly isolated strains; the fluorescent types predominate in stock cultures. The dwarf type tends to dissociate into granular and fluorescent forms.

Differential reactions. The most recent and fullest description of the biochemical characteristics of *A. lignieresi* is that given by Phillips, who examined a large number of strains from lesions in cattle and sheep.[11] All strains fermented glucose, levulose, mannose, xylose, maltose, dextrin, and mannitol within 24 hours, without the production of gas. No fermentation occurred within 14 days with trehalose, inulin, dulcitol, salicin, and inositol. Differences between strains were observed in the reactions with lactose, sucrose, sorbitol, raffinose, arabinose, glycerol, galactose, and rhamnose. Differences between strains were observed in the production of catalase, hydrogen sulfide, unrease, and starch, and in the reduction of methylene blue. All strains grew well.

Cellular morphology. The morphology of the cells of *A. lignieresi* varies, depending upon the medium used and the duration of the incubation period. On primary isolation, the cells are small and rod-shaped and measure 0.5×1 μm. Later, especially on nutrient agar, coccobacillary and diplococcal forms occur. Filamentous forms appear in serum broth, on dextrose or maltose agar, and in old cultures. The intensity of the Gram stain shows considerable variation between individual organisms within the same smear, some staining quite deeply and others being only faintly colored and having the appearance of "ghost" forms. A constant feature of all cultures is that granules are scattered among the rods.

Animal inoculation. Inoculation of animals is not usually employed, since, generally speaking, laboratory animals such as rabbits, guinea pigs, and hamsters are resistant to infection with this organism; however, embryonated chicken eggs have been shown to be susceptible.

Immunology and serology. The most recent and most complete description of the antigenic structure and serology of *A. lignieresi* is that given by Phillips, who examined over 200 strains isolated from lesions of actinobacillosis in cattle and sheep.[13] Through the use of slide and tube agglutination tests and absorption tests, six antigenic types and two subtypes were distinguished by the differences in their heat-stable antigens; over 90% of the strains studied could be fitted into these types. The majority of strains isolated from cattle belonged to one type and most of those from sheep to three other types. Heat-labile antigens common to different antigenic types were found in living and formaldehyde-killed cells, and these antigens appeared to be responsible for the inagglutinability of the living organisms tested with antisera to the heat-stable antigens. Thus, while there are antigenic types, serologic tests do not give clear-cut results on which a diagnosis could be made.[12]

Actinobacillus equuli

Actinobacillus equuli causes acute septicemia, glomerular nephritis, and joint-ill in foals, and it has been reported as an isolate from metritis in swine and from a case of verrucose endocarditis involving a heart valve of a young pig. Wetmore et al. isolated organisms similar to *A. equuli* from swine killed by atomic blast.[18] However, a detailed study of these isolates together with stock cultures of *A. lignieresi* and *A. equuli* led them to conclude that there was no basis for the separate speciation of *A. lignieresi* and *A. equuli,* and they suggested that the use of the taxon *equuli* be discontinued. The isolation of this organism from swine following stress produced by irradiation suggested another possibility: actinobacilli may occur as a commensal in normal swine as well as in cattle. Neither of these organisms is virulent for normal healthy livestock unless given in large doses parenterally.

Joint-ill is an acute infectious disease of newborn animals that occurs in the first few days of life and usually not later than the fourth week. It is a disease of suckling calves and colts and occasionally of lambs. Purulent inflammation of the joints and general pyemia are characteristic symptoms.

A. equuli has also been isolated from suppurative nephritis. The infection originates from a primary infection in some other part of the body. The bacteria reach the kidney through the renal vessels and lodge in the capillary loops in the glomeruli, in the intertubular capillaries, and occasionally in the larger vessels. In small vessels, miliary abscesses arise; in the larger vessels, septic infarcts occur. Bacteria may later pass into the Bowman's capsules and into the renal tubules to produce abscesses there.

In a study of the cause of infections in foals conducted over a 25-year period, researchers found that *A. equuli* caused the death of a larger number of foals than any other microorganism.[2] In addition, evidence was obtained to support the conclusions of earlier workers that the distribution of this organism was wide, that it was commonly present in normal horses, and that it produced infections only when the host resistance had been lowered.[2]

Because joint-ill and suppurative nephritis and metritis in animals may result from infection with a variety of bacteria, diagnosis is dependent upon the isolation and identification of the causative agent. Synovial fluids, blood, and urine and infected tissues are the usual source materials for the isolation of *A. equuli*. The procedures employed are identical to those used for the isolation of *A. lignieresi*. These two organisms are related serologically and also possess similar biochemical properties.[17,18]

Actinobacillus actinomycetemcomitans

In 1912, Klinger isolated an organism from a case of human actinomycosis where he found it in association with the ray fungus.[7] Although it has not been possible to find any convincing report concerning the pathogenicity of this species for animals, the possibility of its presence in bovine actinomycosis or other animal infections cannot be excluded. Since the original observation, the occurrence of this organism in cases of human actinomycosis in association with *Actinomyces israeli* has been confirmed many times and the symbiotic relationship established.

The first human infection in which this organism was the sole infecting agent was reported in 1951.[16] In 1962, the isolation of strains of organisms similar to *A. actinomycetemcomitans* was reported from human patients, the majority of whom had symptoms suggestive of bacterial endocarditis.[6] The occurrence of this organism as part of the human oral flora has also been established. A description is included here because the possibility of its occurrence in animal infections cannot be definitely excluded.

Specimens

Blood, pus from lesions, urine, and pleural fluid have been the source materials used to isolate this organism in human infections.

Laboratory Procedures

Cultures. Reports of isolations of this organism from the cases described by Page and King indicate that a variety of liquid media can be employed.[10] Thioglycollate was frequently mentioned. Media usually employed for the isolation of *B. abortus* would appear to be quite suitable. The use of an atmosphere enriched with 10% CO_2 for incubation is highly recommended.

On rabbit blood agar, there is no reaction in 24 hours but a slight greening occurs later. Colonies, after 24 hours, may be punctate to 0.5 mm in diameter and are usually translucent, smooth, and entire. On prolonged incubation, they may attain a diameter of 2 or 3 mm and some colonies may become quite rough and adherent. In those colonies, an opaque star formation frequently develops in the center of the colony and grows into the agar.[3,4] The optimum temperature for growth is 37°C.

Differential reactions. The suggested media for determining the biochemical activities of this microorganism are: Difco heart infusion broth containing bromcresol purple (BCP) and 1% carbohydrate, and Difco MR-VP broth for MR and VP reactions (Difco Lab., Detroit). The following physiological tests may be performed with the media indicated: urease—Christensen's urea agar; indole—2% tryptone broth or heart infusion broth; H_2S production—TSI agar with lead acetate paper; nitrite—2% Bacto-peptone broth or heart infusion broth with 0.2% potassium nitrite.

The results obtained by King and Tatum were as follows: all strains gave weakly positive catalase reactions, a few strains showed weakly positive reactions with oxidase reagent, and the remainder were negative.[6] The majority of strains fermented glucose, maltose, galactose, levulose, mannose, dextrin, glycogen, and starch, and failed to ferment salicin, arabinose, adonitol, dulcitol, rhamnose, sorbitol, cellobiose, inulin, erythritol, melibiose, melizitose, lactose, sucrose, glycerol, trehalose, raffinose, and occasionally inositol. Both MR and VP reactions were negative. All strains were negative with respect to motility and to urease, gelatinase, and indole production, but they all reduced nitrate to nitrite and produced small quantities of H_2S. From these fermentation tests, King and Tatum established three biochemical groups on the basis of each strain's catalase, xylose, and mannitol reactions.[6]

Actinobacillus actinoides

In 1918, Smith isolated from the lungs of calves suffering from epizootic pneumonia an organism to which he gave the name *B. actinoides*.[15] The condition was found to be common in the second and third months of life, and was characterized by areas of consolidation, focal necroses, and other lesions. On microscopic examination of the lungs, the organisms were seen as slender bacilli at the periphery of necrotic areas, in masses in the alveoli and the alveolar ducts, or in the proliferating epithelium that occupied the smaller bronchioles. The organism was nonpathogenic to laboratory animals but intratracheal injection into calves was sometimes followed by the appearance of small necrotic areas in the lungs, indistinguishable from those observed in the natural disease. Subcutaneous injection into calves causes a large necrotic swelling with caseous contents. Other investigators have shown that although the organism is associated with bronchopneumonia, its etiologic significance is far from convincing.[8] An organism morphologically and culturally indistinguishable from *A. actinoides* has been isolated from the genitalia of bulls affected with seminal vesiculitis.[5]

Specimens

Semen specimens should be collected in the usual manner and shipped to a laboratory immediately, or, if this is not possible, refrigerated. The fragility of this organism and its fastidiousness make it mandatory that the specimens be cultured as soon as possible.

Specimens of affected tissues, e.g. testicle and epididymis, should be obtained and prepared for histologic examination in the usual manner.

Laboratory Procedures

Cultures. Samples of pus and semen should be cultured directly and tissue samples should be homogenized and the homogenate plated. Samples should be inoculated onto plates of heated blood agar (chocolate agar), incubated in a CO_2 atmosphere, and examined daily for growth. After 3 days incubation, small, convex, entire, glistening, translucent colonies, approximately 1.5 mm in diameter, should be seen. The colonies produce a slight greening of the medium. Inoculation of cultures into the condensation water of horse serum slants usually gives a visibly floccular growth in 3–4 days in a CO_2 atmosphere.

Differential reactions. The need for cultivation in a CO_2 atmosphere and the lack of growth in simple media present special problems in determining the biochemical reactions of these strains. Use of peptone water containing carbohydrates, enriched with 5% rabbit serum to encourage growth, and incubation in an atmosphere containing 10% CO_2 are recommended. Following incubation, the tubes should be subjected to a negative pressure to remove the excess CO_2. In addition, sugar fermentations may be determined on sugar-serum agar media containing 3% rabbit serum, 6% low-temperature broth, and 0.25% lysed red blood cells. Incubation is carried out at 37°C in a CO_2 atmosphere. Acid is not produced from dulcite, glucose, lactose, maltose, mannitol, sucrose, or salicin in peptone water serum-enriched media and is produced from glucose only in sugar-serum agar.

Other characteristics of *A. actinoides* are as follows: catalase is not produced, the oxidase reaction is negative, indole and urease are not produced, nitrate is not reduced, and there is no production of hydrogen sulfide in 20% serum-enriched cysteine broth.[5] Growth on chocolate agar (Harber's medium) is excellent and colonies grown on this medium attain a diameter 1.5–2 mm at 48 hours; on serum agar, Filde's digest medium, and fresh ox-blood agar, growth is usually poor.[5]

Actinobacillus seminis

In 1960, Baynes and Simmons in Australia described three natural cases of epididymitis caused by a hitherto unreported bacterium that they placed in the genus *Actinobacillus*.[1] Transmission experiments with cultures of the bacterium and with semen from a naturally infected ram were also described and the role of the causative agent of this pathologic condition was established. Because the bacillus isolated was nonsporeforming, nonmotile, and gram-negative, and required lowered oxygen tension and serum-enriched media for optimal growth, the organism was classified in the genus *Actinobacillus;* in view of its isolation from semen, the specific epithet *seminis* was proposed.

The incidence of ovine epididymitis due to infection with *A. seminis* is not known and the routes by which it spreads have not been established. In 1964, Livingston and Hardy in Texas reported the isolation of a similar organism from the semen of a ram with epididymal infection.[9] Both teams of investigators pointed out the similarity that existed between the disease produced by this organism and that produced by *Brucella ovis* and concluded that it was possible to distinguish between the two diseases only by the use of laboratory procedures.

Specimens

Samples of semen are collected in the usual manner and taken to the laboratory for examination as soon as possible. Specimens of diseased tissue for histopathological examinations are collected and preserved by routine methods. Samples of blood may also be collected for use in both cultural and serologic tests. Semen may be thick and creamy as a result of the presence of numerous leukocytes and cellular debris, gross pathologic changes in testes may also be present.

Gram stains of films of semen show the presence of gram-negative bacilli that occur both inside leukocytes and extracellularly; the bacilli occur in chains or in palisade formation. While the cells of pure cultures are nonacid-fast in smears, occasional organisms retain the stain, especially when they occur intracellularly.

The histopathologic examination of tissues from naturally infected animals conducted by Baynes and Simmons showed atrophy of both testes.[1] The left epididymis showed chronic interstitial fibrosis with no sperm in the ductules. The right epididymis showed interstitial edema and melanosis. In the ductus deferens, chronic inflammatory changes with marked fibrosis and invasion of the mucosa by polymorphs, lymphoid cells, and macrophages were observed.[1]

Laboratory Procedures

Cultures. Semen and pus can be plated directly; tissue samples should be macerated in saline and then samples of the suspension plated. Primary isolation should be carried out on media enriched with serum or blood and incubated at 37°C. The addition of 10% CO_2 to the atmosphere favors growth. After incubation for 24 hours, pinpoint colonies are present on blood; after 48 hours, colonies are 1–2 mm in diameter, convex, round, with an entire margin, and grayish-white; after 4 days, colonies up to 3 mm in diameter, with entire or undulate edges with radial striation, are present. Under micro-aerophilic atmospheric conditions, growth after 4 days incubation consisted of umbonate colonies, 4–5 mm in diameter, with grayish-white centers, transparent periphery, and undulate margins. Colonies are shiny and moist, whereas those grown in an aerobic atmosphere tend to be dull.

Differential reactions. Baynes and Simmons reported that no acid was produced after 4 days incubation from arabinose, xylose, rhamnose, glucose, maltose, lactose, trehalose, raffinose, inulin, dextrin, glycogen, glycerol, adonitol, mannitol, dulcitol, sorbitol, salicin, aesculin, or inositol.[1] After incubation for 28 days, both strains tested showed slight acid production in arabinose, fructose, and trehalose and one strain produced acid from mannitol. Andrade's indicator was employed in these tests. No changes occurred in Ulrich or litmus milk. Urea was not decomposed and indole was not produced. Loeffler's inspissated serum was not liquefied. No growth occurred on potato, alkaline potato, or glycerol potato. Livingston and Hardy, using phenol red broth base, reported all negative fermentation reactions at 21 days.[9] After 28 days of incubation, acid reactions occurred in mannitol, fructose, and arabinose. Trehalose was not fermented by the Texas isolate. Cultures that had been grown for 8 months on artificial media produced acid in 4 days from all of the carbohydrates mentioned.

Cellular morphology. Cells are pleomorphic, gram-negative rods 1–4 μm long and 1 μm in width. In semen films, the bacilli occur in chains or in palisade formation.

Immunology and serology. Baynes and Simmons employed complement fixation as a diagnostic test and reported that it had limited value.[1] Livingston and Hardy, employing the Baynes and Simmons antigen and the CF test, obtained positive results with serum from experimentally infected animals.[9]

It is not possible to make clear-cut recommendations for tests to separate the members of this genus. Differences exist in the ease with which these species are grown and consequently in the results that are obtained in biochemical tests. Generally speaking, there is considerable intraspecies variation in biochemical characteristics as measured by the usual methods, and the optimal conditions for these tests have not been established. Further complications result from the fact that the cultivation of the original isolates under conditions that are suboptimal leads to the selection of variants that grow more readily under these conditions.

The results of recent investigations indicate that there is little basis for the separate speciation of *A. lignieresi* and *A. equuli,* and it is possible that a re-evaluation of the other members of the genus would indicate close biologic affinities between these also.[18]

References

1. Baynes, I.D., and G.C. Simmons. Ovine epididymitis caused by *Actinobacillus seminis* n. sp. *Austral. Vet. J.* 36:454–459, 1960.
2. Dimmock, W.W., P.R. Edwards, and D.W. Bruner. Infections of fetuses and foals. *Ky. Ag. Exp. Sta. Bull.* 509:3–40, 1947.
3. Heinrich, S., and G. Pulverer. Zur aetiologie und mikrobiologie der aktinomykose. II. Definition und praktische diagnostik des *Actinobacillus actinomycetemcomitans. Zentralblatt Bakt. 174:123*–35, 1959.
4. Heinrich, S., and G. Pulverer. Zur aetiologie und mikrobiologie der aktinomykose. III. Die pathogene bedeutung des *Actinobacillus actinomycetemcomitans* unter den begleitbakterien des *Actinomyces israeli. Zentralblatt Bakt.* 176:91–01, 1959.
5. Jones, T.H., K.J. Barrett, L.W. Greenham, A.D. Osborne, and R.R. Ashdown. Seminal vesiculitis in bulls associated with infection by *Actinobacillus actinoides. Vet. Rec.* 76:24–28, 1964.
6. King, E.O., and H.W. Tatum. *Actinobacillus actinomycetemcomitans* and *Haemophilus aphrophilus. J. Infec. Dis.* 111:85–94, 1962.
7. Klinger, R. Untersuchungen uber menschliche Aktinomykose. *Zentralblatt. Bakt.* 62:191–200, 1912.
8. Levi, M.L., and E. Cotchin. *Bacillus actinoides:* Its association with pneumonia in cattle and its relationship to *Streptobacillus moniliformis. J. Comp. Path. Ther.* 60:17–27, 1950.
9. Livingston, C.W., Jr., and W.T. Hardy. Isolation of *Actinobacillus seminis* from ovine epididymitis. *Am. J. Vet. Res.* 25:660–663, 1964.
10. Page, M.I., and E.O. King. Infection due to *Actinobacillus actinomycetemcomitans* and *Haemophilus aphrophilus. New Eng. J. Med.* 275:181–188, 1966.
11. Phillips, J.E. The characterization of *Actinobacillus lignieresi. J. Path. Bact.* 79:331–336, 1960.
12. Phillips, J.E. The incidence of agglutinating antibodies to *Actinobacillus lignieresi* in the sera of normal and infected cattle. *J. Path. Bact.* 90:557–566, 1965.
13. Phillips, J.E. Antigenic structure and seriological typing of *Actinobacillus lignieresi. J. Path. Bact.* 93:463–475, 1967.
14. Smith, H.A., T.C. Jones, and R.D. Hunt. Diseases caused by higher bacteria and fungi: Actinomycosis and actinobacillosis. In *Veterinary Pathology,* Smith, Jones, and Hunt (eds.), pp. 615–620. 4th ed. Lea and Febiger, Philadelphia, 1972.
15. Smith, T. A pleomorphic bacillus from pneumonic lungs of claves simulating actinomycosis. *J. Exp. Med.* 28:333–344, 1918.
16. Thjøtta, T., and S. Dydves. *Actinobacillus actinomycetemcomitans* as the sole infecting agent in a human being. *Acta Path. Microbiol. Scand.* 28:27–35, 1951.
17. Vallee, A., P. Thibault, and L. Second. Contribution a l'étude d'*A. lignieresi* et d'*A. equuli. Ann. Inst. Pasteur* 104:108–14, 1963.
18. Wetmore, P.W., J.F. Thiel, Y.F. Herman, and J.R. Hare. Comparison of selected *Actinobacillus* species with a haemolytic variety of *Actinobacillus* from irradiated swine. *J. Infec. Dis.* 113:186–194, 1963.

40. Campylobacter and Vibrio

Members of the genera *Campylobacter* and *Vibrio* are widely distributed in nature, but few are pathogenic for humans and lower animals. Clinical manifestations include diarrhea, septicemia, meningitis, and abortion, with a relatively low mortality rate in adults.

Two major groups are considered in this chapter: *Campylobacter fetus* and related microaerophilic organisms that commonly inhabit the intestines or genital organs of animals, and *Vibrio parahaemolyticus* and related marine vibrios, some of which are pathogenic for fish and at times produce food-borne infections in humans. Other unidentified organisms of similar morphology frequently inhabit the oral cavity, intestines, and general environment of animals.

The reclassification of *Vibrio fetus* and related microaerophilic vibrios to the genus *Campylobacter* was recommended in 1970 by the IAMS Subcommittee on Taxonomy of Vibrios and adopted in *Bergey's Manual of Determinative Bacteriology,* 8th edition, 1974.

Campylobacter fetus and Related Microaerophilic Organisms

Bovine genital vibriosis is a venereal disease caused by *C. fetus* subsp. *fetus,* an obligate parasite of the mucous membranes of the bovine male and female genitalia.[17] In the bull the organism is localized within the preputial cavity, primarily in the epithelial crypts on the penis and the fornix.[35] It is not invasive and produces no gross lesions or measurable immune response. The infection becomes more firmly established as the bull grows older. *C. fetus* is transmitted to the cow through venereal contact. The organism localizes in the anterior vagina and invades the uterus and commonly the oviducts during the luteal phase, producing a moderate endometritis and salpingitis that persists generally for several weeks to several months. The inflammation is associated with a period of temporary sterility, presumably due to death of the developing embryo.[1] Recognizable abortions, in which placentitis is evident, occur during later stages of gestation (4–7 months) in a minority of instances. The organism may persist in the anterior vagina for prolonged periods, providing a reservoir of infection comparable to that which is maintained in the bull, although with shorter duration. Genital vibriosis is undoubtedly an important cause of breeding failure in cattle. The disease is prevalent wherever breeding practices are not controlled. It has ceased to be the dominant problem in the dairy industry of Europe and the United States since the advent of antibiotics for treatment of semen used in artificial insemination and the use of noncarrier bulls in natural breeding. However, vibriosis is still a significant cause of sterility in beef cattle, where artificial insemination is less common. Effective vaccination procedures are being developed for control of the disease in breeding herds.[19,22] *C. fetus* subsp. *fetus* is not known to infect animals other than the bovine.

Epizootic abortion in sheep is caused by *C. fetus* subsp. *intestinalis*.[17] The disease is characterized by abortion during the latter half of gestation in ewes and frequently affects a large portion of a flock.[10] Infected ewes become unthrifty and emaciated, with up to 5% mortality. Early in an epizootic of ovine vibriosis, the ewes expel premature dead lambs. As ewes come nearer to the end of pregnancy, both living and dead lambs are expelled and many weak lambs die in 1 hour to 5 days after birth. Death is frequently preceded by depression, convulsions, and intermittent periods of unconsciousness and spasms. Wool of the lambs is heavily stained with viscid yellow feces and bile pigments. During the epizootic, severe diarrhea affects the ewes; the feces are black and fetid and contain mucus. The abortion rate frequently runs as high as 50% of the ewes in a flock, in addition to the birth of weak lambs that may or may not survive. Lesions appear on the livers of some lambs similar to that seen in turkeys suffering from infectious enterohepatitis. After aborting, the ewes have a vaginal discharge characterized by viscid, putrid, reddish-brown exudate. Marked edema of the uterine wall with black necrotic maternal colyledons are observed at necropsy. Many sheep become carriers of *C. fetus* after natural or artificial infection. The gallbladder is probably the most important site of *C. fetus* infection in carriers, although the organism frequently can be isolated from the intestines.[15] Transmission is by ingestion of infectious material; bacteremia and placentitis develop, resulting in abortion.[23,29]

C. fetus subsp. *intestinalis* may also cause abortion in cattle during the latter half of pregnancy.[7,17] Such abortions are extremely sporadic, however. They cannot be distinguished grossly or histologically from later abortions caused by *C. fetus* subsp. *fetus*.

Humans may become infected with *C. fetus* and manifest various disease syndromes, which sometimes simulate brucellosis and occasionally include abortion.[27] The causative agent in the great majority of human infections is *C. fetus* subsp. *intestinalis*.[32,40] Septicemia occurs almost invariably in humans, and a number of deaths have been reported due to meningitis and endocarditis.[4] There is some evidence that humans have become carriers because of chronic infection.[36]

Known reservoirs of *C. fetus* in nature include antelope, wild birds, domestic poultry, swine, dogs, and primates. Vibrionic enteritis, hepatitis, abortion, and septicemia occur in some of these animals although others may be incidental carriers without signs of the infection.

Bovine winter dysentery or winter scours previously was presumed to be caused by *C. fetus* subsp. *jejuni*.[24] The disease is characterized by severe diarrhea, frequent passage of dark brown or black feces often containing mucus and blood, and low grade mortality in calves. The anterior portion of the jejunum is the primary locus of infection.

Although organisms identified as *C. jejuni* were isolated from cases of winter scours in early studies, characterization of this agent is woefully inadequate and the role of vibrios in the etiology of this disease must be re-evaluated.

Swine are subject to a contagious form of dysentery designated bloody diarrhea or black scours. *Vibrio coli* is found in abundance in the bowel contents of affected swine and is considered, with some reservations, as the etiologic agent.[13] The disease, apparently worldwide in its distribution, is confined to swine. Transmission occurs by ingestion of infectious materials that have contaminated feed, water, or fomites. The disease usually affects an entire herd with mortality varying widely, occasionally exceeding 50%. Characteristic lesions are confined to the large intestine and consist of generalized congestion, foci of hemorrhage, and eventual erosion of the epithelium, with flaky or granular material and mucus in the feces.

Specimens

Campylobacter subsp. *fetus* (*Vibrio fetus* var. *venerealis*) can be isolated from bovine semen, genital secretions, or aborted fetuses. Samples should be collected in such a manner as to minimize fecal contamination. Since the oxygen in air is toxic to *C. fetus*, the specimens should be cultured on blood agar soon after collection and then must be incubated under microaerophilic atmospheric conditions. If the samples cannot be cultured within 4–6 hours, they should be protected from air by sealing and frozen to $-79°C$ in dry ice.

Semen is collected in an artificial vagina from bulls with low conception rates. Since numerous bacterial species contaminate semen, the samples must be spread over the surface of blood agar to obtain colony separation. About 0.1 ml of semen can be cultured on each plate. Swarming bacteria are occasionally found in semen from certain bulls, however, and the samples from them must be diluted to obtain adequate colony separation on the plate. Blood agar with inhibitory antibiotics enhances *C. fetus* isolation.[19,42]

Preputial samples suitable for bacteriological culture and staining can be collected readily with a plastic pipette and attached rubber bulb as described by Bartlett for procuring samples for *Trichomonas fetus* examination. The greatest numbers of *C. fetus* (and *T. fetus*) are obtained from the glans penis and immediately adjacent preputial membrane. Samples are collected by passing the plastic pipette into the preputial cavity, scraping the surface of the glans penis, and then flushing the material into a test tube containing 5 ml of nutrient broth or sterile physiological saline. No fluid is introduced into the preputial cavity, as introduction of fluid or swabbing will collect extraneous debris from areas with low *C. fetus* populations, thereby increasing the difficulty of cultural isolation of the pathogen.

For cervicovaginal mucus, samples should be taken from heifers and older cows with histories of repeat-breeding by natural service.[21] The organisms infect the uterine glands and mucous membranes. In cows with chronic infections, organisms are found in lower numbers. Mucus for culture should be collected during active estrus. Mucus can be obtained from the cervicovaginal area with a minimum of contamination with an apparatus consisting of two telescoping stainless steel tubes.[18] A rubber diaphragm covers the end of the tubes; this is broken after insertion of the instrument. About 1–2 g of mucus are aspirated into the tubes, which is sufficient for bacteriological culture. Mucus samples should be cultured on blood agar plates soon after collection to minimize the toxic effects of exposure to oxygen. Another sampling method employed with good results is the use of a glass speculum and plastic insemination pipettes.[37] This method has the advantage that mucus can be collected and sent to a diagnostic laboratory in the plastic tubes with ends sealed to protect samples from oxygen. If more than 4–6 hours will elapse prior to culture, tubes should be packed in dry ice.[37]

Mucus agglutination samples intended for use in the tube agglutination reaction should be collected in a manner avoiding excessive contamination with feces. Mucus collected in tubes as described above may be used, providing a sufficient quantity is obtainable, 0.5 g or more. Alternately, a human vaginal tampon of absorbant gauze can be used for this purpose to collect from 0.5 to 2 g of mucus.[26] Infected cows may not produce agglutinins in their genital secretions during the first 30 days after service from an infected bull. The duration of the positive titer ranges from 4–23 months. Mucus agglutinins persist in cows for several weeks after the infection disappears. Mucus that contains blood almost invariably gives a false-positive reaction due to nonspecific agglutinins in blood serum. Antigens used for the mucus agglutination test are very sensitive to serum agglutinins, but estrous mucus usually dilutes the specific agglutinins, so false-negative reactions may occur. Mucus intended for use in the tube agglutination reaction should be collected during the luteal phase of the estrous cycle.

Fetal abortions of cows or ewes resulting from vibriosis present a generally similar appearance. Placental edema, especially in the placentomes, is evident.[23] Wet mounts of placental fluids and abomasal contents are advisable, in that the organism, with characteristic morphology and motility, usually is present in large numbers, making possible a rapid tentative diagnosis. The organisms are best visualized by means of a phase contrast microscope, using the oil immersion objective. *Campylobacter fetus* cells can be separated from abomasal fluid by differential centrifugation, washing in saline, and filtration through 0.65 μm membrane filters for staining with the FA technique.

Laboratory Procedures

Cultures. Blood agar in petri plates is the preferred culture medium for primary isolation of *C. fetus* from moderately contaminated specimens such as genital secretions, semen, or aborted fetuses. Blood agar containing antibiotics is used for culturing highly contaminated materials such as preputial samples and feces.[14,19,38] Filtration of samples through membrane filters (average pore size, 0.65 μm) prior to culture separates *C. fetus* from most contaminating bacteria.[33] *C. fetus* cells in the filtrates may be concentrated by centrifugation and cultured on inhibitory media.[38,42] Blood agar cultures are incubated 3–5 days at 37°C in desiccator jars, using a gaseous mixture consisting of 5% oxygen, 10% carbon dioxide, and 85% nitrogen.[6]

Hemocultures from cases of septicemia in animals and humans are made by inoculating febrile phase blood into semisolid BHI broth. These cultures are incubated up to 10 days at 37°C and examined daily by phase contrast microscopy. The hemocultures are subcultured onto blood agar plates for isolation of *C. fetus*.

Colonies of *C. fetus* on blood agar are 1–3 mm in diameter, round, smooth, entire, raised, translucent, and butyrous, and have a pink cast but are nonhemolytic. In reflected light the colonies appear to have an internal pattern of white filamentous projections extending radially to the periphery. Viewed by transmitted light, *C. fetus* colonies grown on ABA medium are honey colored and variably granular and exhibit a swarming activity when touched with a needle.[6]

Differential reactions. An isolated colony is inoculated into fluid thioglycollate (FTG) semisolid broth, incubated 3 days at 37°C, examined microscopically for contamination, and used as inoculum for differential metabolic tests.

For the catalase test, inoculate 1 ml of culture into a tube (18×150 mm with metal cap) containing fresh FTG semisolid broth. After 3 days incubation, add 10 ml of 3% H_2O_2 solution; place a rubber stopper with a glass capillary tube insert into the opening of the culture tube, invert over a sink, and mark the fluid level. After 20 minutes, measure the amount of fluid displaced by gas. *C. fetus* gives an average catalase reaction of 50 mm with a range of 20–130 mm.

For the hydrogen sulfide test, inoculate 1 ml of culture into a tube (16×150 mm with cotton plug) containing cysteine beef infusion (CBI) semisolid broth. Insert a strip of lead acetate–impregnated filter paper into the tube and replace the cotton plug. Record H_2S production as $-$, T (trace), $+$, $++$, $+++$, or $++++$ after 24 hours and again after 5 days incubation. *C. fetus* subsp. *fetus* is negative at 1 and 5 days, whereas *C.* subsp. *intestinalis* is negative at 24 hours but positive ($++$ or $+++$) at 5 days.

For the salt tolerance test, inoculate 1 ml of culture into tubes (18×150 mm with metal cap) containing FTG semisolid broth with 4% NaCl. Incubate 5 days and examine for growth. Very few strains of *C. fetus* grow at the 2% NaCl level, whereas *C. sputorum* and some vibrio isolates from fetal samples grow well at the 3% and 4% levels.

For the glycine tolerance test, inoculate 1 ml of culture into a tube (18×150 mm with metal cap) containing FTG semisolid broth with 1% glycine. Examine for growth after 5 days. *C. fetus* subsp. *fetus* is inhibited by 1% glycine, whereas *C.* subsp. *intestinalis* grows well in this medium.

For the heat tolerance test, inoculate 1 ml of culture into each of three tubes (18×150 mm with metal cap) containing FTG semisolid broth; incubate one at 25°C, one at 37°C, and one at 42°C for 5 days and examine cultures for growth. *C. fetus* subsp. *fetus* grows at 25–37°C whereas most *C.* subsp. *intestinalis* strains grow at 25–42°C.

Members of the genus *Campylobacter* isolated from the genital and intestinal tracts of animals are nonproteolytic and nonfermentative, although they reduce nitrates to nitrites. Table 40.1 outlines the key metabolic characteristics used to distinguish these organisms.[3,14,32] *Campylobacter fecalis*,[14] *V. coli*,[6,15] and similar organisms from the bovine intestines are included in Table 40.1, although their identity in respect to habitat, pathogenicity, and antigenic structure has not been determined.

Cellular morphology. *C. fetus* cells are curved rods, comma or spiral shaped, 0.3 μm in diameter and 2–10 μm long, motile with a single polar flagellum, gram-negative, and nonsporeforming. Long spiral forms and coccoid cells appear in aging cultures, but certain strains exhibit these characteristics in early growth stages.

Animal inoculation. Rabbits, guinea pigs, hamsters, and mice may be experimentally infected with *C. fetus*, but pathogenicity is limited at best. *C. fetus* subsp. *intestinalis*

Table 40.1. Characteristics of members of the genera *Campylobacter* and *Vibrio* commonly isolated from animals

Species	Natural habitat	Pathogenicity	Catalase	H₂S	Growth tolerance			Pen. Sen.
					Glycine	4% NaCl	42°C	
Campylobacter fetus								
subsp. *fetus* type 1	Bovine GT	Infert., abort.	+	–	–	–	–	+++
subsp. *fetus* subtype 1	Bovine GT	Infert., abort.	+	++	–	–	–	+++
subsp. *intestinalis*	Bovine and ovine INT	Abort.	+	++	++++	–	V	+
Campylobacter sputorum								
subsp. *bubulus*	Bovine and ovine GT	None	–	++++	++++	+	–	++++
Campylobacter fecalis	Bovine and ovine INT	None	+	+++	+++	V	V	++++
Vibrio coli	Swine INT	Dysentery	+	+++	+	–	+	NT

GT, genital tract; INT, intestinal tract; V, variable, some strains positive, others negative; NT, not tested.

can be differentiated from *C.* subsp. *fetus* by its predilection for the gallbladder and intestines of experimentally inoculated animals.[5]

Immunology and serology. The antigens of *C. fetus* and related organisms are many and complex,[3] and no systematic serotyping method has been perfected. Likewise, the problem of serologic diagnosis of vibriosis has not been resolved, mainly because infection with *C. fetus* subsp. *fetus* does not stimulate significant antibody levels in the serum.

Three heat-stable somatic serotypes, designated A, B, and C, have been described for *C. fetus*.[7] Serotype C reportedly occurs only in sheep. Seven heat-labile antigens have been described, which are most likely flagellar (H) antigens, capsular (K) antigens, or combinations of both.

The tube agglutination test is technically very similar to that employed for diagnosing brucellosis. However, most investigators agree that serum titers are not reliable criteria for diagnosing vibriosis. While infection with *C. fetus* subsp. *fetus* does produce some degree of systemic antibody response, it is slight and variable and must be differentiated carefully from the *C. fetus* O-type antibodies present in normal bovine serum.

The protocol for the mucus agglutination test has been described.[26] *C. fetus* subsp. *fetus* strain UM (isolated from a bovine fetus at the University of Maine) is used as the tube antigen by several diagnostic laboratories. It is highly stable, belonging to the major O serotype, and is effective for detecting *C. fetus* agglutinins in vaginal mucus. This strain does not possess the heat-labile K antigen and will therefore produce a false-positive reaction to O-type agglutinins in normal bovine serum. In interpreting the test, complete agglutination at even the lowest dilution (1:25) is considered sufficient for a positive diagnosis for vibriosis. It is, nevertheless, strongly advised that several cows from a herd be tested, and that herd histories and cultural isolation of *C. fetus* be considered in assessing the disease status within the herd.

For widespread application of the FA test, adequate knowledge of the serologic classification of *C. fetus* is essential.[3] It is known that the heat-stable O antigen is the major component in the reaction, in contrast to the stereo interference by the K antigen that occurs in the serum agglutination reaction.[9] Thus a suitable conjugate should include antibody directed toward each of the O serotypes.

Phages specific for *V. coli* and *C. fetus* have been demonstrated; however, at present, phage typing is not used in differentiation.[8]

C. fetus contains an endotoxin quite typical of that found in the cell wall of other gram-negative bacteria.[41] Both *C. fetus* and *C. sputorum* produce mucinase in relatively low concentrations.

Vibrio parahaemolyticus (and Related Marine Vibrios)

This vibrio produces food poisoning and has been found responsible for more than 70% of the outbreaks of acute gastroenteritis in Japan.[34] It has also been identified as the probable cause of mortality in the Chesapeake Bay blue crab.[16] *Vibrio parahaemolyticus* has been isolated from human feces, marine sediments, sea water, and numerous species of sea fish. It enjoys worldwide distribution in coastal waters, where it is found in high numbers only in the summer months. The seasonal occurrence coincides with vibrionic food poisoning incidents.

The organism also has been isolated from skin lesions of bathers in coastal waters of the United States.[39] It is a facultatively halophilic enteropathogen that is transmitted by ingestion of contaminated raw or semicooked sea foods. Symptoms of the disease are severe abdominal pain, vomiting, watery or bloody diarrhea, fever, and chills, and it may be confused with bacillary dysentery. The mortality rate is very low. Pathologic signs include erosion of the jejunum and ileum, catarrh of the stomach, dilation of brain blood vessels, and interlobal hemorrhages in the lungs.[20] The pathogen is identified by hemolysis on blood agar and by biochemical and serologic tests.[20,34,39]

Two closely related halophilic species, *Vibrio alginolyticus* and *Vibrio anguillarum*, share the marine habitat with *V. parahaemolyticus*, but their pathogenicity for humans is doubtful.[31,34] *V. alginolyticus* has also been isolated from stools of patients with gastroenteritis, but the role of this bacterium in foodborne infection needs to be clarified. Cultural and biochemical characteristics of these three species are very similar, and their identity is often confused (Table 40.2).

Vibrio anguillarum originally was associated with red disease of eels and recently has been recognized as a pathogen for other fish species, including codling, finnock, rainbow trout, and salmon.[11] Mortality due to infection with *V. anguillarum* was over 90% in juvenile salmon reared in a single U.S. location during 1968.[11] Numerous outbreaks of disease due to marine vibrios have been recognized in a variety of fish in Europe.[31] The disease is characterized by red necrotic lesions of abdominal muscles, erythema at the base of fins and in the mouth, and hemorrhaging in gills and the intestine. The natural reservoir of *V. anguillarum* is uncertain, but there is evidence that herring or other natural fish populations that are used as fish food may be the source of epizootics in fish hatcheries.[31]

Specimens

Because *V. parahaemolyticus* is a mesophilic organism, relatively low numbers of vibrios are found on fresh chilled fish and shellfish.[25] Therefore, a search for these bac-

Table 40.2. Characteristics of *V. parahaemolyticus*, *V. alginolyticus*, and *V. anguillarum*

	parahaemolyticus	alginolyticus	anguillarum
Disease (human)	Enteritis, wounds	Unknown	None
Disease (fish)	Morbidity	Unknown	Hemorrhagic disease
Colonies (1.5% agar)	Smooth	Swarming	Smooth
Hemolysis	+	−	−
Indole prod.	+	+	−
VP reaction	−	+	+
H$_2$S prod.	−	−	−
Catalase prod.	+	−	+
Nitrate reduc.	+	+	+
Glucose ferm.	+	+	+
Sucrose ferm.	−	+	+
Cellobiose ferm.	−	−	+
Growth in 1% trypticase broth			
With 0% NaCl	−	−	+
With 3% NaCl	+	+	+
With 7% NaCl	+	+	−
With 10% NaCl	−	+	−
At 37°C*	+	+	+
At 42°C	+	+	−
At pH 5	+	+	−
At pH 6–11	+	+	+

*At 0°C all three are negative, at 30°C all three are positive, and at pH 4 all three are negative.

teria in fish and marine products should be made by a suitable enrichment method followed by subculturing for isolation on appropriate solid media. Specimens from fish, seafoods, or other marine products are homogenized in sterile buffered 3% NaCl solution (pH 7.5) and cultured in alkaline peptone broth. Additional methods for isolating marine vibrios from various fish species are described elsewhere.[2,11,16,25]

Stool specimens from patients with symptoms of seafood-borne vibriosis are cultured directly on BTB-salt-teepal agar and salt-starch agar.[2] Seafood products suspected to be the source of human gastroenteritis are cultured by the preenrichment method described above and subsequently plated on inhibitory agar media.[20]

Laboratory Procedures

Cultures. Homogenized specimens of infected or contaminated seafood products are diluted (10^{-1}) in the alkaline peptone medium, which currently is also used for the detection of *V. cholerae* (*comma*) in stools.[25] Broth cultures are incubated 20 hours at 35°C and plated on BTB-salt-teepal agar and salt-starch agar for isolation of marine vibrios. The BTB-salt-teepal agar cultures are incubated in air whereas the salt-starch agar cultures are incubated anaerobically for detection of starch hydrolysis.[2]

Pure cultures of *V. parahaemolyticus* are streaked on blood agar containing 5% human or sheep blood for the detection of hemolysis. Agar media containing blood from various animal species is useful for distinguishing pathogenic *V. parahaemolyticus* from apathogenic marine vibrio species.

Colonies of *V. parahaemolyticus* grown for 24 hours on isolation media are 2–3 mm in diameter, circular, smooth, entire, translucent to opaque, and nonpigmented.[39] Colonies of *V. alginolyticus* are distinguished from *V. parahaemolyticus* and *V. anguillarum* by their tendency to swarm on agar.[34] Colonies that are smooth, transparent, and nonpigmented and that form a halo of precipitate on salt-starch agar are presumed to be marine vibrios.

Differential reactions. Tests used to identify the three major biotypes of marine vibrios,[34] *V. parahaemolyticus, V. alginolyticus,* and *V. anguillarum,* are given in Table 40.2. Salt tolerance, indole production, VP reaction, sucrose fermentation, and hemolysis of blood are the most useful ones.[11,25,34,39] Potentially pathogenic *V. parahaemolyticus* strains are differentiated from related nonpathogenic marine vibrios by hemolysis on hamster, sheep, and human blood. Strains of *V. parahaemolyticus* isolated from wounds exhibit alpha-hemolytic activity on chicken blood, whereas strains from stool specimens exhibit mostly beta-hemolysis; nonpathogenic marine vibrios are nonhemolytic in this system.

Cellular morphology. The marine vibrios described here are gram-negative, rod-shaped cells, 1 μm in diameter and 2–3 μm long, with rounded ends and a single polar flagellum. They are pleomorphic in culture media, varying from straight cells to slightly curved, coccoid, or swollen cells. Bipolar staining is frequently observed when the cells are stained 15 minutes in weak Giemsa solution. Direct smears from the blood of infected animals show that pathogenic vibrios have a thin capsule.[34]

Animal inoculation. Broth cultures of *V. parahaemolyticus* are highly lethal for 3-week-old mice. Inoculation IP of 0.5 ml of 18-hour broth cultures of the vibrio killed almost all of the inoculated mice by septicemia within 24–48 hours.[34] Broth cultures of the organism produce enteritis when inoculated into the ligated loop of rabbit intestines. Although *V. parahaemolyticus* produces acute gastroenteritis after ingestion by human volunteers, no evidence of this condition was observed in feeding experiments with dogs, cats, and monkeys.[34]

Immunology and serology. Vibrio parahaemolyticus possesses flagellar (H-antigen), somatic (O-antigen), and capsular (K-antigen) components.[30] At least 12 O-antigens and 52 K-antigens have been identified and used for typing of marine vibrios.[12] Typing of these organisms by use of the H antigen is not useful due to the small amount detected.[34] At least 26 of the 52 K-serotypes have been isolated from marine and human sources outside Japan.[16] No significant antigenic relationships between *V. paraphaemolyticus* and *V. cholerae (comma)* were found.[34]

Three serotypes of *V. anguillarum* have been identified on the basis of cross-adsorption of the thermostable antigens. Serotype 1 strains were isolated from salmon in the northwest United States, serotype 2 strains were isolated from European fish sources, and serotype 3 strains were isolated from Pacific herring.[31] Serotype 1 vibrio strains are extremely pathogenic for juvenile chinook salmon.[11,31]

Most strains of *V. parahaemolyticus* are believed to be lysogenic. Two bacteriophages isolated from cultures of *V. parahaemolyticus* that were obtained from Pacific oysters produce lysis on 25% of the Japanese strains but do not lyse strains of *V. alginolyticus* or *V. anguillarum.*[2]

References

1. Adler, H.C. Genital vibriosis in the bovine: An experimental study on the influence on early embryonic mortality. *Acta Vet. Scand.* 1:1–11, 1959.
2. Baross, J., and J. Liston. Isolation of *Vibrio parahaemolyticus* from the Northwest Pacific. *Nature* 217:1263–1264, 1968.
3. Berg, R.L., J.W. Jutila, and B.D. Firehammer. A revised classification of *Vibrio fetus. Am. J. Vet. Res.* 32:11–22, 1971.
4. Bokkenheuser, V. *Vibrio fetus* infection in man. I. Ten new cases and some epidemiologic observations. *Am. J. Epidemiol.* 91:400–409, 1970.
5. Bryner, J.H., P.C. Estes, J.W. Foley, and P.A. O'Berry. Infectivity of three *Vibrio fetus* biotypes for gallbladder and intestines of cattle, sheep, rabbits, guinea pigs, and mice. *Am. J. Vet. Res.* 32:465–470, 1971.
6. Bryner, J.H., A.H. Frank, and P.A. O'Berry. Dissociation studies of vibrios from the bovine genital tract. *Am. J. Vet. Res.* 23:32–41, 1962.
7. Bryner, J.H., P.A. O'Berry, and A.H. Frank. Vibrio infection of the digestive organs of cattle. *Am. J. Vet. Res.* 25:1048–1050, 1964.
8. Bryner, J.H., A.E. Ritchie, J.W. Foley, and D.T. Berman. Isolation and characterization of a bacteriophage for *Vibrio fetus. J. Virol.* 6:94–99, 1970.
9. Burda, K. A study of heat-labile superficial somatic antigen of *Vibrio fetus*. Thesis, Cornell University, Ithaca, N.Y., 1966.
10. Carpenter C.M. Researches upon a spirillum associated with abortion in ewes. *Cornell Vet.* 9:191–203, 1919.
11. Cisar, J.O., and J.L. Fryer. An epizootic of vibriosis in chinook salmon. *Bull. Wildlife Dis. Ass.* 5:73–76, 1969.
12. [Committee on the Serological Typing of *Vibrio parahaemolyticus*]. New serotypes of *Vibrio paraphaemolyticus. Jap. J. Microbiol.* 14:249–250, 1970.
13. Doyle, L.P. Dysentery. In *Diseases of Swine,* H.W. Dunne (ed.), pp. 386–390. 2d ed. Iowa State University Press, Ames, 1964.
14. Firehammer, B.D. The isolation of vibrios from ovine feces. *Cornell Vet.* 55:482–494, 1965.
15. Firehammer, B.D., S.A. Lovelace, and W.W. Hawkins, Jr. The isolation of *Vibrio fetus* from the ovine gallbladder. *Cornell Vet.* 52:21–35, 1962.
16. Fishbein, M., I.J. Mehlman, and J. Pitcher. Isolation of *Vibrio parahaemolyticus* from the processed meat of Chesapeake Bay Blue crabs. *Appl. Microbiol.* 20:176–178, 1970.
17. Florent, A. Les deux vibrioses génitales: La vibriose vénérienne due à *V. fetus (venerealis)* et la vibriose d'origine intestinale due à *V. fetus (intestinalis)*. *Vlaams dierg. Tijdschr. Meded.* 3:1–60, 1959.
18. Frank, A.H., and J.H. Bryner. An instrument for collecting samples from the reproductive tracts of cows for bacteriological study. *J. Am. Vet. Med. Ass.* 121:97–98, 1952.
19. Frank, A.H., J.H. Bryner, and P.A. O'Berry. The effect of *Vibrio fetus* vaccination on the breeding efficiency of cows bred to *Vibrio fetus*-infected bulls. *Am. J. Vet. Res.* 28:1237–1242, 1967.
20. Fujino, T., Y. Okuno, D. Nakada, A. Aoyama, K. Fukai, T. Mukai, and T. Ueho. On the bacteriological examination of Shirasu-food poisoning. *Med. J. Osaka Univ.* 4:299–304, 1952.
21. Hoerlein, A.B., and T. Kramer. Cervical mucus for the diagnosis of vibriosis in cattle. *J. Am. Vet. Med. Ass.* 143:868–872, 1963.
22. Hoerlein, A.B., and T. Kramer. Artificial stimulation of resistance to bovine vibriosis: Use of bacterins. *Am. J. Vet. Res.* 25:371–373, 1964.
23. Jensen, R., V.A. Miller, and J.A. Molello. Placental pathology of sheep with vibriosis. *Am. J. Vet. Res.* 22:169–185, 1961.
24. Jones, F.S., M. Occutt, and R.B. Little. Vibriosis (*Vibrio jejuni,* N.Sp.) Associated with intestinal disorders of cows and calves. *J. Exp. Med.* 53:853–863, 1931.
25. Kampelmacher, E.H., D.A.A. Mossel, L.M. van Noorle Jansen, and H. Vincentie. A survey on the occurrence of *Vibrio parahaemolyticus* on fish and shellfish, marketed in the Netherlands. *J. Hyg.* 68:189–196, 1970.
26. Kendrick, J.W. The vaginal mucus agglutination test for bovine vibriosis. *J. Am. Vet. Med. Ass.* 150:495–498, 1967.
27. King, E.O. Human infections with *Vibrio fetus* and closely related vibrio. *J. Infec. Dis.* 101:119–128, 1957.
28. Mellick, P.W., A.J. Winter, and K. McEntee. Diagnosis of vibriosis in the bull by use of the fluorescent antibody technic. *Cornell Vet.* 55:280–294, 1965.

29. Miller, V.A., R. Jensen, and J.J. Gilroy. Bacteremia in pregnant sheep following oral administration of *Vibrio fetus*. *Am. J. Vet. Res.* 20:677–679, 1959.
30. Miwatani, T., S. Shinoda, T. Tamura, and T. Fujino. Antigens of *Vibrio parahaemolyticus*. I. Preparation of specific antisera to somatic antigen and their application in antigen analysis. *Biken's J.* 12:9–15, 1969.
31. Pacha, R.E., and E.D. Kiehn. Characterization and relatedness of marine vibrios pathogenic to fish: Physiology, serology, and epidemiology. *J. Bact.* 100:1242–1247, 1969.
32. Plastridge, W.N., L.F. Williams, and D.C. Trowbridge. Antibiotic sensitivity of physiologic groups of microaerophilic vibrios. *Am J. Vet. Res.* 25:1295–1299, 1964.
33. Plumer, G.J., W.C. Duval, and V.M. Shepler. A preliminary report on a new technic for isolation of *Vibrio fetus* from carrier bulls. *Cornell Vet.* 52:110–121, 1962.
34. Sakazaki, R. *Vibrio parahaemolyticus*, a non-choleragenic enteropathogenic *Vibrio*. *Proc. Cholera Res. Symp.* (HEW) 2:30–34, 1965.
35. Samuelson, J.D., and A.J. Winter. Bovine vibriosis: The nature of the carrier state in the bull. *J. Infec. Dis.* 116:581–592, 1966.
36. Schwartz, R., E. Hirsch, J.E. Mule, and L. Bluestone. Antral mucosal diaphragm clinical and roentgen characteristics, with first reported case of *Vibrio fetus* in human bile. *Am. J. Gastroenterol.* 45:366–373, 1966.
37. Seger, C.L., and H.E. Levy. Collection of bovine cervical mucus with insemination pipettes for the isolation of *Vibrio fetus*. *J. Am. Vet. Med. Ass.* 141:1064–1067, 1962.
38. Shepler, V.M., G.J. Plumer, and J.E. Faber. Isolation of *Vibrio fetus* from bovine preputial fluid, using millipore filters and an antibiotic medium. *Am. J. Vet. Res.* 24:749–755, 1963.
39. Twedt, R.M., P.L. Spaulding, and H.E. Hall. Morphological, cultural, biochemical, and serological comparison of Japanese strains of *Vibrio parahaemolyticus* with related cultures isolated in the United States. *J. Bact.* 98:511–518, 1969.
40. White, F.H., and A.F. Walsh. Biochemical and serologic relationships of isolants of *Vibrio fetus* from man. *J. Infec. Dis.* 121:471–474, 1970.
41. Winter, A.J. An antigenic anlaysis of *Vibrio fetus*. III. Chemical biologic, and antigenic properties of the endotoxin. *Am. J. Vet. Res.* 27:653–658, 1966.
42. Winter, A.J., J.D. Samuelson, and M. Elkana. A comparison of immunofluorescence and cultural techniques for demonstration of *Vibrio fetus*. *J. Am. Vet. Med. Ass.* 150:499–502, 1967.

41. Mycoplasma

The family Mycoplasmataceae includes only those organisms of the genus *Mycoplasma*. The family Acholeplasmataceae likewise includes only one genus, the non-sterol-requiring but *Mycoplasma*-like organisms of the genus *Acholeplasma*. These two families make up the order Mycoplasmatales. Among the *Mycoplasma*-like organisms that have been isolated from animal hosts, there is one other group that should be mentioned, the classification of which is uncertain. This is the so-called T-strain group of organisms, which differ fundamentally from most other mycoplasmas in colony characteristics and optimum medium requirements.

The diagnosis of diseases for which mycoplasmal etiology has been established is a relatively simple task because the search is often limited to one specific mycoplasma or its antibodies. This is especially true with such organisms as *M. gallisepticum, M. mycoides* subsp. *mycoides,* or *M. agalactiae,* where identification is more important for epidemiologic than for clinical purposes. In these cases, serologic procedures are not only the most sensitive diagnostic tools but also the only methods that can be applied practically on a field scale for use in control or eradication programs.

A more complicated problem is posed by those *Mycoplasma* species that have been recognized as pathogens in natural and experimental infections, but whose characteristics, distribution, and epidemiology are not yet clearly understood. Some of these mycoplasmas may turn out to be sufficiently important to justify eradication programs, while others may be considered as facultative or accidental pathogens capable of persisting as part of the "normal" microflora of the host species for long periods of time.

Pathogenic Mycoplasmas of Cattle

Mycoplasma mycoides subsp. *mycoides* is the etiologic agent of contagious bovine pleuropneumonia. The disease, known since at least 1693, was introduced into the United States in 1843 and was eradicated in 1892; the need to control it led to the establishment of the old Bureau of Animal Industry in 1884. The disease is now confined to parts of Africa and Asia but was present in Europe in Spain and Portugal in recent times. It was eradicated from Britain in 1898, South Africa in 1916, Japan in 1932, and Australia in 1973. It only occurs in cattle, and though a similar mycoplasma causes caprine pleuropneumonia, there is no cross-infection between goats and cattle. The mycoplasmas were for some years known as pleuropneumonia-like organisms or PPLO's.

The infection is transmitted from animal to animal by airborne particles, and the incubation period is usually 30–60 days but can be as long as 200 days. Cattle with the acute disease show pyrexia, anorexia, a distressed cough, and rapid, labored respiration. They frequently stand with elbows abducted and head stretched out; copious quantities of froth and discharge exude from the mouth and nostrils. The mortality appears to depend on the strain of *Mycoplasma,* the climate, and the degree of herding; it can be as high as 80% when the organism is highly pathogenic, conditions are hot and humid, and animals are crowded, but the mortality may be as low as 2 or 3% when the organism is of low virulence, conditions are dry, and cattle are sparsely distributed. A proportion of affected animals make a clinical recovery but remain carriers. The lesions in these are necrotic and are walled off by connective tissue, and the mycoplasmas, which can remain viable for many months, are coughed out intermittently. This is the chronic phase of pleuropneumonia.

Lesions comprise pleurisy with extensive fibrinous adhesions, which later become fibrous; copious pleural exudate; and consolidation of lung tissue. The degree of lung involvement varies greatly but, in most instances in affected areas, lobules are orange-pink to deep red and are separated by widely distended interlobular septa; in some, thrombosed vessels can be seen in the gross specimen, and on histologic examination thrombi are seen in almost all cases. Sequestrated necrotic lesions retain the original lung structure, which is also apparent on section. There is usually a small amount of thick yellow exudate between the necrotic mass and the wall and the whole is surrounded by a thick dense connective tissue capsule.

The disease is diagnosed by identifying the typical histology, by detecting complement-fixing antibody to *M. mycoides,* and by confirming the presence of typical organisms either by growing them from lesions or by a precipitin reaction.

Mycoplasma bovigenitalium is a common inhabitant of the "normal" bovine genital tract in both cows and bulls. It may be a cause of vulvovaginitis, infertility, abortion, and mastitis in cows, and it can cause seminal vesiculitis in bulls.[6]

Mycoplasma bovimastitidis (*M. agalactiae* subsp. *bovis*) is the organism that has most frequently been isolated from clinical outbreaks of mycoplasmal mastitis.[6] *M. bovimastitidis* cultures will readily produce a typical severe mastitis when introduced into the udder. In addition, arthritic lesions also have been observed in spontaneous and experimental cases of bovimastitidis infection. However, the organism has been isolated from the respiratory and genital tract of normal-appearing cattle as well.

Recent studies in Europe with *M. bovirhinis* and T-strain–type mycoplasmas indicate that these organisms very likely play a role in bovine pneumonia.[18] Several other species isolated from arthritic lesions in cattle are very likely also pathogenic, but only limited data are available. A total of 14 or more distinct species or serotypes has been recognized from bovine sources.[1]

Pathogenic Mycoplasmas of Sheep and Goats

Mycoplasma agalactiae is the causal agent of contagious agalactia of goats and sheep, a disease that has never been reported in the United States. It is an economically important disease in the Middle East. Contagious caprine pleuropneumonia is caused by *Mycoplasma mycoides* subsp. *capri* (*Mycoplasma capri*). Organisms closely related to *M. capri* have been isolated several times recently in the United States. The exact description of *M. capri* is a matter of confusion because there are apparently cultural, biological, and serologic variants of this organism whose significance is not clearly understood.

Mycoplasma arginini and a wide variety of unidentified mycoplasmas have been isolated from sheep on various occasions.[4] A number of the unidentified strains were isolated from pneumonic lungs, but their pathogenic significance is essentially unknown.

Pathogenic Mycoplasmas of Swine

Mycoplasma hyorhinis causes acute and chronic serofibrionous polyserositis and arthritis in 3–10-week-old swine, and occasionally in young adult swine when they are introduced into an infected herd.[21] Poor management practices or other infections may predispose the animal to the disease. Affected animals evidence roughened hair coats, abdominal tenderness, and lameness of variable intensity. Anorexia, coughing, and moderate temperature elevations also may be seen. At necropsy, serous membranes are coated with serofibrinous exudate and, depending on the stage of the disease, fibrous adhesions may be seen. The synovial membranes are thickened, yellow, and hyperemic. Synovial fluid is increased and serofibrinous in consistency. As the arthritis becomes advanced, synovial membrane changes are more severe and some articular surface damage is observed.

Mycoplasma hyosynoviae causes an acute nonsuppurative arthritis in 3–6-month-old and young adult swine.[19] The disease occurs more frequently in certain genetic lines, especially those with heavy muscling. Stress created by management or environmental change seems to precipitate the disease. The arthritis is characterized clinically by acute lameness of 3–10 days duration in one or more limbs, followed sometimes by intermittent lameness of indefinite duration. Periarticular swelling usually is not observed since joints covered by heavy muscle are more frequently involved. At necropsy, affected joints contain increased serofibrinous to serosanguineous synovial fluid. Synovial membranes are thickened, yellow, and hyperemic. Articular surface damage is usually not seen. Arginine-utilizing mycoplasmas named *Mycoplasma suidaniae* and *Mycoplasma hyoarginini* were described recently. These mycoplasmas seemingly are very similar to *M. hyosynoviae*.

Mycoplasma hyopneumoniae (*M. suipneumoniae*) causes chronic pneumonia in 3–10-week-old swine, which usually persists to adulthood. Although microbiological or serologic evidence is not available, pathology surveys indicate that this disease probably is present in 30–40% of slaughter-weight swine in the United States.[21] Affected swine evidence chronic coughing of variable intensity, roughened hair coats, and reduced growth during the early stage of the disease. Later, the animals may appear quite normal, but in some cases, secondary or coexistent involvement with *Pasteurella mul-*

tocida, *Ascaris suum* larvae, or *Metastrongylus* sp. increases the clinical severity and even results in death. Typically affected lungs have well-demarcated plum-colored or grayish areas of pneumonia, principally in dependent positions of the apical and cardiac lobes.

Two nonsterol-requiring *Mycoplasma*-like organisms that are also species of the Mycoplasmatales, *Acholeplasma granularum* and *Acholeplasma laidlawii*, are found in the nasal cavities of swine.

Pathogenic Mycoplasmas of Mice and Rats

Mycoplasma neurolyticum infection in mice often does not result in clinical disease,[24] which is frequently associated with experimental infections or other stress factors, such as prolonged or repeated inhalation anesthesia, intranasal inoculation of drugs or chemicals, or tumor transplants. Intracerebral passage of viruses and other agents in mice is most often associated with the activation of latent *M. neurolyticum*. As each new passage of an experimental agent is made into stressed mice, the numbers of *M. neurolyticum* increase until the infection ceases to be latent and signs of neurologic disease are superimposed on the signs of the primary agent. Frequently, the appearance of neurotoxocity at this point is erroneously taken as a new clinical manifestation of the experimental disease being studied.

The onset of CNS disease in the mouse is generally first observed as ataxia, occasional backward rotation of the head, and frequent circling inside the cage. As the disease progresses, the mouse may show spastic locomotor activity, finally leading to a rapid rotation on the long axis of the body ("rolling disease"). Paralysis of the hindlegs occurs shortly thereafter and the animal usually becomes comatose as a progressive ascending paralysis develops. Death may occur from 2 to 48 hours after the initial onset of CNS signs. *Mycoplasma neurolyticum* also has been identified as the etiologic agent of epidemics of conjunctivitis affecting some mouse colonies, primarily the young stock. The infection apparently is localized in the conjunctivas and eyelids although neurotoxic strains of *M. neurolyticum* are present and can be transmitted by direct contact with ocular washings.

The epidemiology of *M. neurolyticum* in mouse colonies is not well known. It is thought that mycoplasmas latent in the female are transmitted to ocular and/or respiratory tissues of young mice shortly after birth. From there the organisms reach the brain at somewhere around 4–8 weeks of age, possibly through hematogenous dissemination, or perhaps by passage from the nasopharynx through the middle and inner ear to the brain. After the age of 2 months, *M. neurolyticum* is generally recovered more frequently from the latter sites. During times of host stress, the agent may move to the liver, spleen, and other organs. However, the incidence of *M. neurolyticum* in normal mouse colonies is quite variable and may depend upon the origin of the colony and breeding practices. Some colonies appear to be relatively free of *M. neurolyticum*, but the reasons for their absence are not apparent. *Mycoplasma neurolyticum* has not been recovered from other animals.

Mycoplasma pulmonis is the etiologic agent of infectious catarrh in both mice and rats.[24] This rapidly transmitted but low mortality disease is only one factor in the chronic respiratory disease pattern in rodents, and the infection is latent in many mouse and rat colonies. The disease is frequently unnoticed until rats or mice reach old age or are examined at the end of long-term experiments. The onset of infectious catarrh in mice is associated with respiratory distress, ruffled fur, gradual loss of weight, and a characteristic chattering. Rats with the disease usually do not chatter but do develop an extensive rhinitis. *Mycoplasma pulmonis* is generally localized in the nasal passages both mice and rats at this stage of the infection. Later, the agent moves into the lung and middle ear. Prolonged middle ear infections apparently allow passage of the mycoplasmas to the inner ear, meninges, and brain.

Natural catarrhal infections reach an equilibrium with the host, and this situation may continue for some time. Changes in resistance of the host brought about by experimental infections, other stresses, or through normal aging favor multiplication of *M. pulmonis* and death of the animal from advanced pneumonia. Rats seem to be less capable than mice in controlling the multiplication of the agent in the lungs and frequently develop an acute bronchopneumonia characterized histologically by leukocytic plugs in the bronchi and peribronchial lymphocytic infiltration.

It appears that newborn rats and mice are free of *M. pulmonis* but become infected during the second and third week after birth. Once the mycoplasmas infect the respiratory tract they remain there or in other tissues for the life of the animal. Selective breeding practices may eliminate *M. pulmonis* and other agents involved in chronic respiratory disease of rodents.

Mycoplasma arthritidis is associated with subcutaneous abscesses and joint infections in rats.[24] The lesions are usually confined to the legs. The inciting conditions are not well known but the onset of disease most often follows animal-to-animal passage of murine tumor or other tissue suspensions. Natural spontaneous joint infections are usually seen in only one or two animals in a colony, but at least one epizootic of disease due to *M. arthritidis* has been reported.[14]

The arthritis begins as a redness of the tibiotarsal or radiocarpal joints and may result in a swelling to two or three times the normal size, which may extend to the phalanges. Occasionally the infection then subsides, but more often the joint lesions erupt and discharge purulent fluid. The lesions heal only after constrictive or self-amputation.

Pathogenic Mycoplasmas of Chickens and Turkeys

Mycoplasma gallisepticum is the primary etiologic agent of chronic respiratory disease of chickens and turkeys.[8] The disease in turkeys has also commonly been called infectious sinusitis.

Mycoplasma synoviae commonly causes infectious synovitis in chickens and turkeys.[8] This organism may cause a systematic disease and very likely is carried in the respiratory tract of normal-appearing burds.

Mycoplasma meleagridis occurs almost universally in commercial turkeys,[8] and will produce airsacculitis in turkey poults. Its actual economic importance and pathogenicity under field conditions have not been clearly established.

In addition to the above three species of avian mycoplasmas for which pathogenicity

Mycoplasmas of Humans

The mycoplasmas that have been reported isolated from humans, and that have been characterized and named, are listed in Table 41.1. The only species for which primary pathogenicity has been proven unequivocally is *Mycoplasma pneumoniae*.[12] The T-strain mycoplasma and similar strains are frequently isolated from humans but are of unknown pathogenic significance.

Table 41.1. Species of Mycoplasmatales (some of the names are proposed only)

	Reported host[3]
Acholeplasma	
axanthum	Unknown
granularum	Swine
laidlawii	Multiple hosts and sewage
Mycoplasma	
agalactiae	Goat
anatis	Duck
arginini	Sheep, cattle
arthritidis	Rat, human
bovigenitalium	Cattle
bovimastitidis	Cattle
bovirhinis	Cattle
canis	Dog
caviae	Guinea pig
dispar	Cattle
edwardii	Dog
feliminutum	Cat
felis	Cat
fermentans	Human
gallinarum	Chicken
gallisepticum	Chicken, turkey
gateae	Cat
hominis	Human
hyopneumoniae	Swine
hyorhinis	Swine
hyosynoviae	Swine
iners	Chicken
leonis	Lion
lipophilum	Human
maculosum	Dog
meleagridis	Turkey
mycoides subsp. *mycoides*	Cattle
mycoides subsp. *capri*	Goat
neurolyticum	Mice
orale, type 1	Human
orale, type 2	Human
orale, type 3	Human
pneumoniae	Human
pulmonis	Rodent
salivarium	Human
spumans	Dog
synoviae	Chicken, turkey

Mycoplasmas of Other Host Species and Cell Cultures

Mycoplasmas have been isolated from a variety of other domestic and laboratory animals including dogs, cats, horses, ducks, guinea pigs, and rabbits. The pathogenic significance of these strains has not been determined.

Mycoplasmas also are often isolated from tissue cultures, especially cell lines. These mycoplasmas could be of many origins, some proven and some only suspected. Contamination during handling of cell cultures with oral human mycoplasmas appears to occur fairly frequently. Serum used in cell culture medium appears to be another, but less common, source of *Mycoplasma* contamination. Heat inactivation (56°C for 30 minutes) kills many but usually not all mycoplasmas in contaminated sera. The tissues from which the cells were obtained may be infected, leading to infection of all subcultures. Trypsin, dehydrated animal proteins, or protein derivatives have been suggested as additional sources of contamination, as have hormonal substances that are sometimes added to cell culture media. The subject of mycoplasmas in cell cultures was covered thoroughly in a recent review.[20]

Mycoplasmas also may be found in some virus seed stocks, having been a contaminant of the original sample or of a cell culture used for isolation or propagation of the virus.

Specimens

Collection of specimens for isolation of mycoplasmas should be made as early as possible in the acute phase of the disease, as organisms sometimes disappear from the lesions rather early in the disease. Many times the specimens to be collected must be selected on the basis of clinical signs rather than pathology seen at necropsy. For example, synovial fluid should be collected from animals with a history of acute lameness whether or not lesions are seen. Likewise, brain tissue should be collected from animals with CNS disturbances, and nasal exudate and/or lung materials should be collected from animals with respiratory disease. In addition, samples should be collected from any tissues showing pathologic changes at necropsy, or from body fluids or exudates which are increased in amount or abnormal in appearance. Whenever possible, collection should be made before antibiotic therapy has been initiated. Samples should be taken using strict asepsis where possible, but moderate bacterial contamination can usually be overcome by use of bacterial inhibitors in the isolation media.

If the clinical material to be cultured comes from deep-seated lesions, there is a higher likelihood of obtaining a pure culture of the particular pathogenic *Mycoplasma*. Such material is most likely to be derived from necropsy specimens or specimens from mycoplasmal mastitis or arthritis. However, when attempts are made to isolate mycoplasmas from upper respiratory tissues or genital mucous membranes, a large percentage of the isolates contain more than one species of *Mycoplasma*.

Fluids from lesions are most often collected with syringes and needles or with special applicators. Because cotton and other fibers may contain small amounts of substances toxic for mucoplasmas and because drying is deleterious, it is wise to use swabs only where transfer of the specimen material can be made directly to mycoplasma medium. If a short delay before inoculation is unavoidable, the swab material may be transferred to a small amount of buffered salt solution. For longer storage, freezing with dry ice is recommended, in which case a small amount of noninhibitory protein (e.g. 0.5% bovine serum albumin) should be added. If bacterial inhibitors are desired, the inhibitors used for isolation media may be added. Samples should be kept in tightly closed containers, so that the sublimated CO_2 will not drastically alter the pH of the suspending medium.

Serologic samples are often of value in establishing the involvement of mycoplasmas in disease processes where the organisms disappear from the tissues after the acute phase of the disease. As there are few *Mycoplasma* species that share common antigens, serology is of value only where a given species is suspected and a culture or antigen is available. Care should be taken to collect blood in chemically clean containers to prevent toxic inhibition of growth when metabolic inhibition or colony inhibition tests are to be used. Serum for these tests likewise should not be taken from animals receiving antibiotics, or, if it is necessary, the antibiotic regimen should be noted on the serum samples.

Antibodies to new (i.e. nonlatent) infection with mycoplasmas usually will not develop until 2–4 weeks postinfection, depending on the type of serologic test used. In some cases, antibodies do not appear for 6–10 weeks after infection.[18] Low levels of circulating antibody may be present at the time of appearance of disease when it is caused by activation of a latent *Mycoplasma* infection.

The time period during which specimen collection will be worthwhile varies with the species. *Mycoplasma hyorhinis,* for example, usually persists in synovial fluid and other sites of infection for several weeks after the appearance of disease. In contrast, *Mycoplasma hyosynoviae* usually can be recovered from synovial fluid for only a few days. As a result, many samples collected from arthritic joints are negative. Obviously, samples should be taken as early as possible, and failure to isolate mycoplasmas from clinical material is no assurance that the disease is not partially or wholly of mycoplasmal etiology.

Examination of tissues for gross or histopathological changes is of little value in diagnosing mycoplasmal disease, as the changes are not pathognomonic for infection with these organisms. The small size of mycoplasmas generally precludes the use of light microscopy for visualizing the causative agents in lesions. FA staining of tissue sections or exudates appears to be quite helpful in confirming infection with these agents, but it has been used only to a limited extent.

Microscopic examination of stained cell culture monolayers appears to be of some value in detecting mycoplasmal contamination. Several methods have been described, but most of them have little or no advantage over Giemsa, MGG, or Dienes stains.[17] Some mycoplasma contaminants are extremely difficult to visualize by staining, as the only evidence of their existence is an amorphous, fuzzy layer on the cell membrane. This material can be shown to be *Mycoplasma* antigen by use of FA, when the identity of the infecting strain is known. A failure to demonstrate mycoplasmas in cell cultures by staining should not be accepted as proof of their absence, however, since they are sometimes isolated from cell cultures that show no evidence of contamination with staining methods.

Laboratory Procedures

Cultures. Tissues should be minced and then either ground in a tissue grinder or with abrasive. A 5–10% (W/V) suspension of tissue in buffered saline or broth medium can be prepared for inoculation into broth or directly onto agar plates. As there are toxic or inhibitory substances in some tissue suspensions,[15,24] several different dilutions should be used as inocula. On the basis of work done with one *Mycoplasma* species, it appears that tissue specimens should be diluted in tubes of broth to a 1:250 dilution. Swabs of exudate or tissues often may be plated directly onto mycoplasma agar or twirled in a tube of broth, but swabs that possibly contain a large amount of cellular material or immunoglobulin-rich exudate should also be inoculated in several dilutions.

A number of studies indicate the importance of using a variety of culture media for primary isolation studies. Even though use of one medium may result in isolation of mycoplasmas from a higher number of specimens, those isolates may represent only one part of the mycoplasmal flora. *Mycoplasma* species differ greatly within host species groups, and a medium usually should not be chosen strictly on the basis of its past use with a given host species. In practice, it may be desirable to start with a relatively simple, easily prepared medium, and then use media of increasing complexity as it becomes clear that a suspected or known agent is not being isolated.

Most *Mycoplasma* media have in common a meat infusion or peptone base, supplemented with a yeast product (fresh or dried extract, hydrolysate, or autolysate), plus a lipid-protein-sterol supplement such as animal serum, serum fraction, ascitic fluid, or egg yolk extract. Many media have other growth factors added for the purpose of isolating fastidious strains or increasing antigen yield.

An easily prepared medium that is suitable for growth of a good many avian and mammalian mycoplasmas is Difco Beef Heart Infusion broth or agar (Difco Lab., Detroit), enriched by the addition of 10% swine serum.[9]

A good but more difficult medium to prepare is briefly outlined below. Beef muscle and liver, 100 g of each, plus 120 g of pig stomach, are cut into small pieces and finely ground in a blender. To this, add 1 liter of distilled water and 10 ml of concentrated HCl and incubate at 50°C for 24 hours. Heat the mixture to 80°C, pass it through clarifying filter paper, heat again to 80°C, and hold overnight at 5–10°C. Pass through filter paper, adjust the pH to 7, and then filter-sterilize the broth. This medium was originally developed for growth of *M. mycoides* subsp. *mycoides* antigen.[25] It also is well suited for obtaining high titers of low-passage broth cultures of *M. meleagridis*.[3] Many other worthwhile and special media have been reported in the literature.[10,11,13,16,19,22]

Medium supplements are usually required. In order for all *Mycoplasma* sp. organisms to grow, 10–20% serum (or substitute) must be added or be included in the media formulation. Broth media require more serum than agar media.

Penicillin (200–1000 units) and thallium acetate (1:2000 to 1:4000) are effective bacterial inhibitors that do not normally interfere with growth of mycoplasmas. Other supplements used are yeast extracts, NAD, DNA, glucose, maltose, and cholesterol. The water used must be of tissue culture quality.

There are mycoplasmas that appear to grow better in broth and others that grow better on agar. *M. meleagridis* grows better on agar than in broth but it does grow well in the beef muscle, liver, and pig stomach broth previously mentioned. The use of long agar slants covered with deep columns of broth provides a full spectrum of growth conditions and probably would allow growth of nearly all strains capable of replicating in the medium used.

The T-strain mycoplasmas grow better at low pH (<6.5), and it is generally assumed that all classic (large colony) mycoplasmas grow better at a high pH (>7.5). For isolation purposes with unknown strains, the logical approach is to use a pH near 7, where most mycoplasmas will multiply sufficiently for growth recognition.

Incubation at 37°C under reduced oxygen tension and increased CO_2 (5–10%) favors isolation of most known strains of mycoplasmas. However, there are a few strains that require strict anaerobic conditions.

Mycoplasmas have a characteristic colony appearance, which helps to differentiate them from conventional bacteria. The colony usually associated with mycoplasmas is the so-called "fried egg" colony, which results from a deep-penetrating core or central papillae surrounded by a lighter peripheral growth. There are no mycoplasmas that have such a unique colony morphology that they can be distinguished from all other mycoplasmas, but some have a colony morphology that differentiates them from others usually isolated from the same host species. There are many factors affecting the colony appearance that must be considered, however. Among these are adequacy of the medium, presence of surface moisture, and presence of antibodies or other inhibitory substances. As a rule the so-called T-strain mycoplasmas have small irregular colonies that lack a well-defined center. With certain media, however, even the T-strain colonies become hard to differentiate from those of certain of the classic mycoplasmas.

Growth of mycoplasmas in broth is somewhat characteristic and is occasionally of help in differentiating species. The nature of the growth in broth is also very dependent on the medium being used and should be considered only when using media with which one has had experience. Some strains grow almost undetectably in broth, while others produce a heavy turbidity similar to that of common bacteria. Scant growth can sometimes be more readily detected by swirling the tubes of broth and looking for small curls of sedimented organisms rising from the bottom. A comparison of the turbidity in inoculated broth with that in uninoculated broth also can help in determining the presence of growth. Direct or indirect incandescent or indirect flourescent light can be used for detecting turbidity. Some mycoplasmas have a filamentous form of growth, e.g. *M. mycoides* subsp. *mycoides*, which is visible as a swirl when the tube of liquid culture is shaken.

Differential reactions. Prior to the performance of biochemical and serological tests, mycoplasmas that are to be identified must be purified as single colony isolates. Broth cultures should be filtered through 450 μm filters and then diluted in broth by serial 10-fold dilution. Each dilution is plated to agar. Single colonies are selected, passed in broth, and recloned twice again.

There are several biochemical and other biologic determinations that help to categorize new isolates prior to final identification by serological techniques. The most useful ones are glucose, arginine, or urea utilization, tetrazolium tellurite or methylene blue reduction, phosphatase activity, production of film and spots, hydrolysis of gelatin, digestion of casein and coagulated serum, sensitivity to optochin, and hemolysis of sheep erythrocytes.[2]

Cellular morphology. Mycoplasma organisms vary in morphology from coccoid to filamentous to occasionally ring shaped. There is a variation within most species that is dependent on culture age and medium and there is also a wide variation between species as to the tendency to form filaments and to branch. The organisms lack a cell wall and thus appear to stain gram-negative.

Animal inoculation. Chick embryo yolk sacs provide an excellent growth medium for some but certainly not all *Mycoplasma* species. Some strains kill the embryos after replicating to a certain titer, while others do not. The embryonating egg is not very suitable for isolating unknown strains because of the variability of growth from species to species. Also, some of the avian *Mycoplasma* species are egg-transmitted, which could lead to a false-positive isolation or contamination of an isolate.

Immunology and serology. The final identification of *Mycoplasma* isolants usually is accomplished by serologic tests. The most commonly employed tests are the disc method of growth inhibition and the FA technique.[5,7,11] Disc growth inhibition involves placing filter paper discs saturated with specific *Mycoplasma* antisera onto agar plates previously seeded with broth cultures of the mycoplasmas to be identified. A zone of growth inhibition around the antiserum disc indicates a serologic relationship. In many cases, dilutions of the broth cultures must be used in order to obtain a satisfactory zone of inhibition. Young cultures of high viability should be used, as overgrown cultures may contain too much antigen in relation to the number of viable organisms at the dilution giving the optimum number of colonies.

Immunofluorescence requires some specialized equipment, conjugated antisera, and more experienced personnel, but it has been used by some with considerable success for the identification of animal mycoplasmas. In laboratories already set up for the conjugation and staining procedures, it may well be the method of choice. It is an especially desirable procedure for identifying species in a mixed culture.

The drawback with all serologic identification procedures is the requirement for antisera to reference *Mycoplasma* strains. While these can be produced in rabbits or other laboratory animals by several protocols, the procedures are quite time consuming and great pains must be taken to avoid antimedium antibodies in the antisera. This is a particularly vexing problem with the mycoplasmas because of their tendency to adsorb serum and other medium constituents of an antigenic nature. Commercial antisera to mycoplasmas of host species other than humans are not readily available but presumably will become so as the demand increases.

The serologic detection of *Mycoplasma* infections in human, avian, and cattle species has been studied extensively, and serologic tests are available and are being used for some infections in these hosts. Serological tests for *Mycoplasma* antibodies in other animals are almost entirely in the experimental stage and have not been evaluated sufficiently. An important point to remember concerning mycoplasmas is that there is no sharing of a group antigen. Except in rare cases where antigens are shared, separate serologic tests must be run for each *Mycoplasma* species.

Toxins have been shown to be associated with *M. gallisepticum* infection in turkeys, *M. neurolyticum* infection in mice, and *M. mycoides* subsp. *mycoides* infection in cattle.[13] With the latter organism, IV injection of 0.25–0.5 ml of broth suspension or filtrate (100 μm) into young mice (9–11 g) has been used as an aid in identification of the organism. Typical neurological signs of rolling disease will appear within 5 minutes to 4 hours, depending on the quantity of mycoplasma in the original suspension.

Reference laboratories. At present, *Mycoplasma* species are available in the United States only from individual investigators, the ATCC, or the Research Resources Branch of NIH.

References

1. Al-Aubaidi, J.M., and J. Fabricant. Characterization and classification of bovine *Mycoplasma*. *Cornell Vet.* 61:490, 1971.
2. Aluotto, B.B., R.G. Wittler, C.O. Williams, and J.E. Faber. Standardized bacteriologic techniques for the characterization of *Mycoplasma* species. *Internat. J. Syst. Bact.* 20:35–58, 1970.
3. Barber, T.L., and J. Fabricant. Primary isolation of Mycoplasma organisms (PPLO) from mammalian sources. *J. Bact.* 83:1268–1273, 1962.
4. Barile, M.F., R.A. Del Giudice, T.R. Carski, C.J. Gibbs, and J.A. Morris. Isolation and characterization of *Mycoplasma arginini*, spec. nov. *Proc. Soc. Exp. Biol. Med.* 129:89–494, 1969.
5. Clyde, W.A., Jr. Mycoplasma species identification based upon growth inhibition by specific antisera. *J. Immunol.* 92:958–965, 1964.
6. Cottew, G.S., and R.H. Leach. Mycoplasmas of cattle, sheep, and goats. In *The Mycoplasmatales and the L-phase of Bacteria,* L. Hayflick (ed.), pp. 527–570. Appleton-Century-Crofts, New York, 1969.
7. Ertel, P.Y., I.J. Ertel, N.L. Somerson, and J.D. Pollack. Immunofluorescence of Mycoplasma colonies grown on coverslips. *Proc. Soc. Exp. Biol. Med.* 134:441–446, 1970.
8. Fabricant, J. Avian mycoplasmas. In *The Mycoplasmatales and the L-phase of Bacteria,* L. Hayflick (ed.), pp. 621–641. Appleton-Century-Crofts, New York, 1969.
9. Fabricant, J., and E.A. Freundt. Importance of extension and standardization of laboratory tests for the identification and classification of Mycoplasma. *Ann. N.Y. Acad. Sci.* 143:50–58, 1967.
10. Frey, M.L., D.P. Anderson, and R.P. Hanson. A medium for the isolation of avian Mycoplasmas. *Am. J. Vet. Res.* 29:2163–2171, 1968.
11. Goodwin, R.F.W., and J.E. Pryor. Direct isolation of *Mycoplasma suipneumoniae* on solid medium from pneumonic lesions of swine. *Vet. Rec.* 87:726–727, 1970.
12. Grayston, J.T., H.M. Foy, and G.E. Kenny. The epidemiology of Mycoplasma infections of the human respiratory tract. In *The Mycoplasmatales and the L-phase of Bacteria,* L. Hayflick (ed.), pp. 651–682. Appleton-Century-Crofts, New York, 1969.
13. Hayflick, L. Cell cultures and Mycoplasmas. *Texas Rep. Biol. Med.* 23(suppl. 1):285–303, 1965.
14. Ito, S., K. Imaizumi, Y. Tajima, M. Endo, and R. Koyama. A disease of rats caused by a pleuroneumonia-like organism (PPLO). *Jap. J. Exp. Med.* 27:243–248, 1957.
15. Kaklamanis, E., L Thomas, K. Stravropoulos, I. Borman, and C. Boshwitz. Mycoplasmacidal action of normal tissue extracts. *Nature* 221:860–862, 1969.
16. L'Ecuyer, C. Enzootic pneumonia in pigs: Propagation of a causative Mycoplasma in cell cultures and in artificial medium. *Can. J. Comp. Med.* 33:10–12, 1969.
17. Madoff, S. Isolation and identification of PPLO. *Ann. N.Y. Acad. Sci.* 79:383–392, 1960.
18. Menšik, J., and K. Jurmanová. Occurrence of *Mycoplasma bovirhinis* in connection with pneumonia of calves. *Proceedings of the 10th Conference on Taxonomy of Bacteria and Mycoplasmas,* pp. 10–11. Brno, Czech., Sept. 1970.
19. Ross, R.F., and J.A. Karmon. Heteerogeneity among strains of *Mycoplasma granularum* and identification of *Mycoplasma hyosynoviae,* sp. n. *J. Bact.* 103:707–713, 1970.
20. Stanbridge, E. Mycoplasma and cell cultures. *Bact. Rev.* 35:206–227, 1971.
21. Switzer, W.P. Swine mycoplasma. In *The Mycoplasmatales and the L-phase of Bacteria,* L. Hayflick (ed.), pp. 607–619. Appleton-Century-Crofts, New York, 1969.
22. Taylor-Robinson, D., J.P. Addey, and C.S. Goodwin. Comparison of techniques for the isolation of T-strain mycoplasmas. *Nature* 222:274–275, 1969.

23. Thomas, L. The toxic properties of *M. neurolyticum* and *M. gallisepticum*. In *The Role of Mycoplasmas and L Forms of Bacteria in Disease,* J.T. Sharp (ed.), pp. 104–136. Thomas, Springfield, Ill, 1970.
24. Tully, J.G. Murine mycoplasmas. In *The Mycoplasmatales and the L-phase of Bacteria,* L. Hayflick (ed.), pp. 571–605. Appleton-Century-Crofts, New York, 1969.
25. Turner, A. W., A. D. Campbell, and A. T. Dick. Recent work on pleuro-pneumonia contagiosa bovum in North Queensland. *Austral. Vet. J.* 11:63–71, 1935.

42. Chlamydia

The etiologic agents of the diseases covered by the term chlamydioses are members of the genus *Chlamydia,* family Chlamydiaceae, order Chlamydiales.[17,18,24] They are spherical monmotile gram-negative microorganisms that multiply only within the cytoplasm of host cells by a developmental cycle that is unique among bacteria. The organisms contain both DNA and RNA but vary in the relative amounts of each at different growth stages. All strains of chlamydiae have the same developmental cycle, general morphology, and a common group antigen but may vary in the specificity of cell wall antigens, toxins, and species-differentiating biochemical properties. There are two species,[18] *C. trachomatis,* many strains of which are human pathogens, and *C. psittaci,* various strains of which cause numerous diseases and infections of humans and animals.[9,13,23] The diseases caused by different strains of *C. psittaci* are summarized in Table 42.1.

Specimens

Acute infections. In cases of acute severe chlamydiosis, the specimens to collect at necropsy for the isolation of *C. psittaci* are exudates of hyperemic tissues of diseased organs. For example, in cases of pneumonitis, collect consolidated or inflamed hyperemic portions of lungs; splenohepatopathy, sections of enlarged spleens and livers; airsacculitis, thickened exudate-coated air sacs and free exudate; placentopathy and abortion, hyperemic necrosed placentomes and fetal liver; encephalomyelitis, pericardial exudate and liver; enteritis, intestinal mucosa at the site of vascular congestion and colon contents; conjunctivitis, conjunctival or nasal discharge and conjunctival scrapings; arthritis, purulent synovia from affected joints and exudate from affected tendon sheaths.

Only a small amount of tissue is needed for the isolation of chlamydiae, but it is helpful to collect the tissue aseptically since contaminating bacteria interfere with its growth. If contaminants are unavoidably present, the tissue should be homogenized in phosphate buffered saline (pH 7.2) containing streptomycin sulfate, vancomycin, and kanamycin, each in a concentration of 1 mg/ml. The tissue then can be inoculated into chicken embryos or mice. Recent research has shown that this antibiotic solution effec-

Table 42.1. Diseases caused by different strains of *C. psittaci*

Disease	Host	Signs, lesions, and epidemiologic notes*
Psittacosis, ornithosis	Wild and domestic birds of all ages	Lethargy, hyperthermia, abnormal excretions, lowered egg production, mortality 0–40% depending upon virulence of organism. Fibrinous airsacculitis, pericarditis, peritonitis, perihepatitis, splenohepatopathy. Endemic in psittacine and columbidine birds worldwide. Probably endemic in waterfowl.
Psittacosis	Humans	Malaise, headache, hyperthermia, cough. Pneumonitis, splenitis, occasional meningitis. Less than 1% mortality in treated cases, 20% in untreated cases. Worldwide distribution. Some strains associated with lymphogranuloma venereum and abortion in humans.
Pneumonitis: feline, ovine, bovine, caprine, porcine, lapine, equine, murine	Domestic: cats, sheep, cattle, goats, pigs, rabbits, horses, mice	Conjunctival and nasal mucopurulent discharge, lethargy, signs of pneumonia, hyperthermia. Conjunctivitis, pneumonitis. Rarely fatal. Mortality may occur if there is concurrent infection with viruses, *Mycoplasma,* or *Pasteurella,* as in the case of shipping fever.
Polyarthritis	Lambs, calves	Lameness, swollen carpal or tarsal joints, hyperthermia, lethargy. Fibrinous synovitis, tendonitis, occasional hepatopathy. Variable mortality. Widespread in western U.S.
Encephalomyelitis (Buss disease)	Calves, dogs?	Lethargy, incoordination, hyperthermia, diarrhea, paralysis. Fibrinous perihepatitis, pericarditis, ascites. Endemic in cattle in mid and western U.S.
Placentopathy (epizootic bovine abortion, enzootic abortion of ewes, etc.)	Cattle, sheep, pigs, goats, rabbits, mice	Transient hyperthermia, chlamydemia; abortion late in gestation. Fetal hepatopathy, occasional edema, ascites, tracheal petechiae. Inflammation and necrosis of placentome. Periodically epidemic in Calif. and Ore. cattle. Endemic in sheep worldwide.
Conjunctivitis	Sheep, cats, guinea pigs, cattle, pigs	Vascular congestion and edema of conjunctiva. Mucopurulent discharge. Hyperthermia in cats. Follicular conjunctivitis, keratitis, pannus formation.
Fatal enteritis	Snowshoe hares, muskrats	Bizarre behavior, diarrhea. High mortality in hares. Enteritis, splenomegaly, focal necrosis in liver, septicemia. High mortality in Canadian snowshoe hares in 1959–1961. May be carried by muskrats.
Enteritis	Cattle, sheep	Diarrhea, weakness, and death in newborn. Enteritis. Epidemiology of subclinical intestinal infections in adults not known.
Subclinical intestinal infection	Cattle	No clinical signs. Chlamydial organisms may be recovered from intestinal mucosa and feces of cattle and sheep throughout U.S. Pathogenicity not known, but some sheep strains cause abortion in experimentally infected ewes. Natural infections stimulate production of antibodies.

*With *C. psittaci* many infections are subclinical. The signs and lesions mentioned occur in severe cases.

tively controls the growth of organisms of the genera *Proteus, Escherichi, Pasteurella, Staphylococcus, Streptococcus,* and *Corynebacterium,* while failing to inhibit the growth of *Chlamydia.* Some investigators suggest triturating tissues in solutions containing streptomycin (10 mg/ml) and neomycin (1 mg/ml), or streptomycin (5 mg/ml), tyrothricin (0.02 mg/ml), and sulfadiazine (2 mg/ml), or bacitracin (1000 units/ml). Solutions containing tetracycline, chloromycetin, or penicillin should not be used since these antibiotics inhibit the growth of chlamydiae.

Fecal samples or tissues heavily contaminated with extraneous bacteria should be suspended to a 20% concentration in a streptomycin-vancomycin-kanamycin solution and centrifuged three times at $1000 \times g$ for 30 minutes. At the end of each centrifugation, the middle portion of the supernatant fluid is carefully removed for the next centrifugation step and any floating materials or sediment discarded. After the third centrifugation, the middle layer is removed and inoculated into susceptible chicken embryos, mice, or cell cultures.

When it is desirable to make a diagnosis based on isolation of chlamydiae but necessary to keep the infected individual alive, the following specimens may be taken: for conjunctivitis, conjunctival scrapings; polyarthritis, fluid from swollen joints; severe pneumonitis, tracheal swabs; febrile period, heparinized whole blood and feces. Contaminated specimens should be treated with antibiotics as described previously.

Subclinical infections. In cases of mild or subclinical infections in birds, samples of liver, spleen, kidney, and colon contents should be collected at necropsy for isolation attempts. Chronically infected birds showing no clinical signs usually have enlarged spleens and livers or thickened air sacs. Subclinical infections of the intestinal tracts of mammals—cattle, sheep, mice, muskrats—are common, and the organisms may be isolated from fresh fecal samples according to methods described in "Acute infections" above. Animals with intestinal infections usually develop chlamydial antibodies in low titer.

Gross characteristics of specimens. The presence of chlamydiae in the tissues of susceptible hosts causes inflammation, vascular damage, necrosis, and proliferative response in certain organs. The organisms produce an intense inflammatory response at the sites of their multiplication, depending upon the strain of *Chlamydia.* Thus specimens from acutely diseased animals are likely to be sticky, due to purulent exudates from affected tissues. Involved organs may be enlarged or hemorrhagic or show signs of focal inflammation or necrosis. Specimens from chronically infected animals may appear normal.

Exudates and organ impression smears. The presence of *C. psittaci* organisms in the cytoplasm of cells in fresh exudates or organ impression smears may be detected microscopically, but the investigator should be warned that it is very difficult to distinguish intracellular *Mycoplasma* organisms from *Chlamydia.* The chlamydiae stain differentially, depending upon their stage of growth. The small, infectious form of the organism stains purple with Giemsa stain, red with Macchiavello's and Gimenez's stains, and blue with Casteneda's.[6] The large, dividing form of the organism is blue with Giemsa or Macchiavello's stains and purple with Casteneda's stain. Fresh exudates may also be examined directly in wet mounts using phase contrast optics. At magnifications of 500 diameters or more (with high and dry phase objectives), the organisms can be clearly and easily seen throughout the cytoplasm of mononuclear cells. Use of phase contrast microscopy avoids time-consuming staining procedures and the need for maintaining fresh stocks of stains. It also eliminates artifacts due to the stains.

Storage of specimens. The viability of chlamydiae in tissue specimens may be preserved indefinitely by storage at $-20°C$ or below. Care should be taken, however, that the storage temperature does not fluctuate between 0 and $-20°C$ repeatedly, since chlamydiae are susceptible to inactivation from ice crystal formation. Chlamydiae in heavily infected tissues remains viable for up to 50 days at 4°C but the infectivity titer falls gradually to nil during this period.

Specimens for histopathology. Tissues preserved for histopathology may be fixed in 10% Formalin or in Zenker's solution. While preservation and sectioning of tissues for histopathology is indispensable to the complete description of the cellular changes caused by chlamydiae in any new form of chlamydiosis, or in certain experimental studies, histologic examination of affected tissues serves primarily as a confirmation of microbiological or serologic tests. In some cases, histologic diagnosis is quite difficult; for example, in avian airsacculitis, the cellular changes caused by chalmydiae cannot be distinguished from those caused by mycoplasmas.

Blood for serology. Demonstration of at least a fourfold rise in titer of circulating antibodies by any of several serologic tests provides proof of recent chlamydial infection. Therefore, obtaining sera from serial bleedings during the acute and convalescent stages of disease may play an important role in diagnosis if the etiologic agent cannot be isolated.

Hazards to humans in handling specimens. Most strains of *C. psittaci* excreted by birds and some strains excreted by mammals can cause disease in humans. Humans become infected when they inhale infectious dust or aerosols containing *C. psittaci*. Inhalation of dried excrement from infected birds or mammals, exposure to infectious aerosols created by mechanical manipulation of suspensions of organisms in syringes, pipettes, or other laboratory equipment, and contamination of broken skin with infectious exudates from animals may be hazardous to susceptible humans. Creating aerosols while pipetting fresh sera from chlamydemic animals may be hazardous to serologists.

Laboratory Procedures

Cultivation. The laboratory animals most commonly used for isolation of *C. psittaci* are chicken embryos, mice, and guinea pigs. Cell cultures are less commonly used. All strains of both chlamydial species can be isolated and propagated in the yolk sacs of developing chicken embryos 6 or 7 days old. Strains of *C. psittaci* from birds can be isolated and propagated in young laboratory mice whether the mice are inoculated by the IC, IN, or IP routes. Strains causing lymphogranuloma venereum in humans and certain strains causing severe enteritis or generalized septicemia in mammals can also be propagated in mice.

Highly virulent, lethal strains from birds and strains causing bovine encephalomyelitis or ovine polyarthritis can be isolated in guinea pigs. Guinea pigs are the laboratory animal of choice for bovine and ovine chlamydiae strains because these animals are more susceptible to the growth of small numbers of chlamydiae than are chicken embryos. The strains of chlamydiae causing encephalomyelitis or polyarthritis will not multiply and cause lesions in mice regardless of the numbers of organisms inoculated.

The investigator should be aware that mice and guinea pigs in laboratory colonies may be naturally infected with chlamydiae. At least five strains of *C. psittaci* and Nigg's "murine pneumonitis" strain of *C. trachomatis* have been isolated from the lungs of mice in various laboratory colonies. The organisms are demonstrated by repeated passage of homogenized lungs of carrier animals inoculated into normal mice by the IN route. Infected mice eventually develop a diffuse pneumonitis. Guinea pigs may be naturally infected with a strain of *C. psittaci* that produces conjunctivitis. The organisms are transmitted between animals by contact and may persist indefinitely in breeding colonies.

Chlamydial strains recovered from birds may be adapted to grow well in primary cultures of chick embryo cells or in cell lines derived from mice (L-cells, McCoy cells) and humans (Chang liver and diploid cells).[7,21,22,25] For the initial propagation of chlamydiae from naturally infected tissues, cell cultures are not as susceptible to the growth of small numbers of chlamydiae as are the yolk sacs of chicken embryos.

Strains of chlamydiae from domestic mammals, such as the agents of polyarthritis, abortion, or pneumonitis in cattle and sheep, multiply only to a limited extent in cell cultures, and then only if the ratio of chlamydial infectious units to host cells is very large. The percentage of infected host cells can be greatly increased if suspensions of chlamydiae are centrifuged at $1000 \times g$ for 60 minutes and then placed directly onto a monolayer of host cells growing on the bottom of a flat-bottomed tube.

Chlamydiae are spheroidal organisms that multiply only within the cytoplasm of host cells by means of a multistage developmental cycle. The infectious form is a small, thick-walled, dense organism 0.2–0.3 μm in diameter. This form, once phagocytized, enlarges to a thin-walled, less dense, noninfectious form, 0.9–1 μm in diameter, that multiplies by fission. Second generation cells gradually change to smaller, thick-walled, infectious forms that contain ribosomes and a diffuse nucleus. This process takes place in an intracytoplasmic vesicle whose wall (in the case of *C. psittaci* infection) soon disintegrates, and the organisms are dispersed throughout the host cell cytoplasm. Intracellular microcolonies of chlamydiae may contain hundreds of organisms in all stages of growth. Therefore, in microscopic examination of wet mounts or stained impressions of infected cells, clusters of organisms of various sizes are observed in the cytoplasm of many host cells.

At 37°C incubation, the growth cycle in cell cultures takes 17–48 hours depending on the strain of organism used and the type of cell culture. Recent research has indicated, however, that the optimum temperature for the growth of most chlamydiae in chicken embryos is probably 39°C; the average number of days until the death of embryos inoculated with any of numerous strains of *C. psittaci* was reduced by as much as 3 days by incubation of infected embryos at 39 or 41°C instead of 37°C.[19] Extremely virulent strains, isolated originally from turkeys, muskrats, and gulls, appeared to multiply equally well over an incubation temperature range of 37–41°C.[20] Chlamydiae kill chicken embryos within 3–12 days depending upon the number of organisms inoculated and the strain of organism.

Differential reactions. The two species of *Chlamydia,* as presently defined,[18] are differentiated first on biochemical grounds. A carbohydrate, often labeled glycogen, is formed in intracellular microcolonies of *C. trachomatis* but not in microcolonies of *C. psittaci.*[7] The carbohydrate is visualized by fixing smears of infected cells with cold methanol and then staining the smears for several hours with 5% potassium iodide-iodine. Carbohydrate-containing microcolonies appear dark brown against a light tan background.[7] Second, the growth of all *C. trachomatis* strains in chicken embryos is inhibited by sodium sulfadiazine, at a dosage of 1 mg per embryo, inoculated into the yolk sac separately from the organisms. The degree of inhibition is such that in a duplicate titration the titer (LD_{50}) will be lowered by at least 2 logs as compared to the controls. In contrast, *C. psittaci* strains are not inhibited by sodium sulfadiazine.

All of the strains of *C. trachomatis,* save one, are found in humans. The exception is the murine pneumonitis strain that has often been isolated from laboratory mice. The other strains cause trachoma, inclusion conjunctivitis, lymphogranuloma venereum, urethritis, and occasional subclinical infections of the human genital tract.[9]

Chlamydiae exhibit several catabolic activities that are independent of host cell metabolic systems. For example, concentrated suspensions of chlamydiae that are free of host cells will enzymatically break down isotope-labeled glucose, pyruvic acid, or glutamic acid in the presence of inorganic and organic cofactors and produce labeled carbon dioxide. The organisms are dependent on the host cell, however, for the production of high-energy phosphates to provide the energy for these and other metabolic functions. This is the reason why chlamydiae have been called "energy parasites."[14,15,16]

The fact that *C. trachomatis* strains are sensitive to sulfadiazine suggests that they have a metabolic system for the production of precursors for the vitamin folic acid. As far as it has been tested, the growth of all strains of chlamydiae (except experimental mutants) is inhibited by the presence of tetracycline, chloromycetin, and 5-fluorouracil. Many strains are also sensitive to penicillin and cycloserine.

The cell walls of chlamydiae contain a high proportion of lipid, which makes the organisms susceptible to lipid solvents and detergents. A practical disinfectant for laboratory use is a dilute solution (1:1000) of the quaternary ammonium compound, alkyl-dimethylbenzyl-ammonium chloride, which rapidly inactivates concentrated suspensions of chlamydiae in solutions containing large amounts of protein. Phenol in low concentration is a poor disinfectant by comparison. The organisms are resistant to acid and alkali and survive suspension in 0.1 N NaOH or 0.1 HCl for short periods. Yet purified suspensions of organisms are inactivated within 48 hours in 0.85% NaCl at 37°C. The organisms are killed rapidly at 56°C or above but the exact thermal death time depends upon the amount of protective cellular matter present.

Immunology and serology. Organisms of both species of *Chlamydia* contain an antigenic lipopolysaccharide that is identical in all strains. The antigen is resistant to heat, phenol, and various proteinases but is inactivated by periodate and lecithinase. This group antigen is widely used for the detection of chlamydial antibodies in the sera of infected hosts. The group antigen is prepared from yolk sacs of *Chlamydia*-infected chicken embryos. The crude yolk sac harvest is homogenized and diluted to make a 20–30% suspension in beef heart broth or phosphate buffered saline (pH 7.2). The suspension is boiled for 30 minutes and cooled, and phenol is added to make a final suspension containing 0.5% phenol. The antigen is then ready to use in any of several CF tests. A second method uses ether and acetone to extract the chlamydial antigen from yolk sac homogenates.[8] A third method employs sodium lauryl sulfate extraction followed by repeated acid precipitation to obtain the antigen.[2]

The standard CF test can be used with sera from mammals that have had chlamydial infections. An indirect CF test can be used with sera from birds, since avian sera when reacted with chlamydial antigens normally do not fix guinea pig complement. In this test one CF unit of mammalian chlamydial antiserum is added to make the hemolytic indicator system operative.[11] The direct CF test can, however, be used with avian sera if normal rooster serum is added to help fix the complement.[3]

Usually, CF antibodies appear in birds and mammals within 7–10 days after chlamydial infection. The serologic diagnosis of chlamydial infection in individuals requires proof of at least a fourfold rise in antibody titer. On a group basis, however, if 80% or more of the individuals show titers, and half of the titers are as high as 1:64 or more, this is reasonable evidence that the group, flock, or herd is infected with chlamydiae. Subclinical intestinal infection with chlamydiae of low virulence is common in birds and mammals in the United States. The incidence of serologically positive but apparently asymptomatic individuals in a group, flock, or herd may run as high as 80% for pigeons, 0–80% for sparrows, 20–80% for sheep, 25% for cattle, and 50–75% for turkeys.

The capillary tube agglutination test also may be used to detect chlamydial antibodies in sera.[12] In this test, purified suspensions of chlamydiae are stained with Giemsa solution. The test can easily be conducted in the field and the results compare well with CF tests for antibody detection but not for detection of titer.

The CF test and direct and indirect FA tests may be used to detect chlamydial antigens and thus to identify the organism. The FA tests are more reliable with infected cell cultures than with impression smears or tissues.

In addition, a nonspecific test has been found in which a gram-negative organism, *Bacterium anitratum* (*herellea*), fixes complement in the presence of chlamydial antiserum. This is a unidirectional nonspecific reaction similar to the Weil-Felix reaction in which suspensions of *Proteus vulgaris* OX19 agglutinate with certain antirickettsia sera.

In the chlamydial neutralization tests, the chicken embryos, cell cultures, or mice are protected by the inhibiting effect of the specific antiserum. The success of these tests depends upon the use of high-titered antisera. Because they reflect variations in the specificity of the antigens found in the organisms' cell walls, they have been used to separate "serotypes" among strains of *C. psittaci*. There is strong evidence now that the cell walls of chlamydiae contain a mosaic of antigens that are distinct from the group antigen but are often shared within a group of strains affecting a certain class of animals; for example, human versus mammalian versus avian strains.[10] The specific antigens are detected and separated by a variety of methods (CF, neutralization of toxicity, neutralization of infectivity, FA, and AD tests).[4] Some antigens, however, are apparently shared between the groups of strains. Because of the complexity and sharing of the specific cell wall antigens between strains, no clear-cut serologic classification of the multitide of isolated chlamydial strains has been devised.[5]

Turkeys become skin reactive to detergent extracts of *C. psittaci* about 4 weeks after experimental infection.[1] If a small amount of the extract is inoculated into the wattle skin of birds previously infected with the organisms, a noticeable red swelling of the wattle develops. This allergic response is useful in screen-testing large flocks for exposure to chlamydial infection.

Many strains of *C. psittaci* apparently produce antigenically distinct toxins that are associated with the organisms' cell walls. The lethal effect of the toxin can be measured experimentally by the IV inoculation of mice with homogenates of infected yolk sacs. The lethal effects can be prevented by injection of specific antitoxin from hyperimmunized animals.

Reference laboratories. NADC; Department of Veterinary Microbiology, School of Veterinary Medicine, University of California, Davis; Department of Veterinary Microbiology, College of Veterinary Medicine, Texas A & M University, College Station.

References

1. Benedict, A.A. The intradermal test for epidemiologic studies of turkey· ornithosis. *Am. J. Hyg.* 66:245–252, 1957.
2. Benedict, A.A., and C. McFarland. Direct complement fixation test for diagnosis of ornithosis in turkeys. *Proc. Soc. Exp. Biol. Med.* 92:768–771, 1956.
3. Brumfield, H.P., and B.S. Pomeroy. Direct complement fixation by turkey and chicken serum in viral systems. *Proc. Soc. Exp. Biol. Med.* 94:146–149, 1957.
4. Collins, A.R., and A.L. Barron. Demonstration of group and species specific antigens of chlamydial agents by gel diffusion. *J. Infec. Dis.* 12:1–8, 1970.
5. Fraser, C.E.O. Analytical serology of the Chlamydiaceae. In *Analytical Serology of Microorganisms,* J.P. Kwapinski (ed.), vol. 1, pp. 257–330. Wiley, New York, 1969.
6. Gimenez, D.F. Staining rickettsiae in yolk-sac cultures. *Stain Techn.* 39:135–140, 1969.
7. Gordon, F.B., and A.L. Quan. Occurrence of glycogen in inclusions of the psittacosis-lymphogranuloma venereum-trachoma agents. *J. Infec. Dis.* 115:186–196, 1965.
8. Hilleman, M.R. Studies on lymphogranuloma venereum CF antigens. *J. Immunol.* 59:349–364, 1948.
9. Jawetz, E. Agents of trachoma and inclusion conjunctivitis. *Ann. Rev. Microbiol.* 18:301–334, 1964.
10. Jenkin, H.M. Preparation and properties of cell walls of the agent of meningopneumonitis. *J. Bact.* 80:639–647, 1960.
11. Karrer, H., K.F. Meyer, and B. Eddie. The complement fixation inhibition test and its application to the diagnosis of ornithosis in chickens and ducks. I. Principles and techniques of the test. *J. Infec. Dis.* 87:13–23, 1951.
12. Mason, D.M. A capillary tube agglutination test for detecting antibodies against ornithosis in turkey serum. *J. Immunol.* 83:661–666, 1959.
13. Meyer, K.F. The host spectrum of psittacosis-lymphogranuloma venereum (PL) agents. *Am. J. Ophthalmol.* 63:1225–1245, 1967.
14. Moulder, J.W. *The Psittacosis Group as Bacteria.* Wiley, New York, 1964.
15. Moulder, J.W. The relation of the psittacosis group (Chlamydiae) to bacteria and viruses. *Ann. Rev. Microbiol.* 20:107–130, 1966.
16. Moulder, J.W. A model for studying the biology of parasitism: *Chlamydia psittaci* and mouse fibroblasts (L cells). *Bioscience* 19:875–887, 1969.
17. Page, L.A. Revision of the family Chlamydiaceae Rake (Rickettsiales): Unification of the psittacosis-lymphogranuloma venereum-trachoma group of organisms in the genus *Chlamydia* Jones, Rake and Stearns, 1945. *Internat. J. Syst. Bact.* 16:223–252, 1966.
18. Page, L.A. Proposal for the recognition of two species in the genus *Chlamydia* Jones, Rake and Stearns, 1945. *Internat. J. Syst. Bact.* 18:51–66, 1968.

19. Page, L.A. Influence of temperature on the multiplication of chlamydiae in chicken embryos. In *Trachoma: Proceedings of an International Congress on Trachoma and Allied Diseases, Boston,* pp. 40–51. Excerpta Medica Conference Series 223, Amsterdam, 1971.
20. Page, L.A., and R.A. Bankowski. Factors affecting the production and detection of ornithosis antibodies in infected turkeys. *Am. J. Vet. Res.* 21:971–978, 1960.
21. Pearson, J.W., J.T. Duff, N.F. Gearinger, and M.L. Robbins. Growth characteristics of three agents of the psittacosis group in human diploid cell cultures. *J. Infec. Dis.* 115:49–58, 1965.
22. Piraino, F. Plaque formation in chick embryo fibroblast cells by *Chlamydia* isolated from avian and mammalian sources. *J. Bact.* 98:475–480, 1969.
23. Storz, J. *Chlamydia and Chlamydia Induced Diseases.* Thomas, Springfield, Ill., 1971.
24. Storz, J., and L.A. Page. Taxonomy of the chlamydiae: Reasons for classifying organisms of the genus *Chlamydia,* family *Chlamydiaceae,* in a separate order, *Chlamydiales* ord. nov. *Internat. J. Syst. Bact.* 21:332–334, 1971.
25. Tanami, Y., M. Pollard, and T.J. Starr. Replication pattern of a psittacosis virus in a tissue culture system. *Virology* 15:22–29, 1961.

43. Leptospira

Leptospiras are slender spirochetal bacteria that infect humans and a very wide variety of animals throughout the world. More than 100 antigenically distinct serotypes of pathogenic leptospiras have been isolated.[23]

During the past 20 years, widespread infections have been demonstrated in domestic animals, particularly in the canine, porcine, and ruminant populations, and to a lesser degree in horses and cats. In addition, pathogenic leptospiras are found in both wild and caged mice, rats, hamsters, and guinea pigs, in numerous species of rodents, and in many other wildlife species (skunk, fox, opossum, raccoon, deer, and others).[1] These infections are frequently characterized by localization of the leptospiras in the tubules of the kidneys, where they persist sometimes for the life of the animals, and from where they are shed with the urine, sometimes in enormous numbers. As a result, the organisms pollute surface waters and constitute a source of infection for other animals and humans.[9]

Climatic conditions are important ecological factors in the epidemiology of leptospirosis. Although the disease occurs throughout the world, warm humid conditions increase its incidence since leptospiras survive in water (or soil) for weeks if the pH is neutral or slightly alkaline. Agricultural management and animal husbandry practices also contribute to the spread of leptospirosis. Improper drainage, flooded yards, ponds of stagnant water, and the intermingling of cattle and swine are obvious factors.

For the description of the detailed clinical signs and pathology of leptospiral infections, standard references should be consulted. In cattle and swine, the cardinal clinical sign is abortion. Depending upon breeding practices, signs of leptospirosis may be detected throughout the year.[24] Although most infections are inapparent, leptospiras can cause serious if not fatal infections in dogs, cattle, and swine; these infections are characterized by fever, icterus, hemoglobinuria, oligogalactia, or abortion, as well as periodic ophthalmia in horses.

Young animals are less resistant to leptospiral infections and often die, whereas adult animals usually recover; other factors (sex, breed, and genetic background) apparently have little influence on the outcome of infection.

Specimens

In collecting samples for diagnosis of leptospirosis by direct microscopic examination, the clinician should take suitable precautions to avoid exposure. Potentially infected samples of blood or urine, or tissue from aborted fetuses, should be handled carefully and with proper protective clothing. Glasses should be worn to prevent the accidental inoculation of the eyes with droplets of urine while working with potentially leptospiruric cattle or swine.

Samples of blood for microscopic and cultural examinations should be collected in an aseptic manner with or without the addition of an anticoagulant. If an anticoagulant is used, sodium oxalate (0.5 ml of a 1% solution to 5 ml of blood) is preferred to sodium citrate, which inhibits the growth of leptospiras. Samples of other body fluids (urine, ocular, or cerebrospinal fluids) should be maintained at room temperature and examined as soon as possible. If samples of suspected tissue cannot be examined within a few minutes, they should be refrigerated at about 4°C. Leptospiras may persist in infected tissues for 5 days or longer if refrigerated.

With a little patience, urine can be collected during natural voidings of both cattle and swine. However, the application of tepid water to the prepuce by means of a sponge frequently stimulates urination. Urine can be collected from dogs aseptically by a bladder tap technique.[15] If the sample cannot be examined immediately, 1–2 ml of phosphate buffer (0.02 M) at a pH of 7.2 should be added to neutralize the urine. If the samples will not be examined for several days, Formalin may be added (10%) to preserve the leptospiras for subsequent microscopic examination.

Samples of tissue for histologic examination should be placed in at least 10 volumes of a 10% solution of buffered Formalin or frozen in a dry ice bath for examination with the FA technique. The FA technique has been used in only a few laboratories, though, and is not a routine diagnostic procedure.

A diagnosis of leptospirosis can be made by serologic methods only if the samples are collected at the proper time (Table 43.1). Samples collected during the febrile stage of acute leptospirosis should not contain specific antibodies; therefore, another sample must

Table 43.1. Specimens for the diagnosis of leptospirosis during acute (A) or convalescent (C) stages

Tissue or fluid	Direct microscopic examination A	C	Animal inoculation A	C	Laboratory culture A	C	Histopathology A	C	Serology A	C
Adults										
Blood	+		+		+				+	+
Peritoneal fluid	+		+		+					
Urine		+		+		+				
Ocular fluid		+		+		+				
Liver	+		+		+		+			
Kidney	+	+	+	+	+	+	+	+		
Fetuses (aborted)										
Blood	+		+		+				+	
Liver	+		+		+		+			
Kidney	+		+		+		+			
Urine	+		+		+					

be taken after the first week of disease. Conversion from a negative to a positive serologic status or a significant rise over an initially positive sample is diagnostic. Sera from cows or sows that have recently aborted due to leptospirosis will ordinarily react in high dilutions because the animals had to have been infected 2 or more weeks previously. Special precautions should be taken in the collection, preparation, and transportation of blood samples for the diagosis of leptospirosis because hemolyzed red blood cells or the products of bacterial growth have a detrimental effect on the living leptospiras used in the microscopic agglutination test.

Laboratory Procedures

Direct microscopic, cultural, animal inoculation, and serologic methods can be used in the laboratory diagnosis of leptospirosis (see Table 43.1).[3,10] The direct microscopic examination of samples for leptospiras is complicated by two factors: (1) leptospiras cannot be easily stained by procedures used with other bacteria, and (2) they are so slender that they cannot be seen with the ordinary bright-field microscope. However, leptospiras can easily be seen by dark-field microscopy.

Except in unusual circumstances (heavily parasitized laboratory animals or aborted fetuses, for example), the direct examination of blood or tissue homogenates for leptospiras is not recommended as a routine procedure; it is often successful, however, with urine from animals with profuse leptospiruria. Pseudospirochetes, which may be fibrin strands, are often present in specimens examined microscopically and may be confused with leptospiras. On the other hand, negative results on microscopic examinations do not rule out leptospirosis and the diagnosis always should be confirmed by cultural or serologic procedures.

By the use of staining techniques,[4] leptospiras have been detected in tissue sections of material obtained by biopsy and at necropsy. The Warthin-Starry method, as modified,[5] or Levaditi's method are commonly used. As a positive control, some investigators include a section of an agar plate containing colonies of leptospiras. These methods do not distinguish the leptospiral serotypes, and artifacts simulating *Leptospira* are often seen. As in the case of microscopic examinations, the diagnosis should be confirmed by cultural or serologic tests. However, in case of abortion a diagnosis of leptospirosis is justified by the histologic demonstration of leptospiras in the tissues of an aborted fetus together with the demonstration of a high level of agglutinins in the serum of the dam. The FA procedure has been used to demonstrate leptospiras in the urine and tissue of infected animals, and it promises to become a useful diagnostic tool.[14]

Cultures. Isolation of leptospiras by direct culture or by the use of laboratory animals provides the best evidence for a diagnosis of leptospirosis. Leptospiras may be isolated directly from the blood, urine, or tissues of animals. Using aseptic precautions, a sample of blood is obtained by venipuncture and 1 ml is added to each of two duplicate tubes of culture mediums. At least two types of media should be used (e.g. Stuart's and Fletcher's, or Fletcher's and Ellinghausen and McCullough's). If advisable, 5-fluorouracil may be added to inhibit the growth of contaminating bacteria. After mixing, further decimal dilutions are made through eight tubes of medium using a separate pipette for each dilution. An alternative procedure is to inoculate four or more tubes of each medium

Leptospira

with small inocula, i.e. one drop of blood per 5 ml of medium. The inoculated tubes are incubated at 28–30°C and examined at weekly intervals. Some strains grow rapidly and macroscopic evidence of growth appears in 5–7 days while other strains must be incubated for 30 or even 60 days before growth can be recognized. Before the tubes are discarded as negative, samples of the culture should be microscopically examined for leptospiras.

Procedures for the isolation of leptospiras from urine are similar to those recommended for blood. Because urine from animals usually contains microbial contaminants, it is usually advisable to filter the sample before cultures are made. Urine (1 or 2 ml) is drawn into a small syringe, a sterile Swinney filter-holder equipped with a membrane filter (0.45 μm pores) is attached, and the urine is expelled through the filter into tubes of culture medium.

For the isolation of leptospiras from tissues, the choice of tissue depends upon the stage of the disease (see Table 43.1), but usually liver or kidney are used. Some investigators recommend that Wharton's jelly of the umbilical cord be cultured whenever possible. If the kidney has numerous foci or cellular infiltration, they should be avoided, because they seem to have an inhibitory effect on isolations. One or more small pieces of tissue are removed aseptically, placed in a small disposable syringe, and forcibly expelled into a screw-capped tube containing 10 ml of growth medium. The tissue suspensions are then diluted and incubated as described above.

Essentially, media for the culture of leptospiras consist of dilute solutions of animal serum or serum proteins.[6,13] Most laboratories use rabbit serum to supplement the basal medium but serum from the sheep or cow is also satisfactory if free of specific agglutinins and heated (60°C for 30 minutes). Stuart's and Fletcher's basal media and modified Ellinghausen and McCullough's medium, which contains bovine serum albumin instead of serum, are available from commercial sources.

In order to minimize evaporation of the medium during the extended periods of incubation, the use of screw-capped tubes is recommended. Stock cultures are maintained best in tubes of semisolid (e.g. Fletcher's) medium. Cultures are transferred at monthly intervals using 1 ml of culture for 10 ml of fresh medium.

Tubes of inoculated medium should be examined against a bright light for evidence of leptospiral growth at weekly intervals for at least a month. Negative cultures should be examined under a microscope because the level of growth may be inadequate for macroscopic detection. Visual evidence of leptospiral growth in fluid media consists of a faint to slight turbidity that has a distinctive silky, swirling appearance when the tube is gently shaken. In a semisolid medium such as Fletcher's, leptospiras congregate in a "linear disc" 1–2 cm below the surface. More than one band may develop.

Cox's solid medium in petri dishes has been used to obtain colony growth of leptospiras.[6] Not all strains of leptospiras can be readily colonized. The medium has been used for purification of contaminated cultures, but it is not commonly used for routine isolation or maintenance of stock cultures.

Differential reactions. Compared to most bacteria, leptospiras are biochemically inert, and differential tests in media neither demonstrate their presence nor differentiate the leptospiral serotypes. In vitro, leptospiras are insensitive to the sulfonamides, relatively insensitive to the peptide antibiotics, and sensitive to the tetracycline and macrolide antibiotics.[20] Bacteriophages have not been isolated from leptospiras.

Cellular morphology. Leptospiras are helically coiled organisms 7–40 μm in length and approximately 0.1 μm in thickness. Usually one or both ends are turned back in the shape of a hook.

Animal inoculation. Because of limitations in the present culture methods for the isolation of leptospiras, these techniques cannot completely supplant procedures involving the use of laboratory animals.[19] Gerbils, chinchillas, weanling rabbits, and baby chicks have been used for this purpose, but weanling or young hamsters (30–60 g) and guinea pigs are used most commonly. The suspected material (blood, urine, or tissue suspension) is injected IP into each of three hamsters (0.25–10.5 ml) or guinea pigs (0.5–1 ml) and the animals are observed for 2–3 weeks. Usually, the first manifestation of leptospirosis is fever (39–41°C); icterus may develop and death may occur 6–14 days after exposure. Other investigators rely on losses in body weight as evidence of leptospiral infection. However, some strains of leptospiras may not elicit any clinical signs, although animals are infected. Beginning with the third day after inoculation or whenever signs of disease occur, two or more samples of blood (0.5–1 ml) for culture should be obtained at 2–3-day intervals. Two weeks after inoculation, the animals are killed and the kidneys are removed aseptically; they are triturated and cultured as described above.

Immunology and serology. As with other diseases of microbial origin, serologic tests for the diagnosis of leptospirosis have certain disadvantages and limitations: (1) antibodies are usually not detectable during the first week of disease, (2) antibody titers may be low if animals were treated with antibiotics, and (3) a positive seroreaction does not prove that the illness was due to leptospirosis since the agglutinins may reflect an earlier infection or antigenic stimulation due to active immunization or even passive immunity, e.g. from the ingestion of colostrum.

Serologic evidence of leptospirosis has been obtained with agglutination, CF, hemolytic, and FA techniques.[14,16] Of these, the microscopic agglutination (MA, also known as agglutination lysis) test is the standard procedure, although the time and effort required to maintain stocks of these antigens, their hazards to laboratory personnel, and the laboriousness of the test itself limit its use. Furthermore, the antigens used in the MA test are specific, and it is therefore necessary to use a battery of 12 or more antigens to assure the detection of the antibodies that may be provoked by the large number of diverse serologic types of leptospiras. Pathogenic serotypes of the following serogroups are present in the United States: *australis, autumnalis, ballum, bataviae, canicola, grippotyphosa, hebdomadis, icterohaemorrhagiae, pomona, pyrogenes,* and *tarassovi.*

In an attempt to standardize the technique of the MA test, the following procedures were recommended by the Leptospirosis Committee of the United States Animal Health Association.[17,18] (1) Use Stuart's medium supplemented with sterile rabbit serum. The serum should be from a pool of several rabbits and be tinged with hemoglobin. After the pH value of the serum is checked and adjusted to 7.3–7.5, if necessary, sterilize it by filtration through asbestos or membrane (0.45 μm porosity) filters and store at -20°C until used. Cultures of leptospiras can be maintained in Stuart's medium by subculture at intervals of 5–7 days. For use in the MA test, they should contain between 100 and 300×10^6 leptospiras per ml as determined by nephelometry or by counting in a Petroff-Hausser and Helber counting chamber. If the culture is more dense than desired, dilute it with sterile Stuart's medium. Cultures that contain clumps of leptospiras ("breed nests") or aged cultures (10 days or more) are not suitable. (2) The serum to be tested need not be heat inactivated. Prepare dilutions of 1:5, 1:50, 1:500, 1:5000, and 1:50,000 in phosphate-buffered saline (pH 7.4) using 1 ml serologic pipettes. (An alternate scheme used in some laboratories is to begin with a serum dilution of 1:25 and make fourfold dilutions.) (3) Mix an equal amount (0.1 ml or 0.2 ml) of each serum dilution with each antigen. The final dilutions of serum thus become 1:10, 1:100, 1:1000, 1:10,000, and 1:100,000. The serum and antigen may be mixed by a few seconds of gentle shaking in test tubes, porcelain dishes, or plastic trays. (4) Include an antigen control (equal amount of antigen and diluent) and a positive control (known positive serum diluted as the test serum). (5) Cover to minimize evaporation and incubate at 30°C for 2 hours. (6) Use a microscope providing a magnification of approximately $150\times$ and dark-field illumination to determine the results. (7) With a pipette or a bacteriological loop, begin with the highest dilution and place a small drop of each mixture on a clean glass slide. Do not superimpose a coverslip. Compare the test to the antigen control for clearing (i.e. disappearance) of leptospiras with agglutination into brilliant clumps or balls.

Different results may occur in different laboratories because of differences in the dilution scheme, antigen sensitivities, and interpretations of the reactions. The WHO Expert Group recommended that the "endpoint reaction be defined as the highest final dilution of serum in the serum-antigen mixture in which 50% or more of the cells are agglutinated."[23] Most investigators consider a titer of 1:100 as significant and high titers (1:10,000 or greater) as strongly indicative of recent infection.

The following 15 serotypes have been recommended by the WHO Expert Group for use as antigens in the MA test.[23]

autumnalis	*butembo*	*javanica*	*pyrogenes*
bataviae	*canicola*	*patoc*	*tarassovi* (*hyos*)
borincana	*grippotyphosa*	*pomona*	*wolffi*
bratislava	*icterohaemorrhagiae*		

The numerous pathogenic leptospiras are distinguished by serologic procedures.[8] Whereas definitive culture typing requires elaborate reciprocal agglutinin-absorption tests with many specific antisera and is usually done in reference laboratories, preliminary typing can be accomplished in the diagnostic laboratory. The unknown culture is used as the antigen in the MA test along with antisera to the different leptospiras, and the end titers are determined. The antiserum is produced in rabbits by a series of IV injections at intervals of 5–7 days. Increasing amounts of antigen (0.5–5 ml) are given until high-titered serum is obtained. If the unknown antigen reacts to the same end titer as the homologous antigen, it may be presumed to belong to the same serogroup. Isolates that fail to react to high titers with any of the standard antisera should be referred to typing centers for further identification.

In veterinary diagnostic laboratories, macroscopic tests with killed leptospiras as antigens are used far more frequently than all other tests. Macroscopic plate test antigens developed by Stoenner,[22] and by Galton and her associates,[11] are available commercially (Fort Dodge Lab., Fort Dodge, Iowa; Difco Lab., Detroit). The antigens in both tests are essentially the same and consist of Formalin-fixed cells in select buffer solutions; the antigens are used singly or in pools of three. The tests should be performed as recommended by the manufacturers. Generally, the test consists of placing a loopfull or small drop of serum on a glass plate and adding a drop of antigen.

After the mixture is spread to a diameter of about 1 cm, the plate is rotated 5 or 6 times to mix the serum and antigen and then is incubated in a humidified environment for 6 minutes. After that the plate is removed, rotated 15 times, and read for clumps of agglutinated leptospiras. In positive reactions, small clumps will be clearly visible by indirect illumination.

Results of tests by this procedure on human sera have shown good agreement with titers on the same sera obtained by the MA test. With animal sera, however, there is little correlation of MA titers with the reactions in the macroscopic plate tests.[7]

Although toxins have been demonstrated in leptospiras and in the liver of infected guinea pigs, the role, if any, of these materials in the pathogenesis of leptospirosis is not known.[2,21] Hemotoxins specifically affecting ruminant cells have been found in select serotypes (e.g., *pomona, grippotyphosa, australis*) and may figure in the hemolytic manifestations of disease in ruminants.

Reference laboratory. The WHO and FAO have jointly established several Leptospirosis Reference Laboratories throughout the world. The laboratory in the western hemisphere is WHO/FAO Leptospirosis Reference Laboratory, Walter Reed Army Institute of Research, Walter Reed Army Medical Center, Washington. Proper arrangements should be made before cultures are sent for identification.

References

1. Alston, J.M., and J.C. Broom. *Leptospirosis in Man and Animals*. E. & S. Livingstone, Edinburgh, London, 1958.
2. Arean, V.M., G. Sarasin, and J.H. Green. The pathogenesis of leptospirosis: Toxin production by *Leptospira icterohaemorrhagiae*. *Am. J. Vet. Res.* 25:836–843, 1964.
3. Babudieri, B. Laboratory diagnosis of leptospirosis. *Bull. WHO*, 24:45–58, 1961.
4. Blendon, D.C., and H.S. Goldberg. Silver impregnation stain for *Leptospira* and flagella. *J. Bact.* 89:809–810, 1965.
5. Bridges, C.H., and L. Luna. Kerr's improved Warthin-Starry Technic: Study of the permissible variations. *Lab. Invest.* 6:357–367, 1957.
6. Cox, C.D. Hemolysis of sheep erythrocytes sensitized with leprospiral extracts. *Proc. Soc. Exp. Biol. Med.* 90:610–615, 1955.
7. Crawford, R.P. Evaluation of a plate test for the detection of leptospiral antibodies in bovine serum. *J. Am. Vet. Med. Ass.* 145:683–687, 1964.
8. *Diagnosis and Typing in Leptospirosis*. WHO Technical Report Series no. 113. Geneva, 1956.
9. Galton, M.M. The epidemiology of leptospirosis in the United States with special reference to wild animal reservoirs. *Southwestern Vet.* 13:37–42, 1959.
10. Galton, M.M., R.W. Menges, E.B. Shotts, A.J. Nahmias, and C.W. Heath. *Leptospirosis*. Public Health Service Publication no. 951. U.S. Government Printing Office, Washington, 1962.
11. Galton, M.M., D.K. Powers, A.D. Hale, and R. Cornell. A rapid macroscopic-slide screening test for the serodiagnosis of leptospirosis. *Am. J. Vet. Res.* 19:505–512, 1958.

12. Hanson, L.E., P.R. Schnurrenberger, R.B. Marshall, and G.W. Sherrick. Leptospiral serotypes in Illinois cattle and swine. *Proc. U.S. Livestock Sanitary Ass.* 69:164–169, 1965.
13. Johnson, R.C., and J.B. Wilson. Nutrition of *Leptospira pomona*. *J. Bact.* 80:406–411, 1960.
14. Maestrone, G. The use of an improved fluorescent antibody procedure in the demonstration of Leptospira in animal tissues. *Can. J. Comp. Med. Vet. Sci.* 27:108–112, 1963.
15. Menges, R.W., M.M. Galton, and A.D. Hall. Diagnosis of leptospirosis from urine specimens by direct culture following bladder tapping. *J. Am. Vet. Med. Ass.* 132:58–60, 1958.
16. Randall, R., P.W. Wetmore, and A.R. Warner. Sonic vibrated leptospirae as antigens in the complement fixation test for the diagnosis of leptospirosis. *J. Lab. Clin. Med.* 34:1411–1415, 1949.
17. Roth, E.E. Report of Committee on Leptospirosis. *Proc. U.S. Livestock Sanitary Ass.* 63:140–142, 1959.
18. Roth, E.E., W.V. Adams, B. Greer, G.E. Sanford, K. Newman, and M. Moore. Comments on the laboratory diagnosis of leptospirosis in domestic animals with an outline of some procedures. *Proc. U.S. Livestock Sanitary Ass.* 65:520–534, 1961.
19. Stalheim, O.H.V. Leptospiral lysis by lipids of renal tissue and milk. *J. Bact.* 89:545, 1965.
20. Stalheim, O.H.V. Effects of antimicrobial agents on leptospiral growth, viability, motility, and respiration. *Am. J. Vet. Res.* 27:797–802, 1966.
21. Stalheim, O.H.V. A toxic factor in *Leptospira pomona*. *Proc. Soc. Exp. Biol. Med.* 126:412–415, 1968.
22. Stoenner, H.G. Further observations of leptospiral plate antigens. *Am. J. Vet. Res.* 28:259–266, 1967.
23. World Health Organization Expert Group. *Current Problems in Leptospirosis Research*. Technical Report Series no. 380. Geneva, 1967.
24. *Zoonoses Surveillance, Annual Summary: Leptospirosis.* Report of Chief, Veterinary Public Health Laboratory, National Communicable Disease Center, Atlanta, 1967.

44. Borrelia

This genus of spirochetes is represented by several species of veterinary importance, foremost among which are *B. anserina* of avians, *B. theileri* of cattle and possibly horses, and *B. suilla* and *B. hyos* of pigs, together with some less well-defined organisms that apparently produce disease in other domestic animals and in rodents. Several important members of this genus are the cause of relapsing fever and certain ulcerative conditions in humans. In general, these organisms are transmitted to animals by soft ticks of the genus *Ornithodorus* or *Argas*, but they are also transmitted by other kinds of ticks, various insects, and even by contact or mechanically.[12] These diseases are generally more prevalent in hot dry areas, such as deserts and semideserts, than in high rainfall areas. *Borrelia* infections often occur simultaneously or in association with other infections in their respective hosts.

Borrelia anserina

This organism is the cause of spirochetosis in geese, chickens, turkeys, ducks, and wild birds.[7,10,15] In hot dry areas it is an important disease of the poultry industry, particularly in backyard flocks, but it can also be a problem in commercial flocks, where transmission other than by ticks takes place.[5,16,24] It sometimes occurs simultaneously with *Aegyptionella pullorum*, as both are transmitted by the same vector, *Argas persicus*.[1] An interesting feature of this combination is that spirochetes have a shorter incubation period and are more virulent than the aegyptionellas when they occur independently, but not when they occur together.

In spirochetosis the sick bird shows weakness, paleness, a green diarrhea, which is usually attended by excessive urate evacuation in the feces, fever (42–44°C), and anorexia. Mortality can be high, often exceeding 50% in susceptible birds, and birds of all ages can be affected. In backyard flocks, however, the disease is enzootic and adult birds usually survive the natural disease. The new crop of young chicks, however, is suceptible. Field evidence supported by laboratory findings indicates that if infected ticks feed on immune birds, the organisms they carry can become neutralized.[21] The effect in backyard conditions is a seasonal incidence of the disease in the spring or early summer when the young crop of susceptible chicks is exposed.

Birds dying from the acute form of the disease show a severe anemia and lesions of the spleen and liver.[25] The spleen is often enlarged two to six times in size, and it shows a characteristic mottling where the lymphoid aggregations are more pronounced and stand out as gray nodules, whereas the red pulp is mottled with dark areas, which are actually due to ecchymotic hemorrhages.[22] On section, the cut surface has a cooked appearance, being drier than normal. The liver is also enlarged and shows patchy necrotic areas. Intestinal lesions are mild, but there often is a watery green diarrhea containing urate deposits and causing soiling of the vent feathers. Occasionally, in experimental subjects where only anemia is noted, the red bone marrow is pale and organisms can be found in it.[16]

The disease is generally transmitted by the soft blue tick *Argas persicus,* which hides during the day in cracks of the woodwork or mud walls of the poultry house, usually at a height out of reach of the chickens, who seem to relish the blood-filled ticks. *Culex* mosquitoes, red mites, and probably many other biting insects may transmit the disease in a mechanical way.[5,10] One study has claimed that it can also be spread through the feces or through cannibalism; and it certainly can be spread by contaminated hypodermic needles.[16] The disease has in fact often been seen in outbreaks where no ticks were known to be present.

Specimens

A thin blood film is made and stained with Giemsa or other aniline dye. This is not as good for the diagnosis of spirochetes as the Nigrosin method, but it is a necessary step in order to detect other organisms in the blood, such as aegyptionellas, pasteurellas, etc.

A drop of blood is placed in the center of a second glass slide and a drop of Nigrosin stain placed next to it. A wooden spreader (e.g. a toothpick) is then used to mix the blood with the Nigrosin stain and the mixture is spread as thin as possible. This negative staining has an effect similar to dark-field illumination but the objects are fixed and permanent.[27] The stain can be examined under oil immersion as soon as it is dry (within minutes) and is a most simple but effective test.

For the purpose of isolation of the organisms in culture or by egg inoculation, it is preferable to take heart blood, 2 ml of blood to 3 ml of 2% sterile citrated saline. This should be stored at 4–7°C. If the material is to be freeze-dried, then the blood should be collected in 10% glucose containing 2% sodium citrate, dried as soon as possible, and then stored at −20°C. The freeze-dried material is then reconstituted in distilled water and injected into the yolk sac of 10-day-old embryos. After incubation for about 7 days, the embryos are examined. If positive for living spirochetes, harvested material can then be introduced into susceptible chickens. *Borrelia anserina* has been stored in this way for periods greater than 10 years.

If the chicken or bird is freshly dead from the acute form of the disease, clotted blood can be collected from the heart and placed in 2% citrated saline and then prepared for injection IM into two susceptible chickens, 3–6 weeks of age. When the inoculated chickens' rectal temperatures rise, heart blood can be collected as described above for storage or further processing. Another method, for diagnosing the disease in birds dead from the subacute form, is based on the demonstration of antibodies in the spleen.[19]

Spleen material from the dead bird, which contains neutralizing antibodies, is emulsified and used as antiserum. Suspensions of known *B. anserina* containing an infective dose are then treated with this material, while control suspensions are treated with negative spleen material prepared from a normal susceptible chicken. Both mixtures are then injected into susceptible birds. The test cannot, however, differentiate between antibodies from a previous exposure and those from a current infection.

For serologic work, heart blood is collected in 10 ml amounts from recovered birds for serum harvest.

The bodies of affected birds should also be searched for larvae, which usually attach on the inner side of the legs or wings and remain there for about a week. Adult ticks feed only at night and are hidden during the day. Drops of clotted blood often can be seen either on the skin of the feet and legs or on the perches where the birds roosted. If the infestation with ticks is of long standing, darkened trails of fecal droppings can be seen on the walls leading to their hiding places. The ticks can be stored in either 70% alcohol, or, if needed alive, in screw-capped bottles half filled with cotton and kept at room temperature.

Thin pieces of spleen, liver, red bone marrow, and other organs can be collected in 10% formol-saline. To demonstrate the spirochetes, sections are stained by the Levaditi silver impregnation technique or similar methods.[28]

Laboratory Procedures

Cultures. Growth of *Borrelia* occurs in Noguchi's ascitic fluid–rabbit kidney medium. Artificial media are rarely used for diagnostic work, however, but they do have application in the production of antigens and antisera. The cultures should be incubated at 37°C under anaerobic conditions.

Differential reactions. *Borrelia* are extremely sensitive to most chemicals, even to substances generally considered inocuous, e.g. distilled water, tryptose, peptone, and glycerol. The organisms are highly sensitive to all antibiotics. For storage at 4°C, citrated saline is preferred. For freeze-drying, 10% glucose is used. The common bacteriological differential reactions are not used.

Cellular morphology. The length of the organisms differ from strain to strain and with the duration of the cultivation. *Borrelia* are generally said to have 6 spirals. However, when observed in the blood of hatched chicks that were inoculated as embryos 6–10 days old, the organisms appear in long chains with more than 20 spirals. The *Borrelia* differ from the *Treponema* and *Leptospira* in that they are easily stained with ordinary aniline dyes.

Animal inoculation. Only avian species are susceptible; chickens, turkeys, ducks, geese, and many species of wild birds can be infected. The preferred method of cultivation of *B. anserina* for diagnostic work and vaccine production is the use of embryonating chicken eggs. The organism rapidly multiplies in the embryo but is not highly pathogenic. The main lesion from the infection is an enlarged spleen. The embryonating eggs at 6–10 days of age are inoculated with infectious citrated blood via the CAM, AlC, or YS routes. If allowed to hatch, the chicks may be stunted but otherwise look normal. Such chicks may have blood that is heavily infected with three or four times as many spirochetes as RBC per microscopic field. When such blood is citrated and stored at 4°C overnight, the RBC settle and the fluid portion can be harvested as an antigen with a high concentration of spirochetes.

Young susceptible chickens 3–6 weeks of age are often used for diagnostic work with *B. anserina*. They may be inoculated IM with the specimen material. Blood smears should be made from the chickens daily from the second day after injection. Usually the organisms appear in the blood smears in 3–5 days. Within 1–3 days thereafter, a peak spirochete concentration should be reached. The organisms in the blood tend to clump 1–2 days before recovery begins, and collections of blood should be made before this happens. The spirochetes do not live long after clumping, probably because of the action of antibodies.

Immunology and serology. The usual method for determining immunologic types is by cross-immunity tests in chickens that previously were immunized with vaccines of specific strains or were inoculated with viable organisms and then treated with penicillin after the infection was established. Some workers do not believe that there are true immunologic type differences.[8]

Good vaccines for spirochetosis can be made from infected homogenized embryo tissues. Such vaccines consist of the equivalent of one highly infected embryo (trimmed) per 100 ml of saline. Either 0.05% Formalin, 0.1% betapropriolactone, or 0.0001% Merthiolate are used as inactivants. The vaccine is reported to have a long shelf-life at 4°C storage (at least 10 years). The duration of immunity is sufficiently long for commercial broiler and layer production. The vaccine dose is 0.5 ml IM for adults and 0.25 ml IM for chicks. If infection already has occurred in a flock, each vaccinated chicken should also be given 40,000 i.u. of procaine penicillin (added to the vaccine or given separately). In Russia a phenolized hemolysate vaccine has been used on a large scale in the field with good results.[23] In India a lyophilized Merthiolated vaccine is used successfully.

B. anserina is antigenically distinct from other species of *Borrelia* found in mammals. The immobilization test seems to be reliable.[14,17,19] The AD, agglutination, and precipitin tests do not have confirmed specificity.[16]

Borrelia theileri

This organism was first seen by Theiler in the blood of cattle in South Africa, and it is now known to occur in most parts of Australia.[4,11,26] Unfortunately, there are no reports of its in vitro cultivation or of serologic work. The host range also is not clear. However, in one study, blood taken from an infected donkey was used to transmit the disease to a calf.[13] From studies carried out in Australia it would seem that the equine form of the disease is caused by the same organism, but laboratory proof is lacking.

This is apparently a benign organism that may well be of the "relapsing fever" type, because it is usually found in conjunction with other infections, probably as a secondary infection that flares up in times of stress. Thus Theiler found the organism in the blood of cattle suffering from anaplasmosis, and it has often been seen in the blood of cattle ill from babesiosis, trypanosomiasis, and theileriosis, but seldom in cattle not suffering from another disease. It therefore does not appear to be a primary pathogen. In experimental infections, spirochetemia appears and is accompanied by a brief febrile reaction.[13]

When blood from an Australian bull that showed spirochetemia following recovery from babesia and anaplasma infection was inoculated into another bovine, large numbers of parasites occurred in the recipient's blood after 6 days. Thus the incubation period for the disease seems to be about 5–6 days.[18] The septicemic form of the disease is believed to be transmitted by the ticks *Margaropus decoloratus* (*Boopholus decoloratus*) and *Rhipicephalus evertsi* in South Africa, and by *B. annulatala* and *B. microplus* in Australia.

Various superficial lesions in cattle and horses also have been ascribed to *B. theileri*. One investigator in England stated that spirochetes were constantly present in every case of canker of the foot and "greasy heels" of the horses examined by him. In another case in Australia, spirochetes were found in large numbers in the semen of a stallion, which also showed ulcers and nodular lesions on the lining of the prepuce and the body of the penis.[20] Scrapings from these lesions showed spirochetes morphologically similar to those found in the semen. However, since very little laboratory work has been done on this organism, there is insufficient evidence for incriminating *B. theileri* as the primary cause of superficial lesions in cattle and horses.

Specimens

Blood is collected from the jugular vein in citrated saline for transmission experiments, but the organism's keeping qualities are not well known. Blood smears in thin films are prepared for staining with Giemsa or other aniline dyes. Blood also could be prepared for dark-ground examination or phase contrast microscopy as described for *B. anserina*. The Nigrosin staining method also should be tried. It is recommended that attempts be made to isolate the organism by the same techniques as those used for *B. anserina*, which are described earlier in this chapter.

Borrelia suilla

This organism has been associated with an important, chronic, granulating wound infection of pigs in Australia,[11,26] South Africa,[9] and New Zealand.[20] It may be the same organism as *B. hyos*, but this remains to be proved. It is significant that in both South Africa and Australia, hog cholera is not present, so HCV is not the primary pathogen providing favorable conditions for secondary invasion by *B. suilla*.

The lesions in this condition occur in the skin and soft underlying tissues of pigs. These lesions are ulcerative granulomata that occur most commonly in pigs kept under unhygienic conditions, particularly those where the runs are littered with bones and other objects that can produce wounds. Dirty muddy wallows may be a contributing factor. Castration incisions often are prone to infection but any cutaneous wound or abrasion may become involved, and lesions may even occur on the gums where the teeth are erupting.

The lesions vary in appearance from large tumors to flat undurated ulcers with gross tissue destruction. They may occur anywhere on the body, and if not treated they may become very large and penetrate down to the bone. Some clinicians differentiate the various manifestations—castration infection may be called "scirrhous cord," foot lesions may be termed "foot rot," and intestinal lesions referred to as "pimply gut." The causative organism is generally considered to be *Borrelia suilla,* but secondary infections with *Fusiformis necrophorus, Corynebacterium pyogenes,* streptococci, coliform bacteria, and other organisms are invariably present. Unfortunately this spirochete has not been isolated and studied so that it is not yet known whether it is the primary cause of the disease described above.

Specimens

Scrapings made with a scalpel and stained with Giemsa or any aniline dye reveal the spirochetes in large numbers. These can also be demonstrated with dark-ground illumination or phase contrast microscopy. It is also likely that the Nigrosin staining method described for *B. anserina* would be very effective in demonstrating the presence of these spirochetes. The spirochetes are large and vary from 9 to 26 μm in length; each parasite contains two to six spirals. The organisms may be found in the lymph glands that drain the ulcerative lesions. The disease can be effectively treated with antibiotics such as penicillin.

Borrelia hyos

Theobold Smith first noted this organism, which later was found in association with hog cholera in the United States. The organism has been associated with the production of the "boutons" in Peyer's patches of the intestinal tract and in other ulcerative lesions in hog cholera.[9] Even though many other organisms, such as *Pasteurella suis,* have likewise been incriminated in the HC complex, HCV is regarded as the primary cause of such lesions.

Spirocheta penortha

This organism, which appears to be a *Borrelia,* was first described by Beveridge,[3] and it is apparently an accessory factor in the syndrome of foot rot of sheep, with *Fusiformis nodosus* being the primary pathogen. Other organisms, such as *Sphaerophorus necrophorus* and other unidentified bacteria that are present in the lesions, possibly play a secondary role also. This complex, therefore, resembles the ulcerative granulomas in pigs. The spirochete concerned has not been sufficiently studied to permit its exact classification.

References

1. Ahmed, A.A.S., and M.A. Elsisi. Observations on aegyptionelosis and spirochaetosis of poultry in Egypt. *Vet. Med. J. Giza* 11:139–146, 1966.
2. Al-Hilly, J.N.A. Immunodiffusion agar-gel test for demonstration of *Borrelia anserina* antigen produced by livers of infected chicks. *Am. J. Vet. Res.* 30:1877–1880, 1969.
3. Beveridge, W.I.B. A study of *Spirochaeta penortha* (n.s.p.) isolated from foot-rot in sheep. *Austral. J. exp. Biol. Med. Sci.* 14:307–318, 1936.
4. Callow, L.L. Observations on tick-transmitted spirocaetes of cattle in Australia and South Africa. *Brit. Vet. J.* 123:492–497, 1967.
5. Ciolca, A., I. Tanase, and I. May. Role of the poultry mite, *Dermanyssus gallinae,* in transmission of spirochaetosis. *Arch. Vet.* 5:207–215, 1968 (in Bulgarian).

6. Djankov, I., I. Soumrov, and F. Penev. Agglutinin formation and its relationship to immunity against spirochaetosis in fowls. *Vet. Med. Nauki Sof.* 2:701–708, 1965 (in Bulgarian).
7. Galuzo, I.G., and M.P. Iakunin. Spirochaetosis of birds in nature. *Proc. 1st Internat. Cong. Parasit.* (Rome) 1:405–406, 1964.
8. Hart, L. Spirochaetosis in fowls: Studies on immunity. *Austral. Vet. J.* 39:187–191, 1963.
9. Henning, M.W. *Animal Diseases in South Africa,* pp. 362–367. 3rd ed. Central News Agency, Onderstepoort, South Africa, 1956.
10. Hinshaw, W.R. Spirochaetosis. In *Diseases of Poultry,* H.E. Biester and L.H. Schwarte (eds.), pp. 1308–1314. 5th ed. Iowa State University Press, Ames, 1967.
11. Hungerford, T.G. *Diseases of Livestock,* p. 312. 7th ed. Angus & Robertson, Sydney, 1970.
12. Kapur, H.R. Transmission of spirochaetosis through agents other than *Argas persicus. Indian J. Vet. Sci. Anim. Husbandry* 10:354–360, 1940.
13. Kaschula, V.R. Treponema (Spirochaeta) Theileri transmitted from a donkey to a calf. *J. S. African Vet. Med. Ass.* 19:100–102, 1948.
14. Levaditi, C., A. Vaisman, and A. Hamelin. Les immobilisines actives a l'égard du Spirachaeta gallinarum: Immobilizing antibodies for *Borrelia anserina. Ann. Inst. Pasteur* 83:260–262, 1952.
15. Mathey, W.J., and P.J. Siddle. Spirachaetosis in pheasants. *J. Am. Vet. Med. Ass.* 126:123–126, 1955.
16. McNeil, E., W.R. Hinshaw, and R.E. Kissling. A study of *Borrelia anserina* infection (spirochaetosis) infection in turkeys. *J. Bact.* 57:191–206, 1949.
17. Mehta, M.L., and A.R. Muley. *In vitro* agglutination and immobilization tests for typing antigenically different strains of Borrelia gallinarum. *Indian Vet. J.* 45:1059–1060, 1968.
18. Mulhearn, C.R. A note on two blood parasites of cattle (*Spirochaeta theileri* and *Bartonella bovis*) recorded for the first time in Australia. *Austral. Vet. J.* 22:118–119, 1946.
19. Nobrega, P., and A.S. Reiss. O diagnostico da espiqouitose aviaria em animais mortos. *Arq. Inst. Biol. São Paulo* 18:91–96, 1947.
20. Osborne, V.E., and R.V.S. Bain. Genital infection of a horse with spirochaetes. *Austral. Vet. J.* 37:190–191, 1961.
21. Pavlov, P., I. Dzhankov, and P. Penev. Interaction between blood from spirochaetosis immune fowls and *Borrelia anserinum* in the tick *Argas persicus. Vet. Med. Nauki Sof.* 5:11–16, 1968 (in Bulgarian).
22. Reddy, M.V., P.K. Ramachadran, and S. Ramachadran. Histopathological studies on experimental avian spirachaetosis in chicks. *Indian J. Vet. Sci.* 36:1–12, 1966.
23. Reshetnyak, V.Z. Specific preventive measures against avian spirochaetosis. *Proc. 13th World Poul. Cong.* (Kiev), pp. 420–423, 1966 (in Russian).
24. Rokey, N.M., and V.N. Snell. Avian spirochaetosis (Borellia anserina) epizootios in Arizona poultry. *J. Am. Vet. Med. Ass.* 138:648–652, 1961.
25. Savova-Burdarova, S. Pathological changes in hens experimentally infected with spirochaetes. *Vet. Med. Nauki Sof.* 4:99–104, 1967 (in Bulgarian).
26. Seddon, H.R. *Diseases of Domestic Animals in Australia.* Part 5, *Bacterial Diseases.* Vol. 2, pp. 201–203. Department of Health, Melbourne, 1965.
27. Soliman, M.K., A.A.S. Ahmed, S. el-Amrousi, and I.H. Moustafa. Cytological and biochemical studies on the blood constituents of normal and spirochaete-infected chickens. *Avian Dis.* 10:394–400, 1966.
28. Young, B.J. A reliable method for demonstration of spirochaetes in tissue sections. *J. Med. Lab. Tech.* 26:248–252, 1969.

45. Clostridia

This discussion will be limited to pathogenic *Clostridium* sp. of veterinary importance. To avoid repetition, the text is divided into eight sections: general procedures, *Cl. hemolyticum* and *Cl. novyi*, *Cl. perfringens*, *Cl. septicum*, *Cl. chauvoei*, *Cl. botulinum*, *Cl. tetani*, and *Cl. sordellii* (*Cl. bifermentans*).

General Procedures

Since *Clostridium hemolyticum* is the most fastidious clostridia species of veterinary importance, it is the model for the media and techniques given. Definitive procedures are described in preference to presumptive ones. All of the materials and methods described here may not be applicable to every situation, and the amount of time required for certain techniques may make them a luxury veterinary diagnosticians cannot afford.

Specimens

The tissues selected for bacteriological cultivation should be removed in a reasonably aseptic manner as soon after death as possible. If there is a delay in the preparation of cultures, the specimens should be preserved to prevent growth and invasion of the tissue by contaminating microorganisms. Tissue sections should be a minimum of 7.5 cm sq and preferably 5 cm thick or the thickness of the organ. Each specimen should be placed in a separate plastic bag and frozen, or bagged with powdered sodium borate (borax) and held at about 4°C. Unless tissue fluids are removed aseptically and immediately examined, cultured, or frozen, they are usually of little value because of excessive development of contaminants.

Laboratory Procedures

Cultures. Satisfactory preparation of tissue specimens requires meticulous adherence to accepted bacteriological techniques. Tissue blocks to be cultured are taken from the plastic holding bag, excess sodium borate is removed, and the tissue is placed in a sterile pan. A layer of tissue should be removed from that portion of the block to be cultured. The surface should then be seared with a red hot heavy metal file of similar tool. Five to ten g of tissue is removed aseptically from the seared surface, cut into small pieces, and macerated with sterile sand in a sterile mortar and pestle. The macerated tissue is suspended in 10–15 ml of sterile 0.85% NaCl. Smears of tissue suspension should be prepared, fixed, Gram-stained, and examined microscopically. The tissue suspension is streaked on blood agar and egg yolk agar plates, which are incubated at 36°C both aerobically and anaerobically for 48 hours or more. These plates are then examined for types and numbers of bacteria.

To facilitate the isolation of clostridia, a heat-resistant gradient of the bacteriological flora present in the tissue suspension may be prepared as follows. Tubes of culture medium are heated in a boiling water bath for 10 minutes to eliminate dissolved oxygen; then they are rapidly cooled to about 36°C. About 1 ml of the tissue suspension is inoculated into each of eight or so tubes of culture medium. The inoculated tubes of culture medium are serially heat-treated approximately as follows: (1) unheated, (2) heated at 80°C 5 minutes, (3) heated at 80°C 10 minutes, (4) heated at 80°C 15 minutes, (5) heated at 80°C 20 minutes, (6) heated at 90°C, (7) heated to boiling, (8) boiled 3–5 minutes. The serially heated tubes of culture are cooled rapidly to 40°C and incubated anaerobically at 36°C for 18–72 hours or longer, depending upon the type and quality of the bacterial growth that is desired. Gram-stained smears are prepared from the cultures and examined microscopically to select those most suitable for the inoculation of plating media. Careful preparation and examination of the heat-treated cultures will usually reveal pure or nearly pure populations of bacteria having similar morphologic characteristics to those organisms found in the Gram-stained smears of the original tissue suspension.

To obtain isolated colonies, these cultures are inoculated on both blood agar and egg yolk agar plates. The combination of colony characteristics found on blood agar and egg yolk agar media will frequently give a direction for future work or give tentative identification of the clostridia. Some types of clostridia, such as *Cl. perfringens, Cl. sordelli, Cl. bifermentans,* and *Cl. septicum,* usually grow moderately well on the surface of agar media several weeks old. However, a more otpimum environment for the growth of the bacterium can be obtained from freshly prepared media. Optimum environmental conditions are essential for isolation of the more fastidious clostridia, particularly *Cl. hemolyticum* and *Cl. novyi* type B, and very helpful in the growth of *Cl. chauvoei.*

Exposure to the atmosphere is detrimental to the culture media, as well as to many of the clostridia. Petri plates of freshly prepared agar media exposed to the atmosphere for 20–30 minutes before inoculation have failed to adequately support the growth of *Cl. hemolyticum.* Plating medium held in a water bath for 2–3 hours before it has been poured into petri plates has also failed to support the growth of some of the more fastidious clostridia. The addition of reducing agents to the media will not correct this condition.

Media containing tissue, tissue extracts, egg yolk, or other substances of animal origin are preferred to commercially produced dehydrated media for the propagation of clostridia. Formulas are included in Appendix A for (1) liver-egg-brain medium—for isolation and maintenance cultures; (2) anaerobic deep meat medium—for isolation; (3) papain digest of beef muscle—for toxin production; (4) peptic digest of beef liver—for basal ingredients of prepared media; (5) liver infusion broth—for basal ingredients of prepared media; (6) beef infusion broth—for basal ingredients of prepared media; (7) iron-milk medium—differential medium; (8) coagulated serum; (9) toxin medium—for toxin production.

Media to be used several weeks after preparation and autoclaving keep best when the pH is 6.8 or less. However, if media is to be prepared and frozen, adjust the pH to 7.2 prior to freezing. Tissues for media should be obtained on the killing floor of the slaughterhouse, processed, packaged, and quick-frozen with dry ice as rapidly as possible to retain labile factors, e.g. enzymes. Tissues used in media must be tested for factors inhibtory to clostridial growth. Tissues from animals that prior to slaughter consumed rations containing antibiotics or that had been injected with antibiotics are unsuitable. Eggs for use in making egg yolk agar must come from flocks not on antibiotic feeds and must not be more than 2–3 weeks old. Distilled water used in media preparation must be repeatedly tested for suitability. In those laboratories where anticorrosives, e.g. octadecylamine, are injected into the steam supply to reduce corrosion in the steam-condensate return lines, the anticorrosive agents may be carried over into distilled water obtained by steam condensation. Engineers attempt to produce levels of octadecylamine of 2 ppm in steam condensate, and this amount is markedly inhibitory for clostridia of veterinary importance. Lesser levels of octadecylamine may be even more insidious because only partial inhibition may occur and may not be recognized. Octadecylamine is readily transferred to media during the steam sterilization process. To produce media free from octadecylamine, use an electrically heated autoclave with a distilled water supply known to be free of inhibitory materials. Also, do not produce distilled water by repeated distillation in glass units. Trace growth factors necessary for clostridial growth appear to be removed by this process.

Plating media used for the isolation of heat-treated cultures may be prepared as follows. Commercial dehydrated blood agar base medium (Baltimore Biological Lab.; Difco Lab., Detroit) is prepared and sterilized according to the manufacturer's instructions and then cooled to 47–48°C in a water bath. Sterile bovine blood or yolk from fresh chicken eggs is mixed in the prepared agar medium to give a 5% concentration. Mix by stirring with a sterile pipette; avoid excessive aeration and the formation of air bubbles. As soon as the culture medium is poured, the petri plate is placed on a cold aluminum sheet 5–7 mm in thickness. The medium solidifies within 2–4 minutes and the surface of the medium should be immediately streaked with the culture. The petri plate is inverted, cover down. Several drops of glycerol are placed inside the cover of the petri plate and covered with a filter paper to absorb excess moisture that may accumulate during anaerobic incubation. In order for the filter paper to be held properly in place, the diameter of the paper should be slightly larger than the petri plate. The inoculated plates should be placed in the anaerobic container and an anaerobic environment should be developed as rapidly as possible.

To provide an optimum environment for some of the more fastidious clostridia, particularly *Cl. hemoyticum* and *Cl. novyi*, a subsurface inoculation of the agar medium is recommended. The prepared agar medium is poured into three sterile petri plates. Immediately a loopful of culture is steaked successively through the "soft" agar medium in the three plates. The inoculated medium is solidified and handled as previously described. This method usually provides adequate dilution of the culture for the development of isolated colonies.

There are a number of methods that may produce a suitable anaerobic environment for the cultivation of clostridia. The most common and a relatively efficient method for obtaining anaerobiosis is the reduction of oxygen within the anaerobic jar by hydrogen using a platinum or palladium catalyst, such as the Brewer, McIntosh-Fildes, or Brown anaerobic jar.

After inoculated agar plates or tubes of broth are placed in a Brewer jar, the cover is sealed by a layer of plasticine modeling clay. Anaerobic indicators may be used in glass anaerobic jars. A partially oxidized tube of fluid thioglycollate medium, or a mixture of 9 parts $NaHCO_3$ (about 2 g per tube) and 1 part glucose plus sufficient crystals of methylene blue to make a colored aqueous solution serve as suitable reduction indicators. Indicators also can be purchased commercially. After being closed and sealed the jar is evacuated to a vacuum of about 600 mm of mercury and then refilled with replacement gas. The replacement gas is admitted into the anaerobe jar at a pressure of not more than 1–2 psi. This step is repeated three or more times. The final filling of the jar with the replacement gas should be controlled so that a slight vacuum remains in the container. If excessive vacuum is applied, however, agar medium may be separated from the glass surface of petri plates or a boiling effect may result in liquid culture medium.

When a platinum catalyst is used, it is electrically heated for approximately 20 minutes to activate the reduction of the residual oxygen in the jar to water. This method is quite satisfactory for the growth of clostridia on the surface of agar media.

For the cultivation of fastidious clostridial species such as *Cl. hemolyticum, Cl. novyi,* and *Cl. chauvoei,* hydrogen, or a combination of at least 10% hydrogen with nitrogen and/or carbon dioxide, should be used as the replacement gas after evacuation of the anaerobic container. Carbon dioxide, in appreciable concentration, should always be included in the atmosphere in anaerobic jars, because it is essential for the growth of some of the anerobes found in clinical specimens and because it markedly stimulates the growth of others.[3] If carbon dioxide is not present in the replacement gas, about 2 g methylene blue indicator–carbon dioxide source should be used in every jar. Regardless of what type of replacement gas is used, each tank must be checked for factors inhibitory to growth. Freshly prepared egg yolk agar plates should be streaked with a culture of *Cl. hemolyticum* in the logarithmic growth phase. Anaerobic incubation for 72 hours in an environment of the gas being tested should provide surface colony growth. If hydrogen is not available, use nitrogen or propane, but note that the probability of isolating fastidious clostridia is significantly decreased.

CAUTION: Take steps to protect against the possible explosion of propane, since it is heavier than air and does not dissipate readily. A water pump with a vacuum gauge connected to the system should be used to evacuate anaerobic containers. Unless about 50 lb (344 kPa) of water pressure is exerted at the faucet to which the pump is attached, evacuation of anaerobic containers is very slow or incomplete.

Incubate anaerobically at 36°C for 48 hours; colonies will develop in or on the surface of the agar medium. Longer incubation periods are usually not necessary. "Spreaders," however, e.g. *Cl. septicum,* often cannot be incubated longer than 14–16 hours if one wishes to obtain isolated colonies. The cultures should be quickly examined microscopically, and several of each colony type immediately transferred into tubes of culture media. In order to avoid exposure of anaerobic organisms to the atmosphere longer than necessary, materials and equipment should be prepared prior to opening the anaerobic jars. Examine petri plate cultures carefully for the number and characteristics of colony types; this includes extent and type of hemolysis on blood agar and the extent of precipitation on egg yolk agar plates.

A convenient method of providing an anaerobic atmosphere for occasional screening purposes is the use of commercial gas packs (Difco).

An anaerobic atmosphere is less essential for the growth of clostridia in a liquid medium. In many cases, adequate bacterial growth in liquid medium can be readily attained without special anaerobiosis. The anaerobic environment for bacterial growth in liquid media can be improved by using freshly heat-sterilized media, by the addition of reducing agents, and by the addition of a small concentration (0.05–0.1%) of agar to increase the surface tension and reduce the diffusion of oxygen into the medium.

Differential reactions. Differential media used after isolation of clostridia include glucose, lactose, maltose, sucrose, salicin, iron-milk, and thiogel, and two tubes of beef infusion broth to check for indole production. Indicators for pH should not be added to culture media since they may inhibit the growth of some anaerobes. Acid formation in the culture is determined by use of a spot plate rather than by adding pH indicators directly to the cultures. This method permits additional incubation of the cultures if necessary. Add pH indicator to the depressions in the spot plate, dilute with distilled water, and mix with a loopful of culture. Acid production is indicated by a color change. Bromthymol blue, which is commonly used as a pH indicator, has a pH range of 7.6 (blue color) to 6 (yellow color).

One tube of culture in beef infusion broth is checked for indole production after 5 days incubation; another after 10 days incubation. Kovacs reagent is used, and the formula is as follows: p-dimethyl amino benzaldehyde, 5 g; N-amyl or butyl alcohol, 75 g; concentrated hydrochloric acid, 25 ml. Overlay the culture being tested with a small quantity of Kovacs reagent and wait for a few minutes. A rose color indicates a positive reaction. If the first attempt is negative, mix the contents of the tube and overlay for a second time. Depending upon culture conditions, indole may be produced early and disappear before the end of the 10-day incubation period. Excess nitrates in a medium may give a false-poisitive indole reaction.

Sugars are prepared as sintered glass or Millipore-filtered stock solutions, except glucose, which can be sterilized by autoclaving. The sugar concentrations are 10%, except for salicin, which is about 4%. Fluid thioglycollate medium is used as the base to which the sugars are added.

Efforts to reduce the 10-day incubation period for obtaining biochemical reactions may lead to invalid identification. Techniques permitting more rapid identification of clostridial cultures are gas chromatography and the fluorescent antibody reaction, especially for *Cl. chauvoei, Cl. septicum,* and *Cl. novyi.*

Clostridium hemolyticum and Clostridium novyi

Clostriudium hemolyticum and *Clostridium novyi (oedematiens)* should be studied together because there is a close relationship between their morphologic and cultural characteristics. Strains vary from toxigenic to nontoxigenic (*Cl. novyi* type C). Some strains produce intermediate biochemical reactions. All *Cl. novyi* strains appear to have two somatic antigens in common and one of these is shared with *Cl. hemolyticum*. It has been suggested that *Cl. hemolyticum* should be classified as *Cl. novyi* type D. They are both strict obligate anaerobes and are usually considered the most fastidious of the veterinary pathogenic clostridia. Spore suspensions in a suitable medium held at 5°C or a lower temperature, and spores held in a dry environment, e.g. sand or soil, remain viable for years. Spores of the more resistant strains will survive 30 minutes heating at 95°C.

Clostridium hemolyticum is the etiologic agent of bacillary hemoglobinuria or red water disease, which usually affects cattle and occasionally sheep and has been reported in pigs. The disease has been found mainly in the Rocky Mountain region and along the Gulf of Mexico and has also been reported in other areas of the United States and a number of foreign countries. The highest incidence of bacillary hemoglobinuria is on irrigated or poorly drained land; the disease is rare on dry, open range land. Liver damage from infestation by liver flukes is commonly associated with the disease and is assumed to be a predisposing factor.

The relatively high incidence of *Cl. novyi* in the soil provides a potential source of infection. These microorganisms have been found in apparently healthy animals, particularly in the liver and occasionally in the spleen and kidneys. Physiological changes in the animal may trigger an acute infection. Because *Cl. novyi* and *Cl. hemolyticum* may be part of the normal flora within the animal, the significance of their presence in necropsy material is questionable unless additional supporting evidence is available.

Growth characteristics. The colonies are usually irregularly round, 2–10 mm in diameter, grayish, and semitranslucent, with a ground-glass appearance. The colonies may be slightly raised to umbonate. Subsurface colonies in agar medium are 1 mm in diameter or smaller. On egg yolk agar there is a 4–12 mm zone of discolored, precipitated egg yolk surrounding each colony. On blood agar there is a corresponding, but less discernable, zone of diffuse discoloration of the blood agar, with a 1–3 mm zone of hemolysis beneath and surrounding the colony. Usually *Cl. novyi* type A strains grow more profusely on agar medium than type B strains of *Cl. hemolyticum*. The "pearly sheen" surrounding colonies on the surface of egg yolk agar is produced by epsilon toxin of *Cl. novyi* type A strains and may be used for tentative identification. A misleading but slightly different type of luster may be found surrounding colonies of *Cl. botulinum, Cl. sporogenes,* and some species of bacillus.

Cellular morphology. In general, the clostridia in this group are large gram-positive rods, 3–10 μm long and approximately 1 μm wide, with large oval spores in a subterminal position. Marked variation in the size, shape, and staining of the bacterial cell as well as in the heat resistance of the spore may be found from strain to strain and from one preparation to another of the same strain.

Differential reactions. Clostridium hemolyticum ferments glucose, fructose, and glycerol, produces indole and hydrogen sulfide, and liquifies gelatin but does not digest coagulated albumen. Nitrates are not reduced. Iron-milk remains relatively unchanged. The identity of the organism should be confirmed by neutralization tests of toxin with specific antitoxin, using either a lecithovitellin reaction, hot-cold hemolysis of red blood cells, or mouse inoculations as indicator reactions. Plate or tube agglutination tests with a known positive *Cl. hemolyticum* antiserum may contribute to the identification of the organism and are useful tools in experimental studies. However, agglutination titration of animal sera has limited significance because *Cl. hemolyticum* agglutinins can be found in apparently normal cattle and sheep. Many of these positive agglutination reactions are due to the natural exposure of the animal to maltose-fermenting variants of *Cl. hemolyticum*. The variant differs from the classic virulent strains of *Cl. hemolyticum* in fermenting maltose and it usually produces less beta-toxin. There is a close antigenic relationship. The variant differs biochemically from *Cl. novyi* types A and B in the production of indole. However, in some strains of the variant the formation of indole has been weak or equivocable. The maltose-fermenting variant has been found as the predominant organism in tissues from sheep and cattle, several of which have exhibited typical clinical signs of bacillary hemoglobinuria. It also has been recovered from a number of poorly defined infections of sheep and cattle.

Proper identification of *Cl. novyi* requires extensive examination for all the major characteristics of the group. To illustrate the relationship of the bacterial types within this group, some of their toxigenic and biochemical characterisics are presented in Table 45.1. *Clostridium novyi* alpha-toxin, found in types A and B, is highly lethal for animals, resulting in the formation of marked subcutaneous gelatinous edema. The presence of this toxin can be demonstrated only by its characteristic lethal effect in animals. The toxin can be neutralized by the specific antitoxin. Because some strains of *Cl. novyi* are atypical with regard to metabolic characteristics, it is not always possible to make a definite identification on the basis of culture reactions.[3] The researcher should inoculate experimental animals to demonstrate the species-specific toxin. The beta-toxin, produced by *Cl. novyi* type B and *Cl. hemolyticum,* is a calcium-dependent, hemolytic, necrotizing, lethal lecithinase. Intradermal inoculations of 0.1–0.2 ml of culture filtrate will produce erythema and necrosis of the skin. After several hours incubation at 36°C in the presence of beta-toxin, a suspension of erythrocytes is chilled to approximately 4°C to cause quick lysis. The toxin, as demonstrated by this hot-cold hemolysis, is readily neutralized by the specific antitoxin. A lechitovitellin reaction is indicated by development of an opalescence with gradual formation of a white fattylike layer on the surface of a clear emulsion of egg yolk mixed with culture fluid. This reaction is not specific since the enzymes of a number of clostridial species will hydrolyze egg yolk lecithin at different points on the molecule. The characteristics and magnitude of the reaction of the culture fluid with the egg yolk emulsion are variable, but the activity is neutralized by specific antitoxin. *Cl. hemolyticum* produces up to tenfold more beta-toxin than *Cl. novyi* type B but lecithovitellin reactions of both are neutralized by the antitoxin of either species. A relatively weak lecithovitellin reaction is produced by a lipase or a lecithinase (gamma-toxin) of type A strains but activity is neutralized only by type A antitoxin.

Table 45.1. Major toxins and biochemical reactions of *Clostridium novyi* and *Cl. hemolyticum*

	Cl. novyi types			Cl. hemolyticum
	A	B	C	
Alpha-toxin	+	+	−	−
Beta-toxin	−	+	−	+
Epsilon-toxin	+	−	−	−
Gamma-toxin	+	−	+	−
Lecithovitellin reaction	(+)*	+	−	+
Glucose fermentation	+	+	+	+
Maltose fermentation	+	+	+	−
Lactose fermentation	−	−	−	−
Sucrose fermentation	−	−	−	−
Salicin fermentation	−	−	−	−
Indole production	−	−	−	+
Thiogel liquefaction	+	+	(+)*	+

*Weak reaction.

To produce lecithovitellin, the yolk of one fresh egg is thoroughly emulsified in 200 ml of 0.85% NaCl solution that has been borate buffered (pH 7.4) and contains 0.02 M $CaCl_2$ solution. This emulsion is then centrifuged at approximately $10,000 \times g$ for 10 minutes. The yellow, slightly opalescent, supernatant fluid is filtered through a 0.45 μm Millipore filter. The filtrate is adjusted to an approximate optical density of 0.3 with sterile buffered saline using a Klett colorimeter with a blue filter. The emulsion is relatively stable when stored in the refrigerator and protected from bacterial contamination. Two-tenths of a milliliter of culture filtrate is placed in small test tubes and mixed with various types and quantities of antitoxin. The volume of each tube is adjusted to 1 ml with 0.85% NaCl solution. After the mixtures have been held at room temperature for 1 hour, 1 ml of the egg yolk emulsion is added. The tubes are held at 36°C for 2 hours before reading.

Immunology. Clostridium hemolyticum–adjuvanted bacterins are produced commercially. The duration of immunity in the vaccinated animal is relatively short, Cattle in endemic areas should be revaccinated every 5–6 months. The primary protective antigen in commercially produced preparations appears to be mainly cellular in nature since it has been demonstrated that *Cl. hemolyticum* (beta) toxin cannot be effectively toxoided using Formalin.[2]

Commercially produced *Cl. novyi*–adjuvanted bacterin-toxoids may be combined with preparations from as many as five other clostridial species in a single biologic product. *Clostridium novyi* (alpha) toxin is the principle lethal factor and the primary antigen needed. Since both type A and type B *Cl. novyi* produce alpha-toxin, ample cross-protection can be expected; however, to insure maximum protection both types should be incorporated into commercially produced bacterin-toxoids for use in the United States.

Animal pathogenicity. Guinea pigs inoculated IM with *Cl. hemolyticum* will die within 16–48 hours. There is necrosis and edema of the tissues around the site of inoculation. If death occurs more than 24 hours after inoculation, there is a marked increase in swelling of the infected limb and abdominal region, and a port wine–colored fluid is present. *Cl. hemolyticum* can be readily recovered from the infected tissues.

In infected cattle, appetite, rumination, lactation, and bowel movements usually cease suddenly. The urine is a very dark red or a port wine color, which is entirely due to suspended hemoglobin. At the time when the characteristic hemoglobinuria is first observed, from 30 to 50% of the red cells may have been hemolyzed. If the progressive hemolysis is not arrested promptly, the blood becomes thin, assumes a definite icteric color, and coagulates slowly. Death results from anoxia induced by the rapid and extensive destruction of red cells.

The local focus of infection appears to be in the liver, where propagation of the organism and toxin production take place. At necropsy an anemic infarct 5–20 cm in diameter showing peripheral areas of congestion may be found in the liver. Occasionally multiple infarcts may be found, some with varying degrees of tissue degeneration, which may suggest a chronic infection. The kidneys are covered with petechiae. The small intestine may be intensely hemorrhagic. *Cl. hemolyticum* can be usually seen in gram-stained smears of the liver. The organism can be readily recovered from the infected liver, usually from the spleen, and less frequently from the kidney. In ruminants as well as dogs, bacterial organisms can pass through the intestinal mucosa and gain access to the liver where they may lodge, fully capable of propagating once a nidus of anaerobiosis is provided by fluke infestation.

Many postparturition and wound infections as well as other poorly defined infections appear to be caused by *Cl. novyi*. Clinical symptoms and lesions similar to those noted in cases of anthrax have been reported in swine.[1] Most characteristic is the rather thick layer of clear gelatinous edema. However differentiation must be made clinically from infections caused by *Cl. sordelli,* which also produces a gelatinous edema colored by hemoglobin, and the urine also may contain hemoglobin.

Clostridium perfringens

In the United States, major economic losses of domestic animals are caused by *Cl. perfringens* infections of both type C and type D. These organisms are commonly found in soil samples and in the intestinal tracts of many animals. Type C infections produce enterotoxemia in lambs, young calves, and baby pigs that usually are less than 7 days of age. Type D infections produce enterotoxemia in lambs and adult sheep. A limited number of reports have been made of type D enterotoxemia in cattle. Experimentally, cattle produce a good immunologic response to type C antigens but a poor response to type D antigens. The incidence of *Cl. perfringens* infections in the United States is not known due to a lack of an accurate system for gathering this data as well as failure of some veterinary diagnostic laboratories to support clinical observations with serologic identification using a specific antitoxin.

Specimens

Animals suspected of being affected with enterotoxemia should be necropsied as soon after death as possible. Contents of the small intestine or peritoneal fluid should be collected in glass bottles, chilled in an ice bath to 2–7°C as rapidly as possible, and held at this temperature for toxin-antitoxin neutralization. These precautions are necessary since tissue enzymes as well as heat may rapidly inactivate toxins, especially type C. In many cases of suspected enterotoxemia the toxins can be found in the peritoneal fluid when they cannot be detected in the intestinal contents. While this relationship does not always exist, it does occur in a large enough percentage of cases to make examination of the peritoneal fluid for toxin imperative.

Laboratory Procedures

Cultures. In diagnostic samples, *Cl. perfringens* may be mixed with more fastidious clostridia, e.g. *Cl. hemolyticum* or *Cl. novyi*. After one serial heating series, though, *Cl. perfringens* spores will vegetate more rapidly and overgrow the more fastidious organisms. By subjecting the preparation to a second heating series, after *Cl. perfringens* has vegetated, the researcher may be able to isolate *Cl. hemolyticum* or *Cl. novyi*. The ability of *Cl. perfringens* to vegetate rapidly can be used to eliminate other bacterial contaminants. The mixed culture can be inoculated into a deep meat medium containing a drop of glucose and incubated at 36°C for 4–6 hours. The culture should then be transferred to iron-milk medium, in which *Cl. perfringens* multiplies rapidly, using the milk lactose to produce an acid environment unsuitable for the growth of many of the contaminants. Plating and incubation of the iron-milk culture should provide isolated colonies for selection. Ordinarily *Cl. perfringens* will grow readily in an anaerobic environment when streaked on blood agar plates; colonies are round, smooth, 2–7 mm in diameter, and white or gray in color.

Cellular morphology. *Cl. perfringens* organisms are gram-positive rods, 1–1.8 μm in diameter and 4–10 μm in length. Unfavorable culture conditions may cause marked elongation of the rods as well as the formation of coccoidal-like forms. In a deep meat medium, spores in competition with other organisms may not be formed even after the culture has been subjected to a serial heating series.

Differential reaction. *Cl. perfringens* ferments glucose, lactose, maltose, and sucrose with the production of acid. Most strains fail to ferment salicin. Indole is not formed, gelatin is liquefied, and iron-milk is fermented and clotted with rapid gas production so that the clot is broken. Biochemical differentiation should be supported by a toxin-antitoxin neutralization test using specific antitoxin.

Serology. Toxin preparations should be made by inoculating either a deep meat or general toxin medium with a pure, actively growing culture. Gas formation and considerable growth should become evident after 3–4 hours of anaerobic incubation at 36°C. Two tubes of medium should be inoculated for toxin production. One tube should be incubated anaerobically at 36°C for no longer than 8 hours because beta-toxin produced by type C cultures may be inactivated by longer incubation. After incubation the culture should be centrifuged, filtered, and 0.9 ml of the filtrate mixed with 0.3 ml of specific beta-antitoxin and allowed to react at room temperature for 30 minutes. Then inoculate 0.3 ml of the toxin-antitoxin mixture into the lateral tail veins of three 16–20 g white mice. Postive control mice should be inoculated with an equal quantity of culture filtrate. Usually deaths will occur in 5 minutes to several hours if the preparation is lethal. However, inoculated mice should be held overnight to check for delayed deaths. If mice die within 2 minutes after inoculation, a nonspecific reaction may be the cause of death. If no mice are dead the following morning, the second culture, which was incubated for 16–20 hours, should be centrifuged and its pH adjusted to about 8.4 using 1 N NaOH. Then prepare a 2.5% trypsin solution that is approximately 0.25 g of reagent-grade trypsin per 10 ml of diluent. The diluent should be of the following composition: peptone, 1%; NaCl, 0.25%; distilled water, enough to make 100%. Adjust the pH to 7.2. Autoclave at 121°C for 25 minutes. Store in the refrigerator. Add 1 part of approximately 2.5% trypsin solution to 9 parts of the toxin preparation, mix, and let react 30 minutes. Then set up a toxin-antitoxin neutralization using specific epsilon-antitoxin and inoculate mice as described for beta-toxin. Mouse deaths from epsilon-toxin usually occur more than 6 hours after inoculation. A large proportion of the epsilon-toxin in the preparation may be in a pre-formed state, thus requiring trypsin activation. Commercial trypsin reagents vary in their ability to activate epsilon-toxin, and if the material is not used promptly, the toxin may be destroyed by an excess of trypsin.

Immunology. A bacterin-toxoid is defined as "the toxin growth products of bacterial organisms propagated in suitable medium, containing all or part of the cells or their particulate components from the original culture or a combination of such fractions which have been rendered non-toxic and inactivated without appreciable loss of antigenic value as measured by suitable animal tests. A bacterin-toxoid shall contain cellular antigens and shall stimulate the development of antitoxin."[4] A toxoid is defined as "the sterile, aqueous filtrate resulting from growth of bacterial organisms in a suitable culture medium and which has subsequently been rendered non-toxic without appreciable loss of antigenic value as measured by suitable animal tests. Toxoid shall not be applied to a product which has not had the bacterial cells removed during process."[4] A bacterin is defined as "a suspension of organism, or their particulate components with or without their unevaluated growth products, which have been inactivated by chemical or physical means; and the basic immunizing antigens are believed to be primarily cellular."[4]

Commercial *Cl. perfringens* type C, type D, and combined type C and D bacterin-toxoids are produced. Type C, type D, and combined antitoxins are also produced. Combined antitoxin is often used because veterinarians are not able to secure diagnostic facilities that can provide definitive serologic identification of the type of *Cl. perfringens* causing enterotoxemia.

Vaccination of ewes twice during pregnancy with type C or type D bacterin-toxoid provides passive immunity for lambs either in utero or through the colostrum. Young swine may be similarly protected. Lambs intended to be sent to feedlots should be vaccinated 2–3 weeks prior to the initiation of fattening.

Clostridium septicum

Cl. septicum generally has been associated with wound-type infections. The common name for these infections is malignant edema. Tissues obtained from animals necropsied more than 8 hours after death may become contaminated with *Cl. septicum* from the intestinal tract. In the United States, veterinary diagnostic laboratories seldom are able to necropsy dead animals within 8 hours after death. More often animals have been dead 24–36 hours. Infections caused by *Cl. septicum* do occur in cows whose genital tracts have been traumatized during parturition, in feeder cattle whose briskets are punctured by frayed steel cables supporting feed bunks in the lots, and in vaccinated swine and cattle, with the organism being carried though the skin by the needle. The disease may be confused with blackleg.

Growth characteristics. Cl. septicum is not fastidious as to cultural or anaerobic requirements. On blood agar incubated 14–16 hours at 36°C, colonies may be small to "swarming" and almost translucent to gray in color, with irregular margins, and some may be surrounded by zones of hemolysis up to 4 mm in width. The recommended technique for obtaining isolated colonies when swarming is a problem is to reduce incubation time to 14–16 hours, or even less if necessary.

Cellular morphology. Rods in the logarithmic growth phase are gram-positive. Cells that have been exposed to an acid environment after completion of active growth may be gram-negative and granular in appearance. Cells may be pleomorphic in size and shape and may even become filamentous if inhibitory factors are present in the media. Spores are oval and subterminal.

Differential reactions. Cl. septicum ferments glucose, lactose, maltose, and salicin with acid production. An occasional strain may ferment sucrose. Indole is not formed, thiogel is liquified, and iron-milk is clotted.

Immunology. The antigen used is primarily cellular in nature. Potency of bacterins has been assayed using the amount of toxin as the indicator. This approach has value since *Cl. septicum* is a relatively poor toxin producer and a good yield of toxigenic cells is therefore necessary before an appreciable amount of toxin is formed. *Cl. septicum* bacterins are produced commercially, usually added to biologic products containing one or more additional clostridia.

Clostridium chauvoei

Cl. chauvoei is the causative agent of the disease commonly called blackleg, which in most cases causes considerable myonecrosis. In the United States it causes major economic losses in cattle and minor losses in sheep. The highest incidence occurs in the western Rocky Mountain states but it is apparently endemic in many states. Texts have described the disease as generally occurring in cattle ranging in age from 6 months to 2 years of age; however, younger calves and aged cattle occasionally become infected. Naturally infected animals may not be noticed until they are unable to rise and have swelling of one or more limbs and other muscle groups. Crepitation may or may not be detected beneath the skin over affected muscles. When myonecrosis occurs, usually the organism can be isolated.

Growth characteristics. Colonies on agar plates generally are small, ranging from barely visible to 3 mm in size, and are transparent with irregular edges. Hemolysis may be evident only beneath the colony or may extend a slight distance from the colony edge. It may be necessary to select 6–12 pinpoint-sized colonies and transfer them to boiled and cooled broth media to insure isolation.

Cellular morphology. Organisms are gram-positive when selected during the logarithmic growth phase, 3–8 μm long and 0.6–0.8 μm wide. However, organisms subjected to inhibitory growth factors may be relatively long, spindle shaped, or coccoidal. Rods may contain oval spores that swell the rod and range from central to subterminal in position.

Differential reactions. Good growth occurs in glucose, lactose, maltose, and sucrose and results in fermentation, but salicin is not fermented. Thiogel is liquefied, indole is not produced, and acid and gas are produced, with variable clotting in iron-milk. In those cases where differential biochemical reactions, fluorescent antibody, and gas chromatography procedures still do not provide strain identification, an antigen may be produced for agglutination reactions with specific *Cl. chauvoei* antiserum. (The only commercial supplier is Burroughs Wellcome & Co., Research Triangle Park, N.C.) To prevent autoagglutination, antigen should be prepared from vegetative cells, possibly containing a few spores, which are obtained by short-term growth (6–16 hours). A few strains of *Cl. chauvoei* can be found that apparently possess no agglutinogens.

Immunology. Experimental studies in guinea pigs and cattle indicate that for immunizing purposes cellular antigens are of major importance. Soluble antigens also contribute to the production of a potent biologic product. *Cl. chauvoei* produces a lethal and hemolytic toxin. Immunologic comparison of U.S. strains with those isolated in England show no major antigenic differences. Adjuvanted commercially produced bacterins are available containing *Cl. chauvoei* alone or in combination with as many as four other clostridial organisms. In endemic areas, e.g. the Rocky Mountain states, where calves may be vaccinated just a few days after being born, young animals should be revaccinated when they return from mountain pastures in the fall. Twice-vaccinated bovines are solidly immune for a duration of at least 1 year.

One of the difficulties in experimentally evaluating vaccination effectiveness is that oxygen in a challenge preparation of *Cl. chauvoei* must be at the absolute minimal level that technique will permit or else erratic challenge reults will be found. This has been repeatedly demonstrated experimentally in guinea pigs and cattle.

Clostridium botulinum

Type C *Cl. botulinum* is the only type causing major economic losses in mammals and birds in the United States. Losses occur in ranch-raised mink when food contains the toxin. Extensive losses may occur on game farms where dead pheasants are not picked up promptly. In egg-producing or even broiler operations, losses of birds may sometimes occur under conditions of poor husbandry. Wildlife, e.g. ducks, gulls, loons, and other shore birds, have suffered extensive losses during certain years from type C botulism. These losses occur after the flooding of agricultural lands, resulting in shallow expanses of water, is followed by a period of hot weather during which the toxin develops. *Cl. botulinum* type C is found in the soil of these affected areas.

Since *Cl. botulinum* type C may be isolated from the soil or the intestinal tracts of mammals or birds, assurance that deaths were caused by this organism requires that the toxin be neutralized by specific antitoxin. In the case of contaminated food for mink, suspensions can be made, filtered, and mixed with antitoxin. Since this is a very lethal toxin it may be necessary to dilute the food suspension before mixing with antitoxin. The neutralized suspension and a nonneutralized control preparation can then be inoculated IV into mice. The specific antitoxin may protect the indicator animals, whereas control animals should die. If indicator mice die within 5 minutes after they are inoculated, this may indicate that the toxin was different from the specific antitoxin, that there was an overwhelming amount of toxin in the toxin-antitoxin preparation, or that a nonspecific substance rather than *Cl. botulinum* toxin killed the mice by anaphylactic shock. Depending upon the potency of the specific antitoxin, the toxin preparation may have to be diluted. Mink, pheasants, ducks, or other mammals and birds may be passively protected by inoculating them with specific antitoxin and then challenging them 16 hours later with a toxin preparation. Fly larvae found in dead birds may also be used to challenge passively protected birds.

Growth characteristics. Surface colonies on blood agar range from 4 to 10 mm in diameter and are quite variable from strain to strain except that most produce hemolysis beneath and surrounding the colony. Morphology also varies as strains are subcultured on agar media. Surface colonies on egg yolk agar may exhibit a pearlylike sheen around and on the colony surface. Both surface and subsurface colonies are surrounded by enzyme-altered media.

Cellular morphology. Rods are gram-positive, pleomorphic, and occur singly, in pairs, and occasionally in short chains. Inhibitory physiological conditions may cause the rods to become markedly elongated from their usual length of 3–6 μm. Spore location usually is subterminal, occasionally ranging to central. Because these characteristics are variable, toxin isolation and typing remain the definitive approaches to identification.

Differential reactions. Most strains of type C *Cl. botulinum* ferment glucose, producing acid and gas. Occasional strains may also ferment maltose to a slight degree, whereas other strains may fail to ferment any of the sugars.

Immunology and serology. At the present time botulinum antitoxin types A, B, and C are not being produced for interstate distribution in the United States since an extremely small volume is required annually. *Cl. Botulinum* type C bacterin-toxoid is produced commercially primarily for the vaccination of mink on ranches.

Animal pathogenicity. Adult pheasants ingesting as few as one or two fly larvae from a dead bird infected with *Cl. botulinum* type C may be killed by the toxin. The optimal temperature for the production of *Cl. botulinum* type C toxin is 28–32°C, but toxin also may be elaborated at much lower environmental temperatures. During the 1950s a whale was captured on the West Coast of the United States late on a Friday so that it was not processed for animal food until the following Monday. Unfortunately, this whale carried *Cl. botulinum* type C in its intestinal tract and the tissues became grossly contaminated over the weekend. Meat from this mammal was sold for mink food and caused over 95% mortality in animals that ingested it.

Birds dying of botulism often exhibit limberneck and the feathers are easily removed. Mammals and birds dead from botulism exhibit no pathognomonic lesions, probably because only a small dosage of toxin results in death very quickly. It would appear that *Cl. botulinum* produces some substance that greatly increases the permeability of the intestinal mucosa to the toxin itself since purified toxins are rather poorly absorbed. Toxigenic types are apparently specific except for the two subtypes of type C where cross-reactions occur. The effects of the toxin can be neutralized by the administration of type C antitoxin.

Clostridium tetani

Cl. tetani is commonly found in the intestinal tracts of humans and animals and in the soil, except in some places in the Rocky Mountains of the United States and the Andes of South America. Its absence in certain areas of the Rocky Mountains is interesting since the incidence of other clostridial infections affecting animals is relatively high in the same areas. In England it was experimentally estimated that dust on hospital floors may contain 5000–10,000 *Cl. tetani* organisms per gram. The horse is the domestic animal most susceptible to the effects of tetanus toxin. Cattle, sheep, and swine may also be affected. Guinea pigs or mice are used in the laboratory to assay the potency of antitoxins or toxoids. Susceptibility to toxin is apparently not related to sex or age.

Tetanus usually develops as the result of a wound infection and isolation of *Cl. tetani* can usually be accomplished as previously described. However, tissues for culture must be carefully selected because the nidus of infection may be very small. Although the toxin produced by this organism is several times less toxic than the toxins of *Cl. botulinum*, it is still very lethal. An example occurred in Kansas City in the 1950s when a teenager while chewing on a tiny pebble forced it into a tooth cavity. Tetanus resulted but clinical signs were not quickly recognized since no apparent wound infection had occurred. Death resulted and at autopsy the pebble was found. *Cl. tetani* was isolated from the tooth pulp.

Growth characteristics. Colonies on blood agar may range in size from 2 mm to relatively large and spreading with feathered edges. Hemolysis usually occurs beneath the colony and may extend a small distance beyond the colony.

Cellular morphology. Rods are gram-positive and somewhat pleomorphic, ranging from 2 μm in length to filamentous forms, depending upon the strain and cultural conditions. Most characteristic is the round terminal spore, but laboratory strains may produce few spores.

Differential reactions. The failure of most strains of *Cl. tetani* to ferment sugars, its cellular morphology, and its relatively weak proteolytic action provide partial differentiation. However, this should be augmented by neutralization of toxin with specific antitoxin using guinea pigs or mice as indicator animals.

Immunology. Tetanus antitoxins and toxoids are produced commercially for distribution in the United States. Because many of the veterinary biologic producers also produce human biologics, the standard reagents used and methods employed for potency assaying are essentially those produced or promulgated by the Division of Biologics Standards, NIH. The optimum temperature of incubation for toxin production using Mueller's strain is 33°C. With incubation at 36°C, about one-tenth of this amount of toxin is formed.

Clostridium sordellii (Clostridium bifermentans)

Cl. bifermentans is often found as a contaminant in tissue specimens, is commonly found as part of the intestinal flora, and appears to be widely distributed in the soil.

Nearly all pathogenic strains produce urease; they are commonly referred to as *Cl. sordellii* and are of primary significance in veterinary medicine. Not all *Cl. sordellii* strains are pathogenic, however. The two species cannot be separated on the basis of pathogenicity since some strains of *Cl. sordellii* rapidly lose virulence while other strains are not virulent when first isolated. Biochemical reactions are very similar with the exception that salicin, sorbitol, and mannose are fermented only by *Cl. bifermentans* while urease is produced only by *Cl. sordellii*.

Cl. sordellii is pathogenic for humans, cattle, and sheep. It has been primarily associated with wound infections. A few scattered reports suggest that this organism may be responsible for some enterotoxemia-like disorders in cattle and sheep, particularly in feedlot operations in the western United States, and *Cl. sordellii* has been recovered as part of a mixed bacterial population from necropsied cattle clinically diagnosed previously as cases of blackleg or bacillary hemoglobinuria. There is sufficient evidence to indicate that *Cl. sordellii* is usually a disease-producing agent but only vague information is available concerning its incidence or economic significance. This may be partially due to the failure to isolate and identify the organism from infected animals. Erroneous identification of *Cl. sordellii,* particularly as *Cl. novyi,* has occurred frequently in diagnostic and other laboratories. *Cl. sordellii,* like most other clostridia, should be considered an "opportunist" since optimal environment is necessary for the development of recognizable infection.

Infected tissue specimens should be aseptically collected as described previously. Filtrates from tissue fluids of recently dead animals, particularly from animals with enterotoxemia-like syndromes, should be inoculated intravenously into mice as a test for toxicity. Although *Cl. sordellii* toxin has not been commonly demonstrated in animal tissue, toxin neutralization tests in mice using specific antitoxin for *Cl. sordellii* and *Cl. perfringens* may aid in the tentative diagnosis of the disease. Virulent strains of *Cl. sordellii* produce a highly lethal toxin. Possibly this toxin in animal tissues is difficult to detect due to relatively rapid inactivation by proteolytic enzymes. Morphologic characteristics and the number of organisms in infected tissue, as determined by examination of gram-strained smears, often provide direction for additional diagnostic procedures. Because this organism grows readily with minimal requirements, it may quickly overgrow other organisms in mixed culture or even mask the primary cause of death due to infection with *Cl. hemolyticum* or *Cl. novyi*.

Cl. sordellii grows moderately well in an anaerobic atmosphere at approximately 36°C. If it is thought to be the primary infecting agent, the tissue specimens can be inoculated directly on plating media as previously described. Distinct colony growth on agar medium is usually present within 24 hours, however, the culture should be incubated 48 hours to provide characteristic colony morphology and to permit observation for other bacterial types. Colonies of *Cl. sordellii* are 2–5 mm in diameter and slightly raised with an irregular surface. Bacterial growth at the edge of the colony has a slight tendency to spread, especially along the lines of the streak. The appearance of the colonies seems to be related to the degree of sporulation. Colonies composed of mainly vegetative cells with only a few spores are semiopaque and grayish in color; colonies composed almost entirely of free spores or rods with spores are white and opaque.

Usually a slight zone of hemolysis occurs beneath and surrounding colonies grown on blood agar. On egg yolk agar medium the colonies are usually surrounded by a 5–12 mm diameter zone of precipitation.

Cl. sordellii is moderately proteolytic, readily liquefying thiogel and slowly digesting casein, coagulated egg albumin, and coagulated serum. Milk is clotted and then slowly digested and blackened, and indole is produced. Glucose, maltose, and fructose are fermented. The presence of urease, which is an important factor in the identification of *Cl. sordellii*, can be rapidly determined by covering colonies on the surface of egg yolk agar medium with a small quantity of urea broth medium. If urease is present, the colonies will become an intense pink color within 5–10 minutes due to the alkaline reaction produced by the hydrolysis of urea. Urease can also be determined by placing a heavy suspension of colonies in urea broth medium and incubating at 36°C for 30 minutes or longer. This method requires more time and the color change may be less perceptible.

Virulent strains of *Cl. sordellii* inoculated into guinea pigs may cause death within 12 hours. On necropsy a marked subcutaneous red to dark-red fluid or gelatinous edema is present. Muscles of the abdominal wall are usually dark red. Gas pockets may be found at the site of inoculation. Occasionally, red-colored urine will be found. Commercially produced bacterins are available; however, the effectiveness of these products against *Cl. sordellii* in the field is not fully known.

References

1. Bourne, F.J., and J.B. Kerry. Clostridium oedematiens associated with sudden death in the pig. *Vet. Rec.* 77:1463, 1965.
2. Claus, K.D., and M.E. Macheak. Nonantigenic nature of *Clostridium hemolyticum* toxoid. *Am. J. Vet. Res.* 26:353–356, 1965.
3. Smith, L., and L.V. Holdeman. *The Pathogenic Anaerobic Bacteria*, pp. 301–327. Thomas, Springfield, Ill., 1968.
4. Veterinary Biologics Division. *Nomenclature for Bacterins, Toxoids, and Bacterin-Toxoids.* Biological Products Memo no. 35. ARS, Hyattsville, Md., November 1, 1967.

46. Nonsporeforming Anaerobes

The methods of Hungate have provided the basis for the most thorough anaerobic bacterial studies yet undertaken.[15] These extremely sensitive techniques have been used by several investigators for extensive studies of the rumen flora.[6,8,16] Adaptation of these methods to the study of clinically occurring and normal flora of various animals and humans has demonstrated that our knowledge of anaerobes and their significance is very incomplete.[11,19] The new techniques also have demonstrated that anaerobes occur in about 70% of the organ and soft-tissue abscess infections in humans.[20] In the few comparative studies that have been made, the same species have usually been found in both animal infections and in normal flora.

Infections containing anaerobes can occur in any site in the body. Anaerobic microenvironments in tissue can be produced by tissue damage, swelling, or by microorganisms that biochemically reduce their environment. Anaerobes alone are found in about 25% of human organ and soft tissue infections; facultative species alone are found in another 25% of such infections. Most infections contain one or more species of each.[2,20] The isolation of one species of bacteria (facultative or anaerobic) from an infection often gives microbiologists a false sense of security because they are ignorant of the one or more they did not isolate. Knowledge of these may be most important for proper diagnosis and therapy or for the development of preventative measures.

In addition to the general lack of information concerning the prevalence of obligately anaerobic nonsporeforming bacteria in animal infections, the identification of many species cited in early reports is now in question. Characterization procedures were often inadequate and the organisms described may have been members of any of several distinct species that have now been characterized in detail. Most species found in lesions are part of the normal flora of the intestinal or respiratory tract. Several of these that have been studied experimentally cause infections in pure culture or in combinations that appear to be synergistic. However, not all species of the normal flora (even some of those normally present in high numbers) have been found in lesions.

In animals, the role of the nonsporeforming anaerobes in footrot and in liver infections has been investigated in some detail, but adequate anaerobic culture techniques have generally not been used to examine other types of infections.

Foot Infections of Sheep

Foot infections in sheep are a problem wherever sheep are raised in large numbers. The infections vary in severity and are usually referred to as different disease entities, the same condition having several names.

The etiology of infections of the feet of sheep in Australia has been investigated by experimentally infecting animals with organisms isolated from clinical infections.[11,12,22,25,26,27,28] Results of these studies indicate that most of the infections are caused by more than one organism and that the severity or the type of infection depends on the kinds of organisms present and their properties.

Ovine interdigital dermatitis (OID) is an acute necrotizing infection of the interdigital skin. The skin usually is erythematous and swollen and is often covered with a moist film of gray necrotic material. In severe cases the skin is eroded.[22] OID is associated with an intense epidermal invasion by *Fusobacterium necrophorum* (*Sphaerophorus necrophorus, Fusiformis necrophorus*). Because *F. necrophorum* is part of the normal fecal flora of animals, it is present in the animal environment. Prior skin damage and a moist environment are thought to contribute to the initiation of infection.

Another common bacterial foot infection has been referred to as digital suppuration, foot abscess, or abscess of the lamellar and bulbar region of the foot. Necrotizing infections of the heel have been called infective bulbar necrosis (IBN), and this is considered to be a different disease from suppurative infection of the lamella.[28] IBN occurs most frequently in the hind feet of lambing ewes, but it has been found in sheep of all ages. The results in animals experimentally infected indicate that the disease is caused by *F. necrophorum* and *Corynebacterium pyogenes*. *F. necrophorum* is capable of massive invasion of the intact interdigital skin and appears to be responsible for the necrosis. *C. pyogenes*, however, produces a factor that stimulates the proliferation of *F. necrophorum* in the tissues, and *F. necrophourm* produces a leukocidal toxin that protects *C. pyogenes* from phagocytosis.

Contagious footrot (progressive footrot, virulent footrot) is the most common cause of lameness in sheep and occurs in most sheep-raising areas of the world. Goats are sometimes affected. The disease starts as an infective and inflammatory interdigital dermatitis and spreads into the epidermal matrix of the hoof, resulting in separation of the horn from the underlying soft tissues.

From recent reports it appears that footrot in sheep results from the synergism of several bacteria. Benign and virulent footrot can be regarded as OID complicated by the presence of *Bacteroides nodosus*.[12,27] *C. pyogenes* may add to the severity of the condition.

Infection by *F. necrophorum* is established first, causing inflammation and destruction of the epidermis. In the superficial part of the lesion a growth factor is provided by *C. pyogenes*, but as successive waves of *F. necrophorum* proliferate deeper into the tissue a different growth factor is provided by *B. nodosus* to stimulate *F. necrophorum*. *B. nodosus* multiples slowly between the successive invasive phases of *F. necrophorum*, and a motile fusiform bacillus appears to add to the pathogenesis of footrot by providing a further growth factor for *B. nodosus*.[26,27] Continued multiplication of *B. nodosus* during the periods when deeper invasion by *F. necrophorum* is static produces a sustained irritation that prevents healing. This may account for the more chronic nature of footrot as compared to OID.

The only known natural habitat of *B. nodosus* is infected feet (usually of sheep, sometimes of goats and cattle). The organism survives only a short time outside the animal hoof (2 weeks in soil). It is transmitted from diseased feet to healthy feet by infective organisms shed into soil, bedding, or flooring. Several reports discuss the treatment and eradication of footrot.[3,9]

The degeneration of the horn in footrot is associated with the proteolytic properties of *B. nodosus*.[33] Less proteolytic strains of *B. nodosus* are associated with benign footrot of sheep (also called atypical footrot, nonprogressive footrot, or scald), in which there is no necrosis of the underlying tissues or separation of the hard horn, although the soft horn sometimes is separated.[10] The infection may be chronic; lameness may occur but is not always seen. *F. necrophorum* as well as the less virulent strains of *B. nodosus* can be isolated from the lesion. The proteolytic activity of the strains of *B. nodosus*[10] is determined by streaking a loopful of sedimented cells in a straight line across the surface of a recently poured casein plate and incubating the plate for 4 days in an anaerobic atmosphere.[11] A zone of precipitate develops under the area of confluent growth. Upon continued incubation, the area of precipitation increases and clearing occurs around the area of confluent growth. The width of the clear zone (between the area of confluent growth and precipitate) compared to that of the remaining band of precipitate is used to indicate proteolytic activity. For virulent strains, the ratio is 1.5:4.5 (mean, 2.14:1); for strains from benign footrot, the ratio is 0.25:1 (mean, 0.616:1).

Specimens

Samples for examination should be collected from a recently invaded area after removal of the grossly contaminated material and the superficial necrotic tissue. In Gram-strained smears, *B. nodosus* usually is not the predominant organism, but it generally can be found in an active footrot lesion. Rods are $0.6-0.8 \times 3-10$ μm, single or in pairs, often with enlargements at one or both ends. Enlargements usually are less pronounced in smears from cultures.

Laboratory Procedures

Cultures. Stuart's transport medium kept in ice has been used to hold specimens until they can be cultured in the laboratory.[10] Specimens are then placed in 0.25% sucrose, shaken, and streaked on hoof agar medium. After incubation in an anaerobic atmosphere for 2 days, surface colonies are about 1 mm in diameter, smooth, convex, and butyrous.

The ingredients for hoof agar medium are: 0.5 g Oxoid Lab-Lemco (London) meat extract, 1 g proteose peptone (Difco Lab., Detroit), 0.2 g Difco yeast extract, 0.5 g NaCl, 2 g powdered hoof, 1.5 g Difco Bacto agar in 100 ml water, with final pH adjusted to 7.4.[27] To prepare hoof powder, wash the horn in water, cut in strips 0.5–1 cm wide, dry at 37°C for 4 days, and grind to a powder in a hammer mill.[32]

A similar medium with 5–7% blood instead of powdered hoof has been used for culture of *F. necrophorum*.[22] *F. necrophorum* and other kinds of anaerobes have been isolated from highly contaminated material by the researcher streaking the surface of agar in roll tubes, freshly poured blood agar plates, and egg yolk agar plates, and incubating in an anaerobic atmosphere for 48–71 hours. On blood agar, colonies of *F. necrophorum* incubated for 2–3 days are opaque, convex to umbonate, and entire to erose, and usually are beta-hemolytic on horse or rabbit blood; they produce lipase on egg yolk agar. Cells are gram-negative, $0.4–1 \times 2.5–18$ μm, with rounded or slightly tapered ends; filaments usually are seen. In older cultures, cells are frequently granular and have swellings. For sources where only a few organisms may be expected, inoculate chopped meat and chopped meat glucose medium, incubate in an anaerobic atmosphere for 24–48 hours, and streak on solid agar as described above.

Two selective media are recommended: (1) an agar containing 0.04% sodium azide, 0.0032% brilliant green, 2% yeast extract, and 10% blood; or (2) 100 μg paromomycin and 7.5 μg vancomycin per ml of plating medium.[2,14]

Differential reactions. Some investigators differentiate between *F. necrophorum* and *F. funduliformis (Sphaerophorus funduliformis).*[2,13,24] Strains of *F. necrophorum* are hemolytic, possess a hemogglutinin, and are pathogenic for mice; strains of *F. funduliformis* are hemolytic but do not have the hemagglutinin and are nonpathogenic for mice. In most reports, however, pathogenicity and hemagglutinating properties have not been determined and strains of both "species" have been called both names. In Bergey's 8th edition,[7] "necrophorum" and "funduliformis" are designated as subspecies or phases of *F. necrophorum*.

The necrotizing effect of *F. necrophorum* is thought to be caused by a toxin, or soluble growth product. In addition, most strains produce a lipase and hemolysin. Attempts to immunize animals have not been effective, and in cattle that have extensive liver lesions containing *F. necrophorum* no antibody develops naturally.

Vaccination with Formalin-killed broth cultures of *F. necrophorum* does not control *F. necrophorum* infection but does accelerate the development of lesions by *B. nodosus*.[12]

Other Infections of Mammals Caused by Nonsporing Anaerobes

Liver abscesses in cattle are reported from all parts of the world, but they are particularly prevalent in the United States where animals are rapidly fattened on a diet high in carbohydrate and protein. The condition is most prevalent when the diet is rapidly changed from roughage to high-concentrate feed. Apparently, ulceration of the rumen follows this rapid change. *F. necrophorum*, part of the normal flora of the rumen, is found in the ulcers. Via the hepatic portal vein, the organisms are carried to the liver, where they lodge, multiply, and produce necrosis. *F. necrophorum* can be isolated from most of these abscesses (90–95%), but a small proportion are caused by other organisms.[30] Infected livers may contain up to 70 yellowish-white abscesses that are a few millimeters to several centimeters in diameter; most are on the surface. The animals usually appear healthy, although the livers are enlarged.

Footrot is a common cause of lameness in cattle. Swelling and inflammation develop above the hoof and in the soft part between the claws. This may be followed by the formation of deep abscesses under the horny wall. In advanced cases, the joint within the hoof becomes inflamed and the articular attachments may be destroyed. Usually only one foot is affected.[4]

Bovine footrot is generally thought to be caused by *F. necrophorum*. However, in one study gram-negative nonsporing anaerobes were isolated from only 12 of 32 cattle with infectious footrot, but anaerobic gram-positive cocci were found in a large proportion of the samples.[17] The study suggested that the low prevalence of nonsporing gram-negative anaerobes isolated may have been caused by sampling after the organisms had disappeared or because inappropriate isolation techniques were used. In another study of 108 specimens of bovine footrot, organisms resembling *F. necrophorum* was seen in only 10% of the smears and isolation of *F. necrophorum* was made from only 5% of the samples.[23] Several other species, including *Bacteroides melaninogenicus, C. pyogenes, Bacillus cereus,* clostridia, and streptococci were isolated. Undoubtedly some of the other species were contaminants, but it might be that *B. melaninogenicus* or *C. pyogenes* contributed to the infection, particularly in view of the relationship between *C. pyogenes* and *F. necrophorum* in ovine foot infections.

Calf diphtheria or necrotic laryngitis is a disease characterized by necrosis of the membranes and underlying tissues of the larynx. It occurs mainly in cattle up to 3 years of age. *F. necrophorum* is generally thought to be responsible for the necrosis. The infection is usually associated with predisposing factors such as viral infection or malnutrition.[18]

Navel ill is a disease of calves, foals, and lambs and is characterized by lesions of the joints, liver, or other sites. The infectious agents, including *F. necrophorum,* are transmitted to the newborn via contamination of the umbilical cord.

Infections with *F. necrophorum* have been reported in horses, cattle, pigs, sheep, goats, rabbits, reindeer, buffalo, dogs, cats, apes, and rats.[29] It is reported to be responsible (or is seen in) infections of all parts of the body and most kinds of tissue. However, the identification of the organisms seen, cultured, or reported as *F. necrophorum* is often questionable. *F. necrophorum* infections in humans and animals have been reviewed.[13]

Isolation of *Bacteroides melaninogenicus* from different kinds of abscesses in domestic animals (cats, dogs, cattle, sheep, horses, swine) has been reported.[5] Of 2164 samples examined, *B. melaninogenicus* was recovered from 102; the incidence varied from 1.6% in samples from horses to 12.1% in samples from cats. From 1 to 5 other species were isolated from 100 of the samples containing *B. melaninogenicus*. Reports of *Bacteroides* (either *B. fragilis* or other species of *Bacteroides*) from various kinds of diseases (abscesses, abortion, mastitis), though infrequent, indicate that nonsporing anaerobes other than *F. necrophorum* contribute to animal diseases, probably more frequently than is known, as they do to human diseases.

Liver Granulomas of Turkeys

Liver granulomas occur in up to 20% of the commercial turkeys reaching market age and are a common cause for condemnation of the livers. In this disease, from 1 to 20 or more light-colored spheroid masses having dense fibrous linings surrounding hard caseous cores are tightly embedded in the liver. Many of these granulomas are easily visible on the liver surface. There are no apparent symptoms in the live bird.

Tissue Gram stains of the lesions usually show numerous bacterial cells, often including long filamentous gram-positive cells. Bacterial cells are also evident in crushed specimen smears. Cultures of the lesions often contain one to three species of bacteria. Organisms isolated include *Eubacterium tortuosum,* unidentified species of *Eubacterium, Bacteroides fragilis, B. clostridiiformis, B. hypermegas, Propionibacterium acnes, Streptococcus liquefaciens,* microaerophilic lactobacilli, and obligately anaerobic lactobacilli.

Liver granulomas were investigated in experimental birds in some detail, using one of the bacteria isolated, *E. tortuosum.*[21] Turkeys inoculated IV with *E. tortuosum* developed liver granulomas in 10 days, but no change was noted when this organism was administered orally. However, when a virulent strain of *Streptococcus liquefaciens* was administered orally, liver granulomas developed. Apparently *S. liquefaciens* affects the integrity of the gut wall, particularly in the duodenum, and intestinal bacteria are carried via the blood to the liver where they establish foci of infection. The gut wall itself heals rapidly following the initial tissue damage.

To culture the organisms from the lesions, cauterize the surface, remove a core from the lesion, and place the sample in pre-reduced peptone–yeast extract glucose broth. Incubate 24–72 hours. After growth is apparent, Gram stain and streak on pre-reduced agar.

Liver granulomas containing organisms morphologically similar to those in turkeys have been reported in rabbit colonies; however, no liver lesions were produced experimentally with *E. tortuosum* in guinea pigs or rats.

General Methods
Specimens

Because the gastrointestinal and respiratory tracts, skin, and vagina contain large numbers of anaerobes in the normal or predominant flora, contamination can easily occur during sampling or autopsy. Aseptic technique is essential for collecting diagnostic specimens.

If possible, specimens of abscess material, blood, or spinal fluid should be cultured in pre-reduced media within a few minutes after the sample is taken. If holding or transport is required, tissue, pus, or exudate should be placed in sterile stoppered test tubes flushed with oxygen-free CO_2. These should be held at room temperature until cultured. No transport medium or diluent solution should be used because facultative bacteria that may also be present, or may occur only as specimen contaminants, can quickly overgrow anaerobes. Even pre-reduced media do not have as low an oxidation-reduction potential (are not as chemically reduced) as infection sites; therefore, the growth of facultative or aerotolerant species is favored when specimens are placed in transport solutions.

Careful microscopic examination of the material to be cultured is strongly recommended; it can give an estimate of the number of different kinds of organisms present.

However, direct microscopic examination is not entirely reliable because two species may appear similar, and because pleomorphic forms, common among some species of nonsporeforming anaerobes, may appear to be two different species.

Laboratory Procedures

Cultures. To isolate the bacteria in the same proportions as they occur in the infections, it is necessary to streak from specimen material directly onto anaerobic agar. Both anaerobic and facultative bacteria grow under these conditions. When large numbers of media-adapted organisms are used as inocula, better culture conditions are generally required to isolate organisms (especially anaerobes) from infections than to subculture pure cultures of the same bacteria. However, if the best possible techniques are used for subcultures, characterization is more rapid and reliable.

When exposed to air, media are very rapidly oxidized. The oxidized components inhibit or prevent growth of many anaerobic bacteria. If it is necessary to use plating media, they should be reconstituted, sterilized, and used immediately. Because exposure to air is progressively detrimental, as soon as the agar hardens, plates should be streaked and placed in anaerobe jars equipped with a catalyst. Jars are sealed, evacuated, and flushed four times with gas containing hydrogen and a high concentration of CO_2 (10% H_2, 90% CO_2). Systems that are not evacuated mechanically expose the inoculated media to air for even longer periods and therefore are less satisfactory. Even under ideal conditions, plate and jar methods expose the media to air and many of the more strict anaerobes cannot be isolated. This usually accounts for the reports of "sterile abscesses."

To prevent oxidation of media, a simple and very effective method has been developed based on Hungate's roll tube technique. Media are prepared, tubed, and sterilized under oxygen-free gas in rubber-stoppered tubes (also available commercially, Robbin Lab., Chapel Hill, N.C.). These pre-reduced, anaerobically sterilized (PRAS) media have an oxidation-reduction potential of minus 150 to minus 170 mv. A film of agar medium is made on the inner walls of the stoppered tubes by spinning them while the agar cools. Whenever the stoppers are removed for streaking, picking, or making culture transfers in broth media, air is excluded from the tubes by a gentle stream of oxygen-free CO_2 introduced into the neck of the tube through a flame-sterilized cannula. The agar film is streaked with a stainless steel or platinum loop while the tube is rotating. (Do not use nichrome for anaerobic work; it oxidizes the media.) After the stopper is replaced, the tube is ready for incubation immediately. Individual tubes can be examined without exposing cultures to air. This system is simple and inexpensive but provides superior culture conditions. Specimens of blood frequently contain so few bacteria that direct streaking is not practical. These should be injected (without air) into pre-reduced chopped-meat glucose broth or E medium.[1]

As soon as the specimens or scrapings of the specimens are streaked in roll tubes or on blood agar plates, a direct smear of the original material should be made and then Gram stained. The different morphotypes should be carefully noted so that after incubation representatives of each important type can be sought, and any contaminant organisms not present in the original material can be recognized as such. The remaining specimen material should be placed in pre-reduced chopped meat glucose to serve as a reserve specimen culture in case all the significant types of organisms are not recovered.

After incubation, the roll tube or plate should be examined under a dissecting microscope and each colony type picked to chopped meat glucose medium. Each colony should be picked a second time to a tiny drop of water on a glass slide and stained. All morphotypes in the original material should be represented among the different isolates. Allowance must be made, however, for slight differences in morphology of cells from infections as compared with cells from culture media. If it is possible to pick the same colony a third time, a tube of melted deep agar should also be inoculated to determine aerotolerance.

Differential reactions. The characteristics of the well-described species that can be isolated are mentioned in the keys and tables of the VPI manual.[1] However, not all of the species that will be encountered have been well described. Organisms that are isolated but do not conform to described species should be sent to a reference laboratory. Most of the tests used in the identification of anaerobes are similar to those used for identification of other bacteria; only the culture techniques and media preparation are different. Pre-reduced, anaerobically sterilized media are recommended for ease of culturing. Semisolid agar (stored for not more than 2 weeks) may be used.[31]

The type of metabolic acids produced by different kinds of nonsporeforming anaerobes is a very important characteristic because several of the genera can be differentiated accurately only on this basis. The introduction of simple and rapid gas chromatograph procedures for the analysis of bacterial products in a routine manner has greatly improved the precision of identification of anaerobic bacteria. Approximately 4 ml of glucose broth culture is acidified with 0.2 ml of 50% H_2SO_4–50% H_2O (V/V) and extracted with 1 ml of ethyl ether. After thorough mixing, the ether is allowed to separate and the tube is placed in a freezer until the liquid freezes. The ether is decanted into a separate tube, and dissolved water is removed by adding a small amount of anhydrous Na_2SO_4 or $MgSO_4$. Fourteen microliters of the ether extract are injected onto a 0.6×183 cm column packed with Resoflex (LAC-1-R-296 std. conc. [P], Burrell Corp., Pittsburgh) at 110°C. Alcohols and volatile fatty acids are separated and eluted in 20–40 minutes. They are detected with a thermal conductivity detector and identified by comparing elution time with known standards.[1] This simple procedure is now being used in an increasing number of clinical laboratories.

For analysis of lactic, pyruvic, fumaric, or succinic acids, 1 ml of acidified culture is mixed with 1 ml of BF_3-methanol (14% W/V boron trifluoride methanol, Applied Science Lab., State College, Pa.), and 14 μl of a chloroform extract is injected onto the same column at the same operating conditions. The methyl esters are eluted and detected in 10–15 minutes. The two chromatographic procedures have been described in detail in the VPI manual.[1]

The biochemical, cultural, and morphologic tests used for identification of nonsporeforming anaerobes are similar to those for other bacteria but special precautions are required for some of them.

Colorimetric pH indicators added to medium often are not reliable for measuring acid production in cultures of anaerobic bacteria because the indicators may be chemically reduced by the low oxidation-reduction potentials. Therefore, pH should be measured with glass electrodes or by adding a sterile indicator to the tube at the time the pH is checked. Compare the culture pH with the pH of a similar medium that has been "inoculated" with sterile broth.

Many gram-positive anaerobic bacteria rapidly become gram-negative. Young cultures (12–14 hours) should be stained with Kopeloff's modification of the Gram stain. With this procedure the pH of the stain is controlled and more reliable results are obtained than with Hucker's modification. The presence of any gram-positive cells indicates a gram-positive species.

Esculin hydrolysis is detected by adding a few drops of a 1% aqueous solution of ferric ammonium citrate to a culture in esculin broth medium. Immediate appearance of black color indicates positive hydrolysis.

Gelatin liquefaction is detected by inoculating pre-reduced 12% gelatin (plus 0.5% glucose) and incubating the tube at 37°C for 3–5 days. Incubated tubes and sterile control tubes are chilled at 3–4°C. Failure to solidify indicates complete liquefaction. Melting at room temperature in less than half the time for the control tubes indicates partial digestion.

Starch hydrolysis is detected by the addition of Gram's iodine to starch broth cultures without stirring. Immediate appearance of blue-black color (which may rapidly disappear) indicates that starch remains and has not been hydrolized. Appearance of only slight color indicates partial hydrolysis, and no blue-black color indicates complete starch hydrolysis.

Oxygen tolerance and gas production are detected by inoculating tubes of melted pre-reduced peptone–yeast extract–glucose deep agar (cooled to 45°C) with two to three drops of inoculum. The opening of the tube is covered with a square of flame-sterilized aluminium foil to allow the surface of the agar to oxidize. Growth only below the oxidized layer (in which the resazurin is pink) indicates an obligate anaerobe that does not chemically reduce the medium in which it grows. Growth in the pink area and on the surface indicates a facultative organism. Growth in the pink zone but not on the surface indicates an aerotolerant (less oxygen-sensitive) anaerobe. Many cultures chemically reduce the medium; the resazurin turns colorless again and growth progresses up to but not on the surface. These cultures are obligate anaerobes that reduce the medium.

Gas production is indicated by splits in the agar. If the agar actually separated all the way across the tube, gas production is recorded as $++$. If the agar is broken and plugs of agar are pushed to the lip of the tube, gas production is recorded as $++++$.

Catalase is produced by several species of obligately anaerobic bacteria, but with most catalase-positive species (even facultative species) it is necessary to expose anaerobic surface growth to air for at least 30 minutes before testing for catalase with hydrogen peroxide.

Indole production may be determined from chopped meat culture. Extract with xylene and test with Ehrlich's reagent.

Cellular morphology. Spores in several species of clostridia are difficult to demonstrate. When none are seen in stained smears, all isolates should be tested by placing three to four drops of 5-day chopped-meat glucose culture in pre-reduced starch broth and heating the broth at 80°C for 10 minutes. Growth in the starch broth should be stained to compare with the original culture. Surviving cultures usually are sporeformers and every effort should be made to detect sporing cells microscopically and to determine their location within the cells. No one medium is best for spore production in all species and several should be tried. One excellent test medium is chopped-meat glucose slants incubated at 30°C for 5–21 days.

Some gram-negative species produce heat-resistant spores. Many gram-negative species produce cells with vacuoles that frequently have been mistaken for spores, especially when the presence of spores was not verified with a heat test.

Motility is determined by placing a drop of actively growing (usually 5–6 hours) culture in chopped-meat or peptone–yeast extract broth on a slide under a coverslip and examining immediately with phase or reduced-light bright-field microscopy. To determine the genus that motile gram-negative species belong to, use flagella stains.

References

1. Anaerobe Laboratory. *Outline of Clinical Methods in Anaerobic Bacteriology,* L.V. Holdeman and W.E.C. Moore (eds.). Virginia Polytechnic Institute and State University, Blacksburg, 1972.
2. Beerens, H., and M. Tahon-Castel. *Infections humaines à bactéries anaérobies non toxigènes.* Presses Academies européenes, Brussels, 1965.
3. Beveridge, W.I.B. Footrot of sheep: Its epidemiology and control. *Bull. Off. Internat. Epiz.* 59:1537–1549, 1963.
4. Beveridge, W.I.B. Diseases caused by non-sporing anaerobes: Ovine footrot, necrobacillosis. *Bull. Off. Internat. Epiz.* 67:1–5, 1967.
5. Biberstein, E.L., H.D. Knight, and K. England. *Bacteroides melaninogenicus* in diseases of domestic animals. *J. Am. Vet. Med. Ass.* 153:1045–1049, 1968.
6. Bryant, M.P. Bacterial species of the rumen. *Bact. Rev.* 23:125–153, 1959.
7. Buchanan, R.E., and N.E. Gibbons (eds.). *Bergey's Manual of Determinative Bacteriology.* 8th ed. Williams and Wilkins, Baltimore, 1974.
8. Dehority, B.A. Characterization of several bovine rumen bacteria isolated with a xylan medium. *J. Bact.* 91:1724–1729, 1966.
9. Egerton, J.R., and I.M. Parsonson. Parenteral antibiotic treatment of ovine footrot. *Austral. Vet. J.* 42:97–98, 1966.
10. Egerton, J.R., and I.M. Parsonson. Isolation of *Fusiformis nodosus* from cattle. *Austral. Vet. J.* 42:425–429, 1966.
11. Egerton, J.R., and I.M. Parsonson. Benign foot-rot: A specific interdigital dermatitis of sheep associated with infection by less proteolytic strains of *Fusiformis nodosus. Austral. Vet. J.* 45:345–349, 1969.
12. Egerton, J.R., D.S. Roberts, and I.M. Parsonson. The aetiology and pathogenesis of ovine foot-rot. I. A histological study of the bacterial invasion. *J. Comp. Path.* 79:207–217, 1969.
13. Fiévez, L. *Etude comparée des souches de Sphaerophorus necrophorus isolées chez l'homme et chez l'animal.* Presses Academies européenes, Brussels, 1963.
14. Finegold, S.M. Isolation of anaerobic bacteria. In *Manual of Clinical Microbiology,* pp. 265–279. American Society for Microbiology, Bethesda, Md., 1970.
15. Hungate, R.E. The anaerobic mesophilic cellulolytic bacteria. *Bact. Rev.* 14:1–49, 1950.
16. Hungate, R.E. *The Rumen and Its Microbes.* Academic Press, New York, 1966.
17. Johnson, D.W., A.R. Dommert, and D.G. Kiger. Clinical investigations of infectious foot-rot of cattle. *J. Am. Vet. Med. Ass.* 155:1886–1891, 1969.
18. Mackey, D.R. Calf diphtheria. *J. Am. Vet. Med. Ass.* 152:822–823, 1968.
19. McMinn, M.T., and J.J. Crawford. Recovery of anaerobic microorganisms from clinical specimens in pre-reduced media versus recovery by routine clinical laboratory methods. *Appl. Microbiol.* 19:207–213, 1970.
20. Moore, W.E.C., P. Cato, and V. Holdeman. Anaerobic bacteria of the gastrointestinal flora and their occurrence in clinical infections. *J. Infec. Dis.* 119:641–649, 1969.

21. Moore, W.E.C., and W.B. Gross. Liver granulomas of turkeys: Causative agents and mechanism of infection. *Avian Dis.* 12:417–422, 1968.
22. Parsonson, I.M., J.R. Egerton, and D.S. Roberts. Ovine interdigital dermatitis. *J. Comp. Path.* 77:309–314, 1967.
23. Pérez, J.E., E.A. Padilla, J.D. Rivera Anaya, and A. Torrech. Bacterial flora of foot-rot: Report of findings in 100 cattle. *J. Ag. U. Puerto Rico* 40:118–124, 1956.
24. Prévot, A.R., A. Turpin, and P. Kaiser. *Les bactéries anaérobies*. Dunot, Paris, 1967.
25. Roberts, D.S. The pathogenic synergy of *Fusiformis necrophorus* and *Corynebacterium pyogenes*. I. Influence of the leucocidal exotoxin of *F. Necrophorus*. *Brit. J. Exp. Path.* 48:665–673, 1967.
26. Roberts, D.S. The pathogenic synergy of *Fusiformis necrophorus* and *Corynebacterium pyogenes*. II. The response of *F. necrophorus* to a filterable product of *C. pyogenes*. *Brit. J. Exp. Path.* 48:674–679, 1967.
27. Roberts, D.S., and J.R. Egerton. The aetiology and pathogenesis of ovine foot-rot. *J. Comp. Path.* 79:217–227, 1969.
28. Roberts, D.S., N.P.H. Graham, and J.R. Egerton. Infective bulbar necrosis (heel-abscess) of sheep, a mixed infection with *Fusiformis necrophorus* and *Corynebacterium pyogenes*. *J. Comp. Path.* 78:1–10, 1968.
29. Simon, P.C., and P.L. Stovell. Diseases of animals associated with *Sphaerophorus necrophorus:* Characteristics of the organism. *Vet. Bull.* 39:311–315, 1969.
30. Smith, L.D.S. *Sphaerophorus necrophorus* and liver abscesses in cattle. *Bull. Off. Internat. Epiz.* 59:1517–1526, 1963.
31. Smith, L.D.S., and L.V. Holdeman. *The Pathogenic Anaerobic Bacteria*. Thomas, Springfield, Ill., 1968.
32. Thomas, J.H. A simple medium for the isolation and cultivation of *Fusiformis nodosus*. *Austral. Vet. J.* 34:411, 1958.
33. Thomas, J.H. Proteolytic enzymes produced in liquid media by *Fusiformis nodosus*. *Austral. J. Ag. Res.* 15:417–426, 1964.

47. Mycobacterium

Several species of the genus *Mycobacterium* are economically important, resulting in illness or death in both human and animal populations. They are usually slow-growing, nonmotile rods of variable width and length and are acid fast.

Infections due to mycobacteria are usually characterized by development of the delayed type of hypersensitivity to homologous bacterial products such as tuberculin. The lesions are characterized in most instances by formation of histologically recognizable granulomas, often with giant cells and caseation necrosis.

Most species have a worldwide distribution. There are four species of special importance in veterinary medicine, *Mycobacterium bovis*, *M. avium*, *M. tuberculosis*, and *M. paratuberculosis*. *M. leprae* and *M. ulcerans* are important in human medicine but are not known to cause naturally occuring disease in animals.[5] *M. marinum* causes infection in cold-blooded animals and fish; it has also been isolated from superficial granulomas on the extremities of humans. A rapidly growing soil microorganism, *M. fortuitum*, has been isolated from lesions in humans and animals.

In addition, there are numerous species of so-called atypical mycobacteria that have been divided into four groups depending on pigmentation, response to light, and rate of growth.[7] Group I mycobacteria, or photochromogens, are yellowish when exposed to light. They have seldom been isolated from animals. Group II organisms, or scotochromogens, have yellow pigment. They are common in soil and in water and are seldom associated with lesions in humans or in animals. Group III organisms, the *M. avium–M. intracellulare–M. scrofulaceum* complex, are nonchromogenic or slightly buff-colored. They may be isolated from lesions in humans and animals. Group IV organisms are the rapid growers. They are soil and water forms and are seldom associated with lesions. Some of these unclassified mycobacteria may sensitize animals and humans to tuberculin and thus be a cause of nonspecific tuberculin reactions.

There are other species of mycobacteria that are of less importance in veterinary medicine. These may be found in the soil, in plants, and in warm- and cold-blooded animals. Examples are *M. xenopi*, *M. ulcerans*, *M. phlei*, and *M. gordonae*.[12]

Since many species of the above mycobacteria are pathogenic to humans, adequate precautions should be used in the laboratory and animal rooms. Individuals working with mycobacteria should be tuberculin-tested at 6-month intervals. In the event a positive tuberculin reaction is reported, a thorough examination including chest X ray should be required. An individual who is known to be hypersensitive to tuberculin should receive a chest X ray only, because there is danger in repeated tuberculin testing of hypersensitive individuals. Laboratory workers should remove street clothing and wear laboratory clothing while at work. In addition, they also should wear gloves and gowns when actually working with mycobacteria. All clothing should be removed at the end of the working day and sterilized before being worn again. Each employee should shower before donning his street clothes. Laboratory workers themselves should clean the laboratory each day and not depend on a janitor for this service.

A suitable disinfectant should always be on hand to swab any area that might have become contaminated with mycobacteria (5% phenol in water is a good disinfectant). The animal room should ideally have negative air pressure and a filtered exhaust system. Attendants caring for infected animals should wear rubber gloves and use plastic hoods with an external air supply. This equipment should also be used by individuals inoculating or engaged in necropsy of infected animals. Upon leaving the animal room each individual should change clothing and shower.

In the laboratory, biologic safety hoods with negative pressure and filtered exhaust systems should be used. Mouth pipetting should not be permitted. All contaminated glassware, instruments, gloves, clothing, discarded tissue specimens, and cultures should be placed in covered containers and sterilized in autoclaves.

Specimens

Most specimens submitted for laboratory examination for mycobacteria are usually taken from freshly slaughtered cattle, hogs, or poultry, although tuberculosis can sometimes be found in other species. Examples of animals less frequently affected are sheep, goats, deer, monkeys, elephants, horses, dogs, cats, mink, and various zoo animals.[5] Tissues to be collected are usually those showing a tuberculous lesion, which is usually nodular and consists of a caseocalcarious center surrounded by a fibrous capsule. Lesions may be found in any internal organ, lymph node, or the skin but are not observed in the muscles. The extent and size of the lesions vary. In some instances, there may be only one lesion barely visible to the naked eye in the entire carcass. In other cases, there may be many lesions throughout the carcass. Lesions may involve entire pulmonary lobes and large areas of liver and spleen. Large lesions have usually been formed by the merging of many small lesions. Infected lymph nodes may be several times larger than normal. If the lesion is too large to send to the laboratory, a representative portion should be sent. Bacilli are usually most numerous in the region bordering the inside of the capsule and adjacent to the caseous mass and are seldom found in the center. Therefore, whenever possible, a piece of capsule including some of the purulent matter adjacent to it should be collected.

Sometimes it is necessary to collect tissues for culturing and histopathologic examination from tuberculin reactors that show no gross lesions of the disease on postmortem examination. With such animals, one lymph node each from the head, the thoracic cavity, and the abdominal cavity should be collected for examination. Specimens that are suspected of being tuberculous should be removed from the carcass aseptically, if possible, and placed in small screw-capped specimen jars. Specimens for cultural examination should ideally be chilled and taken to the laboratory without adding a preservative and should be cultured within 24 hours of collection. Inclusion of 2 g of powdered borax to coat the tissue will inhibit surface contaminants if prolonged transit of chilled specimens is necessary. This may be rinsed off in the laboratory with sterile saline. Tissue for histologic examination should be placed in a 10% Formalin solution.

If specimens are obtained from an animal infected in the laboratory, all the precautions described under laboratory procedures should be followed. If specimens are obtained at slaughtering establishments, a face mask, rubber gloves, coveralls, and boots should be worn. Before leaving the slaughtering plant, the operator should place the clothing in a waterproof covered container. The container should be washed with a disinfectant before it leaves the slaughtering plant and sterilized after it returns to the laboratory. The operator should take a shower before donning street clothing.

Specimens for paratuberculosis examination usually are obtained from the intestinal tract of carcasses of animals suspected of harboring *M. paratuberculosis*. The animals most commonly affected are cattle, sheep, and goats although the disease is sometimes observed in other ruminants, e.g. deer and reindeer. Lesions of the disease consist of a thickening of the wall of the small intestine. The thickening is the result of proliferation of epithelioid cells in the mucosa and submucosa. The mesenteric lymph nodes may be enlarged and may present a milky appearance when cut open. A piece of intestine about 2 cm square should be excised just anterior to the ileocecal valve and placed in 10% Formalin solution. In addition, approximately 2 g of intestinal mucosa should be scraped from an adjacent area for culture. The mucosa is placed in a 50 ml round-bottom centrifuge tube with a screw-cap vial and then frozen.

Fecal specimens for culture should be obtained from the rectum and not from the ground. About 20 g of fecal material are collected in a 30 ml specimen jar. These specimens should be taken to the laboratory and cultured within 36 hours after collection.

Laboratory Procedures

Cultures. The procedure for all mycobacteria except *M. paratuberculosis* is as follows. The tissues are removed from the glass jars and placed in sterile petri dishes within the biologic safety hood, where they can be dissected and examined for gross lesions. The central area from each tissue, including the lesions, is cut into small pieces and transferred to a blender jar. (The total quantity should not exceed 25 g.) Fifty ml of nutrient broth containing 0.4% phenol red indicator is added. The mixture is blended for about 2 minutes and then placed in a flask. A Teflon magnetic stirring bar and 100 ml of papain solution (prepared by adding 50 g papain and 0.6 g cystine hydrochloride to 1 liter of distilled water) are added to the blended tissues.[8] Sufficient 4% NaOH to change the phenol red indicator from yellow to red is slowly added. Digestion is continued by placing the flask on a magnetic stirrer for 1 hour at 37°C.

After digestion, 10 ml of pentane is added to the contents, which are then shaken vigorously and allowed to stand for 30 minutes. Mycobacteria released from the tissues during the digestion will be contained in the pentane layer and at the pentane-water interface.[1] All the pentane and the material at the interface should be removed with a sterile pipette, filtered through a double layer of unbleached muslin in a glass funnel, and collected in a 20 × 125 mm test tube. The tube is then placed inside a screw-capped safety capsule and centrifuged at 1630 RCF for 20 minutes. A sediment will form on the bottom of the tube and a pellicle on top. Almost all the liquid separating the sediment and pellicle should be removed with a pipette and discarded. One ml of nutrient broth is then added to the centrifuge tube, which is shaken vigorously to produce a homogenous mixture of sediment and pellicle. This mixture is used to inoculate solid media.

Four tubes of media are each inoculated with four drops of inoculum delivered from a Pasteur pipette. The remaining inoculum is mixed with an equal volume of 0.2% benzalkonium chloride, which suppresses the growth of contaminating organisms. This inoculum is placed on four additional tubes of medium. Stonebrink's is the preferred standard diagnostic medium. Supplementary media that contain more glycerol (e.g. Lowenstein-Jensen) may be used in addition, as these favor the growth of *M. tuberculosis*. The inoculated tubes should be held so that the inoculum flows evenly over the surface of the medium and then the tubes should be placed in a rack in a horizontal position in the incubator for 24 hours at 37°C. The tubes can then be placed in a vertical position for continued incubation. All tubes should be examined weekly for 8 weeks for mycobacterial colonies.

Evidence of growth may be observed as early as 2 weeks. Colonies can be observed for morphology and pigmentation with the aid of a hand lens. *M. bovis* and *M. avium–M. intracellulare–M. scrofulaceum* complex (group III) organisms growing on Stonebrink's medium usually appear as moist, white, convex colonies. *M. tuberculosis* colonies are very dry, rough, flat to raised, and white to buff in color, with irregular edges. Group I colonies are colorless when grown in the dark but pigmented when grown in light. Group II colonies are pigmented when grown in light or darkness. Because *M. avium–M. intracellulare–M. scrofulaceum* complex organisms are difficult to differentiate, animal inoculation may be required. Group IV colonies appear in 6 days or less and pigment is not usually present.

Smears should be prepared from a typical colony in each tube, stained with the Ziehl-Neelson (Z-N) technique and examined for cellular morphology. The dimensions of bacilli vary but they have an average size of about 0.5 μm in width and 2–4 μm in length. A typical colony should also be inoculated into 10 ml of Dubos broth medium (containing albumin and Tween 80) for preparing the inoculum for laboratory animals, and into 10 ml of Proskauer and Beck medium for studying growth characteristics and the niacin test.[3]

Differential reactions. When grown in Proskauer and Beck medium, cells of *M. tuberculosis* and *M. bovis* have a granular (clumped) appearance in transmitted light.[6] Most other mycobacteria have a uniform dispersion of cells when observed in transmitted light. A smear of the bacterial sediment from a Proskauer and Beck culture should be stained by the Z-N technique and examined for cords and for cell morphology. *M. tuberculosis* and *M. bovis* produce cords consistently. This phenomenon is an indicator of virulence and is best described as a parallel alignment of bacterial cells that results in a long serpentine or stringlike formation of the cells.

The presence of niacin in a culture growing in Proskauer and Beck medium can be used to differentiate *M. tuberculosis* from all other mycobacteria. To perform the test for niacin, add 1 ml of 4% aniline in ethyl alcohol to the culture, then add 1 ml of aqueous cyanogen bromide (a deadly poison). The appearance of a yellow color within 5 minutes indicates the presence of niacin.

Animal inoculation. Inoculation is used to differentiate *M. tuberculosis*, *M. bovis*, certain strains of *M. intracellulare*, and *M. avium*. Guinea pigs, chickens, and rabbits approaching maturity are used for this purpose (the chickens must be from a tuberculosis-free flock). About three of each species are used. They are kept for 2 months after inoculation and any that die during this period are examined for evidence of tuberculosis. All surviving animals are killed and examined for evidence of disease at the end of the 2-month period. The pathogenicity of mycobacteria for these species is shown in Table 47.1. Exceptions to this pattern occur especially with the *M. avium–M. intracellulare–M. scrofulaceum* complex.

Table 47.1. Pathogenicity pattern for laboratory animals

Strain	Guinea pig	Rabbit	Chicken
M. bovis	+	+	−
M. tuberculosis	+	−	−
M. avium–M. intracellulare–M. scofulaceum complex (group III)	−	+	+

The inoculum for the animals is prepared from Dubos broth medium. (This medium is prepared in dehydrated form by Digestive Ferments Co., Detroit, and by Becton, Dickinson and Co., Cockeysville, Md. Directions for preparation are given by the manufacturer.) Two ml of the broth culture is placed in a Fitch-Hopkins tube and centrifuged at 2350 RCF for 20 minutes. The bacterial cells are then packed into the bottom of the tube and the net weight of the cells is determined from the calibrations (Fig. 47.1). From these results the weight of bacilli in the remaining broth can be calculated and the desired quantities of bacterial weight for animal inoculation can be prepared by dilution with saline solution. The animals are inoculated IP with 1 ml of suspension, which for guinea pigs and chickens should contain 0.1 mg of bacterial cells per ml and for rabbits 0.01 mg.

The inoculated animals should be closely observed, because they may begin to lose weight and present an unthrifty appearance within a few weeks.

For the diagnosis and cultivation of *Mycobacterium paratuberculosis*, 2 ml of the intestinal mucosa, collected as previously described, is suspended in 30 ml of 2% trypsin solution using either a Ten Broeck tissue grinder or a blender.[9,10] The suspension is adjusted to pH 8.4 with 1% NaOH and shaken for 30 minutes to facilitate digestion. The digest is then centrifuged for 45 minutes at 3000 rpm. The supernatant fluid is discarded and a smear is made from the sediment; the smear should be stained by the Z-N technique and examined for the presence of small acid-fast bacilli. *M. paratuberculosis* appears as a short thick rod measuring about 0.5×1 μm. It is strongly acid fast and often

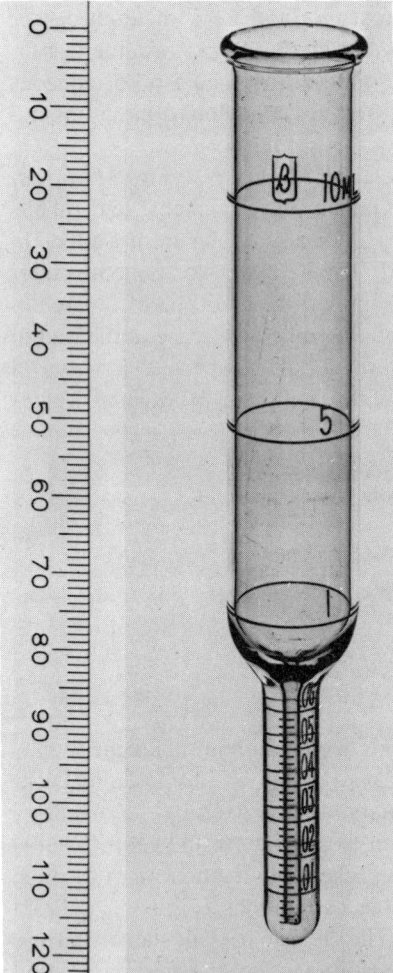

Figure 47.1. Fitch-Hopkins tube. After a 2 ml suspension of mycobacteria in Dubos broth has been centrifuged in a Fitch-Hopkins tube, the level of packed bacterial cells in the stem of the tube may be used to estimate the W/V ratio of the cells in the suspension. The labeled markings on the stem of the tube of .01, .02, .03, .04, .05, and .06 indicate 5, 10, 15, 20, 25, and 30 mg/ml, respectively, of mycobacterial cells in the suspension. The tube is made by Bellco Biological Glassware, Vineland, N.J.

appears in small clumps. This arrangement aids in diagnosis: if the bacillus is found, a tentative positive diagnosis can be made. However, a negative diagnosis cannot be made if it is not found because the bacillus may be present in small numbers.

After making the smear, mix the sediment with 30 ml of a 0.1% solution of benzalkonium chloride for decontamination. This mixture is shaken for 30 minutes and then allowed to stand for 24 hours. The sediment is then pipetted onto four tubes of modified Herrold's medium containing a source of mycobactin, which is necessary for growth of *M. paratuberculosis*. (This product is not commercially made, so it must be prepared by extracting it from *M. phlei* grown on Dorset and Henley's medium.)[2,4] The tubes are laid in a horizontal position in the incubator with the caps loosened to allow the suspending fluid to evaporate. Following a week of incubation of 37°C, the caps are tightened and the tubes placed in a vertical position. Evidence of growth may be observed after 8 weeks incubation, but tubes showing no growth should not be discarded before 12 weeks. Growth is indicated by very small white convex colonies. To determine if these are *M. paratuberculosis*, a typical colony should be inoculated onto another tube of Herrold's medium containing mycobactin and onto a tube containing no mycobactin. A smear also should be made, stained by the Z-N technique, and examined for the presence of typical acid-fast bacilli.

Cultivation of fecal samples is accomplished as follows: approximately 2 g of fecal material is added to 30 ml of distilled water and shaken for 30 minutes. The mixture is then allowed to stand for 30 minutes to allow the larger particles to settle out. Five ml of the supernatant fluid is collected and mixed with 30 ml of 0.3% benzalkonium chloride and allowed to stand for 24 hours. From this point on, the procedure is identical to that used in the cultivation of tissue specimens.

Serology. Strains of *M. avium* and some strains of the atypical unclassified groups I through IV can be identified by their agglutination reaction with type-specific antisera prepared from rabbits.[11,13] The antisera are prepared by inoculating rabbits with the desired strain of mycobacterium. This procedure is not satisfactory for identifying *M. tuberculosis, M. bovis,* and *M. paratuberculosis.* Therefore, most laboratories would not have the volume of work necessary to make this a practical procedure unless a commercial source of antisera were to become available.

Preservation. Cultures of mycobacteria can be kept viable for periods of a year at $-70°C$.[12]

References

1. Diagnostic Service, Animal Health Division, ARS. *A Manual for the Isolation and Typing of Mycobacteria.* U.S. Department of Agriculture, Ames, Iowa, 1971.
2. Dorset, M., and R.R. Henley. *A Synthetic Medium for B. tuberculosis.* Bureau of Animal Industry, USDA, Washington, 1934.
3. Dubos, R.J., F. Fenner, and C.H. Pierce. Properties of a culture of BCG grown in liquid media containing Tween 80 and the filtrate of heated serum. *Am. Rev. Resp. Dis.* 60:66–76, 1950.
4. Francis, J., H.M. Macturk, J. Macinaveita, and G.A. Snow. Mycobactin, a growth factor for *Mycobacterium johnei. Biochem. J.* 55:596–607, 1953.
5. Karlson, A.G. The genus *Mycobacterium.* In *Veterinary Bacteriology and Virology,* I.A. Merchant and R.A. Packer (eds.), pp. 441–465. 7th ed. Iowa State University Press, Ames, 1967.
6. Karlson, A.G., J.K. Martin, and R. Harrington. Identification of *M. tuberculosis* with one tube of liquid medium. *Mayo Clinic Proc.* 39:410–415, 1964.
7. Lester, W., R.F. Corpe, and E.H. Runyon. Status of disease due to unclassified mycobacteria. *Am. Rev. Resp. Dis.* 87:459–461, 1963.
8. Lupe, R.S., W.L. Mallman, and J.A. Roy. *An Enzyme Procedure for the Concentration of Mycobacteria in Low Populations from Tissues.* 4th Semi-Annual Progress Report of the Research Contract with the United States Department of Agriculture, Public Health and Veterinary Pathology, Michigan State University, East Lansing, June 30, 1961.
9. Merkal, R.S., K.E. Kopecky, A.B. Larsen, and J.R. Thurnston. Improvements in techniques for primary cultivation of *Mycobacterium paratuberculosis. Am. J. Vet. Res.* 25:1290–1293, 1974.
10. Merkal, R.S., and A.B. Larsen. Improved methods for primary cultivation of *Mycobacterium paratuberculosis. Am. J. Vet. Res.* 23:1307–1309, 1962.
11. Shaefer, W.B. Serologic identification of the atypical mycobacteria and its value in epidemiological studies. *Am. Rev. Resp. Dis.* 96:115–118, 1967.
12. *Trudeau Mycobacterial Culture Collection Manual.* Trudeau Institute, Saranak Lake, N.Y., 1972.
13. Yoder, W.D., and W.B. Schaefer. Comparison of the seroagglutination test for the pathogenicity test in the chicken for the identification of *M. avium* and *M. intracellulare. Am. Rev. Resp. Dis.* 103:173–178, 1971.

48. Corynebacterium

The typical disease situations in which the corynebacteria are found in animals are characterized by extensive pus formation. Any more specific statement would have to be qualified according to the species of corynebacterium involved and the host species affected. Four species of corynebacteria are recognized as regular animal parasites associated with disease. Their occurrence and involvement in pathologic conditions are summarized in Table 48.1.

Table 48.1. Occurrence and pathogenicity of corynebacteria

Corynebacterium	Principal hosts	Normal reservoir	Disease entities
pyogenes	Cattle, sheep, swine, goats	Mucous membranes	Many purulent processes: bovine mastitis, abortion, arthritis
pseudotuberculosis	Sheep, horses, goats, cattle	Soil	Sheep: caseous lymphadenitis; horses: ulcerative lymphangitis and ventral abscesses
renale	Cattle, sheep	Lower urogenital tract	Cystitis, ureteritis, pyelonephritis
equi	Horses, swine	Equine alimentary tract, soil of corrals	Pneumonia of foals, lymphadenitis of swine

Corynebacteria of undeterminable species are isolated from a variety of disease conditions, usually along with other bacteria. Most prominent among these conditions are purulent infections of uncertain etiology, such as the serositides of cats and dogs, and abscesses developing contiguously in the upper digestive and respiratory tracts. Among the 262 strains of corynebacteria isolated, 99 belong to this anonymous group.

Corynebacterium bovis, which is frequently present in normal cow's milk, has been described on occasions as a possible cause of mastitis.[3] The etiologic agent of human erythrasma, *C. minutissimum,* has also been recovered from sheep and cattle. In sheep it was associated with a moist interdigital dermatitis. A pyelonephritis in swine yielded an anaerobic *Corynebacterium,* which was named *C. suis.*[13]

Corynebacterium pyogenes

C. pyogenes is worldwide in distribution and is found in cattle, sheep, swine, and goats generally, regardless of age or season. Certain special cases should be noted. *C. pyogenes* mastitis, where it is prevalent, is seen predominently in the warm weather months and has as a result sometimes been called summer mastitis. The suggestion that flying insects are involved in the epidemiology seeks to account for this incidence. Similar circumstances have been suspected in a pustular dermatitis of cattle from which *C. pyogenes* is commonly recovered. *C. pyogenes* is most frequently found in association with other bacteria, which are generally assumed to be secondary, although the assumption has not been subjected to rigorous tests. The organisms most frequently found in *C. pyogenes* infections are *Pasteurella* sp., *Escherichia coli*, *Actinomyces* sp., and gram-negative anaerobes, especially *Spaerophorus necrophorous* and *Bacteroides melaninogenicus*. The sources from which *C. pyogenes* is often recovered in pure culture include aborted bovine and ovine fetuses and tissues affected by arthritis and mastitis.

Specimens

The location and nature of the lesion will usually determine the type of specimen collected. Apart from the usual aseptic precautions, refrigeration, and quick shipment, no other special handling is required. In the case of aborted fetuses, the liver and lung appear to be the organs with the greatest number of bacteria. The animal corynebacteria do not present a serious hazard to laboratory workers, but aseptic precautions should be taken with all specimens.[10]

Because of the mixed composition of the normal bacterial flora, it is not clear which characteristics of *C. pyogenes* lesions and exudates are due to the activities of this organism alone. References by researchers to a greenish-white pus of fetid odor and a consistency varying from thick and creamy to thin and fluid strongly suggest that a number of factors are involved. The fetid odor in particular is not consistent with any known metabolic properties or products of *C. pyogenes*, but it is characteristic of the anaerobic components of *C. pyogenes* processes.

The organism is demonstrable in tissue sections from aborted fetuses by means of the Gram-Weigert stain. Here it appears in colonies throughout the liver and spleen, unaccompanied by any pronounced cellular response beyond a mild lymphoreticular reaction.

Laboratory Procedures

Cultures. Routine procedures in the preparation of an inoculum are adequate to assure recovery of *C. pyogenes*. The primary isolation medium should contain some supplement such as serum, blood, ascitic fluid, milk, or tissue fragments. Blood agar is preferred by most people because it reveals the hemolytic activity of the organism in addition to furnishing the necessary nutrients. Specimens can also be inoculated into thioglycolate broth; growth will be satisfactory in this medium if the inoculum contains some tissue constituents. Sometimes gram-negative anaerobic organisms will grow in conjunction with *C. pyogenes*, but the latter can readily be purified by subculture on aerobic media. Like most parasitic facultative anaerobes, *C. pyogenes* will grow well in an atmosphere of 5–10% CO_2, although most strains can be propagated without difficulty in air. The incubation temperature should be near 37°C.

After an incubation period of 24 hours at 37°C on blood agar, minute colonies surrounded by a narrow zone of hemolysis will appear. With blood agar plates of medium thickness it may be difficult to decide whether this is true hemolysis or only the greening effect because the hemolytic action may not have penetrated the total depth of the medium. Careful examination of the colonies under low-power magnification may be necessary. The growth pattern of *C. pyogenes* will be quite reminiscent of that of streptococci, except that the hemolytic zone will be much more narrow relative to the colony size. On further incubation, the colonies and hemolytic zones will enlarge, but the colonies will remain translucent and their diameters remain smaller than 3 mm, especially in unmodified atmospheric conditions. Under 10% CO_2 we have seen colonies of 3 mm diameter on the surface of blood agar plates.

On plates inoculated with a nurse organism for the purpose of isolating *Haemophilus* sp., *C. pyogenes* has been observed growing in a satellite pattern. The substances responsible for inducing this satellitism could not be identified but appear to be related to a serum ingredient acted upon or liberated by the nurse organism. This satellitism was apparent only on media containing serum or serum protein but not on infusion agar or media containing washed RBC.

In broth, *C. pyogenes* causes uniform cloudiness and a granular deposit at the bottom. Again the growth is similar to that of streptococci.

Differential reactions. Properties of *C. pyogenes* that can be used in its identification include the fermentation of lactose, lack of catalase activity, and presence of proteolytic enzymes. In the first two respects its similarity to the streptococci is once more apparent. *C. pyogenes* is one of the very few corynebacteria that ferments lactose. A number of other sugars are fermented, among them maltose and sucrose. (Fermentation patterns are of secondary utility in differentiating corynebacteria, since the patterns often vary, and since few corynebacteria have a vigorous fermentative attack on the usual substrates.) In litmus milk the fermentation of lactose causes a shift toward acidity. This change is usually overshadowed, however, by the effects of proteolysis, which converts the milk into a serumlike fluid with a fine white deposit remaining at the bottom of the tube. Proteolysis can also be demonstrated by inoculation of coagulated serum slants (Loeffler's). A trough will form along the line of inoculation, while large amounts of fluid will accumulate at the bottom of the slant. Gelatin is also liquified.

Erythrocytes are promptly lysed either in agar or fluid media. The latter system is less equivocal, since on agar streak cultures the hemolytic zones often do not involve the entire depth of the medium even after 18–24 hours and therefore need to be differentiated carefully from the alpha (greening) effect. Liberation of hemoglobin in blood broth is an indisputable criterion of beta-hemolysis provided an uninoculated or sham-inoculated control tube remains unhemolysed under identical conditions of incubation.

Cellular morphology. *C. pyogenes* can usually be demonstrated without difficulty in Gram-stained smears of pus and tissue impressions. It appears as a small, almost cocobacillary gram-positive organism that sometimes forms chains. Its characterization as a displaced streptococcus applies not only to its biochemical traits but in some measure to its morphologic properties. Its maximum dimension is 2 μm in the bacillary forms. The gram-positive character is easily lost through aging and sometimes not readily apparent even on direct smear from tissue and exudates. Metachromatic granules, which can be found in most other corynebacteria, are virtually absent. The organism lacks capsules, flagella, and spores.

Animal inoculation. Animal inoculations have not been found useful in the isolation of *C. pyogenes,* although rabbits are susceptible to experimental pyemia, which follows a course similar to the analogous staphylococcal infection. A weak protein toxin, presumably identical with the hemolysin, and demonstrable by mouse inoculation, has been described. It develops satisfactorily in Todd-Hewitt broth.[9]

Immunology and serology. No immunologic or serologic diversity has been described.[7] No specific bacteriophages are known. An indirect FA procedure employing rabbit antiserum and antirabbit–gamma-globulin fluorescent conjugate has been described.[11]

Corynebacterium pseudotuberculosis

C. pseudotuberculosis (*C. ovis*) is associated with chronic purulent conditions, especially abscesses of sheep, horses, goats, and to a lesser degree cattle. The organism is restricted in the United States to the mid and far west, where it is quite common. Of the 262 corynebacterial isolates, 55 are *C. pseudotuberculosis*. There appears to be no special age predisposition. Cases of pseudotuberculosis in sheep and cattle occur throughout the year, but there is a clustering of ovine cases in the spring and early summer that is related to shearing, docking, and marking practices. Ventral abscesses, the most common form of the disease in horses in this country, occur almost entirely between July and January.

Specimens

Pus samples aseptically removed from unopened lesions are quite satisfactory without any special precautions. Organisms will remain viable for weeks and months in pus at average room temperatures. The organism is not inhibited by admixtures of other bacteria, such as *Staphylococcus,* which is often encountered in samples obtained from open lesions.

In ulcerative lymphangitis of horses, where the pus from a lesion is often not of sufficient quantity for aspiration, specimens may be collected on suitable swabs following surface cleansing of the lesion. In view of the widespread incidence of *C. pseudotuberculosis* and the scarcity of reports on human infections, it may be concluded that the organism is of low infectivity for humans.[7]

Diagnostic serology of *C. pseudotuberculosis* infections is not widely practiced, as the significance of antibodies to this organism and its products is not fully known. For such serology as has been reported from various investigations, serum obtained from clotted, unhemolysed blood appears to be satisfactory without special handling.

Exudates obtained from *C. pseudotuberculosis* infection tend to be white to off-white in color and pasty to cheesy in consistency, and they occasionally but not typically contain bloody admixtures. There is no suggestive odor as a rule, because *C. pseudo-*

tuberculosis produces no odoriforous substances nor is it usually found in the company of bacteria that do.

Laboratory Procedures

Cultures. The inoculum is usually pus, necrotic tissue, or exudate from an external lesion. It requires no special preparation. A rather rich medium is needed for prompt and abundant growth of this organism. Supplementation with serum or blood will render most of the common media satisfactory. Blood agar is preferred for isolation from reasonably uncontaminated material. For nasal swabs, fecal specimens, soil, or similar material, a selective medium like potassium tellurite agar is useful. On potassium tellurite agar the growth is a muddy black. The edges of the colony are irregular and the surface pitted.

C. pseudotuberculosis will grow best at 37°C. Ordinary atmospheric conditions are satisfactory. It requires about 36–48 hours for characteristic growth to appear on solid media. On blood agar, growth will appear in 18–24 hours as practically transparent colonies less than 1 mm in diameter. If the streak has a thick portion, a confluent area of growth of an opalescent gray to whitish hue may be discernible. With thin plates, a narrow zone of hemolysis may be evident there. Off-white colonies, 1–2 mm in diameter, with narrow hemolytic zones surrounding them, will be observable on the second day. The surface is comparable to ivory in color and other characteristics. The colonies can be easily pushed around the agar surface without breaking up or leaving trails. They are difficult to pick up, since they do not adhere well to a needle or loop. These characteristics are due to the hydrophobic quality imparted by the high lipid content of their cell walls and evidenced by the impossibility of working them into smooth aqueous suspensions. In broth cultures they typically form a pellicle and granular sediment, leaving the intervening column of liquid almost clear. Flaming a loop or needle charged with *C. pseudotuberculosis* results in sizzling and spattering.

Differential reactions. There is considerable variation among strains of *C. pseudotuberculosis* regarding the kind of carbohydrates they attack. Only glucose broth is unanimously reported as being acidified by all strains. The attack is fermentative and takes several days to produce maximum acidity, which even then is rather mild. Serum additions to the usual carbohydrate broths enhance and accelerate growth.

Urea is hydrolyzed slowly by about 50% of the cultures. The most interesting biochemical test concerns the reduction of nitrates, since this reaction permits a division of the species into two groups based on ecological patterns: cultures recovered from sheep are uniformly negative, while isolates from horses are equally consistent in their reduction of nitrates. Both patterns have been observed in cattle strains.

C. pseudotuberculosis is hemolytic both on blood agar and in blood broth. The hemolytic zone on the former is quite narrow. In broth the liberation of hemoglobin into the supernatant fluid may be slow, requiring several days. The hemolytic capacity may be substantially potentiated by cross-streaking the blood agar culture with the ordinarily nonhemolytic *C. equi*.[5] Where the two organisms intermingle, a very wide zone of clear hemolysis results. Another type of interaction occurs between *C. pseudotuberculosis* and the "hot-cold" hemolysins of *Staphylococcus aureus* and *Clostridium perfringens*. The manifestation of these is suppressed by *C. pseudotuberculosis*.

Cellular morphology. *C. pseudotuberculosis* is probably the most typical of the animal diphtheroids. It shows the characteristic palisading, Chinese letter patterns, and has clubbed, granular, and segmented forms. Young cultures are unequivocally gram-positive and nonacid-fast. Capsules, flagella, and spores are absent, but metachromatic granules are readily demonstrable. Neisser's stain is used for this purpose.

Animal inoculation. For purposes of isolation, neither animal inoculation nor a particularly sensitive method is necessary.

Immunology and serology. No identification method using serologic means is available at present for *C. pseudotuberculosis*. A promising immunologic approach has been described, wherein the dorsal skin of a rabbit is injected ID with mixtures of toxin and serum.[4] Either known toxin with unknown serum or suspected toxin with known antitoxin may be used. In either case, when the homologous pairs are injected, no reaction results. If toxin with heterologous serum is used, a dermal response, consisting mostly of swelling and erythema, takes place.[4] For identification of a strain, the dermal toxicity of the culture supernatant fluid must be demonstrated as well as its neutralization by specific antiserum.

An agglutination test suitable for field diagnostic purposes has been described.[1] Its success hinges on the use of a selected bacterial culture, which, in contrast to the almost universal suspension instability of *C. pseudotuberculosis,* forms a fairly stable suspension, especially in a 5% NaCl solution containing 10–20% normal rabbit serum. No data are available on phage that are specific for *C. pseudotuberculosis*.

C. pseudotuberculosis is naturally pathogenic for sheep, goats, horses, and cattle. One human infection has been reported.[7] Experimentally, rabbits and guinea pigs also are susceptible. In the latter, a purulent infection of the vaginal tunics of the testes can be produced with carefully gauged doses administered IP. With large doses, early death is apt to result due to the action of the exotoxin. The manifestations of the exotoxin include rapid death (in about 24 hours) of guinea pigs, dermal necrosis in many animal species, and in vitro lysis of erythrocytes, particularly when potentiated by *C. equi*. It is assumed that all these manifestations are due to one toxin.[10] Toxic activity is also ascribed to constituents found in crude extracts of surface lipids and to certain intracellular proteins.[2,6] Various methods of producing toxic filtrates have been described. Time of incubation will vary with media, but maximum toxin yield should be gauged to coincide with the lowest pH value attained by the medium in the course of incubation. This value appears to be constant for any one kind of medium. Brain-heart infusion and trypticase soy broths give good yields.[3]

Corynebacterium renale

C. renale is primarily a parasite of the urinary and lower genital tract of ruminants. The diseases with which it is mainly associated are cystitis, ureteritis, and pyelonephritis of cattle and less frequently of sheep. It has also been encountered in dogs, and it has been recovered on rare occasions from nongenitourinary pyogenic processes. The clinical urinary infection preferentially affects mature females around the time of parturition. The organism and the disease it causes are found in both Europe and the Americas. Differences in incidence may be linked to variations in husbandry methods rather than to the frequency of the organism in a given population. Thus, stabled and stanchioned dairy cows appear to be more frequently affected than beef cattle on pasture and range.

Specimens

The usual specimen suspected of containing *C. renale* is urine from a case of cystitis or pyelonephritis. Ideally, and especially in cases showing uncertain clinical manifestations, collection should be made aseptically. In obvious cases the abundance of *C. renale* will make slight contamination a less critical matter. In any case the vulva should be thoroughly cleansed and disinfected and the sample collected in two vials, one to catch the first stream, the second to catch the remainder. If a second portion is collected, the first can be discarded or used purely for noncultural work-up.

Even though unnecessary delay should be avoided, the organism is rather resistant and will survive for a reasonable time in transit. Should quantitative cultures be desired, however, refrigeration and prompt forwarding are mandatory, in order to prevent multiplication of *C. renale* or contaminants in the urine.

The most characteristic feature of urine collected from active cases of pyelonephritis-cystitis is the admixture of unclotted and clotted blood. Usually, intact RBC are found, rather than hemoglobin. A confirmative characteristic is the extremely high pH of the specimens. Ammonia odor, especially if noted in freshly collected samples, adds further circumstantial evidence. Protein levels may vary from ++ to ++++ depending on the degree of renal involvement. A wet mount of sediment will reveal—in addition to bladder epithelium, fibrin shreds, and blood cells—clumps of rod-shaped bacteria.

Laboratory Procedures

Cultures. Usually the clinical picture is sufficiently suggestive that a qualitative culture is all that is required. Also, the clumping habit of the organism renders quantitative culturing more difficult. For qualitative culture, urine is centrifuged at moderate speed for 10 minutes and the sediment streaked on blood agar. For a quick presumptive test, sediment may be planted directly onto a Christensen's urea slant and incubated either at room temperature or 37°C. The pre-formed urease present in the inoculum, provided *C. renale* is the organism involved, will start a shift toward alkaline within 5–60 minutes. *C. renale* will grow on most of the ordinary media, but blood agar is preferred for isolation. Aerobic incubation at 37°C is satisfactory. Although growth under these conditions will be recognizable in 24 hours, its diagnostic features do not become apparent for 36–48 hours. In 18–24 hours the colonies are gray and opaque and about 0.5 mm or less in diameter. As they enlarge to about 1.5 mm, they become yellow-white or gray-white with a dullish surface.

Differential reactions. The most useful differential reaction is extremely rapid urea hydrolysis. Although many other cornyebacteria attack urea, none do so with comparable alacrity. Apart from producing acid (without gas) in glucose broth, the species has no uniform pattern of carbohydrate fermentation. There is neither hemolysis nor proteolysis comparable to that of *C. pyogenes*. A presumably caseinolytic phenomenon, demonstrable in 10% skim milk agar, has been described.[8] In litmus milk, a shift toward the more alkaline occurs, accompanied by deposition of a precipitate and corresponding clearing of the supernatant fluid.

Cellular morphology. This organism is the largest and most bacilliform of the diphtheroid bacteria under consideration, attaining a width of up to 0.7 μm and a length of up to 3 μm. Tapering of the cells toward one end is seen; the tendency to clump, especially in exudates, has already been mentioned. Cells are gram-positive, noncapsulated, nonsporeforming, nonmotile, and nonacid-fast. Metachromatic material is present but not as prominently as in *C. pseudotuberculosis*.

Animal inoculation. A series of experiments have shown the susceptibility of mice and rabbits to IV infection with *C. renale*.[8] Localization takes place in the urinary tract and is ascribed to the organism's ureatropism. No toxins have been found in association with *C. renale*.

Immunology and serology. There are no immunologic or serologic procedures of recognized use. No bacteriophages specific for *C. renale* are known.

Corynebacterium equi

C. equi is a parasite of horses and swine. It is found in many parts of the world and manifests its pathogenic activity mainly as the agent associated with purulent necrotic pneumonia of foals up to about 4 months of age. Systemic involvement is common. Genital infections of mares are also seen, and occasionally adult horses develop the pneumonic condition.[12] In swine it is reported as a frequent inhabitant of the cervical lymph nodes, possibly as a harmless commensal. Although it appears to be able to maintain itself in this environment for long periods of time, it is probably not a true saprophyte but has as its reservoir the mucous membranes of animals.

Specimens

The usual specimens are lesions from the lung or other organs at the time of autopsy, or exudates from the respiratory or genital tracts. No special handling of such samples is necessary in collection and transmittal. Serologic testing of affected or suspected animals is not applicable. The material from the lung lesions is apt to be yellowish-gray and caseopurulent. A Gram stain will reveal pleomorphic gram-positive rods of variable size. Other organisms such as streptococci and actinobacilli are frequently present in the lesions and are sometimes difficult to differentiate morphologically from *C. equi*.

Laboratory Procedures

Cultures. The only special preparation of inocula applicable to *C. equi* is the treatment of contaminated specimens with oxalic acid, to which *C. equi* is reportedly very resistant. Ground-up tissue is suspended in 2.5% oxalic acid, and incubated for up to 20 minutes, and then inoculated into media.

Any of the usual bacteriological media are acceptable for culturing *C. equi,* and growth will occur readily under atmospheric conditions at wide temperature ranges. Large wet colonies develop promptly. They often tend to be elongated in the direction of the streak, and their early appearance is reminiscent of drops of skim milk. Later the pigmentation intensifies and a pink color emerges within a few days. In broth, turbidity is produced throughout.

Differential reactions. *C. equi* appears to be quite inert on the customary differential media. No acid is produced from any carbohydrates. No hemolysis or proteolysis is demonstrable. The only properties readily shown are catalase activity and slow hydrolysis of urea.

Cellular morphology. *C. equi* is gram-positive and pleomorphic. From gross colony characteristics, serologic data, and the appearance of smears, the presence of a capsular or slime layer is strongly implied. However, the morphologic demonstration of such a structure has not been reported. The organism may be partially acid fast. No spores or flagella are present.

Animal inoculation. Injection of suspensions of *C. equi* into tissues usually results in local lesions only, although fatal injections can be made in guinea pigs and mice by the IP route. Exposure IT has been reported to kill mice and produce pneumonia in swine.[14] No toxins of *C. equi* are known.

Immunology and serology. A number of serotypes, determined apparently by surface antigens, exist within the species. Thus isolates from swine are serologically distinct from those of horses, and a number or serotypes of equine derivation have been described. Acid extraction of cells removes type specificity and reveals species specificity.

References

1. Awad, F.I. Serologic investigations of pseudotuberculosis in sheep. I. Agglutination Test. *Am. J. Vet. Res.* 21:251–253, 1960.
2. Cameron, C.M., and L. Buchan. Identification of the protective and toxic antigens of *Corynebacterium pseudotuberculosis*. *Onderstepoort J. Vet. Res.* 33:39–48, 1966.
3. Cobb, R.W., and J.K. Walley. *Corynebacterium bovis* as a probable cause of bovine mastitis. *Vet. Rec.* 74:101–102, 1962.
4. Doty, R.B., H.W. Dunne, J.F. Hokanson, and J.J. Reid. A comparison of toxins produced by various isolates of *Corynebacterium pseudotuberculosis* and the development of a diagnostic skin test for caseous lymphadenitis of sheep and goats. *Am. J. Vet. Res.* 25:1679–1685, 1964.
5. Fraser, G. The effect on animal erythrocytes of combinations of diffusible substances produced by bacteria. *J. Path. Bact.* 88:43–53, 1964.
6. Jolly, R.D. Some observations on surface lipids of virulent and attenuated strains of *Corynebacterium ovis*. *J. Appl. Bact.* 29:189–196, 1966.
7. Lopez, J.F., F.M. Wong, and J. Quesada. *Corynebacterium pseudotuberculosis:* First case of human infection. *Am. J. Clin. Path.* 46:562–567, 1966.
8. Lovell, R. Studies on *Corynebacterium renale*. I. A systematic study of a number of strains. *J. Comp. Path. Ther.* 56:196–204, 1946.
9. Matthews, P.R.J., and J.B. Derbyshire. Observations of the mouse lethal power and serology of Corynebacterium pyogenes. *Res. Vet. Sci.* 4:531–536, 1963.
10. Purdom, M.R., A. Seaman, and M. Woodbine. The bacteriology and antibiotic sensitivity of *Corynebacterium pyogenes*. *Vet. Rev. Annotations* 4:55–91, 1958.
11. Roberts, R.J. Immunofluorescence as an aid to diagnosis of Corynebacterium pyogenes infection. *Vet. Rec.* 79:346–347, 1966.
12. Simpson, R.M. *Corynebacterium equi* in adult horses in Kenya. *Bull. Epiz. Dis. Afr.* 12:303–306, 1966.
13. Soltys, M.A. *Corynebacterium suis* associated with a specific cystitis and pyelonephritis in pigs. *J. Path. Bact.* 81:441–446, 1961.
14. Thal, E., and L. Rutquist. The pathogenicity of *Corynebacterium equi* for pigs and small laboratory animals. *Nord. Vet. Med.* 11:298–304, 1959.

49. Actinomyces

Actinomycosis is a subacute or chronic disease caused by organisms of the genus *Actinomyces*. In humans most cases are associated with *A. israelii* while in cattle and swine *A. bovis* is usually found. The disease has the same basic features in all host species. Recognition of the widespread presence of actinomycosis in dogs is relatively recent; a substantial proportion of purulent conditions involving the body cavities of dogs are associated with *Actinomyces* sp. *A. viscosus* has been identified in several of these. Occurrence of actinomycosis in other animal species is not well documented. The histologic lesions on which some reports are based are not etiologically specific. Only specific cultural identification of the agents permits a diagnosis of actinomycosis, since other microorganisms, including nocardias, actinobacilli, staphylococci, and corynebacteria, are capable of causing indistinguishable lesions.

The *Actinomyces* organisms are microaerophilic pathogens. Actinomycosis is not a transmissible disease in the usual sense of the term. The usual source of infection is considered to be endogenous. Devitalization of tissues through injury or through intercurrent infection with other bacteria is thought to be a precursor to the development of actinomycosis. However, clinical specimens should be handled with the same reasonable care as used with other potentially infectious materials.

The best-known, though not the most frequent, form of actinomycosis in animals is lumpy jaw of cattle caused by *A. bovis*. In this form of the disease, the organism invades and erodes the bony part of the jaw or face, producing a honeycomb of sinuses that eventually form sinus tracts and discharge into the exterior. The organisms may be present on the normal oropharyngeal mucosa and may gain access to the bone via the alveoli or the teeth. The organisms grow in the soft tissues as well, where they form abscesses and granulomas that are generally outwardly identical with lesions in true lumpy jaw. *A. bovis* is found in many purulent processes often in association with other bacterial forms.

Actinomycosis in swine is commonly localized in the mammary gland. Trauma due to the action of the teeth of suckling pigs is thought to provide both the tissue insult and the inoculum necessary for establishing the infection.

A. viscosus has been isolated from cases of canine pleuritis as well as from swine, goats, and hamsters. The source of infection is presumed to have been endogenous. This organism has also been identified in the oral cavities of humans.

Specimens

It is preferable to obtain specimens aseptically from closed abscesses and pleural exudates by aspiration, or from surgically opened or excised lesions. However, pus or exudate from open draining sinuses and tracheobronchial washings can be collected directly in sterile containers or by washing or curetting the walls of sunus tracts. Often, if free-flowing pus with granules is not seen, a gauze pad over the sinus opening will trap pus and granules exuded over a period of time.

Laboratory Procedures

The first laboratory procedure is to search for granules for direct examination and for culturing. Although the formation of granules is characteristic of actinomycosis, they are not always present. Granules are hard, white to yellowish grains that range from barely visible to 5 mm in diameter. When grossly visible, they can be removed from the specimen material with a capillary pipette; when not visible, the specimen can be placed in a sealable flask, diluted with sterile saline, and shaken vigorously to free the granules and permit them to settle to the bottom of the flask where they can be retrieved.

Samples of the granules are placed on a slide with a drop of water or 10% KOH and pressed out gently with a coverslip. Examine under low power for an irregular "clubbed" surface, and under oil immersion for the presence of a mass of delicate filaments in the interior of the granule. The filaments extend into the clubs, but clubs are not always present. If granules were not found, make smears from pus, sputum, or centrifuged sediments from pleural or other body fluids. Stain separate smears of pus or crushed granules with the Gram and acid-fast stains (use Kinyoun's modified acid-fast stain). Examine the slides under oil immersion for gram-positive, nonacid-fast branched filaments, or for pleomorphic, occasionally branched forms of bacillar size.

For a histopathologic demonstration of actinomycosis, use the Brown and Brenn modified Gram stain, and use the Fite-Faraco modified acid-fast stain developed for *Nocardia*. Look for filamentous, branched organisms in the interior of granules, with staining reactions as previously mentioned. With H & E and other common histologic stains, the organism within the granules will not stain, and the granules cannot be distinguished from those caused by other organisms.

Cultures. The ideal inoculum for cultures is prepared from granules that have been washed in sterile saline and crushed. Pleural or other body fluids should be centrifuged and the sediment used for inoculum. Direct inoculation of pus or exudates may be successful if previous examination showed the presence of gram-positive filamentous organisms.

All *Actinomyces* species are microaerophilic to anaerobic, and for primary isolation good anaerobic conditions are needed. The organisms require media rich in nutrients, a pH between 6.8 and 7.2, and incubation at 37°C. The presence of CO_2 greatly stimulates their growth. For a liquid medium, it is preferable to use an enriched, freshly boiled thioglycollate broth. For a solid medium, freshly prepared plates of brain-heart infusion agar are recommended. Tubed media (except thioglycollate) must be under anaerobic seal: pyrogallol and Na_2CO_3. Plate cultures should be incubated in anaerobe jars. Jars without a catalyst (Thomas or Cawe) can be used with a mixture of 95% N_2 and 5% CO_2. Jars with a catalyst can be used with a mixture of 80% N_2, 10% H_2, and 10% CO_2 as follows: a Brewer jar, electrically heated 10 minutes to reactivate catalyst, or a Torbal jar with 37°C catalyst; a Gaspak anaerobe jar (Baltimore Biological Lab. [BBL] 06-200) with disposable H_2-CO_2 generator envelopes (BBL 06-112) can be used also.

In *Actinomyces,* rough (R) and smooth (S) colonies reflect the degree of filamentation. Although all the species can vary from one isolate to another or from one subculture to another, each species has a degree of R or S that is characteristic. *A. bovis* is usually diptheroidal and forms S colonies. Thioglycollate broth cultures have a soft diffuse growth. In 24–48 hours, tiny, smooth, convex, entire, shining "dew drop" colonies are formed. Under the 10× objective of the microscope, the colonies are flat and granular with a granular or denticulate edge. Colonies on agar 7–10 days old are convex, smooth, entire, and soft. Occasionally *A. bovis* is isolated in a rough form and resembles *A. israelii.*

A. israelli is usually very filamentous and produces R colonies. In thioglycollate broth, granular or bread crumb colonies are seen in clear medium. Colonies on agar 24–48 hours old are difficult to see without magnification. With the 10× objective, delicate, branched, filamentous (spider) colonies are visible. Colonies 7–10 days old are heaped and lobulated (molar tooth type) and are formed and embedded in the agar. Sometimes *A. israelii* has a smooth form resembling *A. bovis. A. viscosus* forms filamentous colonies with dense centers after 24–48 hours and these mature into smooth, convex colonies although some strains may have granular colonies. In general, colonies of *Corynebacterium acnes* and *C. pyogenes* are morphologically similar to the S forms of *Actinomyces.*

Differential reactions. Catalase production is the most useful test for separating *Actinomyces* (except *A. viscosus*) from *C. acnes* and other catalase-positive bacteria. To test for catalase, in a drop of 3% H_2O_2 make a slide mount from a culture and add a coverslip; or preferably, pour 3% H_2O_2 over growth on a slant and watch for a stream of small bubbles, which indicates a positive reaction.

Other useful biochemical tests include gelatin liquefaction, reaction in litmus milk, starch hydrolysis, nitrate reduction, sugar fermentation, and determination of O_2 requirements. To assess O_2 requirements, six cotton-stoppered BHI agar slants are inoculated with the same amount of a well-mixed inoculum and incubated at 37°C; two are done anaerobically, two microaerophilically, and two aerobically. Growth is quantitated (0 to ++++) in each tube after 3 and 10 days. The important differences between *A. bovis, A. israelii, A. viscosus, C. acnes,* and *C. pyogenes* are given in Tables 49.1 and 49.2.

Cellular morphology. The *Actinomyces* granules are made up of microcolonies of branching filaments, which terminate at the periphery in characteristic club-shaped endings that are enveloped in precipitate (Gram + filament, Gram − precipitate). The threadlike filaments measure about 0.4–0.5 μm in thickness.

Animal inoculation. Mice or hamsters may be used to demonstrate the pathogenicity

Table 49.1. Biochemical characteristics of *Actinomyces* and *Corynebacterium* species in animal materials

Biochemical tests	*Actinomyces bovis* (S form)	*Actinomyces bovis* (R form)	*Actinomyces israelii* (R form)	*Actinomyces viscosus*	*Corynebacterium pyogenes*	*Corynebacterium acnes*
Catalase	0	0	0	+	0	+
Litmus milk	No change or acid	No change or acid	No change or acid	Acid clot	Clot plus digestion (rapid)	Acid plus clot (slow)
Gelatin liquefaction	0	0	Usually 0	0	+ (rapid)	+ (slow)
Nitrate reduction	Usually 0	0	Usually 0	+	0	Variable
Starch hydrolysis	+	0	Usually 0	0	Variable	0
Acid produced*						
Glucose	+	+	+	+	+	+
Arabinose	Variable	0	+	0	0	0
Glycerol	Variable	0	0	+	Variable	+
Lactose	+	0	+	+	+	0
Maltose	Variable	+	+	+	+	0
Mannitol	Variable	0	+	0	0	Usually 0
Salicin	Variable	0	+	+	+	0
Starch	+	0	0	+	+	0
Sucrose	+	+	+	+	+	0
Xylose	Variable	+	+	−	+	0

*Final readings at 7 days.

Table 49.2. Cultural characteristics of *Actinomyces* and *Corynebacterium* species in animal materials

Growth characteristics	*Actinomyces bovis* (S form, common cause of actinomycosis)	*Actinomyces bovis* (R form, rare cause of actinomycosis)	*Actinomyces israelii* (R form, rare cause of actinomycosis)	*Actinomyces viscosus* (occasional cause of actinomycosis)	*Corynebacterium pyogenes* (common cause of suppurative lesions)	*Corynebacterium acnes* (common skin saprophyte)
Oxygen requirements	Microaerophilic to anaerobic	Microaerophilic to anaerobic	Microaerophilic to anaerobic	Aerobic to microaerophilic	Facultative	Anaerobic
Growth in thioglycollate broth	Soft, diffuse	Rough, lobulated or granular, broth clear	Rough, lobulated or granular, broth clear	Viscous	Soft, diffuse	Soft, diffuse
Microscopic morphology in thioglycollate broth	Diptheroidal X and Y forms, occ. branching	Long, branched filaments	Long, branched filaments	Short, irregularly branched filaments	Diphtheroidal X and Y forms, occ. branching	Diphtheroidal X and Y forms, occ. branching
24–48-hr colony (BHI plate)	Flat, granular, entire	Spider colony	Spider colony	Dense center, filamentous fringe	Flat, granular, entire	Flat, granular, entire
7-day colony (BHI plate)	Convex, smooth	Molar tooth	Molar tooth	Convex, smooth, sometimes pits	Convex, smooth	Convex, smooth
Blood agar plate (BHI agar plus rabbit blood)	No change	No change	No change	No change	No change	Slight beta-hemolysis

of the organisms, but animal inoculation is not routinely used as an aid in the identification of *Actinomyces*.

Immunology and serology. Antigenic differences between *Actinomyces* species have been demonstrated. Both gel diffusion precipitin and FA tests are currently used experimentally as an aid in species identification. There is no routine test for the detection of antibodies in a patient's serum.

References

1. Ajello, L., L.K. Georg, W. Kaplan, and L. Kaufman. *Laboratory Manual for Medical Mycology*. 2d ed. HEW, Atlanta, 1962.
2. Blank, C., and L.K. Georg. The use of fluorescent antibody methods for the detection and identification of Actinomyces species in clinical material. *J. Lab. Clin. Med.* 7:283–293, 1968.
3. Buchanan, R.E., and N.E. Gibbons (eds.). *Bergey's Manual of Determinative Bacteriology*. 8th ed. Williams and Wilkins, Baltimore, 1974.
4. Emmons, C.W., C.H. Binford, and J.P. Utz. *Medical Mycology*. 2d ed. Lea and Febiger, Philadelphia, 1970.
5. Georg, L.K. Diagnostic procedures for the isolation and identification of the etiologic agents of Actinomycosis. *Proc. Internat. Symp. Mycoses,* Pan Am. Health Organ., Sci. Pub. no. 205, pp. 71–81, 1970.
6. Geog, L.K., J.M. Brown, H.J. Baker, and G.H. Cassell. *Actinomyces viscosus* as an agent of actinomycosis in the dog. *Am. J. Vet. Res.* 33:1457–1470, 1972.
7. Georg, L.K., and R.M. Coleman. Comparative pathogenicity of various Actinomyces species. In *The Actinomycetales,* H. Prauser (ed.), pp. 35–45. Internat. Symp. Taxon., Jena, 1968.
8. LeChevalier, H.A., and M.P. LeChevalier. A critical evaluation of the genera of aerobic actinomycetes. In *The Actinomycetales,* H. Prauser (ed.), pp. 393–405. Internat. Symp. Taxon., Jena, 1968.
9. Pier, A.C. The actinomycetes. In *Diseases of Animals Transmitted from Animals to Man,* W. Hubbert, W. McCulloch, and P. Schnurrenberger (eds.), pp. 361–368. Thomas, Springfield, Ill., 1975.
10. Prauser, H. Characters and genera arrangement in the Actinomycetales. In *The Actinomycetales,* H. Prauser (ed.), pp. 407–418. Internat. Symp. Taxon., Jena, 1968.
11. Slack, J., and M.A. Gerencser. Revision of serological groupings of *Actinomyces*. *J. Bact.* 91:2107, 1966.
12. Waksman, S.A. *The Actinomycetes*. Williams and Wilkins, Baltimore, 1959.

50. Dermatophilus

Dermatophilus congolensis, an actinomycete, is the etiologic agent of an exudative dermatitis of several animal species and of humans. The disease, dermatophilosis (cutaneous streptothricosis), is worldwide in distribution.[1,2] In the United States, isolations have been reported from horses, cattle, sheep, deer, a rabbit, and a ground squirrel [8,9] *D. congolensis* has been found only in clinical lesions. Experimental transmission by stable and house flies has been accomplished and ticks have also been implicated in the spread of the disease.[5] Trauma and prolonged wetting by rain appear to be predisposing factors.[6]

Clinical lesions in horses and cattle appear initially as an exudative dermatitis with subsequent formation of scabs and crusts. These may appear as projections from the body surface or may be small and detectable only by palpation. In wet climates the lesions may coalesce and involve extensive areas of the body surface. In sheep, the wool becomes matted from exudation; this condition is called lumpy wool. Another syndrome in sheep caused by *D. congolensis* is known as strawberry footrot; in this condition lesions extend from the coronet to the knee with ensuing encrustation of the affected area.[7]

Although animals sometimes die from complications, they usually recover, often spontaneously, from dermatophilosis. Dry conditions and treatment with dihydrostreptomycin aid in clearing the infection. Laboratory workers should be aware of the infectiousness of *Dermatophilus* for human skin.

Specimens

Exudative crusts can be readily removed, but a pair of forceps should be used to avoid human infection by direct contact. Collected specimens can be placed in a dry container for transport to the laboratory.

Direct microscopic examination for *Dermatophilus congolensis* can be made by placing a small portion of exudative crust in a drop of water on a clean glass slide and then emulsifying the exudate with a small glass rod. After the suspension is air dried, the smear is stained with Giemsa stain and examined microscopically under oil ($\times 950$). Morphologic features of *Dermatophilus* in tissue exudate are depicted in Figure 50.1. Smears obtained in this manner may also be used for FA staining.[3]

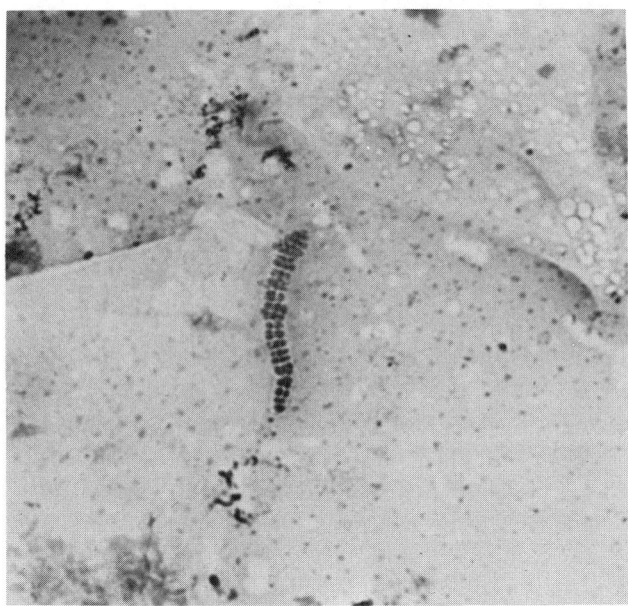

Figure 50.1. *Dermatophilus congolensis* in exudate. Giemsa stain. ×950. (From *Veterinary Bacteriology and Virology*, I.A. Merchant and R.A. Packer (eds.), 7th ed., Iowa State University Press, Ames, 1967.)

Laboratory Procedures

Cultures. For culture, approximately 0.06 g of exudative crust can be ground in a Ten Broeck tissue grinder with 5 ml of sterile 0.15 M PBS solution (pH 7.4). Allow the tissue suspension to stand at room temperature for 1 hour. The supernatant fluid containing motile phase cells can then be withdrawn from the sediment with a syringe, passed through a Millipore Swinney adapter filter (1.2 μm pore size) directly onto the surface of the BHI blood agar medium. Three drops of filtrate is sufficient inoculum. Streak for isolation and incubate at 37°C. Typical colonies of *D. congolensis* will usually appear in 24–48 hours, although plates should be retained for 7 days before discarding.

Dermatophilus congolensis forms tiny (0.5–1 mm) round or irregular colonies on BHI blood agar after 24 hours at 37°C. They are grayish in color, with a granular texture; they are adherent and sunken into the medium and often exhibit beta-hemolysis. The colonies become yellowish or an orange-tan color. Colonies of some fresh isolates become apically mucoid in approximately 72 hours. In 10% serum broth a flocculent growth is obtained in 24 hours at 37°C.

Differential reactions. *D. congolensis* is an aerobe that has the staining and biochemical reactions shown in Table 50.1. Isolates of *D. congolensis* can be maintained in the laboratory in 10% serum broth culture and transferred monthly. Isolates have remained viable for at least 2 years following lyophilization in either skim milk or bovine serum.

Cellular morphology. Microscopic examination of Giemsa-stained smears from colonies 24–48 hours old reveals branched septate hyphae approximately 0.5–1.5 μm in diameter. Subsequently, the filaments increase in diameter (3.5–5 μm), and transverse and longitudinal divisions appear. The hyphae that result are 8–10 cells in width. From each cell a flagellated coccoid zoospore (0.9–1.1 μm) is formed and subsequently released.

Table 50.1. Staining and biochemical reactions of *Dermatophilus congolensis*

Test technique	Reactions
Gram stain	+
Acid-fast stain (Kinyoun)	−
Catalase (H_2O_2)	+
Urease (urea agar)	+
Amylase (Starch agar)	+
Casein hydrolysis (skim milk agar)	+
Liquefaction	
Loeffler's coagulated serum	+ (rarely −)
Gelatin	+ (rarely −)
Peptonization of milk	+
Acid production:	
Glucose	+
Lactose	−
Maltose	+
Sucrose	−
Xylose	−
Fructose	+
Galactose	+ (or variable)

Animal inoculation. Infections can be established in rabbits by clipping the hair from a 13 sq cm area on the back, and, after light scarification, applying 0.3 ml of a suspension of ground exudative crust or 0.3 ml of a 3-day-old 10% serum broth culture.

Immunology and serology. Circulating antibodies can be demonstrated in experimentally and naturally infected cattle by agglutination, AD, and indirect HA techniques.[4] These techniques can be used in the diagnosis of dermatophilosis in addition to cultural and microscopic methods.

Reference laboratory. NADC.

References

1. Ainsworth, G.C., and P.K.C. Austwick. *Fungal Diseases of Animals.* Commonwealth Agricultural Bureau, Farnham Royal, Bucks., Eng., 1959.
2. Gordon, M.A. The genus *Dermatophilus. J. Bact.* 88:509–522, 1964.
3. Pier, A.C., J.L. Richard, and E.F. Farrell. Fluorescent antibody and cultural techniques in cutaneous streptothricosis. *Am. J. Vet. Res.* 25:1014–1020, 1964.
4. Pulliam, J.D., D.C. Kelley, and E.H. Coles. Immunologic studies of natural and experimental cutaneous streptothricosis infections in cattle. *Am. J. Vet. Res.* 28:445–455, 1967.
5. Richard, J.L., and A.C. Pier. Transmission of *Dermatophilus congolensis* by *Stomoxys calcitrans* and *Musca domestic. Am. J. Vet. Res.* 27:419–423, 1966.
6. Roberts, D.S. The life cycle of *Dermatophilus dermatonomus,* the causal agent of ovine mycotic dermatitis. *Austral. J. Exp. Biol. Med.* 39:463–476, 1961.
7. Roberts, D.S. Dermatophilus infection. *Vet. Bull.* 37:513–521, 1967.
8. Schotts, E.B., and T. Kistner. Naturally occurring cutaneous streptothricosis in a cottontail rabbit. *J. Am. Vet. Med. Ass.* 157:667–670, 1970.
9. Wobester, G., and M.A. Gordon. Dermatophilus infection in Columbian ground squirrels. *Bull. Wildlife Dis. Ass.* 5:31–32, 1969.

51. Nocardia

Nocardia are free-living, soil-dwelling bacteria that are capable of acting as primary pathogens or as opportunists in injured or debilitated tissue.[3] The genus *Nocardia* lies at the interface between the funguslike genus *Streptomyces* and the more typically bacterial genus *Mycobacterium*. The classification of a number of these organisms is debatable; whether the *Streptomyces*-like nocardias should be included in *Streptomyces* and whether certain other species should be considered mycobacteria are matters awaiting definitive taxonomic judgments. For the major portion of this section the description of the genus *Nocardia* will be that of the type species, *Nocardia asteroides;* sufficient information will be given to permit identification of two other species of veterinary interest, *N. brasiliensis* and *N. caviae*. Features helpful in generally differentiating these *Nocardia* species from *Actinomyces,* mycobacteria, and *Streptomyces* will be indicated also.[1,2,6]

Nocardiosis is a relatively common infectious disease of animals and of humans. Infection has been recognized in many animal species including domestic mammals, cetaceans, and fish. Prominent among the recognized infections of domestic animals are those in cattle and dogs. Cattle acquire nocardial infections of the mammary gland, respiratory tract, and subcutaneous lymph vessels and nodes. Mammary infection often follows unsanitary teat infusion procedures and results in an acute to chronic mastitis typified by extensive fibrosis, sinus tract formation, and lymphatic or hematogenous dissemination to other organ systems.

Respiratory infection in cattle is usually restricted to foci in the bronchial nodes, although pulmonary dissemination may occur; the infection presumably is the result of inhaling *Nocardia*-laden dust. The subcutaneous form of nocardiosis in cattle forms granulomatous abscesses and ulcers along the peripheral lymphatics and clinically resembles farcy. While this form may result from extension of internal foci, infection through cutaneous wounds of the extremities appears more likely. Canine nocardiosis most frequently occurs as a chronic pulmonary disease. Nocardial mycetomas, proliferative lesions with draining sinus tracts, occasionally develop on the extremities of dogs. Canine pulmonary nocardiosis is typically a disease of young dogs, often involving those with intercurrent distemper infection. Considerable serosanguineous to purulent fluid accumulates in the thoracic cavity; the fluid contains numerous discrete, soft, white, 1–3 mm rice grain–like microcolonies in the sediment. A marked proliferative pleuritis usually is a part of this condition. An indistinguishable syndrome is formed in infections associated with *Actinomyces* sp.

Nocardial mycetomas usually develop on the extremities. Dogs of any age can be involved, and the condition results from local infection through penetrating wounds. The mycetoma develops as a swelling. Sinus tracts form and small (1–3 mm) white, hard, mineralized granules or soft microcolonies appear in the exudate; dissemination to underlying bone or internal organs may occur.

The reaction of tissues to nocardial infection embodies both erosive and proliferative responses. Suppuration, granulomatous reaction, extensive fibrosis, and sinus tract formation are all features of nocardiosis at various stages. Since *Nocardia* is a respiratory pathogen of humans, it should be handled with the usual precautions under a properly ventilated safety hood.

Specimens

Aseptically collected mammary or thoracic exudates, aspirates from closed subcutaneous lesions, and surgical biopsy specimens are ideally suited for cultural and microscopic examinations. Exudates from draining sinus tracts or bronchial aspirates, though contaminated, can be used also. Abscess cavities or sinus tracts should be curetted lightly as higher populations of *Nocardia* are often evident at the periphery of suppurating lesions.

Examine the exudates for granules or microcolonies. If the sample is contaminated, these granules or microcolonies can be removed, rinsed several times in sterile saline, and then emulsified and streaked for isolation. Granules and microcolonies are good sources of the organism, but they are not evident in all exudates or tissue specimens.

Direct examination of specimens is best accomplished by staining air-dried smears by Gram's method and by Kinyoun's acid-fast stain. *Nocardia* in tissue sections are readily demonstrated by the Gram-Weigert technique.

Laboratory Procedures

Cultures. N. asteroides, the type species, grows well on routine bacteriological media including BHI blood agar, tryptose blood agar, Sabouraud's dextrose agar, and potato dextrose agar. Media containing antibiotics should not be used. Good growth is obtained with aerobic incubation at either 25 or 37°C. Colonies 1–2 mm in diameter, grayish white to orange, rough, raised, and adherent to the medium form on BHI (containing 5% bovine blood) after 48–72 hours incubation at 37°C. The colonies become heaped and warty with age; the basal portion develops an orange-tan color that is overlain with varying amounts of powdery white aerial hyphae in some isolates. Some strains produce so few aerial hyphae that the orange color prevails and the aerial hyphae must be demonstrated microscopically. A flakey, waxy pellicle forms on liquid media, as does a granular sediment that may contain fluffy microcolonies approximately 1 mm diameter. Morphologic features of hyphal elements can be conveniently demonstrated in stained smears from 72-hour broth cultures or from specially prepared slide cultures. While fragmentation of filamentous hyphae into rod and coccoid elements is a feature more typical of *Nocardia,* the production of terminal chains of conidia is more typical of *Streptomyces.*

Nocardia strains usually can be preserved on BHI blood agar for months when stored in the refrigerator. However, more permanent preservation is obtained by lyophilizing skim milk suspensions of stock strains. *N. brasiliensis* does not survive for long periods on refrigerated slants and lyophilization or frequent transfer is recommended. Care should be taken to locate the lyophilization apparatus in an enclosed, exteriorly vented room since the procedure creates dangerous aerosols.

Differential reactions. Reactions helpful in identifying nocardias and in differentiating between *N. asteroides, N. brasiliensis,* and *N. caviae* include heat tolerance and ability to decompose nitrogenous substances. Heat tolerance can be tested by exposing organisms from a 72-hour BHI blood agar slant, suspended in 10% serum broth, to a water bath temperature of 60°C for 4 hours; nearly all strains of *N. asteroides* and *N. caviae* grow when subcultured after the heat exposure, while *N. brasiliensis, Mycobacterium fortuitum,* and *M. rodochrous* do not. Also, hemolysis of bovine erythrocytes is usually seen with cultures of *N. brasiliensis* and many strains of *Streptomyces* but not often with *N. asteroides, N. caviae,* or *Nocardia*-like mycobacteria.

Tests for the hydrolysis of casein in skim milk agar and the decomposition of crystals of tyrosine or xanthine suspended in nutrient agar are conducted by making heavy spot inoculations of the test organisms on plates of the appropriate medium, incubating at 37°C, and observing for clearing of the opaque mediums after 14 and 21 days.

The nocardias usually produce acid from glucose but not from arabinose or sorbitol; reaction on mannose is variable. Criteria for identification of *N. asteroides, N. brasiliensis,* and *N. caviae* are summarized in Table 51.1.

Table 51.1. Typical reactions of *Nocardia* and related organisms*

	Nocardia			M. fortuitum	Streptomyces sp.
	asteroides	brasiliensis	caviae		
Gram reaction	+	+	+	†	+
Acid fastness	+	+	+	+	−
Branching filaments	+	+	+	−	+
Aerial hyphae	+	+	+	−	+
Survive 60°C 4 hr	+	−	+	−	+
Decomposition of					
Casein	−	+	−	−	V
Tyrosine	−	+	−	−	+
Xanthine	−	−	+	−	V

* + or − indicates the usual occurrence and is not intended to imply a 100% response; V indicates a variable or inconstant response.
†The reaction of mycobacteria to the Gram stain is atypical.

Cellular morphology. Staining reactions of *N. asteroides, N. brasiliensis,* and *N. caviae* are helpful presumptive criteria for identification. These organisms are strongly gram-positive. The longer filamentous forms may stain unevenly in a beaded fashion. In exudates branching filaments 0.5–1.0 μm in diameter are seen; culture forms vary from branching filaments to rod and coccoid elements. Acid-fastness is best demonstrated in *Nocardia* using a modification of Kinyoun's acid-fast stain; the most important feature of this technique is the use of 1% H_2SO_4 rather than acid-alcohol to decolorize the nonacid-fast elements. Nocardia often appear to be nonacid-fast with techniques employing acid-alcohol. Acid-fastness is most constantly demonstrated on organisms in exudates or those grown in milk. Smears prepared from cultures, particularly old laboratory strains, may show only part of the organisms or segments of the filaments to be acid fast.

Nocardia differ from *Actinomyces* in being free living and aerobic; from *Streptomyces* in fragmentation of the hyphal elements into branching filaments of rod and coccoid elements; and from *Mycobacterium* in being markedly gram-positive and forming branch filaments and aerial hyphae. The three species of *Nocardia* under discussion are also distinguished from *Actinomyces* and *Streptomyces* by their acid-fastness.

Animal inoculation. The demonstration of animal pathogenicity is a useful criterion for the identification of *Nocardia*, particularly *N. asteroides*. Guinea pigs can be used for this purpose. However, many strains are of low virulence and require the addition of 5% gastric mucin in equal parts with a heavy suspension of a 72-hour culture for IP inoculation. Death or the development of granulomatous lesions of the liver, diaphragm omentum, and various abdominal viscera occur within 14 days. *N. brasiliensis* infections, natural or experimental, more frequently develop truly mineralized granules than do *N. asteroides* or *N. caviae;* however, this is not a definitive criterion of differentiation.

Immunology and serology. Culture filtrate antigens of *N. asteroides* have been used to detect cutaneous hypersensitivity, precipitins, and CF antibodies in naturally or experimentally infected animals, but they are not in general use.[4] These antigens can also be used to provide subspecific typing of *N. asteroides*.[5]

Most strains of *Nocardia* are susceptible to a variety of antibiotics, but sulfonamides are recommended for therapy. Laboratory areas can be effectively decontaminated with 2% amphyl solution.

Reference laboratory. NADC.

References

1. Gordon, R.E., and J.M. Mihm. The type species of the genus Nocardia. *J. Gen. Microbiol.* 27:1–10, 1962.
2. Gordon, R.E., and J.M. Mihm. Identification of *Nocardia caviae.* (Erickson) Nov. Comb. *Ann. N.Y. Acad. Sci.* 98:628–636, 1962.
3. Pier, A.C. Nocardiosis in animals. *Proc. U.S. Livestock Sanitary Ass.*, pp. 409–415, 1962.
4. Pier, A.C., J.R. Thurston, and A.B. Larsen. A diagnostic antigen for nocardiosis: Comparative tests in cattle with nocardiosis and mycobacteriosis. *Am. J. Vet. Res.* 29:397–403, 1968.
5. Pier, A.C., and R.E. Fichtner. Serologic typing of *Nocardia asteroides* by immunodiffusion. *Am. Rev. Resp. Dis.* 103:698–707, 1971.
6. Schneidau, J.D., and M.F. Shaffer. Studies on Nocardia and other Actinomycetales. I. Cultural studies. *Am. Rev. Tuberc. Pulm. Dis.* 76:770–788, 1957.

52. Rickettsia

The rickettsias are small rod-shaped organisms that are obligate intracellular parasites. They grow only in living media, they contain both RNA and DNA, they reproduce by binary fission, and they are affected by certain antibiotics. The rickettsias are about 300 nm in diameter. Thus they are larger than chlamydiae (200 nm) and as large as the largest viruses (20–300 nm) and the largest mycoplasmas (50–300 nm), all of which are much smaller than the regular forms of bacteria (1000–2000 nm). In the current classification, rickettsias are considered bacteria.

Diseases caused by the rickettsias are collectively called rickettsioses. Many are zoonoses of importance to veterinary microbiologists concerned with public health. Some cause overt disease in lower animals whereas others, which are pathogenic only for humans, are maintained in cycles that also involve wild animals in nature and in some cases domestic animals. The major rickettsioses of humans, though not of primary interest to veterinarians, will be reviewed briefly to provide some insight into the comparative aspects of rickettsial diseases. Because livestock are extensively involved in the epidemiology of Q fever in humans, the diagnosis of infection—not disease—in domestic animals will be discussed in detail.

Rickettsioses of Humans

As shown in Table 52.1, the human rickettsial diseases are divided into five major groups: spotted fever, typhus fever, scrub typhus, Q fever, and trench fever.[17] All are caused by organisms resembling bacteria, which, with the exception of *Rochalimaea quintana,* are obligate parasites of mammalian or arthropod tissue cells. *Rickettsia prowazeki* and *Rochalimaea quintana* are maintained by primary cycles involving humans and their body louse, *Pediculus humanus,* whereas the remainder are maintained naturally in cycles involving various species of animals and their ectoparasites, chiefly ticks. In those with tick cycles, humans become infected when they accidentally intrude into the natural cycle. *Coxiella burneti* is unique for several reasons. It is unusually resistent to heat, sunlight, and desiccation; it thrives and persists in the placenta and mammary glands of cattle, sheep, and goats; and it is the only rickettsia disseminated to humans chiefly by air. In humans, most species of rickettsias parasitize cells of the reticuloen-

Table 52.1. Major rickettsioses of humans

Disease	Geographic distribution	Causative organism	Major vectors	Primary natural hosts	Preferred experimental hosts
Spotted fever group					
Spotted fever	North and South America	Rickettsia rickettsi	Dermacenter andersoni, D. variabilis, Rhipicephalus sanguineus, Amblyomma americanum, A. cajennense	Many species of feral mammals, chiefly rodents; dogs	Male guinea pigs, Microtus sp., EC eggs*
Siberian tick typhus	Siberia	R. siberica	Dermacentor nuttalli, D. silvarum, D. marginatus, D. pictus, Haemaphsalis concinna, H. punctata	Many species of feral mammals, chiefly rodents	Male guinea pigs, EC eggs
Rickettsial pox	Russia	R. akari	Allodermanyssus sanguineus	Mus sp., Rattus sp.	Mice, EC eggs
North Queensland tick typhus	Australia	R. australis	Ixodes holocyclus	Small marsupials, rats	Mice, EC eggs
Fievre boutonneuse, South African tick-bite fever, Kenya tick typhus, Indian tick typhus	Mediterranean area, Africa, India	R. conori	Rhipicephalus sanguineus, R. appendiculatus, Haemaphysalis leachi, Amblyomma hebraeum	Dogs, small feral mammals	Male guinea pigs, EC eggs
Typhus fever group					
Epidemic typhus	Worldwide (colder climates)	R. prowazeki	Pediculus humans, Amblyomma variegatum, Hyalomma sp.	Humans (cattle, sheep, goats?)	Male guinea pigs, cotton rats, EC eggs
Murine typhus	Worldwide (warmer climates)	R. typhi	Xenopsylla cheopis	Rattus norvegicus	Male guinea pigs, EC eggs
Scrub typhus	Eastern and southern Asia, islands of southwest Pacific	R. tsutsugamushi	Leptotrombidium akamushi, L. deliensis	Many species of small feral mammals, chiefly rodents	Mice, cotton rats, EC eggs
Q fever	Worldwide	Coxiella burneti	Chiefly airborne, also found in many species of ticks	Cattle, sheep, goats, many species of feral mammals	Guinea pigs, hamsters, EC eggs
Trench fever	Europe, North Africa, Mexico	Rochalimaea quintana	Pediculus humanus	Humans	Laboratory-reared body lice, blood agar

*EC eggs, embryonating chicken eggs.

dothelial system, and those of the spotted fever and typhus fever groups, in particular, invade the walls of smaller blood vessels and capillaries. Generally, infection confers a lifelong immunity, but occasionally recrudescence occurs in persons who have had epidemic typhus, and chronic progressive Q fever has presumably resulted in cardiovascular disease.

The diagnosis of rickettsial diseases is based principally on recovery of the causative organism from acute-phase blood in a suitable laboratory host (Table 52.1) or on a fourfold or greater increase in agglutinin or CF antibody titer between acute- and convalescent-phase sera. Several agglutination and toxin neutralization systems have been developed for special research purposes, but the CF test is most commonly used in rickettsial serology of both humans and animals. Each species contains group-distinctive antigens that do not cross-react with antisera for other groups; however, rickettsias of the spotted fever and typhus fever groups share common antigens that cross-react in the CF test only with other members of their respective groups.

Most reliable results are obtained with ether-extracted antigens prepared from yolk sacs of embryonating chicken eggs containing maximal growth of rickettsias. With members of the spotted fever group, except *R. akari*, maximal growth is achieved in 4–5-day-old embryos inoculated with a dose that will kill most of the embryos by the fourth day after inoculation.[22] After inoculation, eggs should be incubated at 33.5°C and held at this temperature for 48 hours after death of embryos before the sacs are harvested. Maximal yields or *R. prowazeki* and *R. typhi* are obtained in 5-day-old embryos inoculated with a dose that will kill 60–70% of the eggs by the eighth or ninth day postinoculation, when incubated at 36.5°C. Best growth of *C. burneti* is obtained when the inoculum is adjusted so that a comparable death rate occurs a day earlier, i.e. by day 7 or 8. Sacs are harvested from surviving eggs and from those in which the embryo has not been dead for more than 6 hours. Infected sacs can be frozen and stored at −20 or −70°C until sufficient quantities are obtained for preparation of a batch of antigen.

Rickettsial antigens are prepared by ether extraction of infected YS. Sacs are first emulsified in a Waring blender with sufficient 0.066 M phosphate-buffered saline, pH 5.8, to make a 20% YS suspension. After the addition of Formalin to a 0.2% concentration, the material is held overnight at 4°C. The YS suspension is then mixed with 1.5 volumes of ether in a separatory funnel, shaken several times during the day, and allowed to separate overnight at 4°C. The liquid that contains the antigen is withdrawn and residual ether removed by vacuum. Antigenic activity is then assayed by cross-box titration against three specific antiserums with suitable controls to evaluate anticomplementary activity of the antigen. If the antigen contains significant anticomplementary activity, it may sometimes be removed by one or more additional ether extractions.

Cultivation of rickettsias in eggs, isolation procedures, and general handling of live rickettsias or infected animals are hazardous. Work with *C. burneti* is particularly so, because it is readily disseminated by air to all occupants in a building. Therefore, persons working with living rickettsias should be vaccinated and adequate containment facilities should be obligatory to prevent escape of organisms into the ambient environment.

Q Fever

This disease is the only rickettsiosis of humans in which livestock are extensively involved. *Coxiella burneti*, the causative organism, occurs typically as a bipolar rod, 0.25×1 μm, that stains red with Macchiavello's stain and bright red with Gimenez.[13] Some observations suggest the existence of a smaller filterable stage, but its true nature has not been clarified. Strains newly isolated from animals and ticks are characteristically in phase I and react only with antibodies in late convalescent-phase sera. Upon repeated passage in embryonating chicken eggs, the organism converts to phase II and reacts with antibodies in early convalescent-phase serum. This organism does not share common antigens with any other known pathogen.

This rickettsia is maintained by a cycle in feral animals and their ticks and by a separate but related airborne cycle in livestock, chiefly cattle, sheep, and goats. After the organism has been inhaled, it localizes and proliferates in the pregnant uterus and mammary glands. Though it may reach concentrations of 10^9 ID_{50} per gram of placenta, abortion or other disease has not been associated with infection in livestock. Neither has the presence of *C. burneti* in milk (usually not greater than 10^2 ID_{50} per ml) been related to mastitis. Because of its unusual resistance to desiccation, *C. burneti* eliminated from animals remains in the soil for months and becomes airborne when wind or human activities disperse it into the atmosphere.

Specimens

Infection rates among herds of dairy cattle and goats can be determined by testing pooled milk samples from the entire herd. Flocks of sheep can be surveyed at lambing season by testing a representative number of placentas from each flock. During a 3-month period after lambing, infected flocks can be identified by testing surface soil (protected by bedding) from lambing pens or corrals.

Laboratory Procedures

Animal inoculation and cultures. Two or more guinea pigs or hamsters per specimen should be inoculated IP (1–2 ml), held separately from animals inoculated with other specimens for 35–40 days, and bled by cardiac puncture. Sera from each animal are then tested against *C. burneti* antigen by CF or agglutination tests. The appearance of antibodies in the postinoculation serum of one or more animals generally indicates presence of *C. burneti* in the original specimen. If desirable, strains can then be established by inoculating 5–6-day embryonating chicken eggs by the YS route with 10% suspensions of spleens from seropositive test animals. These spleens may or may not be enlarged, depending on the pathogenicity of the strain. One or two blind passages in eggs may be necessary before organisms can be seen in YS smears stained by Macchiavello's or Gimenez' methods. After the strain has been well established in eggs, ether-extracted antigens can be prepared and tested against specific anti–*C. burneti* serum containing both phase I and II antibodies. The identity of the rickettsia can also be established by the FA test.

Serology. The prevalence of infection with *C. burneti* among domestic livestock may be determined by examining serum by CF, capillary tube, or radioisotope precipitation

(RIP) techniques. Because these techniques measure different antibodies, complete agreement among them may not be obtained; for example, CF antibodies are associated with the 19 S macroglobulins, whereas antibodies reactive in the RIP test are thought to occur in the 7 S gamma globulins. Furthermore, the rate of antibody response to infection with *C. burneti* and the persistence of antibodies varies in different species of animals.

Infection rates among herds of dairy cattle are most readily determined by testing individual or pooled milk samples by the capillary tube technique.[18] Best results are obtained with fresh whole milk, held at 4–8°C before testing, or with milk preserved with 0.1% Formalin, but whey, skim milk, and frozen whole milk may also be used. The antigen consists of a clarified suspension of hematoxylin-stained phase I *C. burneti*. About one-third of the capillary tube is filled with antigen and the remainder with milk. Tubes are inverted, placed in Plasticine, and incubated either at 37°C for 5 hours or at room temperature for 24 hours before reactions are read. Milk containing agglutinins causes the rickettsias to clump and rise with the cream layer. The intensity of the blue-black color in the cream layer is related to the antibody content, which may be titrated by testing twofold dilutions of milk in physiological saline. Positive reactions in dilutions of milk are recognized by clumps of rickettsias scattered throughout the length of the column.

When sera are tested by the CF test, care should be exercised to prevent contamination or hemolysis before the serum is separated from the clot. More valid results are obtained with freshly drawn serum, because anticomplementary activity in some sera tends to increase with age. Antigen used should be in phase II to assure detection of antibodies in sera of cattle, sheep, and goats. Phase I CF antibodies, which are occasionally found in low titer in sera of infected livestock, are almost always found in association with phase II antibodies. The titer of antibodies considered significant of infection is dependent on the quality of serum and antigen. When antigen and serum controls are free of anticomplementary activity, a titer of 1:8 is considered suggestive and a titer of 1:16 significant of past infection.

The capillary tube test can also be used for detecting antibody in undiluted sera of livestock by the same procedure described for testing milk samples. Positive reactions are similar to those seen in diluted milk samples. Physiological saline used for diluting serums of sheep for titration of antibody content should contain 10% normal bovine serum free of antibodies to *C. burneti*, otherwise titers are reduced. For titrating human and guinea pig serums, the concentration of normal bovine serum in the diluent should be increased to 25% to achieve maximal titers. If sera of good quality are tested, a titer of 1:2 is significant of past infection.

Positive serologic findings by CF or agglutination tests merely indicate past infection with the organism or, in the case of vaccination, a specific response to antigens in the vaccine. Generally, persistent infection in the placenta or mammary glands can be correlated with a high titer of antibodies, but conversely, some livestock, particularly sheep, may have rickettsias in their tissues without a significant antibody titer in their sera.

The RIP test is the most sensitive technique and detects antibodies longer after infection than any other.[23] The antigen for this method contains purified phase I rickettsias labeled with I^{131} by persulfate oxidation. After unbound iodine is removed by washing four times, the antigen is diluted according to the radioactivity desired. Both serum and antigen are diluted in 0.02 M phosphate-buffered saline, pH 7.1, containing 0.002 M EDTA. With a Lang-Levy constriction pipette, 0.4 ml of diluted antigen is added to each of a series of tubes containing an equal volume of serum diluted from 1:32 to 1:32,768. After serum and antigen mixtures are incubated and rotated for 1 hour at 37°C, each tube should receive 0.2 ml of specific anti–gamma globulin diluted by a factor previously determined by titration with a known positive anti–*C. burneti* serum. Incubation and rotation are continued for an hour and the tubes are then held overnight at 4°C. To each tube, 0.5 ml diluent is added and the tubes are then shaken briefly with a cyclo-mixer just before centrifugation in a horizontal head at $175 \times g$ for 10 minutes. Immediately after centrifugation, 0.5 ml supernatant fluid is removed from each tube with constricted pipettes and placed in planchets for counting. The planchets are dried and the radioactivity determined in a planchet-type radiation counting system, preferably one equipped with a Geiger-Müller detector tube. If over 50% of the radioactivity is sedimented, the reaction is considered positive. A titer of 1:32 or greater is considered significant of past infection.

Rickettsioses of Domestic Animals

Salient features of eight major animal rickettsioses considered in this chapter are recorded in Table 52.2. These organisms comprise a heterogenous group whose members share few common characteristics. As far as has been determined, each is immunologically distinct from the others. Although several of these diseases have been studied extensively, the limited host range of these rickettsias has impaired thorough investigations comparable to those done on human rickettsioses. None of these organisms has been cultivated in embryonating eggs, and with the exception of *Cowdria ruminantium, Ehrlichia phagocytophila,* and the organisms recovered from horses with equine erhlichiosis, none causes disease or infection in small laboratory animals.

The extensive endothelial involvement seen in heartwater is comparable to that observed in spotted fever in humans. Tick-borne fever, benign rickettsiosis of sheep and cattle, and ehrlichiosis of dogs and equine species are similar in one aspect—invasion of circulating leukocytes by the causative rickettsia. In tick-borne and equine ehrlichiosis, cells of the granulocyte series are invaded, whereas in the other rickettsioses, lymphocytes and monocytes are affected. *Neorickettsia helminthoeca* invades primarily the lymphoid tissue of dogs, where the organism may be found in reticular cells as morula-like masses or diffusely scattered throughout the cytoplasm. *Colesiota conjunctivae* is limited to the conjunctival epithelium of affected animals.

None of the rickettsias considered in this section can be cultivated in embryonating eggs or cause disease in small laboratory animals. *C. ruminantium* will infect white mice and ferrets but the infections are inapparent. Similarly *E. phagocytophila* has been adapted to guinea pigs and mice but these animals are not useful for demonstrating the organism. Because of the difficulty of preparing suitable antigens, serologic methods for the detection of antibodies to these agents have not been developed. Therefore, diag-

Table 52.2. Major rickettsioses of animals

Disease	Geographic distribution	Causative organism	Major vectors	Primary natural hosts	Preferred experimental hosts
Heartwater	East and South Africa, Sudan	*Cowdria ruminantium*	*Amblyomma hebraeum*, other *Amblyomma* sp.	Sheep, cattle, goats, some wild ungulates; vascular endothelium	Bluetongue-immune sheep, mice
Tick-borne fever, pasture fever	Great Britain, Norway, Finland, Netherlands, India	*Ehrlichia phagocytophila*	*Ixodes ricinus*	Cattle, sheep, goats, wild ungulates; granulocytes	Cattle, sheep, goats
Benign bovine rickettsiosis	North and South Africa	*Ehrlichia bovis*	*Hyalomma excavatum*, other *Hyalomma* sp.	Cattle; lymphocytes, monocytes	Cattle
Benign ovine rickettsiosis	North and South Africa	*Ehrlichia ovina*	*Rhipicephalus bursa*	Sheep; lymphocytes, monocytes	Sheep
Canine ehrlichiosis	East and North Africa, India, Ceylon, Aruba, United States	*Ehrlichia canis*	*Rhipicephalus sanguineus*	Dogs, jackels; lymphocytes, monocytes	Babesia-free dogs
Contagious ophthalmia	Africa, Australia, New Zealand, Europe, North and South America	*Colesiota conjunctivae*	Flies	Sheep, cattle, goats, swine, chickens; conjunctival epithelium	Sheep, cattle, goats, swine, chickens
Salmon poisoning	Northwest United States	*Neorickettsia helminthoeca*	*Nanophyetus salmincola*	Dogs, wild Canidae; reticuloendothelial system, lymph nodes	Dogs

nosis must be based on the reproduction of the disease or by demonstrating the organism in selected tissues or cells stained with Giemsa, MGG, or other appropriate stains. These rickettsias are found only in the cytoplasm of affected cells.

Heartwater

Heartwater is a septicemic infectious disease of cattle, sheep, and goats characterized by high fever, signs of CNS involvement, and high mortality.[3] The causative agent, *Cowdria ruminantium,* also infects a variety of ungulate game animals but does not regularly cause overt disease in them. The severity of the disease varies from the peracute form, characterized by high fever, sudden collapse, and death after a few paroxysmal spasms, to a mild or abortive form. In the most common acute form, a sudden rise in body temperature occurs first. Most animals are depressed and lose their appetite, but some may continue to feed and ruminate. A high-stepping and unsteady gait is a characteristic early sign. Progressive signs of encephalitis appear, including chewing movements, twitching of eyelids, walking in circles, aggressive and blind charges into objects, and final collapse with attendant convulsions, galloping movements, and twitching of muscles.

There are no gross tissue changes pathognomonic of heartwater. Although the name suggests hydropericardium, this result is not always seen in sheep; in cattle, the absence of pericardial fluid is pathognomically significant. Animals that die of the peracute form rarely have gross lesions. Those that survive longer have changes characteristic of a septicemic disease.

The characteristic microscopic changes seen in heartwater are leucostasis, which occurs in all organs, and perivascular infiltration, chiefly in the liver and kidney, and sometimes in the adrenal glands. The organism multiplies profusely in vascular endothelium; the lumen of capillaries may be occluded by swollen epithelial cells containing masses of rickettsias.[9]

Specimens

Diagnosis can be established by demonstration of rickettsias in tissue smears or reproduction of the disease in bluetongue-immune sheep. The organism is most readily demonstrated in the endothelial cells of large vessels (aorta and jugular vein) and capillaries of the brain, especially the gray matter of the cerebrum. Although vascular scrapings can be spread on a slide and stained, equally good results are obtained by staining "squash" smears of brain tissue taken from the cerebral gray matter.[20] A small piece of tissue about the size of a tomato seed is placed on an end of a slide. With a second, spreader slide, the tissue is compressed until it spreads nearly across the width of the slide. The spreader slide is then elevated about 5 degrees and the edge drawn across the other slide. After the smear is air dried and fixed with methyl alcohol, it should be stained with Giemsa stain. Smears should be scanned under low power to find areas rich in capillaries. When stained with Giemsa, the organism appears dark blue while the nuclei of endothelial cells are purple. The organism may be coccoid (0.3 μm diameter), bacillary (0.3 × 0.5 μm), or diplococcoid. Rickettsias are restricted to the cytoplasm and appear singly, in small clumps, or in masses so large that the lumen of a capillary may be occluded by the swollen cell.

Specimens taken 2–4 days after onset of fever are best for demonstration of rickettsias or subinoculation into sheep. Blood may not be infectious after the temperature has returned to normal, and the rickettsias lose their staining properties rapidly in unfixed tissues. Blood should be obtained in sterile containers, defibrinated, and inoculated IV into test animals immediately after withdrawal from the sick animal. *C. ruminantium* is extremely labile and will not survive for more than a few hours in blood at room temperature. However, it has been reported to survive at −70°C for 2 years.[15] When field-autopsied material cannot be inoculated promptly into sheep, the material should be inoculated IP into white mice, which will preserve the organism for later passage in the laboratory.

Laboratory Procedures

Animal inoculation. If diagnosis is to be confirmed by reproduction of the disease in animals, heartwater-susceptible but bluetongue-immune sheep should be inoculated IV because many cattle and sheep may harbor bluetongue virus, which interferes with interpretation of a heartwater reaction.[2] The incubation period of bluetongue is about 5 days, whereas that of heartwater is about 11 days. Test animals should be killed 2–4 days after onset of fever and the organism should be demonstrable in endothelial cells.

If mice were inoculated with specimens collected in the field, spleens should be taken 4–21 days postinoculation, triturated in nutrient broth, and the suspension injected IV into sheep. An incubation period in mice appears to be necessary for a successful transfer from them to sheep. Mice will retain the organism for as long as 90 days without showing signs of disease, but it cannot be maintained in mice by serial passage.

Immunology. One attack of naturally or experimentally induced disease usually provides protection against challenge with the same strain, but this immunity is not complete in all animals. When recovered animals are challenged with different strains, frequently only partial protection occurs. This circumstance suggests a multiplicity of immunologically different strains of the organism in nature. A solid immunity is established naturally by repeated infection, which occurs during continuous exposure to ticks. It should be noted that animals are protected against disease, not infection. When immune domestic animals are bitten by infected bont ticks, they develop sufficient rickettsemia to infect other normal bont ticks feeding on the animal at the same time.

Tick-borne Fever

Tick-borne fever is characterized by sudden rise in temperature and a period of irregular fever that persists 3–5 days in cattle and 10 days in sheep.[24] Animals become listless and suffer considerable weight loss. A sudden drop in milk production is seen in dairy cattle and normal production may not be fully restored after recovery. Febrile relapses may occur 2–4 weeks after the initial attack. In some outbreaks, abortions have occurred among sheep and cattle that are in the last stages of gestation. Where babesiosis, which is also tick-borne, occurs in the same area, the clinical disease may be complicated by concurrent infection with *Babesia*.

Specimens

Although *Ehrlichia phagocytophila* may persist in the blood of some animals for months after the initial febrile attack, the best time to obtain blood samples for the demonstration of rickettsias is during the peak of the initial febrile period of 3–4 days. At that time, appreciable numbers are circulated. The carrier state is extremely variable; most animals free their tissues within a month, whereas some sheep have remained carriers for 2 years. Blood smears may be made at the time of collection or citrated blood samples may be taken in sterile tubes and refrigerated at 4°C, if smears cannot be made promptly. This organism, though labile, usually remains viable in blood stored at 4°C for 7 days, and will survive for several months if the blood is shell-frozen in an alcohol–dry ice bath and stored at $-70°C$.

Giemsa or MGG are excellent stains for demonstrating the organism in blood smears. It can also be identified by the FA technique, but this method does not offer any advantage in ease or certainty of diagnosis.[26] This rickettsia is found chiefly in the granulocytes, although monocytes may also be invaded. The percentage of granulocytes that are infected varies with stage of disease, pathogenicity of the strain, and susceptibility of the host. At the peak of rickettsemia, more than 50% of the granulocytes may be infected by some strains, but others may invade only 6%. At least 100 cells should be examined before a smear can be classified as negative.

Several types of rickettsial bodies are seen in Giemsa-stained smears, sometimes in the same cell.[14] The simplest is a deep purple–staining coccoid or rod-shaped body about 0.5 μm diameter, often situated near the periphery of the cell. The second type is a larger (1.3×2 μm) homogeneously staining body more deeply situated in the cell. Often these appear to fragment into smaller irregularly shaped parts. The third type (morulae) are founded or oval masses that contain numerous distinct bodies that stain deeper blue or purple than the matrix surrounding them.

Laboratory Procedures

Animal inoculation. The disease may be reproduced by IV injection of defibrinated blood taken from animals during the febrile period into susceptible cattle or sheep. The organisms naturally involved in tick-borne fever in sheep and cattle are considered to be different strains of the same organism. They appear to have a degree of specificity, inducing more severe disease in their respective natural hosts. The incubation period varies from 4 to 8 days when animals are exposed to infected ticks, and from 5 to 12 days after inoculation of blood.

Immunology. An attack of tick-borne fever is followed by partial immunity of varying degree and generally of short duration. Most cattle and sheep, in the absence of exposure to ticks, are fully susceptible within 3–6 months after the initial attack. Therefore, the occurrence of tick-borne fever in the same cow on successive seasons is not rare. In areas of heavy tick infestation, however, repeated attacks (exclusive to relapses) are seldom seen.

Strains of *E. phagocytophila* are immunologically heterogeneous.[25,26] There is no apparent cross-immunity between Scottish and Finnish strains. Generally, strains that cause more severe disease are more immunogenic than mild strains.

Benign Bovine and Ovine Rickettsioses

Available reports on bovine and ovine benign rickettsiosis contain only meager information about the nature of the disease.[11] Irregular fever of several weeks duration and low mortality rate were seen. The most prominent lesion is excessive pericardial fluid, comparable to that of heartwater in sheep. Lymphadenopathy and splenomegaly are also consistent changes.

Specimens

Procedures recommended are the same as those outlined for tick-borne fever. Adequate data on survival of these rickettsias in blood specimens are not available. Biopsied tissue from lung, liver, or spleen is suitable for demonstrating the organism in tissue cells, but the organism can be demonstrated readily in monocytes of blood smears as long as the animal is febrile.

The rickettsias are found chiefly in circulating monocytes and in cells (monocytes?) of the lungs, liver, and spleen, especially the first. When stained with Giemsa, they are tinctorially similar to *E. phagocytophila*. The organisms are usually assembled in round colonies from 2 to 10 µm in diameter, but they are seen also as closely packed granules 0.5–1 µm in diameter. Some authors have described "initial bodies" (3–6 µm) that stain a homogeneous red and later separate into elementary bodies by way of a morula stage, the component parts of which stain purple with MGG stain. Monocytes in a blood smear tend to gather at the edge of the smear. The percentage of monocytes that contain rickettsia is lower than that seen in granulocytes in tick-borne fever. Hence, a thorough search should be made before a smear is considered negative.

Laboratory Procedures

Animal inoculation. Blood taken during the febrile period or 10% suspensions of spleen and lung are commonly used to pass the organism in its natural host. After parenteral inoculation of the agent, the incubation period in cattle and sheep is reported to be about 12 days.

Immunology. In both cattle and sheep, chronic infection persists for at least 10 months and recovered animals develop a solid immunity against challenge with the homologous organism. The duration of immunity and the immunologic relationship between *E. bovis* and *E. ovina* have not been explored.

Canine Ehrlichiosis

Ehrlichiosis in dogs is frequently complicated by concurrent infection with *Babesia canis,* because both organisms are transmitted by the same species of tick, *Rhipicephalus sanguineus.*[5,12] The uncomplicated disease is essentially a severe anemia of the normocytic-normochromic type. Onset is signaled by high fever and depression. Progressive weakness, vomition, icterus, splenomegaly, and bilateral mucopurulent ocular discharge with photophobia are seen as the disease progresses. The mortality rate among pups is higher than that in older dogs.

Certain hematologic findings suggest ehrlichiosis in the dog.[12] Monocytosis occurs early in the disease and eosinophils almost disappear from the circulation. As the disease progresses, a profound anemia of the normocytic-normochromic type develops, with attendant depressed values for hemoglobin, packed cell volume, and total erythrocyte counts.

The gross changes regularly seen in canine ehrlichiosis at necropsy include anemia, enlargement of the spleen, liver, and lymph nodes, petechiae on the lungs, and hyperactivity of the bone marrow. Other less constant lesions are hemorrhages and ulcers in the intestinal tract, hydrothorax, and pulmonary edema.

Specimens

Dogs infected with this organism remain carriers for months after recovery from the acute phase. However, the rickettsia is most readily demonstrated in blood smears from 2 to 3 days after the start of the febrile reaction until the end of the attack. If the organism cannot be found in direct smears of blood, smears should be made of the buffy coat of heparinized or citrated blood samples. Because *Ehrlichia* infections, especially of the dog, are often complicated by concurrent infections with *Babesia,* a thorough search should be made also for this organism in erythrocytes. During the febrile period, the organism can also be demonstrated in biopsy material taken from the lungs, liver, or spleen, especially the first. Adequate data are not available on the conditions required for survival of rickettsia in blood samples or tissues taken at autopsy.

Laboratory Procedures

Animal inoculation. Blood withdrawn aseptically for passage should be inoculated promptly into susceptible dogs.

Immunology. Dogs remain carriers for a period of at least 5 months after recovery from an acute attack.[10] Persistence of the organism in the recovered animal can be demonstrated by splenectomy, after which rickettsias again appear in monocytes in the blood. Recovered animals are solidly immune to reinfection.

Contagious Ophthalmia

Colesiota conjunctivae causes an acute purulent conjunctivitis in sheep, cattle, goats, swine, and chickens. The severity of the disease varies from mild cases in which recovery is complete in one week to severe cases complicated by keratitis, vascularization, and occasionally ulceration of the cornea.[4] Most severely affected eyes eventually heal without residual blemish.

The relationships among the organisms causing eye disease in livestock has not been firmly established. In early studies in Australia, contagious ophthalmia was restricted to sheep, whereas in South Africa similar rickettsias also have been associated with conjunctivitis in goats, cattle, swine, and chickens.[16] The strains are host specific and cannot be transferred among species of livestock. Some workers contend that *C. conjunctivae* occurs only in sheep, and that the rickettsias which infect the conjuctivae of other livestock belong to a separate genus.

Specimens

The upper eyelid should be everted and some of the epithelial lining from the inner surface removed by scraping with a scalpel until a tinge of blood appears. Scrapings should be spread on a slide, air dried, and fixed with absolute alcohol before staining.[4] For reproduction of the disease in other sheep, saline washings of the conjunctival sac should be taken during the acute purulent phase.

Several types of inclusions are seen in Giemsa-stained smears. Smears made early in the disease contain many polymorphonuclear leukocytes, and most organisms in the cytoplasm are in the form of small ovals or short rods (0.3×0.5 μm) and stain a uniform purplish-red. As recovery progresses, the polymorphonuclear leukocytes are replaced by lymphocytes and monocytes. Rickettsias seen at this stage are often extracellular, 0.8×1.4 μm and irregular in shape, and stain unevenly. They may form imperfect rings, triangles, or irregularly shaped horseshoes.[7]

Laboratory Procedures

Animal inoculation. The disease may be reproduced by instilling conjunctival washings into the eyes of susceptible animals of the same species in which the natural disease occurred. When the disease affects sheep, it will not spread to cattle in close contact with them. Some breeds of sheep, e.g. the merino, appear to be highly susceptible. The incubation period is about 2–4 days. When one eye is initially affected, the opposite eye will become involved in 3–4 days.

Immunology. From reports of research on the disease in Australia, it appears that sheep develop a solid immunity that persists for at least 100 days.[4] Immunity then begins to wane, and by 250 days after initial infection about 10% of sheep are again susceptible. The persistence of the carrier state in some sheep for over a year and the gradual loss of immunity in others explain the enzootic persistence of the organism in some flocks of sheep.

Some workers have reported that immunity is local and develops only in the eye that has been affected. Others claim to have been able to establish reinfection within 25 days after the initial attack. Immunity in animals other than sheep has not been thoroughly studied.

Salmon Poisoning

Salmon poisoning is an acute febrile disease of dogs that occurs in the northwestern United States within the geographic distribution of *Goniobasis plicifera silicula,* a snail that is the intermediate host of the vector fluke, *Nanophyetes salmincola*. Dogs acquire the disease only by eating trout or salmon containing the encysted cercariae of this fluke. Hence the presence of ova of this fluke in the feces of a dog with high fever along with other clinical signs of salmon poisoning is highly suggestive. The diagnosis can be confirmed by demonstrating the organism in lymph-node biopsy tissue obtained during the febrile period.

The initial signs are high fever, depression, and inappetence. As the temperature drops gradually after the second or third day, the eyelids become edematous and the eyes appear sunken. Rapid weight loss, complicated by vomition and diarrhea with blood-tinged feces, is seen by the fifth to seventh day. At this time, the temperature may be normal and the dog appear brighter, but the apparent improvement is temporary. As the disease progresses, the temperature becomes subnormal and death ensues in 24–48 hours. Most untreated cases terminate fatally. The most prominent gross change seen at necropsy is the tremendous enlargement of the lymph nodes, particularly those of the abdominal cavity.[8] In some cases, the ileocecal and mesenteric nodes may be enlarged three- to sixfold. Somatic nodes are also affected but not to this degree. Nodes are usually edematous and yellow with white foci representing cortical follicles. Thymus, tonsils, and spleen are slightly to moderately enlarged. Solitary lymph follicles and Peyer's patches along the intestinal tract are usually noticeably enlarged. Hemorrhages are frequently found in the lungs and intestinal tract, and many animals have petechiae of the gastrointestinal mucosa. The contents of the small intestine may vary from bile-stained mucus to blood-tinged watery fluid.

Microscopically, lymph node changes are prominent; there is marked and regular depletion of small lymphocytes and hyperplasia of reticuloendothelial cells in the cortex and medulla. Occasionally, the cortex may contain large foci of necrosis around which neutrophils are numerous. The sinuses may contain an increased number of large macrophages and erythrocytes. Rickettsias are found in reticuloendothelial cells of sinuses and the parenchyma. Changes similar to those in lymph nodes are seen also in the thymus, tonsils, and lymphoid follicles of the intestine. The splenic follicles rarely contain necrotic foci but often show central hemorrhage.

In dogs and foxes, flukes are found embedded in villi or duodenal glands of the intestine, but their presence does not stimulate an inflammatory reaction. Small foci of macrophages and neutrophils, often necrotic, are frequently found in the connective tissue of the lamina propria. Cellularity of the lamina propria may also be increased, especially by plasma cells and some neutrophils. Centrolobular lipidosis of the liver is common in foxes but rare in dogs. A moderate mononuclear infiltration of the interlobular connective tissue of the liver is seen in both foxes and dogs.

Leptomeningitis, characterized by accumulations of mononuclear cells, is most intense over the cerebellum. Other commonly seen lesions include exudative and proliferative cellular changes in the sheaths of small and medium-sized blood vessels of the cerebrum, and focal collections of the glia of mesenchymal cells (so-called glial nodules). The urogenital system is usually free of lesions, except for a few small hemorrhages beneath the epithelium of the bladder. Small areas in alveolar walls of the lungs are occasionally thickened by an accumulation of mononuclear and neutrophilic leukocytes.

Specimens

Shortly after the onset of fever, rickettsias can be demonstrated in cells of lymph nodes. Suitable material is most readily obtained by aspirating cells from the mandibular lymph node with a syringe, or by other methods of biopsy. Tissue smears should be fixed promptly with methyl alcohol for staining. Blood obtained during the febrile period contains the organism, but not in sufficient quantity to enable detection by direct microscopic examination. Feces should also be collected for examination for fluke ova.

The rickettsias are labile but will survive in frozen whole tissue stored at −70°C for at least 6 months and will withstand lyophilization. In Giemsa-stained material, the organisms appear as purple coccoid or coccobacillary bodies, about 0.3 µm in diameter, which are scattered or arranged in compact plaques in the cytoplasm of reticular cells and macrophages.[19]

Laboratory Procedures

Animal inoculation. The organism can be passed in dogs by inoculation of blood taken during the febrile phase or with suspensions of spleen. The incubation period varies from 6 to 12 days.

Immunology. Very few dogs recover from the naturally acquired disease without specific antibiotic therapy. Those that recover after treatment with sulfonamides or other antibiotics are solidly immune against reinfection.

Equine Ehrlichiosis

Equine ehrlichiosis is a distinct disease entity occurring among horses in California. The disease was first described in 1961;[15] since then 5 cases have been reported, all from the foothills on both sides of the Sacramento Valley. The information presented here was derived from these cases and from pathogenetic studies conducted on 43 horses and 4 burros.

The infections were characterized by fever, anorexia, depression, edema of the legs, and ataxia. Experimentally, the incubation period varied from 1 to 9 days, with a mean of 2.5 days when the inoculum was fresh blood and 6.4 days when the inoculum was frozen blood. Onset of fever was sudden and persisted for 5–6 days. During the febrile period the rickettsialike inclusions could be demonstrated in granulocytes and they reached peak numbers about the second or third day of fever, when 25–30% of the granulocytes contained inclusions. During this period, depression was often pronounced, and some animals appeared to be in a stupor. Prominent hematologic changes included thrombocytopenia, elevated plasma icterus index, decreased packed cell volume, and marked leukopenia involving first lymphocytes and then granulocytes. Subcutaneous edema of the legs, which began from the second to sixth day of fever, appeared first at the metacarpal and metatarsal regions and sometimes ascended to the midshaft of the radius and 15–20 cm above the hock. At necropsy, petechial and ecchymotic hemorrhages and edema in the affected areas of the legs were regularly seen. Some horses had increased quantities of peritoneal and pericardial fluid. Jaundiced tissues were often seen and orchitis was often present in mature males.

Histologically, vasculitis of small arteries and veins is seen, and it is characterized by swelling of the endothelium and smooth muscle cells, thromboses, and perivascular infiltrations of monocytes and lymphocytes.[15] Vessels of the legs, ovaries, testes, and pampiniform plexus are chiefly affected.

Specimens

Blood specimens for diagnostic purposes should be obtained aseptically during the febrile period, preferably 3–5 days after onset of fever. Blood smears to demonstrate the rickettsia are best made with flesh blood; however, citrated samples may be taken in sterile tubes and refrigerated at 4°C for later examination. Fresh whole blood should be used for subinoculation into susceptible horses; defibrinated blood sealed in glass ampules and stored at −70°C remains infectious for long periods but the incubation period is prolonged.

Diagnosis is principally based on demonstrating typical inclusion bodies in granulocytes that are contained in blood smears stained with Giemsa or Wright-Leishman stains.[15,21] With these stains, the inclusion bodies appear deep blue to pale blue-gray. They may vary from small darkly stained bodies about 200 nm in diameter to large granular structures about 5 µm in diameter, which represent a cluster of many small bodies. The percentage of neutrophils parasitized varies with the stage of disease, but the mean maximum is 36% (0.5%–73%).

Laboratory Procedures

Animal inoculation. Blood taken during the febrile phase may be used to reproduce the disease in susceptible horses. Young horses under 2 years of age do not regularly develop clinical signs other than fever. Sheep, goats, and dogs are susceptible, as judged by the appearance of parasitized granulocytes, but clinical signs attending infections in these species are mild or absent.

Immunology. Recurrence of the disease in recovered animals has not been observed and the results of challenge experiments suggest that one attack confers immunity. Each of seven horses reinoculated with an infectious dose of blood at 2.5–20 months after the initial attack was resistant to reinfection, as judged by the absence of clinical signs and inclusion bodies in their circulating leukocytes.[15]

Jembrana Disease

In December 1964, a disease that was at first thought to be rinderpest occurred in the Jembrana district on the island of Bali, Indonesia. The disease affected both cattle and buffalos and within 8 months spread throughout Bali.[1,6] The Jembrana district lost more than 60% of its bovine population (about 19,284 animals).[3] It was estimated that 40,000 animals had died on Bali by September 1967.[3] Young cattle, sheep, and goats appeared to be unaffected. New but less severe outbreaks of the disease occurred in April 1972 and mid-1974.[6]

Clinical signs of the disease were anorexia, fever (40–42°C), generalized lymphadenopathy, nasal discharge, salivation, anemia, constipation (febrile stage), diarrhea (after pyrexia), and blood sweating.[6] Hemorrhages were sometimes seen in vaginal mucosa, at the base of tongue, and in the anterior chamber of the eyes.

Postmortem findings were generalized lymphadenopathy, numerous hemorrhagic areas in various tissues, and splenic enlargement (three- to fourfold).[6] Rickettsialike intracellular organisms were found in white blood cells and in cells from biopsies of prescapular lymph nodes in some animals during the febrile stage.[6] The disease was transmitted to normal cattle and male guinea pigs (orchitis and peritonitis) by inoculation of tissue suspensions. The histopathological findings differed from those of rinderpest.

References

1. Adiwinata, R.T. Some informative notes on a rinderpest-like disease on the island of Bali. *Bull. Off. Internat. Epiz.* 69:7–14, 1968.
2. Alexander, R.A. Heartwater: The present state of our knowledge of this disease. In *17th Report of the Director of Veterinary Services and Animal industry,* pp. 89–150. Onderstepoort, Union of South Africa, 1931.
3. Anon. Jembrana disease: A rickettsial infection of cattle. Editorials *Austral. Vet. J.* 52:53, 1976.
4. Beveridge, W.I.B. Investigations of contagious opthalmia of sheep, with special attention to the epidemiology of infection by Rickettsiae conjunctivae. *Austral. Vet. J.* 18:155–164, 1942.
5. Bool, P. H., and P. Sutmoller. Ehrlichia canis infections in dogs in Aruba (Netherlands Antilles). *J. Am. Vet. Med. Ass.* 130:418–420, 1957.
6. Budiarso, T., and S. Hardjosworo. Jembrana disease in Bali cattle. Letters to the editor. *Austral. Vet. J.* 52:97, 1976.
7. Coles, J.D.W.A. A rickettsia-like organism in the conjunctiva of sheep. *Rep. Vet. Res. S. Afr.* 17:172–189, 1931.
8. Cordy, D.R., and J.R. Gorham. The pathology and etiology of salmon disease in the dog and fox. *Am. J. Path.* 26:617–637, 1950.
9. Cowdria, E.V. Studies on the etiology of heartwater. *J. Exp. Med.* 42:231–274, 1925.
10. Donatien, A., and F. Lestoquard. Sur la persistence de Rickettsia canis dans l'organisme du chien, après guérison. *Bull. Acad. Med.* 114:857–859, 1935.
11. Donatien, A., and F. Lestoquard. Etat actuel des connaissances sur les rickettsioses animales. *Arch. Inst. Pasteur Algeria* 15:142–187, 1937.
12. Ewing, S.A., and R.G. Buckner. Manifestations of babesiosis, ehrlichiosis and combined infections in the dog. *Am. J. Vet. Res.* 26:815–828, 1965.
13. Gimenez, D.F. Staining rickettsiae in yolk-sac cultures. *Stain Tech.* 39:135–140, 1964.
14. Gordon, W.S., A. Brownlee, D.R. Wilson, and J. McLeod. The epizootiology of louping ill and tick-borne fever with observations on the control of these sheep diseases. In *Aspects of Disease Transmission by Ticks,* D.R. Arthur (ed.), pp. 1–28. Zoological Society of London. 1962.
15. Gribble, D.H. Equine ehrlichioses. *J. South Vet. Med. Ass.* 155:462–469, 1969.
16. Henning, M.W. *Animal Diseases in South Africa,* p. 879. Central News Agency, Onderstepoort, South Africa, 1949.
17. Horsfall, F.L., Jr., and I. Tamm. *Viral and Rickettsial Infections of Man,* p. 1282. 4th ed. Lippincott, Philadelphia. 1965.
18. Luoto, L. A capillary agglutination test for bovine Q fever. *J. Immunol.* 71:226–231, 1953.
19. Philip, C.B., W.J. Hadlow, and E.H. Lyndahl. Studies on salmon poisoning disease of canines. I. The rickettsial relationships and pathogenicity of Neorickettsia helmintheca. *Exp. Parasit.* 3:336–350, 1954.
20. Purchase, H.S. A simple and rapid method for demonstrating *Rickettsia ruminantium* (Cowdry, 1925) in heartwater brains. *Vet. Rec.* 36:413–414, 1945.
21. Stannard, A.A., D.H. Gribble, and R.H. Smith. Equine ehrlichiosis: A disease with similarities to tick-borne fever and bovine petechial fever. *Vet. Rec.* 84:149–150, 1969.
22. Stoenner, H.G., D.B. Lackman, and E.J. Bell. Factors affecting the growth of rickettsias of the spotted fever group in fertile hens' eggs. *J. Infec. Dis.* 110:121–128, 1962.
23. Tabert, G.C., and D.B. Lackman. The radioisotope precipitation test for study of Q fever antibodies in human and animal sera. *J. Immunol.* 94:959–965, 1965.
24. Tuomi, J. Studies in epidemiology of bovine tick-borne fever in Finland and a clinical description of field cases. *Ann. Med. Exp. Biol. Fenn.* 44(suppl. 6):1–62, 1966.
25. Tuomi, J. Experimental studies on bovine tick-borne fever. III. Immunological strain differences. *Acta Path. Microbiol. Scand.* 71:89–100, 1967.
26. Tuomi, J. Experimental studies on bovine tick-borne fever. IV. Immunofluorescent staining of the agent and demonstration of antigenic relationship between strains. *Acta Path Microbiol. Scand.* 71:101–108, 1967.

PART FOUR: MYCOLOGY

53. Aspergillus

Members of the genus *Aspergillus* are involved in several diseases of domestic animals. They are generally considered to be saprophytes whose excursions as animal pathogens are opportunistic. Numerous species of birds have been affected by the respiratory disease, avian aspergillosis.[1,6] This disease occurs in both an acute and a chronic form, often causing severe economic losses in the poultry industry. The acute form of avian aspergillosis occurs primarily in young birds and is usually fatal. The lungs and air sacs of affected birds contain discrete whitish foci of caseation; when these lesions are aerated they may develop green powdery areas where the invading fungus has sporulated. The chronic form of the disease usually involves adult birds and is characterized by the development of large consolidated areas of the lungs, liver, and other organs and by airsacculitis with fibrinocaseous plaques or by green powdery areas on the serosal surface. This disease is caused primarily by *A. fumigatus;* it is important in poultry breeding stock and occurs frequently in captive water birds, especially penguins.

A second disease associated with members of the genus *Aspergillus,* particularly *A. fumigatus,* is bovine mycotic abortion.[4] Presumably, spores from bedding, hay, and other feedstuffs become airborne and enter via the respiratory tract; the gravid uterus becomes involved following hematogenous dissemination from pulmonary foci. The disease is asymptomatic in the dam except for the act of abortion. The placenta usually possesses thickened and necrotic cotyledons. Occasionally, skin lesions are observed in the fetus.[5]

Systemic aspergillosis in mammalian species generally resembles that of adult birds.[3] Lesions occur in the lungs, liver, gut, and occasionally other organs. This infrequently reported disease is usually caused by opportunistic *A. fumigatus* infections. Aspergillosis is not considered a serious hazard to the health of laboratory personnel.

In addition to these mycoses, certain members of the genus *Aspergillus* are prominent producers of mycotoxins. For information concerning these toxins, see Chapter 66.

Specimens

Lesion materials as free from contamination as possible should be collected. Scrapings of lesion debris and exudate, as well as tissues, are placed in sterile containers for transport to the laboratory and representative portions of lesions are placed in 10% Formalin for histopathologic processing. In the case of mycotic abortion, 15–20 ml of stomach contents are collected in a sterile vial and the entire placenta (regardless of contamination by soil, manure, bedding, etc.) is placed in a plastic bag for transport to the laboratory. Tissues to be submitted to a laboratory for mycological examination should be packed in ice.

Diagnosis by direct microscopic examination is often impossible since definitive fungal elements may not be visible in the preparation. Scrapings or small pieces of lesion material can be emulsified on a glass slide in a few drops of Parker 51 (P-51) stain and placed under a coverslip for examination under medium magnification (400–500×) and reduced light. Negative or thick preparations should be placed in a moist chamber at room temperature for several hours or overnight and re-examined. This time period allows for clearing of the tissues and staining of the hyphae; fungal elements can be observed as blue-stained structures. Fetal stomach contents are centrifuged (approximately $3000 \times g$ for 10 minutes) and a portion of the sediment is used to make a P-51 preparation for microscopic examination.

Wash heavily contaminated placentas with tap water before shipping to the laboratory or before selecting materials for examination. The placentomes should be examined for exudation and necrosis, and the intercotyledonary chorioallantoic membrane should be examined for edema and thickened areas. If fetal skin lesions are observed, scrapings can be examined microscopically following staining with P-51 stain.

Hyphae of *Aspergillus* species treated with P-51 stain generally appear as blue-stained, septate, dichotomously branched structures approximately 2–4 µm in diameter with the hyphal walls generally parallel, as opposed to the contorted swollen hyphae observed in mucormycosis (see Chapter 61).

Following Formalin fixation, paraffin embedding, and sectioning, stain the tissues with H & E, which is quite useful in demonstrating most hyphal forms of *Aspergillus* species in tissues. The Gomori-Gridley stain is useful in demonstrating fungal elements that might go undetected by the H & E stain. In this procedure the fungal hyphae stain a bright-pink to deep-rose color and the tissue stains yellow. In tissue sections, the *Aspergillus* hyphae are dichotomously branched, septate, and 2–4 µm in diameter, and possess parallel walls. Other periodic acid–Schiff stains or the Gomori methenamine silver stains can also be used satisfactorily on tissue sections.

Laboratory Procedures

Cultures. A specific etiologic diagnosis requires isolation of the agent by culture for identification. After searing the surface of lesion material with a hot spatula, carefully grind aseptically excised pieces in saline solution in a Ten Broeck tissue grinder (avoid motor-driven blenders if possible). The ground tissue is streaked on the surfaces of duplicate Sabouraud's dextrose agar slants and incubated, one slant at 27 and the other at 37°C. Portions of lesion scrapings or of the sediment from fetal stomach contents are streaked directly on the surface of Sabouraud's dextrose agar slants and incubated as above. The cultures should be examined daily and portions of fungal colonies should be

Aspergillus

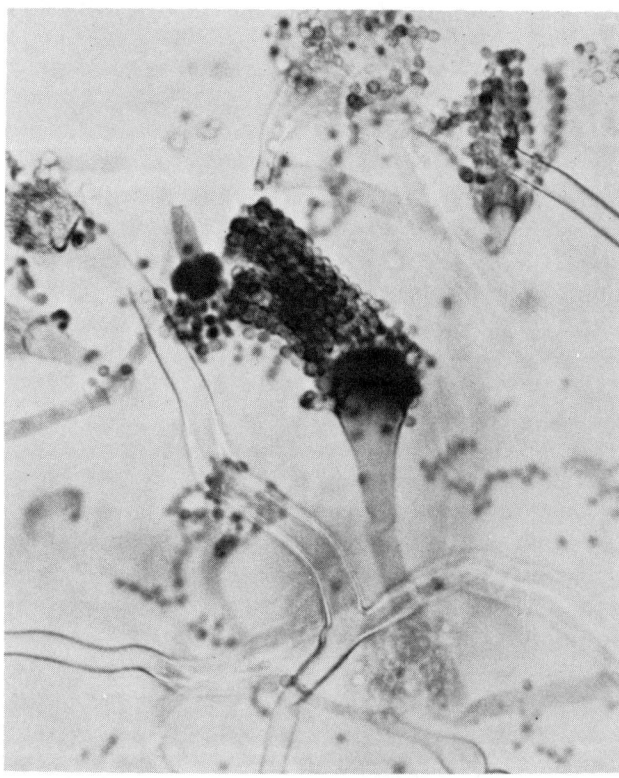

Figure 53.1. *Aspergillus fumigatus*, vesicle, single row of sterigmata and chains of conidia arising from distal pole of conidiophore. ×500.

transferred to fresh media. Subcultures of such isolates can be preserved by covering them to a depth of 2 cm with sterile mineral oil.

For light-microscopic examination of the *Aspergillus* organisms from culture, a small portion of the colony containing fruiting structures is picked aseptically and placed on a clean glass slide in a drop of suitable mounting medium such as lactophenol cotton blue. Tease the fungal elements apart, add a coverslip, and examine the preparation.

Characterization and identification. The species identity of *Aspergillus* is based on the morphology of the spore-bearing structure (conidiophore), color and morphology of the spore, and colony characteristics. However, a number of organisms that produce sexual spores also possess asexual fruiting structures comparable to the structures of *Aspergillus*. These organisms are frequently called *Aspergillus,* although they are properly classed as ascomycetes under the genera *Eurotium, Sartorya,* or *Emericella* (for example, *Aspergillus nidulans* is properly called *Eurotium nidulans*), according to the morphology of their cleistothecia.[2] Despite the Botanical Rules of Nomenclature, most investigators use the generic term *Aspergillus* for both the perfect (sexual) and imperfect (asexual) organisms and classify them largely on the basis of their imperfect structures.

Two of the more prominent members of the genus *Aspergillus* are *A. fumigatus* and *A. flavus;* the latter is a producer of mycotoxins as well as an opportunistic pathogen.

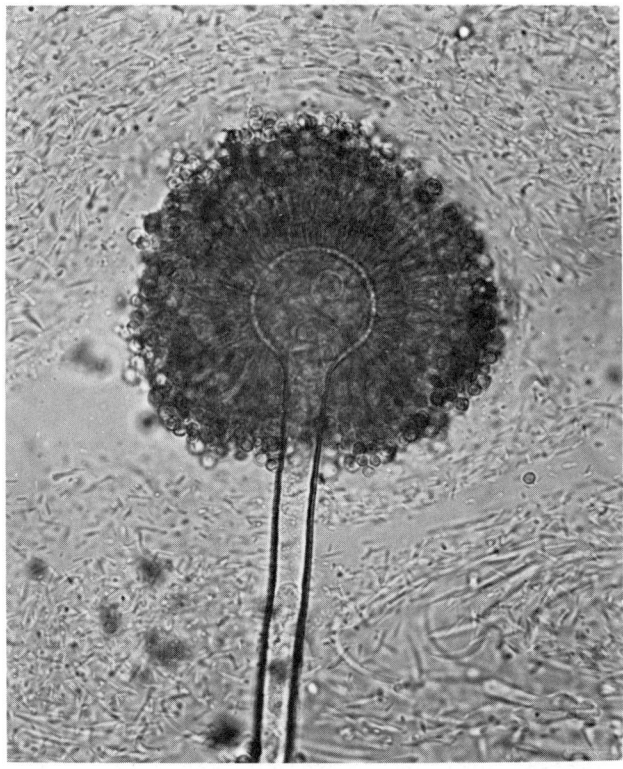

Figure 53.2. *Aspergillus flavus*, vesicle, double row of sterigmata and spores arising from all parts of the conidia. ×500.

The general morphologic and cultural characteristics of these two organisms are summarized below.

In *A. fumigatus,* conidia are blue-green to green, becoming gray-green with age. At 37°C, growth is rapid, with colonies becoming 1–2 mm in diameter in 24–48 hours. Young colonies may be entirely white but develop blue-green centers as pigmented conidia are formed. Colonies are flat, spreading, usually powdery to velvety in appearance, but may be feltlike or floccose. The reverse side of the colony is usually colorless.

Microscopically, the conidiophores are short and smooth walled, bearing a terminal flask-shaped vesicle. Conidial heads are erect, with parallel chains of conidia forming compact, well-defined columns. The vesicle is 20–30 μm in diameter with a single layer of sterigmata covering the upper half. Conidia arise from the sterigmata and are connected to form chains and a columnar mass of spores (Fig. 53.1). Usually these masses break up quite easily in making a slide preparation. The conidia are echinulate and globose and are approximately 2–3 μm in diameter. Sexual reproduction has not been described for this species.

In *Aspergillus flavus,* young white colonies develop shades of citrine yellow through various shades of green to a deep green as the pigmented conidia mature. Colonies develop best at 25–27°C, reaching a diameter of approximately 5–6 cm in 10 days. Colonies possess low-growing mycelia, often submerged, forming aerial conidiophores with

Aspergillus

conidia, giving the young colony a velvety appearance. Many isolates of this organism produce sclerotia that are globose and 1 mm in diameter, and change in color from white through brown to black with age. The reverse side of the colony is usually colorless.

Microscopically, the conidiophores are short, with coarsely roughened heavy walls. Conidial heads are erect, with radiating chains of conidia. Sometimes the radiating chains are in compact, poorly defined columns. Vesicles are globose, varying in size, but usually 25–50 μm in diameter with one or two layers of sterigmata covering the entire surface (Fig. 53.2). Conidia arise from the sterigmata, forming chains, which sometimes form loosely compacted columns. Conidia are green, usually globose, echinulate, and approximately 3–6 μm in diameter.

References

1. Ainsworth, G.C., and P.K.C. Austwick. *Fungal Diseases of Animals*. Commonwealth Agricultural Bureau, Farnham Royal, Bucks., England, 1959.
2. Alexopoulos, C.J. *Introductory Mycology*. 2d ed. Wiley, New York, 1962.
3. Austwick, P.K.C. The presence of *Aspergillus fumigatus* in the lungs of dairy cows. *Lab. Invest.* 11:1065–1072, 1962.
4. Chute, H.L. Diseases caused by fungi. In *Diseases of Poultry*, M.S. Hofstad, B.W. Calnek, C.F. Helmbolt, W.M. Reid, and H.W. Yoder, Jr. (eds.), pp. 448–462. 6th ed. Iowa State University Press, Ames, 1972.
5. Cysewski, S.J., and A.C. Pier. Mycotic abortion in ewes produced by *Aspergillus fumigatus*: Pathologic changes. *Am. J. Vet. Res.* 29:1135–1151, 1968.
6. Raper, K.B., and D.I. Fennell. *The Genus Aspergillus*. Williams and Wilkins, Baltimore, 1965.

54. Blastomyces

North American blastomycosis, caused by the fungus *Blastomyces dermatitidis*, has been reported in humans, dogs, cats, horses, and sea lions. The infection is characterized by the formation of suppurative and granulomatous lesions in any part of the body, with a predilection for the lungs and skin. The causative organism has a sexual or perfect form named *Ajellomyces dermatitidis*. This organism should be considered a serious laboratory hazard and should be handled with care. The use of cotton-stoppered slants, well-ventilated safety hoods, and culture surfaces wet with sterile saline before opening is recommended.

Signs of blastomycosis in an animal include fever, anorexia, weakness, depression, loss of weight, nasal and eye discharge, chronic cough, and dyspnea. Multiple cutaneous abscesses or tumorlike masses in the skin may be present. Chest radiographs may show lung lesions and a dense mass at the bifurcation of the trachea. The signs in any individual may vary, depending on where the organism has localized. The lungs are almost always involved, and frequently lymph nodes and the skin are too. At times, the eyes, brain, joints, and bones may also be involved.

The lungs usually show a diffuse distribution of grayish-white nodules that are firm in consistency, easily incised, and not calcified. Some lung lesions are soft with necrotic centers. The lymph nodes most commonly involved are those at or near the bifurcation of the trachea. The skin lesions in most cases are multiple cutaneous and subcutaneous abscesses. The lesions appear to start as small papules, which become pustular. The abscess contents are usually gray, thick, and mucopurulent.

Causative organisms in lesions are either found free or in macrophages, as yeastlike cells, 8–15 μm in diameter, with double-contoured walls. The yeast cells may be spherical or budding (extruding a daughter cell) (Fig. 54.1).

The suspected endemic area for blastomycosis in the United States, based on 1461 human and 376 canine cases, appears to be similar to the endemic area for histoplasmosis. The area of high incidence appears to be in the Mississippi and Ohio river basins, including the states of Louisiana, Mississippi, Arkansas, Tennessee, Kentucky, West Virginia, Illinois, and Wisconsin; and in North Carolina, a central Atlantic state.

Canine blastomycosis is most frequent in male sporting dogs or hounds under 4 years

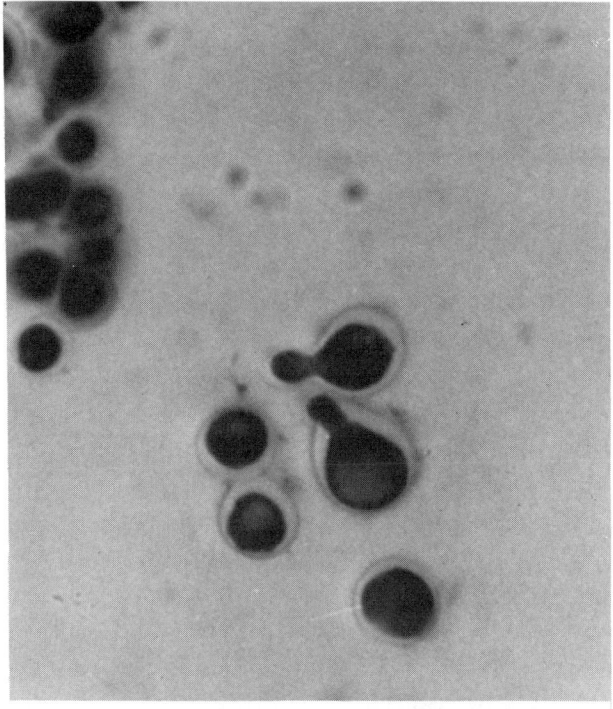

Figure 54.1. *Blastomyces dermatitidis* yeast phase cells. ×900.

of age.[8] The annual incidence for proven canine cases in Arkansas varied from 5.1 to 8.6 per 100,000. The seasonal incidence appeared to be greatest during the fall.

There has been no evidence to indicate that blastomycosis is transmitted from human to human, animal to human, or animal to animal.[10] It seems more likely that animals and humans are infected by airborne means from a common source in nature, such as soil.[3] Among canine cases studied, there was no evidence that the dog was a hazard to human health. If a dog has skin lesions, people having contact with it should take the usual precautions to prevent the introduction of the infectious pus into cuts or open sores.

Specimens

Specimens should be obtained from animals that were ill or were destroyed because of an acute or chronic pulmonary disease, and from animals with a systemic disease where the diagnosis has not been clearly established. Specimens from diseased tissues, usually lung, bronchial lymph node tissues, and skin, should be collected.

The tissues (1 cm squares or larger) can be collected in two screw-capped 50 ml jars. One jar should contain 20 ml of sterile buffered cysteine-saline solution with 25 μg of chloromycetin per ml. Portions of lung tissue and bronchial lymph nodes should be placed in this jar; these tissues are used for FA studies and culture. The second jar should contain 30 ml of 10% Formalin. Portions of involved lung tissue, enlarged bronchial or mediastinal lymph nodes, tumorlike masses, or ulcerated areas in the skin, liver, spleen, and adrenal tissues should be placed in the jar so that histopathologic studies can be done. Also, blood specimens should be collected for the serologic tests.

After preliminary diagnosis of blastomycosis based on signs and chest radiographic findings, one should attempt to isolate the fungus or demonstrate the organism in smears or tissue sections. Pus from skin lesions, draining lymph nodes, or biopsy material from enlarged prescapular or popliteal lymph nodes should be examined by making a wet mount with lactophenol cotton blue mounting fluid or KOH-ink stain. The diagnosis is confirmed if budding yeast cells 8–15 μm in diameter with a thick refractile wall are found.

Almost any tissue may be examined by using the FA technique, but lung and bronchial lymph node tissues should be examined routinely. At necropsy, two impression smears should be made of each tissue. The slides are allowed to dry and then fixed in undiluted acetone solution for 10 minutes. The direct method technique may be used with *Histoplasma* conjugate.[12] The bluish-white autofluorescence of yeast cells of *Blastomyces dermatitidis* that occurs with *Histoplasma* conjugate has proved to be satisfactory for presumptive diagnosis. Specific fluorescent antiglobulins for the detection and identification of *B. dermatitidis* yeast-phase cells have been reported and have been found reliable in the demonstration of the yeast form in clinical materials.[4] A nonadsorbed conjugate is generally used for screening clinical materials.

The histopathologic examination of biopsy or necropsy tissues may be done following staining with H & E or Bauers (periodic acid–Schiff) stains.[6] Lung, lymph node, skin, or other affected tissues should be examined routinely.

Laboratory Procedures

Cultures. Small portions (1–2 g) of each tissue (in the culture jar) are placed in a sterile mortar; sterile sand is added and the tissues are ground. Then sterile buffered cysteine-saline solution is added to make an approximate 10% suspension and the tissues are mixed well. A 0.5 ml portion of the suspension is inoculated on one slant of Sabouraud's dextrose agar containing cyclohexamide and chloramphenicol (C & C), and on two BHI blood agar slants.[2] Cultures are incubated at room temperature (25°C) and are held for at least 1 month before being discarded. Cultures can be examined by making a wet mount using lactophenol cotton blue mounting fluid.

Cellular morphology. The fungus *Blastomyces dermatitidis* occurs in tissues and on blood agar at 37°C in the yeast phase, and on Sabouraud's dextrose agar at room temperature in the mycelial or mold phase. The yeast phase is found in tissues and pus from cutaneous lesions as thick-walled spherical or budding cells 8–15 μm in diameter.

On Sabouraud's glucose agar at room temperature, the yeast phase converts to the mycelial phase. The fungus grows slowly, often in concentric waves, producing a white, cottony, aerial mycelium that becomes tan to brown with age. Microscopically, fully developed cultures show numerous oval to round conidia, 3–4 μm in diameter, attached to the hyphae near septa. Other round to pyriform conidia, 4–5 μm in diameter, are borne on lateral sterigmata of varying lengths. In old cultures, many chlamydospores 7–18 μm in diameter are developed. A mycological diagnosis is established by converting the mycelial phase to the yeast phase to demonstrate the characteristic budding yeast cells

8–15 μm in diameter. Conversion can be done with cottonseed agar medium or Kelley's medium.[5,15]

Blastomycosis caused by *B. dermatitidis* has been commonly called North American blastomycosis, but since the disease has been found outside North America, the *B. dermatitidis* form is now being called simply blastomycosis. South American blastomycosis, caused by *Paracoccidioides brasiliensis*, should be called paracoccidioidomycosis. This organism differs from *B. dermatitidis* in that the yeast form has multiple buds. Cryptococcosis, caused by *Cryptococcus neoformans*, has been called European blastomycosis. This organism, when typical, has a large capsule. Some forms of *Coccidioides immitis*, the cause of coccidioidomycosis, may be confused with *B. dermatitidis*. In tissues, *C. immitis* may be larger in size (spherules or sporangie range from 5 to 200 μm in diameter) than *B. dermatitidis*.

Animal inoculation. Mice may be inoculated IP with 1 ml of a 10% tissue suspension. After 1 month, the mice are necropsied and 0.5 ml of the combined liver and spleen tissue suspension of each mouse is cultured on the same media as used for direct culture. If hamsters are available they may be used instead of mice.

Immunology and serology. Because of clinical similarities, overlapping areas of endemicity, and antigenic cross-reaction between *Blastomyces* and *Histoplasma*, it is recommended that comparative serologic and cutaneous hypersensitivity tests employing antigens from both organisms be used. Additional comparative tests with antigens from *Coccidioides*, *Mycobacterium*, and *Nocardia* are also suggested.

Two serologic tests are commonly used for the diagnosis of blastomycosis: the AD test and the CF test.[14] Sera are tested by the AD test with undiluted blastomycin concentrated 10 times and with histoplasmin concentrated 10 times.[1,13] Precipitins appear during the early course of infection.

Sera are tested also by the CF test with a *Blastomyces dermatitidis* yeast-cell suspension and with histoplasmin and a *Histoplasma capsulatum* yeast-cell suspension.[13]

The standard or micro 50% CF methods may be used. Information concerning the serologic tests and the antigens can be obtained from the reference laboratories.

The CF tests have not been adequately evaluated for animals. For humans there are limitations in using the CF tests for the diagnosis of histoplasmosis and blastomycosis: the organisms share a common antigen, and sera from cases of chronic pulmonary histoplasmosis and blastomycosis frequently give negative CF tests. However, the percentage of false-positive CF tests is low, and the CF test yields results far more rapidly than culture methods. If cultures were used exclusively, many cases would not be diagnosed and early diagnosis would be uncommon.

A review of serologic data from human cases of chronic pulmonary histoplasmosis and blastomycosis revealed that when the homologous antigens were used, a titer of 1:32 or greater was recorded for 68% of the histoplasmosis cases, while only 9% of the blastomycosis cases had titers of this magnitude.[11] Ten percent of the histoplasmosis cases and 64% of the blastomycosis cases had negative tests. The titers were greater for the homologous antigens for 84% of the histoplasmosis cases but only for 22% of the blastomycosis cases. The best solution to the problem is to perform the CF test with antigens of both fungi and also perform the test on serial serum specimens.[14]

Blastomycin, a culture filtrate prepared from the mycelial phase of *B. dermitidis,* has been used as a skin test antigen. The blastomycin skin test has been regarded as unsatisfactory by investigators who have used the test on human patients. The test on dogs may be used as a diagnostic aid, and it has been shown to have some value as an epidemiologic tool.[9]

Animals should be skin-tested with standardized lots of blastomycin and histoplasmin at the same time.[7] The two antigens should be of equivalent potency so that the size of the two reactions can be compared. The antigens for animals must be more concentrated than those used for humans, and frequently the undiluted culture filtrate must be concentrated to be of value. Generally blastomycin is used undiluted while histoplasmin is diluted 1:10 for large animals and 1:10 to 1:1000 for dogs. Intradermal injections of 0.1 ml of each antigen are made approximately 7–8 cm apart, and reactivity in the form of induration (5 mm or greater) and erythema are assessed after 48 hours. Where reaction to both antigens occurs, the homologous reaction is considered to be the reaction with greater induration. Frequently in canine blastomycosis the reaction to blastomycin is twice the diameter of the reaction to histoplasmin.

Reference laboratories. Ecological Investigations Program, CDC, Kansas City, Kansas; Mycology Laboratory, CDC, Atlanta, Ga.

References

1. Abernathy, R.S., and D.C. Heiner. Precipitation reactions in agar in North American blastomycosis. *J. Lab. Clin. Med.* 57:604–611, 1961.
2. Ajello, L., L.K. George, W. Kaplan, and L. Kaufman. *Laboratory Manual for Medical Mycology.* Public Health Service Pub. 994. U.S. Government Printing Office, Washington, 1963.
3. Denton, J.F., and A.F. DiSalvo. Isolation of *Blastomyces dermatitidis* from natural sites at Augusta, Georgia. *Am. J. Trop. Med. Hyg.* 13:716–722, 1964.
4. Kaplan, W., and L. Kaufman. Fluorescent antiglobulins for the detection and identification of *Blastomyces dermatitidis* yeast-phase cells. *Mycopathol. Mycol. Appl.* 19:173–180, 1963.
5. Kelley, W.H. A study of the cell and colony variations of *Blastomyces dermatitidis. J. Infec. Dis.* 64:293–296, 1939.
6. Kligman, A.M., and H. Mescon. The periodic-acid–Schiff stain for the demonstration of fungi in animal tissues. *J. Bact.* 60:415–421, 1950.
7. Menges, R.W. The histoplasmin skin test in animals. *J. Am. Vet. Med. Ass.* 119:69–71, 1951.
8. Menges, R.W. Blastomycosis in animals: A review of an analysis of 116 canine cases. *Vet. Med.* 55:45–54, 1960.
9. Menges, R.W., M.L. Furcolow, L.A. Selby, H.R. Ellis, and R.T. Habermann. Clinical and epidemiologic studies on seventy-nine canine blastomycosis cases in Arkansas. *Am. J. Epidemiol.* 81:164–179, 1965.
10. Menges, R.W., R.T. Habermann, L.A. Selby, H.R. Ellis, R.F. Behlow, and C.D. Smith. A review and recent findings on histoplasmosis in animals. *Vet. Med.* 58:331–338, 366 1963.
11. Newberry, W.M., F.E. Tosh, I.L. Doto, and T.D.Y. Chin. The complement fixation antibody test in the diagnosis of chronic pulmonary histoplasmosis and blastomycosis. *J. Chronic Dis.* 20:303–309, 1967.
12. Porter, B.M., B.K. Comfort, R.W. Menges, R.T. Habermann, and C.D. Smith. Correlation of fluorescent antibody, histopathology, and culture on tissues from 372 animals examined for histoplasmosis and blastomycosis. *J. Bact.* 89:748–751, 1965.
13. Schubert, J.H., H.J. Lynch, Jr., and L. Ajello. Evaluation of the agar-plate precipitin test for histoplasmosis. *Am. Rev. Resp. Dis.* 84:845–849, 1961.
14. Turner, C., C.D. Smith, and M.L. Furcolow. The efficiency of serologic cultural methods in the detection of infection with histoplasma and blastomyces in mongrel dogs. *Sabouraudia* 10:1–5, 1972.
15. Weeks, R.J. A rapid, simplified medium for converting the mycelial phase of *Blastomyces dermatitidis* to the yeast phase. *Mycopathol. Mycol. Appl.* 22:153–156, 1964.

55. Candida

Candida are mycelial yeasts that reproduce asexually by budding (forming blastospores) and that form elongated mycelial structures; both true mycelia and pseudomycelia (elongated buds) are formed. The genus *Candida* is comprised of a relatively large number of species, several of which are of importance in veterinary medicine. *Candida albicans* is by far the most prominent pathogen of the genus, but other species—*C. guilliermondii, C. krusei, C. parapsilosis, C. pseudotropicalis, C. stellatoides* (considered by many as a variant of *C. albicans*), and *C. tropicalis*—are encountered occasionally as pathogens. *Candida* species are distributed widely in nature and have been isolated from the skin and mucous membranes of normal animals and humans, as well as from plant materials, including tree sap and fruit, and from the soil. While *Candida albicans* is a known pathogen of humans, it is not considered hazardous if handled in the laboratory with usual care.

Candidiasis (moniliasis) is an acute to chronic disease of the skin and mucous membranes; it occasionally becomes systemic. Factors that predispose an animal to infection include broad spectrum antibiotic therapy (especially involving tetracyclines), debilitating diseases, and anticancer and immunosuppressant regimes. The young are usually more susceptible than the mature. Infection occurs in the skin and mucous membranes of poultry, cattle, horses, swine, dogs, cats, and humans. Prominent disease syndromes include crop mycosis (thrush) of broiler age chickens and young turkeys, esophagitis and gastritis of young swine, bovine mastitis, and superinfection of the uterus of the cow and mare following antibiotic therapy. The disease appears as a pseudomembranous, necrotizing process with the production of a caseous exudate on the affected surface. A toxic substance, canditoxin, appears to augment the pathogenicity of *C. albicans*.

Specimens

The specimens from which *Candida* can usually be isolated are exudates from skin and mucous membranes. The upper alimentary tract of mammals and birds is a frequent source. Skin and nails are often involved, and *Candida* occurs in urinary tract infections, mastitis, and septicemia. Swabs, scrapings, urine, feces, and blood should be submitted for culture. They are treated identically to their bacteriological counterparts.

The gross appearance of a candidal exudate varies with its tissue of origin. On the mucous membranes of the mouth, esophagus, cardiac region of the stomach, and vagina, the exudate is often thick, crumbly, white and caseous. Skin and nail involvement produces dry flaky areas; acute candidiases of the skin may produce erythematous areas with vesiculation and necrotic patches on the skin surface. Exudates from mastitis and metritis are typically purulent.

Exudates are smeared on microscope slides for Gram staining or mixed with 10% KOH for the preparation of wet mounts. The latter are preferable when the specimen contains much keratinized material as in skin and nail scrapings and when an abundance of microorganisms is expected. Gram-stained smears are more helpful when sparsely populated specimens are examined. Because *Candida* is normally present in the environment and on the skin and mucous membranes, care must be taken in assessing the significance of these organisms in clinical specimens. The caseous exudates from skin and mucous membranes usually team with budding yeast cells and mycelial or pseudomycelial elements. Mastitis and metritis exudates are often sparsely populated with definitive forms, among which blastospores predominate. These are oval and approximately 2×5 μm in size; the pseudomycelial elements are substantially longer. All forms are strongly gram-positive.

Specimens taken for histopathology should be cut with care so as not to dislodge the surface exudates; Formalin fixation and staining of sections with Gridley's fungal stain or Brown and Brenn's Gram stain is satisfactory.

Laboratory Procedures

Cultures. When fluid specimens such as milk, urine, and uterine exudate are cultured, concentration by centrifugation—consistency permitting—is advisable. *Candida* grows well on blood agar or Sabouraud's agar; selective media such as Sabouraud's with C & C can be used for isolating it from contaminated specimens. Either room temperature or 37°C is satisfactory for the propagation of *Candida*. The organisms grow under ordinary atmospheric conditions or increased carbon dioxide tension. No growth occurs in an anaerobic environment.

Preservation of *Candida* cultures can be accomplished for 6 months or longer by refrigeration on Sabouraud's dextrose agar slants covered with plastic caps. More permanent preservation is obtained by lyophilization of a skim milk suspension of the culture or the immersion of its surface under sterile mineral oil and storage at room temperature.

Candida grown on blood agar plates produced gray to white, raised, glistening colonies within 48 hours incubation at 37°C; the consistency is soft and creamy. A similar type of growth appears on Sabouraud's dextrose agar where a dense, white, raised creamy growth appears within 48 hours at either 37°C or room temperature.

Differential reactions. Metabolic criteria used for specific identification of *Candida* species include fermentative reactions in beef extract broth that contains 1% glucose, lactose, maltose, or sucrose, plus bromthymol blue indicator. Sugar fermentation tests are incubated for 10 days at 37°C and observed for production of acid and gas. Reactions typical of *C. albicans* and five other species that have been associated with animal diseases are given in Table 55.1.

Candida

Table 55.1. Sugar fermentation and sugar assimilation reactions of Candida

	Fermentation			
	Glucose	Lactose	Maltose	Sucrose
C. albicans	AG	–	AG	±A
C. guilliermondii	±A	–	–	±AG
C. krusei	AG	–	–	–
C. parapsilosis	AG or A	–	±A	±A
C. pseudotropicalis	AG	AG	–	AG
C. tropicalis	AG	–	AG	AG

	Assimilation				
	Glucose	Lactose	Maltose	Sucrose	Raffinose
C. albicans	+	–	+	+	–
C. guilliermondii	+	–	+	+	+
C. krusei	+	–	–	–	–
C. parapsilosis	+	–	+	+	–
C. pseudotropicalis	+	+	–	+	+
C. stellatoides	+	–	+	–	–
C. tropicalis	+	–	+	+	–

A, acid; G, gas; ±, variable reaction.

In addition to sugar fermentation reactions, it is often necessary to test the sugar assimilation ability of *Candida* cultures. The assimilation test is conducted by providing a source of selected sugars (10% solutions of glucose, lactose, maltose, sucrose, and raffinose) at intervals on the surface of a pour plate of the isolate; five equidistant spots of sugar crystals can be placed on a plate (see Auxanographic Technique in Appendix A). The test is observed for the appearance of halos of growth about the sugar source after incubation at room temperature for 24–72 hours (Table 55.1). In both the fermentation tests and the assimilation test it is absolutely necessary to have a pure culture and one that has been depleted of stored sugars. For these reasons the isolated strain should be passed three times on beef extract agar before being used in the above tests.

Among a large number of tests proposed for the presumptive identification of *C. albicans* is a useful and quick procedure involving germ tube formation in a serum medium. Cultures from Sabouraud's dextrose or potato dextrose agar are inoculated into tubes of sterile bovine or human serum. After 1–2 hours incubation at 37°C, the oval yeast cells of *C. albicans* cells produce distinct cylindrical outgrowths or germ tubes.

The pathogenic yeasts can be differentiated by growth characteristics on cornmeal infusion agar plus 1% Tween 80. This enhances the formation of a pseudomycelium (*Candida*), a mycelium (*Geotrichum* and *Trichosporon*), and chlamydospores. Some yeasts do not produce a mycelium (*Cryptococcus*). The presence or absence of blastospores and arthrospores also helps in the determination (Fig. 55.1).

Cellular morphology. The blastospores of *C. albicans* are oval and approximately 2×5 μm; the pseudomycelial elements are substantially longer. All forms are strongly gram-positive. There are several rapid presumptive screening tests to differentiate *C. albicans* from other *Candida* species.

Morphologic features are determined on cut-streak–inoculated cornmeal agar–coated slide cultures. Clusters of blastospores and chlamydospores usually appear in 5–7 days when *C. albicans* preparations are incubated at room temperature. The morphologic fea-

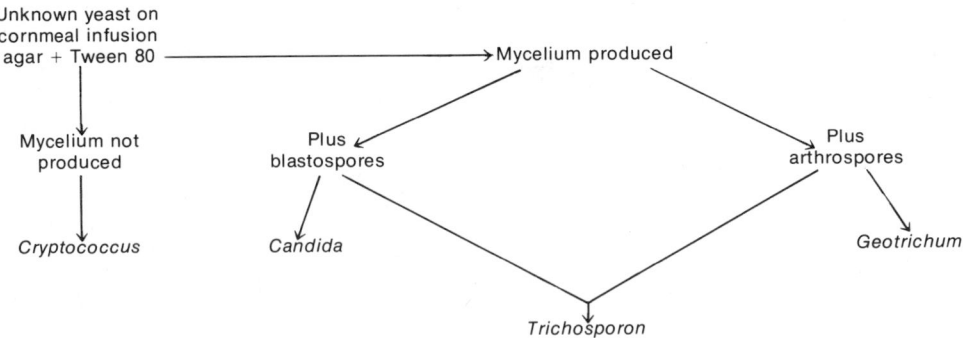

Figure 55.1. Differentiation of pathogenic yeasts. *Cryptococcus neoformans* has growth at 37 and 25°C, capsule formation, animal pathogenicity, and nitrate assimilation and is urease positive. *Candida* has a pseudomycelium and blastospores.

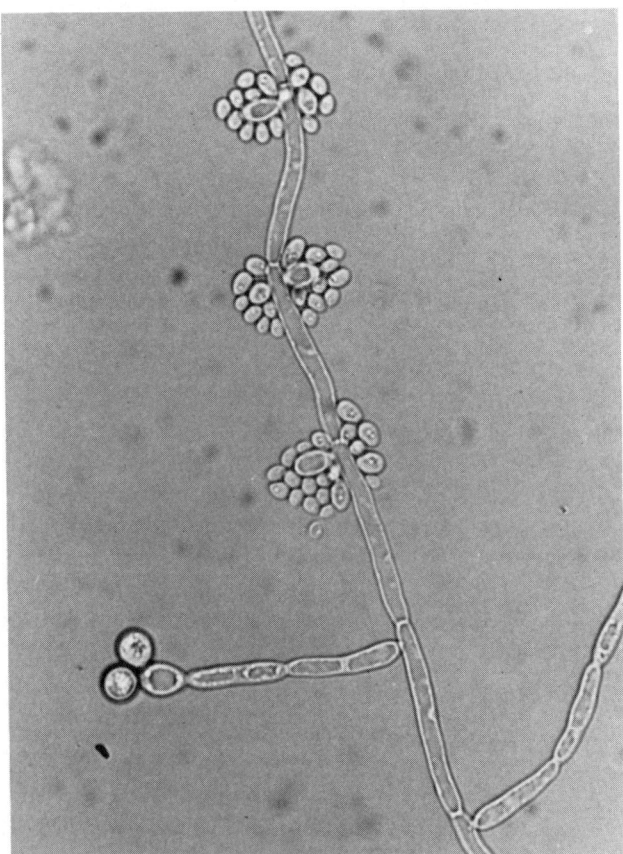

Figure 55.2. *Candida albicans* pseudomycelia with clusters of blastospores at septa and terminal chlamydospores. ×500. (Reprinted by permission from I.A. Merchant and R.A. Packer, *Veterinary Bacteriology and Virology,* 7th ed., Iowa State University Press, Ames, 1967.)

Table 55.2. Morphologic features of *Candida* on cornmeal agar

- *C. albicans:* 2–5 µm oval budding blastospores located in spherical clusters at septa of pseudomycelium. Chlamydospores, 8–15 µm with thick walls, found on terminal mycelial projection after incubation at 25°C.
- *C. guilliermondii:* 2–3 µm budding blastospores in small spherical clusters at septa of fine pseudomycelium.
- *C. krusei:* Elongate pseudomycelial elements forming crosses at septa.
- *C. parapsilosis:* Mixed fine and giant mycelial strands. Blastospores singly or in short chains at septa.
- *C. pseudotropicalis:* Elongate pseudomycelial elements that readily disorient from tandem to parallel association.
- *C. stellatoides:* Similar to *C. albicans*.
- *C. tropicalis:* Blastospores randomly distributed along mycelium or in irregular clusters. Chlamydospores can be seen infrequently.

tures of *C. albicans* and six other *Candida* species are summarized in Table 55.2. The demonstration of chlamydospores as well as typical configurations of blastospores and pseudomycelia is necessary to the identification of *C. albicans* (Fig. 55.2).

Animal inoculation. Although rabbits can be infected fatally with IV injection of *C. albicans,* animal inoculation is not used in the identification of *C. albicans* or other *Candida* species.

Immunology and serology. Serologic procedures are not used widely to detect infection by *Candida,* since agglutinins are present in the sera of a high percentage of normal individuals. *Candida* antigens have been used as a skin test for immunologic competence in humans. The FA test has been applied to diagnosis of candidiasis but is not used widely and lacks definite specificity. No specific toxins useful for identification have been recognized, but an antigenic substance, canditoxin, has been associated with pathogenicity in *C. alibicans.*

Reference laboratory. Mycology Unit, CDC.

References

1. Ajello, L., L.K. Georg, W. Kaplan, and L. Kaufman. *Laboratory Manual for Medical Mycology.* 2d ed. U.S. Department of Health, Education and Welfare, Atlanta, Ga., 1962.
2. Winner, H.I., and R. Hurley. *Candida Infection.* E. & S. Livingstone, London, 1966.

56. Coccidioides

The pathogenic fungus *Coccidioides immitis* is dimorphic; it has one form (spherule) when living in tissue and another (mold) when in its free-living state in soil (or on most culture media). Its presence in soil is geographically restricted to certain regions of low rainfall and high mean annual temperature. Such desert areas are found in parts of California, Arizona, New Mexico, Texas, Nevada, and Utah. Mexico and South America also contain infective foci. Spontaneous infection of animals having no history of residence in an endemic area is unlikely.

Coccidioides has a potential for infecting any mammal. Dogs, cattle, and humans are affected in greatest numbers, but the disease has occurred spontaneously in other domestic species and in a variety of zoo and wild animals including rodents. Between 5 and 20% of cattle from southern Arizona feedlots have coccidioidal lesions at slaughter,[7] but the bovine disease is benign, and lesions can be trimmed off with little or no loss of carcass value; up to 45% of dogs and approximately 90% of human residents of endemic areas show evidence of infection.

Human infection rates are highest during the summer, but the disease develops in dogs at a higher rate during the cool months of the year. Animals of all ages are susceptible, but the disease tends to affect the young more seriously. Males of several species are less resistant than females. Negro and Filipino people more commonly develop serious disease, and this is also true of the boxer breed of dogs.

Most coccidioidal infections are incurred by inhalation of airborne arthrospores. Infection via wounds is rare and difficult to prove. Clinical diagnosis of the disease is uncommon in animals other than the dog. Canine coccidioidomycosis may begin with nonspecific signs, such as fever, poor or intermittent appetite, weight loss, diarrhea, and coughing.[9] Uncomplicated primary infections often resolve themselves before a diagnosis is established. Among dogs or other animals that are unable to contain the disease, the organism may spread to and cause lesions in nearly any organ in the body. Granulomatous lesions of the lungs and associated lymph nodes are frequently encountered during meat inspection of cattle, sheep, and swine from endemic areas; such lesions must be differentiated from those caused by mycobacterial infection.

At necropsy of disseminated cases, granulomas may be observed in nearly all tissues,

Coccidioides

except those of the gastrointestinal tract and female reproductive tract; bone lesions occur frequently in the dog. Liquid exudate may be plentiful in pleural, pericardial, and sometimes abdominal cavities.

Specimens

There are only two types of specimens to consider in identifying *Coccidioides* in lesions: affected tissue and exudate. Sinuses draining infected bones or joints, lymph nodes, and skin are most likely to yield samples for culture identification of the fungus. Exudate from sinuses and cerebrospinal fluid may be aspirated or otherwise collected in sterile vials for microbiological examination. Biopsy specimens or postmortem specimens should be divided in two, one portion preserved in 10% Formalin, the other placed in a sterile container for culture. The lesions of coccidioidomycosis resemble those of several other fungal and bacterial processes; dignosis can be accomplished by microscopic demonstration of typical mature spherules in tissue sections or wet mounts or by culture identification.

For culturing exudates, generous amounts (up to 30 ml) are preferred, but it is often possible to culture the fungus from a cotton swab soaked with exudate. Occasionally, antibiotic-treated sputum, bronchial aspirates, gastric washings, or feces may yield the organism upon culture or animal inoculation. Unfixed tissues and exudates for microbiological use keep well for a day or two at 4°C and can be shipped with an ice can, but if the material must be held for a longer time, it should br frozen with dry ice. Special care should be taken to prevent leakage from specimens containing viable organisms; they should be sealed in a metal can that is in turn protected by a mailing tube. The parasitic form of *C. immitis* will produce infections if inoculated via cuts or punctures. Use care and wear gloves. Also, leaked specimens, if allowed to dry, may permit growth and sporulation and therefore constitute a serious health hazard. Fixed tissues should be wrapped in Formalin-soaked gauze, sealed in a plastic bag, and packaged.

For serologic testing, 5 ml of clear Merthiolated serum (1:10,000) collected from a fasted patient should be submitted.

Heat-fixed and stained smears prepared from coccidioidal lesions are of no value. Wet mounts under a coverslip provide the best means for preliminary evaluation. Exudates may be examined undiluted or after dilution in saline followed by centrifugation. Scrapings from lesions may be dispersed in a drop of water, 10% KOH, or lactophenol cotton blue solution. The operator should learn to distinguish between spherules and fat droplets, air bubbles, and large mononuclear phagocytes. The objective of the search is the doubly contoured, nonbudding, tissue-phase spherule containing endospores measuring between 20 and 200 μm. If simpler methods are unsuccessful, there is an FA method that provides specific identification of *Coccidioides* in smears and may be resorted to.[6]

Capable pathologists experience little difficulty in identifying *Coccidioides* in tissue sections stained routinely with H & E. Even where organisms are scarce, the characteristic granulomatous tissue reaction provides stimulus for careful search. Three special stains are of great assistance.[2] The Gomori methenamine silver method stains most fungi brown to black, providing enough contrast that organisms are easily located in sections. Cellular detail is usually obscured, but size, shape, and the presence of buds and endospores can be evaluated. The PAS stain provides good contrast without obscuring cell morphology, and the usual counterstain also permits good visualization of the accompanying tissue reactions. Another common and useful method is the Gridley fungus stain. Control slides should always be included with diagnostic sections as a check on stain efficacy. Search for fungus elements in tissue must be reasonably diligent.

Laboratory Procedures

Cultures. Uncontaminated specimens require no special preparation and may be transferred directly to Sabouraud's dextrose agar by standard methods. Contaminated clinical specimens can be inoculated on media containing C & C. Specimens so heavily contaminated that overgrowth occurs on selective media may be pretreated by the addition of 1000–10,000 units of penicillin and 1000 units of streptomycin to each ml of specimen, followed by incubation at 37°C for an hour before inoculation. This method is used for treating all soil specimens from which isolation of *Coccidioides* is being attempted.

Exudate is usually diluted to an appropriate volume (1 ml for IP injections in mice) and used without treatment for animal inoculation, but contaminated specimens (e.g. soil) should be pretreated with penicillin and streptomycin (P & S).

To assure maximum opportunity for isolation, numerous tubes of media should be inoculated, especially if wet-mount search of exudate or lesion scrapings has been unsuccessful. Transfer of cultures is easily handled by cutting a square of agar bearing mycelia and transporting this to fresh media with a wire loop. Arthrospore inoculum can be prepared by wetting the culture with sterile physiological saline, agitating with a loop, and aspirating the fluid suspension with a syringe and needle.

Mature cultures of *C. immitis* form spores that readily aerosolize and constitute a severe laboratory hazard. It is strongly recommended that suspect cultures be handled under a properly ventilated safety hood. Flooding culture slants by injecting sterile saline through the cotton stopper before opening the culture tube minimizes aerosolization.

Sabouraud's dextrose agar is the basic medium for culturing *C. immitis*. Two other media are useful, one for the inhibition of saprophytic fungi[4] and the other to provide more voluminous growth over shorter periods of incubation for antigen production. The first medium is Sabouraud's dextrose agar with C & C added. The second medium, commonly referred to as glucose-yeast extract (GYE) agar, consists of 2% glucose, 1% yeast extract, and 1.5 or 2% agar. GYE broth (agar omitted) is the medium used for coccidioidin production by the toluene lysis method.

Medical mycologists usually recommend either 25 or 30°C for incubation; however, room temperature is satisfactory, and the ordinary incubator temperature (37°C) has no inhibiting effect. Test tube slants of solid media with cotton closures are recommended and are safer than petri dishes. Be very cautious when opening culture tubes; use a microbiological safety hood. Liquid cultures for antigen production are agitated during incubation. Various rates of gentle reciprocation or rotation have been used, but violent shaking that might lead to breakage of containers must be avoided.

Test tube cultures will keep for many months if sealed or flooded with sterile mineral oil to retard dessication of the medium. Inoculation of sporulated cultures into dry sterile soil has permitted recovery of the organism after 4 years without subculture and transfer; spores have survived much longer this way than in lyophilized preparations. In addition, lyophilization of *C. immitis* creates hazardous aerosols. In contrast to simple maintenance, the preservation of either arthrospores or sperules at a high level of viability for any length of time is much more difficult.

Cultures may be killed with 0.5% Formalin. The various coccidioidins used as antigens are preserved after filtration by the addition of 1:1000 aqueous Merthiolate to a final concentration of 1:10,000.

Unless affected by high (above 1 mg/ml) levels of cyclohexamide in the medium, *Coccidioides* produces visible colonies on solid media within 3–4 days. Arthrospores form at 4–7 or more days, although colonies continue to grow and sporulate vigorously for a much longer time. Very early growth is moist and membranous, but characteristic cottony-white aerial mycelia appear promptly afterward and spread to form a white mat that often has a patchy or moth-eaten appearance. The back side of most colonies soon turns yellow to brown and the mycelium also colors with age. Numerous variations in appearance have been described.[3]

Differential reactions. Only one species, *Coccidioides immitis,* is recognized. Identification is based on recognition of typical parasitic and saprophytic phase morphology in tissues, smears, and cultures, on animal inoculation, and on serologic tests. The colony and the arthrospores of *C. immitis* in mold form may superficially resemble those of *Geotrichum* sp.; morphologic differentiation is made by the fact that the arthrospore chains of *Geotrichum* are not intermittent, blank spaces do not occur between the spores, the spores of *Geotrichum* are often much longer than wide, and the free spore does not have tabs of blank hyphae attached, as do *Coccidioides* spores. If confusion still exists, *Coccidioides* is readily differentiated from *Geotrichum* by animal inoculation; *C. immitis* will produce spherules in tissue while *Geotrichum* will not.

Cellular morphology. *C. immitis* is a dimorphic fungus; it has separate mold and tissue forms. The vegetative colony (mold form) is composed of a branched septate mycelium. Short intermittent chains of spores are formed when alternate segments of terminal hyphae form thick-walled, somewhat biconvex arthrospores (2.4×5 μm) that separate easily, leaving tags of the empty segments attached to the individual spore (Fig. 56.1). When inhaled or otherwise introduced into the tissues of a susceptible animal, arthrospores and nonsporulated mycelial segments round up to form the parasitic (tissue form) spherule. By progressive enlargment (20–80 and up to 200 μm) and progressive cytoplasmic cleavage, the maturing spherule becomes filled with endospores 2–5 μm in diameter (Fig. 56.1). Mature endospores develop directly into spherules, often doing so while still enclosed by the capsule of the parent sporangium (spherule). *Coccidioides* spherules do not form buds; a false impression of budding is sometimes created by the side-by-side development of spherules from endospores or from still-attached neighboring arthrospores.

Animal inoculation. Saline suspensions of minced tissue, exudates, or soil suspensions pretreated as indicated are injected into the peritoneal cavity of young laboratory mice. After 4 weeks mice are killed and examined for gross lesions, from which wet mounts and tissue sections are prepared. If the inoculum contained only a few organisms

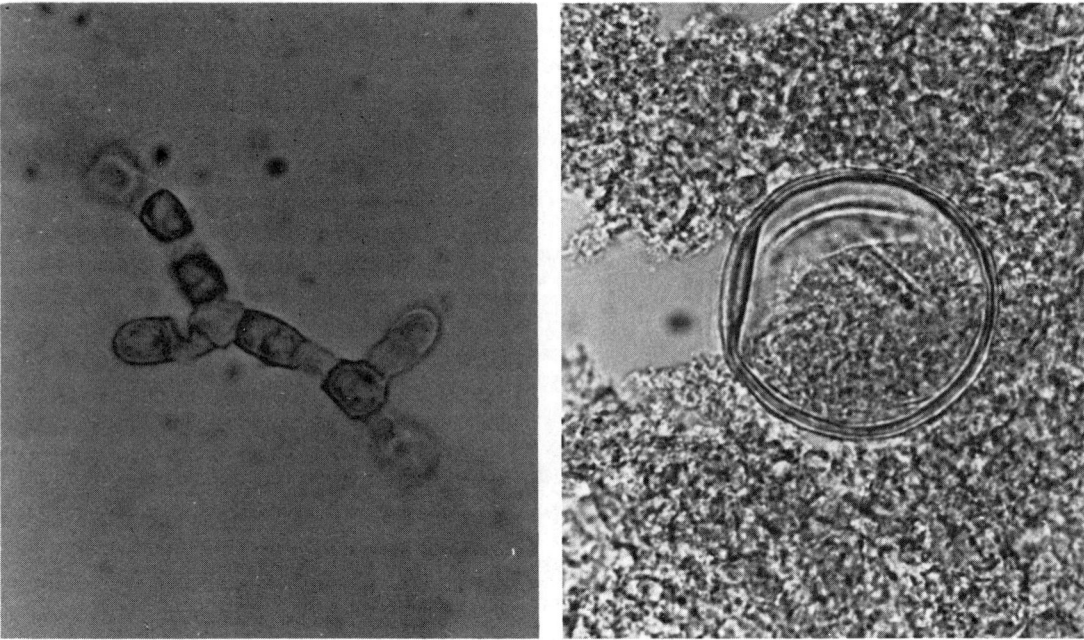

Figure 56.1. *Coccidioides immitis:* left, intermittent chain of arthrospores of mold form ×900; right, spherule in exudate ×2! (Reprinted by permission from I.A. Merchant and R.A. Packer, *Veterinary Bacteriology and Virology,* 7th ed., Iowa Sta University Press, Ames, 1967.)

of a relatively avirulent strain, gross lesions may not be apparent, but in this case the liver and spleen should be minced and inoculated on media.

Mice inoculated IP with a highly virulent strain or a large number of viable fungus particles will lead to the formation of lesions in thoracic and other tissues. These may be preserved by freezing for the preparation of FA control slides, laboratory demonstration materials, and so forth.[6]

Culture identification is greatly facilitated by animal inoculation in the production and recognition of the characteristic parasitic phase. Culture tubes are wet with sterile saline and opened with extreme caution. A fragment of the mycelium is recovered for microscopic examination. If fungus morphology is characteristic (keep in mind the wide variation possible in growth and sporulation characteristics), the fungus mat is then disturbed with the inoculation loop to loosen arthrospores and hyphal fragments. A suspension of this material is aspirated with a hypodermic syringe and injected IP into mice in 1 ml amounts, usually four mice per culture. Needles should be changed after aspiration and between each injection to avoid creating superficial lesions. Take care to avoid spraying droplets into the air or contaminating the animals' hair. Intratesticular inoculation of guinea pigs has been recommended as a relatively quick means of producing abscesses containing spherules.

The NAMRU strain of mouse is considerably more suceptible than most ordinary commercial stock. Young animals are are preferred, as a degree of resistance develops with age. Pathogenicity of *Coccicioides* for mice is mediated by strain virulence, dose, and route of inoculation. Most mice will survive a 4-week holding period after IP inoculation, but many die if inoculated by IN or IV routes.

Immunology and serology. Previous or current infection of sufficient duration leads to a delayed hypersensitive reaction when properly prepared and standardized culture filtrate (coccidioidin) is injected ID. Coccidioidin is usually prepared in asparagine medium,[11] but products of the toluene lysis method are also active.[8] Animals are seldom sensitive to diluted coccidioidin. Tests with cattle or dogs are performed by injecting 0.1 ml of undiluted coccidioidin into the dermis and checking for induration at 24 and 48 hours in dogs and at 96 hours in cattle. The clipped neck area, inside the flank fold, and inside the ear are test sites that have been used. Reactions 5 mm or more in diameter are considered positive. Cross-reaction in patients infected by other systemic fungi must be considered, but coccidioidin is quite specific. It is less likely to evoke a confusing reaction in a histoplasmosis patient than is histoplasmin in a coccidioidomycosis or blastomycosis patient. Differentiation is often possible after the injection of a battery of two or more test antigens (e.g. coccidioidin, histoplasmin, etc.) at the same time in different sites. Generally, the reaction to the specific antigen is largest. A negative test may indicate that the animal has not been exposed, that exposure is so recent that dermal sensitivity has not developed, or that the animal is so seriously affected that it is anergic. An initial negative test followed by conversion to positive on a subsequent test provides good diagnostic evidence of recent infection. Tests must be performed with care and be properly interpreted.

The CF test is a standard diagnostic aid in coccidioidomycosis although results often vary widely between different laboratories; evaluation is best made by those familiar with this problem. The CF test antigen is coccidioidin, either prepared in asparagine medium, by the toluene lysis technique, or with a neopeptone dialysate medium.[1] The quantitative Kolmer CF test with overnight incubation at 4°C is recommended. CF antibody titers provide the most convincing evidence of infection short of fungus identification. Although moderate titers may persist for years in a clinically recovered animal, the test is seldom performed unless there is strong physical evidence of active infection. A dog with a titer of 1:32 to 1:64 on initial testing may be considered seriously affected and in danger of disseminating the disease, if this has not already occurred. Increase in titer on successive tests indicates increasingly serious disease, while a drop in titer signals recovery unless it is obvious that there is no physical improvement, in which case it may indicate developing anergy.

The tube precipitin test is useful in the early stages of coccidioidal infection.[10] The precipitin antibody appears earlier in the course of infection than CF antibody but also disappears earlier. Coccidioidin (0.2 ml) from a batch that has been shown to have precipitin reactivity is combined in undiluted, 1:10, and 1:40 dilutions with 0.2 ml of clear undiluted serum and incubated at 37°C in 7×70 mm test tubes. Tubes are examined daily for 5 days by attempting to spin a button of precipitate off the bottom of the tube. An AD test has been developed that with appropriate antigens will yield results comparable to the standard CF and tube precipitin tests.[5] A latex particle slide test for precipitin antibody is available commercially (Hyland Division, Travenol Lab., Los

Angeles). The production of toxin by *Coccidioides* has yet to be conclusively established.

Reference laboratories. Mycology Laboratory, CDC; Department of Animal Pathology, College of Agriculture, University of Arizona, Tucson; Diagnostic Services, NADC.

References

1. Ajello, L., K. Walls, J.C. Moore, and R. Falcone. Rapid production of complement fixation antigens for systemic mycotic diseases. *J. Bact.* 77:753–756, 1959.
2. Ambrogi, L.P. *Manual of Histologic and Special Staining Technics.* 2d ed. U.S. Armed Forces Institute of Pathology. McGraw-Hill, Blakiston Div., New York, 1960.
3. Friedman, L., D. Pappagianis, R.J. Berman, and C.E. Smith. Studies on *Coccidioides immitis:* Morphology and sporulation capacity of forty-seven strains. *J. Lab. Clin. Med.* 42:439–444, 1953.
4. Georg, L.K., L. Ajello, and M.A. Gordon. A selective medium for the isolation of *Coccidioides immitis. Science* 114:387–389, 1951.
5. Huppert, M., J.W. Bailey, and P. Chitjian. Immunodiffusion as a substitute for complement fixation and tube precipitin tests in coccidioidomycosis. In *Coccidioidomycosis,* L. Ajello (ed.). University of Arizona Press, Tucson, 1967.
6. Kaplan, W., and M.K. Clifford. Production of fluorescent antibody reagents specific for the tissue form of *Coccidioides immitis. Am. Rev. Resp. Dis.* 89:651–658, 1964.
7. Maddy, K.T. Coccidioidomycosis in animals. *Vet. Med.* 54:233–242, 1959.
8. Pappagianis, D., C.E. Smith, M.T. Saito, and G.S. Kobayashi. Preparation and property of a complement fixing antigen from mycelia of *Coccidioides immitis.* In *Proceedings of a Symposium on Coccidioidomycosis.* U.S. Public Health Service Pub. No. 575, 1957.
9. Reed, R.D. Diagnosis of disseminated canine coccidioidomycosis. *J. Am. Vet. Med. Ass.* 128:196–201, 1956.
10. Smith, C.E., M.T. Saito, and S.A. Simons. Pattern of 39,500 serologic tests in coccidioidomycosis. *J. Am. Vet. Med. Ass.* 160:546–552, 1956.
11. Smith, C.E., E.G. Whiting, E.E. Baker, H.G. Rosenberger, R.R. Beard, and M.T. Saito. The use of coccidioidin. *Am. Rev. Tuberc.* 57:330–360, 1948.

57. Cryptococcus

Cryptococcus neoformans is a common cause of infection in humans, particularly of the CNS and lungs, and is also well recognized as a disease agent in lower animals.[1,8] It causes cryptococcosis, which is also known as torulosis, torula meningitis, European blastomycosis, and Busse-Buschke's disease. Host reports in the literature concern mastitis in cattle and central nervous infections in cats, but from the wide variety of hosts reported it is apparent that no mammal can be considered insusceptible. The disease in cats is predominantly seen in mature animals, 5 years or older.[13] The disease in all these animals most often originates as a subacute or chronic infection of the nasal passages, mouth, or lungs, causing granulomatous lesions, abscesses, or tumorous, often myxomalike, masses, and of the CNS, where it gives rise to meningitis or to cystic or granulomatous lesions of the brain. It may become generalized, affecting lymph nodes, kidneys, liver, skin (usually with subcutaneous granulomatous swellings), and other organs. Lesions have eroded the bones in some instances. In reported cases of mastitis the infection involved only the mammary glands and their lymph nodes.

C. neoformans and cryptococcosis are of worldwide prevalence.[6] The microorganism seems almost ubiquitous in the environment (although it is doubtful that it occurs on or in the normal human or animal body), especially in dust containing much organic matter.[12] It has been isolated from (nonpasteurized) cows' milk, the juice of peaches, soil, certain plants, and notoriously from pigeon droppings, but also in droppings of other birds. The usual route of infection is by inhalation of yeast-laden dust, but some facial lesions of cats may be a result of primary cutaneous inoculations.

C. neoformans does not constitute a major health hazard to laboratory personnel so long as ordinary precautions are observed. Mouth pipetting and flaming of unrinsed loops should be avoided.

Specimens

Specimens include CSF, tracheobronchial washings, urine, blood, pus and other exudates, and biopsy tissue. Relatively voluminous and dilute specimens, such as CSF and urine, should be centrifuged (10 minutes at $1500 \times g$) in order to concentrate yeast cells in the sediment, which can then be used for direct examination and culture (save the supernatant fluid for serology!) Pus should be aspirated if possible; specimens from granulomatous ulcers should be obtained by swabbing the edges.[4]

Blood serum, CSF, and urine should be examined serologically for evidence of cryptococcal capsular polysaccharide antigen, and serum also for anticryptococcal antibody. Samples should be drawn preceding specific therapy as well as at relatively frequent intervals (1 week) thereafter, since a single pretreatment specimen may provide a presumptive diagnosis, and since changes in titer are closely related to the prognosis.

Grossly, clues may be provided by the sometimes mucoid or gelatinous aspect of granulomatous lesions or, in case of mastitis, stringiness of the exudate. Affected organs often have a slimy appearance, with tissue structure distorted by the presence of a jellylike substance.

Direct microscopic examination of clinical specimens is, as with other mycoses, extremely important in suspected cryptococcosis. A wet India-ink mount is the classic and preferred method for demonstrating the encapsulated yeastlike cells in CSF and other fluids, and in squash preparations of tissues such as those of the brain. A stain that is applicable in wet mounts is lactophenol cotton blue. In any of these materials the fungus appears as spherical to ovoid, usually single-budding, moderately thick-walled, yeastlike cells, mostly 4–7 μm in diameter, surrounded by very wide gelatinous capsules. Care must be taken to distinguish *C. neoformans* from "encapsulated" artifacts, which occur especially in spinal fluid. The latter are generally irregular in size or lack the sharply outlined cell wall, and the border of the "capsule" is not well-defined.

Specimens for histopathology may be fixed and embedded in the usual manner. Impression films of freshly cut, unfixed tissue may also be used. The H & E is usually adequate to demonstrate cryptococci, which may occur free, singly, or in gelatinous masses, or within giant cells. The purple-staining cell walls are surrounded by the unstained capsule. In granulomatous lesions, small intracellular forms of *C. neoformans* in giants cells or histiocytes may resemble *Histoplasma capsulatum,* and certain forms resemble *Blastomyces dermatitidis,* which, however, buds on a broad base and has no capsule. Excellent special strains for *Cryptococcus* are the Grocott-Gomori silver methenamine technique, the Gridley fungus stain, and mucicarmine, which helps differentiate this organism from nonencapsulated pathogenic yeasts by staining the inner portion of the capsule as well as the cell wall. In stained sections the normally spherical cells of *C. neoformans* often appear punched-in or football-shaped.

Lesions of the skin, subcutaneous tissues, or bone show either a mass of yeastlike cells with chronic inflammation and numerous giant cells, or no cellular reaction. In the brain there may be tumorlike masses of fungi with or without much cellular reaction, or a chronic inflammatory reaction with giant cells and scar tissue and many other types of cells, including macrophages, lymphocytes, and eosinophils.

Laboratory Procedures

Cultures. Voluminous liquid specimens should be concentrated by centrifugation. If the specimen is heavily contaminated, for example, when taken from an open cutaneous or mucosal lesion, enrichment by incubation with antibiotics, preceding inoculation of isolation media, is advisable. Inoculate all tubes or plates in duplicate. Use routine mycological culture media: (1) Sabouraud dextrose agar (the antibiotics chloramphenicol, 1 mg/ml, or P & S may be added to Sabouraud's medium to inhibit contaminants but do *not* add cycloheximide, to which *C. neoformans* is relatively sensitive); (2) a beef infusion–blood agar. A tube of beef infusion–peptone broth, in addition, may yield growth where only a few microorganisms are present. A specific and valuable selective-differential medium for this organism, especially useful for heavily contaminated specimens, is nigerseed-creatine agar with diphenyl.[11]

Incubate two tubes or plates of medium 1 and 2 above, aerobically, at each of the two recommended temperatures, i.e. "room temperature" (22–27°C) and 35–37°C. Colonies generally appear within 2–4 days, but primary media should be held at least 2 weeks before results are considered negative. Most strains of *C. neoformans* will grow to some extent at temperatures as low as 4°C and as high as 41°C.

Specimens should be cultured as soon as possible. If inoculation of media is delayed, specimens should be kept refrigerated. Stock cultures are readily preserved on agar slants under refrigeration, and may be kept indefinitely (at least 12 years) at room temperature under sterile mineral oil. Most strains of *C. neoformans* are killed by exposure to 60°C for 10 minutes or 2% Formalin for 18 hours (in either case, they retain their antigenicity). Cultures are also killed by contact for 15 minutes with any of the following common disinfectants: Zephiran 10%, hydrogen peroxide 3%, ethyl alcohol 70 and 95%, and normal sodium hydroxide.[10]

Colonies are convex, smooth, characteristically mucoid but sometimes pasty, and white to cream, often becoming tan. (*Rhodotorula*, a genus which is very rarely involved in animal infection, and then as a terminal invader, produces red, pink, or orange colonies and consists of ovoid to spherical, budding, yeastlike cells.)

Differential reactions. Table 57.1 summarizes the reactions that are useful in the identification of *C. neoformans*.

Table 57.1. Reactions that are useful for identifying *C. neoformans*

Morphology: budding yeast cells 4–7 µm; no mycelium produced.

Growth at 25 and 37°C	+
Urease positive	+
Animal pathogenicity	+
Capsule formation	+
Nitrate assimilation	+

Cellular morphology. The cells of *C. neoformans* in culture are similar to those seen on direct examination, being spherical to ovoid, variably encapsulated, gram-positive, nonacid-fast, and mostly 4–7 µm in diameter but ranging from 2 to 15 µm or more. Reproduction is by budding on a narrow isthmus, generally singly, occasionally in short chains. There are no spores or flagella. Mycelia are rarely formed, but sometimes short filaments resembling either germ tubes or pseudohyphae are seen in young nonmucoid colonies on primary isolation. In old cultures, bizarre thick-walled cells often occur. The size of the capsule, best visualized in India ink mounts, varies among strains in vitro, although all strains form large capsules in vivo. The diameter of the encapsulated organism may be three times that of the naked cell, or it may be only slightly greater. Certain nonpathogenic species of *Cryptococcus* are indistinguishable morphologically from *C. neoformans*.

Animal inoculation. *C. neoformans* is the only species of cryptococcus known to be pathogenic for laboratory mice when inoculated IC by the following procedure, and this trait will confirm identification of the species. An approximate 1:500 (wet, packed cell volume) suspension of cells from a 2–3-day-old culture on Sabouraud dextrose agar is made in physiological saline. By means of a 26-gauge needle with a 0.25 in (6–7 mm) shank, 0.02–0.04 ml of this suspension is injected in the posterior quandrant of the brain, lateral to the median line, of each of four 18–20 g mice. Death occurs usually in from 7 to 10 days, often sooner, and is preceded by marked swelling of the cranium. The latter sign is an indication for the researcher to sacrifice the animal. If death or cranial enlargement has not intervened, two mice are sacrificed after 2 weeks and the remainder 2 weeks later. The top of the skull is excised and affected areas of the brain, usually soft and gelatinous, are examined by means of squash preparations of India ink for presence of encapsulated yeastlike cells, which confirm the pathogenicity. As an alternative to the preferred IC method, 0.5 ml of a 1:100 suspension may be administered IP, with death and/or brain lesions ensuing in 2–3 weeks. Gelatinous masses may be found in the abdominal cavity and lungs, as well as the brain.

As an alternative, or supplement, to mouse inoculation, isolates may be tested for their ability to assimilate certain substrates. The information obtained is called an auxanogram (see Appendix A for directions).

Immunology and serology. Skin tests with cell wall antigen (not commercially available) are positive in most active human cases but also in many with no known cryptococcal infection, possibly on account of past exposure.[9]

At least four serologic types of capsular antigen (A, B, C, and D) have been distinguished, but typing is not diagnostically or therapeutically useful, and the epidemiology of cryptococcosis is just beginning to be explored. Blood serum and CSF (the supernatant fluid of a centrifuged specimen is sufficient) of suspect animals may be tested for the presence of polysaccharide antigen, which indicates active infection, by means of the latex slide agglutination test with antibody-coated particles, in which antigen titer correlates with severity of infection.[3,5] An alternative procedure is the CF test for antigen.[2] The FA test also may be used.[7] In non-CNS human cases, in very early stages of CNS infection, and in amphotericin B–treated cases, serum antigen is usually absent or diminished in titer, and antibody may then often be detected by means of an agglutination test using whole killed yeast cells as antigen.

Reference laboratories. New York State Department of Health, Albany; CDC; NADC. Serologic tests for cryptococcosis are performed by the last two laboratories. Specimens are accepted by the CDC laboratory only through referral by state health department laboratories.

References

1. Barron, C.N. Cryptococcosis in animals. *J. Am. Vet. Med. Ass.* 127:125–132, 1955.
2. Bennett, J.E., H.F. Hasenclever, and B.S. Tynes. Detection of cryptococcal polysaccharide in serum and spinal fluid: Value in diagnosis and prognosis. *Trans. Ass. Am. Physicians* 77:145–150, 1964.

3. Bloomfield, N., M.A. Gordon, and D.F. Elmendorf, Jr. Detection of *Cryptococcus neoformans* antigen in body fluids by latex particle agglutination. *Proc. Soc. Exp. Biol. Med.* 114:64–67, 1963.
4. Conant, N.F., D.T. Smith, R.D. Baker, J.L. Callaway, and D.S. Martin. *Manual of Clinical Mycology.* 2d ed. Saunders, Philadelphia, 1954.
5. Gordon, M.A., and D.K. Vedder. Serologic tests in diagnosis and prognosis of cryptococcosis. *J. Am. Med. Ass.* 197:961–967, 1966.
6. Littman, M.L., and L.E. Zimmerman. *Cryptococcosis.* Grune and Stratton, New York, 1956.
7. Marshall, J.K., L. Iverson, W.C. Eveland, and A. Kase. Application and limitations of the fluorescent antibody stain in the specific diagnosis of cryptococcosis. *Lab. Invest.* 10:719–728, 1961.
8. Merchant, I.A., and R.A. Packer. *Veterinary Bacteriology and Virology.* 7th ed. Iowa State University Press, Ames, 1967.
9. Muchmore, H.G., F.G. Felton, E.R. Rhoades, and S.B. Salvin. Delayed skin hypersensitivity in man with a new cryptococcus antigen. *Am. Rev. Resp. Dis.* 90:310, 1964.
10. Simon, J. *In vitro* inhibition of mixed strains of *Cryptococcus neoformans* isolated from cattle. *Am. J. Vet. Res.* 16:394–396, 1955.
11. Staib, F., and H.P.R. Seeliger. Zur selektivzuchtung von *Cryptococcus neoformans. Mykosen* 11:267–272, 1968.
12. Swatek, F.E., J.W. Wilson, and D.T. Omieczynski. Direct plate isolation method for *Cryptococcus neoformans* from the soil. *Mycopathol. Mycol. Appl.* 32:129–140, 1967.
13. Wilkinson, G.T. *Diseases of the Cat.* Pergamon, Oxford, 1966.

58. Dermatophytes

The dermatophytes or ringworm fungi are among the oldest known agents of infectious disease.[1] They are also the only fungal pathogens of domestic animals that are truly contagious.[1] Seven species of dermatophytes are commonly associated with skin lesions in domestic animals: *Microsporum canis,* the *M. gypseum* complex, *M. nanum,*

Table 58.1. Features of the main dermatophytes of domestic animals

Imperfect state	Main hosts*	Identifying characteristics	Perfect state	Vitamins required
Microsporum canis	Cat, dog (horse, pig, cow, sheep, donkey)	Macroconidia	*Nannizzia* sp.	Unknown
M. gallinae	Chicken (pig, dog)	Colony morph., especially pigmentation; micromorph.	Unknown	Unknown
M. gypseum complex	Dog, horse, cat, pig, donkey, cow, chicken	Macroconidia; spore mating to form perfect state	*N. incurvata* and *N. gypsea*† for *sensu lato;*‡ *N. fulva* for *M. fulvum*	Unknown
M. nanum	Pig (cow)	Macroconidia	*N. obtusa*	Unknown
Trichophyton equinum	Horse (dog)	Colony morph.; microconidia	Unknown	Nicotinic acid needed except var. *autotrophicum* found in Australia and New Zealand
T. mentagrophytes	Dog, cat, horse, cow, sheep, pig, chicken, goat, donkey	Colony morph.; microconidia of var. *quinckeanum*	*A. benhamiae*	Unknown
T. verrucosum	Cow (horse, pig, donkey, cat, sheep, dog, goat, chicken)	Slow growth; improved at 37°C; colony morph.; chlamydospores	Unknown	All strains need thiamine, some need inositol

*Parentheses mean that the animal is susceptible but not the main host.
†As yet, *Nannizzia incurvata* and *N. gypsea* have only been reported from cats and dogs.
‡The *sensu lato* var. of *M. gypseum.*

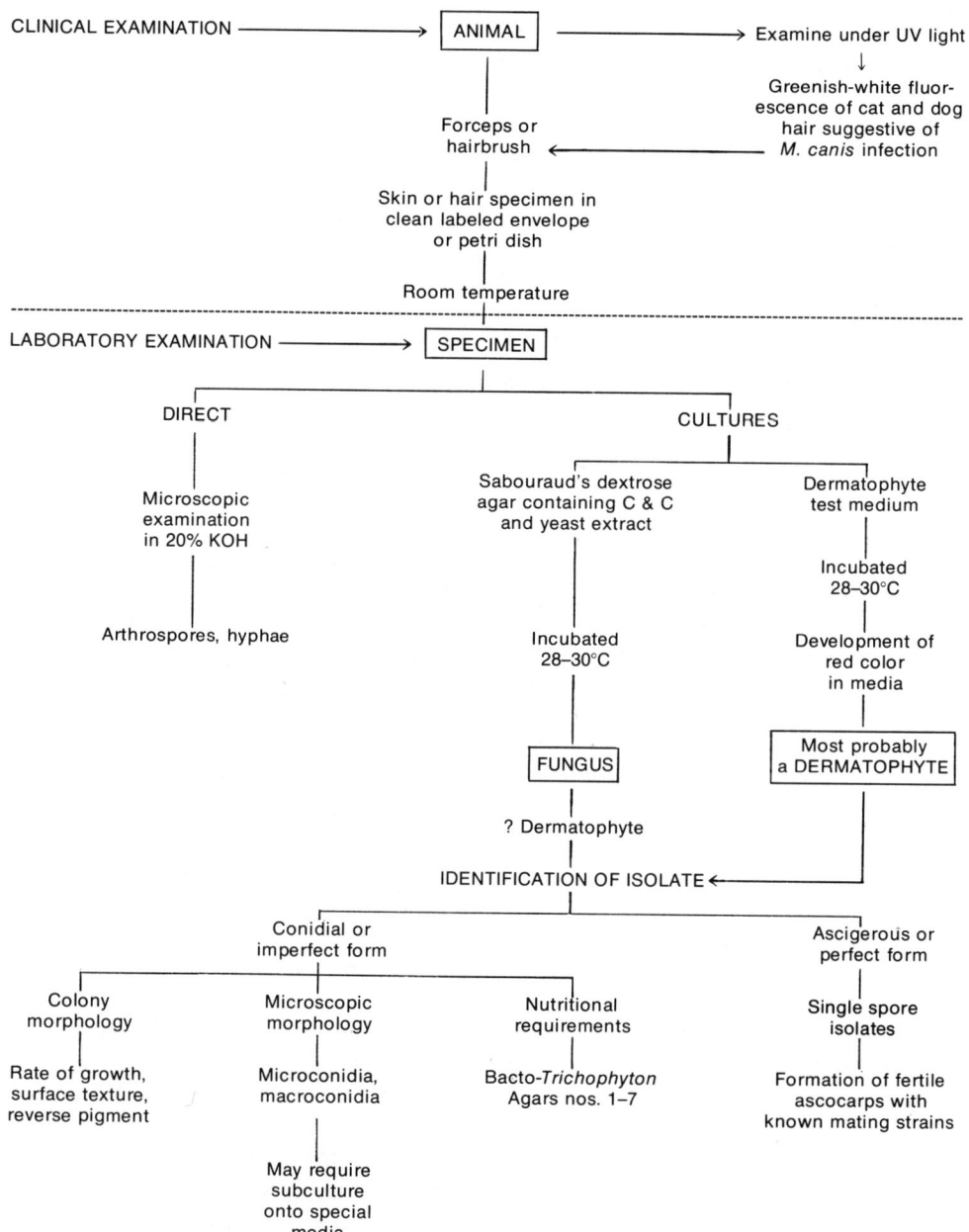

Figure 58.1. Methods for examining suspect ringworms

M. gallinae, Trichophyton mentagrophytes, T. equinum, and *T. verrucosum.*[39] The main features of these fungi are shown in Table 58.1, and a summary of the methods employed in the collection and examination of clinical materials is given in Figure 58.1.

Specimens

Animals should be examined for areas of hair loss, erythema, scaling, or thick crusts. Lesions are usually circular and are most frequently seen on the head of the animal near the eyes, nose, or mouth.[24] Occasionally the infection is more widespread, and then it often involves the friction areas (saddle and harness area in horses, neck in cattle).[39]

Specimens of hair plus skin are plucked from lesions using a pair of forceps. With small animals, lesions may be inconspicuous or consist of faint areas of scaling and hair loss. In such cases examination under a UV light in a darkened room may help in the detection of infected areas (see below under *M. canis*). When dealing with large animals, thick crusts should be removed and specimens taken from the borders of the lesions. Small bits of crusts (containing infected hairs) should be obtained for study from as many areas or lesions as practical. Until isolation techniques are attempted, all specimens should be kept dry in a clean labeled envelope or in a petri dish at room temperature.

Scrapings should *never* be placed in closed containers such as screw-topped tubes or jars. In such a container the specimens remain moist and contaminating bacteria and saprophytic fungi will grow on the hairs and skin scrapings, thus making the isolation of pathogenic fungi more difficult. Spores of dermatophytes are resistant to drying and will remain viable in a specimen for many months. It is advisable to accompany specimens with data concerning the species and age of the animal, the location and character of the lesions, and any evidence of human contagion.[12]

The "hairbrush" technique developed by Mackenzie is particularly suitable for sampling large areas of the body of animals in which no apparent lesions occur.[30] A sterilized brush (toothbrush for small animals, hairbrush for larger animals) is stroked over the entire coat of the suspect animal and then sealed in a clean paper bag. On arrival at the laboratory, the brush is removed from the bag and the bristles pressed directly into a plate of Sabouraud's dextrose agar containing antibiotics and yeast extract. If the researcher taps on the brush, any skin or hair fragments adhering to the bristles are dropped onto the agar surface. After removal of the brush, the skin or hair fragments can, if necessary, be partially pushed into the agar with sterile forceps.[30] The plate is then incubated at 30°C in the usual manner.

In most cases, confirmation of a dermatophyte infection can be made by the demonstration of characteristic fungal elements in a wet mount of the lesion scrapings. Hair stubs or hairs that show small grayish-white collars at their base are most apt to be infected. A clump of hairs or some of the skin scrapings are placed in a drop of 10–20% KOH on a clean glass slide. A coverslip is added and the slide gently heated (do not boil) over a Bunsen burner or microscope lamp. A blue ink colorant (KOH-ink stain) may be added to the KOH to facilitate demonstration of the fungal elements in clinical specimens. After a few minutes the slide is placed between two sheets of blotting paper, and if one gently pushes down on the coverslip, excess KOH is removed. This also

Dermatophytes

squashes out the preparation to a certain extent. The preparation is then examined under the low and high dry powers of the microscope (with the light reduced) for the presence of fungal elements. Fungal hyphae and arthrospores should be visible in the skin and along the hair shafts.

Laboratory Procedures

Cultures. Sabouraud's dextrose agar (2% agar) at pH 5.6 is the standard medium used for the isolation of the ringworm fungi from clinical materials. This medium is available in powdered form from several commercial sources. However, for the isolation of fungi from heavily contaminated sources such as animal hair and skin scrapings, best results are obtained by the inclusion of C & C (0.5 mg/ml of each) and yeast extract (0.3%). In this highly selective medium the chloramphenicol (chloromycetin) inhibits the growth of most contaminating bacteria; the cycloheximide (actidione) suppresses the growth of many saprophytic fungi; the yeast extract provides additional vitamins, particularly of the B complex, which are essential for the growth of some of the more fastidious dermatophytes. The characteristics of the ringworm fungi are not changed by these antibiotics but their isolation is greatly facilitated.

Plates of media are more satisfactory than tubed slopes. A 9 mm petri dish should contain at least 25–30 ml of medium. After pouring, the plates are dried at 37°C overnight before use. The advantages of plates are: a number of specimens from one animal can be placed on a single plate; saprophytic contaminants can be cut from the plate as they appear; and the resulting dermatophyte growth can be viewed microscopically for the development of characteristic conidia while still on the plate. (The term aleuriospore can be used in place of conidium.) Initial isolations should not be attempted on tubed slopes and certainly not on slopes in tightly screw-topped containers.

Inoculations are made by placing small clumps of hair or skin scrapings (using sterile forceps) on the surface of the medium. These are pushed partially into the agar. The inoculated medium is incubated at 28–30°C. A feathery fernlike fringe of radiating hyphae will be visible around the inoculum within 2–6 days depending on the species concerned. After 7–10 days, the fungal growth is usually well advanced and suitable for subculturing onto other media. Inoculated media that do not show growth should be incubated for 21 days before being discarded as negative.

On Sabouraud's dextrose agar, most colonies rapidly become pleomorphic and the characteristic conidial and pigment production is lost. For this reason many additional media have been formulated for the investigation of microscopic and macroscopic features of dermatophyte growth. Of these media, the most useful are potato dextrose agar and lab-lemco agar. On potato dextrose agar, aerial growth and pigmentation are reduced but characteristic conidia are produced in abundance. On lab-lemco agar, pigmentation is marked although again aerial growth is limited. Subculture onto these two media is only necessary when isolates cannot be identified satisfactorily on the primary isolation medium.

Recently a new culture medium, dermatophyte test medium or DTM, has been devised for the simplified diagnosis of dermatophyte infection.[45] Isolation results can be evaluated by a color change in an indicator incorporated in the medium. The color change (yellow to red) relies on the fact that during growth dermatophytes and some other fungi produce a rise in pH of the medium. Most saprophytic contaminants tend to lower the pH and do not change the yellow color of the medium. A positive (red) color reaction is only presumptive evidence that a dermatophyte is present. Specific identification of dermatophyte isolants, which is important to prediction of the source of infection, must be accomplished by microscopic examination of culture material and nutritional tests.

Microscopic preparations to show conidia are easily made with transparent "sticky" tape. Common stationery mending tapes can be used (e.g. Scotch tape, Sellotape, etc.). To make a slide, tear off about 8 cm of tape and clasp each end between the thumb and forefinger. The middle portion of the sticky side of the tape is then gently touched onto the colony with one thumb. With *Microsporum* colonies, samples should be obtained from the central area, while with *Trichophyton* cultures the tape should be touched onto the colony more toward the periphery. The tape is then pressed sticky side down on a slide with a drop of lactophenol cotton blue stain and examined microscopically. The tape selectively removes branches of aerial hyphae bearing conidia and avoids the taxonomically unimportant vegetative hyphae.

Several satisfactory methods are available for the maintenance of dermatophyte stock cultures. The simplest technique is the storage of cultures in baskets or racks at room temperature. However, drying of the plates with accompanying death of the culture is fairly rapid, and to maintain stocks, subcultures must be made every 3–4 weeks. Even cultures kept at 5–10°C in the refrigerator or cold room slowly dry out and must be subcultured every 6–10 weeks. Cotton-stoppered tubed slopes may remain viable for longer times than plates and if kept in the cold room may need subculturing only every 4 months. However, with constant subculturing most dermatophytes become pleomorphic and lose many of their characteristic microscopic and macroscopic features.

Several methods have been developed for the maintenance and survival of fungal cultures without the need for subculturing every 3–4 months, but most of these procedures have some disadvantages with certain groups of fungi. Such methods include lyophilization (only of use with freely sporulating fungi and it also creates potentially dangerous aerosols), freezing ($-20°C$ or slightly lower), the use of a mineral oil overlay, the use of feathers as substrate, or simply the use of distilled water as a maintenance medium. With dermatophytes, the most satisfactory method of long-term conservation is Al-Doory's modification of Castellani's water method.[7] Here hyphae/spores are scraped off the surface of an actively growing culture and suspended in 10–15 ml of sterile distilled water containing small pieces (1–2 cm long) of autoclaved horse hair.[7] After shaking, the tubes are incubated at around 25°C for a week or so and then left at room temperature. Viability without pleomorphism appears to be maintained for at least 3 years with most species of *Microsporum, Trichophyton,* and *Epidermophyton.*[7]

Microsporum canis

Microsporum canis is the most common cause of ringworm in cats and dogs. Other domestic animals from which the fungus has been isolated are horses, pigs, and sheep. *M. canis* has also been recovered from lesions in a variety of wild animals, of which monkeys and members of the cat genus (*Felis*) are most important. This zoophilic fungus appears to have worldwide distribution, although it is uncommon in equatorial Africa, Central Europe, and Eastern Asia. It is frequently transmitted to humans.[12,22,31,39]

Although *M. canis* was first isolated from dogs, it is apparently much more common in cats. In the United States, *M. canis* is responsible for about 98% of ringworm in cats and 66% in dogs.[24] Young animals are infected most frequently. Infections in dogs have a well-defined seasonal incidence with a peak in the fall and winter (October to February), but the incidence in cats is poorly defined.[24] There is, however, some evidence that many of the cat infections occur in autumn. These facts may indicate that temperature and humidity and other environmental factors play an important part in the spread of *M. canis* infections. Purebred Persian and Siamese appear more prone to ringworm infection than other breeds or common cats.[39]

The clinical manifestations of *M. canis* infection in cats are often inconspicuous, and attention may first be drawn to an infected animal by the development of lesions in a human contact.[12] The absence of clinical signs of infection is particularly common in cats 1 year old and older.[25] Kittens exhibit lesions more frequently and these vary from mild, noninflammatory, scaly, bare patches showing broken hairs to a more inflammatory reaction leading to crust formation. The face, ears, and paws are sites usually affected and infection of the claws has been seen. In severe cases, there may be a more generalized infection with scaling and hair loss on several parts of the body. Infected hairs can remain viable at room temperature for over 300 days. The fact that infected hairs may show a characteristic greenish fluorescence under long-wave UV light (Wood's light) has greatly facilitated the diagnosis of infection in apparently normal animals. The fluorescence is associated with a metabolite produced in the hair by the invading fungal elements. Among the dermatophyte infections of veterinary importance, only *M. canis* causes fluorescence under UV light; serum, ointments, and so forth may result in false fluorescence. Fluorescence may be used as a guide to select hairs, scales, and so on for cultural or microscopic examination.

In the dog, as in the cat, infections may be perceptible only with the aid of the UV light. More commonly, however, definite lesions are visible. These vary from clearly defined areas of scaling to discrete circular areas with hair loss and peripheral vesiculation. Broken hair stumps may be visible within the lesion, especially towards the edge. In severe cases, thick crusts may be formed or the infection may be generalized, with scaling, erythema, and loss of hair over widespread areas.

In *M. canis* infections, the hair is covered with a sheath of very small spores. These spores are 2–3 μm in diameter and usually cannot be seen clearly unless examined under the high power of the microscope. The spores (arthrospores) are packed together tightly in a mosaic over the surface of the hair, but if they are dislodged, branching mycelial filaments may be visible in the interior of the hair (Fig. 58.2A, B).

Growth characteristics. In the following paragraphs details of colonial and microscopic characteristics of ringworm fungi refer to growth on Sabouraud's dextrose agar plates containing yeast extract (with or without C & C) incubated at 30°C unless specifically stated otherwise.

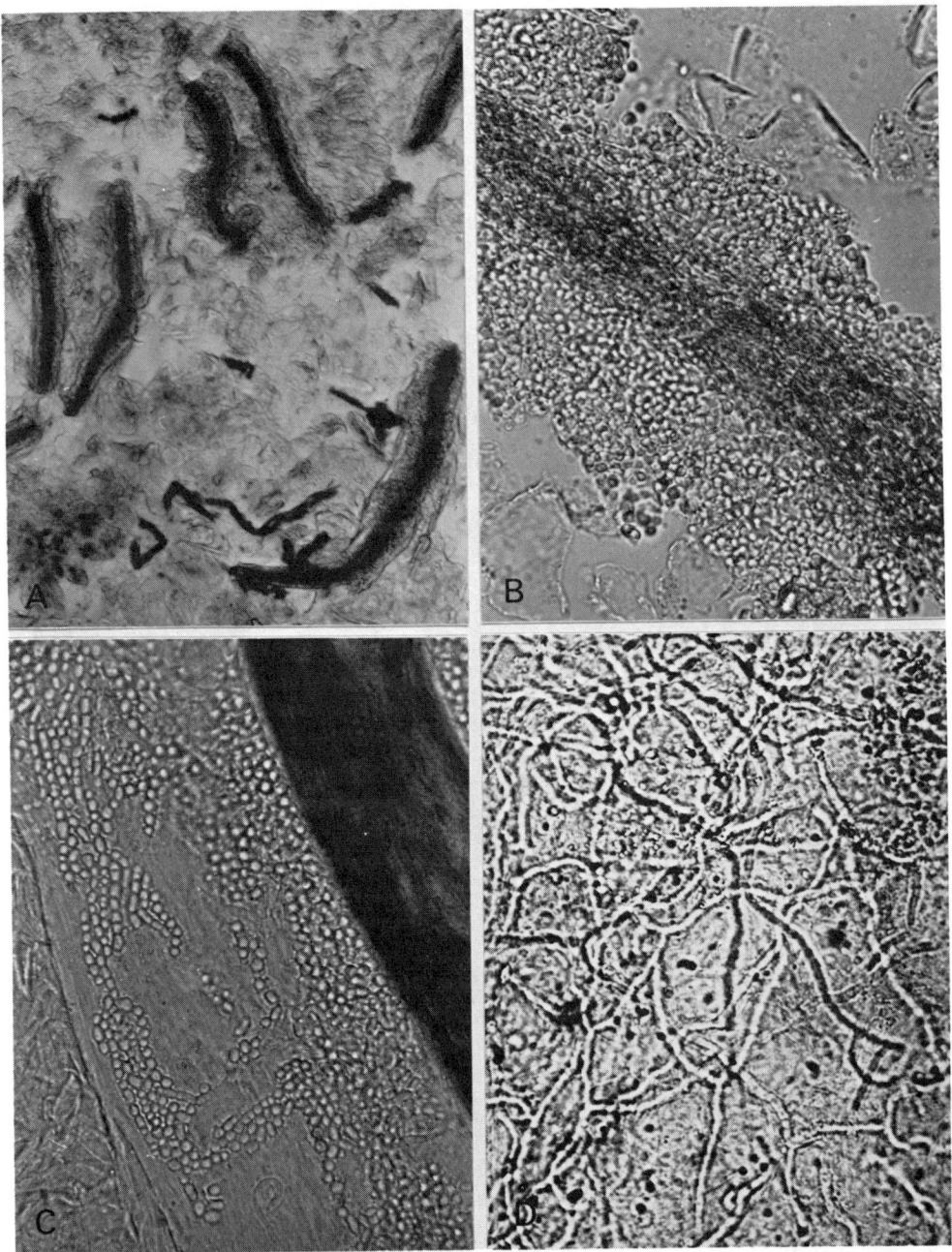

Figure 58.2. Dermatophyte parasitic morphology (KOH preparations). A, *M. canis* cat lesion. Note hair stubs surrounded by a mosaic of arthrospores, which are difficult to discern at this low magnification. ×30 approx. B, high power of A. The mosaic of spores surrounding the hair can be clearly seen. ×335 approx. C, *T. verrucosum*-infected cow hair. The preparation has been squashed slightly to reveal the chains of arthrospores surrounding the hair. ×300 approx. D, *M. nanum* hyphae in pig skin scales. ×400 approx.

M. canis colonies first appear as a flat, waxy, thin, strongly radiating growth. A buff, granular to downy area gradually develops at the center where macroconidia are formed. A yellowish pigment may be present in the peripheral area. Continued incubation results in the production of patches of dense, fluffy, whitish to pale buff, aerial mycelium that eventually grow over the whole colony (Fig. 58.3A). The colony reverse usually is pigmented amber to orange, the pigment becoming dull in older cultures. Some isolates have little or no reverse pigmentation and dysgonic strains also occur. The latter are slow growing, waxy, and brownish, and are usually confined to a very small area around the hair stump. These are not stable, however, and on subculture usually give rise to more typical *M. canis* colonies. On potato dextrose agar, the pigment of the colony reverse is lemon-yellow.

Differential reactions. *M. canis* has no special vitamin requirement.[15] The rapid production of typical fusiform macroconidia on potato dextrose agar or rice grains allows the differentiation of *M. canis* from the closely related anthropophilic *Microsporum audouinii* and zoophilic *Microsporum distortum*. *M. audouinii* grows very poorly on rice while *M. distortum* typically produces highly distorted macroconidia (Fig. 58.4B).

British and European writers distinguish *M. canis* isolates taken from horses as a separate species, *Microsporum equinum*. However, the production of colonies with a pinkish grooved surface and of macroconidia that are smaller in size than those of *M. canis* is not considered by American authors sufficient to warrant separation as a distinct species. As the perfect state of *M. canis* (*Nannizzia* sp.) has now been found, this argument should soon be clarified.[20]

Cellular morphology. In culture, thick-walled, multiseptate, spindle-shaped, spiny (echinulate) or rough-walled macroconidia (macroaleuriospores) are usually abundant at the center of the colony (Fig. 58.4A). Ends of the macroconidia remain narrow and relatively thin walled. Microconidia are rarely seen on Sabouraud's dextrose agar; when they occur they are smooth walled and clavate and are borne along the sides of the hyphae. Production of conidia is enhanced on potato dextrose agar or on cooked polished rice; both media are useful in the identification of strains that show no or poor conidial formation on Sabouraud's dextrose agar.

Microsporum gypseum

Microsporum gypseum is the name now used for the imperfect (conidial) state of *Nannizzia gypsea* and *Nannizzia incurvata*.[42] A closely related species *Microsporum fulvum* (imperfect state of *Nannizzia fulva*) will be included in this section as previous literature does not permit separations of *M. fulvum* from the commoner *M. gypseum* forms.[19]

M. gypseum infections in both animals and humans have been recorded only sporadically in the literature. Domestic animals that have been found infected include dogs, horses, cats, pigs, a donkey, and a chicken.[34] The fungus has also been recovered from the hair of a wide variety of apparently normal small wild animals. *M. gypseum* has a worldwide distribution in the soil (particularly in warmer areas) where it exists as a free-living agent. It is from this geophilic habitat that most animal infections occur. In the United States, *M. gypseum* causes 24% of the ringworm in dogs and 1% of the ring-

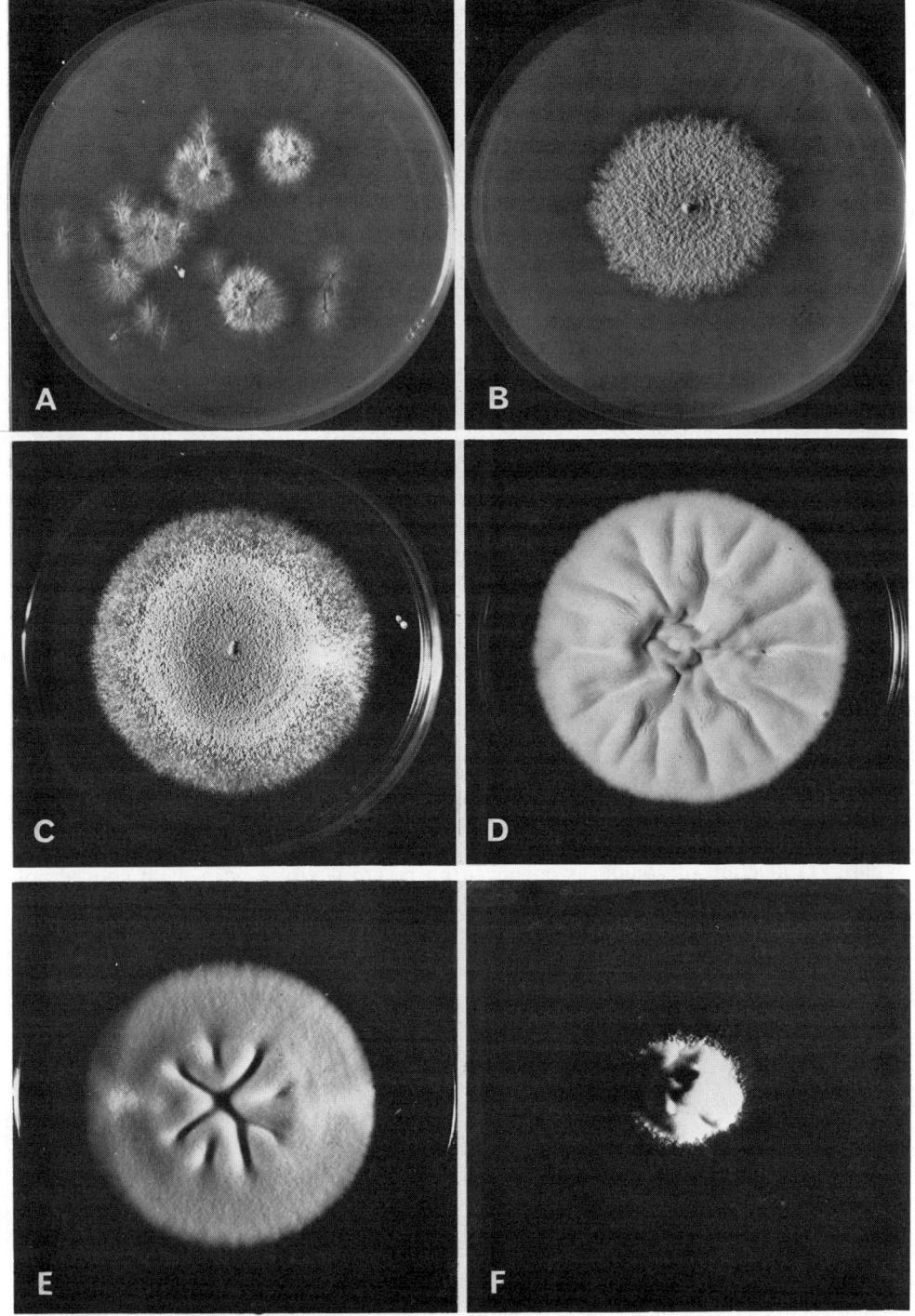

Dermatophytes

worm in cats.[24] It has also been isolated from horses in the United States and elsewhere where it may result in ringworm epizootics.[23] In dogs, *M. gypseum* shows a well-defined seasonal incidence with infections occurring mainly in the summer and fall. Most infections occur at less than 1 year of age.

In small animals, *M. gypseum* lesions are usually circular and show scaling, loss of hair, erythema, and occasional suppuration. A raised peripheral vesicular area may be present. Scattered discrete lesions over the body and foot pads may occur but often a single lesion on the head or leg is the only sign of infection. In horses, lesions develop thick crusts, which later fall off leaving alopecic areas and giving the animal a rather characteristic moth-eaten appearance. However, those lesions do not differ markedly from the more common *Trichophyton equinum* lesions.

Mere isolation of *M. gypseum* from skin or hair specimens is of little value unless accompanied by microscopic evidence (KOH mount) of the parasitic nature of the fungus by demonstrating hair invasion. This species often exists on the hair of animals as a harmless transient from its natural habitat, the soil. Microscopic examination of scrapings on KOH preparations reveals a septate branching mycelium and masses of arthrospores of various sizes. Infected hairs contain mycelial filaments in their interiors. On the surface of the hairs are irregular masses of large spores, some of which are in chain formation. The arthrospores are quite variable in size, ranging from 5 to 8 μm. They are much larger than the arthrospores formed by *M. canis*.

Growth characteristics. On Sabouraud's dextrose agar, *N. incurvata* forms spreading, flat, finely granular, buff to orange colonies with a reddish-brown reverse pigment that becomes ocherous-amber as the colony matures. The colony of *N. gypsea* is similar to *N. incurvata* but it is more coarsely granular and it has a rosy-buff to cinnamon reverse pigment. This pigment usually occurs in uneven radiating patches giving the reverse of the colony a marbled appearance. Colonies of *N. fulva* are much denser than those of the other two species, with a downy to granular buff-colored aerial growth and white cottony periphery. Reverse pigment is a uniform reddish-yellow.

Differential reactions. *M. gypseum* and *M. fulvum* have no special vitamin requirements.[15] Characteristic macroconidia are produced abundantly on all media.[4] These species cannot be differentiated from each other morphologically; mating experiments are necessary to distinguish between them.

Cellular morphology. Microscopically all the species are seen to produce enormous numbers of symmetrical, cylindrical to ellipsoidal, rough, thin-walled, multiseptate macroconidia (Fig. 58.4C). A few elongated clavate microconidia may be present. *N. fulva* produces predominantly cylindrical macroconidia with tapering ends and a rounded

---

Figure 58.3. Dermatophyte colony morphology (all cultures grown on Sabouraud's dextrose agar plates incubated at 30°C unless otherwise stated). A, colonies of *M. canis* on primary isolation medium (contains antibiotics). Note waxy, strongly radiating growth in young colonies and more downy aerial growth in older colonies. Incubated for 8 days. B, colony appearance of *M. gypseum*. This isolate closely resembles *Nannizzia gypsea*. Incubated for 10 days. C, colony appearance of *T. mentagrophytes*. In older cultures the peripheral growth becomes thin and cottony. Incubated for 10 days. D, colony appearance of *T. mentagrophytes* var. *quinckeanum* after 18 days incubation. E, colony appearance of *T. equinum* after 18 days incubation. F, colony appearance of *T. verrucosum* after 21 days incubation. ×1.25 approx.

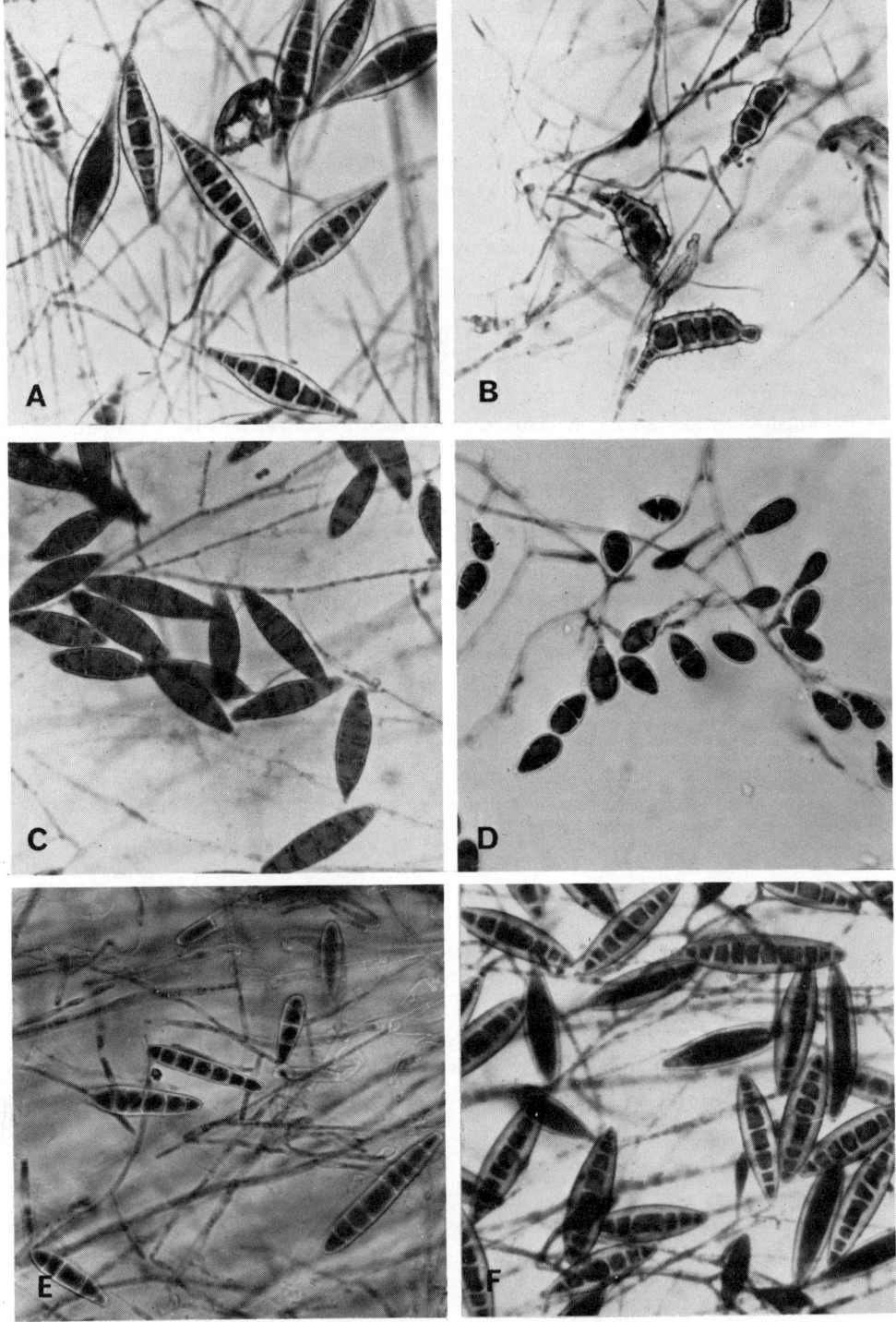

apex, while those of *N. gypsea* and *N. incurvata* are more ellipsoidal and occasionally have slender whiplike appendages arising from the apical cell.[8]

M. gypseum is the conidial or imperfect state of at least two distinct species—*Nannizzia incurvata* and *Nannizzia gypsea*. Stockdale has suggested the use of the name *Microsporum gypseum* var. *sensu lato* for the *Microsporum* state of either species as it is impossible to decide from Bodin's original description of *Achorion gypseum* whether his isolate was the conidial state of *N. incurvata* or *N. gypsea*. Both species are probably of worldwide distribution in soil. *N. incurvata* has been recorded from humans, a dog, and a cat, and *N. gypsea* from humans, a dog, and three cats. Both species are heterothallic, and gymnothecia are formed by culturing compatible mating strains together on soil and keratin, or cornmeal agar with 0.5% glucose and powdered child's hair, or modified Alphacel medium.[46]

N. fulva is the ascigerous state of *M. fulvum*.[42] This species is probably of worldwide distribution in soil and has been recorded only from humans.[5,43] *N. fulva* is heterothallic and ascocarps are formed by culturing compatible mating strains together on natural unautoclaved soil and horse hair or modified alphacel medium. *N. fulva* appears to be markedly less pathogenic for rabbits than either *N. incurvata* or *N. gypsea*. Members of the *M. gypseum* group must be distinguished from morphologically similar geophilic species, such as *M. fulvum, M. racemosum, M. ripariae, M. amazonicum, M. boullardii,* and *M. praecox*.

Microsporum nanum

Microsporum nanum appears to be a relatively common parasite of pigs although the first infections were only diagnosed a few years ago. Infected animals have been found in Kenya, the United States, Cuba, Australia, and New Zealand but it appears likely that *M. nanum*-infected pigs will be found wherever swine are raised. Surveys in the United States have revealed that about 27% of the farms visited housed pigs with ringworm, with the numbers of animals affected ranging from 5 to 70% of the herd.[10,17] *M. nanum* has been classed as a geophilic dermatophyte, as it grows and sporulates in soil.[6] A limited number of human infections have been recorded.

Lesions vary from circular to very irregularly outlined areas often covering large areas of the shoulders and flank. These noninflamed areas have a red cast and frequently develop brownish crusts. The crusts are especially prominent at the periphery of the lesion where they form a prominent band. Infection is limited to the skin; hair is not invaded. There is usually no apparent alopecia or pruritis. Irregular areas of apparently healthy skin may occur within the affected areas. Small circular red-crusted pustules on the back of the ears are often the first signs of infection. The disease appears to be more prevalent in adult pigs although all ages from 8 weeks upward have been found affected.

In pigs, lesions are best scraped with a blunt instrument (scalpel), rather than plucked

Figure 58.4. *Microsporum* saprophytic microscopic morphology. A, macroconidia of *Microsporum canis*. ×315. B, macroconidia of *M. distortum*. Note conspicuous verrucae, a characteristic of the *Microsporum* genus (best seen when isolates are grown on more natural media such as hair). ×500. C, macroconidia of *M. gypseum*. ×315. D, macroconidia of *M. nanum*. ×375. E, macroconidia of *M. gallinae*. ×315. F, macroconidia of the geophilic *M. cookei*. ×315.

with forceps, and the skin scales collected in a petri dish. Scraping reveals a reddened skin surface. In KOH preparations of infected material, a dense network of branched septate fungal hyphae about 3 μm in diameter is usually visible (Fig. 58.2D).

Growth characteristics. Colonies of *M. nanum* on Sabouraud's dextrose agar resemble a somewhat slightly pleomorphic *M. gypseum.* They develop as white, cottony, spreading colonies that on ageing become granular to velvety with a finely radiating margin. The surface is buff to tan while the undersurface of the colony, at first yellow, becomes brownish-red.

Differential reactions. M. nanum has no apparent special nutritional requirement. As with *M. canis* and *M. gypseum,* characteristic macroconidia are produced on rice grains.

Cellular morphology. The characteristic macroconidia of this species are produced abundantly on Sabouraud's dextrose agar. They are clavate to egg shaped, usually unicellular or with one septum but rarely with two to three septa, with thin rough walls (Fig. 58.4D). Slender whiplike appendages may arise from the apical cell. Microconidia are rare, being clavate and borne laterally on the hyphae.

M. nanum is the conidial or imperfect state of *Nannizzia obtusa.*[9] This species is heterothallic and ascocarps are obtained by culture of compatible mating strains on soil and hair. Gymnothecia are produced sparsely and take 10–12 weeks to mature.[6]

Microsporum gallinae

Microsporum gallinae (formerly *Trichophyton gallinae*) is the cause of ringworm in poultry but has also been recovered from lesions in a dog, a number of wild birds, a monkey, and humans.[18] Although apparently sporadic in nature, the organism has been recovered from poultry in the United States, South America, Great Britain, Europe, New Zealand, and Australia.[21,29,39]

M. gallinae infection in poultry results in the production of a powdery white scaliness on the comb, wattles, or any affected area of the skin. Later, thick white crusts may form in the affected area (''white comb'' or favus of chickens). The feathers are not invaded by the fungus although infected skin scales may be found at the base of the feathers.

Growth characteristics. This fungus produces rapidly growing downy white colonies that often develop irregular radial folds or irregular folding over the entire surface. With age, a light pink to buff color develops in the aerial growth. A characteristic dark strawberry-red pigment that diffuses into the agar is formed on the reverse of the colony. Cultures readily become pleomorphic and fluffy and lose their characteristic pigment production.

Differential reactions. This organism, which does not appear to have any special nutritional requirements, has in the past been confused with *Trichophyton megninii.* However, these two species differ on several counts, of which the absolute requirement for 1-histidine (Bacto-*Trichophyton* Agar no. 7) by *T. megninii* is the most outstanding.[13]

Cellular morphology. Numerous small, pyriform to elongated microconidia are produced along the hyphae or in clusters. Macroconidia are generally rare but when produced appear as oval or elongated, usually smooth- but occasionally rough-walled, multiseptate, spatulate structures (Fig. 58.4E). The development of verrucose macroconidia (best seen on wort agar) by this fungus is the reason why this formerly *Trichophyton* species has been transferred to the *Microsporum* genus. Compare the structure of *M. gallinae* with that of the geophilic *M. cookei* (Fig. 58.4F).

Trichophyton mentagrophytes

Trichophyton mentagrophytes is a common worldwide fungus that exists in at least two distinct zoophilic varieties—the common granular *T. mentagrophytes* (*T. mentagrophytes* var. *mentagrophytes*) and *T. mentagrophytes* var. *quinckeanum*.[2] A number of other varieties of *T. mentagrophytes* exist including *T. mentagrophytes* var. *interdigitale* and *T. mentagrophytes* var. *nodulare*.[44] Although the "hedgehog fungus" was originally included as a variety of *T. mentagrophytes* (var. *erinacei*), it is now regarded as a distinct species, *Trichophyton erinacei*.[37]

T. mentagrophytes infections occur among a wide variety of animals. Surveys indicate that small pets, especially dogs, and many wild animals, particularly rodents, are important reservoirs of this parasitic fungus. It has been isolated from the following domestic animals: dogs, horses, cats, cows, sheep, pigs, rabbits, and poultry, as well as from fur-bearing animals (chinchillas, squirrels, foxes, muskrats), laboratory animals (guinea pigs, mice, rats, hamsters), and a host of large and small wild animals (kangaroos, monkeys, opossums, porcupines, hedgehogs, hares, and various species of rats and mice).[11] A feature of the isolations from small wild and laboratory animals was the apparent absence of skin lesions on many occasions. While *T. mentagrophytes* var. *quinckeanum* is primarily a parasite of wild mice, it has also been recovered from horses, dogs, cats, sheep, cattle, and poultry.[27] Human infections with both varieties have been recorded on numerous occasions, particularly in rural areas where it is felt that rodents play an important epidemiologic role. While *T. mentagrophytes* has a worldwide distribution, var. *quinckeanum* has been isolated only in Canada, Europe, Northern Africa, and Australia.

Lesions due to *T. mentagrophytes* occur most commonly on the head, near the mouth and eyes, or at the base of the tail but may appear anywhere on the body (e.g. the girth of horses).[21] These appear as irregularly defined areas of hair loss with considerable scaling and inflammation and usually crust formation. Pustules may form at the edges of lesions, and suppuration beneath the crusts is common. With var. *quinckeanum*, the crusts form yellowish concave cuplike structures (favic crusts or scutulae), which in wild mice may reach such proportions as to render the animal blind or unable to open its jaws. It is important to remember that infections may be clinically inapparent. Infected hairs show a sheath of smallish spores 3–5 μm in diameter that may be in chains but are usually packed in a mass around the hair. Parasitized hairs do not fluoresce under the UV light.

Growth characteristics. Since the two varieties of *T. mentagrophytes* differ markedly, they will be described separately.

With *T. mentagrophytes* (granular form or var. *mentagrophytes*), growth on Sabouraud's dextrose agar is rapid. Colonies are generally flat and spreading with a coarsely granular cream to buff or tan-colored surface (Fig. 58.3C). Reverse pigmentation develops to a deep red-brown with most strains.

With *T. mentagrophytes* var. *quinckeanum*, colonies are at first fluffy, white, and dome shaped, often with a well-defined fringe of radiating surface mycelium. After about 10 days incubation, the center of the colony becomes depressed and folded and the aerial mycelium in this area may become creamy or pinkish in color (Fig. 58.3D). Reverse pigmentation is usually limited to a faint yellow but may deepen to a brownish-yellow as the culture matures. Incubation of cultures in a CO_2 (candle) jar may stimulate the production of a purplish-red reverse pigment.

Differential reactions. Neither variety appears to have any special nutritional requirements and both grow well on Bacto-*Trichophyton* Agar no. 1. On this media, colonies of var. *quinckeanum* show a central craterlike folding while those of var. *mentagrophytes* remain flat. Microconidia of var. *quinckeanum* tend to be more regularly spherical on this media. With most strains of both varieties, urea dextrose slopes rapidly become red, indicating the production of the enzyme urease. This allows their differentiation from *T. erinacei* and *T. rubrum*, which are negative on this medium after 4 days.[35] *T. mentagrophytes*, unlike *T. rubrum*, does not produce red pigment on potato dextrose or lab-lemco agars.

In certain circumstances *T. mentagrophytes* may be confused with *T. simii*, a dermatophyte apparently restricted geographically to India where it has been recovered from animals (especially chickens and monkeys), humans, and soil.[44] *T. simii* differs from *T. mentagrophytes* on a number of points, the most helpful of which is the micromorphology. In comparison to *T. mentagrophytes*, *T. simii* produces enormous numbers of macroconidia that degenerate rapidly to form intercalary chlamydospores. The microconidia of *T. simii* are generally elongated and are formed mainly along the hyphae.[44]

T. mentagrophytes is the conidial state of *Arthroderma benhamiae*.[3] This species is also heterothallic and fertile gymnothecia are obtained by the culture of compatible mating strains on sterile soil and horse hair or modified Alphacel medium. Ascocarps may take 10–12 weeks to mature. As fertile gymnothecia were produced by mating the tester strains of *A. benhamiae* with what was then known as *T. quinckeanum*, the proper designation of the etiologic agent of mouse favus is now considered to be *T. mentagrophytes* var. *quinckeanum*.[27] In a similar manner, var. *nodulare* and var. *interdigitale* have been shown to be true varieties of *T. mentagrophytes* in that they mate with either the + or − strains of *A. benhamiae*. Conversely, var. *erinacei* was eliminated as a variety of *T. mentagrophytes* because of its inability to form a perfect stage with tester strains of *A. benhamiae*.[41]

Cellular morphology. Again the two varieties differ.

With *T. mentagrophytes* (granular), masses of spherical to slightly pyriform micro-

---

Figure 58.5. *Trichophyton* saprophytic microscopic morphology. A, micro- and macroconidia as seen in most *Trichophyton* species. This is the granular zoophilic variety of *T. mentagrophytes*, which has circular microconidia. ×375. Inset a ×650. B, microconidia of *T. mentagrophytes* var. *quinckeanum*. ×375. Inset b ×650. C, microconidia of *T. equinum*. ×375. Inset c ×650. D, hyphae and chlamydospores of *T. verrucosum*. This is the usual morphology seen on Sabouraud's dextrose agar. The chlamydospores become more numerous in cultures incubated at 37°C. ×650. E, macroconidia of the geophilic *T. ajelloi*. Microconidia are scarce in this species. ×325. F, conidia of the geophilic *T. terrestre*. Note broad base where spores are attached to the hyphae. ×575.

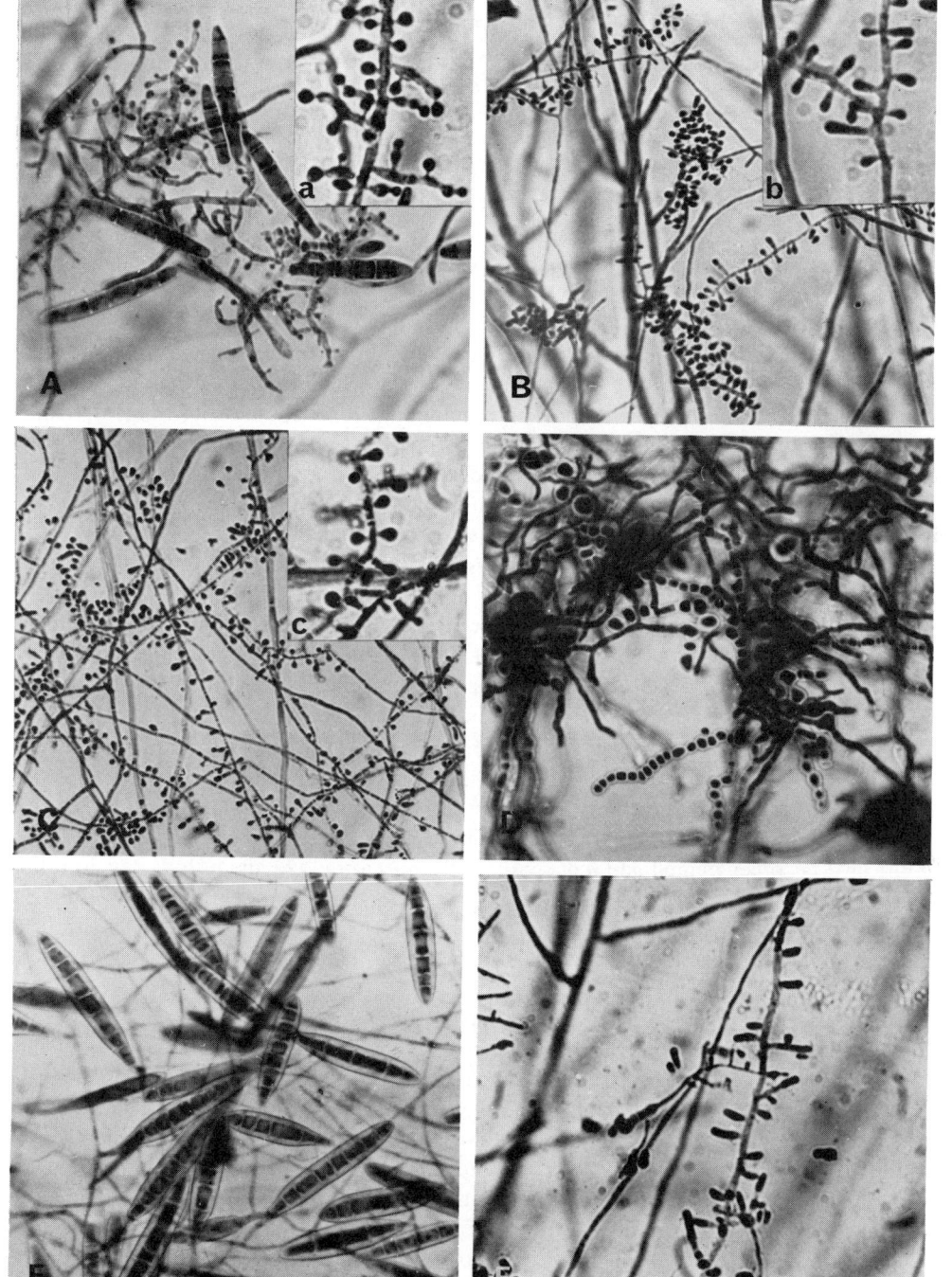

conidia can be seen both in clusters ("en grappe") and along the hyphae ("en thyrse") (Fig. 58.5A). Cigar-shaped, smooth, thin-walled, multiseptate macroconidia and spiral hyphae are usually numerous.

With *T. mentagrophytes* var. *quinckeanum*, microscopic examination reveals the production of pyriform to elongated microconidia singly along the hyphae or clusters (Fig. 58.5B). Macroconidia are not as conspicuous as in the granular variety. Where present these are cigar shaped, thin walled, smooth, and multiseptate. Immature forms often show tapered ends. Production of macroconidia can be stimulated by growing the fungus on a more natural substrate such as potato dextrose agar, wheat grains, or bran agar.

Trichophyton equinum

Trichophyton equinum, the usual causal agent of equine ringworm, exists in two distinct varieties. Isolates of the fungus from the United States, South America, Europe, and South Africa show a specific growth requirement for nicotinic acid (niacin), while those from New Zealand and Australia appear to be less exacting nutritionally and grow equally as well with or without the addition of this vitamin.[38,40] These strains not requiring nicotinic acid have been designated a separate variety, *T. equinum* var. *autotrophicum*. At present var. *autotrophicum* appears limited to Australia and New Zealand. Although *T. equinum* is regarded essentially as an equine fungus, it has been recovered from a dog and humans in close contact with infected horses.

Although all ages have been found to be affected, colts and yearlings appear most susceptible. The disease is characteristic of large stables, and a number of epizootics have occurred in army establishments and in racing stables where infection is undoubtedly spread by brushes, combs, and saddle gear.[28]

Infected horses usually present a number of ringworm plaques. Isolated lesions are scattered over the hind quarters and shoulders while others are grouped together in the saddle area (girth itch) where they tend to become confluent.[33] Lesions first appear as a swelling that can be felt through the hair. These areas gradually become visible as hair in the area becomes matted and a dry gray scurfiness forms. As the lesions develop, the scurfiness becomes more marked and hairs begin to fall out. A peripheral swelling is usually present at this stage. Finally a thick crust forms, which slowly cracks and lifts leaving a relatively clean alopecic area of epidermis. The bald areas give the animal a typical moth-eaten appearance.

Fungus-infected skin reveals branched hyphae and arthrospores as seen in all types of ringworm infection. The interior of infected hairs contains hyphae while on the outside are found chains of rather large arthrospores 3–8 μm in diameter.[16] These spores frequently appear rectangular in shape. Direct microscopic examination of KOH-treated material from infected horses may be unreliable in diagnosing dermatophyte infection as definitive forms often are not evident. Cultures are often obtained from scrapings that on direct microscopic examination appeared free of fungal infection.

Growth characteristics. The features of *T. equinum* and *T. equinum* var. *autotrophicum* are similar. Colonies are at first dome shaped, downy, and white, but become flattened with a softly folded velvety center after about 9 days (Fig. 58.3E). This central area may develop a cream to buff color. Reverse pigment is initially a bright yellow or even lemon-yellow but later turns a deep red-brown, especially under the center. In cultures incubated at lowered temperatures (or in young cultures placed in the refrigerator), a reddish-yellow brown pigment may form around the submerged peripheral growth.

Differential reactions. Isolates of *T. equinum* from countries other than New Zealand or Australia have an absolute nutritional requirement for nicotinic acid, as in Bacto-*Trichophyton* Agar no. 4. *T. equinum* var. *autotrophicum* does not show this nutritional requirement and grows equally well on Bacto-*Trichophyton* Agar no. 1 and no. 5.[40] On Agar no. 1, colonies of var. *autotrophicum* closely resemble those of the granular form of *T. mentagrophytes*. Both varieties of *T. equinum* are urease positive.[40]

Cellular morphology. Microscopically, microconidia are abundant but vary notably in shape and size. They range from almost spherical forms attached to the hyphae by short delicate sterigmata to more elongate clavate forms attached directly to the hyphae. Oval to pyriform types appear to predominate (Fig. 58.5C). Macroconidia, which are typically of the *Trichophyton* type, are rare in most strains but are occasionally found in others.

Trichophyton verrucosum

Trichophyton verrucosum is the main etiologic agent of ringworm in cattle but has also been recovered from horses, pigs, sheep, dogs, a cat, a donkey, a goat, and poultry and is a common cause of human ringworm in rural areas.[14,26] Based on colony morphology the fungus has been divided into a number of varieties—var. *album,* var. *discoides,* and var. *ochraceum*.[36]

Ringworm of cattle occurs largely in calves, although it is often seen in adult animals.[32] Epizootics occur commonly among very young animals. In the United States, most herd infections occur in the winter and early spring, but no significant seasonal incidence has been found in Great Britain. A survey carried out in Gouda, Holland, during one winter showed 2.5% of 3174 cattle to be infected. Infected animals were found in 27 (16%) of the herds visited and *T. verrucosum* was the only pathogen isolated. Infected scabs have been shown to remain viable at room temperature for up to 4.5 years.

Lesions in cattle range from discrete areas of slight scaling and hair loss to clearly circumscribed plaques 3–10 cm in diameter covered with grayish-white asbestoslike crusts that may become very thickened. Lesions are noticeably most numerous and severe in calves. The site of infection is usually the head around the eyes and muzzle and frequently the neck, but other parts of the body may be affected. In calves, large areas over the top of the head, back, and rump may be covered with thick crusts. In an active lesion, the crust is firmly attached and when forcibly removed, moist bleeding areas remain. Pus may be found under the crusts, and if pruritus is present, raw areas are seen. Around the edge of the lesion and in the crust itself stubs of broken-off infected hairs may be found. When a lesion begins to heal, the thick crust is lost and dry scaly gray patches with hair loss are left.

The examination of skin scrapings or fragments of the crust reveals branching hyphae and chains of arthrospores as seen in all types of ringworm infections. The interior of the hair may show hyphae and on the outside of the hair there is usually a characteristic thick sheath of large arthrospores 5–10 μm in diameter (Fig. 58.2C).

T. verrucosum is a slow-growing fastidious dermatophyte and may not become visible around the inoculum until after 7–10 days incubation. Incubation at a higher temperature (37°C) may hasten the growth, as will supplementation of the medium with thiamine.

Growth characteristics. This slow-growing species produces small, heaped, folded buttonlike colonies (Fig. 58.3F). In var. *album* the colonies are at first glabrous and waxy but usually develop a white powdery or velvety surface with age. Two other variants occur: a flat yellow glabrous colony (var. *ochraceum*) and a flat, slightly downy, gray-white colony (var. *discoides*). On blood agar base with yeast extract, colonies are usually flatter and more spreading.

Differential reactions. All strains show a nutritional requirement for thiamine (Bacto-*Trichophyton* Agar no. 4), while some strains require inositol (Bacto-*Trichophyton* Agar no. 3) as well. Unlike other dermatophytes (except for *T. erinacei*) growth of *T. verrucosum* is usually enhanced at 37°C.

Cellular morphology. Usually only a thin irregular mycelium with chlamydospores is produced (Fig. 58.5D). In cultures grown at 37°C, these chlamydospores are very numerous and form heavy chains. On blood agar base plus yeast extract (or thiamine), tear-shaped microconidia may be arranged along the hyphae; less frequently, there may be macroconidia with a rather characteristic rat-tail or string-bean shape. Photographs of geophilic *T. ajelloi* and *T. terrestre* have been included for comparison (Fig. 58.5E, F).

References

1. Ainsworth, G.C., and P.K.C. Austwick. *Fungal Diseases of Animals*. 2d ed. Commonwealth Agricultural Bureau, Farnham Royal, Eng., 1973.
2. Ajello, L., L. Bostick, and S.L. Cheng. The relationship of *Trichophyton quinckeanum* to *Trichophyton mentagrophytes*. Mycologia 60:1185–1189, 1968.
3. Ajello, L., and S.L. Cheng. The perfect state of *Trichophyton mentagrophytes*. Sabouraudia 5:230–234, 1967.
4. Ajello, L., L.K. Georg, W. Kaplan, and L. Kaufman. *Laboratory Manual for Medical Mycology*. Public Health Service Pub. no. 994. HEW, Washington, 1963.
5. Ajello, L., and A.A. Padhye. Dermatophytes and the agents of superficial mycoses. In *Manual of Clinical Microbiology*, E.H. Lennette, E.H. Spaulding, and J.P. Truant (eds.). 2d ed. American Society for Microbiology, Bethesda, Md., 1974.
6. Ajello, L., E. Varsavsky, O.J. Ginther, and G. Bubash. The natural history of *Microsporum nanum*. Mycologia 56:873–884, 1964.
7. Al-Doory, Y. Survival of dermatophyte cultures maintained on hair. Mycologia 60:720–723, 1968.
8. Conant, N.F. A statistical analysis of spore size in the genus *Microsporum*. J. Invest. Dermatol. 4:265–278, 1941.
9. Dawson, C.O., and J.C. Gentles. The perfect states of *Keratinomyces ajelloi* Vanbreuseghem, *Trichophyton terrestre* Durie & Frey and *Microsporum nanum* Fuentes. Sabouraudia 1:49–57, 1961.
10. Dodd, D.C., R.W. Newlin, and G.R. Niksch. Infection of swine with *Microsporum nanum*. J. Am. Vet. Med. Ass. 146:486–489, 1965.
11. Emmons, C.W., C.H. Binford, and J.P. Utz. *Medical Mycology*. 2d ed. Lea and Febiger, Philadelphia, 1970.
12. English, M.P. The epidemiology of animal ringworm in man. Brit. J. Dermatol. 86(suppl. 8):78–82, 1972.
13. Georg, L.K. Cultural and nutritional studies of *Trichophyton gallinae* and *Trichophyton megnini*. Mycologia 44:470–492, 1952.

14. Georg, L.K. *Animal Ringworm in Public Health*. Public Health Service Pub. no. 727. HEW, Washington, 1960.
15. Georg, L.K., and L.B. Camp. Routine nutritional tests for the identification of dermatophytes. *J. Bact.* 74:113–121, 1967.
16. Georg, L.K., W. Kaplan, and L.B. Camp. Equine ringworm with special reference to *Trichophyton equinum*. *Am. J. Vet. Res.* 18:798–810, 1957.
17. Ginther, O.J., and L. Ajello. The prevalence of *Microsporum nanum* infection in swine. *J. Am. Vet. Med. Ass.* 146:361–365, 1965.
18. Gordon, M.A., and G.N. Little. *Trichophyton (Microsporum) gallinae* ringworm in a monkey. *Sabouraudia* 6:207–212, 1968.
19. Gordon, M.A., U. Pérrin, and G.N. Little. Differences in pathogenicity between *Microsporum gypseum* and *Microsporum fulvum*. *Sabouraudia* 5:366–370, 1967.
20. Hasegawa, A., and K. Usui. The perfect state of *Microsporum canis*. *Jap. J. Vet. Sci.* 36:447–449, 1974.
21. Jungerman, P.F. and R.M. Schwartzman. *Veterinary Medical Mycology*. Lea and Febiger, Philadelphia, 1972.
22. Kaplan, W., L.K. Georg, and L. Ajello. Recent developments in animal ringworm and their public health implications. *Ann. N.Y. Acad. Sci.* 70:636–649, 1958.
23. Kaplan, W., J.L. Hopping, and L.K. Georg. Ringwrom in horses caused by the dermatophyte, *Microsporum gypseum*. *J. Am. Vet. Med. Ass.* 131:329–332, 1957.
24. Kaplan, W., and M.S. Ivens. Observations on the seasonal variations in incidence of ringworm in dogs and cats in the United States. *Sabouraudia* 1:91–102, 1961.
25. Keep. J.M. A survey of *Microsporum canis* infection of cats in Sydney. *Austral. Vet. J.* 39:330–332, 1963.
26. Klokke, A.H. Report of a systemic survey of animal ringworm in humans and cattle. *Dermatologica* 127:220–223, 1963.
27. Le Touche, C.J. Mouse favus due to *Trichophyton quinckeanum* (Zopf) Macleod and Muende: A reappraisal in the light of recent investigations. *Mycopathol. Mycol. Appl.* 13:33–47, 1960.
28. Londero, A. T., O. Fischman, and C.D. Ramos. An epizootic of *Trichophyton equinum* infection on horses in Brazil. *Sabouraudia* 3:14–15, 1963.
29. Londero, A.T., O. Fischman, and C.D. Ramos. *Trichophyton gallinae* in Brazil. *Sabouraudia* 3:233–234, 1964.
30. Mackenzie, D.W.R. "Hairbrush diagnosis" in detection and eradication of non-fluorescent scalp ringworm. *Brit. Med. J.* 2:363–365, 1963.
31. Marples, M.J. The ecology of *Microsporum canis* Bodin, in New Zealand. *J. Hyg.* 54:378–387, 1956.
32. McPherson, E.A. A survey of the incidence of ringworm in cattle in Northern Britain. *Vet. Rec.* 69:674–679, 1957.
33. McPherson, E.A. The influence of physical factors on dermatomycosis in domestic animals. *Vet. Rec.* 69:1010–1013, 1957.
34. Okoshi, S., and A. Hasegawa. *Microsporum gypseum* isolated from feline ringworm. *Jap. J. Vet. Sci.* 29:195–199, 1967.
35. Philpot, C. The differentiation of *Trichophyton mentagrophytes* from *T. rubrum* by a simple urease test. *Sabouraudia* 5:189–193, 1967.
36. Rebell, G., and D. Taplin. *Dermatophytes: Their Recognition and Identification*. Rev. ed. Dermatology Foundation of Miami, 1970.
37. Rippon, J.W. *Medical Mycology: The Pathogenic Fungi and the Pathogenic Actinomycetes*. Saunders, Philadelphia, 1974.
38. Smith, J.M.B. An unusual dermatophyte from horses in New Zealand. *Sabouraudia* 5:124–125, 1966.
39. Smith, J.M.B. Superficial and cutaneous mycoses. In *Diseases Transmitted from Animals to Man*, W.T. Hubbert, W.F. McCulloch, and P.R. Schnurrenberger (eds.). 6th ed. Thomas, Springfield, Ill., 1975.
40. Smith, J.M.B., R.D. Jolly, L.K. Georg, and M.D. Connole. *Trichophyton equinum* var *autotrophicum*: Its characteristics and geographical distribution. *Sabouraudia* 6:296–304, 1968.
41. Smith, J.M.B., and M.J. Marples. *Trichophyton mentagrophytes* var *erinacei*. *Sabouraudia* 3:1–10, 1963.
42. Stockdale, P.M. The *Microsporum gypseum* complex (*Nannizzia incurvata*). Stockd., *N. gypsea* (Nann.) comb. nov., *N. fulva* sp. nov. *Sabouraudia* 3:114–126, 1964.
43. Stockdale, P.M. Fungi pathogenic for man and animals. I. Diseases of the keratinized tissues. In *Methods of Microbiology*, vol. 4, C. Booth (ed.). Academic Press, London, 1971.

44. Stockdale, P.M., D.W.R. Mackenzie, and P.K.C. Austwick. *Arthroderma simii* sp. nov., the perfect state of *Trichophyton simii* (Pinoy) comb. nov. *Sabouraudia* 4:112–123, 1965.
45. Taplin, D., N. Zaias, G. Rebell, and H. Blank. Isolation and recognition of dermatophytes on a new medium (DTM). *Arch. Dermatol.* 99:203–209, 1969.
46. Weitzman, I., and M. Silva-Hutner. Non-keratinous agar media as substrates for the ascigerous state in certain members of the Gymnoascaceae pathogenic for man and animals. *Sabouraudia* 5:334–340, 1967.

59. Geotrichum

The genus *Geotrichum* contains a single species, *G. candidum*. The organism is a mycelial yeastlike fungus that is distributed in nature as a saprophyte on vegetation and in the soil. The role of *G. candidum* as a pathogen is insecure in that it often appears as an opportunist.[2] Geotrichosis is seen most often as an involvement of mucosal surfaces, including the enteric canal. Intestinal infection in cats and calves and mammary infections in cattle are seen occasionally, and there has been some association with cutaneous lesions in dogs and swine. Systemic geotrichosis occurs as a complication of pulmonary infection.

Geotrichum is not a notable hazard in the laboratory as long as it is handled with the usual precautions. Strains that produce extensive aerial hyphae should be handled under a properly ventilated hood.

Specimens

Because of the prevalence of *G. candidum* as a saprophyte, both microscopic and cultural demonstration of the organism in lesion material and exudates is important.[1] Air-dried smears are made from skin scrapings, mucosal swabbings, and milk. Culture specimens are often contaminated and may require the use of antibiotics in Sabouraud's dextrose agar (e.g. chloramphenicol 0.05 mg/ml), but the use of cycloheximide is not recommended as it inhibits the growth of *Geotrichum* and other yeastlike fungi. *Geotrichum* will grow also on bacteriological media such as blood agar. Stock cultures can be preserved for several months on screw-capped slants in a refrigerator or for longer periods when the culture is immersed under sterile mineral oil at room temperature. The organism is susceptible to nystatin, a fungistatic antibiotic.

Histologic specimens are fixed in Formalin, sectioned in the usual manner, and stained with Gridley's fungus stain, Gram-Weigert stain, or Gomori's methenamine silver stain.

Laboratory Procedures

Cultures. *Geotrichum* grows very rapidly when streaked on Sabouraud's dextrose agar and incubated at room temperature or 37°C. Isolation of pure culture material is best accomplished from the periphery of isolated spreading colonies. Animal inoculation is not used for isolation or identification. The isolated fungus is examined microscopically in a wet mount prepared with lactophenol cotton blue. Cornmeal agar slide cultures as used with *Candida* can be used for morphologic studies of *Geotrichum*.

Cellular morphology. The identification of *Geotrichum* is essentially morphologic. The colony develops rapidly on Sabouraud's medium as a spreading, flat, largely submerged mycelium. The surface of the colony can vary from soft, glistening, and yeast-like, to dry and flat, to cottony with aerial hyphae. In fluid media, *Geotrichum* forms a dry surface pellicle. The organism is strongly gram-positive.

Microscopic morphology consists of a true mycelium with frequent septations. The mycelium fragments readily into chains of elongate, rectangular to barrel-shaped arthrospores approximating 3–5 μm × 5–15 μm. The arthrospores occasionally bud at the corner of the spore, and they are in a continuous chain as opposed to the arthrospores of the mold form of *Coccidioides immitis,* which appear in intermittent chains alternating with blank spaces in the hyphae. Features differentiating *Geotrichum* from other mycelial yeasts are discussed in Chapter 55.

References
1. Conant, N.F., D.J. Smith, R.D. Baker, J.L. Callaway, and D.S. Martin. *Manual of Clinical Mycology.* Saunders, Philadelphia, 1954.
2. Emmons, C.W., C.H. Binford, and J.P. Utz. *Medical Mycology.* 2d ed. Lea and Febiger, Philadelphia, 1970.

60. Histoplasma

The genus *Histoplasma* is comprised of three species of medical importance. *Histoplasma capsulatum* is the agent of histoplasmosis of animals and of humans in the United States; *H. farciminosum* causes a condition known as epizootic lymphangitis of horses in Europe, Africa, and Asia; *H. duboisii* is a species apparently limited to Africa where it causes histoplasmosis of humans.

Histoplasma capsulatum is a dimorphic fungus that has a mold and a yeast (tissue) form. The mold form reproduces by the production of asexual conidia in the soil.[7] *Histoplasma capsulatum* in the mold form constitutes a very high hazard in the laboratory. The fungus should be handled only under a properly ventilated hood. Aerosolization of spores can be minimized if the fungus is grown in cotton-stoppered tubes and sterile saline is injected through the stopper until the mold is submerged and thoroughly wetted before the culture tube is opened.

Histoplasmosis is a chronic granulomatous disease with a variety of clinical manifestations. It can vary from a benign infection of the lungs, which heals, leaving calcified areas in parenchyma and hilar nodes, to a disseminated, progressive, and eventually fatal condition. The clinical similarity to tuberculosis is apparent.[4,5] Most mammals appear to be susceptible to infection, and natural cases have been reported in dogs, cattle, swine, and horses, as well as numerous wild species.[6,8,12]

Distribution of histoplasmosis is worldwide.[19] Some researchers estimate that the fungus resides in the soil of nearly all river valleys in the temperate and tropical zones of the world between 45° north and 45° south. In the United States the infection is prevalent in residents of the central valley of the Mississippi and its tributaries; in the Champlain, St. Lawrence, and Hudson River valleys; the Susquehanna, Delaware, and Potomac River valleys, and the major river valley areas of central and east Texas. It has been estimated that in the United States alone, 30,000,000 persons are infected with the fungus and that about 500,000 acquire the infection each year.

Only incomplete data are available on the incidence in animals. The disease has been reported in dogs, mostly in endemic areas.[13] In cattle the incidence of skin test reactors varied from 0 to 30% according to location. In a similar survey of horses, sheep, and swine in central Missouri, reactor rates were 72, 32, and 1.5%, respectively. Surveys in humans and animals revealed the substantial incidence of infected individuals and the very wide margin between *Histoplasma* infection and clinical disease.

Histoplasma capsulatum is dimorphic: while in its natural habitat the fungus is in its filamentous (mold) phase, but it converts to the yeast phase when parasitizing an animal host.[13,14] The disease is not transmissible between infected animals, but birds and bats can carry the spores in their intestinal tract. The droppings of birds and bats provide favorable substrates for fungal growth.

Epizootic lymphangitis caused by *H. farciminosum* is typified by chains of draining ulcers along cutaneous lymphatics of the extremities (e.g. neck and legs) of infected horses. The exudates discharged from these lesions are highly infectious and this infection is readily transmitted by direct or indirect contact within groups of horses.

The disease caused by *H. duboisii* resembles that caused by *H. capsulatum* in the United States except that the yeast or tissue form of *H. duboisii* is much larger than that of *H. capsulatum*. Infections by *H. duboisii* are not currently considered to be a veterinary problem and the organism will not be considered further here.

Specimens

Specimens should be obtained from animals, particularly dogs, affected by acute or chronic pulmonary disease and any systemic diseases typified by emaciation and chronic enteritis where the diagnosis has not been clearly established. Specimens from diseased tissues, usually lung, bronchial, mediastinal, mesenteric, or cervical lymph nodes, liver, spleen, adrenal, and currettage from intestinal ulcers, should be collected.

Specimens for *H. capsulatum* culture examination should not be frozen; this often kills the fungal elements. The tissues (1–2 cm squares or larger) can be collected in two screw-capped 30 ml jars. One jar should contain 20 ml of sterile buffered cysteine-saline solution with 25 μg of chloromycetin per ml. Portions of lung, bronchial, mediastinal, or cervical lymph nodes, liver, spleen, and adrenal are placed in the jar. These tissues are used for FA studies and culture.

The second jar should contain 30 ml of 10% Formalin. Duplicate portions of the affected tissues should be placed in this jar for histopathologic studies.

Blood also is collected in the usual manner for serologic tests.

At the present time, suspicion of histoplasmosis in an animal is based on clinical signs, chest radiographic findings, and serologic tests. This is followed by attempts to isolate the fungus or demonstrate the organism in tissue or body fluids.

Impression smears of organs and films of exudates are stained with Giemsa stain and examined for the presence of *Histoplasma* cells within macrophages.[10] The yeast cells are 1–4 μm in diameter and have a central or polar nucleus and a heavy cell wall that suggests a capsule. The organism has the same appearance in sections. The histopathologic examination of biopsy or necropsy tissues may be done following staining with H & E or Gridley's fungus stain. Lung, lymph nodes, liver, spleen, and adrenal gland are examined routinely.

Histoplasma

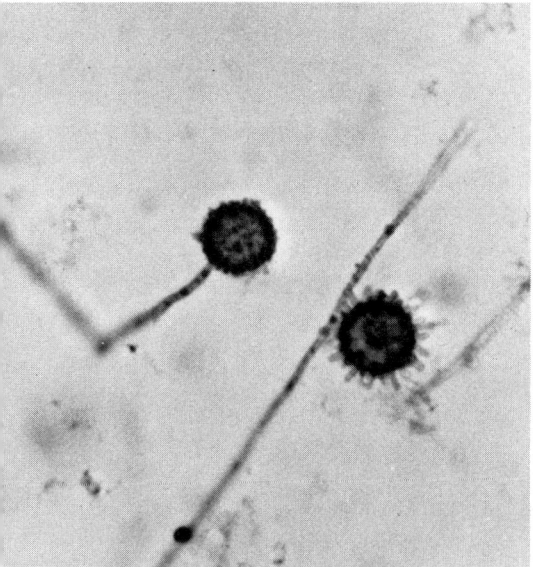 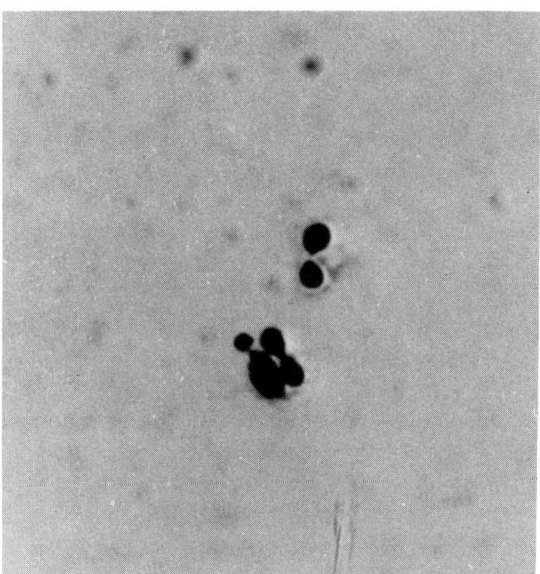

Figure 60.1. *Histoplasma capsulatum:* left, tuberculate macroconidia of mold phase, ×500; right, yeast phase cells, ×900.

Laboratory Procedures

Cultures. Small portions (1–2 g) of each tissue (in the culture jar) are placed in a sterile mortar, sterile sand is added, and the tissues are ground. Then sterile buffered cysteine-saline solution is added to make an approximately 10% suspension, and the tissues are mixed well. A 0.5 ml portion of the suspension is inoculated on cotton-stoppered slants of Sabouraud's dextrose agar, Sabouraud's dextrose with C & C, and two tubes of BHI blood agar.[2] The Sabouraud's tubes and one BHI blood agar tube are incubated at room temperature (25°C), the other BHI blood agar tube is incubated at 37°C; all are held for at least 1 month before being discarded. Cultures can be examined by making a wet mount in lactophenol cotton blue mounting fluid. Stringent precautions must be taken at all times against respiratory exposure of laboratory personnel to the mycelial phase.

Cellular morphology. The fungus *Histoplasma capsulatum* is dimorphic and occurs in tissues or in BHI blood agar culture at 37°C in the yeast phase, and in soil or in Sabouraud's dextrose agar cultures at room temperature in the mycelial phase (Fig. 60.1). The yeast phase is found in tissues as a nucleated oval body 1–4 μm in diameter in mononuclear cells and occasionally in polymorphonuclear cells.

At room temperature *H. capsulatum* develops a white fluffy colony. The aerial mycelium is typically fine and silky. Most isolates grow slowly, requiring at least 10–14 days incubation before the development of a distinct colony. After several weeks, however, the entire surface of the slant is covered with the growth and the colony may develop a buff to tan color. Sporulation is usually associated with the tan coloration. Morphologic studies of the mold are conducted in teased wet mounts or slide cultures under lactophenol cotton blue.

The spores of the mycelial phase of *H. capsulatum* are of two types: microconidia and macroconidia. The small spores or microconidia usually appear first. They are sessile or stalked, round to pyriform structures that measure 2–6 μm in diameter. Most of the microconidia are smooth but a few may be echinulate. Some of the microconidia may be double-celled or have buds; such conidia are capable of producing one or more secondary microconidia. Later, most cultures develop large round or pyriform macroconidia. They measure 7–25 μm in diameter and have a thick wall. The macroconidia (also known as chlamydospores) usually have a tuberculated surface. The tubercles (fingerlike or spiny projections) are 1–8 μm in length and are of various lengths on a single spore. Although tuberculate macroconidia have been described as characteristic of *H. capsulatum*, and these spores are necessary to establish a mycologic diagnosis, all isolates of this fungus do not produce these spores, and other fungi (e.g. *Sepedonium* sp.) produce very similar structures. However, *Sepedonium* is not dimorphic nor is it pathogenic for animals as is *H. capsulatum*. For this reason both the yeast phase and the mold phase of *H. capsulatum* must be demonstrated for definitive identification.

Histoplasma farciminosum, the agent of epizootic lymphangitis in horses, resembles *H. capsulatum* in its tissue phase and its dimorphism in culture. The average diameter of the parasitic form is reported to be larger (3-5 μm) and occasionally reaches 15 μm. It is found as singly budding yeast cells within macrophages, and it can be differentiated from *H. capsulatum* with certainty only by culture. The organism grows best on rich infusion base media supplemented with blood and glucose. Ordinary blood agar and Sabouraud's agar have been described as suboptimal and unsuited for purposes of isolation. The yeast form consists of spherical and oval budding cells similar in size to the cells of the tissue phase. The mold phase contains septate hyphae but lacks tuberculate and other kinds of distinctive macrospores. It has been described as "mycelia sterila."

The interconversion between yeast and mold phase appears to be governed by different factors than those operative on other dimorphic fungi. Both phases of *H. farciminosum* are expressed in cultures at temperatures below 30°C on optimal media and can be maintained at that temperature. Conversion of the mycelial to the yeast phase has been achieved by propagation of the mold form on ordinary blood agar at 37°C and under 15–20% CO_2. Preservation of mold phase cultures is done by immersing the culture surface in sterile mineral oil and storing at 25°C. Yeast phase cultures must be kept on BHI blood agar and transferred frequently. *H. capsulatum* is susceptible to the fungicidal antibiotic, amphotericin B. Decontamination of laboratory surfaces can be effected with 2% Amphyl.

Animal inoculation. Three white Swiss mice are each inoculated IP with 1 ml of a 10% tissue suspension. After 1 month, the mice are necropsied and 0.5 ml of the combined liver and spleen tissue suspension of each mouse is cultured on the same media as used for direct culture. If hamsters are available they may be used instead of mice.[2]

Immunology and serology. The two serologic tests commonly used for the diagnosis of histoplasmosis are the AD and the CF tests. Either the standard or micro 50% CF method can be used.

Frequently, it will be advantageous to test one serum sample for antibodies to several fungal agents. In the AD test, sera are tested for histoplasmosis with histoplasmin concentrated 10 times and for blastomycosis with undiluted blastomycin concentrated 10 times.[1,18] This test appears to be most useful during the acute phase of the illness, and it appears to be satisfactory for the diagnosis of canine histoplasmosis.

Because of antigenic differences between mycelial and yeast phase antigens, in the CF test, sera are tested for histoplasmosis with histoplasmin and a *Histoplasma capsulatum* yeast cell suspension, and for blastomycosis with a *Blastomyces dermatitidis* yeast cell suspension.[17] Information concerning all the serologic tests and antigens can be obtained from the reference laboratories.

The CF tests have not been adequately evaluated for animals. For humans there are limitations in using the CF test for the diagnosis of histoplasmosis and blastomycosis.[16] The organisms share a common antigen; thus sera of persons with histoplasmosis frequently show positive CF reactions with antigen prepared from *Blastomyces dermatitidis*. Also, sera of a significant proportion of persons with chronic pulmonary histoplasmosis and blastomycosis give negative CF tests. However, the percentage of false-positive CF tests is low, and the CF test yields results far more rapidly and frequently than culture methods.

Cross-reactions of CF antibodies between antigens of *H. capsulatum* and *B. dermatitidis* present problems in diagnosis. In one study the titers were greater for the homologous antigens for 84% of the histoplasmosis cases and only 22% of the blastomycosis cases. The best solution to the problem is to perform the CF test with antigens of both fungi and also perform the test upon serum specimens.

FA staining of air-dried, acetone-fixed preparations of spleen, lymph nodes, and other specimens is a fast and reliable adjunct to diagnosis in laboratories equipped for this technique. However, conjugates available at present lack absolute specificity.[9]

Histoplasmin, a culture filtrate prepared from the mycelial phase of *H. capsulatum*, has been used as a skin test antigen. The histoplasmin skin test has been regarded as satisfactory by investigators who have used the test on human patients. The test on animals may be used as a diagnostic aid, and it has been shown to be useful as an epidemiologic tool. It should be kept in mind that in areas where the histoplasmin sensitivity rates are high, apparently healthy animals may have a positive reaction.

Animals should be skin-tested with standardized lots of histoplasmin, blastomycin, and coccidioidin at the same time. The antigens should be of equivalent potency so that the size of the reactions can be compared. The antigens for animals must be more concentrated than those used for humans, and frequently the undiluted culture filtrate must be concentrated to be of value.

The skin tests should be done as follows: 0.1 ml each of undiluted blastomycin and coccidioidin are routinely injected ID into separate areas on the side of the neck (cattle) or on the inside of the thigh (dogs); 0.1 ml of histoplasmin diluted 1:10 (cattle) to 1:100 (dogs) is injected in a similar fashion using tuberculin syringes with 0.25 in to 0.5 in (0.64-1.27 cm) 26-gauge needles.[11] The tests are read at 48 hours and a reaction is called positive when there is a definite induration of 5 mm or more in diameter. The histoplasmin and blastomycin reactions are compared; a specific reactor is one that reacted only to or more markedly to the specific than to the cross-reacting or nonspecific antigen. Frequently, but not always, canine histoplasmosis cases will show a reaction in millimeters of induration that is double the blastomycin reaction.

To concentrate the skin test antigens, pour the undiluted antigen (100 ml) into seamless cellulose dialyzing tubing (flat diameter of 44 mm). The tubing is then tied at both ends to seal it and then is suspended in front of a fan at room temperature. The evaporation period varies depending on the concentration desired. From 100 to 80 ml ($2\times$) takes about 12 hours and from 100 ml to 10 ml ($9\times$) takes 4 days. The tubing is marked so that when the final volume is reached it will be the exact concentration desired. The final volume is then filtered through a Seitz filter (type ST-1 L-6) with a 0.5 μm filter pad and bottled.

Reference laboratories. Ecological Investigations Program, CDC, Kansas City, Kansas; Mycology Laboratory, CDC, Atlanta, Ga.

References

1. Abernathy, R.S., and D.C. Heiner. Precipitation reactions in agar in North American blastomycosis. *J. Lab. Clin. Med.* 57:604–611, 1961.
2. Ajello, L., L.K. Georg, W. Kaplan, and L. Kaufman. *Laboratory Manual for Medical Mycology.* Public Health Service Pub. no. 994. U.S. Government Printing Office, Washington, 1963.
3. Awad, F.I. Studies on epizootic lymphangitis in the Sudan. *J. Comp. Path.* 70:457–463, 1960.
4. Darling, S.T. A protozoan general infection producing pseudotubercles in the lungs and focal necrosis in the liver, spleen, and lymph nodes. *J. Am. Med. Ass.* 46:1283–1285, 1906.
5. DeMonbreun, W.A. The cultivation and cultural characteristics of Darling's Histoplasma capsulatum. *Am. J. Trop. Med.* 14:93–125, 1934.
6. DeMonbreun, W.A. The dog as a natural host for *Histoplasma capsulatum. Am. J. Trop. Med.* 19:565–587, 1939.
7. Emmons, C.W. Isolation of *Histoplasma capsulatum* from soil. *Public Heath Rep.* 64:892–896, 1949.
8. Emmons, C.W., D.A. Rowley, B.J. Olson, C.F.T. Mattern, J.A. Bell, E. Powell, and E.A. Marcey. Histoplasmosis: Occurrence of inapparent infection in dogs, cats, and other animals. *Am. J. Hyg.* 61:40–44, 1955.
9. Kaufman, L., and S. Blumer. Development and use of a polyvalent conjugate to differentiate *Histoplasma capsulatum* and *Histoplasma duboisii* from other pathogens. *J. Bact.* 95:1243–1246, 1968.
10. Kligman, A.M., and H. Mescon. The periodic-acid-Schiff stain for the demonstration of fugi in animal tissues. *J. Bact* 60:415–421, 1950.
11. Menges, R.W. The histoplasmin skin test in animals. *J. Am. Vet. Med. Ass.* 119:69–71, 1951.
12. Menges, R.W., M.L. Furcolow, R.T. Habermann, and R.J. Weeks. Epidemiologic studies on histoplasmosis in wildlife. *Envir. Res.* 1:129–144, 1967.
13. Menges, R.W., M.L. Furcolow, L.A. Selby, H.R. Ellis, and R.T. Habermann. Clinical and epidemiologic studies on 79 canine blastomycosis cases in Arkansas. *Am. J. Epidemiol.* 81:164–179, 1965.
14. Menges, R.W., M.L. Furcolow, L.A. Selby, R.T. Habermann, and C.D. Smith. Ecologic studies of histoplasmosis. *Am. J. Epidemiol.* 85:108–119, 1967.
15. Menges, R.W., R.T. Habermann, L.A. Selby, H.R. Ellis, R.F. Behlow, and C.D. Smith. A review and recent findings on histoplasmosis in animals. *Vet. Med.* 58:331–338, 1963.
16. Newberry, W.M., F.E. Tosh, I.L. Doto, and T.D.Y. Chin. The complement fixation antibody test in the diagnosis of chronic pulmonary histoplasmosis and blastomycosis. *J. Chronic Dis.* 20:303–309, 1967.
17. Porter, B.M., B.K. Comfort, R.W. Menges, R.T. Habermann, and C.D. Smith. Correlation of fluorescent antibody, histopathology, and culture on tissues from 372 animals examined for histoplasmosis and blastomycosis. *J. Bact.* 89:748–751, 1965.
18. Schubert, J.H., H.J. Lynch, Jr., and L. Ajello. Evaluation of the agar-plate precipitin test for histoplasmosis. *Am. Rev. Resp. Dis.* 84:845–849, 1961.
19. Sweaney, H.C. *Histoplasmosis.* Thomas, Springfield, Ill., 1960.

61. Phycomycetes

The phycomycoses are caused by a diverse group of lower fungi that have been generally grouped under the heading Phycomycetes. Recent taxonomic proposals have placed nearly all of the phycomycetes that are opportunistic pathogens of domestic animals in the taxonomic class Zygomycetes. The phycomycoses have in common the development of suppurative lesions that contain broad, irregular, relatively aseptate hyphae; these hyphae usually stain well with H & E or PAS-CB.[20] The taxonomic position of the pathogenic members (or purported members) of phycomycete classes is shown in Table 61.1. The agents of coccidioidomycosis and rhinosporidiosis have been classified as phycomycetes by a few authorities but they are not considered in this chapter. (*Coccidioides immitis* is discussed in Chapter 56, but *Rhinosporidium seeberi* is not considered further because, while it is presumed to be a fungus, it has not been cultured.) In this chapter the two terms mucormycosis and entomophthoromycosis have been used to designate conditions caused by zygomycetes in the orders Mucorales and Entomophthorales respectively.

Table 61.1. Pathogenic phycomycetes

Class: Zygomycetes
  Order: Mucorales
    Family: Mucoraceae
      Genera: *Absidia, Mucor, Rhizopus*
    Family: Mortierellaceae
      Genera: *Mortierella, Hyphomyces?*

  Order: Entomophthorales
    Family: Entomophthoraceae
      Genus: *Entomophthora*
    Family: Basidiobolaceae
      Genus: *Basidiobolus*

Class: Chytridiomycetes
  Order: Chytridiales
    Family: not assigned
      Genus: *Coccidioides*

Mucormycosis

Mucormycosis is an opportunistic fungal infection that usually occurs in the presence of lowered or altered host resistance and that may affect any organ of the body.[13,18] Details on some recorded infections and names of the fungi for which adequate proof of a pathogenic role has been established are listed in Table 61.2. A fungus, *Hyphomyces destruens,* that has been recovered from chronic proliferative inflammatory lesions of the skin and mucous membranes of horses is included in the list, as it appears that the orga-

Table 61.2. Some recorded phycomycoses of animals

Hosts	Pathology*	Fungi isolated
Cow	a,b,c,d,e,f,g,m	1,2,6,8,9,10,11,12, 13,14,16,17,18,20
Horse	a,b,c,d,j,k,l	3,4,5,13,14,15
Sheep	a,b,d,m	13
Dog	b,c,d,h	1
Mule	k,l	4,5
Chicken	b,d,i,m	7,19
Okapi	b,d	1
Guinea pig	c	1,2
Mink	k	1
Mouse	j	1
Buzzard	i	7
Waterfowl	i	13

a, abortion; b, ulcers of GI tract; c, enlarged lymph nodes; d, granulomatous foci of organs; e, acute pneumonia; f, bronchitis/tracheitis; g, brain lesions; h, abdominal mass; i, respiratory disease; j, SC lesions; k, cutaneous ulcers; l, nasal polyps and granulomas; m, bone lesion.

1, *A. corymbifera;* 2, *A. ramosa;* 3, *Basidiobolus* sp.; 4, *E. coronata;* 5, *H. destruens;* 6, *Mortierella wolfii;* 7, *M. hygrophila;* 8, *M. polycephala;* 9, *M. zychae;* 10, *Mucor circinelloides;* 11, *M. dispersus;* 12, *M. hiemalis;* 13, *M. pusillus;* 14, *M. racemosus;* 15, *M. spinosus;* 16, *R. arrhizus;* 17, *R. cohnii;* 18, *R. microsporus;* 19, *R. oryzae;* 20, *R. stolonifer.*

*In addition, phycomyceses infections causing ulcers of the GI tract have been diagnosed, on the basis of histopathologic evidence without isolation of the fungi, in the cat, rabbit, goat, gazelle, buffalo, *Macaca mulatta,* and *Mandrillus sphinx.*

nism may in fact be a *Mortierella* species,[4] although recent observations suggest that a more likely taxonomic position is in the genus *Pythium.*[6,16] No reliable information is available on the epidemiology of mucormycosis but infection appears to follow ingestion of or wound contamination by hyphae or spores from moldy feeds.[18]

Pathologically, mucormycosis has several different results, including (1) erosion or ulceration of the alimentary tract or skin; (2) enlargement and/or calcification of lymph nodes, causing tumoruous swellings; (3) granulomatous foci involving internal organs; (4) encephalitis; and (5) placentitis, mycotic abortion, and acute pneumonia.[3,15] While it appears that animals of all ages are attacked, infection is most common in young domestic animals and captive wild animals.[1,14,17] Pregnancy, local tissue damage and devitalization, and prolonged antibacterial therapy appear to be factors that predispose to infection.

Specimens

Specimens of organs containing suspect lesions should be collected in a sterile container and transferred as soon as possible to the laboratory. For mailing purposes, specimens are best inoculated onto suitable media before shipment rather than being sent in the sterile container (Fig. 61.1). A second set of specimens should be placed in 10% Formalin for histologic examination. Scrapings or biopsy material from the necrotic areas are usually adequate for mycological examination. In the case of mycotic abortion, placentas are the most satisfactory specimens. (In only about one in four cases of placental infection are fungal elements present in the stomach contents of the fetus.) In cattle, mycotic abortion caused by their organisms is often followed by an acute mycotic pneumonia.

Material for direct and culture examinations should be obtained from necrotic foci. Placental material should be dissected from the maternal tissue and from the bases of the fetal villi. For preliminary investigation, suspect tissue should be mounted directly in a

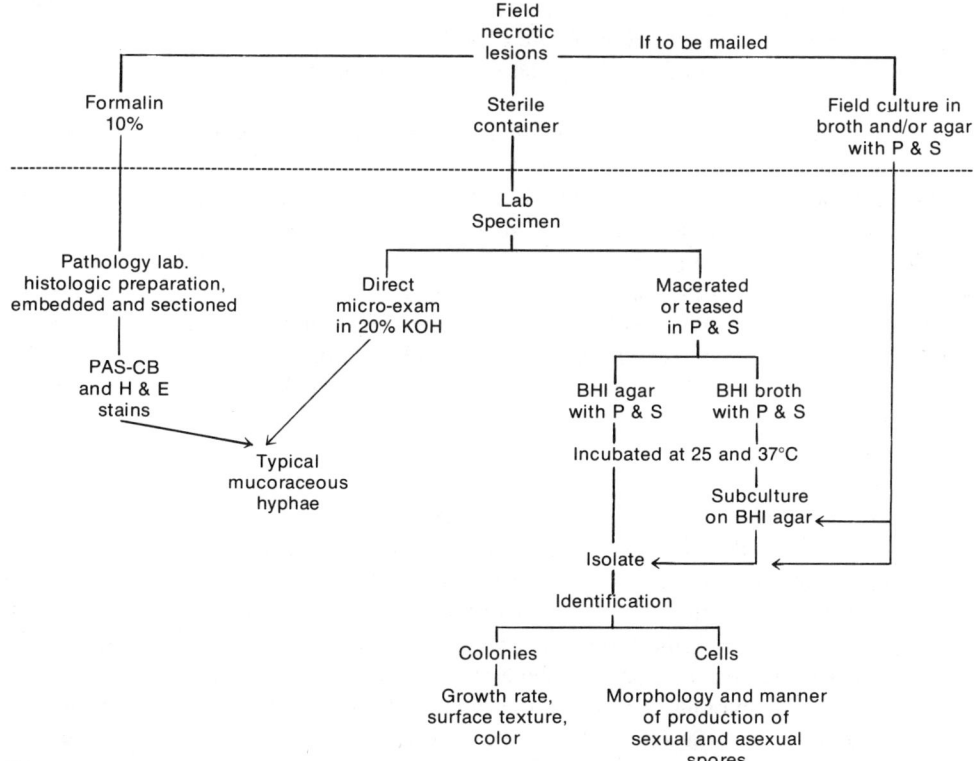

Figure 61.1. Methods for examination of lesions suspected of phycomycosis. P & S, mixture of penicillin (100 units/ml) and streptomycin (100 µg/ml) or chloramphenicol (0.05 mg/ml). Instead of BHI agar, 2% malt extract agar plus P & S can be used.

drop of 20% KOH solution with teasing out and gentle warming before the application of the coverslip.[2] This wet mount is then viewed under the microscope with the light reduced. A useful staining method is to make supplementary mounts in a solution of equal parts of P-51 stain and 20% KOH. Mucoraceous hyphae generally stain rapidly, but most fungi stain if the preparation is kept moist overnight. Hyphae of phycomycetes appear as broad, irregular-sized strands 2–8 µm wide, with few septa and frequent bulbous swellings. Cytoplasmic fat globules may be prominent, especially with *Mortierella* species. Hyphal elements are often found along blood vessels but they may be missed unless the material is thoroughly examined.

Specimens for histopathology, after fixation in 10% Formalin, are embedded and cut in the usual manner. While mucoraceous hyphae usually stain adequately with H & E, specific fungal stains such as Gridley or Grocott's modification of Gomori's methenaminesilver stain are recommended.[20] Where possible, separate histologic specimens should be stained routinely by both H & E and Gridley stains. Only by this method will lesions be screened adequately for possible fungal participation.

In sections, mucoraceous hyphae are characteristically 2–8 µm wide, freely branching, and irregular in outline. Hyphae are usually scattered throughout the necrotic foci but are most numerous at the periphery and about small arterioles that may be present in the larger foci. In chronic lesions, numerous hyphal swellings and even cross walls may be visible, although septa are not regarded as a mucoraceous feature. The intercalary and/or terminal swellings may be up to 50 µm in diameter, and the thin hyphal walls frequently display internal thickenings that stain intensely with Gridley's, PAS-CB, or Gomori's stains. These thickenings are particularly pronounced on the walls of the swollen portions. In open lesions, sporangiophores and sporangia may occur. Species of *Mucor, Rhizopus, Absidia,* and *Mortierella* enter and proliferate in arterial vessels and the resulting thrombi influence the histopathology. Zones of necrosis are found around the hyphae and infected vessels. Neutrophils and eosinophils are usually numerous. *Hyphomyces destruens* evokes a severe host reaction, and hyphae are usually encased by amorphous eosinophilic sleeves, a reaction that is also a typical feature of entomophthoromycosis.

Laboratory Procedures

Cultures. One of the features of mucormycosis is the difficulty that has been experienced in isolating the etiologic fungus. Even when hyphae are abundant in direct microscopic examination, culture techniques may fail.[1] Most of the pathogenic mucoraceous fungi grow well at 37°C on a sugarless medium. Isolations can be made on (1) BHI blood agar, (2) malt extract, or (3) Sabouraud's dextrose agar to which antibiotics have been added (e.g. chloramphenicol, 0.05 mg/ml, or a mixture of streptomycin, 100 µg/ml, and penicillin, 100 units/ml). Of these media the first two are probably the best. While firm yellowish necrotic material taken from a lesion after searing may be plated directly onto the medium, a more satisfactory techique is dissection (under binocular microscope) of fungal elements from tissue near the margin of the lesion followed by washing in sterile saline or an antibacterial solution (as above) before inoculation. Macerated portions or blocks of tissue from the lesion can also be placed in BHI broth containing antibiotics and, when fungal growth is evident, transferred onto solid medium. Wherever possible, both solid and liquid techniques should be attempted. When large pieces of tissue are present, the surface can be seared and pieces of caruncle 3–4 mm in diameter cut out and placed directly on the surface of the agar or in the broth medium.

Bovine, ovine, and equine placentas normally become grossly contaminated with bacteria and saprophytic fungi. The chief difficulty lies in deciding whether an isolate is of causal significance or is simply a contaminant. Very careful comparison of the hyphae seen in the direct examination with those of the isolate must be made to ascertain the significance of their presence. Histologic examination is essential to demonstrate the characteristic hyphae and associated inflammatory response. In some cases it may be necessary to dissect individual lengths of hyphae from pathologic specimens and observe their continued growth in culture. It is advisable to incubate inoculated media at 37 and 25°C, as some significant species, e.g. *Mucor racemosus,* fail to grow at the higher temperature. Fungal growth is usually well advanced after 24 hours.

Subcultures are most satisfactorily preserved by the use of mineral oil overlays or in distilled water suspensions. In the first method, actively growing cultures on tubed media (slants or butts) are covered with a good grade of sterilized heavy mineral oil. As long as the whole agar surface is covered, oiled cultures will remain viable without further attention for several years. To transfer a fungus from an oiled culture, draw out a portion of the fungus on the agar substratum through the oil with a long inoculating needle. Excess oil is drained off along the inside of the tube and the inoculum transferred to a fresh agar plate or slope.

With the water method, hyphae or spores are scraped off the surface of an actively growing culture and suspended in 15–20 ml of sterile distilled water in a screw-topped container. Fungal elements remain viable in the water for several months or even years. Subcultures are obtained by removing small fragments of hyphae and spores with a loop or pipette and inoculating onto a suitable medium. Both methods eliminate the need for continuous subculturing.

The serologic demonstration, by the AD technique, of precipitating antibodies in the sera of cattle has been found to be an extremely useful aid in the diagnosis of *Mortierella wolfii* abortion.[6]

Cellular morphology. Phycomycetes are identified by the manner of spore production. Unfortunately it is often difficult to induce this spore production on such substrates as potato dextrose agar. A nonenriched "hay-extract" agar has been found satisfactory for initiating spore development in many species including those of the genus *Mortierella.* The following is a list of the morphologic features of the main genera of the order Mucorales that have been found associated with mucormycosis. As identification of the genera at a species level is a highly specialized field, cultures for further identification and confirmation should be sent to a recognized mycological institute such as the Northern Utilization Research and Development Division Laboratory, Peoria, Ill.; the Mycology Unit, CDC; or the Commonwealth Mycological Institute, Ferry Lane, Kew, Surrey, Eng.

Rhizopus species

Macroscopic features. Growth is rapid and voluminous. The mycelium is long fibred, coarse, and woolly; it is white, becoming gray and sprinkled with many black or brown dots (sporangia) as it matures.

Microscopic features. The mycelium is nonseptate and colorless. The sporing structure consists of long stalks (sporangiophores) surmounted by spherical sporangia. Sporangia are dark walled and when mature are filled with spherical hyaline spores and a columella. Sporangiophores are unbranched and are clustered at nodes opposite root-like rhizoids along a horizontal runner or stolon (Fig. 61.2).

Absidia species[9,12]

The macroscopic and microscopic features of *Absidia* are similar to those of *Rhizopus,* but the sporangia arise along the internodes of the arching stolon instead of the nodes. The sporangia are slightly pear shaped instead of round and the columella is prominent, protrudes deeply into the sporangium, and has a peaked apex (Fig. 61.2).

Mucor species[7,10,18]

Macroscopic features. The colony grows rapidly, with a fluffy aerial mycelium that is at first white, later gray to brown.

Microscopic features. The mycelium is nonseptate, colorless, and without rhizoids (a few septa may be visible in the old mycelium). Sporangiophores arise singly from the mycelium, forming a thick erect tuft. The sporangiophore may be either unbranched or branched, with spherical, many-spored sporangia on all the branch ends (Fig. 61.2). Columellae are always present and may bear remnants of the sporangial wall after spores have been released (Fig. 61.2).

Mortierella species

Macroscopic features. The mycelium is submerged or closely apposed to the surface of the agar, so that the amount of aerial mycelium is much less than in most genera of the Mucorales. Tufts of aerial mycelium may appear with age.

Miscroscopic features. Sporangiophores are erect, simple, or branched and usually taper to a hairlike tip on which the sporangium is borne (Fig. 61.2). Sporangia are round and lack a columella. The sporangial wall is delicate and usually only a remnant remains after the sporangiospores are released (Fig. 61.2). Conidia (stylospores) are round, unicellular, and echinulate (spiked). These occur at the tips of simple or branched conidiophores. Zygospores are surrounded at maturity with a thick layer of closely woven hyphae.

Hyphomyces destruens (*Pythium* or *Mortierella* sp.)

The macroscopic and microscopic features are similar to *Mortierella* species. In the past, various workers failed to induce sporulation in their isolates, perhaps because of too rich a medium. However, it has recently been demonstrated, by placing portions of colonies in sterile water containing small pieces of sterilized rotted corn silage, that

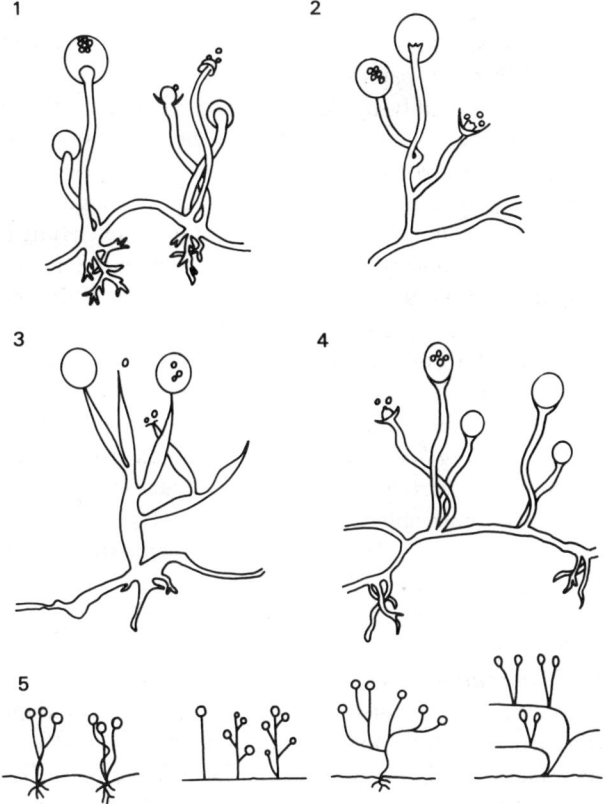

Figure 61.2. Drawings of microscopic features of phycomycete genera important in mucormycosis: 1, micromorphology of *Rhizopus* species; 2, micromorphology of *Mucor* species; 3, micromorphology of *Absidia* species; 4, micromorphology of *Mortierella* species; 5, (left to right), growth habits of *Rhizopus, Mucor, Mortierella,* and *Absidia* species.

biflagellate zoospores are formed; they arise from the cleavage of protoplasmic masses emitted from undifferentiated filamentous sporangia.[3]

Entomophthoromycosis

Entomophthormycoses infections caused by fungi belonging to the order Entomophthorales are primarily diseases of the subcutaneous tissues and the nasal mucosa. Unlike mucormycosis, entomophthoromycosis occurs in otherwise healthy individuals.[10] The characteristic histologic picture of an eosinophilic granuloma with hyphae surrounded by a collar of eosinophilic granular material differentiates these diseases from the mucormycoses, in which the prominent features are infarction and infiltration of blood vessels by the fungus.

Two genera have been incriminated in entomophthoromycosis of animals, *Basidiobolus* and *Entomophthora*. Infection by *Basidiobolus ranarum* (*B. haptosporus*) has been described; it occurred in the leg of a horse.[19] Lesions were characterized by indurated masses that extended widely between skin and muscle fascia. Infection by *Entomophthora coronata* in the nostrils, nasal mucosa, and lips of several horses and a mule has been described.[5,11] The lesions are limited to nasal polyps and granulomas. The localization of these lesions in the head structures is in contrast to the lesions of *Hyphomyces destruens,* which are found in many parts of the body.

The mode of infection of *E. coronata* is probably by the inhalation of spores, which then invade the nasal mucosa. The fungus occurs in soil and decaying vegetation and can infect insects.[10] Warm climates appear to favor infection.[8]

In entomophthoromycosis, numerous small irregular yellowish areas of coagulation necrosis are scattered through a very vascular granulation tissue. With Gridley's fungal stain, large (4–8 μm wide) branching mucoraceous hyphae can be seen within the necrotic foci. Bulbous hyphal swellings (up to 12 μm diameter) may also be visible, while the hyphae are usually surrounded by an amorphous, granular, eosinophilic sheath.

Specimens are collected by biopsy or after surgical removal of the lesions. Tissue containing yellow necrotic foci are sought for mycological and histologic examinations. Direct examination and isolation procedures are similar to those already described for mucormycosis. Both *E. coronata* and *Basidiobolus* species can be isolated from specimens by implanting small portions from the necrotic foci onto media such as malt extract of Sabouraud's glucose agar (containing antibacterial agents). Hyphal growth around the inoculum usually becomes visible in 2–3 days at 30°C. Characteristics of the two fungal species are given below.

Entomophthora coronata

Macroscopic features. In culture, *E. coronata* grows rapidly reaching a diameter of 6 cm within 48 hours at 30°C. The colorless to yellowish-white colony is at first flat and waxy but quickly produces radial and irregular folds and a white bloom on the surface, which represents surface hyphae and short conidiophores. The surface of the petri dish lid facing the colony or the wall of the tube facing the slant is covered in 24–36 hours by a gray film of conidia that have been forcibly discharged from the tips of the conidiophores. These conidia may replicate or produce hyphae on the nonnutritive dish surface.

Microscopic features. Hyphae vary in dimensions between 6 and 15 μm. They contain droplets and granules of varying size, which are apparently fat, glycogen, and other metabolites. Many germinated spores and older hyphae appear empty and these structures are separated by septa from the viable portions. Conidiophores emerge from hyphal segments near the surface of the medium. They are phototropic and discharge conidia toward a light source. Conidiophores are $8–12 \times 60–90$ μm, bulge slightly in the midportion, and taper toward the tip. The conidium originates as a spherical enlargement at the tip of the conidiophore (Fig. 61.3). The tip of the conidiophore extends into the young spore as a columella. At maturity the almost spherical spore (basal papilla were attached to conidiophores) is forcibly discharged. Diameters of the primary spores are 36–44 μm; secondary spores, formed by replication, are smaller. Occasionally conidia extrude a material that forms hairlike appendages over their entire surface (Fig. 61.3). Although brittle and noncellular, these appendages are considered to be related to the type of multiple germination by replication that is frequently observed with this fungus.

Conidia on a nonnutritive surface may sporulate by producing one or a number of

Phycomycetes

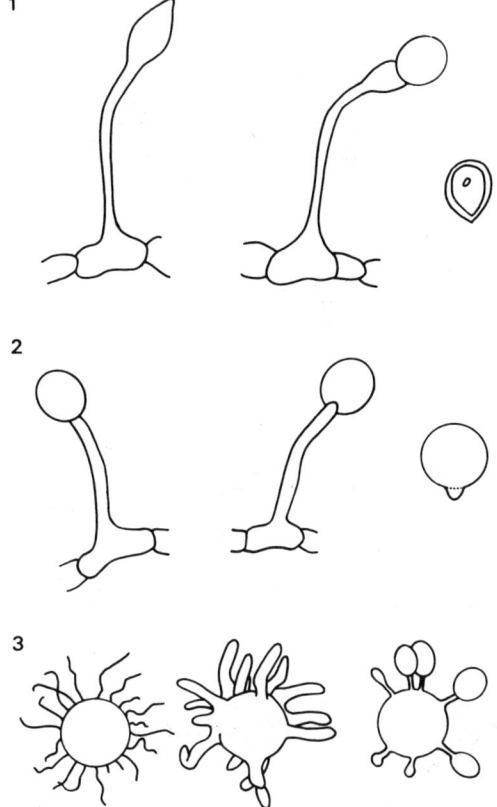

Figure 61.3. Drawings of microscopic features of the genera *Entomophthora* and *Basidiobolus*: 1, formation of *Basidiobolus* conidia; 2, formation of *Entomophthora* conidia; 3, *Entomophthora* conidia showing (left to right) hairlike appendages, multiple germination tubes, and secondary conidial formation.

short tubes that become conidiophores and bear secondary conidia (Fig. 61.3). Germination of conidia on a nutritive surface may be by single or multiple germination tubes (Fig. 61.3).

Basidiobolus species (*B. haptosporus*)

Macroscopic features. The colony develops rapidly as a thin sheet of mycelium on the surface of the agar. The surface is at first gray to pale yellow and waxy. However, it soon develops a short while aerial mycelium.

Microscopic features. Large numbers of chlamydospores and zygospores are usually produced along the hyphae. On the zygospore surface, the two short copulation tubes appear as beaks or protuberances. The zygospore has a thick smooth wall but it is entirely enclosed within the mother cell.

Asexual reproduction is by sporangiospores. The short slender erect sporangiophore develops a club-shaped tip. From this structure a terminal bud develops that enlarges to form a pear-shaped sporangium. The sporangium is uninucleate and is discharged forcibly from the sporangiophore, along with a fragment of the sporangiophore (Fig. 61.3). Spores develop later in this structure.

References

1. Ainsworth, G.C., and P.K.C. Austwick. *Fungal Diseases of Animals.* 2d ed. Commonwealth Agricultural Bureau, 1973. Farnham Royal, Eng.,
2. Ajello, L., L.K. Georg, W. Kaplan, and L. Kaufman. *Laboratory Manual for Medical Mycology.* Public Health Service Pub. no. 994. HEW, Washington, 1963.
3. Austwick, P.K.C., and J.W. Copland. Swamp cancer. *Nature* 250:84, 1974.
4. Bridges, C.H., and C.W. Emmons. A phycomycosis of horses caused by *Hyphomyces destruens. J. Am. Vet. Med. Ass.* 138:579–589, 1961.
5. Bridges, C.H., W.M. Romane, and C.W. Emmons. Phycomycosis in horses caused by *Entomophthora coronata. J. Am. Vet. Med. Ass.* 140:673–677, 1962.
6. Carter, M.E., D.O. Cordes, M.E. diMenna, and R. Hunter. Fungi isolated from bovine mycotic abortion and pneumonia with special reference to *Mortierella wolfii. Res. Vet. Sci.* 14:201–206, 1973.
7. Cordes, D.O., and E. H. Shortridge. Systemic phycomycosis and aspergillosis of cattle. *New Zealand Vet. J.* 16:65–80, 1968.
8. Dawson, C.O. Phycomycosis in animals in the tropics. *Ann. Soc. Belge Med. Trop.* 52:357–364, 1971.
9. Emmons, C.W. Phycomycosis in man and animals. *Rivista Patologia Vegetale* 4:329–377, 1964.
10. Emmons, C.W., C.H. Binford, and J.P. Utz. *Medical Mycology.* 2d ed. Lea and Febiger, Philadelphia, 1970.
11. Emmons, C.W., and C.H. Bridges. *Entomophthora coronata,* the etiologic agent of phycomycosis of horses. *Mycologia* 58:307–312, 1961.
12. Ftizpatrick, H.M. *The Lower Fungi, Phycomycetes.* McGraw-Hill, New York, 1930.
13. Greer, D.L. Fungi of phycomycosis. In *Manual of Clinical Microbiology,* E.H. Lennette, E.H. Spaulding, and J.P. Truant (eds.). 2d ed. American Society for Microbiology, Bethesda, Md., 1974.
14. Jungerman, P.F., and R.M. Schwartzman. *Veterinary Medical Mycology.* Lea and Febiger, Philadelphia, 1972.
15. Migaki, G., K.A. Langheinrich, and F.M. Garner. Pulmonary mucormycosis (phycomycosis) in a chicken. *Avian Dis.* 14:179–183, 1970.
16. Rippon, J.W. *Medical Mycology: The Pathogenic Fungi and the Pathogenic Actinomycetes.* Saunders, Philadelphia, 1974.
17. Smith, J.M.B. Diseases of laboratory animals—mycotic. In *Handbook of Laboratory Animal Science,* E.C. Melby and N.H. Altman (eds.), vol. 2. CRC Press, Cleveland, 1974.
18. Smith, J.M.B. The investigation of opportunistic mycoses? A review. *Pathology* 8:29–41, 1976.
19. Williams, A.O. Pathology of phycomycosis due to *Entomophthora* and *Basidiobolus* species. *Arch. Path.* 87:13–20, 1969.
20. Young, B.J. Staining of fungal hyphae in tissue sections. *J. Med. Lab. Technol.* 25:343–346, 1968.

62. Prototheca

Prototheca is classified among the achlorophyllic algae in the family Chlorellaceae. There are a number of species within the genus and several species have been incriminated in diseases of domestic animals and humans.[3,6]

Prototheca portoricensis has been isolated in England from a cow with bovine mastitis.[1] Another species, *P. zopfii*, has been used in artificial transmission studies of bovine mastitis. This organism was grown from the secretions of an inflamed udder and subsequently used for intracisternal infusion into two cows. One of the two cows developed acute mastitis; the other cow had a chronic infection. Even after a dry period of 2.5 months, the alga could be demonstrated in the milk. *Prototheca* has been isolated from several cows with a mastitis problem in the United States. In 1959 the organism was isolated in Florida from several cows in a milking herd with mastitis. Recently, a number of cows in a 100-cow herd in Ohio were proven infected with *Prototheca*.[5] Thirty of the cows were removed from the herd because of reduced milk production and lack of response to treatment. *Prototheca* was the only organism isolated from the affected cattle. When it was used to experimentally infect a cow, an acute mastitis developed and the cow was "dry" in 3 days.

Pathogenicity for guinea pigs has been demonstrated using an isolate from potatoes, *P. ciferrii*.[8] As early as 1930, *P. portoricensis* was isolated from the stools of human patients suffering from sprue.[2] However, it was uncertain whether this organism was the cause of the disease. *P. segbwema* was isolated as the causative agent of a spreading skin lesion on the inside of a human patient's foot. *P. wickerhamii* has been cultured from and demonstrated in ulcerating papules of the skin of the lower leg of another human patient.[4,7]

Specimens

Milk samples obtained from cows with mastitis can be collected in small vials for transport to the laboratory. Direct microscopic examination for *Prototheca* can be made by smearing a small drop of milk or other exudate on a glass slide. After the smear is well dried, it may be stained with Newman-Lampert milk stain or with Giemsa stain and examined under oil.

Laboratory Procedures

Cultures. Exudate or milk can be streaked on a plate for isolation of *Prototheca*. The organisms grow well on tryptose blood agar with 5% defibrinated calf blood, Sabouraud dextrose agar, potato dextrose agar, cornmeal agar, and yeast malt agar.[9] They will not grow on media containing cycloheximide. Plates should be incubated at both 27 and 37°C. Growth usually occurs quite rapidly, and a white, opaque, dry, yeastlike colony is formed that obtains an approximate diameter of 4 mm in 3 days.

Prototheca segbwema has been shown to be sensitive to nystatin, amphotericin B, brilliant green, gentian violet, and copper sulphate. It was not sensitive to griseofulvin at 50 μg per ml incorporated into peptone glucose agar.

Cellular morphology. There are a number of species of this genus and the morphology varies slightly with the species. In culture, cystlike structures are formed that are approximately 20–30 μm in diameter. Internal division takes place in the cystlike structure, and there may be numerous uninucleate daughter cells formed and subsequently released by rupture of the cyst wall. Each of the daughter cells then may eventually form a cystlike structure and repeat the cycle.

Prototheca apparently has lost the ability to produce chloroplasts and pyrenoids and behaves as a saprophyte. It was originally described as a funguslike organism and later placed among the algae. The cell wall of this organism is made of cellulose and lacks chitin. In tissue, the organism stains only faintly with H & E and is PAS positive.

References

1. Ainsworth, G.C., and P.K.C. Austwick. A survey of animal mycoses in Britain: Mycological aspects. *Trans. Brit. Mycol. Soc.* 38:369–386, 1955.
2. Ashford, B.K., R. Ciferri, and L.M. Dalmau. New species of Prototheca and variety of same isolated from human intestine. *Arch. Protistenk.* 70:619–638, 1930.
3. Chodat, R. Monographies d'algue en culture pure. *Beit. Kryptogamenfl. Schweiz* 4:121–130, 1913.
4. Davies, R.R., H. Spencer, and P.O. Wakelin. A case of human protothecosis. *Trans. Roy. Soc. Trop. Med. Hyg.* 58:448–451, 1964.
5. Frank, N., L.C. Ferguson, R.F. Cross, and D.R. Redman. Prototheca, a cause of bovine mastitis. *Am. J. Vet. Res.* 30:1785–1794, 1969.
6. Heidrich, H.J., W. Renk. *Diseases of the Mammary Glands of Domestic Animals*, L.W. Van den Heever (trans.). Saunders, Philadelphia, 1967.
7. Klintworth, G.K., B.F. Fetter, and H.S. Nielson. Protothecosis, an algal infection: Report of a case in man. *J. Med. Microbiol.* 1:211–216, 1968.
8. Negroni, P., and R. Blaisten. Estudio morfologico y fisiologica de una neuva especie de *Prototheca: Prototheca cifferrii* n. sp. aislada de epidermis de papa. *Mycopathol. Mycol. Appl.* 3:94–104, 1941.
9. Tubaki, K., and M. Soneda. Cultural and taxonomical studies on *Prototheca*. Nagaoa 6:25–34, 1959.

63. Sporotrichum

Sporotrichosis is a subacute or chronic disease of humans and various species of lower animals caused by the dimorphic fungus *Sporotrichum schenckii*.[1] The disease is usually limited to the skin and subcutaneous tissues; occasionally the deeper tissues are involved. Sporotrichosis is worldwide in distribution, occurring sporadically, as a rule, in both temperate and tropical regions.[4,5] *Sporotrichum schenckii* exists as a saprophyte in nature. It has been isolated from soil and from plant and plant products. Infections usually follow injuries to the skin that become contaminated with elements of the fungus. The disease in humans characteristically appears as a linear series of subcutaneous nodules along the course of the lymphatic vessels that drain the area of a primary lesion. The nodules eventually break down, forming suppurating ulcers. This syndrome usually characterizes the disease in horses, mules, and donkeys, the animals most commonly found to have sporotrichosis. Sporotrichosis has also been recognized in dogs. In this species the classic lymphangitic form has been recognized as well as a disseminated form confined to the skin or involving the bones and internal organs. Sporotrichosis has also been described in rats and mice. In rodents the lesions appeared as subcutaneous nodules that broke down to form suppurating ulcers.

Specimens

Pus and exudate from ulcerated lesions should be collected with a sterile loop for preparation of smears and inoculation of culture tubes. Pus from unopened subcutaneous nodules can be collected with a sterile needle and syringe, and tissue can be obtained by biopsy from one of the nodules. In cases of suspected pulmonary sporotrichosis, washings are obtained by bronchoscopy.

Smears are made from some of the pus, exudate, and washings for direct microscopic examination. The remainder of the specimen should be cultured. A portion of the biopsy tissue is fixed promptly in 10% Formalin for sectioning. The remainder should be used for direct microscopic examination and culture.

Sporotrichosis is not a transmissible disease in the usual sense. However, in rare cases the disease has been contracted by humans working with infectious materials. Therefore, reasonable care should be exercised when collecting or handling such materials.

Because of the paucity of *S. schenckii* cells in lesions, the direct microscopic examination of clinical materials by conventional methods is usually of little value in the diagnosis of sporotrichosis. The FA technique, however, is of great value for the detection of *S. schenckii* in smears of clinical materials.[3] Moreover, the added dimension of serologic specificity afforded by this procedure enables identification of this fungus with a high degree of accuracy. In clinical materials *S. schenckii* is yeastlike and appears in the form of round or oval single or budding cells.

Tissues are fixed and sectioned by conventional histopathologic procedures. With ordinary histologic stains, *S. schenckii* cells are usually difficult to find. The use of PAS or methenamine silver (Gomori) stains, as well as the FA technique, facilitates demonstration of these organisms, since with these stains they are more clearly delineated from tissue elements.

Laboratory Procedures

Cultures. Whether organisms are detected in clinical materials or not, culture studies should be carried out. *S. schenckii* is a dimorphic organism appearing in a mycelial form when grown at room temperature (25°C) and in a yeastlike form when grown at 37°C on an enriched medium or in animal tissue. Demonstration of the two forms is necessary for definitive identification of this fungus. For isolation of the mycelial form of *S. schenckii*, clinical specimens are inoculated on Sabouraud's dextrose agar containing C & C. These cultures are incubated at room temperature (25°C). For isolation of the yeastlike form, clinical materials should be inoculated on an enriched medium such as BHI agar and incubated at 37°C.

Morphologic characteristics. The mycelial form grows rapidly on Sabouraud's dextrose agar with C & C. Within 3–7 days, moist white colonies appear that soon develop irregularly wrinkled or folded surfaces, particularly at the center of the colonies. The colonies may remain moist, leathery, and wrinkled, or a fine grayish velvety growth may appear at the outer borders. The color of mature colonies varies from cream through brown to black.

Microscopic examination of the mycelial form reveals a fine (2 μm diameter), branched, septate, hyaline mycelium. Conidia are produced in abundance and vary in morphology. Thin-walled, pyriform to elongate conidia (1.5–3×3–6 μm) usually appear first. As the cultures mature, somewhat larger, round to ovoid, relatively thick-walled spores are produced. Some isolates form pyramidal or conical-shaped spores. Two sporulation patterns occur: (1) Conidia are borne in small groups at the tips of conidiophores. Each spore is attached to the conidiophore by a short delicate sterigma. (2) Conidia are borne individually on delicate sterigmata along the sides of the hyphae, forming a sleevelike pattern. Pigment that may be present in spores gives *S. schenckii* colonies their dark color.

The yeast form develops rapidly when grown on enriched medium at 37°C. Yeast-form colonies of *S. schenckii* are characteristically soft and cream colored. Microscopically the growth is composed of round or oval, single or budding cells (up to 10 μm in diameter) or as elongated budding cells (1–3×3–10 μm) often referred to as cigar shaped.

Definitive identification of *S. schenckii* isolates should rest on the demonstration of both mold and yeast forms. Consequently, if only the mycelial form has been isolated, attempts should be made to convert it to the yeast form. Such conversion may be accomplished by subculture of the isolate on an enriched medium such as BHI agar and incubation at 37°C. It may be necessary to make several serial transfers on such a medium before complete conversion is accomplished. If conversion cannot be accomplished in vitro, animal inoculation may be necessary. Mice can be used for this purpose. A dense 0.2-ml suspension of the mycelial culture in physiological saline is injected intratesticularly into several mice. After a period of 1–2 weeks, orchitis is produced. Gram-stained smears of the purulent material will reveal the numerous characteristic yeast-like cells when conversion has occurred. Mice can also be given IP injections of 1 ml of a dense suspension of the mycelial culture. After a period of 1–2 weeks the mice are sacrificed and smears of lesions in the abdominal cavity are stained by the Gram method. These preparations are examined for the presence of the yeastlike cells of *S. schenckii*. The identification of yeast-form cultures can be confirmed by their conversion to the mycelial form. This can be accomplished by subculture on a simple medium such as Sabouraud's dextrose agar and incubation at room temperature (25°C).

Animal inoculation. Animal inoculation is generally not necessary for isolation of *S. schenckii*. Mice are susceptible.

Immunology and serology. Yeast-form cultures of *S. schenckii* can be identified by means of the FA technique. Agglutinins, precipitins, and CF antibodies can be demonstrated in sera of experimentally infected and vaccinated animals. However, the value of serologic tests for the diagnosis of natural infections in animals remains to be determined.

Persons infected with *S. schenckii* develop delayed cutaneous hypersensitivity to antigens prepared from this organism. Due to the persistence of this hypersensitivity for long periods of time the skin test is of limited value for diagnosis of active disease. Litttle is known regarding the development of delayed hypersensitivity in naturally infected animals.

Reference laboratory. CDC.

References

1. Ainsworth, G.C., and P.K.C. Austwick. *Fungal Diseases of Animals.* Review Series no. 6. Commonwealth Bureau of Animal Health, Commonwealth Agricultural Bureau, Farnham Royal, Bucks., Eng., 1959.
2. Ajello, L., L.K. Georg, W. Kaplan, and L. Kaufman. *Laboratory Manual for Medical Mycology.* Public Health Service Pub. no. 994. HEW, Washington, 1963.
3. Kaplan, W., and A. Gonzalez. Application of the fluorescent antibody technique to the rapid diagnosis of sporotrichosis. *Lab. Clin. Med.* 62:835–841, 1963.
4. Norden, A. Sporotrichosis: Clinical and laboratory features and a serologic study in experimental animals and humans. *Acta Path. Microbiol. Scand.*, suppl. 89, 1951.
5. Brown, R. Sporotrichosis infection in mines of the Witwatersrand: A symposium. *Proc. Transvaal Mine Med. Officer's Ass.* (Transvaal Chamber of Mines, Johannesberg, S. Afr.), 1947.

64. Trichosporon

Trichosporon species are widely distributed mycelial yeastlike fungi that occasionally occur as pathogens of animals. *Trichosporon cutaneum* is seen in infections of the hair shaft of humans and lower primates and this and other species are encountered occasionally in bovine mastitis.[1] The organism is not considered to be hazardous in the laboratory when handled with the usual care.

Specimens

Skin scrapings, hair, and mammary exudates are prepared for microscopic examination under 10% KOH (skin and hair) or air-dried smears for Gram staining (exudates). The microscopic morphology of the culture is best assessed by examination of slide cultures as described in Chapter 55.

Laboratory Procedures

Cultures. Specimens are streaked over the surface of Sabouraud's dextrose agar and incubated at room temperature. The fungus grows fairly rapidly, forming soft, creamy to tan colonies that become wrinkled and tenacious to leathery with age. These organisms are sensitive to cycloheximide.

Cellular morphology. The elements of *Trichosporon* are gram-positive. Exudates contain yeastlike arthrospores $2-4$ μm $\times$ $4-9$ μm. The colony is comprised of true mycelial elements $2-4$ μm in diameter, arthrospores, and blastospores. *Trichosporon cutaneum* does not ferment sugars. Features differentiating *Trichosporon* from other mycelial yeast pathogens are listed in Chapter 55.

References
1. Ajello, L., L. K. Georg, W. Kaplan, and L. Kaufman. *Laboratory Manual for Medical Mycology.* Public Health Service Pub. no. 994. HEW, Washington, 1963.

65. Fungi Associated with Tumors or Wartlike Lesions

Mycetoma

The term mycetoma implies a tumor or swelling of fungal origin. Traditional usage includes under this classification pathologically similar lesions of actinomycotic and nocardial etiology;[3] these have been dealt with in Chapters 49 and 51. Mycetomas caused by true fungi are called eumycotic in distinction to the actinomycotic mycetomas.[4] The terms maduromycosis and maduromycetoma are also used to describe these conditions.[5]

A large variety of saprophytic fungi have been found associated with eumycotic mycetoma in humans, including *Aspergillus* and *Penicillium* sp. In the United States the most common species involved is *Allescheria boydii*. In animals the disease has been reported but only rarely; there are less than 20 cases on record.[2] The species of fungi implicated were *Helminthosporium spiciferum, Curvularia geniculata,* and *Allescheria boydii*.

Specimens

Eumycotic mycetomas are the result of granulomatous and pyogenic processes. Samples are apt to be biopsy or surgical specimens. In cases where sinus tracts have developed to the outside, exudates can be collected on bandages or swabs. Attempts can be made to aspirate pus with syringe and needle.

Exudates collected from mycetomas contain typically small concentrations: "grains" made up of varying proportions of fungal elements and cementing substances. Their color is consistent according to the fungus involved, yellowish or whitish-gray for *Allescheria boydii,* black for *Curvularia* and *Helminthosporium* and other dematiacious species. When mounted in 10% KOH under a coverslip, the grains are seen to consist of septate hyphae, 2 μm or more in width, and chlamydospores. The identifiable fungal constituents tend to occupy the peripheral portion of the granule while the center is made up of amorphous material.

Tissues intended for histopathologic studies are fixed in the usual manner and may be stained with H & E or one of the PAS procedures.

Laboratory Procedures

Cultures. In case of solid tissue specimens or samples obtained under sterile precautions from closed cavities, no special preparation is necessary. Exudates obtained from draining tracts should be mixed with sterile saline containing antibacterial agents. Ajello et al. recommend penicillin (5000 units/ml) and streptomycin (500 μg/ml) or chloramphenicol (0.05 mg/ml).[1] The mixture is incubated overnight and centrifuged the next day to sediment the grains. These can then be inoculated.

The fungi so far identified as causes of mycetoma in animals readily grow on ordinary laboratory media including blood, infusion, and tryptose agar as well as Sabouraud's. If antimicrobic substances are to be included, cycloheximide should not be one of them since the fungi involved may be sensitive to it.

The fungi in question grow at 37°C and lower temperatures. Some fungi associated with human eumycotic mycetoma have more specific temperature preferences, such as 30 or 37°C. Suspect cultures are therefore incubated at both these temperatures. In view of the very rudimentary nature of current knowledge regarding eumycotic mycetoma in animals, it may be well to follow the same procedures.

The fungi seen in animal mycetomas are normal inhabitants of the inanimate environment. Their preservation poses little problem. Cultures can be stored for years under a layer of sterile mineral oil. They are readily sterilized by heat and the usual fungal disinfectants.

Cellular morphology. Allescheria boydii is a rapidly growing fungus producing a fluffy mycelium that is whitish-gray and turns darker with age. It has been aptly compared with singed cotton. The reverse side is a darker gray to black. Microscopically the thallus consists of broad hyaline hyphae bearing pyriform single-celled conidia, with dimensions averaging about 6×8 μm. They are borne singly or in clusters. Many strains are capable of sexual reproduction, especially on media like cornmeal or potato dextrose agar. Spherical perithecia, several hundred microns in diameter and visible to the naked eye as tiny black dots in the culture, are formed and, when mature, dehisce, liberating their ascospores. Some mycologists reserve the name *A. boydii* for sexually reproducing strains, while they call those not demonstrably capable of doing so *Monosporium apiospermum.*

Curvularia and *Helminthosporium* are very similar fungi. They grow rapidly on ordinary laboratory media, producing velvety to cottony colonies of dark pigmentation—brown, gray, or black.[1] Microscopic examination reveals dark-colored dematiaceous septate hyphae with groups of characteristic conidia borne on the terminal portion of conidiphores of variable length. The spore-bearing portion changes direction at each point where a spore is attached so that it assumes the appearance of a gnarled tree limb. The multicellular spores of *Helminthosporium* are straight and symmetrical while those of *Curvularia* are distorted and bent due to the disproportionate enlargement of one of the central cells.

Animal inoculation. There is no reliable way of producing eumycotic mycetoma in experimental animals, nor are the agents associated with this condition ordinarily pathogenic for laboratory species. Experimental animals have not been used in the diag-

Chromomycosis

Chromomycosis or chromoblastomycosis is another subcutaneous chronic fungal disease caused by a number of saprophytic dematiaceous fungi. It differs from mycetoma in that (1) the process appears to be entirely granulomatous, suppuration occurring only as a bacterial complication following ulceration; (2) grains are not found in the exudate; (3) the primary disease is practically always confined to subcutaneous tissues; (4) the disease is characterized typically by proliferative lesions resembling warts and even epidermoid carcinomas; (5) the fungal elements in tissue are thick-walled, nonstaining, septate, dividing sclerotia; and (6) the etiologic agents are all closely related mycologically.

A recent review stated that no verified case of chromomycosis in lower animals has been recorded. There is, however, at least one report of an equine case in which both the pathology and mycology are consistent with chromomycosis.[6] Other cases, based largely on morphologic studies of the lesions, are very strongly suggestive of the condition.

Specimens

Specimens are nodular, verrucous, or ulcerated skin lesions or portions thereof. Scrapings may be examined in 10% KOH mounts. Tissue blocks are fixed and processed like other histopathologic specimens. In H & E preparation the granulomatous nature of the lesion will be apparent. The fungal components, predominantly yeastlike sclerotic bodies and occasionally hyphal fragments, will be unstained but will be recognizable by their heavy black-brown to yellowish walls. They are identical in appearance regardless of the species of fungus involved.

Laboratory Procedures

Cultures. The specimens are cultured like other skin scrapings. In view of the frequently heavy bacterial admixtures and the indifference of the causative agents to cycloheximide, C & C agar should be used for culturing surface material. Incubation at room temperature is recommended. Growth is quite slow and results at first in glabrous, darkly pigmented, waxy or tarry colonies, which eventually, sometimes only on subcultures, become pubescent. Some forms produce a dark soluble pigment that diffuses into the medium.

Cellular morphology. Microscopically, growth consists of the heavily contoured dematiaceous hyphae, which give rise to one or more of three types of sporulation: (1) An urn- or vaselike conidiophore is called a phialide. Spores are liberated at the mouth of the vase where they aggregate in variably sized clusters. (2) A single pointed unbranched conidiophore gives rise to conidia that arrange themselves around the tip and along the distal portion of the conidiophore, rather like the bristles of a bottle brush. This is called the acrothecal type of sporulation. (3) Branching conidiophores bear chains of conidia that in turn may branch; this is called the cladosporial type.

The sporulation patterns have been used for various determinations. One school (CDC manual) holds that all cultures showing phialide sporulation exclusively should be called *Phialophora*.[1] Similarly, those with only the cladosporial type are assigned to the genus *Cladosporium,* while those with mixed types are designated *Fonsecaea*. Another school (Emmons et al.) calls all strains sporulating via phialides *Phialophora,* whether other forms of sporulation are present or not.[3] All are agreed that those exhibiting only the cladosporial type should be placed in the genus *Cladosporium*. The one isolate from the authentic animal case was reported to be *Hormodendrum,* a synonym of *Cladosporium.*

Animal inoculation. There are no immunologic procedures in routine use at present, and inoculation of experimental animals is not helpful in the study and diagnosis of chromomycosis.

Reference laboratory. Mycology Section, CDC.

References
1. Ajello, L., L.K. Georg, W. Kaplan, and L. Kaufman. *Laboratory Manual for Medical Mycology.* Public Health Service Pub. no. 994. HEW, Washington, 1963.
2. Brodey, R.S., H.F. Schryver, M.J. Deubler, W. Kaplan, and L. Ajello. Mycetoma in a dog. *J. Am. Vet. Med. Ass.* 151:442–451, 1967.
3. Emmons, C.W., C.H. Binford, and J.P. Utz. *Medical Mycology.* 2d ed. Lea and Febiger, Philadelphia, 1970.
4. Jang, S.S., and J.A. Popp. Eumycotic mycetoma in a dog caused by *Allescheria boydii. J. Am. Vet. Med. Ass.* 157:1071–1075, 1970.
5. Kurtz, H.J., D.R. Finco, and V. Perman. Maduromycosis (*Allescheria boydii*) in a dog. *J. Am. Vet. Med. Ass.* 157:917–921, 1970.
6. Simpson, J.G. A case of chromoblastomycosis in a horse. *Vet. Med. Small Anim. Clinic* 61:1207–1209, 1966.

66. Mycotoxins

The mycotoxins are fungal metabolites that can produce pathologic responses in humans and other animals.[1,2,13] These metabolites occur in foodstuffs that have been infested during life or during storage by toxigenic fungi.[23] When ingested in sufficient quantity, the toxins cause clinical disease, reduced productivity, and other less dramatic but economically important responses such as reduced weight gains and alterations of immunity.

Despite the early knowledge of ergotism and of poisonous fleshy fungi, little scientific attention has been focused on other mycotoxins until recent years. The present concern over mycotoxins has been emphasized because some (notably aflatoxin and sterigmatocystin) can be carcinogenic.

The mycotoxicoses discussed in this chapter are some of those that have been studied for a number of years and have occurred as natural outbreaks causing considerable economic loss (Table 66.1).

Aflatoxicosis

The discovery of a related group of mycotoxins that caused widespread deaths of turkey poults in Great Britain in 1960 began a voluminous literature on the metabolites (aflatoxins) produced by *Aspergillus flavus* and *A. parasiticus*.[19] These toxins have been produced on a variety of substrates under a variety of conditions and have been extracted and purified by a number of procedures. Peanut meal, cottonseed meal, corn, and other concentrates have been prominent sources of intoxication.[8,11]

The aflatoxins are hepatotoxins that are dicoumarin derivatives capable of carcinogenesis.[24] The four major aflatoxins, B_1, B_2, G_1, and G_2, are named for their fluorescence (B, blue; G, green) under long-wave UV light and their R_f values on thin-layer chromatograms (TLC). The aflatoxins are soluble in methanol and chloroform; they are heat stable and nonantigenic. Criteria important for their identification are listed in Table 66.2. Another important aflatoxin is M toxin, a metabolite of aflatoxin B_1, which occurs in the urine or milk of animals being fed aflatoxins and in many crude preparations of aflatoxins. This toxin has a blue-violet fluorescence under UV light and has a lower R_f value than aflatoxin G_2.

Table 66.1. Mycotoxicoses: well-defined disease, mycotoxin(s) known

Condition	Mycotoxin(s)	Animals affected	Major effects	Major sources
Aflatoxicosis	Aflatoxins	Poultry, swine, cattle	Centrilobular necrosis, hemorrhage, bile duct cell proliferation, hepatoxic	*Aspergillus flavus, A. parasiticus*
Facial eczema	Sporodesmin	Sheep, cattle	Hepatotoxic, bile duct occlusion, photosensitivity	*Pithomyces chartarum*
Slobber factor	Slaframine	Cattle, sheep	Excessive salivation, lacrimation, frequent defecation, dyspnea	*Rhizoctonia leguminicola* on clover hay
Ergotism	Ergot alkaloids	Cattle, sheep	Gangrenous necrosis of extremities	*Claviceps purpurea* (sclerotia)
Paspalum staggers	Ergotlike alkaloids, lysergic acid amides	Cattle, sheep, horses	Ataxia, tremors, nervousness	*Claviceps paspali* (sclerotia)
Estrogenism	Zearalenone (F-2)	Swine	Uterotropic, swollen vulva, enlarged mammae and prepuce	*Fusarium roseum, F. oxysporum, F. tricinctum, F. moniliforme*
Mold nephrosis	Ochratoxin (citrinin?)	Swine	Nephrotoxic, some liver changes	*Aspergillus ochraceus, Penicillium viridicatum*

A number of animal species are susceptible in varying degrees to aflatoxins (dog, pig, cow, duckling, turkey poult, pheasant, quail, chicken, guinea pig, rabbit, rat, hamster, ferret, mink, monkey, rainbow trout, and Coho salmon). Sheep and mice are relatively resistant to the aflatoxins.

The primary effect of aflatoxicosis is liver damage. Acute aflatoxicosis typically results in hepatic necrosis and widespread hemorrhages; chronic aflatoxicosis typically results in bile duct hyperplasia and portal fibrosis.

Aflatoxicosis is confirmed by demonstrating aflatoxins in feed or M toxin in urine specimens as well as by finding typical hepatopathy in affected animals. Aflatoxins can be demonstrated in feed specimens by bioassay in ducklings or by TLC. Feed containing aflatoxin and fed *ad libitum* to day-old white Pekin ducklings for approximately 10 days often causes death after 9 or more days; typical hepatic changes including necrosis or biliary hyperplasia are seen in dead or surviving ducklings.

Table 66.2. Physical characteristics of aflatoxins*

Aflatoxin	Molecular formula	Molecular weight	Melting point	Ultraviolet (265 nm)	Absorption (362 nm)	Fluorescence (nm)	Approx. R_f†
B_1	$C_{17}H_{12}O_6$	312	268–269	13,400	21,000	425	0.37
B_2	$C_{17}H_{14}O_6$	314	286–289	11,000	20,800	425	0.52
G_1	$C_{17}H_{12}O_7$	328	244–246	10,000	16,100	450	0.28
G_2	$C_{17}H_{14}O_7$	380	237–240	11,200	19,300	450	0.23

*Partially adapted from Schoental.[19]
†Silica gel HR, analytical thin-layer plate, chloroform–methanol–formic acid (97:2:1).

Mycotoxins

Analysis of aflatoxins in mixed feeds is more difficult than in most grains. Therefore, when dealing with such feeds the mixed feed method can be used. For analysis of aflatoxins in grains the multimycotoxin method can be used. Both are described below.

Mixed feed method (adapted from Pons et al.[17]). Finely grind mixed feed and place 50 g in a 1-liter Erlenmeyer flask. Add 70 ml of 0.1 N HCl to wet the sample. Then add 200 ml of acetone, 10 mg of Celite (Analytical Filteraid, Johns-Manville, Denver), and 150 ml of CH_2Cl_2 (methylene chloride) *in that order*. Shake for 1 hour. Filter the extract through Whatman #1 paper (Whatman Co., Maidstone, Kent, Eng.) into an evaporation flask. Repeat the extraction with 200 ml acetone plus 150 ml CH_2Cl_2. Filter and combine extracts in the evaporation flask. Evaporate extracts to dryness. Redissolve in 20 ml acetone and 60 ml H_2O, then add 20 ml of 20% lead acetate containing 0.3% glacial acetic acid. Add 5 g of filter aid and filter into a 125 ml Erlenmeyer flask; note the volume of filtrate. Place the filtrate in a 500 ml separatory funnel and partition twice with equal volumes of CH_2Cl_2. Collect the bottom phase and evaporate to dryness. Weigh and transfer to a 4-dram (15 ml) vial. This material is then used for column chromatography.

Column chromatography. Column size is approximately 40 cm × 2.5 cm. Place a small amount of glass wool in the bottom (if the column has a fritted glass disc the glass wool is unnecessary). Add CH_2Cl_2 until the column is one-third full. Then add 5 g of acidic alumina (activity grade I) to the column. Slurry 15 g of Silica gel into the column (Silica gel, Mallinckrodt cc-4, 100–200 mesh). Dry 2 hours at 110°C and then add 1% H_2O. Next, wash the sides of the column with some additional CH_2Cl_2. Allow to settle and then add 2 cm of anhydrous granular sodium sulfate to the top of the column. Drain the excess CH_2Cl_2 until the solvent reaches the top of the column. Add the extract to the column and allow the column to drain until the extract reaches the top of the sodium sulfate.

Multimycotoxin method (adapted from Eppley et al.[7,8,9]). This procedure can be used for detection of aflatoxins, ochratoxin, zearalenone, and T-2 toxin (a trichothecene) in grains. Grind the sample (fine grind); add 50 g of sample to a 500 ml Erlenmeyer flask; then add 25 ml of distilled water, 25 g diatomaceous earth, and 250 ml chloroform. Shake for 1 hour. Filter through Whatman #1 filter paper and collect the first 50 ml of chloroform filtrate. Add 150 ml hexane. Place this mixture on the column (see column chromatography above) and allow to elute; add 150 ml of benzene to wash the column (none of these eluates need to be saved). Then (1) elute for zearalenone with 250 ml acetone-benzene (5:95) (save); (2) elute the column with 150 ml anhydrous ether and then with 150 ml methanol-chloroform (3:97) for both T-2 and aflatoxins (save); (3) elute for ochratoxin with 250 ml glacial acetic acid–benzene (1:9) (save).

Concentrate each eluate to dryness and redissolve in 0.5 acetonitrile-benzene (2:98). Ochratoxin may require vigorous agitation. Spot 5, 10, and 20 μl spots on TLC plates (Silica gel G-HR) including appropriate internal and external standards (see above). Develop plates in 97:2:1 chloroform–methanol–formic acid. Visualize aflatoxin and ochratoxin under long-wave UV light; ochratoxin fluoresces yellow (R_f about 0.35–0.4). Zearalenone fluoresces yellow under short-wave UV light (R_f about 0.5).

Zearalenone, when sprayed with anisaldehyde spray reagent, is orangish-brown; T-2 is pink. (Spray with anisaldehyde spray reagent and heat the plates 10 minutes at 30°C. Watch the plates during the heating process. To make anisaldehyde spray reagent, mix 70 ml methanol, 10 ml glacial acetic acid, 5 ml H_2SO_4, and 0.5 ml p-anisaldehyde.) Ochratoxin subjected to ammonia fumes fluoresces blue under UV light. Aflatoxins sprayed with 25% H_2SO_4 and placed under long-wave UV light fluoresce yellow.

Column chromatography. Place glass wool in the bottom of the column and then add 5 g anhydrous sodium sulfate. Fill the column one-half full with chloroform; then add 10 g of Silica gel (0.05–0.2 mm). (Activate Silica gel by drying 10 g for 1 hour at 105°C; cool in a dessicator and then add 1% water and mix thoroughly [Brinkmann Institute Silica gel 60, 70-230 mesh ASTM].) Wash the sides with 20 ml of chloroform and allow the Silica gel to settle. Then remove excess chloroform from the column with a pipette until there is 5 cm of chloroform above the silica gel. Then add 15 g of sodium sulfate to the column (carefully). Draw off chloroform to the top of the sodium sulfate.

Analysis of urine samples for aflatoxin M toxin. Urine from animals that are suspected to have died from, or to have been affected by, acute aflatoxicosis can be collected and examined for the presence of M toxin by the following method: (1) mix 30 ml of urine with 45 ml of absolute methanol in a 250 ml separatory funnel; (2) extract three times with 55 ml volumes of chloroform (forms the bottom layer in the separatory funnel) and combine the two chloroform extracts; (3) reduce the volume of the chloroform extracts by evaporation and transfer to a 4-dram (15 ml) vial; (4) dry on a steam bath and add 0.5 ml of acetonitrile-benzene (2:98 V/V); and (5) conduct TLC according to the procedure for analysis of aflatoxin in mixed feeds, using M toxin as the standard.

Not all isolates of *A. flavus* and *A. parasiticus* are toxigenic; they can be tested for this property by the following procedure. Three 1-liter Erlenmeyer flasks containing 75 g of polished rice and 30 ml of distilled water each are held at room temperature for 1 hour and then autoclaved, cooled, and inoculated with 1 ml of a spore suspension of the organism. Rice cultures are incubated at 28°C on a shaker (250 rpm) for 5 days. Each culture is then extracted three times with 350 ml volumes of chloroform with constant agitation for 4 hours. The extract from each culture is evaporated to a 5 ml volume and then spotted on an analytical TLC plate or tested in ducklings as described earlier.

Some physical characteristics of the four major aflatoxins are shown in Table 66.2.

Zearalenone Toxicosis

Zearalenone (F-2) is an estrogenic metabolite produced by *Fusarium roseum, F. oxysporum, F. tricinctum,* and *F. moniliforme.* Swine given feed containing 1–5 ppm of zearalenone will show a syndrome characterized by hypertrophy of the vulva, vaginal and rectal prolapse, preputial enlargement, and precocious enlargement of the mammary gland.[16] Infertility, reduced litter size, and weak piglets are also effects attributed to zearalenone.

The organisms will produce the metabolite when grown on moist corn for 2 weeks at 25–28°C followed by 8 weeks at 12°C. For analysis or zearalenone in feed and grains, the multimycotoxin method already described can be used. Ultraviolet absorption spectra of the toxin possess maximal absorption peaks at 314, 247, and 236 nm. Its melting point lies between 163 and 165°C.

Toxicity of extracts from suspect feeds can be assessed by injecting extracts in propylene glycol IM in weanling, virgin, female rats. Increased uterine weight occurs when approximately 350 μg of toxin is administered over a period of 7 days.

Trichothecene Toxicoses

The largest group of chemically related mycotoxins is the tricothecenes. Several fungi produce these compounds; however, the predominant organisms are of the genus *Fusarium*. About 27 of these occur naturally and several are thought to be involved in *Fusarium* toxicoses. Certain organisms can produce more than one trichothecene and the same trichothecene can be produced by more than one organism (Table 66.3).

Table 66.3. Fungi known to produce trichothecenes

Family and genera	Trichothecenes produced
Hypocreaceae	
Hypocrea	Trichodermin, trichodermal
Calonectria	Calonectrin, deacetylcalonectrin
Moniliaceae	
Cephalosporum	Crotocin
Trichoderma	Trichodermin, trichodermol (roridin C)
Trichothecium	Trichothecin, crotocin
Dematiaceae	
Stachybotrys	Roridin E; two other 12,13-epoxy-Δ9-trichothecenes
Tuberculariaceae	
Dendrochium	Verrucarin A
Myrothecium	Verrucarins, roridins
Fusarium	Diacetoxyscirpenol; T-2 and HT-2; nivalenol; fusarenon; solaniol; 4β-15-diacetoxy-3α,7α-dihydroxy-12,13-epoxytrichothec-9-en-8-one; 4β,8α,15-triacetoxy-12-13-epoxytrichotec-9-en-3α,7α-diol

The trichothecenes produce dermal necrosis when sufficient quantities are applied to the shaved skin of a rat or rabbit. Trichothecenes can produce bone marrow depression and necrotic lesions of the mouth, stomach, and intestines accompanied by diarrhea or rectal hemorrhage. In chickens, hysteroid seizures, impaired righting reflex, and abnormal wing positioning are also seen. These organisms also have been incriminated in such diseases as moldy corn toxicosis in cattle and alimentary toxic aleukia in humans and may be involved in syndromes characterized by emesis and refusal of corn by swine.[5]

Although the trichothecenes have proved to be difficult to isolate in sufficient purity for easy detection with TLC, the multimycotoxin method has been used for analysis of T-2 toxin, one of the trichothecenes.

A screening method for the presence of trichothecenes in feeds employs the use of the dermal necrosis test. Grind 100 g of sample and add 30 ml of water; extract three times with 250 ml of ethyl acetate in a Waring blender for about 5 minutes each time. Filter extracts, pool, and evaporate to dryness. Redissolve in 10 ml of ethyl acetate. Apply approximately 5 μl of extract to shaved skin on a rat or a rabbit. In rabbits, 0.005 or 0.01 μg of T-2 toxin in 2 μl of ethyl acetate produced dermal toxicity in 48 hours. In this same study 0.04 μg of T-2 in 2 μl of ethyl acetate gave reliable sensitivity in rats.[14,15] If dermal toxicity occurs in a sample and difficulty in TLC analysis is encountered, a sample should be submitted to a laboratory where gas chromatography–mass spectra analysis can be performed.

Stachybotryotoxicosis

Stachybotrys atra, a cellulolytic fungus, produces a metabolite that has caused severe illness and death of horses fed stored moldy hay or straw.[10] Human beings, cattle, swine, and sheep are also susceptible to the toxin; natural outbreaks have occurred in cattle.

Animals ingesting sublethal amounts of the toxin for extended periods develop excessive salivation, congestion of the mucous membranes of the eyes and mouth, inflammation and edema of the subcutaneous tissue of the lips, cracks of focal necrosis of lips and oral mucosa, progressive thrombocytopenia, leukopenia, agranulocytosis, and increased prothrombin time (Table 66.4). Diarrhea and dehydration frequently occur, as does enlargement of mucosal lesions. Death may result, with extensive hemorrhages and necrosis throughout the body. When an animal ingests large quantities of toxic substrate, a peracute form of the disease is produced wherein death precedes other signs.

For determining toxicity of isolates of *S. atra,* the organism can be cultured on 200 g of oats, moistened, and incubated in shake culture at 25°C for 3 weeks. Toxigenic strains usually produce death in mice fed the culture for approximately 7 days. Culture can be extracted with ether and tested for dermal toxicity as previously described. Samples of suspect feed should be handled in the same manner as those for examination for trichothecenes.

Table 66.4. Mycotoxicoses: well-defined disease, toxin(s) problematic

Condition	Mycotoxin(s)	Animals affected	Major effects	Major sources
Leucoencephalomalacia	*Fusarium moniliforme* toxin	Horses	Liquefactive necrosis	*Fusarium moniliforme*
Alimental toxic aleukia	Trichothecenes (?), poaefusarin, sporofusarin	Humans	Dermal and GI necrosis, hematopoetic depression	*Fusarium* sp. (?)
Stachybotryotoxicosis	Trichothecenes (?)	Horses, humans	Hematopoetic depression, stomatitis, dermatitis, sudden death	*Stachybotrys atra* (*S. alternans*), black sooty mold
Vomition-refusal	Trichothecenes (?)	Swine	Emesis, refusal of feed	*Fusarium* sp. (?)
Yellow rice disease	Leutoskyrin, citreoviridin, islanditoxin, cyclochlorotine, citrinin	Humans	Nephropathy, cirrhosis, nervous and circulatory disorders	*Penicillium* sp.

Mycotoxins

Table 66.5. Mycotoxicoses: mycotoxins without a disease

Condition	Mycotoxin(s)	Animals affected	Major effects	Major sources
?	Sterigmatocystin	?	Hepatotoxic	*Aspergillus versicolor, A. nidulans, A. flavus, A. rugulosus, Bipolaris* sp.
?	Rubratoxin	?	Hepatotoxic	*Penicillium rubrum, P. purpurogenum*
?	Penicillic acid	?	Carcinogenic (?), skin tumors	*Penicillium* sp., *Aspergillus* sp.
?	Citrinin	?	Nephrotoxic	*Penicillium citrinum*
?	Tremorgens	?	Tremors	*Penicillium* sp., *Aspergillus fumigatus, A. flavus*
?	Some trichothecenes	?	Dermal necrosis	*Fusarium* sp., *Myrothecium* sp., *Hypocrea* sp., *Calonectria* sp., *Cephalosporium* sp., *Trichoderma* sp., *Trichothecium* sp., *Dendrochium* sp.

Rubratoxicosis

Rubratoxin B is known to be produced by *Penicillium rubrum* and *P. purpurogenum;* both organisms will produce the toxin when grown on corn. Both of these organisms have been found in moldy grains causing intoxications of domestic animals; however, rubratoxin has not been demonstrated conclusively in feeds or grains. Rubratoxin is difficult to demonstrate in grains, as present methods of analysis are not very sensitive (Table 66.5).

Rubratoxin is a hepatotoxin and produces hepatic degeneration, centrolobular necrosis, and hemorrhage of the liver and intestine. Experimental animals given rubratoxin develop prolonged clotting times.

The organisms can be tested for rubratoxin production by growing them on a modified Raulin-Thom solution (see Appendix A) for 12–14 days at 27°C in Povitsky bottles containing 350 ml of medium. The medium is filtered and concentrated 4.5 times and the pH is adjusted to 1.5 with concentrated HCl. The medium is then extracted with diethyl ether in a liquid-liquid extraction apparatus for 48 hours. White platelike crystals of rubratoxin will be present in the ether reservoir; if no crystals are present, allow the reservoir to slowly evaporate for 48 hours and check for crystal formation on the wall of the reservoir. Crystals may be collected by filtration and washed with additional ether or hexane. Rubratoxin is readily soluble in acetone.

Detection of rubratoxin corn (adapted from Hayes and McCain[12]). Grind a sample of the corn until it can pass a 20-mesh screen. Place 100 g of the sample in a 500 ml Erlenmeyer flask and add 300 ml of ethyl acetate. Stopper the flask and shake overnight to 24 hours at 350 rpm. Filter the extract through Whatman #1 filter paper and collect the filtrate in an evaporator flask. Evaporate the contents of the flask to a volume of 20 ml (if this is to be used for TLC at a later time, wrap in aluminum foil and store at 4°C).

Spot one 5, two 10, and one 20 µl quantities of sample extract on a TLC plate. Silica gel G-25 plates work well. *All spotting of rubratoxin should be done under a stream of nitrogen to prevent oxidation.* Include an external standard on the plate and an internal standard on one of the 10 µl spots of the sample. The standard should be of sufficient concentration to provide 5 µg of rubratoxin on each spot. Develop the plates in an unlined tank containing chloroform–methanol–glacial acetic acid–water (80:20:1:1 V/V). Allow the solvent front to migrate about 16 cm from its origin and remove the plate from the tank. Allow the plates to air dry and place immediately in an oven at 200°C for 10 minutes. View the plates under long-wave UV. Rubratoxin will have a greenish fluorescence and an approximate R_f of 0.75. The plates can subsequently be sprayed with 2',7'-dichlorofluorescein; under long-wave UV, rubratoxin will then be a bright yellow-green fluorescent spot on a fluorescent yellow-green plate.

Ochratoxicosis

The ochratoxins are produced primarily by *Aspergillus ochraceus* and *Penicillium viridicatum,* with the possibility that the latter organism may be the more important producer, as it competes much better with other fungi under storage conditions (see Table 66.1).

Porcine nephropathy has occurred in swine fed grains naturally contaminated with ochratoxin and the disease has been reproduced with ochratoxin-contaminated grain given at levels found in naturally contaminated grain. The disease is characterized by a necrosis of the tubular epithelium of the kidney and by intestinal fibrosis. Fatty change also occurs in the liver. Ochratoxins can be determined in grains using the multimycotoxin method.

Analysis of urine for ochratoxin. Extraction should be conducted soon after urine is collected or the urine should be frozen. Acidify a 50 ml urine sample to pH 2 with concentrated HCl. In a 250 ml separatory funnel extract the urine sample twice with 75 ml volumes of chloroform. Evaporate the chloroform extract to dryness and redissolve in 2 ml benzene-acetonitrile (98:2). Spot on a TLC plate 5, 10, and 20 µl of sample. Use the same plates and solvents used for ochratoxin in the multimycotoxin method.

Facial Eczema

A toxic metabolite of *Pithomyces chartarum (Sporodesmium bakeri)*, a saprophytic fungus, is known to cause hepatitis and a photosensitivity disease of sheep and cattle known as facial eczema.[6,21] The hepatotoxic substance produces necrosis of liver tissue, which results in accumulation of phylloerythrins in the bloodstream and subsequent photosensitization of the animals. The fungus grows on dead plant parts and produces an abundance of spores under appropriate environmental conditions. The spores and mycelium of the fungus contain the toxin and these fungal elements are ingested by the animal while grazing.

A simple presumptive test known as the beaker test has been used for assessment of possible toxicity to pasture grasses.[3] The beaker test is carried out as follows: a 50 g portion of ground grass is extracted with 100 ml of acetone. The acetone extract is placed on a two-piece column chromatogram, the upper portion containing alumina, the lower portion containing absorptive carbon. More acetone is run through the column and the first 75 ml of eluate is discarded. The second 75 ml aliquot is collected in a beaker and allowed to evaporate to dryness. A positive test is indicated by a white deposit on the beaker wall.

The beaker test substance and the toxic principle of *P. chartarum* are not the same; the test substance is a presumptive indication of toxin because both are produced by the fungus. The mere presence of *P. chartarum* on grasses or other substrates does not indicate that the substrate is toxic. Also, some care must be taken in interpretation of the beaker test as not all samples that are positive by this test are toxic and vice versa. Suspected toxic grasses can be assayed for toxicity in 120 g guinea pigs. About 2 kg of toxic pasture grass should be collected for each guinea pig used in the assay. The pasture grass should be extracted with ether. The extract from 2 kg of grass is poured over a 3-week supply of normal guinea pig diet ration. After the ether has evaporated, the ration is fed for 3 weeks and a normal diet is fed during the fourth week; at the end of this period the guinea pig is sacrificed and observed for pathologic changes of the liver, including proliferation of the bile ducts, areas of noninflammatory hepatic necrosis, and some portal fibrosis.

Isolates of *P. chartarum* can be tested for toxigenicity by growing the organisms on 200 ml of potato-carrot medium for 7 days at 25°C. The culture is homogenized in a Waring blender and extracted four times with equal volumes of anhydrous ether.[22] The extract from a 200 ml culture can be assayed in a guinea pig in the same manner used for the extracts of pasture grass. In assaying for toxicity, sufficient substrate or culture should be extracted to test several guinea pigs. The toxic substance, sporodesmin, has been purified and is water soluble.

Slaframine

Rhizoctonia leguminicola, an organism that causes blackpatch disease on legumes, is also known to produce a toxic metabolite, slaframine, which causes excessive salivation, lachrymation, diarrhea, and frequent urination in cattle when ingested.[4] The clinical signs can be reproduced in guinea pigs fed toxin; the toxin is a histaminelike alkaloid whose effects resemble those of parasympathomimetic drugs and can be counteracted by antihistamines or atropine. Cattle, swine, sheep, chickens, rats, and mice are also sensitive to the toxic factor; however, ruminants seem to be less reactive to the toxin than other animals (see Table 66.1).

Toxigenic strains of this organism produce toxin when grown in still cultures at 27°C for 30 days in a medium containing 20 g soybean meal, 20 g glucose, 5 g $CaCO_3$, and 5 g corn steep liquor per liter of distilled water. Blended fungal mycelium and medium are used to bioassay the organisms for toxigenicity.

Bioassay of the salivation factor can be accomplished in guinea pigs by administering 10 ml of a test suspension by stomach tube to a 200–300 g guinea pig. The animal should be observed for salivation every 10–20 minutes for 5–6 hours.

The toxic metabolite from *R. leguminicola* has been extracted and purified. The material has an R_f value of 0.35 when chromatographed on Whatman #1 paper in butanol–acetic acid–water (120:30:50); an orange spot is obtained when treated with Dragendorff's reagent and a gray spot is obtained when treated with iodoplatinate.[18]

Ergotism

The classic disease ergotism has been known since the middle ages, when epidemics occurred in Europe that caused both gangrenous and convulsive forms (see Table 66.1).

The ergot fungus, *Claviceps purpurea,* invades the female portion of the parasitized plant and replaces the ovary with a mass of fungal tissue called a sclerotium. The sclerotia often contain quantities of ergot alkaloids sufficient to cause the typical disease when ingested. No attempt will be made here to review this disease; however, a method for extraction and detection of ergot alkaloids is given.

Extraction and detection of ergot alkaloids. Remove the ergot from the grain sample and grind to a powder. Mix 2.5 g of ergot powder with 0.3 g sodium bicarbonate and add water until a crumbly paste is obtained. Extract with 100 ml diethyl ether (shake for 1 hour and decant extract). Repeat three times. Combine extracts (approximately 400 ml). Partition into 10 ml of 1% tartaric acid. (Repeat three times using 10 ml of 1% tartaric acid each time). Collect tartaric acid extracts and bring volume to 50 ml with 1% tartaric acid. This may be analyzed by qualitative color change or by TLC as follows: (1) Remove 5 ml of solution and add 10 ml of Van Urk's reagent with $FeCl_2$. (Van Urk's reagent contains 0.125% paradimethylaminobenzaldehyde in 65% H_2SO_4. Add 0.1 ml of 5% $FeCl_2$ solution per 100 ml of Van Urk's reagent.) If ergot alkaloids are present the solution will turn blue in 3 minutes. (2) For TLC, remove 10 ml of tartaric acid solution and adjust to pH 8.5 with ammonium hydroxide. Extract with equal portions of chloroform. Remove the chloroform layer and evaporate to dryness. Dissolve in 0.5 ml chloroform. Spot 5, 10, and 20 μl on a Silica gel G plate. Include known ergot alkaloids as standards. Develop the plate in ethyl acetate–dimethylformamide–ethanol (13:1.9:1 V/V) until the solvent front is 1 cm from the top of the plate. Examine for blue fluorescence of some alkaloids under UV light (250 nm). Nonfluorescent alkaloids can be detected by spraying the plate with 3.5% paradimethylaminobenzaldehyde in concentrated HCl.

Sterigmatocystin

Sterigmatocystin is a naturally occurring hepatotoxic compound closely related to the aflatoxins and is produced by *Aspergillus versicolor, A. nidulans, A. flavus, A. rugulosus,* and *Bipolaris* sp. (see Table 66.5).

Detection of sterigmatocystin in grains (adapted from Stack and Rodricks[20]). Finely grind a 50 g sample and place it in a 500 ml Erlenmeyer flask. Add 180 ml acetonitrile plus 20 ml 4% KCl solution (V/V). Shake for 30 minutes to 1 hour. Filter through Whatman #1 paper and collect 180 ml of filtrate. Place filtrate in a 250 ml separatory funnel and add 50 ml hexane. Shake and allow layers to separate. Discard hexane layer (top layer). Repeat with a second 50 ml volume of hexane. Add 25 ml H_2O and 50 ml $CHCl_3$ to the bottom layer and shake. Allow layers to clear and collect the bottom layer in a 250 ml Erlenmeyer flask. Add another 25 ml $CHCl_3$ to the H_2O layer and shake.

When the bottom layer clears, add it to the Erlenmeyer flask. Add a few silicon carbide (SiC) boiling chips and evaporate to near dryness; then transfer with $CHCl_3$ through filter paper into a 4-dram (15 ml) vial. Evaporate to dryness on a steam bath under a stream of nitrogen. Seal the vial and save for TLC.

Thin-layer chromatography. Dissolve the sample saved for TLC in 1 ml of benzene. Spot one 1, two 5, and one 10 μl samples on a plate. Use an external standard and an internal standard on one of the 5 μl spots (standard should contain approximately 100 μg sterigmatocystin per ml of benzene). Spot on Silica gel N-HR plates. Develop in a lined equilibrated tank containing benzene–acetic acid–methanol (95:5:5 V/V). Remove the plate from the tank and allow the solvent to evaporate. Then spray the plate with $AlCl_3$ solution (20 g $AlCl_3 \cdot 6H_2O$ grade in 100 ml ethanol). Place the plate in an oven at 80°C for 10 minutes. Examine the plate under short-wave UV for bright yellow fluorescent sterigmatocystin. If no spots are seen on the sample, it contains less than 100 μg sterigmatocystin per kg.

Diseases Suspected of Being Mycotoxic

Fescue foot, ryegrass, and bermudagrass poisoning sometimes occur after livestock are pastured on or fed hay from these grasses. While mycotoxins have been suspected as the cause of the diseases, thus far all efforts to find specific mycotoxins have failed (Table 66.6).

Table 66.6. Mycotoxicoses: diseases suspected of being mycotoxic

Condition	Mycotoxin(s)	Animals affected	Major effects	Major sources
Fescue foot	?	Cattle	Necrosis of feet and other appendages	Fescue hay or pasture
Ryegrass	?	Horses, cattle	Neurological signs	Ryegrass hay or pasture
Bermudagrass poisoning	?	Cattle	Neurological signs	Bermudagrass hay or pasture

References

1. Brook, P.J., and E.P. White. Fungus toxins affecting mammals. *Ann. Rev. Phytopath.* 4:171–194, 1966.
2. Ciegler, A., S. Kadis, and S. Ajl. *Microbial Toxins.* Vol. VI, *Fungal Toxins.* Academic Press, New York, 1971.
3. Clare, N.T. The beaker test as an indicator of facial exzema toxicity. *New Zealand Soc. Anim. Prod. Proc.* 19:69–76, 1959.
4. Crump, M.H., E.B. Smalley, J.N. Henning, and R.E. Nichols. Mycotoxicosis in animals fed legume hay infested with *Rhizoctonia leguminicola. J. Am. Vet. Med. Ass.* 143:996–997, 1963.
5. Curtin, T.M., and J. Tuite. Emesis and refusal of feed in swine associated with *Gibberella zeae*–infected corn. *Life Sci.* 5:1937–1944, 1966.
6. Dodd, D.C. The pathology of facial eczema. *New Zealand Soc. Anim. Prod. Proc.* 19:48–52, 1959.
7. Eppley, R.M. Screening method for zearalenone, aflatoxin and ochratoxin. *J. Ass. Off. Anal. Chem.* 51:74–78, 1968.
8. Eppley, R.M., L. Stoloff, and A.D. Campbell. Collaborative study of "a versatile procedure for assay of aflatoxins in peanut products" including preparatory separation and confirmation of identity. *J. Ass. Off. Anal. Chem.* 51:67–73, 1968.
9. Eppley, R.M., L. Stoloff, M.W. Truckses, and C.W. Chung. Survey of corn for *Fusarium* toxins. *J. Ass. Off. Anal. Chem.* 57:632–635, 1974.

10. Forgacs, J., W.T. Carll, A.S. Herring, and W.R. Hinshaw. Toxicity of *Stachybotrys atra* for animals. N.Y. Acad. Sci. Trans. 20:787–808, 1958.
11. Goldblatt, L.A. *Aflatoxin*. Academic Press, New York, 1969.
12. Hayes, A.W., and H.W. McCain. A procedure for the extraction and estimation of rubratoxin B from corn. *Food Cosmet. Toxicol.* 13:221–229, 1975.
13. Hesseltine, C.W. Mycotoxins. *Mycopathol. Mycol. Appl.* 39:371–383, 1969.
14. Kadis, S., A. Ciegler, and S. Ajl. *Microbial Toxins*. Vol. VII, *Algal and Fungal Toxins*. Academic Press, New York, 1971.
15. Kadis, S., A. Ciegler, and S. Ajl. *Microbial Toxins*. Vol. VIII, *Fungal Toxins*. Academic Press, New York, 1972.
16. Mirocha, C.J., C.M. Christensen, and G.H. Nelson. Estrogenic metabolite produced by *Fusarium graminearum* in stored corn. *Appl. Microbiol.* 15:497–503, 1967.
17. Pons, W.A., A.F. Cucullu, and L.S. Lee. Determination of aflatoxins in mixed feeds. *Proc. 3d Internat. Cong. Food Sci. Tech.* (Washington), pp. 705–711, 1970.
18. Rainey, D.P., E.B. Smalley, M.H. Crump, and F.M. Strong. Isolation of salivation factor from *Rhizoctonia leguminicola* on red clover hay. *Nature* 205:203–204, 1965.
19. Schoental, R. Aflatoxins. *Ann. Rev. Pharmac.* 7:343–356, 1967.
20. Stack, M., and J.V. Rodricks. Method for analysis and chemical confirmation of sterigmatocystin. *J. Ass. Off. Anal. Chem.* 54:86–90, 1971.
21. Synge, R.L.M., and H.P. White. Sporodesmin: A substance from *Sporodesmium bakeri* causing lesions characteristic of facial eczema. *Chem. Indus.,* pp. 1546–1547, 1959.
22. White, E.P. Chemical extraction and fractionation of the toxin. *New Zealand Soc. Anim. Prod. Proc.* 19:64–68, 1959.
23. Wogan, G.N. *Mycotoxins in Foodstuffs*. M.I.T. Press, Cambridge, 1965.
24. Wogan, G.N. Chemical nature and biological effects of the aflatoxins. *Bact. Rev.* 30:460–470, 1966.

APPENDIXES

A. Media, Reagents, and Special Techniques

Alkaline Peptone Broth. The ingredients are peptone 5 g, glucose 5 g, NaCl 5 g, Teepal (Shell, Netherlands) 1 ml, methyl violet 2 mg, dist. H_2O 100 ml. Adjust to pH 8.5, sterilize, and dispense.

Alsever's Solution. The solution contains glucose 2.05 g, sodium citrate 0.8 g, citric acid 0.055 g, NaCl 0.42 g, dist. H_2O 100 ml. Autoclave at 10 lb (68.94 kPa) pressure for 10 minutes. The solution is used as an anticoagulant diluent for collecting and sometimes washing RBC. Blood is added at the volume of 10–20 ml per 50 ml of the solution.

Ammonium Nitrate Agar, see Casein Agar

Anaerobic Deep Meat Medium. Obtain beef muscle tissue from carcass at the slaughterhouse as soon after killing as possible. Dissect out and discard fat, connective tissue, blood vessels, and nerves. Grind muscle tissue and defat by placing in boiling water for about 1 minute. Mix 25 ml of 1 N NaOH solution with 975 ml dist. H_2O and a pound (454 g) of the ground beef. Adjust pH to 7.2–7.4. Heat to about 90°C with constant stirring. Cool mixture and then filter through cheesecloth to separate the ground meat from the beef infusion. Obtain 16×125 mm screw-capped tubes and add about 2.5 cm of ground meat per tube. Determine the quantity of beef infusion needed for the tubes and then add to it the following: polypeptone 3%, yeast extract 0.5%, NaCl 0.5%. Adjust the pH to 7.4–7.6. Then fill the tubes about two-thirds full with the beef infusion and additives.

Place the filled tubes in baskets in water and heat to boiling and hold for 10 minutes to drive off trapped gas. Place caps on tubes one-fourth turn less than tight and then place in autoclave for 25 minutes at 121°C. When autoclave is opened, tighten caps and chill media in cold water. (See also Liver-Egg-Brain Stock Culture Medium.)

Andrade's Base for Carbohydrate Fermentation. Dissolve 5 g of beef extract, 10 g of Bacto-peptone, and 5 g of NaCl in 900 ml of dist. H_2O. Adjust pH to 7.2 with 4% NaOH. Autoclave for 30 minutes and filter through cotton or filter paper (an extra quantity should be made to assure a yield of 900 ml). Add 10 ml of Andrade's indicator solution (see below). Autoclave for 20 minutes.

To 100 ml of dist. H_2O that has been autoclaved for 30 minutes, add 10 g of desired carbohydrate and autoclave 12 minutes (arabinose and xylose must be sterilized by filtration). Add the 100 ml of sterile carbohydrate solution and 100 ml of sterile equine serum aseptically to the 900 ml of broth. Dispense aseptically into sterile tubes.

Andrade's Indicator. Combine acid fuchsin 0.5 g, dist. H_2O 100 ml, and 4% NaOH 16 ml. If after several hours the fuchsin is not sufficiently decolorized, add an additional 1 or 2 ml of alkali.

Auxanographic Technique for Differentiating Species of Cryptococcus. For media, use Sabouraud's dextrose agar slants; yeast nitrogen base (YNB), $10\times$ strength (Difco, Detroit), in 2 ml amounts; yeast carbon base (YCB), $10\times$ strength (Difco), in 2 ml amounts; washed agar, 2%, in 18 ml amounts.

The method for carbohydrate assimilation follows. For each culture (unknowns plus standard *C. neoformans* and *C. diffluens*) prepare 48-hour growth on Sabouraud slants. Suspend growth on each slant in 5 ml saline and centrifuge; wash into two 5 ml portions of saline and resuspend in another 5 ml. During this procedure, melt the agar. To each of duplicate tubes of 2 ml YNB (add no sugar!), add 0.1 ml of cell suspension; pour into sterile petri dish; add a tube of cooled molten agar and mix well. Harden by cooling 2 hours or more. With small spatula, dust crystals of pure carbohydrates in distinct piles on the surface of the agar; five equidistant spots may be placed on a plate. Incubate plates right side up at 25°C. Read at 48 and 96 hours.

For controls, use (1) agar plus 0.1 ml inoculum in YNB; no carbohydrate; (2) agar plus 0.1 ml inoculum in 2 ml saline; no carbohydrate. If growth occurs in either of these, the test is not valid.

For nitrogen assimilation do as above but: (1) use YCB in place of YNB; (2) in place of carbohydrates add crystals of KNO_3 and peptone to opposite halves of each dish. Growth of *C. neoformans* should occur with peptone but not with KNO_3.

Basal Mineral Medium (BMM). This medium is used for carbon assimilation studies. The ingredients are: $(NH_4)_2SO_4$ 2 g, $NaH_2PO_4 \cdot H_2O$ 0.5 g, K_2HPO_4 0.5 g, $MgSO_4 \cdot 7H_2O$ 0.2 g, $CaCl_2 \cdot 2H_2O$ 0.1 g, H_2O 1000 ml.

The respective carbon sources are added to the basal medium to give a final concentration of 0.03 M. Each medium is adjusted to a pH of 6.5 ± 1. The ingredients, excluding agar, are made up as a twofold concentration and are sterilized by Seitz filtration. This is brought up to normal concentration by adding the appropriate volume of sterile melted 3.2% agar; this mixture is dispensed into sterile tubes for making slants. The basal medium must be supplemented with methionine for growth of *Pseudomonas maltophilia* and with pantothenate, biotin, and cyanocobalamin for growth of *P. diminuta*.

Beef Extract Agar. This medium can be used for the purification of *Candida* isolants and the depletion of stored sugar. The ingredients are beef extract 3 g, peptone 10 g, NaCl 5 g, agar 25 g, dist. H_2O 1000 ml.

Prepare as slants in screw-capped tubes. Final pH should be 7.4 after autoclaving.

Beef Extract Broth. The medium contains beef extract 3 g, peptone 10 g, NaCl 5 g, BTB 0.04 g, dist. H_2O 1000 ml.

After the dye is in solution adjust pH with 1 N NaOH and 1 N HCl until neutrality is reached. The medium can be filter-sterilized or autoclaved at 120°C for 15 minutes. The basal medium is used for sugar fermentation tests and as inoculum for sugar assimilation test. Fermentation tests are prepared by adding filter-sterilized stock solutions of glucose, lactose, maltose, and sucrose to autoclave-sterilized aliquots of the beef extract basal medium. The final fermentation medium should contain 1% of the test sugar in beef extract broth that contains 0.004% BTB indicator. The final pH should be 7.2. After inoculation, the fermentation tests are covered with 1–2 cm of sterile petroleum jelly and observed for the production of acid and/or gas after incubation for 10 days at 37°C. (Smith fermentation tubes can be used but petroleum jelly plugs are recommended to detect gas formation.) An uninoculated control tube of each sugar should be prepared and incubated as a check on sterility and as a color reference for pH change.

Beef Infusion Agar. The formula is the same as for beef infusion broth, except that agar is added at the rate of 20 g/L of infusion. Autoclave and filter through cotton or several layers of milk filter disks. Autoclave again and dispense.

Beef Infusion Broth. Add ground defatted beef to dist. H_2O at the rate of 1 lb/L (454 g/L). Allow to stand overnight at 4°C. Cook 1 hour at 80–90°C, allow to stand 2 hours, and filter through muslin. Add 10 g of Bacto-peptone and 5 g of NaCl per liter of infusion. Adjust pH to 7.6 with 4% NaOH and autoclave. Filter through cotton or filter paper, dispense, and autoclave again.

Beef Infusion Broth (Stock for Anaerobes). Use beef muscle obtained directly from the killing floor. It should have had vessels, nerves, and connective tissue removed and been thoroughly defatted, ground, packaged in tinfoil, and then quick-frozen, using dry ice. Store in a freezer until used.

Add 1 liter of water per pound of ground defatted beef muscle. *Do not change proportions.* Let stand overnight in a stainless steel kettle in a walk-in cooler. The following morning place in a steam kettle and heat for 1 hour at 80–90°C, stirring occasionally. Cover and let stand for approximately 2 hours. Strain through a double layer of muslin. Adjust pH to 6.6–6.8 (it must remain on the acid side of neutrality but not lower than pH 6.6).

To store, add broth to screw-capped 500 ml polyethylene bottles until three-fourths filled. Freeze and store frozen for extended use.

Beef Infusion Broth (Tubes for Anaerobes). Make up a working solution of beef infusion in the following proportions: beef infusion stock (anaerobes) 500 ml, dist. H_2O 500 ml, 10 g polypeptone (Baltimore Biological Lab.) 1%, 5 g NaCl 1%, 0.5 g cysteine hydrochloride 0.05%. Dissolve into solution. Adjust pH with NaOH (not stronger than 5 N) to 7.2–7.4. Filter through a layer of diatomaceous earth. Tube in 16×125 mm screw-capped tubes in approximately 10 ml amounts (approximately two-thirds full) and place caps on tubes loosely. Autoclave 25 minutes at 121°C. Tighten caps and chill media in cold water.

Bicarbonate Agar. This medium must be prepared fresh because the bicarbonate breaks down upon storage. Dissolve $NaHCO_3$ in distilled water and sterilize the solution by filtration through a filter that will retain bacteria. Add the proper amount of solution to melted (45°C) agar made from soybean peptone and pancreatic digest of casein to a final concentration of 0.7% $NaHCO_3$. The pH of the medium is about 8 and need not be adjusted. (See Chapter 36.)

Bismuth Sulfite (BS) Agar. This agar is used for the isolation of *Salmonella* sp. It contains beef extract 5 g, peptone (polypeptone or Bacto) 10 g, glucose 5 g, disodium phosphate 4 g, ferrous sulfate 0.3 g, BS indicator 8 g, agar 20 g, brilliant green 0.025 g, dist. H_2O 1000 ml.

Blood Agar. Prepare BHI agar (Bacto B418, Difco, Detroit) according to label instruction. Autoclave 360 ml BHI agar in 500 ml Erlenmeyer flask and cool to 50°C in water bath. Add 40 ml fresh defibrinated blood (of species recommended or similar to host in question) and pour 20 ml of medium per petri plate. Allow surface of agar to dry before use. Blood agar plates may be stored up to 3 weeks at 5°C.

Blood Agar with Antibiotics, Selective. The ingredients are BHI agar 360 ml, fresh defibrinated blood 40 ml, novobiocin (Albamycin, Upjohn, Kalamazoo, Mich.) 2000 µg, bacitracin (Lilly, Indianapolis) 4000 units, mycostatin (Squibb, New York) 20,000 units. Mix antibiotics with blood and add to sterilized BHI agar at 50°C. Pour 20 ml of medium per petri plate. Final antibiotics concentration per ml of blood agar is 5 µg novobiocin, 10 units bacitracin, 50 units mycostatin.

Blood Agar Base. As with potato dextrose agar, this medium is available commercially in a dehydrated state from Difco Laboratories (Detroit) and Baltimore Biological Laboratories. This medium enriched with 0.3% yeast extract is suitable for initiating spore production in *Trichophyton verrucosum*. Caps of screw-topped containers should be loose during incubation.

Brain-Heart Infusion (BHI) Agar with Chloramphenicol. Prepare as for Sabouraud's dextrose agar except that 37 g BHI broth (Baltimore Biological or Difco) and 20 g agar are substituted for Sabouraud's agar.

Brain-Heart Infusion Blood Agar. The ingredients are BHI broth 37 g, agar 20 g, dist. H_2O 900 ml. The pH should be 7.6. Sterilize in autoclave at 15 lb (103.42 kPa) pressure for 10 minutes, cool to 56°C, then add 1000 ml of citrated blood and pour plates or tubes. When Actidione (cyclohexamide) is added, subtract the volume from the total volume of water. Penicillin and streptomycin can be added, but only after the media has cooled to 45°C.

Brain-Heart Infusion Broth with Chloramphenicol. The medium contains 0.2% glucose. The composition is BHI broth (Baltimore Biological or Difco), chloramphenicol 0.05 mg/ml. Suspend 37 g BHI broth in 1000 ml dist. H_2O. Heat to boiling. After removal from heat, add 50 mg chloramphenicol suspended in 10 ml of 95% alcohol. Dispense in 15 ml amounts into 50 ml conical flasks. Add cotton stoppers and autoclave at 121°C (15 lb [103.42 kPa]) for 15 minutes.

Brilliant Green (BG) Agar. This agar is used for the isolation of *Salmonella* sp. It contains yeast extract 3 g, peptone (polypeptone or proteose no. 3) 10 g, NaCl 5 g, lactose 10 g, sucrose 10 g, phenol red 0.08 g, agar 20 g, BG 12.5 mg, dist. H_2O 1000 ml.

Brilliant Green Sulfa Agar. Use the same formula as for BG agar with the addition of 1 g/L of sulfapyridine. *S. gallinarum* apparently will not grow in this medium.

CAUTION: BG is toxic for many organisms, including some of the enteric organisms.

Bromthymol Blue–Salt–Teepal Agar. The composition is as follows: beef extract 0.3 g, peptone 1 g, sucrose 1.5 g, NaCl 3 g, agar 1.5 g, Teepal (Shell, Netherlands) 0.1 ml, BTB 0.008 g, dist. H_2O 100 ml. Adjust to pH 7.8.

Candle Jar. Any large can or jar can be used. Place inoculated cultures in the container; add a lighted candle; seal the container with a tight-fitting lid. The candle burns for a few seconds, providing an atmosphere of about 6–8% CO_2 in the container. Place the sealed container in the appropriate incubator.

Carbohydrate Fermentation Broth Base. The preferred basal medium for enteric organisms is that of Edwards, employing Andrade's indicator. This is because some enteric organisms have the ability to reduce (make colorless) many indicators such as phenol red and BCP. Nevertheless, laboratories that examine a variety of families of microorganisms may wish to use one of the dehydrated fermentation broth bases available commercially that contain one of the above indicators.

Edwards' formula is as follows: peptone 10 g, meat extract 3 g, NaCl 5 g, Andrade's indicator 10 ml, dist. H_2O 1000 ml. Adjust to pH 7.1–7.2. Carbohydrates are added in concentrations of 1%; with a few exceptions they can be added before sterilization. The medium is tubed with inverted insert tubes and sterilized at 121°C for 15 minutes. Remove from the autoclave as soon as the pressure is down and then cool rapidly in a cold water bath. Lactose, sucrose, maltose, arabinose, and xylose (10% in dist. H_2O) are sterilized by filtration and added to previously sterilized basal medium. Examine inoculated media daily. Note production of acid (pink color) and the volume of gas produced by aerogenic cultures. If acid has not been produced in 1 week, seal the tubes and hold for 30 days, examining at 3-day intervals. VP-positive organisms revert from pink to colorless in glucose. Salmonellae often revert from pink to colorless in dulcitol after 1 or 2 days.

Carbonate-Bicarbonate Buffer, see Chapter 5, page 87

Casein Agar. The medium contains casamino acid, vitamin free (Difco-Bacto) 2.5 g, dextrose (Difco-Bacto) 40 g, $MgSO_4$ 0.1 g, KH_2PO_4 1.8 g, agar (Difco-Bacto) 20 g, dist. H_2O 1000 ml. Adjust to pH 6.8. To make ammonium nitrate agar the formulation is the same except that 1.5 g NH_4NO_3 is substituted for the casamino acid. These media are used in examining dermatophyte nutritional requirements. Nutritional tests help in the identification of *Trichophyton equinum* and *T. verrucosum* and allow the differentiation of *Microsporum gallinae* from *T. megninii*.

The various test agars are obtained by adding the required vitamins to the basal casein or ammonium nitrate media. Final concentrations of vitamins should be: casein-thiamine agar 200 µg/L, casein-inositol agar 50 mg/L, casein-thiamine-inositol agar 200 µg/L and 50 mg/L, casein–nicotinic acid agar 2 mg/L, ammonium nitrate–histidine agar 30 mg/L. The ingredients are heated to boiling and then autoclaved at 121°C (15 lb [103.42 kPa]) for 12 minutes. After cooling to 50°C, the medium is poured into sterile petri dishes. The medium can be dispensed in screw-topped containers before autoclaving, in which case the tubes are left to harden in a slanted position after sterilization.

The inoculum can be taken from cultures grown on any of the usual isolation media. It is important, however, to take only a fragment, in order to avoid carrying over an excess of the nonvitamin-free isolation medium. The caps of screw-topped containers should be loosened during incubation.

Chapman-Stone Medium. The formula is yeast extract 2.5 g, tryptone 10 g, gelatin

30 g, d-mannitol 10 g, NaCl 55 g, dipotassium phosphate 5 g, ammonium sulfate 75 g, agar 15 g. Dissolve in 1000 ml dist. H_2O by boiling; sterilize in an autoclave. The medium is commercially available.

Chocolate Agar. Chocolate agar is prepared either by heating blood agar to 100°C for 10 minutes or by heating blood agar plates in an oven at 65°C for 1 hour.

Citrate Agar. The medium contains NaCl 5 g, magnesium sulfate 0.2 g, monoammonium phosphate 1 g, dipotassium phosphate 1 g, sodium citrate 2 g, agar 15 g, BTB 0.08 g, dist. H_2O 1000 ml. Slant medium with short butt, long slant. Inoculate lightly with a straight wire. Never inoculate the medium just after withdrawing the wire from a medium containing a carbohydrate. A safe procedure is to suspend the organism in saline and inoculate from the suspension. Growth on the medium, as indicated by development of a blue color, is a positive test for utilization of citrate as the sole source of carbon.

Citrate Anticoagulant Solution. Dissolve 10 g of sodium citrate in 100 ml dist. H_2O. Sterilize in the autoclave. Dispense at 1 ml/10ml of blood.

Coagulated Serum Medium. Add about 2 ml of normal horse serum to a tube of beef infusion broth and place in boiling water for 10 minutes to coagulate.

Cornmeal Infusion Agar. The agar is used for morphologic studies with *Candida* species. Melt agar (Tween 80 may be added to 1% final concentration to enhance pseudomycelium and chlamydospore formation), flow 1 ml over the surface of a sterile glass microscope slide, and let solidify. Cut-inoculate two streaks of the test isolant along the long axis of the slide and cover a portion of these streaks with a sterile 22 sq mm coverslip; place on supports in a moist incubation chamber (i.e. a petri dish lined with wet filter paper); incubate at room temperature and microscopically examine periodically after 3–10 days. This agar is commercially available.

Cottonseed Agar. This agar can be used for the conversion of the mycelial phase of *Blastomyces dermatitidis* to the yeast phase. Note that no one method will convert all strains of the fungus. An inoculum of mycelium is placed on fresh slants of cottonseed agar. The culture is incubated at 37°C. Growth, which usually appears in 3–4 days as moist colonies around the mycelium, is transferred to fresh agar slants (fresh medium should be warmed to 37°C before inoculation). This procedure is repeated until complete conversion is accomplished. The ingredients of cottonseed agar are glucose 20 g, agar 18 g, pharmamedia 20 g, dist. H_2O QS 1000 ml.

Cysteine Beef Infusion (CBI) Semisolid Medium. This medium is composed of beef infusion broth 100 ml, cysteine-HCl 20 mg, agar 100 mg. Dispense 8 ml per 16×150 mm culture tube. Insert cotton plug and sterilize.

Cysteine-Saline Solution. The contents are NaCl 8.5 g, cysteine HCl 1 g, deaminized H_2O 1000 ml. Adjust pH to 6.5 with 2 N KOH. Obtain sterile 2 ml ampules containing 0.5 g Chloromycetin (Parke Davis, Detroit). From ampules add 0.1 ml to 1000 ml of cysteine-saline solution to get 25 μg/ml of Chloromycetin. Place 20 ml of the final solution in each culture jar needed; then sterilize in autoclave for 10 minutes at 20 lb (137.9 kPa) pressure. (See Chapter 60.)

Decarboxylase Test Medium Base. Basal medium is divided into four equal parts, one of which is tubed without the addition of any amino acid and used as a control tube. The remaining three parts have 1% L-lysine dihydrochloride, 1% L-argenine monohydrochloride, and 1% L-ornithine dihydrochloride added respectively. Final pH should be 6. Sterilize at 121°C for 10 minutes. Inoculate lightly, then layer with mineral oil. A control tube is inoculated for each culture. The tubes give an early yellow (acid) reaction due to glucose fermentation. Decarboxylation of lysine results in cadaverine. Dihydrolysis of arginine results in urea and putrescine. Decarboxylation of ornithine results in putrescine. Cadaverine and putrescine are toxic amines called ptomaines, and they are basic in reaction; therefore, the medium is purple when they are present.

The basal medium formula is peptone 5 g, beef extract 5 g, BCP (1.6%) 0.625 ml, cresol red (0.2%) 2.5 ml, glucose 0.5 g, pyridoxal 5 mg, dist. H_2O 1000 ml. Adjust pH to 6.

Deoxycholate Agar. This agar is used for isolation of *Escherichia coli* and *Klebsiella*. It contains peptone (Bacto or polypeptone) 10 g, lactose 10 g, sodium deoxycholate 1 g, NaCl 5 g, dipotassium phosphate 2 g, ferric citrate 1 g, sodium citrate 1 g, agar 15 g, neutral red 0.03 g, dist. H_2O 1000 ml.

Dermatophyte Test Medium. Ingredients must be obtained from the sources indicated below. Substitution with other brands may change the specificity and effectiveness of the medium. The composition is phytone (papaic digest of soya meal and agar agar, Baltimore Biological Lab.) 10 g, glucose 10 g, agar agar 20 g, phenol red solution 40 ml, 0.8 M HCl 6 ml, cycloheximide (Actidione, Upjohn, Kalamazoo, Mich.) 0.5 g, gentamicin sulfate (Garamycin, Microbiology Department, Schering Corp., Bloomfield, N.J.) 100 μg/ml, chlortetracycline HCl (Aureomycin, Lederle Lab., Pearl River, N.Y.) 100 μg/ml, dist. H_2O 1000 ml. Add the phytone, glucose, and agar to the 1000 ml dist. H_2O and boil to dissolve the agar. Add 40 ml of phenol red solution while stirring (phenol red solution: 0.5 g Difco-Bacto phenol red dissolved in 15 ml 0.1 N NaOH made up to 100 ml with glass-distilled H_2O). Adjust pH of media with 6 ml 0.8 M HCl added while stirring. Dissolve 0.5 g cycloheximide in 2 ml acetone and add to hot medium while stirring. Dissolve gentamicin sulfate in 2 ml glass-distilled H_2O and add to medium while stirring. Autoclave at 12 lb (82.73 kPa) pressure for 10 minutes and cool to approximately 47°C. Dissolve chlortetracycline in 25 ml sterile glass-distilled H_2O in sterile flask. Add to medium while stirring. Dispense 8 ml amounts in sterile 30 ml screw-capped bottles and cool on slant. The final pH of the media is pH 5.5 ± 0.1 and should be yellow in color. For maximum shelf life, store in a refrigerator.

After inoculation of skin or hair specimens, incubate at 22–30°C with the caps loose. A change in color of the indicator from yellow to red within 14 days is a positive reaction.

Dextrose Broth with Chloramphenicol. Prepare as for BHI broth except that 23 g Bacto-dextrose broth (Difco) is substituted for the BHI broth. The glucose concentration of this medium is 0.5%.

Dorset and Henley's Medium. This medium contains L-asparagine 14 g, potassium phosphate dibasic (anhydrous) 1.42 g, sodium citrate·2 H_2O 0.9 g, magnesium sulfate·7 H_2O 1.5 g, ferric citrate 0.3 g, glucose 10 g, glycerol 50 ml, zinc sulfate (1%

stock solution) 2.7 ml, copper sulfate (1% stock solution) 0.4 ml, calcium chloride (1% stock solution) 6.7 ml, cobalt nitrate (1% stock solution) 0.13 ml, dist. H_2O QS 1000 ml final volume.

Dissolve each ingredient separately in small quantities of water. Gently heat to dissolve asparagine and ferric citrate. Dispense in 100 ml amounts in 300 ml Erlenmeyer flasks. Use nonabsorbent soft cotton plugs covered with aluminum foil. Sterilize at 116–118°C for 25 minutes. The medium is used for *Mycobacterium phlei* production.

E Medium (VPI Anaerobe Laboratory). The medium contains rumen fluid 30 ml, glucose 0.05 g, maltose 0.05 g, soluble starch 0.05 g, peptone 0.05 g, yeast extract 0.05 g, $(NH_4)_2SO_4$ 0.05 g, resazurin solution 0.4 ml, salts solution 50 ml, dist. H_2O 20 ml, L-cysteine–HCl · H_2O 0.05 g. Dissolve one resazurin tablet (about 11 mg, Allied Chemical Cat. 506) in 44 ml dist. H_2O to make the solution. The salts solution contains $CaCl_2$ (anhydrous) 0.2 g, $MgSO_4$ 0.2 g, K_2HPO_4 1 g, KH_2PO_4 1 g, $NaHCO_3$ 10 g, NaCl 2 g, dist. H_2O 1000 ml. Dissolve the $CaCl_2$ and $MgSO_4$ before adding the other salts.

Eagle's Minimum Essential Medium (MEM). All components are in mg/L. The amino acids used are L-arginine 105, L-cystine 24, L-glutamine 292, L-histidine 31, L-isoleucine 52, L-leucine 52, L-lysine 58, L-methionine 15, L-phenylalanine 32, L-threonine 48, L-tryptophane 10, L-tyrosine 36, L-valine 46. The vitamins are Ca pantothenate 1, choline chloride 1, folic acid 1, i-inositol 2, niacinamide 1, pyridoxal · HCl 1, riboflavin 0.1, thiamine · HCl 1. The carbohydrate is glucose 1000. The indicator is phenol red 20. The salts are NaCl 6800, KCl 400, $CaCl_2$ 200, $MgCl · 6H_2O$ 200, $NaH_2PO_4 · H_2O$ 140, $NaHCO_3$ 2200.

Earle's Balanced Salt Solution (BSS). For a 1 × solution the ingredients in g/L of dist. H_2O are as follows: NaCl 6.8, KCl 0.4, $CaCl_2$ 0.2, $MgSO_4 · 7H_2O$ 0.2, NaH_2PO_4 0.125, $NaHCO_3$ 2.2 (prepared as a sterile 8.8% stock solution and added at the time of use), glucose 1, phenol red (1% solution) 1.6 ml (2 ml may be used if a deeper red color is desired).

Egg Yolk Medium. Dissolve commercial dehydrated beef heart infusion (Difco, Detroit) 25 g in 1000 ml dist. H_2O. Sterilize in autoclave for 15 minutes at 15 lb (103.42 kPa) pressure (121°C). The pH of the medium should be about 7.4. Aseptically separate five egg yolks and clarify by centrifugation. Mix 5 parts of the egg yolks with 95 parts of the medium (broth). Add glucose 0.1 g and NaCl 1.5 g and then sterilize the medium by Seitz filtration.

Ellinghausen and McCullough's Medium, Modified. Make separate stock solutions of the following, dissolving each in 100 ml of dist. H_2O; ammonium chloride 25 g, $ZnSO_4 · 7H_2O$ 0.4 g, $CaCl_2$ and $MgCl_2 · 6H_2O$ 1 g each, $FeSO_4 · 7H_2O$ 0.5 g, $CuSO_4 · 5H_2O$ 0.3 g, Tween 80 (polysorbate 80) 10 ml, thiamine 0.5 g, vitamin B_{12} 0.02 g.

Prepare the basal medium as follows: Na_2HPO_4 1 g, KH_2PO_4 0.3 g, NaCl 1 g, stock solution of ammonium chloride 1 ml, stock solution of thiamine 1 ml, dist. H_2O 995 ml. Adjust pH to 7.4 and sterilize in autoclave at 15 lb (103.42 kPa) pressure (121°C) for 20 minutes.

For the albumin–fatty acid supplement, slowly and with careful stirring (to avoid foaming) add 20 g of bovine albumin, fraction V to 100 ml dist. H_2O. Then slowly add with constant stirring the following stock solutions: calcium and magnesium chloride 2 ml, zinc sulfate 2 ml, copper sulfate 0.2 ml, ferrous sulfate 20 ml, vitamin B_{12} 2 ml, Tween 80 25 ml. Adjust to pH 7.4 and add dist. H_2O QS 200 ml final volume. Sterilize by Seitz filtration (porosity of 0.45 μm). The supplement can be stored at 4°C or frozen until needed.

For the complete medium, aseptically add 1 part of supplement to 9 parts of basal medium. Distribute in desired amounts in tubes or flasks. (See Chapter 43.)

Enteric Organisms, Strip Test Papers and Tablets. In laboratories where isolation of many genera of enterics is infrequent and where a large compliment of biochemical media and reagents is impractical, consideration should be given to the use of strip test papers (General Diagnostics Div., Warner-Chilcott, Morris Plains, N.J.) and dehydrated tablets (Key Scientific Products Co., Los Angeles). These are always ready and are convenient to use, take up little space, have a storage life, and are generally reliable. Accuracy can always be tested with known positive and negative reactors. This should be done, as the paper strip tests were reported to give false positives for the lysine decarboxylase reaction and false negatives in urease tests with *Citrobacter* and *Enterobacter*.

Eosin Methylene Blue (EMB) Agar. The formula is peptone (Bacto or gelysate) 10 g, lactose 5 g, sucrose 5 g, dipotassium phosphate 2 g, agar 13.5 g, eosin Y 0.4 g, methylene blue 0.065 g, dist. H_2O 1000 ml.

Erysipelothrix Selective Broth. Prepare broth base as follows. In 1000 ml of 0.1 M phosphate buffer solution (12.02 g of Na_2HPO_4 and 2.09 g of KH_2PO_4 per liter of dist. H_2O), dissolve 3 g of beef extract, 15 g of Bacto-tryptose, and 5 g of NaCl. Filter through cotton or filter paper and autoclave. Add 5% sterile serum (equine, bovine, etc.) and 400 μg/ml of kanamycin, 50 μg/ml of neomycin, and 25 μg/ml of vancomycin. Dispense aseptically and keep at 4°C until used. Do not use if stored longer than 2 weeks.

Ferric Chloride Reagent. The ingredients are ferric chloride 10 g, dist. H_2O 100 ml.

Filter Test Techniques. Laboratory room or biohazard cabinet air filters, especially the HEPA type, may be tested for integrity and filtering efficiency by means of the cold DOP, hot DOP, sodium flame, methylene blue, bacterial spores, or virus tests. All of the tests use the test material as an aerosol of dispersed particles upstream from the filter and then sample the particles in the air downstream from the filter. The tests are conducted in duct rigs designed to control the air flow. The DOP tests employ particles of dioctylphthalate ($C_{24}H_{39}O_4$) detected by a scattered light photometer. The sodium flame test uses crystals of NaCl detected by the yellowing of a hydrogen flame as measured on a photosensitive cell. The methylene blue test employs particles of the dye detected and measured by comparing upstream and downstream dye stains on white filter paper. The bacterial spores test generally involves *Bacillus subtilis* or other nonpathogens as the test agents and the organisms are retrieved from the downstream air on agar plates, or by drawing air through a Millipore filter or a fluid trap. The virus test may employ a bacteriophage, a plant virus, or an animal virus of low or no human hazard, and the virus particles may be retrieved by drawing air through a Millipore filter or a fluid trap, or by the use of small animals or birds that are readily infected by inhalation of the virus aerosol. The hot DOP, methylene blue, sodium flame, and cold DOP tests give mean particle sizes of about 0.3, 0.4, 0.6, and 0.7 μm respectively.

Fletcher's Semisolid Medium. The formula is peptone 0.3 g, beef extract 0.2 g, NaCl 0.5 g, agar 1.5 g, dist. H_2O 920 ml. Suspend ingredients in cold water and heat to boiling to dissolve. Autoclave at 121°C for 15 minutes. Cool the medium to 56°C and add sterile rabbit serum to a final concentration of 8–10%. Dispense in sterile screw-capped tubes in 5–10 ml amounts. Inactivate the whole medium by placing the tubes in a water bath at 56°C for 1 hour on two successive days. The pH value should be 7.4–8. (See Chapter 43.)

Fluid Thioglycollate (FTG) Semisolid Medium. Prepare fluid thioglycollate medium according to bottle directions (BBL 01-140, Baltimore Biological Lab.). Dispense 9 ml per 18 × 150 mm culture tube. Add metal cap to tube and sterilize in autoclave.

Fluid Thioglycollate Semisolid Medium with Inhibitors. Prepare as above, but add either 1% glycine or 3.5% NaCl to inhibit growth of contaminants and permit growth of desired organisms (e.g. *Campylobacter* or *Vibrio* sp.).

5-Fluorouracil Medium for Leptospira. Dissolve 5-fluorouracil 1 g in 25 ml of dist. H_2O containing 2 ml of 2 N NaOH. Then add phosphate-buffered water (0.02 M, pH 7.4) QS 100 ml final volume. Check pH and sterilize by Seitz filtration. Store at 4°C. This solution serves as a selective agent for the growth of leptospirae and may be added to any leptospiral medium (e.g. Fletcher's, Stuart's, or Ellinghausen and McCullough's media) just prior to their use. Add 0.1 ml of the solution to each 5 ml of medium so there will be a final concentration of 200 ug/ml of 5-fluorouracil. Mix by gentle shaking.

The chemical is also available commercially in 10 ml ampules containing 500 mg. The ampule solution can be diluted with 40 ml of sterile dist. H_2O to provide a final concentration of 10 mg/ml (Hoffman La Roche, Nutley, N.J.).

Glucose Broth (MR-VP Medium). The ingredients are buffered peptone or polypeptone 7 g, dipotassium phosphate 5 g, glucose 5 g, dist. H_2O 1000 ml. An incubation period of 48 hours at 37°C is usually sufficient for the methyl red test. If results are not clear-cut, repeat at 25 and 37°C, incubating for 5 days. (See Methyl Red Reagent.) The VP test can be run after 48 hours. Add 1 ml of O'Meara's reagent to 1 ml of culture. Shake. Return to incubator and read in 2 hours.

Glucose-Cysteine Blood Agar. For solution A, use beef extract 0.6%, peptone (Difco) 2%, NaCl 1%. For solution B, use agar 3% in dist. H_2O. Autoclave solutions A and B separately. For use, add cysteine-HCl 0.1% to solution A at a temperature of not more than 30°C. Adjust to pH 7 with 2 N NaOH. Melt solution B and add to A while molten. Sterilize at 15 lb (103.42 kPa) pressure for 20 minutes. Add 5 ml sterile 50% glucose solution and 4 ml of sterile defibrinated rabbit or human blood per 100 ml. Pour in petri dishes and allow to solidify. (See Chapter 33.)

Gram-Negative (GN) Broth. This medium is used for the isolation of *Shigella* and *Salmonella*. It contains peptone (polypeptone) 20 g, glucose 1 g, d-mannitol 2 g, sodium citrate 5 g, sodium deoxycholate 0.5 g, dipotassium phosphate 4 g, monopotassium phosphate 1 g, NaCl 5 g, dist. H_2O 1000 ml.

Ground Beef and Liver Mixture. Fresh lean beef should be finely ground and defat-

Media, Reagents, and Special Techniques

ted by adding it to a container of boiling water in small amounts. The beef should be boiled only long enough to melt the fat—approximately 1 minute so that the outside of the particles are slightly cooked. This will also facilitate future handling. The defatted beef should then be removed, drained, and mixed in equal parts with fresh beef liver finely ground.

Obtain 16 × 125 mm screw-capped tubes; to each tube add a large chunk of oyster shell and a 1–2 cm rolled piece of fine steel wool that has been acid cleaned. The oyster shell should be small enough so that it can be easily removed when washing the tubes. Steel wool must be acid cleaned in dilute HCl. Acid-cleaned steel wool *cannot* be stored, as oxidation and crumbling occurs rapidly. Add to the tubes containing oyster shell and steel wool 1–2 cm of the ground beef and liver mixture. Then dispense to each tube 8–10 ml of the previously prepared liver-egg-brain stock culture medium. Place the uncapped tubes in baskets and place them in boiling water. Boil 10–12 minutes to drive off entrapped gases. Replace caps, but loosen one-quarter turn before placing in the autoclave. Autoclave 35 minutes at 121°C. Do not exhaust autoclave but let it cool normally. Tighten caps and chill media in cold water after removing from the autoclave. (See also Anaerobic Deep Meat Medium.)

Hanks' Balanced Salt Solution (BSS). For a 1× solution the ingredients in g/L of dist. H_2O are as follows: NaCl 8, KCl 0.4, $CaCl_2$ 0.14, $MgSO_4 \cdot 7H_2O$ 0.2, $Na_2HPO_4 \cdot 12H_2O$ 0.12, KH_2PO_4 0.06, $NaHCO_3$ 0.35 (prepared as a sterile 2.8% stock solution and added at the time of use), glucose 1, phenol red (1% solution) 1.6 ml (2 ml can be used if a deeper red color is desired).

Composition of Hanks' and Earle's BSS

Component	Concentration (g/L) in 1X solution	
	Hanks' BSS	Earle's BSS
NaCl	8.00	6.80
KCl	0.40	0.40
$CaCl_2$	0.14	0.20
$MgSO_4 \cdot 7H_2O$	0.20	0.20
$Na_2HPO_4 \cdot 12H_2O$	0.12	
NaH_2PO_4		0.125
KH_2PO_4	0.06	
$NaHCO_3$	0.35*	2.20†
Glucose	1.00	1.00
Phenol red (1% sol.)	1.60 ml‡	1.60 ml

*Prepared as a 2.8% stock solution and added at the time of use.
†Prepared as an 8.8% stock solution and added at the time of use.
‡If a somewhat deeper red color is preferred, 2 ml can be used instead.

Heart Infusion Broth Containing 1% Carbohydrate and 0.15% BCP. Sufficient Bacto heart infusion broth (Difco) to give a final concentration of 2.5% is dissolved in dist. H_2O. A 1% alcoholic solution of BCP is added in a sufficient quantity to give a final concentration of 0.15%. The medium is sterilized at 121°C for 15 minutes. Carbohydrate solutions are prepared as concentrated solutions and sterilized separately either by autoclaving at 121°C for 12 minutes or by filtration through sintered filters of the

Morton type or through Millipore filters. The concentrated sterile solutions are added in sufficient quantities to give a final concentration of 1%.

Because the growth of actinobacilli is enhanced by the presence of serum in the medium, more reliable fermentation reactions can be obtained by using basal media containing 5% sterile serum. The optimal pH of media used for determining the fermentative ability of antinobacilli has not been determined and it is suggested that if possible the tests be conducted in duplicate or triplicate using media with different initial pH levels. Media usually employed for other biochemical tests should generally be satisfactory for characterization of actinobacilli, providing they support growth. Incubation in an atmosphere containing 5% CO_2 is recommended.

Heparin Anticoagulant Solution. Prepare a solution of 4 mg (400 units) of heparin in 10 ml of sterile physiological saline (0.85% NaCl in dist. H_2O). Dispense at 0.3 ml/10 ml of blood.

Herrold's Medium. This medium has been modified for the culture of *Mycobacterium paratuberculosis*. The ingredients are peptone 9 g, NaCl 4.5 g, agar 15.3 g, beef extract 2.7 g, dist. H_2O 870 ml, mycobactin 150 mg (in 4 ml ethanol), glycerol 27 ml, malachite green (2% solution) 5 ml, and 6 egg yolks.

Mix all ingredients except egg yolks and dye using enough heat to dissolve the agar. Cool to 60°C and adjust to pH 7.5 with 1 N NaOH. Pour into an aspirator bottle and sterilize at 121°C for 25 minutes. Cool to 56°C and add the 6 egg yolks and dye. The egg yolks are prepared as follows. Scrub the eggs in warm detergent water and rinse with clear water. Let them air dry on a towel; then soak in isopropyl alcohol for 30 minutes. Dry between layers of sterile towels. Crack shell at one end with sterile forceps, make a hole, and remove and discard egg white with sterile forceps. Break yolk with forceps and twirl to mix. Pour mixed egg yolk into aspirator bottle. Mix gently on magnetic stirrer. Add malachite green solution with sterile pipette. When the medium is complete, dispense aseptically into 20×125 mm screw-capped tubes in 9 ml amounts. Allow medium to harden in slant position.

Hydrogen Sulfide (H_2S) Test, see TSI Agar

Indole Test, see Kovac's Reagent and Tryptone Water

Iron Milk Medium. Add a small ball of acid-cleaned steel wool to each tube of whole or skimmed milk. Do not use homogenized milk. Autoclave at 15 lb (103.42 kPa) pressure for 15–18 minutes. This may produce some caramelization of milk sugars but it is necessary to destroy bacilli, whose growth becomes evident only after incubation at 36°C. The addition of 0.05% cysteine-HCl to the medium will speed up the production of acid, clotting, and digestion.

Kelley's Medium. This is an excellent medium for the conversion to or the maintenance of the yeast phase of *Blastomyces dermatitidis* at 37°C. It contains Bacto-peptone 10 g, glucose 10 g, NaCl 5 g, beef extract 3 g, Bacto-agar 20 g, dist. H_2O 980 ml. Dissolve the ingredients in the water by heating, cool to 50°C, and add 20 ml of a hemoglobin solution (5 ml of blood plus 15 ml of dist. H_2O). Dispense 17 ml into 25×150 mm test tubes, sterilize for 25 minutes at 15 lb (103.42 kPa) pressure, and slant.

Kolmer Saline, see Chapter 5, page 62

Kovac's Reagent. The formula is amyl or isoamyl alcohol 50 ml, paradimethylaminobenzaldehyde 3.3 g, HCl (conc.) 17 ml. Dissolve aldehyde in alcohol. Slowly add acid. *Store in refrigerator.* This reagent is used in the indole test (see Tryptone Water).

Lab-Lemco Agar. Suspend 5 g glucose, 20 g agar, and 2.5 g lab-lemco in 1000 ml dist. H_2O. Heat to boiling. After dispensing into cotton-stoppered tubes, autoclave at 121°C (15 lb [103.42 kPa]) for 15 minutes. Allow to cool in a slanted position. Tubes are inoculated in the usual manner. After incubation at 28–30°C for 10–15 days, the reverse side pigment production is studied. If screw-topped containers are used, the tops should be loose during incubation as pigment production requires an adequate supply of air.

Latex Slide Agglutination Test for Cryptococcal Antigen. The test is performed according to the method of Bloomfield et al. (see Reference 3, Chapter 57), but we recommend that sera be inactivated by heating at 56°C for 30 minutes and that CSF be placed in a boiling water bath for 10 minutes before testing in order to eliminate nonspecific reactions. A ++ reaction even in undiluted inactivated serum or CSF is presumptive evidence of cryptococcal infection. A rise in titer indicates progressive disease, while a falling titer is evidence of reduction of the host cryptococcal population.

Latex particles are available commercially from Dow Chemical Co., Bioproducts Center, Midland, Mich., and from Difco, Detroit. The stock latex suspension is approximately a 1:20 dilution of the material (10% solids) supplied by Dow. The "maximally-reactive" PBS dilution of globulin is determined by box titration of serial dilutions, to each of which has been added an equal volume of stock latex (refrigerated overnight after mixing), against dilutions of a positive control serum or CSF.

Liver-Egg-Brain Stock Culture Medium. The egg-brain mixture is prepared by adding one egg yolk, from eggs obtained from a flock not on antibiotic feeds, to approximately 200 g of calf brain and approximately 25 ml of liver broth. This is minced to a fine pourable mixture in a mechanical blender. This egg-brain base can also be prepared in larger quantities, dispensed in containers in 100 ml amounts, and kept frozen until needed. To 100 ml of the egg-brain mixture, add liver broth 350 ml, Bacto-peptone 3.5 g, dist. H_2O 550 ml. The pH should be about 7.6–7.8.

Liver Infusion Broth. Liver broth is produced by chopping liver finely, adding 1 liter of water per pound of liver, and letting it all infuse overnight in a covered kettle in the refrigerator. The next morning cook slowly but *do not stir* until the liver has coagulated. If the liver is stirred while being cooked, fine particles get into suspension, which is very difficult to clarify. Add 0.5% NaCl and then decant off or siphon off supernatant fluid. Clarify supernatant fluid by filtering through a layer of diatomaceous earth. For extended use, freeze and store.

Lysine Iron (LI) Agar. The formula is peptone (Bacto or gelysate) 5 g, yeast extract 3 g, glucose 1 g, L-lysine 10 g, ferric ammonium citrate 0.5 g, sodium thiosulfate 0.04 g, BCP 0.02 g, agar 15 g, dist. H_2O 1000 ml. Slant and inoculate like TSI. This medium must be examined in 24 hours. A purple butt indicates decarboxylation of L-lysine. A yellow butt indicates that lysine is not attacked. Blackening along the line of the stab indicates H_2S production. It is not uncommon to find cultures of *Salmonella* that have purple slants with the butt of the medium lighter in color. Careful observation will show that the indicator is not yellow but has been reduced to the colorless state.

MacConkey's Agar. The agar contains the following: peptone 17 g, proteose peptone 3 g, lactose 10 g, bile salts mixture 1.5 g, NaCl 5 g, agar 13.5 g, neutral red 0.03 g, crystal violet 0.001 g, dist. H_2O 1000 ml. Bring water to boil to dissolve ingredients. Sterilize in autoclave; pour plates after cooling to 48°C. Allow agar to solidify with plate lids slightly open to insure a dry surface. The final pH should be 7.1. (See Chapters 25 and 31.)

MacConkey's Agar Fortified with 1% Dextrose. Use the formula above and add dextrose 10 g. If a dehydrated commercial agar is used, the following formulation would apply: Bacto–MacConkey's agar 50 g, dist. H_2O 1000 ml, dextrose 10 g. Dissolve agar according to bottle directions, then add the dextrose and sterilize in autoclave for only 15 minutes at 121°C. Remove promptly from autoclave and pour petri plates.

Magnification Formulas. When dealing with photographs of viral, bacterial, or fungal disease agents, the following formulas can be used to determine the magnification, object size, or expected photo print size of the object:

$$\text{Magnification} = \frac{\text{print size in mm} \times 10^6}{\text{object size in nm}}$$

$$\text{Object size in nm} = \frac{\text{print size in mm} \times 10^6}{\text{magnification}}$$

$$\text{Print size in mm} = \text{magnification} \times \text{object size in nm} \times 10^{-6}$$

Malt Extract Agar with Chloramphenicol. Prepare as for Sabouraud's dextrose agar except that 48 g of malt agar (Difco or Baltimore Biological)—increased to 2% agar content—is substituted for the Sabouraud's dextrose agar.

Malt Extract (2%) Broth with Chloramphenicol. Prepare as for BHI broth except that 20 g of malt extract broth (Difco or Baltimore Biological) is substituted for the BHI broth. The pH of this medium is around 4.7, which helps inhibit bacterial contaminants.

Medium 199. All components are in mg/L. The amino acids used are DL-alanine 50, L-arginine 70, DL-aspartic acid 60, L-cysteine 0.1, L-cystine 20, DL-glutamic acid 150, L-glutamine 100, glycine 50, L-histidine 20, hydroxy-L-proline 10, DL-isoleucine 40, DL-leucine 120, L-lysine 70, DL-methionine 30, L-phenylalanine 25, L-proline 40, DL-serine 50, DL-threonine 60, DL-tryptophane 20, L-tyrosine 40, DL-valine 50. The vitamins are p-aminobenzoic acid 0.05, biotin 0.01, Ca pantothenate 0.01, choline chloride 0.5, folic acid 0.01, i-inositol 0.05, niacin 0.025, niacinamide 0.025, pyridoxal·HCl 0.025, pyridoximine·HCl 0.025, riboflavin 0.01, thiamine·HCl 0.01, vitamin A 0.1, ascorbic acid 0.05, α-tocopherol phosphate 0.01, calciferol 0.10, menadione 0.01. The nucleic acid derivatives are adenine 10, guanine·HCl 0.3, hypoxanthine 0.3, thymine 0.3, uracil 0.3, xanthine 0.3, adenylic acid 0.2. The carbohydrates are 2-deoxy-D-ribose 0.5, glucose 1000. Miscellaneous components are sodium acetate 50, Tween 80 5, cholesterol 0.2, glutathione 0.05, adenosine triphosphate 10, phenol red 20. The salts are NaCl 6800, KCl 400, $CaCl_2$ 200, $MgSO_4 \cdot 7H_2O$ 200, $NaH_2PO_4 \cdot H_2O$ 140, $Fe(NO_3)_3 \cdot 9H_2O$ 0.1, $NaHCO_3$ 2200.

Methyl Red (MR) Reagent. This reagent is added to glucose broth for the methyl red test. The ingredients are methyl red 0.1 g, ethyl alcohol (95%) 300 ml, dist. H_2O 200 ml. Dissolve dye in alcohol, then add water. Use one drop per ml of culture.

Motility Test Medium (A). The ingredients are tryptose 10 g, NaCl 5 g, agar 5 g. Add the ingredients to 1000 ml of cold distilled water and heat to boiling to dissolve medium completely. Distribute in tubes and autoclave at 15 lb (103.42 kPa) for 15 minutes. Allow to cool in upright position. Final pH should be 7.2. To use, inoculate medium by stabbing in center. Incubate at proper temperature for organism and examine at 8, 24, and 48 hours. Motility is manifested by a diffuse zone of growth spreading from the zone of inoculation. (See Chapter 36.)

Motility Test Medium (B). The formula is beef extract 3 g, peptone 10 g, NaCl 5 g, agar 4 g, dist. H_2O 1000 ml. Inoculation of 0.4% agar medium will detect motility in cultures that may appear nonmotile by the hanging drop method. Stab the agar column to a depth of 3–5mm and incubate at 37°C. (See Chapter 25.)

Mycoplasma Media

Medium 1. An easily prepared medium that is suitable for growth of a fair number of avian and other animal mycoplasmas is Difco beef heart infusion broth or agar, respectively, enriched by the addition of 10% swine serum. The basal media are prepared according to the directions of the manufacturer (Difco, Detroit), autoclaved, and cooled below 50°C. The enrichments are warmed to 45°C before addition to the agar medium.

Medium 2. Ten percent fresh or fresh-frozen yeast extract is sometimes added to medium 1 to enhance its nutritional value for many strains of mycoplasmas.

Medium 3. This medium consists of Difco PPLO broth or agar supplemented with 20% horse serum and 10% fresh yeast extract. It supports good growth of most human and many animal mycoplasmas and is very widely used.

Medium 4. Difco heart infusion broth 25 g or agar 40 g, plus 10 g of Difco yeast extract and 10 g of Difco proteose peptone no. 3 are added to 1000 ml of dist. H_2O. The pH is adjusted as desired and the medium is autoclave-sterilized for 15 minutes at 121°C. Serum and other supplements are added to the medium after it has cooled. For agar the components are combined at about 45°C. This medium does not appear to support growth of *M. pneumoniae* but does support good growth of other human and many animal mycoplasmas.

Medium 5. Albimi *Mycoplasma* medium base (Pfizer Diagnostics, Flushing, N.Y.) can be purchased as either broth or agar and prepared according to the manufacturer's directions. It supports the growth of a wide range of human and animal *Mycoplasma* species.

Medium 6. This and the following media are more difficult to prepare than the preceding media but have unique value for isolation or propagation of one or more species of mycoplasmas. Fresh beef hearts are trimmed of most of the fat, ground, and infused for 16–18 hours at 4°C in distilled deionized H_2O (500 g/L). The mixture is heated 30 minutes at 93–95°C in a boiling H_2O bath, clarified with gauze and a Whatman GF/A or 934 AH glass-filter pad (Whatman Co., Maidstone, Kent, Eng.), and supplemented with 0.5% NaCl, 0.5% Difco bacteriological mucin, and 0.2% Difco hemoglobin. Approximately 0.5% Celite (Analytical Filteraid, Johns-Manville, Denver) is added to facilitate clarification. The mixture is stirred for 1 hour at room temperature. It is heated again to 93–95°C for 3 minutes and clarified as before. Before sterilization, the infusion is supplemented with 1% Difco peptones (0.3% casamino acids, 0.3% neopeptone, 0.1% casitone, and 0.1% tryptone). This medium was developed for use with *M. hyosynoviae* and supports good growth of many other species as well.

Medium 7. Beef muscle and liver, 100 g of each, plus 120 g of pig stomach are cut into small pieces and finely ground in a blender or meat grinder. One liter of dist. H_2O plus 10 ml of conc. HCl are added with stirring and the suspension is incubated at 50°C for 24 hours. After being heated to 80°C, the mixture is filtered through clarifying filter paper. It is again heated to 80°C and then held overnight at 5–10°C. The cold broth is put through filter paper and the pH adjusted as desired before it is filter-sterilized. This medium was originally developed for growth of *M. mycoides* antigen. It is uniquely well suited for obtaining high titers of low-passage broth cultures of *M. meleagridis*.

Medium 8. This medium consists of 40 parts of Hanks' BSS, 30 parts of Hartley's digest broth (Colab Labs, Glenwood, Ill.), 20 parts of heat-inactivated pig serum from antibody-free pigs, 10 parts of 5% labtalbumin hydrolysate, and 0.5 parts of yeast extract. The Hanks' solution and the lactalbumin hydrolysate are autoclaved and the other components are filter-sterilized. For solid medium, the agar is autoclaved in the Hanks' solution and combined with the other components at 56°C. This medium and medium 9 are among the few formulations that support growth of *M. hyopneumoniae*.

Medium 9. Difco PPLO broth 21 g, Difco lactalbumin hydrolysate 5 g, gastric mucin 5 g (Nutritional Biochemical Corp., Cleveland), and Difco yeast extract 0.1 g are dissolved in 1 liter of dist. H_2O. Heat-inactivated (56°C for 30 minutes) pig serum (20%) from *Mycoplasma*-free swine is added and the medium is sterilized by filtration.

Nigerseed-Creatinine Agar. The ingredients are nigerseed (*Guizotia abyssinica*), pulverized, 50 g, dist. H_2O 1000 ml, glucose 20 g, KH_2PO_4 1 g, $MgSO_4$ 0.5 g, creatinine 1 g, agar 15 g. Boil pulverized nigerseed in 1000 ml dist. H_2O for 20 minutes, filter through gauze, and reconstitute to 1000 ml. Then add other ingredients and after dissolving sterilize in autoclave at 110°C for 30 minutes.

For a selective medium for *Cryptococcus* add an antifungal solution: diphenyl 1 g dissolved in absolute ethyl alcohol 20 ml. Then add antibacterials: penicillin 20 units, streptomycin 40 units, chloramphenicol 1 mg (all per ml). Pour plates and incubate at 26°C. For use, streak plates with specimen material. Growth can be noted in about 4 days. (This description is adapted from F. Staib and H.P.R. Seeliger, Zur Selektivzüchtung von Cryptococcus neoformans, *Mykosen* 11:267–272, 1968.)

Noguchi's Ascitic Fluid–Rabbit Kidney Medium. The medium contains aseptically collected ascitic fluid (or rabbit serum) 1.5 parts, Ringer solution 4.5 parts, agar (2%) 1 part. To improve medium, small pieces of rabbit kidney, with total weight of not more than 1 g/30 ml, can be added. The surface of the medium should be covered with a layer of sterile mineral oil. (See Chapter 44.)

Nutrient Gelatin. The formula for nutrient gelatin is as follows: beef extract 0.3%, Bacto-peptone 0.5%, gelatin 12% in dist. H_2O. A comparable medium can be obtained commercially. Sterilize at 121°C for 12 minutes. Remove from autoclave as soon as pressure is down. Cool rapidly in ice-water bath. Inoculate with straight wire. Incubate at 25°C for enteric organisms.

Ortho-Nitrophenyl-B-D-Galactoside (ONPG) Reagent. The ingredients are ONPG 80 mg, dist. H_2O 15 ml, buffer (formula below) 5 ml. Store reagents at 4°C. If it crystallizes, heat in 37°C water bath until crystals dissolve. Discard reagent if it becomes yellow.

The buffer formula is $NaH_2PO_4 \cdot H_2O$ 6.9 g, 5 N NaOH 7.5 ml, dist. H_2O 40 ml (adjust pH to 7), dist. H_2O QS 50 ml.

The procedure is: add 1% lactose to any agar medium (blood agar base, nutrient agar) that will support good growth of the culture. Inoculate a lactose agar plate with a broth culture and incubate overnight at 37°C. Wash growth from agar surface with 1 ml of saline and remove to a 13×100 mm tube. Add 0.2 ml toluene and shake. Incubate 0.5 hours at 37°C. Add 1 ml ONPG reagent and return to incubator. Examine at 0.5, 1, and 3 hours. Development of a yellow color is a positive result and indicates the presence of the enzyme, B-galactosidase.

Oxalate, Carbolic Acid, and Glycerol (OCG). This is an anticoagulant and preservative solution. The ingredients are potassium oxalate 5 g, carbolic acid 5 g, dist. H_2O 500 ml, glycerol 500 ml.

Oxalate, Phenol, and Glycerol (OPG). The same solution as OCG but using the name phenol instead of carbolic acid.

Oxidation-Fermentation (OF) Basal Medium. The formula is Bacto-tryptone 2 g, NaCl 5 g, dipotassium phosphate 0.3 g, agar 2 g, BTB 3 ml, dist. H_2O 1000 ml. Adjust pH to 7.1. Dissolve by boiling. Dispense in 100 ml amounts. Sterilize 15 minutes at 121°C. To one 100 ml portion, aseptically add 10 ml of sterile 10% carbohydrate solution. Mix and dispense 4 ml amounts in sterile 13×100 mm culture tubes. Inoculate duplicate tubes by stabbing. Cover one tube with a layer of sterile mineral oil or petroleum jelly. Incubate at 37°C for 48 hours. Acid in sealed and open tubes indicates fermentation.

Packer's Medium. Prepare a tryptose agar base containing 1.5% Bacto-tryptose, 0.3% beef extract, 0.5% NaCl, and 1.8% agar in dist. H_2O. Heat to dissolve and filter through cotton or several layers of milk filter discs. Autoclave and add 4 ml of crystal violet stock solution, 25 ml of sodium azide stock solution (see below), and 50 ml of sterile equine serum or blood per liter. Dispense into plates or slants.

Stock solutions of crystal violet and sodium azide are made in dist. H_2O at concentrations of 0.25% and 4%, respectively, and are autoclaved. A comparable medium can be obtained commercially (Bacto–azide violet blood agar base, Difco, Detroit).

Papain Digest of Beef Muscle. One kg of frozen chopped beef muscle is thawed, mixed with 1 liter of dist. H_2O, and held overnight at 5°C. One liter of warm (70°C) dist. H_2O is added. The mixture is warmed to 62–64°C and then 2 g of papain is added. The mixture is digested for 2 hours with the temperature maintained at 62–64°C and the pH at 7–7.4. The digest is partially clarified by passing through gauze mesh and by centrifugation. The partially clarified digest is adjusted to pH 8 and then heated to boiling for approximately 5 minutes to precipitate insoluble phosphates. The digest is cooled in an ice bath and then filtered through a layer of diatomaceous earth. The pH of the digest is adjusted to 7.4 with dilute HCl, and 0.4% NaCl is added.

Penicillin Agar. Dissolve crystalline penicillin G in dist. H_2O and sterilize by filtration through a filter that will retain bacteria. Add the proper amount of solution to melted (45°C) agar made from soybean peptone and pancreatic digest of casein to achieve a final concentration in the medium of 10 units/ml.

Peptic Digest of Beef Liver. One kg of chopped fresh or frozen beef liver and 5 g of pepsin are mixed with 900 ml of dist. H_2O containing 20 ml of conc. HCl. After 1.5 hours of digestion at 55°C, dilute HCl is slowly added until pH 2.5 is obtained. After 18 hours digestion, the digest is centrifuged and the supernatant fluid is passed through a layer of diatomaceous earth. The filtrate is adjusted to neutrality with NaOH solution. The clarified digest is heated to boiling to inactivate the enzyme. After cooling, the pH is adjusted to 7.3. The digest is placed in plastic containers and frozen. The prepared medium contains 2 parts liver digest, 1 part dist. H_2O, and 1% trypticase (Baltimore Biological Lab.).

Peptone Water containing 1% Carbohydrate and 1% Andrade's Indicator. The final concentration of ingredients in the basal medium is as follows: peptone 1%, NaCl 0.05%. Andrade's indicator is prepared by adding 1 N NaOH to a 5% solution of acid fuchsin until the color becomes yellow. The medium is sterilized at 121°C for 15 minutes.

Perfect Stage Production by Modified Alphacel Medium. The medium contains Alphacel (nonnutritive cellulose) 20 g, $MgSO_4 \cdot 7H_2O$ 1 g, KH_2PO_4 1 g, $NaNO_3$ 1 g, Hunt's tomato paste (grocery item) 10 g, Beech-nut baby oatmeal (grocery item) 10 g, agar 18 g, dist. H_2O 1000 ml. The pH is adjusted to 5.6 with NaOH and the suspension is autoclaved at 121°C for 20 minutes. After cooling to 50°C, the medium is dispensed into sterile petri dishes and allowed to harden.

Small cubes cut from single spore cultures (one + strain and one − strain) grown on any of the usual dermatophyte media for 10 days at 23°C are placed side by side in the center of a petri dish containing the above medium. The plates are then incubated at 23°C for 1 month and the development of fertile gymnothecia is observed.

Phenolphthalein Diphosphate Medium. For the nutrient agar the ingredients are beef extract 3 g, peptone 5 g, NaCl 8 g, agar 15 g. For the phenolphthalein diphosphate solution, a stock solution of approximately 0.01 M phenolphthalein diphosphoric acid is prepared in dist. H_2O and sterilized by Seitz filtration. Such a solution has a pH of 2 and is therefore easily hydrolyzed. It becomes relatively stable, however, when diluted 1 in 5 or more in a buffered medium at pH 7.4. A similar solution of the sodium salt of phenolphthalein phosphate gives equally satisfactory results.

To prepare the medium; suspend 31 g of nutrient agar in 1000 ml cold dist. H_2O and heat to boiling to dissolve the medium completely. Autoclave for 15 minutes at 15 lb (103.42 kPa) pressure (121°C). Cool to about 50°C in a water bath and mix 49 parts of the autoclaved melted agar with 1 part of the phenolphthalein diphosphate solution to give a final concentration of 0.01 g phenolphthalein diphosphoric acid per 100 ml nutrient agar. Mix well and pour into petri dish. When plates are ready for use, streak with staphylococci culture.

Media, Reagents, and Special Techniques

To read the plates, incubate overnight (16–18 hours) at 37°C; then hold the inoculated plates over an open bottle of ammonia. Phosphatase-positive colonies become bright pink, others remain unchanged. (See Chapter 28.)

Phosphate Buffer (0.2 M). Prepare solution A as follows: monobasic sodium phosphate ($NaH_2PO_4 \cdot 2H_2O$) 31.2 g, dist. H_2O 1000 ml. Prepare solution B: dibasic sodium phosphate ($Na_2HPO_4 \cdot 7H_2O$) 53.65 g, dist. H_2O 1000 ml. Mix varying amounts of solutions A and B to obtain desired pH. Check solution with a potentiometer and adjust if necessary with NaOH or HCl. Sterilize in the autoclave.

Solution A	Solution B	pH
39 ml	61 ml	7.0
28 ml	72 ml	7.2
19 ml	81 ml	7.4

Phosphate Buffer Solution (0.1 M). Dissolve 12.02 g of Na_2HPO_4 and 2.09 g of KH_2PO_4 in dist. H_2O sufficient to make 1 liter of solution (pH 7.5).

Potassium Cyanide Medium Base. The formula is proteose peptone no. 3 3 g, disodium phosphate 5.64 g, monopotassium phosphate 0.225 g, NaCl 5 g, dist. H_2O 1000 ml. The basal medium is sterilized at 121°C for 15 minutes, then chilled in an ice-water bath. Then 0.5 g KCN is dissolved in 100 ml chilled sterile dist. H_2O and 15 ml of this solution is added to 100 ml of basal medium. The medium is tubed in 1 ml amounts in sterile tubes (use an automatic pipetting device) and quickly stoppered with corks coated with paraffin. Refrigerate at once. Discard unused tubes after 30 days. Inoculate with one loopful of a 24-hour tryptone water culture grown at 37°C. Growth means a positive test.

Potassium Tellurite Agar. The ingredients are: (1) Bacto–tryptose blood agar base 33 g, dist. H_2O 1000 ml. Heat to dissolve, then tube in 20 ml amounts. Sterilize in autoclave at 15 lb (103.42 kPa) for 15 minutes. (2) Potassium tellurite 5 g, dist. H_2O 100 ml. Dissolve and Seitz filter. (3) Defibrinated bovine blood. To pour plates, melt agar base in tubes and cool to 50°C. Then add 1 ml of the tellurite solution and 1 ml of blood, mix thoroughly, and pour contents of each tube into a petri dish.

Potato-Carrot Medium. Boil 100 g each of sliced carrots and potatoes for 5 minutes in 500 ml of water. Strain off juice, add 20 g of glucose to the juice, and bring total volume to 1000 ml. Sterilize by autoclaving.

Potato Dextrose Agar. This medium is available commercially in a dehydrated form from Difco, Detroit, and Baltimore Biological Lab. The agar content is usually increased to 2% to insure a firm dry surface. If the medium is in a screw-topped tube or jar, the tops should be left loose during incubation. This medium is used to induce conidia production in dermatophytes. It is adequate for nearly all species except *Tricophyton verrucosum*.

Proskauer and Beck Medium, Modified. The ingredients are L-asparagine 5 g, potassium phosphate monobasic 5 g, potassium sulfate 5 g, glycerol 20 ml, dist. H_2O 930 ml, magnesium citrate 1.5 g, horse serum (sterile) 50 ml.

Dissolve L-asparagine by heating in part of the water until clear. Dissolve each of the next two chemicals in small amounts of water separately. Add to asparagine mixture; add glycerol and rest of water. Mix thoroughly. Adjust pH to 7 with 10 N NaOH. Now add the 1.5 g of magnesium citrate. Mix until in solution. Pour into aspirator bottle with attachment for aseptic dispensing. Sterilize in autoclave at 121°C for 20 minutes. Cool to 50°C and aseptically add the sterile horse serum. Dispense aseptically into 20×125 screw-capped test tubes in 4 ml amounts. Incubate at 37°C to check sterility.

Raulin-Thom Solution. The formula is glucose 50 g, tartaric acid 2.6 g, ammonium tartrate 2.6 g, ammonium monohydrogen phosphate 0.4 g, potassium carbonate 0.25 g, magnesium carbonate 0.25 g, ammonium sulfate 0.16 g, zinc sulfate · $7H_2O$ 0.06 g, ferrous sulfate · $7H_2O$ 0.06 g. Add 2.5% malt extract for rubratoxin production.

Rice Grains, Polished. This medium is particularly useful for stimulating macroconidial production in *Microsporum* species other than *M. audouinii*, which produces only negligible growth on this medium. The technique is as follows: half-fill a glass petri dish with polished rice. Add sufficient water to moisten all the grains. Autoclave at 121°C for 15 minutes. The fungus to be examined is inoculated directly onto the surface of the rice, as for any other medium. After 7–10 days incubation at 30°C, the resulting growth is examined for conidial production using the cellotape method.

Sabouraud's Dextrose Agar. This agar contains neopeptone 10 g, Bacto-dextrose 10 g, Bacto-agar 20 g, dist. H_2O 1000 ml. It should have a pH of 5.6. Sterilize in autoclave at 15 lb (103.42 kPa) pressure for 10 minutes. When Actidione (cyclohexamide) is added, subtract the volume from the total volume of water.

Sabouraud's Dextrose Agar containing Cycloheximide, Chloramphenicol, and Yeast Extract. The medium contains Sabouraud's dextrose agar (2% agar content), cycloheximide (Actidione, Upjohn, Kalamazoo, Mich.) 0.5 mg/ml, chloramphenicol (Chloromycetin, Parke Davis, Detroit) 0.05 mg/ml, and yeast extract (Difco, Detroit) 0.3%. Suspend 65 g dehydrated Sabouraud's dextrose agar (to which has been added 5 g agar and 3 g yeast extract) in 1000 ml dist. H_2O. Heat to boiling. After removal from heat, add chloramphenicol (50 mg suspended in 10 ml 95% ethyl alcohol) to medium. Add cycloheximide solution (500 mg in 10 ml of acetone). Autoclave at 118°C for 10 minutes. Allow to cool to 50°C and pour into sterile petri dishes, using approximately 25 ml per 9 mm dish. Incubate plates at 37°C overnight. Store in refrigerator until required. Note that some mycotic organisms cannot tolerate Chloromycetin.

Salmonella-Shigella (SS) Agar. This agar was developed by Difco (Detroit) for the isolation of the named organisms. It contains Bacto–beef extract 5 g, proteose peptone 5 g, Bacto-lactose 10 g, Bacto–bile salts no. 3 8.5 g, sodium citrate 8.5 g, sodium thiosulfate 8.5 g, ferric citrate 1 g, Bacto-agar 13.5 g, Bacto–brilliant green 0.33 mg, Bacto–neutral red 25 g, dist. H_2O 1000 ml.

Salt-Starch Agar. The ingredients are soluble starch 0.5 g, peptone 0.3 g, yeast extract 0.1 g, NaCl 5 g, agar 1.5 g, dist. H_2O 100 ml. Adjust to pH 7.5, sterilize, and dispense.

Selective Medium for Focal Isolation of Yersinia pseudotuberculosis. This medium contains peptic digest of sheep's blood 10 ml, novobiocin (0.2%) 2 ml, erythromycin (0.2%) 0.5 ml, mycostatin (50,000 units/ml) 0.8 ml, crystal violet (0.1%) 0.5 ml. Add to 200 ml melted trypsinized meat agar at 50°C just before pouring plates.

Selenite-F Broth. This is an enrichment medium for the isolation of *Salmonella* sp. It contains peptone (polypeptone) 5 g, lactose 4 g, sodium phosphate 10 g, sodium acid selenite 4 g, dist. H_2O 1000 ml.

Skin-Test Antigen Concentration Method. The undiluted antigen (100 ml) is poured into seamless cellulose dialyzing tubing (flat diameter of 44 mm). The tubing is tied at both ends to seal it and is then suspended in front of a fan at room temperature. The evaporation period varies depending on the concentration desired. From 100 ml to 80 ml ($2\times$) takes about 12 hours, and from 100 ml to 10 ml ($9\times$) takes 4 days. The tubing is marked so that when the final volume is reached it is the exact concentration desired. The final volume is then filtered through a Seitz filter (type ST-1, L-6) with a 0.5 μm filter pad and then bottled.

Sodium Azide–Crystal Violet Blood Agar. The following materials are used: blood agar base (Difco B45 or equivalent) 40 g, sodium azide 0.2–0.5 g (the higher concentration may be needed if contamination with enteric bacteria is extreme), crystal violet (0.1% solution) 2 ml (variation in bacteriostatic action among batches of crystal violet may require minor adjustments to content), dist. H_2O, for a total of 1000 ml; and citrated or defibrinated sheep blood 50 ml.

Dissolve the sodium azide in 20–30 ml dist. H_2O. Disperse the sodium azide and crystal violet solutions in the total volume (1000 ml) of cool water and suspend the blood agar base in it. Bring this material to boil, adjust to pH 7, distribute in stoppered flask(s), and sterilize in autoclave at 121°C for 15 minutes. Cool the medium to 40–50°C and aseptically add the 5% quantity of sterile blood. Pour the plates to a depth of approximately 3 mm.

Staphylococcus Medium 110. This medium contains yeast extract 2.5 g, tryptone 10 g, gelatin 30 g, lactose 2 g, d-mannitol 10 g, NaCl 75 g, dipotassium phosphate 5 g, agar 15 g. Dissolve in 1000 ml dist. H_2O by boiling; sterilize in autoclave. The medium is available commercially in dehydrated form (Difco, Detroit).

Stonebrink's Medium. The following equipment should be prepared and sterilized: 1 screw-capped flask (250 ml), 1 aspirator bottle (2 liters) with magnetic stirring bar within and a small bell-type filling attachment on a rubber hose for dispensing aseptically into tubes, 1 large funnel lined with two layers of unbleached muslin and covered with huck towel (muslin taped in place) and then wrapped in paper and taped to sterilize, 2 quart jars with Osterizer blender tops sterilized in inverted position, 1 glass rod to stir eggs in funnel, 1 beaker (250 ml), 140 screw-capped round-bottomed tubes (20×125 mm), 4 towels.

The ingredients are sodium pyruvate (sodium salt–pyruvic acid) 5 g, potassium phosphate monobasic KH_2PO_4 2 g, sodium phosphate monobasic NaH_2PO_4 10 g, crystal violet 100 mg, malachite green 800 mg, dist. H_2O 400 ml, fresh eggs (approximately 20) 800 ml.

Mix sodium pyruvate and potassium phosphate in 300 ml of water until completely dissolved. Place in the aspirator bottle. Slowly add sodium phosphate until pH 6.5 is reached. Mix the crystal violet and malachite green in 100 ml of water until completely dissolved. Place in the screw-capped flask and sterilize at 121°C for 20 minutes. Cool to room temperature. Add dye mixture to the salt mixture in the aspirator bottle.

Wash the eggs with a brush in warm detergent water, rinse in clear water, and lay out on a towel to dry. Then soak in 75% isopropyl alcohol for 30 minutes. Dry by inserting between layers of sterile towels. Dip the top of a sterile beaker in alcohol and burn off the alcohol to sterilize. Break the eggs on the sterile edge of the beaker and drop into sterile blender jars. Mix gently on blender base, just enough to homogenize egg mixture but not enough to cause air bubbles. Filter the eggs through sterile muslin in the funnel and into the aspirator bottle. Keep the cotton-gauze plug from the bottle sterile while it is not in place. When the eggs have been filtered, replace the cotton-gauze plug in the aspirator bottle and mix gently but thoroughly on the magnetic stirrer until the medium is evenly blended. Dispense in 9 ml amounts in the sterile tubes. Inspissate for 40 minutes at 80°C with the tubes in slant position. Cool and incubate at 37°C for 48 hours in slant position so that excess moisture will be reabsorbed by the medium.

Stuart's Medium, Modified. The formula is NaCl 1.93 g, ammonium chloride 0.34 g, magnesium chloride 0.19 g, asparagine 0.13 g, disodium phosphate 0.666 g, monopotassium phosphate 0.087 g, glycerol (optional) 5 ml, dist. H_2O 995 ml. Dissolve each ingredient separately in 100 ml dist. H_2O. Mix the ingredients and add dist. H_2O QS 1000 ml. Autoclave at 121°C for 15 minutes. Allow medium to cool. Add 100 ml of sterile rabbit serum, previously inactivated in water bath at 56°C for 30 minutes, and dispense in desired amounts in tubes or flasks. The pH of this medium should be 7.4–7.6.

Tellurite-Glycine Medium. The ingredients are yeast extract 6.5 g, tryptone 10 g, soytone 3.5 g, d-mannitol 5 g, glycine 10 g, dipotassium phosphate 5 g, lithium chloride 5 g, agar 17.5 g. Suspend the ingredients in 1000 ml dist. H_2O and stir to boiling point. Sterilize in autoclave 15 minutes at 15 lb (103.42 kPa) pressure (121°C). Cool to about 50°C and add 2 ml of Chapman tellurite solution for each 100 ml of the sterile medium, using aseptic precautions. Do not heat medium after addition of tellurite. The final pH should be about 7.2. Sterile Chapman tellurite solution is commercially available (Difco, Detroit).

Tetrathionate Broth. This is an enrichment medium for isolation of *Salmonella* sp. It contains peptone (proteose peptone or polypeptone) 5 g, bile salts 1 g, calcium carbonate 10 g, sodium thiosulfate 30 g, dist. H_2O 1000 ml. Add 10 ml of 1:1000 solution of brilliant green dye per liter of medium.

Thiosulfate Citrate Bile-Salts Sucrose (TCBS) Agar. This medium is composed of the following: yeast extract 0.5 g, beef extract 0.5 g, NaCl 1 g, sodium thiosulfate 1 g, peptone 1 g, sodium citrate 1 g, oxgall 0.5 g, sodium cholate 0.3 g, ferric citrate 0.1 g, sucrose 1.5 g, BTB 0.004 g, thymol blue 0.004 g, agar 1.5 g, dist. H_2O 100 ml. Adjust to pH 9.2.

Todd Hewitt Broth. This broth contains beef heart infusion 500 g, neopeptone 20 g, glucose 2 g, NaCl 2 g, disodium phosphate 0.4 g, sodium carbonate 2.5 g, dist. H_2O 1000 ml. Sterilize in autoclave for 15 minutes at 15 lb (103.42 kPa) pressure. The final pH should be 7.8. (See Chapter 48.)

Toxin Medium. This medium contains phytone (Baltimore Biological Lab.) 3%, Bacto-peptone 1%, trypticase (BBL) 0.5%, soluble starch 0.1%, Na_2HPO_4 0.4%, beef infusion QS for selected volume. Adjust the pH of the medium to 7.8 with 5 N NaOH. Add a small piece of acid-washed steel wool to each container or tube. Autoclave at 121°C for 25 minutes.

Triple Sugar Iron (TSI) Agar. The formula for TSI agar is as follows: beef extract 0.3%, yeast extract 0.3%, peptone 1.5%, proteose peptone 0.5%, glucose 0.1%, lactose 1%, sucrose 1%, ferrous sulfate 0.02%, NaCl 0.5%, sodium thiosulfate 0.03%, agar 1.2%, phenol red 0.0024% in dist. H_2O. A comparable medium can be obtained commercially. Prepare in tubes slanted at a high angle to form deep butts. To inoculate, stab the butt and streak the slant. A yellow butt indicates fermentation of glucose. A yellow slant indicates fermentation of lactose and/or sucrose. Blackening indicates H_2S production. If the color of the medium is unchanged, glucose has not been fermented. By definition, the organism is thus excluded from Enterobacteriaceae.

Tryptone Water. This is used for the indole test. The formula is tryptone or trypticase 15 g, NaCl 5 g, dist. H_2O 1000 ml. Sterilize at 121°C for 15 minutes. Test for indole with Kovac's reagent.

Tryptose Agar. The formula is the same as for tryptose broth, except that 18 g of agar per liter is added. Heat the preparation to melt the agar and filter through cotton or several layers of milk filter discs. Autoclave and dispense. To make tryptose blood or serum agar, add 5% whole blood or serum aseptically before dispensing. A comparable medium can be obtained commercially (Difco, Detroit).

Tryptose Broth. Dissolve 3 g of beef extract, 15 g of Bacto-tryptose, and 5 g of NaCl in 1000 ml dist. H_2O. Adjust pH to 7.6 with 4% NaOH. Filter through cotton or filter paper, dispense, and sterilize by autoclaving.

Tryptose Phosphate Broth. This broth contains tryptose 20 g, glucose 2 g, NaCl 5 g, disodium phosphate 2.5 g. Dissolve the ingredients in 1000 ml dist. H_2O, distribute in tubes or flasks, and autoclave for 15 minutes at 121°C. The final pH should be about 7.3.

Tryptose Serum Broth. Add 5%–10% sterile serum (equine, bovine, etc.) aseptically to tryptose broth after autoclaving.

L-Tyrosine Medium for Identification of Nocardia. The formula is L-tyrosine 0.5 g, nutrient agar 100 ml. Melt sterile agar, allow to cool, and add L-tyrosine powder. Mix to suspend evenly. Pour petri plates.

Urea Agar Base. The formula is peptone 1 g, NaCl 5 g, glucose 1 g, monobasic potassium phosphate 2 g, phenol red 0.012 g, urea 20 g, dist. H_2O 100 ml. Dissolve 15 g agar in 900 ml dist. H_2O and sterilize at 121°C for 15 minutes. Cool sterilized agar to 50°C. Add 100 ml of 20% urea solution that has been filter-sterilized. Dispense in sterile tubes and slant. Inoculate by streaking the slant. Development of a red color is a positive reaction.

Veronal-Buffered Saline, see Chapter 5, page 62

Violet Red Bile (VRB) Agar. The formula is Bacto–yeast extract 3 g, Bacto-peptone 7 g, Bacto–bile salt no. 3 1.5 g, Bacto-lactose 10 g, NaCl 5 g, Bacto-agar 15 g, Bacto–neutral red 0.03 g, Bacto–crystal violet 0.002 g, dist. H_2O 1000 ml.

Voges-Proskauer (VP) Reagent. The materials are KOH 20 g, creatine 0.15 g, dist. H_2O 50 ml. Dissolve KOH in water, then add creatine. Store in refrigerator. Make new reagent every 2 weeks. (See Glucose Broth.)

Voges-Proskauer Test, see Glucose Broth and Methyl Red Reagent

Xanthine Medium for Identification of Nocardia. The ingredients are xanthine 0.04 g, nutrient agar 100 ml. Melt sterile nutrient agar, allow to cool, and add xanthine powder. Mix thoroughly to suspend evenly and dispense 30 ml aliquots into 9 cm petri plates.

Xylose Lysine (XL) Base Agar. The medium is used for enteric organisms. It contains agar 15 g, lactose 7.5 g, sucrose 7.5 g, xylose 3.75 g, L-lysine–HCl 5 g, NaCl 5 g, yeast extract 3 g, phenol red (1% solution) 8 ml, dist. H_2O 1000 ml. Sterilize at 121°C for 15 minutes. Cool to 50°C. Add 20 ml of solution A (see below) and 25 ml of a 10% sodium deoxycholate solution. Adjust pH to 6.9 and pour. Solution A contains sodium thiosulfate 34%, ferric ammonium citrate 4%, dist. H_2O QS for volume selected. XL agar is used for quantitative work with enteric organisms. Brilliant green should be added (XLBG) for isolation of *Salmonella* from food and deoxycholate should be added (XLD) for isolation of *Shigella* from feces. The XLD agar permits growth of most salmonellae and eliminates the problem of brilliant green toxicity.

Yeast Cell Agglutination Test for Cryptococcal Antibody. A washed suspension of Formalin-killed, whole, 2-day-old yeast cells is heated at 56°C for 0.5 hours and adjusted to 15×10^6 cells per ml of saline containing 0.1% Formalin. Serial twofold saline dilutions of serum, in 0.5 ml volumes, are mixed with 0.5 ml of antigen, shaken 2 minutes, incubated at 37°C for 2 hours, and refrigerated at 4°C for 72 hours, with intermediate readings at 2, 24, and 48 hours. Tests must always be accompanied by controls of reacting and nonreacting serum.

Yeast Nitrogen Base. The basal medium is used for the sugar assimilation test. Place in a petri dish 2 ml of a saline suspension (moderate density, cloudy but not opaque) of yeast cells harvested from third passage in beef extract broth, add 1.5 ml of 10-fold concentration of yeast nitrogen base (i.e. 10 times the concentration indicated on directions accompanying the product), and add 13.5 ml of melted, partially cooled 2% agar. Swirl sufficiently to mix all ingredients; let solidify. Place sterile paper assay discs (commercial assay discs, blotter or bibulous paper discs) at designated points on the surface after barely saturating them with 20% solutions of the test sugars. Incubate at room temperature and read for sugar assimilation (halos of opaque growth around the test discs) after 24–72 hours. This base is commercially available (Difco, Detroit).

Yersinia pseudotuberculosis Selective Medium, see Selective Medium for Focal Isolation of Yersinia pseudotuberculosis

B. Stains

Barbeito-Lopez Trichrome Stain. This is a connective tissue stain that is also used to stain bacteria, e.g. *Haemophilus*. The regular histopathologic techniques should be used to process the specimen, from Formalin fixation through embedding in paraffin. Cut sections at 6 μm and mount on slides. Then carry slides through routine solutions back to hydration in dist. H_2O. The staining procedure is as follows: (1) stain in acetic fuchsin solution for 30 seconds to 1 minute; (2) wash vigorously in tap water to remove excess solution; (3) fix color in acetic Formalin solution for up to 3 minutes, place sections in Coplin jar containing the solution, agitate, and renew solution after four or five uses (the color changes from red to pale violet); (4) wash in tap water; (5) stain in molybdic acid–aniline blue–methyl orange solution 30 seconds to 1 minute; (6) wash in tap water rapidly; (7) dehydrate (rapidly), clear, and mount. Disregard the color clouds that appear in the 95% alcohol. Cell nuclei and bacteria stain violet red, cytoplasm green to pale blue, reticulum fibers deep blue, collagen brilliant green, and RBC brilliant orange.

For the acetic fuchsin solution, use carbol fuchsin solution (see Ziehl-Neelson stain) 10 ml, glacial acetic acid 0.2 ml, dist. H_2O 100 ml. For the acetic Formalin solution, use Formalin (37–40%) 4 ml, glacial acetic acid 0.2 ml, dist. H_2O 100 ml.

For the molybdic acid–aniline blue–methyl orange solution, add 1 g of molybdic acid to 100 ml of dist. H_2O in a 250 ml Erlenmeyer flask; shake vigorously and heat gently for 5 minutes. Add 0.5 g of water-soluble aniline blue and dissolve. Add methyl orange in excess until a deposit forms in the bottom of the flask. Filter.

(This description is adapted from J. Barbeito-Lopez, Technical Section, *Am. J. Clin. Path.* 16:53–56, 1946.)

Castaneda's Stain. The formula is: phosphate buffer (Leishman buffer) (pH 7) 95 ml, neutral formaldehyde solution 5 ml, methylene blue (Effler's aged solution) 10 ml. Smears are stained for 2–5 minutes, washed, and counterstained for 10 seconds with 0.2% aqueous safranin solution. This is the Rivers and Berry formulation. Bedson and Bland used Borrel blue 10 ml, and Lépine recommended azur II as a 1% solution in 0.5% phenol in water.

Erichrome Black Counterstain for FA Test. For the chelating agent, use N,N-dimethylformamide 200 ml, dist. H_2O 80 ml, aluminum chloride (0.1 M) 40 ml, acetic acid (1 M) 40 ml; adjust to pH 5.2 with NaOH (1 M); add dist. H_2O QS 400 ml total.

For the staining solution, use Erichrome black A (Nutritional Biochemicals Corp., Cleveland) 0.628 g, N,N-dimethylformamide 80 ml; add 400 ml of chelating agent *slowly* while shaking (shelf-life 2 months at 4°C).

To stain: (1) prepare slide of bacterial culture, dry, and heat fix; (2) fix in ethyl alcohol (95%) for 15 minutes; (3) rinse with PBS solution and air dry; (4) add 0.05 ml of FITC-conjugated specific antiserum and incubate 30 minutes in a moist chamber at 37°C; (5) rinse several times with PBS; (6) counterstain with the Erichrome black staining solution for 5–10 seconds; (7) wash immediately with dist. H_2O; (8) dry and apply coverslip with mounting fluid (Fluormount, Edward Gurr Ltd., West London, Eng., or Difco FA mounting fluid, Difco, Detroit); (9) examine using a BG-12 primary filter with a blue-absorbing secondary filter. This procedure is particularly recommended for *Campylobacter* and *Vibrio* sp.

Giemsa Stain, see May-Grünwald-Giemsa Stain

Gimenez Stain. Carbol–basic fuchsin stock solution contains: basic fuchsin (10% in 95% ethanol W/V) 100 ml, aqueous phenol (4% V/V) 250 ml, dist. H_2O 650 ml. Dye content should be 94% (Cert. no. 51, Color Index no. 42500, Matheson, Coleman, and Bell, Norwood, Ohio). Before first use, store stock solution 48 hours at 37°C; thereafter store at room temperature (shelf-life stability is about 10 months).

Sodium phosphate-buffered solution (PBS), 0.1 M, pH 7.45, contains: 0.2 M NaH_2PO_4 3.5 ml, 0.2 M Na_2HPO_4 15.5 ml, dist. H_2O 19 ml.

Carbol–basic fuchsin working solution is: 4 ml stock solution with 10 ml phosphate buffer, filtered just before each use (shelf-life about 40 hours). For all *Chlamydia* and *Rickettsia* (except *R. tsutsugamushi*) stain as follows: (1) air-dry a thin film of infected yolk sac tissue on slide free of yolk fluid and fix with heat, (2) cover with fuchsin working solution 2 minutes and then wash thoroughly, (3) cover with malachite-green oxalate 0.8% solution for 6–9 seconds, (4) wash, (5) repeat malachite-green stain 6–9 seconds (6) wash and dry slide. The *Chlamydia* and *Rickettsia* stain bright red, tissue cells greenish blue, and background slightly green.

For *R. tsutsugamushi* the procedure is the same for the first two steps. Then (3) cover with about five drops of $FeNO_3 \cdot 9H_2O$ 4% solution for about 2 seconds and then wash immediately, (4) counterstain with fast green FCF (Fisher Scientific, Pittsburgh) 0.5% solution for 15–30 seconds, (5) wash and dry slide. *Rickettsia* stain reddish black, the background green.

Gomori-Gridley Stain. Five solutions are needed: (1) chromic acid—4 g dissolved in 100 ml dist. H_2O; (2) Coleman's Feulgen reagent—heat 200 ml dist. H_2O to boiling, remove from heat and add basic fuchsin 1 g, cool and filter, add sodium metabisulfite 2 g and 10 ml of 1 N HCl, let bleach for 24 hours and then add activated carbon (decolorizing, Norit A, Pfanstiehl, Arthur H. Thomas, Philadelphia) 0.5 g, shake for about a minute, filter through coarse paper, and store in refrigerator (the filtrate should be colorless); (3) acid rinse—sodium metabisulfite (10% solution) 6 ml, 1 N HCl 5 ml, dist. H_2O 100 ml; (4) aldehyde-fuchsin solution—basic fuchsin 1 g, ethyl alcohol (70%) 200 ml, paraldehyde 2 ml, conc. HCl 2 ml; then allow solution to stand at room temperature for

3 days until a deep blue color develops and store at 4°C, but warm to room temperature and filter before use; (5) Counterstain—metanil yellow 0.25 g, dist. H_2O 100 ml, glacial acetic acid 2 drops.

To stain: (1) fix, dehydrate, embed, section, mount on slide, deparaffinize, and rehydrate the specimen to dist. H_2O; (2) place in chromic acid solution (no. 1) for 1 hour (oxidizer); wash in running tap water 5 minutes; (3) place in Coleman's solution (no. 2) for 15 minutes; (4) rinse in three changes of acid rinse (no. 3) and wash 15 minutes in running tap water; (5) place in aldehyde-fuchsin solution (no. 4) for 15–30 minutes; (6) rinse off excess stain with 95% ethyl alcohol and rinse in water; (7) counterstain lightly with metanil yellow solution (no. 5) for 1 minute and rinse in water; (8) dehydrate through 95% and absolute ethyl alcohol; (9) clear in xylene; and (10) mount with coverslip in Permount (Fisher Scientific, Pittsburgh) or equivalent. This staining procedure is especially useful for histologic examination of mycotic specimens.

Gram Stain. The reagents should be prepared as follows: (1) Make a 0.25% aqueous crystal violet solution by grinding the crystals in a mortar and pestle and then filtering to obtain a stock solution. Prepare a 1.25% $NaHCO_3$ solution. Mix equal parts of stock crystal violet and the sodium bicarbonate solution prior to placing on the fixed smear. (2) Use 0.1 N NaOH to make a 2% iodine solution by grinding crystals in a mortar and pestle and then filtering to obtain a working solution. (3) The decolorizer is 95% ethyl alcohol. (4) Use 2.5% safranin dissolved in 95% ethyl alcohol to make the stock solution of the counterstain. For use, dilute the stock solution 1:10 with dist. H_2O. Gram-staining reagents are buffered to an alkaline pH to facilitate rapid staining in seconds. Iodine crystals are used in preference to KI since the latter stains more slowly and tends to change to an acid pH with age.

Gram Stain, Hucker's Modification. For solution A, use crystal violet (90% dye content) 2 g, ethyl alcohol (95%) 20 ml. For solution B, use ammonium oxalate 0.8 g, dist. H_2O 80 ml. Mix solution A with solution B. For Gram's modification of Lugol's solution, use iodine 1 g, KI 2 g, dist. H_2O 300 ml. For the counterstain, use safranin O (2.5% solution in 95% ethyl alcohol) 10 ml, dist. H_2O 100 ml.

To stain: (1) immerse smears 1 minute in ammonium oxalate crystal violet, (2) wash in tap water for not more than 2 seconds, (3) immerse 1 minute in the iodine solution, (4) wash briefly in tap water, (5) decolorize 30 seconds with gentle agitation in 95% ethyl alcohol and blot dry, (6) counterstain 10 seconds in the safranin solution, (7) wash in tap water, (8) dry and examine. Gram-positive organisms stain blue, gram-negative organisms red.

Gram Stain, Kopeloff-Beerman Modification. For solution A, use gentian or crystal violet 1 g, dist. H_2O 100 ml. For solution B, use $NaHCO_3$ 1 g, dist. H_2O 20 ml. Before staining, mix 1.5 ml of solution A with 0.4 ml of solution B. For the iodine solution, use iodine 2 g, 1 N NaOH (40.01 g/L) 10 ml. After iodine is dissolved, add dist. H_2O QS 100 ml. For the counterstain, use basic fuchsin (90% dye content) 0.1 g, dist. H_2O 100 ml.

To stain: (1) dry thinly spread films in the air without heat; (2) apply alkaline gentian violet solution and allow to stay on slide 5 minutes or more; (3) rinse with the iodine solution; (4) cover with fresh iodine solution, let stand 2 minutes or longer, and drain off; (5) decolorize in ether and acetone (1 vol. of ether to 1 vol. of acetone), adding to the slide drop until practically no color comes off in the drippings (usually about 10 seconds); (6) dry in the air; (7) counterstain 5 seconds in basic fuchsin solution; (8) wash in tap water; (9) dry and examine. Gram-positive organisms stain blue, gram-negative organisms red.

Grocott-Gomori Methenamine Silver Nitrate Stain. For the silver stain working solution, make separate stock solutions in dist. H_2O of each of the following chemicals: chromic acid 5%, sodium bisulfite 1%, borax 5%, silver nitrate 10%, methenamine 3%, gold chloride 0.1%, sodium thiosulfate 2%. Then make stock solution A: borax 5% solution 8 ml, dist. H_2O 100 ml, and stock solution B: silver nitrate 10% solution 7 ml, methenamine 3% solution 100 ml. For fresh use, mix equal parts of solutions A and B. Make the counterstain stock light-green solution as follows: Light Green SF Yellowish (Arthur H. Thomas, Philadelphia) 0.2 g, dist. H_2O 100 ml, glacial acetic acid 0.2 ml. For each use make a fresh light-green working solution as follows: light-green stock solution 10 ml, dist. H_2O 50 ml.

To stain histopathologic specimens that have gone through the routine procedure from fixation to mounted slides of sections and then have been carried back to hydration with dist. H_2O: (1) oxidize in 5% chromic acid for 1 hour; (2) wash in running tap water; (3) rinse in 1% sodium bisulfite for 1 minute to remove residual chromic acid; (4) wash in running water 5–10 minutes; (5) wash in three or four changes of dist. H_2O; (6) place in silver stain solution in oven (58–60°C) for 30–60 minutes (when section turns yellowish-brown use paraffin-coated forceps to remove slide from silver nitrate solution; dip slide in distilled water and check with microscope for adequate silver impregnation; fungi should be dark brown in color at this stage); (7) rinse in six changes of dist. H_2O; (8) tone in 0.1% gold chloride for 2–5 minutes; (9) rinse in dist. H_2O; (10) remove unreduced silver with 2% sodium thiosulfate for 2–5 minutes; (11) wash in tap water; (12) counterstain with light-green working solution for 1 minute; (13) wash, dehydrate, clear, and mount coverslip.

India Ink Wet Mount. This technique is used to demonstrate bacterial capsules. Place a loopful of dilute bacterial specimen adjacent to a loopful of Indian ink on a glass slide. Gently mix and add a coverslip. Examine the preparation using oil immersion. The capsules will appear as clear halos around the bacteria. Because the bacterial cells remain unstained with this technique, the illumination must be reduced to render them visible. India ink particles clump when mixed with sputum or acid materials or when touched with a hot needle. With this technique, mycotic cells, e.g. *Cryptococcus,* can be visualized in thick fluid mounts such as exudate, pus, and bronchial washings.

Koster's Stain. Place 5 parts of saturated aqueous safranin O freshly mixed with 2 parts of 4% NaOH on slide for 1.5 minutes, wash and destain with 0.1% H_2SO_4 for 10–20 seconds, wash and counterstain with 1.5% aqueous methylene blue for 10 seconds. *Brucella* organisms stain cherry red against a blue background.

Lactophenol Cotton Blue Mounting Solution. The formula is: phenol crystals (melted) 20 g, lactic acid 20 g, glycerol 40 g, cotton blue (Poirrier's blue) 0.05 g, dist. H_2O 20 ml. This solution is used for preparing mounts of fungal cultures for study.

Leifson's Flagellar Stain. For solution A, use basic fuchsin (certified for flagella staining) 0.6 g, ethyl alcohol (95%) 50 ml. Shake and let stand overnight to dissolve. For solution B, use NaCl 0.75 g, tannic acid 1.5 g, dist. H_2O 100 ml. Combine solutions A and B and mix thoroughly. The stain is ready for use and should remain satisfactory for about 1–2 months when stored at 4°C. A precipitate develops on storage and it should not be disturbed when the stain is used.

The staining procedure is as follows. (1) Smears for flagellar staining can be made from growth on plates by using a light suspension in dist. H_2O, taking care that only bacterial growth and none of the agar is carried into the suspension. More satisfactory preparations can be obtained with a Formalinized washed cell suspension of the organism from an overnight culture in a nonglucose-containing broth. To prepare the cell suspension, add 0.25 ml of Formalin to 5 ml of culture, mix, and allow to stand for 15 minutes. Add an equal portion of dist. H_2O to the tubes, mix, and centrifuge. Decant the supernatant fluid carefully. Add dist. H_2O, mix, and recentrifuge. Decant as before, resuspend the organism in 1–2 ml dist. H_2O, and then dilute to a barely turbid suspension. (2) It is essential that clean and grease-free slides be used for flagellar staining. Concentrated sulfuric acid saturated with potassium dichromate can be used to clean the slides. Immediately prior to use, the slides must be polished with a soft cotton cloth and then flamed well in the blue flame of a Bunsen burner, keeping the side to be used next to the flame. A smokey or yellow flame ruins the slides. (3) To prepare a smear for staining, place prepared slide with one end resting on an applicator stick to tilt the slide slightly. Place a 3 mm loopful of suspension on the slide and allow the drop to run to the other end of the slide. Allow to air dry. (4) Place the slide on a staining rack and add 1 ml of stain warmed to room temperature. Staining is not complete until a metallic sheen has formed on the surface of the stain. This can take from 6 to 12 minutes depending on the age of the stain. It is advisable to prepare fresh stain if the staining time exceeds 12 minutes. (5) Wash the stained slide with tap water without tilting the slide to flush the stain off. Air dry and examine. (6) If counterstain is desired, use a 1:10 dilution of Loeffler's methylene blue (see below) after washing off the flagellar stain.

Lentz Rabies Stain, Modified, see Chapter 20, Rabies virus

Loeffler's Alkaline Methylene Blue Stain. For solution A, use methylene blue (90% dye content) 0.3 g, ethyl alcohol (95%) 30 ml. For solution B, use dilute potassium hydroxide (0.01%) 100 ml. Mix solutions A and B.

To stain: (1) fix smears with gentle heat; (2) flood smears with stain for 1–2 minutes; (3) wash lightly, dry, and examine.

Macchiavello Stain. Prepare a thin film of yolk sac tissue free of yolk fluid on a slide, air dry, and fix with heat; cover with 0.25% aqueous basic fuchsin (filtered) for 5 minutes and drain; cover with 0.5% citric acid solution and wash immediately; counterstain with 1% aqueous methylene blue for 20–40 seconds, rinse, and dry. *Rickettsia* stain bright red against a blue background. *R. tsutsugamushi* can not be stained by this technique. Most bacteria stain blue, but some retain the red fuchsin color.

May-Grünwald-Giemsa (MGG) Stain. Mix equal parts of 0.5% aqueous eosin Y and 0.5% aqueous methylene blue. Filter and dry the precipitate. Wash the dried precipitate with water and redry. The May-Grünwald working solution consists of 1 g of the precipitated dye in 400 ml methanol.

Giemsa stain is prepared by dissolving 3 g of azur II–eosin and 0.8 g of azur II in 250 ml of pure anhydrous glycerol at 60°C. With the solution held at the same temperature, add 250 ml absolute methyl alcohol. The solution is filtered after it has been held overnight at room temperature. Commercially prepared Giemsa stain is a satisfactory substitute for the preceding preparation.

To stain: (1) fix smears promptly for 3 minutes in methyl alcohol; (2) cover for 3 minutes with May-Grünwald working solution; (3) add an equal amount of distilled water and allow to stand for 1 minute; (4) drain without rinsing; (5) cover for 12 minutes with dilute Giemsa stain (15 drops to 10 drops of distilled water); (6) differentiate by agitating in distilled water for about 5 seconds and checking the smear under microscope; repeat step 6 if necessary.

Neisser's Granule Stain. For solution A, use methylene blue 1 g, ethanol (95%) 20 ml, glacial acetic acid 50 ml, dist. H_2O 1000 ml. Mix until dye is dissolved. For solution B, use crystal violet 1 g, ethanol (95%) 10 ml, dist. H_2O 300 ml. For solution C, use chrysoidin 2 g, hot dist. H_2O 300 ml. Filter after dissolving.

Prepare slide from bacterial culture. Cover slide for 10 seconds with a mixture of 2 parts of solution A and 1 part of solution B and wash slide. Stain for 10 seconds with solution C. Wash briefly, or not at all, and then blot dry. This stain will allow demonstration of metachromatic granules. (See Chapter 48.)

Nigrosine Stain. The formulation is: nigrosine (water soluble, Edward Gurr Ltd., West London, Eng.) 10 g, dist. H_2O 100 ml. Boil for 30 minutes; add as a preservative 0.5 ml Formalin (37%). Filter twice through double filter paper and store in screw-capped 5 ml bottles (Corning Glass, Corning, N.Y.) at 4°C. Place a drop of specimen blood on a slide and then a drop of stain. Mix the two together with a toothpick and air dry. This negative stain gives the effect of dark-field examination, and the slide can be retained as a record. (See Chapter 44.)

Parker-51 (P-51) Stain. Mix equal parts of 20% KOH and P-51 superchrome blue-black ink. This ink is no longer available commercially but the dye is available directly from the Parker Pen Co., Janesville, Wis. Also, the specific colorant is available from Fuller Pharmaceutical Co., Minneapolis, Minn. (See Chapter 53.)

Periodic Acid–Schiff—Celestin Blue—Picric Acid Stain. For Schiff's reagent, dissolve 1 g of basic fuchsin in 100 ml of boiling dist. H_2O. Cool to 50°C and filter. Add 2 g of sodium metabisulphate and 20 ml of 1 N HCl. Stopper tightly and store in darkness overnight. Add 300 mg finely powdered activated charcoal, shake for 1 minute, and filter. The solution should be clear light yellow or colorless. It will keep for several months in the refrigerator. Discard if a pink tint appears.

For celestin blue, either solution A or B can be used. For solution A, a saturated solution of celestin blue in dist. H_2O is used. Place a knifepoint of stain in a test tube half-filled with dist. H_2O and shake vigorously for 30 seconds. This solution deteriorates rapidly and loses its staining properties in about 2 days. For solution B, dissolve 2.5 g iron alum overnight in 50 ml dist. H_2O; add 0.25 g of celestin blue and boil for 3 minutes.

Cool, filter, and then add 7 ml of glycerol. This solution keeps for some weeks but should be discarded when it loses its bright blue color.

To stain, fix specimens in 10% buffered neutral Formalin. Cut paraffin sections of 5 μm or less in thickness. Dewax sections and take down to dist. H_2O. Oxidize with 1% aqueous periodic acid for 5 minutes only. Rinse in water. Stain with Schiff's reagent for 15 minutes. Wash in running water for 10 minutes. Stain with freshly filtered celestin blue solution for 10 minutes. Rinse in water. Differentiate with (1) saturated aqueous picric acid for 30 seconds followed by (2) saturated alcoholic (absolute) picric acid for 30 seconds. Complete dehydration with absolute alcohol for 30 seconds. Clear in two changes of xylol and mount in DPX (BDH Chemicals, Poole, Dorset, Eng., or Merck, Rahway, N.J.). Fungal hyphae stain red or blue-gray, nuclei green-blue, background yellow. Note that Schiff-positive components (glycogen, mucoproteins, connective tissue) can be removed or their staining reaction reduced in lesions by pretreating sections as follows: take sections to water; digest at 40°C for 10 minutes in a solution containing 0.5 g pepsin, 1 ml conc. HC1, and 43 ml H_2O; wash well in running water; then stain (PAS-CB) as described above. Fungal hyphae are not greatly affected and become more clearly recognizable.

Polychrome Methylene Blue Stain. For solution A, use methylene blue (90% dye content) 0.3 g, ethyl alcohol (95%) 30 ml. For solution B, use dilute aqueous KOH (0.01% W/V in dist. H_2O) 100 ml. Mix solutions A with B and allow the mixture to ripen for several months (aeration will hasten the ripening). Use undiluted as a simple stain, staining for 2–3 minutes.

Seller's Rabies Stain, see Chapter 20, Rabies Virus

Wayson's Stain. Dissolve separately and then combine: basic fuchsin, 0.2 g/10 ml ethyl alcohol, and methylene blue, 0.2 g/10 ml ethyl alcohol. Add to phenol 5% in 200 ml dist. H_2O. Prepare smear and heat fix. Cover with stain for about 2–4 seconds; wash immediately and examine.

Ziehl-Neelsen–Acid-Fast Stain. For solution A, use basic fuchsin 0.3 g, ethyl alcohol 10 ml. For solution B, use phenol 5 g, dist. H_2O 95 ml. Mix solutions A and B and filter the mixture through filter paper. The mixture is known as carbol fuchsin. For the acid-alcohol, use conc. HCl 3.2 ml, 95% ethyl alcohol 97 ml. For methylene blue (alkaline), first make solution A—methylene blue 0.3 g, 95% ethyl alcohol 30 ml. Then make solution B—KOH 0.01 g, dist. H_2O 100 ml. Mix solutions A and B.

To stain: (1) immerse the smear from 3 minutes in steaming carbol fuchsin, (2) rinse in dist. H_2O, (3) decolorize in acid-alcohol until only a suggestion of pink color remains (2–3 minutes), (4) wash in dist. H_2O, (5) counterstain for 2 minutes with methylene blue solution, (6) wash in dist. H_2O and dry. Examine with the oil immersion lens of a microscope. Acid-fast organisms stain red.

Abbreviations

AAV	Adeno-associated virus
ABA	Albimi *Brucella* agar
ACS	American Chemical Society, Columbus, Ohio
AD	Agar (gel) diffusion (test)
A-D group	Alkalescena-dispar group of *E. coli*
ADR	Arthropod-borne (Animal) Disease Research (Laboratory), Denver
ADV	Aleutian disease virus (of mink)
AG	Arthrogryposis
AHS	African horsesickness
AHV	Allerton herpesvirus
AIB	Avian infectious bronchitis
AlC	Allantoic cavity (route)
AmC	Amnionic cavity (route)
APHIS	Animal and Plant Health Inspection Service (USDA), Washington
APT	Antibody production test
Arbo	Arthropod-borne (arbovirus)
ARS	Agricultural Research Service (USDA), Washington
ASF	African swine fever
ASTM	American Society for Testing and Materials, Philadelphia
ATCC	American Type Culture Collection, Rockville, Md.
AV	Akabane virus
AV_2	Amnionic variant (human amnion cell line)
BAI	Bureau of Animal Industry (formerly of the USDA), Washington
BB	Brown bullhead (cell cultures)
BBL	Baltimore Biological Laboratories
BCG	*Bacillus* Calmette Guerin (attenuated *Mycobacterium bovis*)
BCP	Bromcresol purple (medium)
BD	Borna disease
BEF	Bovine ephemeral fever
BEK	Bovine embryonic kidney (cells)
BEV	Bovine enterovirus
BG	Brilliant green (agar)
BGS	Brilliant green sulfa (agar)
BHI	Brain-heart infusion (agar, usually with blood or broth)
BHK	Baby hamster kidney (cells)

Abbreviations

BHM	Bovine herpes mammillitis
BK	Bovine kidney (cells)
BMM	Basal mineral medium
BPS	Bovine papular stomatitis (virus disease)
BPV	Bovine parvovirus
BS	Bismuth sulfite (agar)
BSA	Bovine serum albumin
BS-C-1	Biological Standards *Cercopithecus* #1 (African green monkey kidney cell line)
BSS	Balanced salt solution (Hanks', Earle's, etc.)
BT	Bluetongue (disease)
BTB	Bromthymol blue (medium)
BTC	Bovine tracheal cells
BUDR	5-bromo-2'-deoxyuridine (DNA inhibitor)
BVD-MD	Bovine viral diarrhea–mucosal disease
CA	Croup-associated (virus)
CAM	Chorioallantoic membrane (route for embryonating eggs)
CAMP	Christie, Atkins, and Munch-Petersen (test)
CB	Celestin blue (stain) (may be added to PAS stain: PAS-CB)
CBI	Cysteine beef infusion (medium)
CBPP	Contagious bovine pleuropneumonia
C & C	Cycloheximide and chloramphenicol (inhibitors used in mycology)
CCVD	Channel catfish virus disease
CD	Canine distemper
CDC	Center for Disease Control (HEW), Atlanta, Ga. (formerly National Communicable Disease Center)
CEF	Chick embryo fibroblast (cell cultures)
CEK	Chick embryo kidney (cells)
CELO	Chick embryo lethal orphan (virus)
CF	Complement fixation (test)
CHV	Canine herpesvirus
C-J	Creutzfeldt-Jakob (disease)
CMF	Calcium-magnesium–free (solution)
CNS	Central nervous system
COFAL	Complement fixation avian leukosis (test)
CP	Chemically pure
CPE	Cytopathic effect (of viruses)
CRFK	Crandell feline kidney (cell line)
CRH	Cottontail rabbit herpesvirus
CSF	Cerebrospinal fluid
CSIRO	Commonwealth Scientific and Industrial Research Organization, Australia
CVS	Challenge virus standard (rabies virus strain)
DCF	Direct complement fixation (test)
DEAE	Diethylaminoethyl (dextran)
DGV	Dextrose-gelatin-Veronal (solution)
Dist.	Distilled (water)
DNA	Deoxyribonucleic acid
DNase	Deoxyribonuclease (enzyme that digests DNA)
DOP	Dioctylphthalate (aerosolized to test HEPA filters)
DP	Duck plague
DPI	Days postinoculation (or exposure to infection)

DS	Double-stranded (RNA or DNA)
DTM	Dermatophyte test medium
EAV	Equine arteritis virus
EBTr	Embryonic bovine tracheal (cell line)
ECBO	Enteric cytopathic bovine orphan (viruses)
ECHO	Enteric cytopathic human orphan (viruses)
ED_{50}	Effective dose 50% (titer)
EDTA	Ethylenediaminetetraacetic (acid) (versene)
EEE	Eastern equine encephalomyelitis
EEV	Equine encephalomyelitis viruses (EEEV, WEEV, VEEV)
EFV	Ephemeral fever virus
Eh	Electrical (potential) hydrogen (oxidation-reduction potential of anaerobic media expressed in minus millivolts)
EHD	Epizootic hemorrhagic disease (of deer)
EIA	Equine infectious anemia
EID_{50}	Embryo infecting dose 50% (titer)
EM	Electron microscope
EMB	Eosin methylene blue (agar)
EMC	Encephalomyocarditis
END	Exaltation of Newcastle disease (virus test)
ERV	Equine rhinopneumonitis virus
ESB	*Erysipelothrix* selective broth
FA	Fluorescent antibody (test)
FCS	Fetal calf serum
Fc_3Tg	Feline (diploid) tongue (cell line)
FFIT	Fluorescent focus inhibition test
FITC	Fluorescein isothiocyanate (conjugate for FA)
FK	Feline kidney (cells)
FMD	Foot-and-mouth disease
FP	Fowl plague
FPL	Feline panleukopenia
FPRV	Feline picorna respiratory virus
FR	Feline rhinotracheitis
FRA	Fluorescent rabies antibody (test)
FTG	Fluid thioglycollate (medium)
FUDR	5-fluoro-2'-deoxyuridine, floxuridine (DNA inhibitor)
g	Gram
g	Gravity (centrifugation)
GAL	*Gallus* adeno-like (virus of *Gallus domesticus*)
GAM	N-acetyl-b-d glucosaminidase (enzyme test)
GI	Gastrointestinal (tract)
GN	Gram-negative (stain result or broth)
GP	Gram-positive (stain result); also used for Guinea pig
GPCMV	Guinea pig cytomegalovirus
GT	Genital tract
GUR	b-glucuronidase (enzyme test)
GYE	Glucose-yeast extract (agar)

Abbreviations

H-1	Hamster osteolytic virus–1
HA	Hemagglutination (test) or hemagglutinin (antigen)
HAd	Hemadsorption (test)
HADEN	Hemadsorbing enteric (virus) (also known as BPV)
HAdI	Hemadsorption inhibition (test)
HAP	Hamster antibody production (test)
HC	Hog cholera (virus)
HCA	Hog cholera antigen
HE	Hydranencephaly
H & E	Hematoxylin and eosin (stains for histology)
HeLa	Helen La-- (patient's name, cervical carcinoma, cell line)
Hep-2	Human epidermoid #2 (carcinoma of larynx, cell line)
HEPA	High efficiency particulate air (filter)
HEW	Health, Education, and Welfare (U.S. Department of), Washington
HI	Hemagglutination inhibition (test)
HLH	Hanks' (BSS and) lactalbumin hydrolysate
HSA	Human serum albumin
HSV	Herpes simplex virus
HVs	*Herpesvirus saimiri*
HVT	Herpesvirus of turkeys
IAb	Intra-abdominal (route)
IAm	Intra-amnionic (cavity or sac route)
IAMS	International Association of Microbiological Societies, Geneva
IBN	Infective bulbar necrosis (of sheep)
IBR	Infectious bovine rhinotracheitis
IBV	Infectious bronchitis virus (avian)
IC	Intracerebral (route)
ICF	Indirect complement fixation (test)
ICTV	International Committee on the Taxonomy of Viruses, Geneva
ID	Intradermal (route)
ID_{50}	Infective dose 50% (titer)
IEOP	Immunoelectroosmophoresis
IgA	Immunoglobulin alpha (antibody class)
IgG	Immunoglobulin gamma (antibody class)
ILT	Infectious laryngotracheitis (avian)
IM	Intramuscular (route)
IN	Intranasal (route)
INT	Intestinal tract
IO	Intraocular (route)
IP	Intraperitoneal
IT	Intratracheal
i.u.	International units; also used for Immunizing units
IV	Intravenous (route)
JBEV	Japanese B encephalitis virus
JD	Joest-Degen (inclusion bodies)
KB	Karl Bis---- (patient's name, oral epidermoid carcinoma, cell line)
KCN	Potassium cyanide (medium)
KIA	Kligler's iron agar

LD_{50}	Lethal dose 50% (titer)
LE	Lactalbumin-Earle's (BSS)
LI	Lysine iron (agar)
LIV	Louping ill virus
LL	Lymphoid leukosis; also used for Lymphoid leukemia
$LLC-MK_2$	Lilly Laboratory culture–monkey kidney 2 (cell line)
$LLC-RK_1$	Lilly Laboratory culture–rabbit kidney 1 (cell line)
LLO	Localized lesion only (at inoculation site)
LLV-F	Friend's leukemia virus (MuLV Friend helper of SFFV)
LLV-R	Rauscher's leukemia virus (MuLV Rauscher helper of SFFV)
LN	Lymph node
LS	Lipid-soluble (antigen) (found in poxviruses)
LVV	Liverpool vervet (green monkey) virus
M	Molar (solution)
MA	Microscopic agglutination (test) (e.g. for *Leptospira*)
MaC	MacConkey's (agar)
MAP	Mouse antibody production (test)
MCF	Malignant catarrhal fever
MD	Marek's disease; also used for Mucosal disease
MDBK	Madin-Darby bovine kidney (cell line)
ME	Micrencephaly
MEM	Minimum essential medium (Eagle's solution of nutrients and salts)
MGG	May-Grünwald-Giemsa (stain)
MI	Metabolic inhibition (test)
MK	Monkey kidney (cells)
MLD	Minimum lethal dose (titer)
MLV	Modified live virus (vaccine)
MP	Mouse protection (test)
MR	Methyl red (reaction or medium)
MRD	Measles, rinderpest, distemper (group of viruses)
MR-VP	Methyl red–Voges-Proskauer (medium or test)
MS	Monkey stable (kidney cell lines)
MuLV	Murine leukemia virus
MVC	Minute virus of canines (parvovirus)
MVEV	Murray Valley encephalitis virus
MVM	Minute virus of mice (parvovirus)
N	Normal (solution); also used sometimes for Negative (result)
NAD	Nicotinamide adenine dinucleotide (precursor of the V-factor)
NADC	National Animal Disease Center (USDA), Ames, Iowa
NAS	National Academy of Sciences, Washington
NCI	National Cancer Institute, Bethesda, Md.
ND	Newcastle disease
Neg.	Negative
NF	Nonfermentative (bacteria)
NI	Neutralization index (VN test result)
NIAID	National Institute of Allergy and Infectious Diseases, Bethesda, Md.
NIH	National Institutes of Health, Bethesda, Md.
NMB	Normal mouse brain
NP	Nonproducer (cells, test); also used for Nucleoprotein (antigen found in poxviruses)
NPV	Neethling poxvirus (lumpy skin disease)

Abbreviations

NRC	National Research Council (NAS), Washington
NT	Not tested
OCG	Oxalate (potassium), carbolic acid, and glycerol (anticoagulant, preservative)
OCT	Optimum cutting temperature (compound, trade name)
OF	Oxidation-fermentation (medium)
OFBM	Oxidation-fermentation basal medium
OID	Ovine interdigital dermatitis
ONPG	Ortho-nitrophenyl-beta-d-galactopyranoside (reaction or medium)
OP	Oesophageal-pharyngeal (fluid)
OPG	OCG using the name phenol instead of carbolic acid
P-51	Parker-51 (superchrome blue-black ink used as a stain)
PAGMK	Primary African green monkey kidney (cells)
PAS	Periodic acid–Schiff (stain)
PAS-CB	Periodic acid–Schiff—celestin blue (stain)
PBS	Phosphate-buffered saline (solution)
PD_{50}	Protective dose 50% (titer)
Pen. Sen.	Penicillin sensitive
PEV	Porcine enterovirus
PF	Potentiating factor
PHV	Pigeon herpesvirus
PI-3	Parainfluenza-3
PIADC	Plum Island Animal Disease Center (USDA), Greenport, N.Y.
PK-15	Porcine kidney–15 (cell line)
PL	Psittacosis-lymphogranuloma (group of *Chlamydia*)
PM	Phenotypic mixing (test)
Pos.	Positive
PPLO	Pleuropneumonia-like organism (*Mycoplasma*)
PPR	Peste des petits ruminants (viral disease of goats and sheep)
PPV	Porcine parvovirus
PR	Plaque reduction (test)
PRAS	Prereduced anaerobically sterilized (medium with an Eh of minus 150 millivolts or lower)
PRK	Primary rabbit kidney (cells)
PrV	Pseudorabies virus
P & S	Penicillin and streptomycin (inhibitor, antibiotic solution)
PV	Panton-Valentine (leukocidin *Staphlococcus* test)
PVA	Polyvinyl alcohol (fixative)
PVB	Paramyxovirus Bangor (isolated from a finch in N. Ireland)
PVT	Paramyxovirus turkeys (isolated from turkeys in Ontario and Wisconsin)
PVY	Paramyxovirus Yucaipa (isolated from chickens in California)
Q fever	Query (not Queensland) fever (a febrile rickettsial infection)
QS	Quantum satis, quantity sufficient (to make a given volume)
RAP	Rat antibody production (test)
RBC	Red blood cells
RCF	Relative centrifugal force (equal to $11.1 \times RN^2$, where R is radius, N is thousands of revolutions per minute)
RDE	Receptor-destroying enzyme (from *V. cholerae*)
RECC	Rat embryo cell cultures

Reo	Respiratory-enteric-orphan (reovirus)
R_f	Rate front (movement of band, i.e. *rate*, divided by movement of advancing *front*) (used with TLC)
RIF	Resistance-inducing factor (to neoplastic transformation) (test)
RIP	Radioisotope precipitation (test)
RK	Rabbit kidney (cells or cell line)
R & M	Reed and Muench (method for calculating 50% endpoints, titer)
RMB	Rabies mouse brain (suspension)
RNA	Ribonucleic acid
RNase	Ribonuclease (enzyme that digests RNA)
RNP	Ribonucleoprotein (soluble antigen)
RSV	Rous sarcoma virus
RTD	Routine test dilution
RU	Rubella (German measles virus)
RV	Rinderpest virus; also used for Rat virus
RVF	Rift Valley fever
S	Svedberg (units, sedimentation coefficient of particles)
SA4	Simian *aethiops* (monkey virus) (viruses are numbered SA4 to SA8)
SA-CV	Sodium azide–crystal violet (agar, usually blood)
SAT	Southern African Territories (3 types of FMDV)
SC	Subcutaneous (route)
SCMV	Swine cytomegalovirus
SEK	Swine embryo kidney (cells)
Ser.	Serum
SFFV	Spleen focus-forming virus
SK	Swine kidney (cells)
S-K	Spearman-Kärber (method for calculating 50% endpoints, titer)
SMEDI	Stillbirth, mummification, embryonic death, and infertility (porcine enterovirus group classification)
SMSV	San Miguel sea lion virus
SMV	Spider monkey virus
SN_{50}	Serum neutralization 50% (titer)
SPA	Sheep pulmonary adenomatosis (Jaagsiekte)
SPF	Specific pathogen–free (animals)
SS	*Salmonella-Shigella* (agar)
SV40	Simian virus (isolates are numbered SV2 to SV49)
SVD	Swine vesicular disease
Tb	Tbilisi (strain of *B. abortus* bacteriophage)
TC	Tissue culture
$TCID_{50}$	Tissue culture infecting dose 50% (titer)
TGE	Transmissible gastroenteritis (of swine)
TLC	Thin-layer chromatograms
TME	Transmissible mink encephalopathy
TRBC	Total red blood cells (count)
TSA	Trypticase-soy agar
TSB	Trypticase-soy broth
TSI	Triple sugar iron (agar)
TWBC	Total white blood cells (count)

Abbreviations

USDA	United States Department of Agriculture, Washington
UV	Ultraviolet (radiation)
VEE	Venezuelan equine encephalomyelitis
Vero	African green monkey kidney cell line
VES	Vesicular exanthema of swine
VIA	Virus infection–associated (antigen, test) (for FMD)
VN	Virus neutralization (test)
VN_{50}	Virus neutralization 50% (titer)
VP	Voges-Proskauer (reaction or medium)
VPI	Virginia Polytechnic Institute (manual), Blacksburg, Va.
VR	Virus repository (precedes numbers for ATCC viral listings)
VRB	Violet red bile (agar)
VS	Vesicular stomatitis
V/V	Volume/volume
WBC	White blood cells
WD	Wesselsbron disease (viral infection)
WEE	Western equine encephalomyelitis
WHO	World Health Organization (United Nations), Geneva
WM1	Wild mouse no. 1 (murine leukemia virus)
W/V	Weight/volume
XC	Experimental code (newborn rat uterine sarcoma cell line originally induced by benzpyrene and inoculation of chicken Rous sarcoma cells; the cell line continues to carry the RSV-C genome) (communication from Dr. Jan Svoboda, Prague)
XL	Xylose lysine (agar)
XLBG	Xylose lysine brilliant green (agar)
XLD	Xylose lysine deoxycholate (agar)
YCB	Yeast carbon base (solution for mycology)
YNB	Yeast nitrogen base (solution for mycology)
YS	Yolk sac (route)
Z-N	Ziehl-Neelsen (staining technique)

Index of Scientific Names

Absidia sp., 639, 642, 644, 645
  corymbifera, 640
  ramosa, 640
Acholeplasma sp., 472
  granularum, 475, 477
  laidlawii, 475, 477
Achorion gypseum, 621
Achromobacter sp., 368, 371, 377
  lwoffii, 371
Acinetobacter sp.; 371
Actinobacillus sp., 411, 452-460, 682
  actinoides, 452, 457, 458
  actinomycetemcomitans, 452, 456, 457
  equuli, 452, 455, 560
  lignieresi, 452-455, 460
  seminis, 452, 458-459
Actinomyces sp., 545, 553-558, 563, 565
  bovis, 452, 553, 555-557
  israeli, 456, 553, 555-557
  viscosus, 553, 555-557
Aedes sp., 309
  aegypti, 193, 196
Aedex vexans, 326
Aegyptionella pullorum, 502
Ajellomyces dermatitidis, 588
Alcaligenes fecalis, 368, 377, 406
Allescheria boydii, 655, 656
Allodermanyssus sanguineus, 567
Amblyomma sp., 567, 572
Anaplasma marginale, 451
Aotus trivirgatus, 166, 271
Argas persicus, 502, 503
Arizona sp., 349-351, 358-366
  hinshawii, 359
Arthroderma benhamiae, 610, 624
Arvicanthus sp., 325
Ascaris suum, 475
Aspergillus sp., 583-587, 655, 665
  flavus, 586, 659, 660, 662, 665, 668

  fumigatus, 585-587, 665
  nidulans, 585, 665, 668
  ochraceus, 660, 666
  parasiticus, 659, 660, 662
  rugulosus, 665, 668
  versicolor, 665, 668
Ateles geoffroyi, 160
Aviadenovirus sp., 112
Avipoxvirus sp., 284, 285

Babesia canis, 574, 576, 577
Bacillus sp., 437-444
  anthracis, 437-444
  brevis, 440
  cereus, 437, 439-442, 530
  circulans, 440
  licheniformis, 440
  megaterium, 440-442
  mycoides, 440
  pumilus, 440
  sphaericus, 440
  subtilis, 437, 440, 679
Bacterium anitratum, 368, 377, 491
Bacteroides
  clostridiiformis, 531
  fragilis, 530, 531
  hypermegas, 531
  melaninogenicus, 530, 545
  nodosus, 527-529
Basidiobolus sp., 639, 645, 647
  haptosporus, 645, 647
  ranarum, 645
Bipolaris sp., 665, 668
Blastomyces dermatitidis, 588-592, 606, 637, 676, 682
Boopholus
  annulata, 506
  decoloratus, 506
  microplus, 506

Index of Scientific Names

Bordetella sp., 368, 404-407
  bronchicanis, 368, 377
  bronchiseptica, 368, 404-407
  parapertussis, 404, 406
  pertussis, 404, 406
Borrelia sp., 502-508, 686, 700
  anserina, 502, 503, 505, 507
  hyos, 502, 506
  penortha, 507
  suilla, 502, 506, 507
  theileri, 502, 505, 506
Bos
  indicus, 226
  taurus, 226
Brucella sp., 395-403, 406, 698
  abortus, 98, 395-402, 456
    strains 19 and 544, 401
  canis, 395, 396, 398-400, 402
  melitensis, 395-398, 400, 402
  neotomae, 400
  ovis, 395-400, 458
  suis, 395, 398, 400, 402

Calonectria sp., 663, 665
Campylobacter sp., 461-471, 680, 696
  fetus
    subsp. *fetus*, 461-467
    subsp. *intestinalis*, 462, 465, 466
    subsp. *jejuni*, 462, 463
  fecalis, 465, 466
  sputorum, 466, 467
Candida sp., 593-597, 672, 676
  albicans, 593, 595-597
  guilliermondii, 593, 595, 596
  krusei, 593, 595, 596
  parapsilosis, 593, 595, 596
  pseudotropicalis, 593, 595, 596
  stellatoidea, 593, 595, 596
  tropicalis, 593, 595, 596
Capripoxvirus sp., 282-284, 290
Carrasius auratus, 156
Cephalosporium sp., 663, 665
Cercopithecus sp., 159, 207, 292, 297
  aethiops, 165, 261
Chlamydia sp., 485-493, 696
  psittaci, 485, 486, 488-492
  trachomatis, 485, 489, 490
Citrobacter sp., 349-351, 679
  freundii, 365
Cladosporium sp., 658
Claviceps
  paspali, 660
  purpurea, 660, 668
Clostridium sp., 99, 509-525
  bifermentans, 509, 523, 524
  botulinum, 509, 514, 521-523
  chauvoei, 509, 510, 512, 513, 520
  hemolyticum, 509-518, 524
  novyi, 509-518, 524
  perfringens, 69, 509, 510, 517-519, 549
  septicum, 509, 510, 513, 519, 520
  sordellii, 509, 510, 517, 523-525
  sporogenes, 514
  tetani, 509
Coccidioides sp., 639
  immitis, 94, 453, 591, 598-604, 639
Colesiota conjunctivae, 571, 572, 577
Comamonas terrigena, 368, 377
Connochaetes
  gnu, 139
  taurinus, 139
Corynebacterium sp., 426, 487, 544-552, 700
  acnes, 555-557
  bovis, 544
  equi, 544, 548-552
  minutissimum, 544
  pseudotuberculosis, 544, 547-549, 551
  pyogenes, 393, 507, 527, 530, 544-547, 551, 555-557
  renale, 549-551
  suis, 544
Cowdria ruminantium, 571-574
Coxiella burneti, 566-571
Cricetus aureatus, 232
Cryptococcus sp., 595, 605-609, 686, 698
  diffluens, 672
  neoformans, 591, 596, 605-609, 672
Culex sp., 193, 309, 503
  tritaeniorhynchus, 326
Culicoides sp., 187, 193
  brevitarsis, 326, 328
  pallidipennis, 187
  variipennis, 187, 197
Curvularia geniculata, 655, 656

Damaliscus
  albifrons, 192
  korrigum, 139
Dendrochium sp., 663, 665
Dermacenter sp., 567
Dermatophilus congolensis, 559-561

Edwardsiella sp., 349
  tarda, 350, 351, 365
Ehrlichia
  bovis, 572, 576
  canis, 572, 576, 577
  ovina, 572, 576
  phagocytophila, 571, 572, 575, 576
Elaphurus davidianus, 139
Emericella sp., 585
Enterobacter sp., 349, 361, 679
  aerogenes, 350, 362, 367
  cloache, 350, 367
  hafnia, 350, 351, 365, 367
  liquefaciens, 350, 367
Entomophthora coronata, 640, 645, 646
Eperythrozoon coccoides, 451

Index of Scientific Names

Epidermophyton sp., 614
Erysipelothrix sp., 314, 429-436
  insidiosa, 393, 426
  rhusiopathiae, 429-436
Erythrocebus patas, 158, 204
Escherichia coli, 26, 349-357, 361, 362, 420, 487, 545, 677
  serologic classification, 356
  A-D group, 354
Eubacterium tortuosum, 531
Eurotium nidulans, 585

Fonsecaea sp., 658
Francisella sp., 413-424
  novicida, 422, 423
  tularensis, 413, 415, 422, 423
Fusarium sp., 663-665
  moniliforme, 660, 662, 664
  oxysporum, 660, 662
  raseum, 660, 662
  tricinctum, 660, 662
Fusiformis
  necrophorus, 507, 527
  nodosus, 507
Fusobacterium
  funduliformis, 529
  necrophorum, 527-530

Galleria melonella, 232
Gallus domesticus, 704
Gazella thompsonii, 139
Geotrichum candidum, 595, 601, 631, 632
Gibberella zeae, 669
Goniobasis plicifera silicula, 578
Guizotia abyssinica, 686

Haemaphsalis sp., 567
Haemobartonella sp., 449-451
  bovis, 449
  canis, 449
  felis, 449-451
  muris, 449
Haemophilus sp., 393, 408-412, 546, 695
  aegyptius, 410
  agni, 411
  aphrophilus, 410
  citreus, 410
  ducreyi, 410
  gallinarum, 410, 411
  hemoglobinophilus, 410
  hemolyticus, 410
  influenzae, 410, 411
  ovis, 410
  paragallinarum, 409, 410
  parahaemolyticus, 410, 411
  parinfluenzae, 410
  paraphrophilus, 410
  parasuis, 409, 410, 411
  piscium, 410
  putoriorum, 410
  somnus, 411
  suis, 409, 410
Helminthosporium spiciferum, 655, 656
Herellea sp., 368
  vaginicola, 368, 377
Herpesvirus sp., 126-166
Histoplasma sp., 590, 591, 633
  capsulatum, 94, 95, 591, 606, 633-638
  duboisii, 633, 634
  farciminosum, 633, 634, 636
Harmodendrum sp., 658
Hyalomma sp., 567, 572
Hydromys chrysogaster, 268, 271
Hylobates lar, 165, 166
Hyphomyces destruens, 640, 642, 644, 646
Hypocrea sp., 663, 665

Ictalurus
  nebulasus, 156
  punctatus, 157
Isoodon macrourus, 268
Ixodes sp., 567, 572

Klebsiella sp., 348-351, 353, 361, 677
  ozaenae, 367
  pneumonia, 367
  rhinoscleromatis, 367

Lactobacillus acidophilus, 26
Lepomis
  macrochiris, 156
  microlopis, 156
Leporipoxvirus sp., 285-289
Leptospira sp., 96, 101, 494-501, 504, 680
  australia, 498, 500
  autumnalis, 498, 499
  ballum, 498
  bataviae, 498, 499
  borincana, 499
  bratislava, 499
  butembo, 499
  canicola, 498, 499
  grippotyphosa, 498, 499, 500
  hebdomadis, 498
  icterohaemorrhagiae, 498, 499
  javanica, 499
  patoc, 499
  pomona, 498, 500
  pyrogenes, 498, 499
  tarassovi (*hyos*), 498, 499
  wolffi, 499
Leptotrombidium sp., 567
Lepus
  europaeus, 287
  timidus, 287
Listeria monocytogenes, 393, 425-428
Lyssavirus sp., 301

Macaca sp., 261, 289, 292, 293, 297
  cyclopsis, 159
  fuscata, 159
  irus, 159, 261
  mulatta (*rhesus*), 159, 208, 261, 640
Mandrillus sphinx, 640
Margaropus decoloratus, 506
Mastadenovirus sp., 112
Melomys lutillus littoralis, 268
Metastrongylus sp., 475
Microsporum sp., 614, 690
  amazonicum, 621
  audouinii, 617, 690
  boullardii, 621
  canis, 610, 612, 614-617, 619-622
  cookei, 623
  distortum, 617, 621
  equinum, 617
  fulvum, 610, 617, 622
  gallinae, 610, 612, 621, 622, 675
  gypseum, 610, 617-622
  nanum, 610, 621, 622
  praecox, 621
  racemosum, 621
  ripariae, 621
Microtus sp., 567
Mima sp., 368, 372, 377
  duplex, 371
  polymorpha, 368, 371, 377
Monosporium apiospermum, 656
Moraxella sp., 368, 377, 445-448
  bovis, 445-448
  duplex, 372
  lacunata, 445
  liquefaciens, 445, 447
Morone saxatilis, 156
Mortierella sp., 639, 640, 642-645
  hygrophila, 640
  polycephala, 640
  wolfii, 640, 642
  zychae, 640
Mucor sp., 639, 640, 642-645
Mus sp., 567
  booduga, 268, 271
Mycobacterium sp., 98, 537-543, 562, 591
  avium, 537, 540, 541, 543
  bovis, 537, 540, 541, 543
  fortuitum, 537, 564
  gordonae, 537
  intracellulare, 537, 540, 541
  leprae, 537
  marinum, 537
  paratuberculosis, 537, 539, 541-543, 682
  phlei, 537, 542, 678
  rodochrous, 564
  scrofulaceum, 537, 540, 541
  tuberculosis, 537, 540, 541, 543
  ulcerans, 537
  xenopi, 537

Mycoplasma sp., 47, 229, 472-484, 487, 685, 686
  agalactiae, 472-474, 477
  arginini, 474, 477
  arthritidis, 476, 477
  bovigenitalium, 473, 477
  bovimastitidis, 473, 477
  bovirhinis, 473, 477
  gallisepticum, 472, 476, 477, 483
  hyoarginini, 474
  hyopneumoniae, 474, 686
  hyorhinis, 474, 479
  hyosynoviae, 474, 479, 686
  meleagridis, 476, 477, 480, 686
  mycoides
    subsp. *mycoides*, 472, 473, 477, 480, 483, 686
    subsp. *capri*, 474, 477
  neurolyticum, 475, 483
  pneumoniae, 477, 685
  pulmonis, 475-477
  suidaniae, 474
  synoviae, 476, 477
  T-strain organisms, 472, 473, 481
Myrmecophaga tridactyla, 277
Myrothecium sp., 663, 665

Nannizzia sp., 610, 617
  fulva, 610, 619, 621
  gypsea, 610, 617, 619, 621
  incurvata, 610, 617, 619, 621
  obtusa, 610, 622
Nanophyetes salmincola, 572, 578
Neisseria sp., 371
Neorickettsia helminthoeca, 571, 572
Nocardia sp., 562-565, 591, 693
  asteroides, 562-565
  brasiliensis, 562, 564, 565
  caviae, 562, 564, 565

Odocoileus virginianus, 197, 211
Ondatra zibetica, 24
Ornithodorus sp., 502
Orthopoxvirus sp., 276-278
Oryctolagus cuniculus, 155, 156, 287

Papio doguera, 261, 263
Paracoccidioides brasiliensis, 591
Paracolobactrum sp., 349, 350, 359
Parapoxvirus sp., 278-282
Pasteurella sp., 215, 229, 314, 413-424, 487, 545
  anatipestifer, 413, 415, 418, 419
  gallinarum, 413, 415, 418
  hemolytica, 213, 413, 415-417
  multocida, 213, 413-418, 420, 475
  pestis, 419
  pneumotropica, 413, 415, 417, 418
  pseudotuberculosis, 421
  septica, 413
  suis, 507

Index of Scientific Names

Pasteurella sp. *(cont.)*
 tularensis, 422
 ureae, 416
Pectobacterium sp., 349, 350
Pediculus humanus, 566, 567
Penicillium sp., 655, 664, 665
 citrinum, 665
 purpurogenum, 665
 rubrum, 665
 viridicatum, 660, 666
Pestivirus sp., 311, 318
Phialophora sp., 658
Phycomycetes sp., 95
Pithomyces chartarum, 660, 666, 667
Propionibacterium acnes, 531
Proteus sp., 349, 353, 361, 390, 487
 mirabilis, 350, 362
 morganii, 350, 362
 rettgeri, 350, 362
 vulgaris, 350, 362, 491
Prototheca
 ciferri, 649
 portoricensis, 649
 segbwema, 649
 wickerhamii, 649
 zopfii, 649
Providencia sp., 349-351
 alcalifaciens, 350, 362
 stuartii, 350, 362
Pseudomonas sp., 353, 373-379
 acidovorans, 373-376
 aeruginosa, 373-378
 alcaligenes, 368, 374-377
 cepacia, 373, 374, 376
 diminutia, 373, 374, 376, 377, 672
 florescens, 373, 375, 376, 378
 mallei, 373-376, 378
 maltophilia, 373, 374, 376, 377, 672
 multivorans, 374
 pseudoalcaligenes, 373-376
 pseudomallei, 373-376, 378
 putida, 373, 375, 376
 putrefaciens, 373, 374, 376, 377
 stutzeri, 373, 374, 376, 377
Pythium sp., 640, 644

Rattus sp., 268, 567
 alexandrinus, 268
 natalensis (Mastomys), 232
 norvegicus, 268, 567
Rhinosporidium seeberi, 639
Rhipicephalus
 bursa, 572
 evertsi, 506
 sanguineus, 572, 576
Rhizoctonia leguminicola, 660, 667
Rhizopus sp., 639, 640, 642, 644, 645
Rhodotorula sp., 607

Rickettsia sp., 96, 566-582, 696, 699
 akari, 567, 568
 australis, 567
 conori, 567
 prowazeki, 566-568
 rickettsi, 567
 siberica, 567
 tsutsugamushi, 567, 696, 699
 typhi, 567, 568
Rochalimaea quintana, 566, 567

Saimiri sciureus, 159, 160, 165
Salmonella sp., 47, 314, 349-351, 353, 358-366, 673, 674, 680, 683, 690-692
 arizona, 359
 choleraesuis, 360, 364
 gallinarum, 359, 360, 363, 364, 369
 paratyphi, 363
 pullorum, 360, 363, 369
 typhimurium, 360, 369, 370
 typhisuis, 351, 361, 363, 364
Sarotorya sp., 585
Sciurus carolinses, 288
Sepedonium sp., 636
Serratia sp., 349-351, 367
Setonix brachyurus, 298
Shigella sp., 349-351, 354, 357, 358, 363, 680, 690
 flexneri, 351
Sphaerophorus necrophorus, 507, 527, 529, 545
Spirocheta penortha, 507
Sporotrichum schenckii, 651-653
Stachybotrys atra, 664
Staphylococcus sp., 380-388, 487, 547, 688
 aureus, 380-386, 393, 409, 453, 549
 epidermis, 380-385
Streptococcus sp., 389-394, 487
 agalactiae, 390-393
 canis, 392
 dysgalactiae, 390, 392, 393
 equi, 390, 392
 equinus, 389, 392
 equisimilis, 389, 392, 393
 faecalis, 389, 392, 409
 lactis, 389, 392
 liquefaciens, 531
 pyogenes, 389, 391, 392, 394
 suis, 390, 392
 uberis, 390-393
 zooepidemicus, 389, 392
Streptomyces sp., 562, 564, 565
Sylvilagus
 braziliensis, 287
 floridanus, 155

Taeniorrhynchus fuscopennatus, 269
Taurotragus oryx, 139
Treponema sp., 504

Trichoderma sp., 663, 665
Trichomonas fetus, 463
Trichophyton sp., 624, 627
  ajelloi, 624, 628
  equinum, 612, 619, 624, 626, 675
  erinacei, 623, 624, 628
  gallinae, 622, 623
  megninii, 622, 675
  mentagrophytes, 612, 619, 623, 624
  rubrum, 624
  simii, 624
  terrestre, 624, 628
  verrucosum, 616, 619, 624, 627, 628, 674, 675, 689
Trichosporon sp., 595
  cutaneum, 654
Trichothecium sp., 663, 665

Vesiculovirus sp., 299
Vibrio sp., 461-471, 680, 696
  alcaligenes, 368
  alginolyticus, 467-469
  anguillarum, 467-469
  cholerae (*comma*), 69, 71, 468
  coli, 463, 467
  fetus, 461 (genus changed to *Campylobacter*)
  parahaemolyticus, 461, 467-469
  percolans, 368

Xenopsylla cheopis, 567

Yersinia sp., 413-424
  enterocolitica, 421
  pestis, 413, 415, 419-421
  pseudotuberculosis, 413, 415, 420, 422, 690, 694

General Index

Abortion
  Akabane viral, 326, 329
  arizonal, 359
  bovine mycotic, 583
  brucellar, 395
  chlamydial, 486
  corynebacterial, 545
  enzootic ovine, 486
  epizootic bovine, 486
  equine arteritis viral, 321
  hog cholera viral, 311, 312
  klebsiellar, 366
  leptospiral, 495
  listerial, 425
  mucosal disease (BVD-MD) viral, 318, 319
  mycoplasmal, 473
  panleukopenia viral, 236
  parvoviral, 241
  phycomycosal, 640
  porcine enteroviral, 255
  pseudomonal, 373
  rhinopneumonitis viral, 129
  Rift Valley fever viral, 325
  vibrial, 461-464
  Wesselsbron disease viral, 310
Abscesses, 373, 380, 389, 408, 452, 526, 553, 554, 563
Acid-fast
  bacilli, 541, 542, 564, 565
  stain, 701
Acridine orange staining, 103
Acriflavin test, 398
Actinobacillosis, 452
Actinomycosis, 452, 453, 456, 553-558
Actinomycotic mycetoma, 655
Adeno-associated viruses, 231, 244-247
Adenoviruses, 69, 70, 112-118, 245
Aflatoxicosis, 659-662
African horsesickness, 26, 192-196

African swine fever, 26, 69, 311, 330-333
Agar diffusion slides, 434, 435
Agar overlay, cell cultures, 56, 57
Air filter tests, 28, 679, 680
AK virus, 269
Akabane virus, 326-329
Alastrim, 273-277
Allantoic cavity, inoculation, 48
Allantoic fluid harvest, 51
Allerton herpesvirus, 143, 283
Alpaca, brucellosis, 396
Alphaviruses, 309
Alpine goat, chamois papilloma, 205, 207
Amnionic fluid harvest, 51
Amnionic route, 48
Anaerobes, chromatographic identification, 533
Anaerobic atmosphere, techniques, 512, 532, 554, 555
Anaplasmosis, 505, 506
Animal diseases transmissible to humans, 24, 25
Antelope: bluetongue, 188; vibrial reservoir, 462
Anthrax, 24, 193, 225, 437-444, 517
Antibiograms, 385
Antibiotic treatment of specimens, 38, 44, 485, 487
Antibiotics, cell cultures, 54, 55, 58
Anticoagulant solutions, 671, 678, 682, 687
Antigens O, K, and H explained, 354-356, 466, 469
Aquariums, erysipelas, 429
Arboviruses, 70
Arthritis, 374, 395, 408, 430, 455, 474, 476, 488, 545
Arthropod-transmitted diseases, 187, 193, 196, 197, 299, 307, 309, 325, 326, 330, 333, 338, 419, 422, 502, 506, 559, 566-582
Arthus-type ocular hypersensitivity, 114
Arvicanthus, Rift Valley fever reservoir, 325
Ataxia, feline, 236
Atomic blast deaths, 455
Atrophic rhinitis, 404

Aujeszky's disease, 131
Australian T virus, 120
Autoclave sterilization, 98
Auxanogram, 608, 672
Avian, *see also* Chicken
  adenovirus (CELO), 47, 112
  airsacculitis, 352, 476, 485, 488, 583
  aspergillosis, 853
  coryza, 408
  encephalomyelitis, 47, 248
  enteroviruses, 248
  erythroblastosis, 168
  hemangioma, 168
  infectious bronchitis, 69, 119-123, 147
  infectious laryngotracheitis, 146-148
  influenza viruses (fowl plague), 201
  leukosis, 47, 167-176, 340
  mycoplasmosis, 47, 476, 477
  myeloblastosis, 168
  nephroblastoma, 168
  ophthalmia, contagious, 577, 578
  osteopetrosis, 168
  phycomycosis, 640
  pox subgroup, 284, 285
  sarcoma, Rous, 168, 174
  tuberculosis, 537, 541

Babesiosis, 505, 506, 576
Baboon: encephalomyocarditis, 268; enteroviruses, 261
Bacillary hemoglobinuria, 514
Bacterin-toxoid for milk vaccination, 519, 522
Bacteriophage
  Bacillus, 443
  Bordetella, 406
  Brucella tbilisi, 401
  Erysipelothrix rhusiopathiae, 435
  Escherichia coli, 357
  Listeria, 427
  Pseudomonas, 378
  Staphylococcus, 385
  Vibrio, 469
Badger, distemper, 221
Balanced salt solutions compared, 681
Barbary sheep, bluetongue, 188
Bassariscus, distemper, 221
Bat: histoplasmosis, 634; vampire, rabies reservoir, 301
Beagle breed of dogs, brucellosis, 395
Beaudette virus, 122
Bermudagrass poisoning, 669
Besnoitia protozoan infection, 26
Bighorn sheep, bluetongue, 187
Binturong, distemper, 221
Biologic inactivation, 101
Bison, brucellosis, 396
Black death, 419
Black scours, 463
Blackleg, 520

Blackpatch, disease of legumes, 667
Blastomycosis, 588
Blesbuck, bluetongue and heartwater carrier, 192
Blood agar technique, 381
Blue pus, 375
Bluetongue, 187-192, 196-198, 327, 328
Bollinger bodies, 285
Borna disease, 26, 338-339
Botryomycosis, 453
Botulism, 521-523
Boutonneuse fever, 25
Bovine, *see also* Cattle
  adenoviruses, 112, 113
  benign rickettsiosis, 572, 576
  contagious ophthalmia, 572, 577, 578
  enteroviruses, 258, 259
  ephemeral fever, 307, 308
  genital vibriosis, 461
  herpes mammillitis, 142, 143
  infectious keratoconjunctivitis, 445
  infectious petechial fever, 26
  lumpy skin disease, 274, 283
  mycotic abortion, 583
  papilloma, 205, 206
  papular stomatitis, 24, 274, 278-280
  parvovirus, 232, 243, 244
  pleuropneumonia, 26, 472-474, 477
  pseudopox, 274, 281
  shipping fever, 212
  vibriosis, 461
  viral diarrhea–mucosal disease, 44, 225, 314, 315, 318-321
Boxer breed of dogs, coccidioidomycosis, 598
Brilliant green dye toxicity, 369
Bromodeoxyuridine, DNA inhibitor, 102, 103, 273
Bronchopneumonia, 457
Brucellosis, 24, 395-403
Bubonic plague, 419
Budgerigar, Marek's disease, 143
Buffalo
  brucellosis, 396
  Jembrana, 581
  malignant catarrhal fever, 139
  parainfluenza, 212, 213
  pasteurellosis, 413
  rinderpest, 226
Buffer solutions, 62, 63, 87, 90, 681, 687, 689
Buffett murine leukemia virus, 177
Buffy-coat cell cultures, 331, 335, 336
Bush pig, African swine fever carriers, 331
Buss disease, 486
Busse-Buschke's disease, 605
Butter, putrid deterioration, 374
Buzzard, phycomycosis, 640
B-virus of macaques, 24, 159-165

Calf diphtheria, 530
Caliciviruses, 248
California encephalitis, 25

General Index

Camelpox, 26
Camel: brucellosis, 396; rinderpest, 226
Canary: Marek's disease, 143; pseudotuberculosis, 421
Canarypox, 274, 284
Candidiasis, 593
Canine, *see also* Dog
  adenovirus, infectious hepatitis, 114, 115
  blastomycosis, 588, 603, 637
  brucellosis, 395, 400
  coccidioidomycosis, 599, 603
  distemper, 212, 219-225
  ehrlichiosis, 571, 572, 576, 577
  herpesvirus, 134-136
  histoplasmosis, 637
  laryngotracheitis, 114
  nocardiosis, pulmonary, 562
  papilloma, 205, 206
  parvovirus, 232
Capripoxviruses, 282, 283
Capsules, bacterial, 442, 698
Carbon dioxide incubation, cell cultures, 55, 56
Carcinogenesis, 659, 665
Cardiovirus group, 270
Carnivore: canine distemper, 221; rabies, 301
Carr Zilber virus, 169
Cat, *see also* Feline
  blastomycosis, 588
  bordetellosis, turbinate atrophy, 404
  candidiasis, moniliasis, 593
  chlamydial conjuctivitis, 486
  corynebacterial abscesses, 544
  cryptococcosis, 605
  geotrichosis, 631
  haemobartonellosis anemia, 449
  melioidosis, 374
  mycoplasmosis, 477
  pseudorabies, 131
  ringworm, 610
  salmonellosis, 758
Cat bite pasteurellosis, 413
Cat scratch disease, 25
Cat use for enterotoxin detection, 384
Catalase reaction technique, 555
Catfish herpesvirus, channel, 156-158
Cationic stabilization, 105
Cattle, *see also* Abortion, Bovine, *and* Mastitis
  actinobacillosis, 452
  actinomycosis, 553
  aflatoxicosis, 659
  Akabane, 326-329
  anaplasmosis, 505
  anthrax, 437
  babesiosis, 505
  bacillary hemoglobinuria, 514
  Bermudagrass poisoning, 669
  blackleg, 520
  bluetongue, 187-191
  brucellosis, 395
  Buss disease, 486
  calf diphtheria, 530
  candidiasis, 593
  chlamydial infections, 486
  coccidioidomycosis, 598, 604
  corynebacterial infections, 544
  cowpox, 24, 273-277
  ergotism, 668
  facial eczema, 666, 667
  fescue foot, 669
  foot-and-mouth disease, 24-26, 225, 248-253, 263, 269, 299
  footrot, 530
  haemobartonellosis, 449
  heartwater, 26, 571, 572
  hemorrhagic septicemia, 413
  Ibaraki disease, 196, 197
  infectious bovine rhinotracheitis, 127-129
  Jembrana disease, 581, 582
  joint ill, 455
  listeriosis, 425
  liver abscesses, 530
  lumpy jaw, 553
  malignant catarrhal fever, 138-142
  mucosal disease–bovine viral diarrhea, 318-321
  mycoplasmal infections, 472-474
  navel ill, 530
  parainfluenza, 212-216
  paratuberculosis, 539
  paspalum staggers, 660
  pasture fever, 572
  phycomycosis, 640
  pseudorabies, 131
  pustular vulvovaginitis, 127
  Q fever, 566-571
  Rift Valley fever, 325, 326
  rinderpest, 225-228
  ringworm, 610
  salmonellosis, 359
  seminal vesiculitis, 473
  theileriosis (spirochetosis), 26, 505
  tick-borne fever, 571, 572
  tuberculosis, 538
  vesicular stomatitis, 249, 299-301
  Wesselsbron disease, 24, 26, 310, 311
  winter dysentery, 462
Ceiling temperature, 275
Cell cultures, techniques, 52-59, 293
Cells in suspension, 53, 57
CELO, avian adenovirus, 112
Central European encephalitis, 24
Centrifugation techniques, 44, 45, 110
Cerebellar hypoplasia, 234
Chamois papilloma, 205-207
Chemical inactivation, 99-101
Chicken, *see also* Avian
  botulism, 521
  candidiasis, moniliasis, 593
  cholera, fowl, 413

Chicken (cont.)
  coli granuloma, 352
  diphtheria, fowl, 285
  favus, 622
  fowlpox, 25, 274, 284, 285
  GAL viruses, 112
  Marek's disease, neural lymphomatosis, 143-146
  Newcastle disease, 147, 212, 216-219
  N-virus infection, 200
  ornithosis, 486
  Ote adenovirus, 112
  plague, fowl, 26, 200
  pullorum disease, 359
  ringworm, 610
  roup, 285
  spirochetosis, 502
  synovitis, infectious, 476
  thrush, 593
  trichothecene toxicosis, 663
  typhoid, fowl, 359
  Yucaipa, 212
Chicken pox (human), 24
Chimpanzee
  adenovirus, 112, 116
  chicken pox, 24
  encephalomyocarditis, 268
  enteroviruses, 260
  molluscum contagiosum, 289
Chinchilla
  pseudomonal enteritis, 373
  pseudotuberculosis, 421
  ringworm, 623
Chinese letter patterns, pseudotuberculosis, 549
Chipmunk, sylvatic plague, 419
Chlamydial
  antiserum nonspecific test, 491
  infections, 486
  stain, 487
Chloramphenicol (Chloromycetin), 590
Chloroform sensitivity, 104
Chorioallantoic
  membrane harvest, 52
  route, 49
Chromatography, 103, 104, 661, 662, 669
Chromomycosis, 657
Classification of pathogens, human risk, 24-26
Clostridial infections, 509
Cloven-hooved animals, foot-and-mouth disease, 248-253
Coagulase reaction, 382
Coati-mundi: distemper, 221; feline panleukopenia, 236
Coccidioidal granuloma, 453
Coccidioidin skin test, 603
Coccidioidomycosis, 591, 598
Coccidiosis, 229
Codfish: pseudomonad contamination, 374; vibriosis, 467
Coe virus, 74

Cold-blooded animals
  equine encephalomyelitis, 309
  erysipelas, 429
  pseudomonad infection, 374
  salmonellosis, 359
  tuberculosis, 537
Colibacillosis and granuloma, 351, 352
Columbia-SK virus, 269
Columbidine birds, ornithosis, 486
Conjunctivitis, 445, 475, 486, 487, 489, 571, 572
Connecticut serotype of avian bronchitis virus, 122
Contagious
  agalactia of sheep, 26, 474
  bovine pleuropneumonia, 26, 472
  ecthyma (Orf), 26, 229, 274, 278-280
  ophthalmia, 571, 572, 577, 578
  pustular dermatitis, 280
Contaminants
  in cell cultures, 44, 155, 232, 240, 260, 478
  in eggs, 47, 359
  in virus seed stocks, 244, 245, 478
Continuous cell lines, 56
Corneal ulcers, 445
Coronaviruses, 119-125
Coryza, avian, 408
Cottontail rabbit herpesvirus, 155, 156
Cowpox, 273-277
Coxsackie B-5 virus, 102, 253, 261
Coyote: distemper, 212, 221; rabies, 301
Crab, Chesapeake Bay blue, vibriosis, 467
Cremation, anthrax carcasses, 438
Croup-associated virus, 212
Cryptococcosis, 591, 605
Cutaneous streptothricosis, 559
Cycloheximide (Actidione), 590
Cytomegaloviruses, 158

Deer
  bluetongue, 188
  brucellosis, 396
  dermatophilosis, 559
  fibroma, 205, 206
  foot-and-mouth disease, 248-253
  hemorrhagic disease, 197, 198
  leptospirosis, 494
  malignant catarrhal fever, 139
  paratuberculosis, 539
  rhinotracheitis, 127
Densonucleosis virus, 231
Dental defects, 232-234
Deoxycholate sensitivity, 105
Dermatophilosis, 24, 559
Dermatophytoses, 25
Dialysis technique (skin test antigen), 691
Diarrhea, bloody, 463
Diphtheroids, 549
Diplornaviruses, 187
Diseases exotic to U.S., 26
Disinfectants, 99-101, 442, 490

General Index

DNA and RNA differentiation tests, 102-104, 273
Dog, *see also* Canine
  aflatoxicosis, 659, 660
  African horsesickness, 194
  candidiasis, 593
  chlamydial encephalomyelitis, 486
  chromomycosis, 657, 658
  coccidioidomycosis, 598
  ehrlichiosis, 572, 576, 577
  fusobacterial abscesses, 530
  haemobartonellosis, 449
  hemorrhagic disease of pups, 39
  kennel cough, 114
  leptospirosis, 494
  mycetoma, 655
  mycoplasmosis, 477
  parainfluenza, 213
  parvovirus infection, 231, 232
  pasteurellosis, 417
  phycomycosis, 640
  pseudorabies, 131
  rabies, 301-307
  ringworm, 610
  salmon poisoning, 572, 579
  sporotrichosis, 651
Dog bite pasteurellosis, 413
Donkey
  African horsesickness, 194
  equine encephalomyelitis, 309, 310
  equine infectious anemia, 333-338
  ringworm, 610
  sporotrichosis, 651
  theileriosis, 505
Duck
  botulism, 521
  hepatitis, 248
  influenza, 201
  Marek's disease, 143
  mycoplasmosis, 477
  new duck disease, pasteurellosis, 418
  plague, virus enteritis, 148-150
  spirochetosis, 502
Dwarfism, runting, 232-234

East African forest rat (Rift Valley fever reservoir), 325
East Coast fever, 26
Eastern equine encephalomyelitis, 24, 309
ECHO viruses, 74, 248
Ectromelia, 273, 274
Edema disease of swine, 357
Eel, vibriosis (red disease), 467
Egg or vertical transmission, 170, 177, 301, 346, 359, 482
Ehrlichiosis of dogs, 572, 576, 577
Eland, malignant catarrhal fever, 139
Electron microscopy, 106-108, 279, 280
Elephant, tuberculosis, 538

Elk: bluetongue, 188; brucellosis, 396; malignant catarrhal fever, 139
Embedding media for EM, 107
Embryonating eggs techniques, 47-52
Emesis and refusal of feed, 663
Encephalomyocarditis, 24, 268-272
Endothelioma, 169
Endotoxin, 357
Energy parasites, 490
Englebreth-Holm virus, 169
Enteric organisms, 349-370
Enteritis, fatal (of snowshoe hare), 486
Enterotoxin detection, 357, 384
Enteroviruses, 248, 255, 258, 260
Entomophthoromycosis, 645, 646
Enzootic abortion of ewes, 25, 486
Eperythrozoa, 449
Epididymitis, 458
Epizootic
  bovine abortion, 486
  hemorrhagic disease of deer, 197, 198
  lymphangitis, 633, 634, 636
Equine, *see also* Horse
  corynebacterial infections, 544, 547, 551
  ehrlichiosis, 580, 581
  encephalomyelitis viruses, 24, 309, 310
  infectious anemia, 193, 333-338
  infectious arteritis, 44, 193, 321-324
  influenza, 199, 201
  papilloma, 205, 206
  parainfluenza, 213-216
  piroplasmosis, 324, 325
  pneumonitis, 486
  rhinopneumonitis, abortion disease, 129-131
  rhinovirus infection, 254, 255
  ringworm, girth itch, 626
  ulcerative lymphangitis, 547
Ergotism, 660, 668
Erysipelas, 311, 429
Erysipeloid, 24, 429
Erythroblastosis, avian, 168
Essential lipid determination, 104
Estrogenism, 660
Ether sensitivity, 104
Eumycotic mycetoma, 655
European blastomycosis, 605
Exaltation of Newcastle disease virus, 313, 316, 317, 319

F virus, 269
Facial eczema, 660, 666
Factors V and X, *Haemophilus* growth, 408-411
False glanders, 373
Favus of chickens, 622
Favus of mice, 624
Fecal specimens, bacterial concentration technique, 431
Feed change, roughage to concentrate, 529
Feed testing, 361, 660-669

Feline
  infectious anemia, 449
  panleukopenia, 232, 236-240
  picorna respiratory viruses, 266-268
  pneumonitis, 486
  rhinotracheitis, 136-138
Ferret: African horsesickness, 194; distemper, 212, 221; polyoma, 205
Fescue foot, 669
Feulgen reaction, 275
Filter test techniques, 679
Filtration, size determination, 44, 108-110
Fish
  erysipelas, 421
  nocardiosis, 562
  tuberculosis, 538
  vibriosis, 467
Fitch-Hopkins tube, 542
Flagellar stain, 699
Flavivirus, 309
Fluke, liver, 514
Fluke, rickettsial vector, 578, 579
Fluorescence of ringworm, 615
Fluorocarbon technique, 44
Fly larva, botulism, 522
Food
  poisoning, 359, 380, 384, 437, 467, 521
  spoilage, 374
Foot abscess, 527
Foot-and-mouth disease, 24-26, 225, 248-253, 263, 269, 299
Footrot
  of cattle, 529, 530
  of sheep, 507, 527, 559
Fossa, distemper, 221
Fowl, *see* Chicken
Fox
  bordetellosis, 404
  brucellosis, 396
  distemper, 212, 221
  encephalitis, 114
  leptospirosis, 494
  rabies, 301
  ringworm, 623
  salmon poisoning, 579
Freezing of organisms, 95-97
Friend helper murine leukemia virus, 177
Fruit, mycotic, 593, 605

GAL 1, 3, 4, avian adenoviruses, 112
Gazelle, malignant catarrhal fever, 139
Genital infections, 366, 408, 425, 457, 458, 461-463, 490
Geotrichosis, 631
Gerbil, leptospirosis, 498
Germ tube formation, 595, 607
Giant anteater, monkeypox, 277
Giant forest hog, African swine fever carrier, 331
Gibbon, herpes simplex, 161

Glanders, 24, 373
Glomerular nephritis, 455
Goat, *see also* Ovine *and* Sheep
  African horsesickness, 192
  caprine pneumonitis, 486
  Kata, 229
  papilloma, 205, 206
  pasture fever, 572
  pleuropneumonia, 473
  pox, 26, 274, 282
  pseudofarcy, 26, 373
  Q fever, 566
  ringworm, 610
  scrapie, 345
  tick-borne fever, 573
Goose
  duck plague, 148
  Marek's disease, 143
  spirochetosis, 502
Gram stain, 697
Granules, bacterial, stain, 700
Granuloblastosis, 168
Gross murine leukemia virus, 177
Guinea fowl, Newcastle disease, 216
Guinea pig
  aflatoxicosis, 569
  bordetellosis, 404
  chlamydial conjunctivitis, 486
  cytomegalovirus infection, 152, 153
  leptospirosis, 494
  moraxellosis, 445
  parainfluenza, 213
  pasteurellosis, 417
  phycomycosis, 640
  polyoma, 205
  salivary gland virus, 152, 153
  yersinial infection, 421
Gull, botulism, 521

Haddock, pseudomonad spoilage, 374
HADEN virus, 243
Haemobartonellosis, 449
Hair and hide anthrax danger, 438
Hairbrush technique for ringworm, 612
Hairy shaker lambs, 319
Hamster
  actinomycosis, 554
  encephalomyocarditis, 268
  leukemia, 182
  osteolytic H virus (H-1), 232
  papilloma and polyoma, 205, 206
  parainfluenza, 213
  pasteurellosis, 417
  ringworm, 623
Hanks' and Earle's BSS compared, 681
Hares vs. rabbits, 287
Harris sarcoma virus, 169
Hazards, occupational, *see* Safety
Heartwater, 26, 571

General Index

Heat inactivation, 97, 98, 105
Hedgehog, ringworm, 623
Hemadsorbing enteric virus, 243
Hemagglutinating encephalomyelitis of pigs, 119
Hemagglutinating viruses, 69, 70
Hemangioma, avian, 168
Hematocrit levels for mice, 184
Hemin solution, 409
Hemolysin, antisheep, 63
Hemolytic patterns, 391
Hemorrhagic
  disease of deer, 197
  disease of pups, 39
  fevers, 24, 25
  septicemia, 413
Herpes simplex virus, 158, 161-165
Herpes zoster virus, 127, 159, 160
Herring, vibriosis, 467
Histochemical tests, 102
Histologic specimens, 40
Histoplasmosis, 591, 603, 633
Hog cholera (swine fever), 26, 311-318, 330
Hong Kong influenza virus, 199
Horse, *see also* Equine
  actinobacillosis, joint ill of foals, 455
  African horsesickness, 192-196
  anthrax, 437
  blastomycosis, 588
  Borna disease, 338, 339
  chromomycosis, 657, 658
  dermatophilosis, 559
  epizootic lymphangitis, 633, 634, 636
  glanders, 374
  histoplasmosis, 633
  leucoencephalomalacia, 664
  moniliasis, 593
  navel ill, 530
  paspalum staggers, 660
  phycomycoses, 640
  pink eye, 321
  pseudotuberculosis, 547
  sporotrichosis, 651
  stachybotryotoxicosis, 664
  streptococcal pharyngitis, 389
  tetanus, 523
  theileriosis (spirochetosis), 26, 505
  ventral abscesses, 547
  vesicular stomatitis, 249, 299-301
Horsepox, 24
Human, *see also* Food poisoning *and* Zoonoses
  alastrim (mild smallpox), 273-277
  alimentary toxic aleukia, 663
  anthrax, 437
  botulism, 521
  brucellosis, undulant fever, 396
  bubonic plague, 419
  Buss-Buschke's disease, cryptococcosis, 605
  candidiasis, 593
  cat and dog bite pasteurellosis, 413
  chandipura virus, 300
  chicken pox (herpes zoster virus), 24
  coccidioidomycosis, 598
  Creutzfeldt-Jacob disease, 345, 348
  enteroviruses, 248
  epidemic typhus, 567
  erysipeloid, 429
  eumycotic mycetoma, 655
  herpes simplex and zoster viruses, 127, 158-165
  histoplasmosis, 591, 633
  influenza, 199-203
  kuru, 345, 348
  leprosy, 527
  lymphogranuloma venereum, 486, 488, 490
  measles (rubeola), 24, 212, 220, 227
  molluscum contagiosum, 289, 290
  moraxellosis, corneal ulcers, 445
  mumps, 24, 212
  otitis media, 374
  papilloma (warts), 204-206
  parainfluenza viruses 1-4, 212, 213
  pathogens, classification for risk, 24-26
  pertussis (whooping cough), 404
  pharyngoconjunctival fever, 116
  pseudomonal infections, 373, 374
  psittacosis, 485, 486
  Q fever, 566-571
  reoviruses, 292
  rubella (German measles), 318
  salmonellosis, 359
  tanapox, 289, 290
  tetanus, 523
  tick typhuses and fevers, 566, 567
  trachoma, 485, 490
  tuberculosis, 537, 538
  vaccinia and variola, 273-277
  yaba and yaba-like pox, 289, 290
  yellow rice disease, 664
Hungate's roll tube technique, 532
Hyena, distemper, 221

Ibaraki virus, 196, 197
Ilheus, 24
Immunoelectrophoresis, 91
Immunoglobulins (IgG, IgM), 427
Impression smears, 42
Inactivation of microorganisms, 97-101
Incinerator exhaust air sterilizing temperature, 97
Inclusion bodies, 112-114, 116, 129, 227, 285, 305
Incubation cell cultures, 53
Incubation of eggs, 47, 51, 189
Indicator for pH change, 58, 59
Infectious
  bovine rhinotracheitis, 127-129
  bronchitis, avian, 119-122
  bulbar paralysis, 131
  canine hepatitis, 114
  catarrh of mice and rats, 476
  feline enteritis, 236

Infectious (cont.)
  laryngotracheitis, avian, 154
  serositis, 418
  sinusitis, 476
Infective bulbar necrosis, 527
Influenza viruses
  avian, equine, human, porcine, 199-201
  pandemic of 1918-1919, 200
  WHO designations, 203
Innisfail virus, 269
Interferon, 101, 127, 150, 214, 300
Intracerebral route, 51
Intravenous route, 50
Iridovirus, 330

Jaagsiekte, 348
Jackal: distemper, 221; ehrlichiosis, 572
Japanese B encephalitis, 214
Jembrana disease, 581, 582
Jenner's smallpox immunity, 276
Joest-Degan bodies, 338
Johne's Disease, 539
Joint ill of neonates, 455
Juncopox, 284

K virus of mice, 205, 206
Kangaroo
  foot-and-mouth disease, 249, 252
  ringworm, 623
Kata, 229
Kennel cough, 114
Keratoconjunctivitis, 427
Kilham's rat virus, 232
Kinkajou, distemper, 221
Knopvelsiekte, 283
Kolmer saline diluent for CF test, 62, 63
Kyasanur Forest disease, 24

Lactogenic immunity, 125
Lancefield
  antigen preparation, 394
  groups of Str., 391, 392
Laryngotracheitis, 146, 153
Leporipoxviruses, 285-289
Leptomeningitis, 579
Leptospirosis, 24, 494
Leucoencephalomalacia, 664
Leukemia
  murine, 176-186
  viruses of cats, chickens, hamsters, rats, 182
Leukocidal toxin, 527
Leukosis, avian, 167-176
Lion: distemper, 221; mycoplasmosis, 477
Listerial silage contamination, 425
Listeriosis, 425
Liver abscesses, 529
Liver granulomas of turkeys, 530
Liverpool vervet virus, 158
Lizard, pseudomonad infection, 373

Llama, brucellosis, 396
Loon, botulism, 521
Louisiana pneumonitis, 25
Louping ill, 24, 26
Lumpy
  jaw, 553
  skin disease, bovine, 26, 283, 284
  wool, 559
Lymphadenitis, 544
Lyophilization, 95, 97
Lyssavirus, 301

Macrophage cell culture technique, 221
Mad itch, 131
Maduromycetoma and maduromycosis, 655
Maedi, 340-344
Magnification formulas, 684
Maitland cell cultures, 53
Malignant
  catarrhal fever, 44, 138-142
  edema, 519
  lymphoma, 155
Marburg virus disease, 24
Marek's disease virus, 143-146
Marten, distemper, 221
Mastitis, 351, 366, 373, 380, 389, 416, 473, 544, 562, 593, 605, 649
Mastomy, polyoma, 205
Measles, 24, 212, 225, 227
Meat and fish handling, erysipeloid, 429
Media
  for bacteria and fungi, Appendix A
  for cell cultures, 54, 55
  for mycoplasmas, 480, 481
  for salmonellae, 369
Medusa head colony, 439
Meerkat, distemper, 221
Melioidosis, 24, 373
Mengo virus, 269
Meningoencephalitis of feedlot cattle, 411, 425
2-Mercaptoethanol treatment to depolymerize IgM antibodies, 427
Milk contamination, 389, 605
Milk sample technique, 380
Milker's nodules, 24, 281
Mink
  aflatoxicosis, 560
  botulism, 521, 522
  brucellosis, 396
  canine distemper, 221
  enteritis, 236-240
  phycomycosis, 640
  pseudomonal pneumonia, 373
  transmissible mink encephalopathy, 344
  vaccination for botulism, 522
Minute virus of canines and mice, 232
Mokola virus disease, 24, 301
Mold nephrosis, 660
Moloney murine leukemia virus, 177

General Index

Mongoloidism, 232, 233
Mongoose: distemper, 212; encephalomyocarditis, 268; rabies reservoir, 301
Moniliasis, 593
Monkey, see also Simian
  alastrim, 273-277
  encephalomyocarditis, 268
  fatal exanthematous disease, 158
  herpes simplex, tamarinus, and zoster, 158-160
  Liverpool vervet virus, 158
  measles, 24, 212
  pox, 273-277
  saimiri infection, 158
  salivary gland virus, 24, 158
  shigellosis, 357
  spider monkey virus, 159-161
  tanapox, 289, 290
  trichosporosis, 654
  tuberculosis, 537
  varicella (chicken pox), 127, 158
  variola (smallpox), 273-277
  Yaba-like pox and Yabapox, 289, 290
Montana lung disease, 341
Moose: bluetongue, 188; brucellosis, 396
Mouse, see also Murine
  bordetellosis, 404
  catarrh, infectious, 476
  chlamydial abortion, 486
  diabetes-like disease, 269
  favus, 624
  haemobartonellosis, 449
  hepatitis, 119
  K virus infection, 205, 206
  leptospirosis, 494
  minute virus of mice, 232
  mycoplasmal encephalopathy, 475, 477
  papilloma and polyoma, 205, 206
  phycomycosis, 640
  pneumonia of mice, 213
  pox, 273-277
  pseudotuberculosis, 421
  Rift Valley fever, 325
  ringworm, 623
  rolling disease, 475, 483
  salmonellosis, 359
  sylvatic plague, 419
Mucormycosis, 640
Mucosal disease (bovine viral diarrhea), 318-320
Mulberry heart disease, 269
Mule, see Donkey and Horse
Mummification, fetus, 236, 240, 255, 318
Murine, see also Mouse
  ectromelia, 274
  encephalomyocarditis, 268
  leukemia, 176-186
  parainfluenza, 212
  pneumonitis, 486
  reovirus, 292
  rickettsioses, 572

sporotrichosis, 651
typhus, 24, 567
Murray Valley encephalitis, 24
Muskrat
  fatal enteritis, chlamydiosis, 486
  Omsk hemorrhagic fever, 25
  ringworm, 623
Mycetoma, 655
Mycoplasmas
  of animals, 475
  in cell cultures and eggs, 47, 478
  in virus seed stocks, 478
Mycotoxins, 659-670
Myeloblastosis, avian, 168
Myxoma viruses, myxomatosis, 274, 286, 287

NAD precursor, 408
Nagana, 26
Nairobi sheep disease, 24, 26
Navel ill, 530
Neethling poxvirus, 283
Negative staining for EM, 106
Negri bodies, 304-306
Nephroblastoma, avian, 168
New duck disease, 418
Newcastle disease, 24-26, 47, 73, 212, 216-219
Nigrosine negative stain technique, 503
Nocardiosis, 562
Nonsporeforming anaerobes, 526
Nucleic acid determination, 102-104, 273
N-virus, 200

Occupational hazard, see Safety
Ochratoxicosis, 666
Octadecylamine in dist. H_2O and steam, 511
Okapia, phycomycosis, 640
Omsk hemorrhagic fever, 24
Ontario disease, 256
Ophthalmic bleeding technique for mice, 184
Opossum
  adenovirus, 112
  bordetellosis, 404
  leptospirosis, 494
  ringworm, 623
Orbiviruses, 187-198
Orchitis, 395
Orf, 24, 274, 278-280
Organ cultures, 57, 58
Ornithosis, 25, 486
Orphan viruses, 112, 292
Orthomyxoviruses, 199-203
Orthopoxviruses, 273-278
Ortlieg virus, 269
Osteopetrosis, avian, 168
Otter, distemper, 221
Ouchterlony gel diffusion, see Tests
Ovine, see also Sheep
  benign rickettsiosis, 572, 576
  interdigital dermatitis, 527

Ovine (cont.)
  polyarthritis, 486
  vibriosis, 462
Oysters, vibriosis, 469

Panda, distemper, 221
Papovaviruses, 204-211
Paracoccidioidomycosis, 591
Parainfluenza
  PI-1, 2, 4 of humans, 212
  PI-3 of cattle and humans, 74, 75, 212-216
  PI-5 of dogs, 213
Paramyxoviruses, 212-230
Parapoxviruses, 278-284
Paratuberculosis, 541
Parvoviruses, 231-247
Paspalum staggers, 660
Pasteurellosis, 311
Pasteurization, 98
Peaches, mycotic, 605
Penguin, aspergillosis, 583
Penicillin and other antibiotic additives
  cell cultures, 54, 58
  mycoplasmal media, 480
  mycotic media, 600, 607, 642, 656
Periodic ophthalmia, 494
Persian cat, ringworm, 615
Peste des petits ruminants, 26, 229, 230
Pestivirus, 311, 318
pH
  adjusted solutions, 689
  indicators: bromthymol blue, 513; phenol red, 58, 59
Phage, see Bacteriophage
Phase variation, salmonellae, 366
Pheasant
  aflatoxicosis, 660
  avian leukosis, 168, 169
  botulism, 521
  laryngotracheitis, 146
  Marek's disease, 143
  spirochetosis, 502
Photodynamic inactivation, 98
Picornaviruses, 248-272
Pig, see also Porcine and Swine
  acholeplasmal infection, 477
  actinobacillosis, 452
  actinomycosis, 553
  aflatoxicosis, 659, 660
  bacillary hemoglobinuria, 514
  coccidioidomycosis, 599
  corynebacteriosis, 544, 545
  emesis and corn refusal, 663
  enterotoxemia, 517
  foot-and-mouth disease, 248-253
  footrot, 507
  genital papilloma, 205, 206, 208
  hemorrhagic septicemia, 413
  hog cholera, 311-317

Hong Kong influenza, 199
mycoplasmal arthritis, pneumonia, and polyserositis, 474, 477
ochratoxicosis, 666
pox (vaccinia virus), 290
pseudorabies, 131
pseudotuberculosis, 421
rinderpest, 226
ringworm, 610
scirrhous cord, 507
streptococcic lymphadenitis, 390
Talfan, 255-257
Teschen disease, 255-257
transmissible gastroenteritis, 123-125
turbinate atrophy, 404
vesicular stomatitis, 249, 299, 300
zearalenone toxicosis, 660, 662
Pig, wild, San Miguel sea lion virus, 263
Pigeon
  cryptococosis, 605
  erysipelas, 435
  herpesvirus, 153-155
  Marek's disease, 143
  ornithosis, 486
  pox, 154, 274, 284
  pseudotuberculosis, 421
Pink eye (EAV), 321
Plague, bubonic and sylvatic, 24, 419
Plant juice contamination, 605
Pleuropneumonia-like organisms, 473
Pneumoencephalitis, avian, 212
Pneumonitis, 486
Poliovirus, 25
Polyoma viruses
  K virus of mice, 205, 206, 208
  of rats and mice, 205, 206
Porcine, see also Pig and Swine
  adenoviruses, 115, 116
  cytomegalovirus, 150
  enteroviruses, 255-258
  estrogenism, 660
  lymphadenitis, 255
  parainfluenza, 213
  parvoviruses, 232, 240-243
  polioencephalomyelitis, Talfan, 255
  tuberculosis, 538
Porcupine, ringworm, 623
Porpoise, erysipelas urticaria, 429
Potatoes, protothecal algae, 649
Potentiating factor (VN test), 163
Poxviruses, 70, 273-291
Prairie dog, sylvatic plague, 419
Preservation
  cell cultures, 58
  fungi, 614
  microorganisms, 94-97
Primary cell cultures, 53-55
Pseudocowpox, 274, 279, 281
Pseudofarcy, 26

Pseudorabies virus, 131-134
Pseudotuberculosis, 421, 422
Psittacosis, 25, 486
Ptomaine, 677
Pyelonephritis, 544, 549

Q fever, 25, 566-571
Quail
  aflatoxicosis, 660
  bronchitis, 112
  pasteurellosis, 418
Quokka, reovirus, 297

Rabbit and hare, 287
  bordetellosis (turbinate atrophy), 404
  Borna disease, 338, 339
  brucellosis, 396
  chlamydial abortion, 486
  cottontail herpesvirus, 155, 156
  dermatophilosis, 559
  hare fibroma, 274, 286, 288
  lapine pneumonitis, 486
  myxomatosis, 285-287
  oral papilloma and polyoma, 205, 206
  pox, 273-277
  ringworm, 623
  Shope papilloma, 205, 206
  Shope's fibroma, 274, 286-288
  snuffles, 413
  squirrel fibroma, 274, 286, 288
  sylvatic plague, 419
  tularemia, 422
  vacuolating virus, 205, 206
  virus III, 127
Rabies
  stains, 305, 306
  virus, 24, 301-307
Raccoon
  bordetellosis, 404
  distemper, 221
  encephalomyocarditis, 268
  feline panleukopenia, 236
  leptospirosis, 494
Radiation inactivation, 99
Radioactive iron ($^{59}FeCl_3$), 184, 185
Radioisotope labeling, 103, 104
Ranikhet disease, 216
Rat
  aflatoxicosis, 660
  bordetellosis, 404
  catarrh, infectious, 476
  encephalomyocarditis, 268-272
  haemobartonellosis, 449
  hamster osteolytic H virus, 232
  Kilham's rat virus, 232
  leptospirosis, 494
  leukemia, 182
  melioidosis, 373
  mycoplasmal arthritis, 476
  pasteurellosis, 417
  polyoma, 70, 205
  rickettsioses, 572
  ringworm, 623
  salmonellosis, 359
  sporotrichosis, 651
  sylvatic plague, 419
Ratbite fever, 24
Rauscher helper virus, 177
Ray fungus, 453, 456
Receptor-destroying enzymes and chemicals, 69, 70, 199, 202
Red blood cells
  counts, total, mice, 184
  parasites, 449
  standard concentration for HA, 71, 72, 295
  suitability test for HA, 276
Red water disease, 514
Reindeer: brucellosis; 395; paratuberculosis, 539
Relapsing fevers, 24
Reoviruses, 70, 292-298
Respiratory syncytial virus, 213
Rhabdoviruses, 299-308
Rickettsial
  antigen technique, 570, 571
  pox, 24
  stains, 696, 699
Rickettsioses, 566, 567, 572
Rida, 345
Rift Valley fever, 24, 26, 310, 311, 325, 326
Rinderpest, 26, 225-228, 581
Ringtail, feline panleukopenia, 236
Ringworm fungi, 25, 610-630
RNA polymerase block, 267
Rocky Mountain spotted fever, 24
Rodent parvoviruses, 232-236
Rolling disease of mice, 475, 483
Rosettes, actinobacillosis, 453
Rous sarcoma virus, 168, 174
Rous-associated viruses, 169, 174
Routine procedures for unknowns, 41-46
Rubin's lymphoid leukosis virus, 169
Rubratoxicosis, 665, 666
Rumen ulcers, feedlot, 529
Russian spring-summer encephalitis, 24
Ryegrass sickness, 669

S (soluble) antigen (RNA), 199
SA6, cytomegalovirus, green monkey, 158
SA8, African green monkey virus, 159, 160
Safety, lab, 22-34
  anthrax, 438
  Brucella, 396
  Chlamydia psittaci, 488
  Coccidioides immitis, 600
  erysipeloid, 429
  Histoplasma, 633, 635
  inactivation, 97-98
  lyophilization, 94

Safety (cont.)
  mycobacteria, 538
  propane, 512
St. Louis encephalitis, 24
Salivary gland virus
  of guinea pigs, 152, 153
  of monkeys, 24, 158
Salivation (slobber) factor, 660, 667
San Miguel sea lion virus, 249, 263, 264
Salmon
  aflatoxicosis, 660
  rickettsial reservoir (poisoning), 571, 572
  vibriosis, 467
Salmonellosis, 24, 311
Salpingitis of hens, 352
Sarcoma, avian, 168, 174
Schmidt Ruppin virus, 169
Scrapie, 345-348
Seal and sea lion
  blastomycosis, 588
  pox, 274, 279, 281
  ringworm, 623
  San Miguel sea lion virus, 249, 263, 264
Sedimentation coefficients, 44, 45
Seminal vesiculitis, 457
Sendai influenza, 24
Septicemia, 357, 374, 378, 380, 408, 413, 416, 421, 443, 462
Sheep, see also Goat and Ovine
  agalactia, contagious, 26, 474
  Akabane, 326
  anthrax, 437
  bacillary hemoglobinuria, 514
  bluetongue, 187-191
  Borna disease, 338, 339
  brucellosis, 395
  chlamydial infections, 486
  clostridial infections, 514, 517, 520, 524
  coccidioidomycosis, 598
  contagious footrot, 527
  epizootic abortion, 486
  erysipelas, 429
  facial eczema, 666, 667
  foot-and-mouth disease, 248-253
  heartwater, 26, 571, 572
  Ibaraki disease, 196, 197
  maedi, 340-344
  malignant catarrhal fever carriers, 138, 139
  melioidosis, 373
  mucosal disease (BVD), 318-321
  ophthalmia, contagious, 577, 578
  Orf, contagious ecthyma, 24, 274, 278-280
  paratuberculosis, 539
  peste des petits ruminants, 26, 229-230
  phycomycosis, 640
  pseudorabies, 131
  pseudotuberculosis, 547
  pulmonary adenomatosis, 348
  Q fever, 566

  rinderpest, 226
  ringworm, 610
  scrapie, 345-348
  sheeppox, 26, 274, 282
  Wesselsbron disease, 310
  vesicular stomatitis, 24, 225, 249
  visna, 340-344
Shellfish, vibriosis, 469
Shipping fever, 212
Shope rabbit papilloma virus, 205, 206
Shope's fibroma, 274, 286-288
Shrew, carrier of rabies-like mokola virus, 24, 301
Siamese cat, ringworm, 615
Sideroleukocytes, 334
Simian, see also Monkey
  adenoviruses, 116
  aethiops viruses, 158-160
  B-virus, 24, 159-165
  cytomegalovirus, 158
  enteroviruses, 260-263
  herpesviruses, 158-166
  reoviruses, 297
  virus 40, vacuolating, 204-207
Skunk
  bordetellosis, 404
  distemper, 212, 221
  leptospirosis, 494
  rabies reservoir, 301
Slaframine, 660, 667
Sleeper syndrome of feedlot cattle, 411
SMEDI viruses, 255
Snail, intermediate host, rickettsial vector fluke, 572, 578
Snake: pseudomonad septicemia, 373; western equine encephalomyelitis, 310
Snuffles, 413
Sparrow
  ornithosis, 486, 491
  pseudotuberculosis, 421
  pox, 284
Specimens
  legal responsibility, 41
  selection and packaging, 40
  for specific diseases and hosts, 39
Spider monkey virus, 159-165
Spirochetosis, 502
Spleen focus-forming virus, 171, 181
Spores, bacterial, 438, 439, 514
Sporotrichosis, 651
Sprue, 649
Squirrel
  encephalomyocarditis, 268
  fibroma, 274, 286, 288
  ringworm, 623
  sylvatic plague, 419
  vaccinia, 277
Stachybotryotoxicosis, 664
Stains for EM, 107, 108
Standardbred horse, equine arteritis, 321

General Index

Staphylococcal infections, 380
Staphylococcal phage typing, 385
Starling, starlingpox, 284
Steam, inhibitors in, 511
Sterigmatocystin, 665, 668
Strawberry footrot, 559
Streptococcal infections, 389
Streptomycin (inhibitor), 54, 55, 485, 600, 607, 686
Stress activation of latent infections in mice, 475; in cattle, 505
String of pearls phenomenon, 441
Sulfur granules, actinobacillosis, 453
Summer mastitis, 545
Suslik, rinderpest, 227
Suspension cell cultures, 57
Swamp fever, 333
Swan: duck plague, 148; Marek's disease, 143
Swine, *see also* Pig *and* Porcine
  African swine fever, 330-332
  anthrax, chronic, 437
  brucellosis, 395, 400
  chlamydial infections, 486
  contagious ophthalmia, 577, 578
  cytomegalovirus, 150-152
  edema disease of swine, 357
  encephalomyocarditis, 268
  erysipelas urticaria, 429
  fever (hog cholera), 311
  histoplasmosis, 633
  influenza, 24, 408
  listeriosis, 494
  mold nephrosis, 660
  polyserositis, 408
  pox, 274, 290, 291
  pseudofarcy (melioidosis), 26, 373
  salmonellosis, 358
  San Miguel sea lion virus infection, 249, 263, 264
  SMEDI virus infections, 255
  spirochetosis, 506, 507
  vesicular disease, 24, 26, 249, 253, 254
  vesicular exanthema of swine, 249, 263-266
  vibrionic dysentery, 463
Sylvatic plague, 419
Symbiotic relationships, 177, 244, 456, 527, 528, 546

Talfan, 255-257
Tanapox, 274, 289, 290
Tape technique for fungi, 614
Teschen disease, 26, 255-257
Tests
  acetylmethylcarbinol, 375
  acriflavin, 398
  agar (gel) diffusion, 90, 91, 384, 416; VIA, 251
  agglutination, 355, 382, 385, 399, 405
  air filter (HEPA), 28, 679, 680
  antibiotic sensitivity, 384
  antibody production (parvoviruses), 234
  Anton rabbit eye test (listeriosis), 427

  assimilation of sugars, 595
  back-challenge, 45
  bacteriostatic effect (basic fuchsin and thionin), 399
  biochemical (viruses), 102-105
  biophysical (viruses), 105-111
  CAMP, streptococcal, 393
  capillary tube agglutination, 491, 569, 570
  catalase, 465, 555
  ceiling temperature, 275
  coagulase, 383, 385
  complement fixation, 61-69, 190, 491, 570
  complement fixation avian leukosis, 170-173
  cross-transfusion, 336
  crystal violet, 384
  cytotoxic, 182
  dermal toxicity or necrosis, 40, 663
  disc growth inhibition, 482
  DNA and RNA differentiation, 102-104, 273
  exaltation of Newcastle disease virus, 313, 316, 317, 319
  fluorescent antibody, 43, 84-90, 303-305, 312, 313, 332, 333, 339, 435, 695
  fluorescent focus inhibition, 305
  fluorescent rabies antibody, 302-305
  germ tube yeast, 595
  glycine, 465
  heat tolerance, 465
  hemadsorption and hemadsorption inhibition, 74, 75
  hemagglutination and hemagglutination inhibition, 69-74, 295, 331
  hematopoietic transformation, 174
  Hotis, 393
  hydrogen sulfide, 399, 465
  indole (Kovac's reagent), 414, 513, 682
  indophenol oxidase, 349
  Lancefield's grouping, 392
  latex slide agglutination, 603, 608, 683
  mallein, 378
  methyl red, 684
  methyl red–Voges-Proskauer, glucose broth, 680
  microscopic agglutination, 498, 499
  motility, 354, 685
  mouse protection, 434
  mucous agglutination, 464, 466
  neutralization (VN), 75-84, 163, 182-184
  niacin, 541
  nonproducer, 170-173
  nonspecific chlamydial and rickettsial, 491
  Panton-Valentine leukocidin, 383
  passive hemagglutination, 384
  pH lability, 105
  phage and pyocin, 378
  phage typing, 384, 385, 401
  phenotypic mixing, 172, 173
  plaque reduction, 133
  precipitation, 384, 434
  Quellung, 367

Tests (cont.)
  radioisotope precipitation, 569-571
  reactivation or resurrection of poxvirus, 276, 277
  resistance-inducing favtor, 168, 170, 171, 173
  salt tolerance, 465
  skin, 378, 492, 538, 592, 603, 608, 637, 638
  slide agglutination, 355, 356, 367, 382, 420
  sodium hippurate, 393
  spleen antibody, 504
  spot plate pH indicator for anaerobes, 513
  sugar assimilation, 595
  suitability of RBC for hemagglutination, 276
  toxicity of brilliant green dye, 369
  toxin-antitoxin neutralization, 518, 519
Tetanus
  absence at high mountain altitudes, 523
  on hospital floors, 523
  in tooth cavity, 523
  organisms in dust, 523
Theileriosis, 26, 505, 506
Thoroughbred horse, equine arteritis, 321
Thrush, 593
Thylaxovirus group, 167
Tick-borne fever, 571, 572
Tissue culture techniques, 52-59, 293
Titer calculation in VN tests, 75-84
Togaviruses, 309-324
Topi, malignant catarrhal fever, 139
Torula meningitis, 605
Transmissible
  gastroenteritis of swine, 123
  mink encephalopathy, 344, 345
Transplantation immunity, 180
Tree sap, mycotic, 593
Tremblent du mouton, 345
Trichothecene toxicoses, 663
Trout: aflatoxicosis, 660; vibriosis, 467
Trypanosomiasis, 193, 505, 506
Trypsinization of cell cultures, 54, 55
T-strain organisms, 472, 473, 477, 481
Tsutsugamushi, 24
Tuberculosis, 24, 537, 633
Tularemia, 24, 413, 422
Turbinate atrophy, 404
Turkey
  aflatoxicosis, 660
  airsacculitis, 352, 476, 583
  arizona infection, 359
  aspergillosis, 583
  bordetellosis, 404
  erysipelas, 429
  infectious sinusitis and synovitis, 476
  influenza, 201
  Marek's disease, 143
  moniliasis (thrush), 593
  mycoplasmosis, 476, 477
  Newcastle disease, 212, 216-219
  ornithosis, 486; skin test, 492
  pasteurellosis, 418, 421
  pox, 274, 284

  reovirus infection, 297
  salmonellosis, 359
  spirochetosis, 502
  tuberculosis, 338
  Yucaipa, 212
Typhus fever, 566, 567

Ultracentrifugation, 110
Ultrasonic inactivation, 99
Ultraviolet radiation sterilization, 98
Ultraviolet technique for ringworm, 615
Unclassified viruses, 330-339
Undulant fever, 395
Unknowns, routine procedures for, 41-46
Uranyl acetate stain, 107, 108

V factor, 408-411
Vaccinia, 273-277
Vacuolating viruses, 204-207
Varicella virus, 127, 158
Variola, 273-277
Venereal disease, 461, 490
Venezuelan equine encephalomyelitis, 24, 309
Verrucose endocarditis, 390, 455
Vertical transmission, 170, 177, 301, 346, 359, 482
Vesicular exanthema of swine, 26, 249, 263-266
Vesicular stomatitis, 24, 225, 249, 299-301
Vibriosis, 461
Vicuna, brucellosis, 396
Virus III of rabbits, 127
Visceral lymphomatosis, 168
Visna, 340-344
Vitamin E–selenium deficiency, 269

Warthog, African swine fever carrier, 331
Weasel: distemper, 212, 221; rabies reservoir, 301
Weil-Felix reaction, 451, 491
Wesselsbron disease, 24, 26, 310, 311
West Nile fever, 24
Western equine encephalomyelitis, 24, 309
Whale
  botulism food poisoning, 522
  nocardiosis, 562
  San Miguel sea lion virus, 249, 263, 264
Wharton's jelly cultured, leptospirosis, 497
White blood cell counts, total
  mice, 184
  rabbits, 155
Whooping cough, 404
Wildebeest, malignant catarrhal fever carrier, 139
Wilm's tumor, 168
Winter scours, 462, 463
Wolf: distemper, 212, 221; rabies, 301
Wool handling, anthrax, 438
Wooden tongue, 452

X factor, 408-411

Yaba and Yaba-like pox, 274, 289, 290
Yak: brucellosis, 396; rinderpest, 226
Yale-SK poliovirus, 269

General Index

Yellow fever, 24, 25
Yellow rice disease, 664
Yolk sac
　harvest, 52
　route, 50
Yucaipa virus, 212

Zearalenone toxicosis, 660, 662, 663
Zebra, African horsesickness, 194
Zoo, effect of erysipelas, 429
Zoonoses, 24, 25
Zoospore, 560
Zwoegerziekte, 341

Library of Congress Cataloging in Publication Data
(For library cataloging purposes only)

National Research Council. Subcommittee on Standardized
    Methods for Veterinary Microbiology.
  Manual of standardized methods for veterinary microbiology.

  Bibliography: p.
  Includes indexes.
  1. Veterinary microbiology—Technique—Standards.
I. Cottral, George E. II. Title.
QR49.N37   1978   636.089′601′028   77-90900
ISBN 0-8014-1119-X

RAYMOND H. FOGLER LIBRARY